Second Edition

ADVERSE DRUG INTERACTIONS

A Handbook for Prescribers

Second Edition

ADVERSE DRUG INTERACTIONS

A Handbook for Prescribers

Edited by

Lakshman Delgoda Karalliedde, MBBS, DA, FRCA

Honorary Visiting Professor in Anaesthesiology
Faculty of Medicine, Peradeniya, Sri Lanka

Formerly, Visiting Senior Lecturer
Department of Public Health Sciences
King's College, London, UK

Consultant Medical Toxicologist
Health Protection Agency, UK

Simon F.J. Clarke, MBChB, DA, FRCS, Ed, FCEM

Consultant Emergency Physician
Frimley Health Foundation Trust
Frimley Park Hospital, UK

Ursula Gotel, BPharmHons, IP, GPhC, MRPharmS

Senior Pharmacist Emergency Medicine
Guy's and St Thomas' NHS Foundation Trust, London, UK

Janaka Karalliedde, MBBS, MRCP, PhD

Clinical Senior Lecturer
Cardiovascular Division
Faculty of Life Science & Medicine
King's College, London, UK

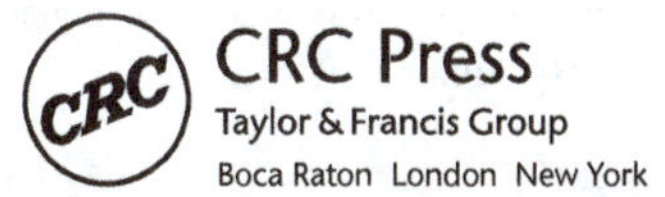

CRC Press is an imprint of the
Taylor & Francis Group, an **informa** business

CRC Press
Taylor & Francis Group
6000 Broken Sound Parkway NW, Suite 300
Boca Raton, FL 33487-2742

Printed on acid-free paper
Version Date: 20160223

International Standard Book Number-13: 978-1-4822-3621-7 (Paperback)

Visit the Taylor & Francis Web site at
http://www.taylorandfrancis.com

and the CRC Press Web site at
http://www.crcpress.com

Contents

Acknowledgments

We have obtained a considerable volume of valuable information from the following sources and acknowledge the editors, contributors, and publishers with gratitude.

British National Formulary. Available at: https://www.medicinescomplete.com/about/subscribe.htm. Accessed on 2015.

Electronic Medicines Compendium, Summary of Product Characteristics (on-line search of manufacturers' SPCs). Available at: https://www.medicines.org.uk/emc/latest-medicines-updates. Accessed on 2015.

Hansten PD, Horn JR. *Top 100 Drug Interactions*. CreateSpace Independent Publishing Platform, CreatesPace Amazon, North Charleston, SC, 2015.

Liverpool HIV Pharmacology Group. Available at: http://www.hivdruginteractions.org/Interactions.aspx. Accessed on 2015.

Martindale: The Complete Drug Reference. Available at: https://www.medicinescomplete.com/mc/martindale/current/. Accessed on 2015.

Stockley. Available at: https://www.medicinescomplete.com/about/subscribe.htm. Accessed on 2015.

We have attempted to indicate the main sources of references in each section within the space available to us.

LK acknowledges the advice, guidance, and continued support of Barbara Norwitz and Jill Jurgensen of Taylor & Francis Group and thanks Dilini Eriyagama and Sidantha Karalliedde for technical assistance and Ajayakumar Anandibhai Patel (B Pharm, King's College, London) for providing necessary information.

Abbreviations

%	Percentage
↓	Reduce (s/d)
↑	Increase (s/d)
$<$	Less than
$>$	More than
5HT	5-Hydroxytryptamine
ABCB1	ATP-binding cassette, sub-family B Member 1. Gene encoding Pgp
ACE	Angiotensin-converting enzyme
ACh	Acetylcholine
ADE	Adverse drug event
ADH	Antidiuretic hormone
ADI	Adverse drug interaction
AIDS	Acquired immune deficiency syndrome
APTT	Activated partial thromboplastin time
ATP	Adenosine triphosphate
AUC	Area under the concentration–time curve
AV	Atrioventricular
BCG	Bacille Calmette-Guerin
BCRP	Breast cancer resistance protein
BP	Blood pressures
BSL	Blood sugar level
BZD	Benzodiazepine
CAR	Constitutive androstane receptor
CHM	Commission on Human Medicine
CHMP	Committee for Medicinal Products for Human Use
CK	Creatine kinase
Cl^-	Chloride ion
CNS	Central nervous system
C_{max}	Highest concentration reached (the peak)
COMT	Catechol-*O*-methyltransferase
CSF	Cerebrospinal fluid
CSM	Committee on Safety of Medicines
CYP	Cytochrome P450
ECG	Electrocardiogram
f	The free, unbound fraction of the drug
FBC	Full blood count
FDA	Food and Drug Administration
GABA	Gamma-amino butyric acid
GBL	Gamma butyrolactone
GHB	Gamma hydroxybutyrate
GTN	Glyceryl trinitrate
H2	Histamine 2 receptor
HbA1c	Glycated hemoglobin
HCO_3	Bicarbonate ion
HIV	Human immunodeficiency virus
HR	Heart rate
IL	Interleukin
INR	International normalised ratio
K^+	Potassium ion
LFT	Liver function test
MAO	Monoamine oxidase
MAOI	Monoamine oxidase inhibitor
MATE	Multi-antimicrobial extrusion protein
MDMA	Methylenedioxymethamphetamine
MDRP	Multidrug resistance protein. A transporter protein related to Pgp
MIC	Minimum inhibitory concentration
MDR	As MDRP
MSG	Monosodium glutamate
Na^+	Sodium ion
NAT	*N*-acetyltransferase
NG	Nasogastric
NICE	National Institute for Health and Clinical Excellence
NJ	Nasojejunal
NMDA	*N*-methyl-D-aspartate
NNMT	Nicotinamide *N*-methyltransferase
NNRTI	Nonnucleoside reverse transcriptase inhibitor
NRTI	Nucleoside reverse transcriptase inhibitor
NSAID	Nonsteroidal anti-inflammatory drug
NTCP	Na^+ taurocholate cotransporting polypeptide

OATP	Organic anion transporting polypeptide
OCT	Organic cation transporter
OTC	Over-the-counter
PDE-5	Phosphodiesterase 5
PEG	Percutaneous enteral gastrostomy
PEJ	Percutaneous enteral jejunostomy
Pgp	P-glycoprotein
pH	Concentration of H^+ ion
PI	Protease inhibitor
PO	Oral administration
PPI	Proton pump inhibitor
PR	Pulse rate
PRN	As required (pro re nata)
PXR	Pregnane X receptor
RF	Renal function
RNA	Ribonucleic acid
RR	Respiratory rate
SNP	Single nucleoside polymorphism
SNRI	Serotonin–norepinephrine (nor-adrenaline) reuptake inhibitor
SSRI	Selective serotonin reuptake inhibitor
TCA	Tricyclic antidepressant
TFT	Thyroid function test
TMT	Cytosolic thiol methyltransferase
$T_{>MIC}$	Cumulative percentage of a 24-hour period that the concentration is above MIC
TPMT	Thiopurine methyltransferase
TSH	Thyroid-stimulating hormone
U&E	Urea and electrolytes
UDPGT	Uridine diphosphate glucuronosyltransferase
UGT	As UDPGT

Preface

Simon F.J. Clarke and Lakshman Delgoda Karalliedde

The search for finite causes and predictability of adverse drug interactions (ADIs) has a strong resemblance to the unraveling of critical information by the fictional sleuths Hercule Poirot and Sherlock Holmes. It is becoming clear that the different permutations of genetic alterations within and between different population groups mean that ethnicity has to be considered for correct dosing of many medications. What next for the sleuths of science?

How can clinicians integrate this new information in a logical way to reduce the risk of unwanted effects of individual drugs (side effects) and the combination of different drugs (ADIs)?

Clinical guidelines have been developed to reduce variation in practice and improve patient safety. However, in the context of complex therapies that involve multiple variable factors and patients with multiple comorbidities, clear guidelines are difficult to develop.

The conclusion that guideline developers have to maintain a balance between producing clear and relatively short recommendations and avoiding glossing over the complexity of the real world[1] could not be more forthright.

Though we see some light at the end of the tunnel, one source being individualized prescribing, there are many obstacles to overcome:

- Is there even a remote possibility that individualized prescribing would be the norm for over half of the global population in the next 50 years?
- How are the required costs to be met by economies in an environment of lack of funds, poor infrastructure, and social inequality?
- As important allele frequencies have been reported to vary between different ethnic groups it is becoming increasingly important to determine dosing strategies for specific populations. This has progressed in countries with diverse populations such as Singapore, Korea, China and America.
- How much do we know with any certainty of the traditional or herbal medicines that have become popular due to accessibility, affordability, and availability causing adverse interactions with allopathic prescriptions? Do we have sufficient knowledge of pharmacokinetics and pharmacodynamics of these traditional medications? Do we have any right to prevent people from prioritizing their medications when health services are increasingly burdened by the cost of drugs? Is there a global responsibility to encourage "therapeutic pluralism," a concept proposed by Broom and Tovey,[2] in societies struggling with the economics of allopathic medicines by concentrating pharmacokinetic (PK) and pharmacodynamic (PD) studies on traditional medicines?
- Inter-population allele frequency discrepancies, particularly between American, European and other cohorts, are large to necessitate communities, regions within large countries, and countries in Asia such as Korea and China where there are large populations with characteristic allele frequencies contrasting to other countries to determine specific therapeutic dosing strategies for their population groups.[3,4]

A handbook has limited scope and space for detail. Our intention is to provide information to busy prescribers in a user-friendly form to ensure that they minimize the risk of harm to patients by ADI, many of which are entirely predictable. However, it is more than a simple list of interactions; we have attempted to provide an overview of the diverse and complex influences that link the mechanisms of interactions with their clinical effects. Prescribing certainly is not "elementary, my dear Watson"!

REFERENCES

1. Dumbreck S et al. Drug-disease and drug-drug interactions: Systematic examination of recommendations in 12 UK national clinical guidelines. *BMJ* 2015;350:h949.
2. Broom A, Tovey P. Therapeutic pluralism? Evidence, power and legitimacy in UK cancer services. *Sociology of Health Illness* 2007 May;29(4):551–569.
3. Meenagh A et al. Frequency of cytokine polymorphisms in populations from Western Europe, Africa, Asia, the Middle East and South America. *Human Immunology* 2002;63:1055.
4. Visentainer JEL, Sell AM, da Silva GC, Cavichioli AD, Franceschi DSA, Lieber SR, de Souza CA. TNF, IFNG, IL6, IL10 and TGFB1 gene polymorphisms in South and Southeast Brazil. *International Journal of Immunogenetics* 2008;35:287–293.

Easy Reference Guide to Drugs

Seneka Abeyratne

This index of drug names serves as a link to the drug interaction (DI) tables (Parts 1 through 18). A drug shown in column 1 may interact adversely with one or more drugs in the corresponding categories shown in column 4. For specific information, the relevant part of the book (as shown in columns 2 and 3) may be consulted.

Drug (primary)	Page	Part of the Book	Category	Subcategory (drug groups only)
abacavir	851, 858, 861	10. Drugs to treat infections	Antivirals	
abatacept	530	3. Anticancer and immunomodulating drugs	Other immunomodulating drugs	
acarbose	620–623	5. Antidiabetic drugs	Acarbose	
ace inhibitors	45–54	1. Drugs acting on the cardiovascular system	Antihypertensives and heart failure drugs	
acebutolol	112	1. Drugs acting on the cardiovascular system	Beta-blockers	
acetaminophen	See paracetamol	7. Analgesics		
acetazolamide	163–165	1. Drugs acting on the cardiovascular system	Diuretics	Carbonic anhydrase inhibitors
aclarubicin	394–395	3. Anticancer and immunomodulating drugs	Cytotoxics	
adalimumab	530–531	3. Anticancer and immunomodulating drugs	Other immunomodulating drugs	
adefovir	868	10. Drugs to treat infections	Antivirals	
adenosine	2	1. Drugs acting on the cardiovascular system	Antiarrhythmics	
adrenergic neurone blockers	54–59	1. Drugs acting on the cardiovascular system	Antihypertensives and heart failure drugs	
agalsidase	964	13. Metabolic drugs		
ajmaline	2–3	1. Drugs acting on the cardiovascular system	Antiarrhythmics	
alcohol	1024–1030	17. Miscellaneous	Miscellaneous pharmaceuticals	
alendronate	674	6. Other endocrine drugs	Bisphosphonates	
alfentanil	709, 712	7. Analgesics	Opioids	
alfuzosin	65	1. Drugs acting on the cardiovascular system	Antihypertensives and heart failure drugs	Alpha-blockers

(*Continued*)

Drug (primary)	Page	Part of the Book	Category	Subcategory (drug groups only)
alimemazine	942	12. Respratory drugs	Antihistamines	
aliskiren	60–62	1. Drugs acting on the cardiovascular system	Antihypertensives and heart failure drugs	
alitretinoin	583	3. Anticancer and immunomodulating drugs	Other immunomodulating drugs	
ALL	394, 530	3. Anticancer and immunomodulating drugs	Cytotoxics Other immunomodulating drugs	
allopurinol	49, 718–719, 1023	1. Drugs acting on the cardiovascular system	Antihypertensives and heart failure drugs	Ace inhibitors antigout drugs
		8. Musculoskeletal drugs	Antigout drugs	
		17. Miscellaneous	Miscellaneous pharmaceuticals	
almotriptan	328–333	2. Drugs acting on the central nervous system	Antimigraine drugs	5-HT1 agonists-triptans
alpha-blockers	62–67	1. Drugs acting on the cardiovascular system	Antihypertensives and heart failure drugs	
alprazolam	366, 368, 371	2. Drugs acting on the central nervous system	Anxiolytics and hypnotics	Benzodiazepines
alprostadil	985	15. Drugs used to treat the urinary system	Drugs used for urinary retention	
aluminum	913–914	11. Drugs acting on the gastrointestinal tract	Antacids	
amantadine	338–339	2. Drugs acting on the central nervous system	Anti-Parkinson's drugs	
ambrisentan	85	1. Drugs acting on the cardiovascular system	Antihypertensives and heart failure drugs	Vasodilator anti-hypertensives
amiloride	170, 171	1. Drugs acting on the cardiovascular system	Diuretics	Potassium-sparing diuretics and aldosterone antagonists
aminoglutethimide	524	3. Anticancer and immunomodulating drugs	Hormones and hormone antagonists	
aminoglycosides	756–758	10. Drugs to treat infections	Antibiotics	
aminophylline	951	12. Respratory drugs	Bronchodilators	Nonselective beta-agonists
aminosalicylates	916	11. Drugs acting on the gastrointestinal tract	Antidiarrheals	

(*Continued*)

Drug (primary)	Page	Part of the Book	Category	Subcategory (drug groups only)
aminosalicylates	532	3. Anticancer and immunomodulating drugs	Other immunomodulating drugs	
amiodarone	4–11	1. Drugs acting on the cardiovascular system	Antiarrhythmics	
amitriptyline	269, 270, 274, 276, 277	2. Drugs acting on the central nervous system	Antidepressants	Tricyclic antidepressants
ammonium chloride	988	15. Drugs used to treat the urinary system	Drugs used for urinary retention	urinary alkalinization
amphetamines	215, 998–1000	1. Drugs acting on the cardiovascular system		
		16. Drugs of abuse	Sympathomimetics	
amphotericin	804–805	10. Drugs to treat infections	Antifungal drugs	
ampicillin	769, 770	10. Drugs to treat infections	Antibiotics	
amprenavir	894, 895	10. Drugs to treat infections	Protease inhibitors	
amyl nitrite	1004	16. Drugs of abuse		
anagrelide	1008	17. Miscellaneous	Miscellaneous pharmaceuticals	
anakinra	533	3. Anticancer and immunomodulating drugs	Other immunomodulating drugs	
anastrazole	524	3. Anticancer and immunomodulating drugs	Hormones and hormone antagonists	
angiotensin ii receptor antagonists	67–73	1. Drugs acting on the cardiovascular system	Antihypertensives and heart failure drugs	
anion exchange resins	181–184	1. Drugs acting on the cardiovascular system	Lipid-lowering drugs	
antacids	912–913, 1020	11. Drugs acting on the gastrointestinal tract		Minerals and vitamins
		17. Miscellaneous	Miscellaneous pharmaceuticals	
antiemetics	916	11. Drugs acting on the gastrointestinal tract	Antidiarrheals	
antihistamines	1064–1065	18. Over-the-counter/ online drugs and remedies	Analgesics	
antimuscarinics	916	11. Drugs acting on the gastrointestinal tract	Antidiarrheals	
apixaban	598–600	4. Anticoagulants	Apixaban	
apomorphine	347, 349, 350	2. Drugs acting on the central nervous system	Anti-Parkinson's drugs	Dopaminergics

(*Continued*)

Drug (primary)	Page	Part of the Book	Category	Subcategory (drug groups only)
aprepitant	279–281	2. Drugs acting on the central nervous system	Antiemetics	
arifenacin	342	2. Drugs acting on the central nervous system	Anti-Parkinson's drugs	Antimuscarinics
aripiprazole	355, 357, 359–361	2. Drugs acting on the central nervous system	Antipsychotics	
arsenic trioxide	395–396	3. Anticancer and immunomodulating drugs	Cytotoxics	
artemether with lumefantrine	821–823	10. Drugs to treat infections	Antimalarials	
asparaginase	396	3. Anticancer and immunomodulating drugs	Cytotoxics	
aspirin	92–98, 1067	1. Drugs acting on the cardiovascular system	Antiplatelet drugs	
		18. Over-the-counter/online drugs and remedies	Drugs for prevention of heart disease	
astemizole	942–944	12. Respratory drugs	Antihistamines	
atazanavir	873, 875, 877, 879–881, 888, 890–893, 896, 897, 902, 905, 906	10. Drugs to treat infections	Protease inhibitors	
atomoxetine	376–378	2. Drugs acting on the central nervous system	CNS stimulants	
atorvastatin	188, 189, 191	1. Drugs acting on the cardiovascular system	Lipid-lowering drugs	Statins
atovaquone	823–824	10. Drugs to treat infections	Antimalarials	
atropine	340–342	2. Drugs acting on the central nervous system	Anti-Parkinson's drugs	Antimuscarinics
avasimibe	185	1. Drugs acting on the cardiovascular system	Lipid-lowering drugs	
axitinib	397–398	3. Anticancer and immunomodulating drugs	Cytotoxics	
azathioprine	533–537	3. Anticancer and immunomodulating drugs	Other immunomodulating drugs	
azimilide	11–12	1. Drugs acting on the cardiovascular system	Antiarrhythmics	

(Continued)

Drug (primary)	Page	Part of the Book	Category	Subcategory (drug groups only)
azithromycin	761, 767, 1020	17. Miscellaneous	Miscellaneous pharmaceuticals	Antibiotics
		10. Drugs to treat infections	Antibiotics	
azoles	809, 812	10. Drugs to treat infections	Antifungal drugs	Azoles
baclofen	726–729	8. Musculoskeletal drugs	Skeletal muscle relaxants	
bambuterol	950	12. Respratory drugs	Bronchodilators	Beta-2 agonists
barbiturates	286–296, 1023	2. Drugs acting on the central nervous system	Antiepileptics	Antiepileptics
		17. Miscellaneous	Miscellaneous pharmaceuticals	
basiliximab	537	3. Anticancer and immunomodulating drugs	Other immunomodulating drugs	
benazepril	48	1. Drugs acting on the cardiovascular system	Antihypertensives and heart failure drugs	Ace inhibitors
bendamustine	398–399	3. Anticancer and immunomodulating drugs	Cytotoxics	
benzbromarone	719	8. Musculoskeletal drugs	Antigout drugs	
benzodiazepines	365–366	2. Drugs acting on the central nervous system	Anxiolytics and hypnotics	
bepridil	132	1. Drugs acting on the cardiovascular system	Calcium channel blockers	
betaxolol	112, 119	1. Drugs acting on the cardiovascular system	Beta-blockers	
bevacizumab	537–538	3. Anticancer and immunomodulating drugs	Other immunomodulating drugs	
bexarotene	399	3. Anticancer and immunomodulating drugs	Cytotoxics	
bicalutamide	524	3. Anticancer and immunomodulating drugs	Hormones and hormone antagonists	
bisoprolol	112	1. Drugs acting on the cardiovascular system	Beta-blockers	
bisphosphonates	674, 675	6. Other endocrine drugs	Bisphosphonates	
bleomycin	399–400	3. Anticancer and immunomodulating drugs	Cytotoxics	
bortezomib	400–401	3. Anticancer and immunomodulating drugs	Cytotoxics	

(*Continued*)

Drug (primary)	Page	Part of the Book	Category	Subcategory (drug groups only)
bosentan	84–86, 88, 90, 91	1. Drugs acting on the cardiovascular system	Antihypertensives and heart failure drugs	Vasodilator anti-hypertensives
bosutinib	402–405	3. Anticancer and immunomodulating drugs	Cytotoxics	
brentuximab vedotin	538	3. Anticancer and immunomodulating drugs	Other immunomodulating drugs	
bromocriptine	344, 345, 350, 356	2. Drugs acting on the central nervous system	Anti-Parkinson's drugs Antipsychotics	Dopaminergics
bupivacaine	746	9. Anesthetic drugs	Anesthetics—Local	
bupropion	383–386	2. Drugs acting on the central nervous system	Drug dependence therapies	
buspirone	373	2. Drugs acting on the central nervous system	Anxiolytics and hypnotics	
busulfan	405–407	3. Anticancer and immunomodulating drugs	Cytotoxics	
cabazitaxel	407–408	3. Anticancer and immunomodulating drugs	Cytotoxics	
cabergoline	344, 346	2. Drugs acting on the central nervous system	Anti-Parkinson's drugs	Dopaminergics
caffeine	953	12. Respratory drugs	Bronchodilators	Nonselective beta-agonists
calcium	915, 1016–1017	11. Drugs acting on the gastrointestinal tract	Antacids	Minerals and vitamins
		17. Miscellaneous	Miscellaneous pharmaceuticals	
cannabis	992–998	16. Drugs of abuse		
capecitabine	408, 439–441	3. Anticancer and immunomodulating drugs	Cytotoxics	
capreomycin	756	10. Drugs to treat infections	Antibiotics	
captopril	48, 50	1. Drugs acting on the cardiovascular system	Antihypertensives and heart failure drugs	Ace inhibitors
carbamazepine	296–305, 1023	2. Drugs acting on the central nervous system	Antiepileptics	Antiepileptics
		17. Miscellaneous	Miscellaneous pharmaceuticals	
carbimazole	675	6. Other endocrine drugs	Carbimazole	
carboplatin	490	3. Anticancer and immunomodulating drugs	Cytotoxics	

(*Continued*)

Drug (primary)	Page	Part of the Book	Category	Subcategory (drug groups only)
carisoprodol	729	8. Musculoskeletal drugs	Skeletal muscle relaxants	
carmustine	408	3. Anticancer and immunomodulating drugs	Cytotoxics	
carvedilol	112, 119, 122	1. Drugs acting on the cardiovascular system	Beta-blockers	
caspofungin	817, 818	10. Drugs to treat infections	Antifungal drugs	Azoles
cefpodoxime	758	10. Drugs to treat infections	Antibiotics	
cefuroxime	758	10. Drugs to treat infections	Antibiotics	
celecoxib	689–692, 695, 698, 700	7. Analgesics	Nonsteroidal anti-inflammatory drugs (NSAIDS)	
centrally acting antihypertensives	74–81	1. Drugs acting on the cardiovascular system	Antihypertensives and heart failure drugs	
cephalosporins	759	10. Drugs to treat infections	Antibiotics	
certolizumab pegol	538	3. Anticancer and immunomodulating drugs	Other immunomodulating drugs	
chloral hydrate	374	2. Drugs acting on the central nervous system	Anxiolytics and hypnotics	
chlorambucil	408–409	3. Anticancer and immunomodulating drugs	Cytotoxics	
chloramphenicol	794	10. Drugs to treat infections	Other antibiotics	
chlordiazepoxide	368	2. Drugs acting on the central nervous system	Anxiolytics and hypnotics	Benzodiazepines
chlormethiazole	374	2. Drugs acting on the central nervous system	Anxiolytics and hypnotics	
chlormethine	409	3. Anticancer and immunomodulating drugs	Cytotoxics	
chloroquine	824	10. Drugs to treat infections	Antimalarials	
chloroquine/ hydroxychloroquine	823	10. Drugs to treat infections	Antimalarials	
chlorphenamine	941	12. Respratory drugs	Antihistamines	
chlorpheniramine	942	12. Respratory drugs	Antihistamines	
chlorpromazine	356, 358, 361, 363	2. Drugs acting on the central nervous system	Antipsychotics	
chlorpropamide	658, 663	5. Antidiabetic drugs	Sulfonylureas	
chlorzoxazone	729	8. Musculoskeletal drugs	Skeletal muscle relaxants	

(*Continued*)

Drug (primary)	Page	Part of the Book	Category	Subcategory (drug groups only)
cholestyramine	916	11. Drugs acting on the gastrointestinal tract	Antidiarrheals	
cholestyramine	1023	17. Miscellaneous	Miscellaneous pharmaceuticals	Lipid-lowering drugs
cibenzoline	12–13	1. Drugs acting on the cardiovascular system	Antiarrhythmics	
ciclosporin	539–556	3. Anticancer and immunomodulating drugs	Other immunomodulating drugs	
cidofovir	868	10. Drugs to treat infections	Antivirals	
cilostazol	199–201	1. Drugs acting on the cardiovascular system	Peripheral vasodilators	
cimetidine	916–929	11. Drugs acting on the gastrointestinal tract	H2 receptor blockers	
cinacalcet	1008–1009	17. Miscellaneous	Miscellaneous pharmaceuticals	
ciprofloxacin	772- 776, 1020–1021	17. Miscellaneous	Miscellaneous pharmaceuticals	Antibiotics, minerals and vitamins
		10. Drugs to treat infections	Antibiotics	
cisplatin	489–491	3. Anticancer and immunomodulating drugs	Cytotoxics	
cladribine	409	3. Anticancer and immunomodulating drugs	Cytotoxics	Cisplatin
clarithromycin	761–763, 765–769	10. Drugs to treat infections	Antibiotics	
clindamycin	795	10. Drugs to treat infections	Other antibiotics	
clodronate	674	6. Other endocrine drugs	Bisphosphonates	
clofarabine	410	3. Anticancer and immunomodulating drugs	Cytotoxics	
clomipramine	270, 274, 276	2. Drugs acting on the central nervous system	Antidepressants	Tricyclic antidepressants
clonidine	74–78, 80	1. Drugs acting on the cardiovascular system	Antihypertensives and heart failure drugs	Centrally acting antihypertensives
clopidogrel	98–101	1. Drugs acting on the cardiovascular system	Antiplatelet drugs	
clozapine	353, 355–357, 360–364, 1023	2. Drugs acting on the central nervous system	Antipsychotics	Antipsychotic drugs
		17. Miscellaneous	Miscellaneous pharmaceuticals	

(*Continued*)

Drug (primary)	Page	Part of the Book	Category	Subcategory (drug groups only)
cobicistat	862–866, 868, 870–873	10. Drugs to treat infections	Antivirals	
cocaine	747, 1003–1004	9. Anesthetic drugs	Anesthetics—Local	
		16. Drugs of abuse		
codeine	701, 709, 712	7. Analgesics	Opioids	
colchicine	720–721	8. Musculoskeletal drugs	Antigout drugs	
colesevelam	183	1. Drugs acting on the cardiovascular system	Lipid-lowering drugs	Anion exchange resins
colestipol	1023	17. Miscellaneous	Miscellaneous pharmaceuticals	Lipid-lowering drugs
colistin	795–796	10. Drugs to treat infections	Other antibiotics	
colony-stimulating factors	1009	17. Miscellaneous	Miscellaneous pharmaceuticals	
conivaptan	675–676	6. Other endocrine drugs	Conivaptan	
corticosteroids	556–561, 563–566, 916, 1021,	11. Drugs acting on the gastrointestinal tract	Antidiarrheals	Anticancer and immunomodulating drugs
		17. Miscellaneous	Miscellaneous pharmaceuticals	
		3. Anticancer and immunomodulating drugs	Other immunomodulating drugs	
cortisone	1021	17. Miscellaneous	Miscellaneous pharmaceuticals	Anticancer and immunomodulating drugs
co-trimoxazole	786–789	10. Drugs to treat infections	Antibiotics	
coumarins	600–611	4. Anticoagulants	coumarins	
crisantaspase	410	3. Anticancer and immunomodulating drugs	Cytotoxics	
crizotinib	411–413	3. Anticancer and immunomodulating drugs	Cytotoxics	
cyclobenzaprine	729	8. Musculoskeletal drugs	Skeletal muscle relaxants	
cyclophosphamide	414–416	3. Anticancer and immunomodulating drugs	Cytotoxics	
cycloserine	796	10. Drugs to treat infections	Other antibiotics	
cyproheptadine	941, 943	12. Respratory drugs	Antihistamines	
cytarabine	416	3. Anticancer and immunomodulating drugs	Cytotoxics	
dabigatran	611–613	4. Anticoagulants	dabigatran	

(Continued)

Drug (primary)	Page	Part of the Book	Category	Subcategory (drug groups only)
dabrafenib	417–419	3. Anticancer and immunomodulating drugs	Cytotoxics	
dacarbazine	420	3. Anticancer and immunomodulating drugs	Cytotoxics	
dalfopristin	801, 802	10. Drugs to treat infections	Other antibiotics	
danazol	970	14. Obstetrics and gynecology		
dantrolene	730	8. Musculoskeletal drugs	Skeletal muscle relaxants	
dapsone	796	10. Drugs to treat infections	Other antibiotics	
daptomycin	797	10. Drugs to treat infections	Other antibiotics	
darifenacin	340–342	2. Drugs acting on the central nervous system	Anti-Parkinson's drugs	Antimuscarinics
darunavir	884, 891–893, 896, 898, 905	10. Drugs to treat infections	Protease inhibitors	
dasatinib	420–423	3. Anticancer and immunomodulating drugs	Cytotoxics	
daunorubicin	423	3. Anticancer and immunomodulating drugs	Cytotoxics	
DDP-4 inhibitors	632	5. Antidiabetic drugs	Dipeptidyl peptidase-4 (DDP-4) inhibitors (gliptins)	
deferasirox	1009–1010	17. Miscellaneous	Miscellaneous pharmaceuticals	
deferoxamine	1010	17. Miscellaneous	Miscellaneous pharmaceuticals	
derivatives	651	5. Antidiabetic drugs	Sodium-glucose co-transporter 2 (SGLT-2) inhibitors (gliflozins)	
desipramine	270, 273, 276	2. Drugs acting on the central nervous system	Antidepressants	Tricyclic antidepressants
desmopressin	676–677, 984	15. Drugs used to treat the urinary system	Drugs used for urinary retention	
		6. Other endocrine drugs	Desmopressin	
desvenlafaxine	264	2. Drugs acting on the central nervous system	Antidepressants	Serotonin norepinephrine reuptake inhibitors
dexamethasone	557–559, 562	3. Anticancer and immunomodulating drugs	Other immunomodulating drugs	

(*Continued*)

Drug (primary)	Page	Part of the Book	Category	Subcategory (drug groups only)
dexamfetamine	216	1. Drugs acting on the cardiovascular system	Sympathomimetics	
dextromethorphan	704, 708	7. Analgesics	Opioids	
diazepam	366–371	2. Drugs acting on the central nervous system	Anxiolytics and hypnotics	Benzodiazepines
diazoxide	84–88, 90, 91	1. Drugs acting on the cardiovascular system	Antihypertensives and heart failure drugs	Vasodilator anti-hypertensives
diclofenac	692	7. Analgesics	Nonsteroidal anti-inflammatory drugs (NSAIDS)	
didanosine	851–856, 859, 860	10. Drugs to treat infections	Antivirals	
diflunisal	692	7. Analgesics	Nonsteroidal anti-inflammatory drugs (NSAIDS)	
digitoxin	151–163	1. Drugs acting on the cardiovascular system	Cardiac glycosides	
dihydrocodeine	709	7. Analgesics	Opioids	
dihydroergotamine	326, 327	2. Drugs acting on the central nervous system	Antimigraine drugs	Ergot derivatives
dihydropyridines	128, 133, 144, 148	1. Drugs acting on the cardiovascular system	Calcium channel blockers	
diltiazem	128, 130–132, 134, 142, 144, 145, 147–150	1. Drugs acting on the cardiovascular system	Calcium channel blockers	
dinoprostone	981	14. Obstetrics and gynecology	Alprostadil	
dipyridamole	101–103	1. Drugs acting on the cardiovascular system	Antiplatelet drugs	
disopyramide	13–16	1. Drugs acting on the cardiovascular system	Antiarrhythmics	
disulfiram	386–387	2. Drugs acting on the central nervous system	Drug dependence therapies	
dobutamine	213	1. Drugs acting on the cardiovascular system	Sympathomimetics	
docetaxel	424–426	3. Anticancer and immunomodulating drugs	Cytotoxics	
dofetilide	16–19	1. Drugs acting on the cardiovascular system	Antiarrhythmics	

(*Continued*)

Drug (primary)	Page	Part of the Book	Category	Subcategory (drug groups only)
dolutegravir	862, 864, 865, 867, 869–872	10. Drugs to treat infections	Antivirals	
domperidone	281–283	2. Drugs acting on the central nervous system	Antiemetics	Dopamine receptor antagonists
donepezil	218, 387, 389, 390	2. Drugs acting on the central nervous system	Antidementia drugs Parasympathomimetics	
dopamine	211	1. Drugs acting on the cardiovascular system	Sympathomimetics	
doxapram	960	12. Respratory drugs	cystic fibrosis therapies	
doxepin	273, 274	2. Drugs acting on the central nervous system	Antidepressants	Tricyclic antidepressants
doxorubicin	426–429	3. Anticancer and immunomodulating drugs	Cytotoxics	
doxycycline	790–793	10. Drugs to treat infections	Antibiotics	
dronedarone	19–22	1. Drugs acting on the cardiovascular system	Antiarrhythmics	
duloxetine	261–263, 984	2. Drugs acting on the central nervous system	Antidepressants	Serotonin norepinephrine reuptake inhibitors
		15. Drugs used to treat the urinary system	Drugs used for urinary retention	
dutasteride	984	15. Drugs used to treat the urinary system	Drugs used for urinary retention	alpha-blockers
efavirenz	836–838, 840–842, 844–847, 849, 850	10. Drugs to treat infections	Antivirals	
eletriptan	328–333	2. Drugs acting on the central nervous system	Antimigraine drugs	
eliglustat	964–966	13. Metabolic drugs		
eltrombopag	1011–1012	17. Miscellaneous	Miscellaneous pharmaceuticals	
elvitegravir	869, 870	10. Drugs to treat infections	Antivirals	
elvitegravir (ritonavir boosted)	862, 864, 865, 867	10. Drugs to treat infections	Antivirals	
emtricitabine	853, 860	10. Drugs to treat infections	Antivirals	
enalapril	48, 49	1. Drugs acting on the cardiovascular system	Antihypertensives and heart failure drugs	Ace inhibitors

(Continued)

Drug (primary)	Page	Part of the Book	Category	Subcategory (drug groups only)
enflurane	742	9. Anesthetic drugs	Anesthetics—General	
enfuvirtide	872	10. Drugs to treat infections	Antivirals	
enoximone	207	1. Drugs acting on the cardiovascular system	Selective phosphodiesterase inhibitors	
entacapone	345, 349, 350	2. Drugs acting on the central nervous system	Anti-Parkinson's drugs	Dopaminergics
epinephrine	745	9. Anesthetic drugs	Anesthetics—Local	
epirubicin	429–431	3. Anticancer and immunomodulating drugs	Cytotoxics	
eplerenone	171	1. Drugs acting on the cardiovascular system	Diuretics	Potassium-sparing diuretics and aldosterone antagonists
epoetins	1012–1013	17. Miscellaneous	Miscellaneous pharmaceuticals	
ergometrine	326	2. Drugs acting on the central nervous system	Antimigraine drugs	Ergot derivatives
ergotamine	326, 327	2. Drugs acting on the central nervous system	Antimigraine drugs	Ergot derivatives
erlotinib	431–433	3. Anticancer and immunomodulating drugs	Cytotoxics	
ertapenem	759	10. Drugs to treat infections	Antibiotics	
erythromycin	761–763, 765–767	10. Drugs to treat infections	Antibiotics	
erythromycin	768, 769	10. Drugs to treat infections	Antibiotics	
escitalopram	256, 258	2. Drugs acting on the central nervous system	Antidepressants	Selective serotonin reuptake inhibitors
esomeprazole	See proton pump inhibitors			
estramustine	433	3. Anticancer and immunomodulating drugs	Cytotoxics	
estrogens	971–978	14. Obstetrics and gynecology		
etanercept	566	3. Anticancer and immunomodulating drugs	Other immunomodulating drugs	
ethambutol	797, 1021	17. Miscellaneous	Miscellaneous pharmaceuticals	Minerals and vitamins
		10. Drugs to treat infections	Other antibiotics	
ethosuximide	305–306	2. Drugs acting on the central nervous system	Antiepileptics	

(*Continued*)

Drug (primary)	Page	Part of the Book	Category	Subcategory (drug groups only)
etidronate	674	6. Other endocrine drugs	Bisphosphonates	
etoposide	434–435	3. Anticancer and immunomodulating drugs	Cytotoxics	
etravirine	836, 837, 839–842, 844, 845, 847–849	10. Drugs to treat infections	Antivirals	
everolimus	435–437	3. Anticancer and immunomodulating drugs	Cytotoxics	
exemestane	438	3. Anticancer and immunomodulating drugs	Cytotoxics	
ezetimibe	185	1. Drugs acting on the cardiovascular system	Lipid-lowering drugs	
famotidine	919, 922, 924	11. Drugs acting on the gastrointestinal tract	H2 receptor blockers	
fampridine	566	3. Anticancer and immunomodulating drugs	Other immunomodulating drugs	
febuxostat	721	8. Musculoskeletal drugs	Antigout drugs	
felodipine	131	1. Drugs acting on the cardiovascular system	Calcium channel blockers	
fentanyl	701, 702, 708, 709, 712	7. Analgesics	Opioids	
festerodine	341, 342	2. Drugs acting on the central nervous system	Anti-Parkinson's drugs	Antimuscarinics
fexofenadine	941, 942, 944	12. Respratory drugs	Antihistamines	
fibrates	185–187	1. Drugs acting on the cardiovascular system	Lipid-lowering drugs	
finasteride	984	15. Drugs used to treat the urinary system	Drugs used for urinary retention	Alpha-blockers
fingolimod	567	3. Anticancer and immunomodulating drugs	Other immunomodulating drugs	
flecainide	22–26	1. Drugs acting on the cardiovascular system	Antiarrhythmics	
fluconazole	805, 806, 808–810, 813, 814, 816–818	10. Drugs to treat infections	Antifungal drugs	Azoles

(*Continued*)

Drug (primary)	Page	Part of the Book	Category	Subcategory (drug groups only)
fludarabine	438	3. Anticancer and immunomodulating drugs	Cytotoxics	
fluoride	1017	17. Miscellaneous	Miscellaneous pharmaceuticals	Minerals and vitamins
fluorouracil	438–442	3. Anticancer and immunomodulating drugs	Cytotoxics	
fluoxetine	247, 249, 252, 254–257	2. Drugs acting on the central nervous system	Antidepressants	Selective serotonin reuptake inhibitors
flupentixol	356	2. Drugs acting on the central nervous system	Antipsychotics	
fluphenazine	356, 359	2. Drugs acting on the central nervous system	Antipsychotics	
flutamide	524	3. Anticancer and immunomodulating drugs	Hormones and hormone antagonists	
fluticasone	562	3. Anticancer and immunomodulating drugs	Other immunomodulating drugs	
fluvoxamine	245, 247, 249, 250, 252, 254–258	2. Drugs acting on the central nervous system	Antidepressants	Selective serotonin reuptake inhibitors
folic acid	442	3. Anticancer and immunomodulating drugs	Cytotoxics	
folinate	442	3. Anticancer and immunomodulating drugs	Cytotoxics	
fondaparinux	613	4. Anticoagulants	Fondaparinux	
fosamprenavir	877, 884, 888, 889, 891–894, 898	10. Drugs to treat infections	Protease inhibitors	
foscarnet sodium	868	10. Drugs to treat infections	Antivirals	
fusidic acid	797	10. Drugs to treat infections	Other antibiotics	
gabapentin	306	2. Drugs acting on the central nervous system	Antiepileptics	
galantamine	218, 387–389	2. Drugs acting on the central nervous system	Antidementia drugs	
gefitinib	442–444	3. Anticancer and immunomodulating drugs	Cytotoxics	
gemcitabine	444–445	3. Anticancer and immunomodulating drugs	Cytotoxics	

(*Continued*)

Drug (primary)	Page	Part of the Book	Category	Subcategory (drug groups only)
gemfibrozil	185, 186	1. Drugs acting on the cardiovascular system	Lipid-lowering drugs	Fibrates
gentamicin	756	10. Drugs to treat infections	Antibiotics	
gestrinone	970	14. Obstetrics and gynecology		
glatiramer acetate	568	3. Anticancer and immunomodulating drugs	Other immunomodulating drugs	
glipizide	656, 662, 1021	17. Miscellaneous	Miscellaneous pharmaceuticals	antidiabetic drugs
		5. Antidiabetic drugs	Sulfonylureas	
GLP-1 analogues	632, 633	5. Antidiabetic drugs	Glucagon-like peptide-1 (GLP-1) analogues	
glucagon	677	6. Other endocrine drugs	Glucagon	
glycoprotein IIb/IIIa inhibitors	103–105	1. Drugs acting on the cardiovascular system	Antiplatelet drugs	
glycopyrronium	340	2. Drugs acting on the central nervous system	Anti-Parkinson's drugs	Antimuscarinics
gold	568–569	3. Anticancer and immunomodulating drugs	Other immunomodulating drugs	
golimumab	569	3. Anticancer and immunomodulating drugs	Other immunomodulating drugs	
grapefruit juice	1032–1043	17. Miscellaneous	Fruit juices	
griseofulvin	818–820	10. Drugs to treat infections	Antifungal drugs	Azoles
guanfacine	378	2. Drugs acting on the central nervous system	CNS stimulants	
H2 receptor antagonists	1066	18. Over-the-counter/online drugs and remedies	Drugs acting on the gastrointestinal tract	
H2 receptor blockers	1023	17. Miscellaneous	Miscellaneous pharmaceuticals	
hallucinogens	1004	16. Drugs of abuse		
haloperidol	355–357, 359, 361–364, 387	2. Drugs acting on the central nervous system	Antipsychotics Drug dependence therapies	
halothane	736, 740–742	9. Anesthetic drugs	Anesthetics—General	
heparins	613–615	4. Anticoagulants	Heparins	
herbal drugs	1045–1060	17. Miscellaneous	Herbs	
hirudins	615	4. Anticoagulants	Hirudins	

(Continued)

Drug (primary)	Page	Part of the Book	Category	Subcategory (drug groups only)
histamine	569–570	3. Anticancer and immunomodulating drugs	Other immunomodulating drugs	
hydroxycarbamide	445	3. Anticancer and immunomodulating drugs	Cytotoxics	
hydroxyzine	940, 941, 944	12. Respratory drugs	Antihistamines	
hypnotics	1067	18. Over-the-counter/online drugs and remedies	Drugs acting on the centra l nervous system	
hypoglycemic drugs	1023	17. Miscellaneous	Miscellaneous pharmaceuticals	Minerals and vitamins
ibandronate	674	6. Other endocrine drugs	Bisphosphonates	
ibuprofen	692	7. Analgesics	Nonsteroidal anti-inflammatory drugs (NSAIDS)	
ibutilide	27–28	1. Drugs acting on the cardiovascular system	Antiarrhythmics	
idarubicin	445–446	3. Anticancer and immunomodulating drugs	Cytotoxics	
ifosfamide	446–449	3. Anticancer and immunomodulating drugs	Cytotoxics	
iloperidone	359	2. Drugs acting on the central nervous system	Antipsychotics	
iloprost	87	1. Drugs acting on the cardiovascular system	Antihypertensives and heart failure drugs	Vasodilator anti-hypertensives
imatinib	449–456	3. Anticancer and immunomodulating drugs	Cytotoxics	
imipenem with cilastatin	760	10. Drugs to treat infections	Antibiotics	
imipramine	270, 274, 276, 277	2. Drugs acting on the central nervous system	Antidepressants	Tricyclic antidepressants
indinavir	873, 875, 877, 879–882, 892, 893, 895, 901, 905	10. Drugs to treat infections	Protease inhibitors	
indomethacin	689, 699	7. Analgesics	Nonsteroidal anti-inflammatory drugs (NSAIDS)	
indoramin	62	1. Drugs acting on the cardiovascular system	Antihypertensives and heart failure drugs	

(*Continued*)

Drug (primary)	Page	Part of the Book	Category	Subcategory (drug groups only)
infliximab	570–571, 916	11. Drugs acting on the gastrointestinal tract	Antidiarrheals	
		3. Anticancer and immunomodulating drugs	Other immunomodulating drugs	
insulin	633–641	5. Antidiabetic drugs	Insulin	
interferon	572	3. Anticancer and immunomodulating drugs	Other immunomodulating drugs	
interferon alfa	571	3. Anticancer and immunomodulating drugs	Other immunomodulating drugs	
interferon beta	572	3. Anticancer and immunomodulating drugs	Other immunomodulating drugs	
interferon gamma	572–573	3. Anticancer and immunomodulating drugs	Other immunomodulating drugs	
interleukin-2	573–574	3. Anticancer and immunomodulating drugs	Other immunomodulating drugs	
ipilimumab	574	3. Anticancer and immunomodulating drugs	Other immunomodulating drugs	
ipratropium	340–342	2. Drugs acting on the central nervous system	Anti-Parkinson's drugs	Antimuscarinics
irbesartan	70	1. Drugs acting on the cardiovascular system	Antihypertensives and heart failure drugs	Angiotensin II receptor antagonists
irinotecan	457–461	3. Anticancer and immunomodulating drugs	Cytotoxics	
iron	1017	17. Miscellaneous	Miscellaneous pharmaceuticals	Minerals and vitamins
isoflurane	736, 742	9. Anesthetic drugs	Anesthetics—General	
isoniazid	797–798	10. Drugs to treat infections	Other antibiotics	
itraconazole	806–817	10. Drugs to treat infections	Antifungal drugs	Azoles
ivabradine	179–180	1. Drugs acting on the cardiovascular system	Ivabradine	
ivacaftor	959–960	12. Respratory drugs	cystic fibrosis therapies	
kaolin	915	11. Drugs acting on the gastrointestinal tract	Antidiarrheals	
ketamine	740, 741, 743	9. Anesthetic drugs	Anesthetics—General	
ketanserin	81–83	1. Drugs acting on the cardiovascular system	Antihypertensives and heart failure drugs	
ketobemidone	702	7. Analgesics	Opioids	

(*Continued*)

Drug (primary)	Page	Part of the Book	Category	Subcategory (drug groups only)
ketoconazole	806–815	10. Drugs to treat infections	Antifungal drugs	Azoles
ketoprofen	692	7. Analgesics	Nonsteroidal anti-inflammatory drugs (NSAIDS)	
ketotifen	943	12. Respratory drugs	Antihistamines	
labetalol	115	1. Drugs acting on the cardiovascular system	Beta-blockers	
lamivudine	853–855	10. Drugs to treat infections	Antivirals	
lamotrigine	307	2. Drugs acting on the central nervous system	Antiepileptics	
lanreotide	525	3. Anticancer and immunomodulating drugs	Hormones and hormone antagonists	
lansoprazole	See proton pump inhibitors			
lapatinib	461–464, 921	11. Drugs acting on the gastrointestinal tract	H2 receptor blockers	
		3. Anticancer and immunomodulating drugs	Cytotoxics	
laronidase	966	13. Metabolic drugs		
laxatives	929	11. Drugs acting on the gastrointestinal tract		
leflunomide	574–577	3. Anticancer and immunomodulating drugs	Other immunomodulating drugs	
letrozole	525	3. Anticancer and immunomodulating drugs	Hormones and hormone antagonists	
levamisole	831–832	10. Drugs to treat infections	Other antiprotozoals	
levodopa	343–345, 347–351	2. Drugs acting on the central nervous system	Anti-Parkinson's drugs	Dopaminergics
levofloxacin	773, 1021	17. Miscellaneous	Miscellaneous pharmaceuticals	Minerals and vitamins
		10. Drugs to treat infections	Antibiotics	
lidocaine	743, 744, 746, 747	9. Anesthetic drugs	Anesthetics—Local	
linagliptin	631	5. Antidiabetic drugs	Dipeptidyl peptidase-4 (DDP-4) inhibitors (gliptins)	
linezolid	228, 230	2. Drugs acting on the central nervous system	Antidepressants	Monoamine oxidase inhibitors

(*Continued*)

Drug (primary)	Page	Part of the Book	Category	Subcategory (drug groups only)
lisinopril	48	1. Drugs acting on the cardiovascular system	Antihypertensives and heart failure drugs	Ace inhibitors
lithium	219–224	2. Drugs acting on the central nervous system	Antidementia drugs	
lixisenatide	632	5. Antidiabetic drugs	Glucagon-like peptide-1 (GLP-1) analogues	
lofexidine	387	2. Drugs acting on the central nervous system	Drug dependence therapies	
lomitapide	187	1. Drugs acting on the cardiovascular system	Lipid-lowering drugs	
lomustine	464	3. Anticancer and immunomodulating drugs	Cytotoxics	
loop diuretics	165–170	1. Drugs acting on the cardiovascular system	Diuretics	
lopera mide	915	11. Drugs acting on the gastrointestinal tract	Antidiarrheals	
lopinavir	873, 877, 880, 885, 886, 889, 891–894, 896–898, 902, 905, 906	10. Drugs to treat infections	Protease inhibitors	
loratadine	943, 944	12. Respratory drugs	Antihistamines	
lorazepam	366, 368	2. Drugs acting on the central nervous system	Anxiolytics and hypnotics	Benzodiazepines
lorcaserin	334–335	2. Drugs acting on the central nervous system	Antiobesity drugs	
losartan	68	1. Drugs acting on the cardiovascular system	Antihypertensives and heart failure drugs	Angiotensin II receptor antagonists
lovastatin	189	1. Drugs acting on the cardiovascular system	Lipid-lowering drugs	Statins
macrolides	760, 761, 763–765	10. Drugs to treat infections	Antibiotics	
macrolides	767–769	10. Drugs to treat infections	Antibiotics	
magnesium	913–915, 1017–1018	11. Drugs acting on the gastrointestinal tract	Antacids	Minerals and vitamins
		17. Miscellaneous	Miscellaneous pharmaceuticals	

(*Continued*)

Drug (primary)	Page	Part of the Book	Category	Subcategory (drug groups only)
maprotiline	275	2. Drugs acting on the central nervous system	Antidepressants	Tricyclic antidepressants
maraviroc	862–867, 869	10. Drugs to treat infections	Antivirals	
mebendazole	832	10. Drugs to treat infections	Other antiprotozoals	
mefenamic acid	692, 693	7. Analgesics	Nonsteroidal anti-inflammatory drugs (NSAIDS)	
mefloquine	825–826	10. Drugs to treat infections	Antimalarials	
megestrol	525	3. Anticancer and immunomodulating drugs	Hormones and hormone antagonists	
meglitinide	642	5. Antidiabetic drugs	Meglitinide derivatives	
melatonin	374	2. Drugs acting on the central nervous system	Anxiolytics and hypnotics	
meloxicam	690	7. Analgesics	Nonsteroidal anti-inflammatory drugs (NSAIDS)	
melphalan	465	3. Anticancer and immunomodulating drugs	Cytotoxics	
memantine	218	2. Drugs acting on the central nervous system	Antidementia drugs	
mepacrine	832	10. Drugs to treat infections	Other antiprotozoals	
meprobamate	374	2. Drugs acting on the central nervous system	Anxiolytics and hypnotics	
mercaptopurine	465	3. Anticancer and immunomodulating drugs	Cytotoxics	
meropenem	759	10. Drugs to treat infections	Antibiotics	
mesna	466	3. Anticancer and immunomodulating drugs	Cytotoxics	
metformin	624–631	5. Antidiabetic drugs	Metformin	
methadone	387, 701, 702, 709–711	2. Drugs acting on the central nervous system	Drug dependence therapies	
		7. Analgesics	Opioids	
methenamine	798	10. Drugs to treat infections	Other antibiotics	
methocarbamol	730	8. Musculoskeletal drugs	Skeletal muscle relaxants	
methotrexate	467–475	3. Anticancer and immunomodulating drugs	Cytotoxics	

(*Continued*)

Drug (primary)	Page	Part of the Book	Category	Subcategory (drug groups only)
methoxsalen	1013–1014	17. Miscellaneous	Miscellaneous pharmaceuticals	
methyldopa	75, 77	1. Drugs acting on the cardiovascular system	Antihypertensives and heart failure drugs	Centrally acting antihypertensives
methylenedioxymeth-amphetamine	1001–1003	16. Drugs of abuse		
methylphenidate	216	1. Drugs acting on the cardiovascular system	Sympathomimetics	
methysergide	327	2. Drugs acting on the central nervous system	Antimigraine drugs	Ergot derivatives
metoclopramide	281–283	2. Drugs acting on the central nervous system	Antiemetics	Dopamine receptor antagonists
metoprolol	110–112, 115, 118, 120	1. Drugs acting on the cardiovascular system	Beta-blockers	
metronidazole	799–800	10. Drugs to treat infections	Other antibiotics	
mexiletine	28–31	1. Drugs acting on the cardiovascular system	Antiarrhythmics	
mianserin	271	2. Drugs acting on the central nervous system	Antidepressants	Tricyclic antidepressants
mibefradil	130, 134	1. Drugs acting on the cardiovascular system	Calcium channel blockers	
miconazole	811	10. Drugs to treat infections	Antifungal drugs	Azoles
midazolam	366–369, 371	2. Drugs acting on the central nervous system	Anxiolytics and hypnotics	Benzodiazepines
mifamurtide	577	3. Anticancer and immunomodulating drugs	Other immunomodulating drugs	
mifepristone	971	14. Obstetrics and gynecology		
milrinone	207	1. Drugs acting on the cardiovascular system	Selective phosphodiesterase inhibitors	
minoxidil	87	1. Drugs acting on the cardiovascular system	Antihypertensives and heart failure drugs	Vasodilator anti-hypertensives
mirabegron	341, 984–985	2. Drugs acting on the central nervous system	Anti-Parkinson's drugs	Antimuscarinics
		15. Drugs used to treat the urinary system	Drugs used for urinary retention	
mirtazapine	235–236	2. Drugs acting on the central nervous system	Antidepressants	

(Continued)

Drug (primary)	Page	Part of the Book	Category	Subcategory (drug groups only)
mitomycin	475–476	3. Anticancer and immunomodulating drugs	Cytotoxics	
mitotane	476	3. Anticancer and immunomodulating drugs	Cytotoxics	
mitoxantrone	477	3. Anticancer and immunomodulating drugs	Cytotoxics	
mivacurium	750, 752, 754	9. Anesthetic drugs	Muscle relaxants—Nondepolarizings	
mizolastine	940, 941, 943, 944	12. Respratory drugs	Antihistamines	
moclobemide	231, 234	2. Drugs acting on the central nervous system	Antidepressants	Monoamine oxidase inhibitors
modafinil	378–382	2. Drugs acting on the central nervous system	CNS stimulants	
monoamine oxidase inhibitors	224–235	2. Drugs acting on the central nervous system	Antidepressants	
montelukast	945	12. Respratory drugs	asthma prophylaxis	Leukotriene receptor antagonists
moracizine	31–32	1. Drugs acting on the cardiovascular system	Antiarrhythmics	
morphine	702, 705–707, 711	7. Analgesics	Opioids	
moxisylyte	201	1. Drugs acting on the cardiovascular system	Peripheral vasodilators	
moxonidine	78	1. Drugs acting on the cardiovascular system	Antihypertensives and heart failure drugs	Centrally acting antihypertensives
mycophenolate	577–580	3. Anticancer and immunomodulating drugs	Other immunomodulating drugs	
nalidixic acid	772	10. Drugs to treat infections	Antibiotics	
naloxone	702	7. Analgesics	Opioids	
nandrolone	678	6. Other endocrine drugs	Nandrolone	
naproxen	692, 699	7. Analgesics	Nonsteroidal anti-inflammatory drugs (NSAIDS)	
natalizumab	581	3. Anticancer and immunomodulating drugs	Other immunomodulating drugs	
nateglinide	641–650	5. Antidiabetic drugs	Meglitinide derivatives	

(*Continued*)

Drug (primary)	Page	Part of the Book	Category	Subcategory (drug groups only)
nefazodone	247–249, 257, 258	2. Drugs acting on the central nervous system	Antidepressants	Selective serotonin reuptake inhibitors
nefopam	688	7. Analgesics	Nefopam	
nelarabine	477	3. Anticancer and immunomodulating drugs	Cytotoxics	
nelfinavir	894, 895, 897, 899, 901	10. Drugs to treat infections	Protease inhibitors	
neomycin	756, 757	10. Drugs to treat infections	Antibiotics	
neostigmine	388, 389	2. Drugs acting on the central nervous system	Parasympathomimetics	
nevirapine	837, 840, 842, 845, 847–850	10. Drugs to treat infections	Antivirals	
nicardipine	131	1. Drugs acting on the cardiovascular system	Calcium channel blockers	
nicorandil	202–204	1. Drugs acting on the cardiovascular system	Potassium channel activators	
nicotinic acid	187	1. Drugs acting on the cardiovascular system	Lipid-lowering drugs	
nifedipine	131, 137, 140, 145	1. Drugs acting on the cardiovascular system	Calcium channel blockers	
niflumic acid	692	7. Analgesics	Nonsteroidal anti-inflammatory drugs (NSAIDS)	
nilotinib	478–481	3. Anticancer and immunomodulating drugs	Cytotoxics	
nitisinone	966–967	13. Metabolic drugs		
nitrates	196–198	1. Drugs acting on the cardiovascular system	Nitrates	
nitrazepam	368	2. Drugs acting on the central nervous system	Anxiolytics and hypnotics	Benzodiazepines
nitrofurantoin	801, 1021	17. Miscellaneous	Miscellaneous pharmaceuticals	Minerals and vitamins
		10. Drugs to treat infections	Other antibiotics	
nitrous oxide	736	9. Anesthetic drugs	Anesthetics—General	
nizatidine	923, 928	11. Drugs acting on the gastrointestinal tract		
nnrtis	835, 836, 839–846, 849, 850	10. Drugs to treat infections	Antivirals	

(*Continued*)

Drug (primary)	Page	Part of the Book	Category	Subcategory (drug groups only)
norfloxacin	773, 775	10. Drugs to treat infections	Antibiotics	
nortriptyline	270, 274, 277	2. Drugs acting on the central nervous system	Antidepressants	Tricyclic antidepressants
nsaids	1063–1064	18. Over-the-counter/online drugs and remedies	Analgesics	
ntacids	1065–1066	18. Over-the-counter/online drugs and remedies	Drugs acting on the gastrointestinal tract	
nucleoside reverse transcriptase inhibitors	851, 852, 857–859	10. Drugs to treat infections	Antivirals	
octreotide	524	3. Anticancer and immunomodulating drugs	Hormones and hormone antagonists	
ofloxacin	774, 1021	17. Miscellaneous	Miscellaneous pharmaceuticals	Minerals and vitamins
		10. Drugs to treat infections	Antibiotics	
olanzapine	358, 359, 362, 363	2. Drugs acting on the central nervous system	Antipsychotics	
omeprazole	See proton pump inhibitors			
ondansetron	284–286	2. Drugs acting on the central nervous system	Antiemetics	5-HT3 antagonists
opioids	1064	18. Over-the-counter/online drugs and remedies	Analgesics	
oral contraceptives	972	14. Obstetrics and gynecology		
oral retinoids	583	3. Anticancer and immunomodulating drugs	Other immunomodulating drugs	
orlistat	335–337	2. Drugs acting on the central nervous system	Antiobesity drugs	
oxazepam	366, 368	2. Drugs acting on the central nervous system	Anxiolytics and hypnotics	Benzodiazepines
oxcarbazepine	308–309	2. Drugs acting on the central nervous system	Antiepileptics	
oxytocin	978	14. Obstetrics and gynecology		
paclitaxel	481–484	3. Anticancer and immunomodulating drugs	Cytotoxics	

(*Continued*)

Drug (primary)	Page	Part of the Book	Category	Subcategory (drug groups only)
pancreatin	930	11. Drugs acting on the gastrointestinal tract		
pancuronium	753	9. Anesthetic drugs	Muscle relaxants—Nondepolarizings	
panitumumab	582	3. Anticancer and immunomodulating drugs	Other immunomodulating drugs	
paracetamol	713–715, 1064	7. Analgesics	Paracetamol	
		18. Over-the-counter/online drugs and remedies	Analgesics	
parecoxib	689, 695	7. Analgesics	Nonsteroidal anti-inflammatory drugs (NSAIDS)	
parenteral bronchodilators	945	12. Respratory drugs	Bronchodilators	
paroxetine	247, 249, 250, 254–257	2. Drugs acting on the central nervous system	Antidepressants	Selective serotonin reuptake inhibitors
pasireotide	525	3. Anticancer and immunomodulating drugs	Hormones and hormone antagonists	
pazopanib	484–487	3. Anticancer and immunomodulating drugs	Cytotoxics	
pegvisomant	678	6. Other endocrine drugs	Pegvisomant	
pemetrexed	487	3. Anticancer and immunomodulating drugs	Cytotoxics	
penicillamine	582–583, 967, 1021	13. Metabolic drugs		Anticancer and immunomodulating drugs
		17. Miscellaneous	Miscellaneous pharmaceuticals	
		3. Anticancer and immunomodulating drugs	Other immunomodulating drugs	
penicillin V	769	10. Drugs to treat infections	Antibiotics	
penicillins	770	10. Drugs to treat infections	Antibiotics	
pentamidine	833	10. Drugs to treat infections	Other antiprotozoals	
pentamidine isetionate	832	10. Drugs to treat infections	Other antiprotozoals	
pentazocine	704, 708	7. Analgesics	Opioids	
pentostatin	488	3. Anticancer and immunomodulating drugs	Cytotoxics	

(Continued)

Drug (primary)	Page	Part of the Book	Category	Subcategory (drug groups only)
pentoxifylline	201–202	1. Drugs acting on the cardiovascular system	Peripheral vasodilators	
pergolide	347	2. Drugs acting on the central nervous system	Anti-Parkinson's drugs	Dopaminergics
perphenazine	363	2. Drugs acting on the central nervous system	Antipsychotics	
pethidine	701, 705, 708, 710, 712	7. Analgesics	Opioids	
phenelzine	226, 227, 232	2. Drugs acting on the central nervous system	Antidepressants	Monoamine oxidase inhibitors
phenobarbitone	292–293	2. Drugs acting on the central nervous system	Antiepileptics	Barbiturates
phenoperidine	705	7. Analgesics	Opioids	
phenothiazine	351–358, 364	2. Drugs acting on the central nervous system	Antipsychotics	
phentolamine	985	15. Drugs used to treat the urinary system	Drugs used for urinary retention	
phenytoin	309–321, 435, 1023	2. Drugs acting on the central nervous system	Antiepileptics	Antiepileptics
		17. Miscellaneous	Miscellaneous pharmaceuticals	
		3. Anticancer and immunomodulating drugs	Cytotoxics	
pimozide	351–353, 355–358, 360, 361, 363	2. Drugs acting on the central nervous system	Antipsychotics	
pindolol	116	1. Drugs acting on the cardiovascular system	Beta-blockers	
pioglitazone	665–672	5. Antidiabetic drugs	Thiazolidinediones (glitazones)	
piperacillin	770	10. Drugs to treat infections	Antibiotics	
piracetam	390	2. Drugs acting on the central nervous system	Parasympathomimetics	
pirfenidone	961	12. Respratory drugs		
piroxicam	690, 692	7. Analgesics	Nonsteroidal anti-inflammatory drugs (NSAIDS)	
pixantrone	488	3. Anticancer and immunomodulating drugs	Cytotoxics	

(*Continued*)

Drug (primary)	Page	Part of the Book	Category	Subcategory (drug groups only)
pizotifen	333	2. Drugs acting on the central nervous system	Antimigraine drugs	
platinum compounds	489–493	3. Anticancer and immunomodulating drugs	Cytotoxics	
polystyrene sulfonate resins	1014	17. Miscellaneous	Miscellaneous pharmaceuticals	
ponatinib	493–495	3. Anticancer and immunomodulating drugs	Cytotoxics	
porfimer	495	3. Anticancer and immunomodulating drugs	Cytotoxics	
posaconazole	805, 807, 811, 812, 816	10. Drugs to treat infections	Antifungal drugs	Azoles
potassium	1018–1019	17. Miscellaneous	Miscellaneous pharmaceuticals	Minerals and vitamins
potassium acetate	989	15. Drugs used to treat the urinary system	Drugs used for urinary retention	urinary alkalinization
potassium citrate	989	15. Drugs used to treat the urinary system	Drugs used for urinary retention	urinary alkalinization
potassium iodide	680	6. Other endocrine drugs	Thyroid hormones and iodine	
potassium-sparing diuretics and aldosterone anta gonists	170–174	1. Drugs acting on the cardiovascular system	Diuretics	
pramipexole	348, 349	2. Drugs acting on the central nervous system	Anti-Parkinson's drugs	Dopaminergics
prasugrel	105–106	1. Drugs acting on the cardiovascular system	Antiplatelet drugs	
prednisone	558, 1021	17. Miscellaneous	Miscellaneous pharmaceuticals	Anticancer and immunomodulating drugs
		3. Anticancer and immunomodulating drugs	Other immunomodulating drugs	
prilocaine	744	9. Anesthetic drugs	Anesthetics—Local	
primaquine	827	10. Drugs to treat infections	Antimalarials	
primidone	1023	17. Miscellaneous	Miscellaneous pharmaceuticals	Antiepileptics
probenecid	722–723	8. Musculoskeletal drugs	Antigout drugs	
probucol	188	1. Drugs acting on the cardiovascular system	Lipid-lowering drugs	

(*Continued*)

Drug (primary)	Page	Part of the Book	Category	Subcategory (drug groups only)
procainamide	32–34	1. Drugs acting on the cardiovascular system	Antiarrhythmics	
procaine	743, 744, 746, 747	9. Anesthetic drugs	Anesthetics—Local	
procarbazine	495–499	3. Anticancer and immunomodulating drugs	Cytotoxics	
procyclidine	340, 341	2. Drugs acting on the central nervous system	Anti-Parkinson's drugs	Antimuscarinics
progestogens	978–981	14. Obstetrics and gynecology		
proguanil	827, 828	10. Drugs to treat infections	Antimalarials	
promethazine	942	12. Respratory drugs	Antihistamines	
propafenone	35–40	1. Drugs acting on the cardiovascular system	Antiarrhythmics	
propantheline	342	2. Drugs acting on the central nervous system	Anti-Parkinson's drugs	Antimuscarinics
propranolol	111, 112, 114–116, 122	1. Drugs acting on the cardiovascular system	Beta-blockers	
protease inhibitors	873–878, 882–892, 896, 897, 900–905	10. Drugs to treat infections	Protease inhibitors	
proton pump inhibitors	1023	17. Miscellaneous	Miscellaneous pharmaceuticals	
pyrazinamide	801	10. Drugs to treat infections	Other antibiotics	
pyridostigmine	388, 389	2. Drugs acting on the central nervous system	Parasympathomimetics	
pyrimethamine	828–829	10. Drugs to treat infections	Antimalarials	
quinidine	40–45	1. Drugs acting on the cardiovascular system	Antiarrhythmics	
quinine	829–831	10. Drugs to treat infections	Antimalarials	
quinolones	771–776	10. Drugs to treat infections	Antibiotics	
quinupristin	801, 802	10. Drugs to treat infections	Other antibiotics	
raloxifene	678, 982	14. Obstetrics and gynecology	Alprostadil	
		6. Other endocrine drugs	Pegvisomant	

(*Continued*)

Drug (primary)	Page	Part of the Book	Category	Subcategory (drug groups only)
raltegravir	863, 866, 868, 870, 872	10. Drugs to treat infections	Antivirals	
raltitrexed	500	3. Anticancer and immunomodulating drugs	Cytotoxics	
ramipril	48	1. Drugs acting on the cardiovascular system	Antihypertensives and heart failure drugs	Ace inhibitors
ranitidine	916, 917, 923, 924, 928, 929	11. Drugs acting on the gastrointestinal tract	H2 receptor blockers	
ranolazine	204–206	1. Drugs acting on the cardiovascular system	Ranolazine	
rasagiline	344–346, 348, 351	2. Drugs acting on the central nervous system	Anti-Parkinson's drugs	Dopaminergics
reboxetine	236–238	2. Drugs acting on the central nervous system	Antidepressants	
regorafenib	500–501	3. Anticancer and immunomodulating drugs	Cytotoxics	
repaglinide	641–650	5. Antidiabetic drugs	Meglitinide derivatives	
retinoids	583–584	3. Anticancer and immunomodulating drugs	Other immunomodulating drugs	
rifabutin	776–785	10. Drugs to treat infections	Antibiotics	
rifampicin	776–785	10. Drugs to treat infections	Antibiotics	
rilpivirine	834, 836, 838, 840, 841, 844, 848	10. Drugs to treat infections	Antivirals	Nonnucleoside reverse transcriptase inhibitors (NNRTIS)
riluzole	390	2. Drugs acting on the central nervous system	Parasympathomimetics	
rimonabant	337	2. Drugs acting on the central nervous system	Antiobesity drugs	
risedronate	674	6. Other endocrine drugs	Bisphosphonates	
risperidone	355, 357, 358, 360, 361, 363	2. Drugs acting on the central nervous system	Antipsychotics	
ritonavir	873, 875–877, 879, 880–882, 884–886, 888–902, 904–906	10. Drugs to treat infections	Protease inhibitors	

(*Continued*)

Drug (primary)	Page	Part of the Book	Category	Subcategory (drug groups only)
rituximab	584	3. Anticancer and immunomodulating drugs	Other immunomodulating drugs	
rivaroxaban	615–616	4. Anticoagulants	rivaroxaban	
rivastigmine	219, 389	2. Drugs acting on the central nervous system	Antidementia drugs	
rizatriptan	330, 332	2. Drugs acting on the central nervous system	Antimigraine drugs	
roflumilast	960–961	12. Respratory drugs	phodphodiesterase type 4 inhibitors	
ropinirole	344, 349	2. Drugs acting on the central nervous system	Anti-Parkinson's drugs	Dopaminergics
ropivacaine	745	9. Anesthetic drugs	Anesthetics—Local	
rosiglitazone	667–669	5. Antidiabetic drugs	Thiazolidinediones (glitazones)	
rosuvastatin	189–191	1. Drugs acting on the cardiovascular system	Lipid-lowering drugs	Statins
ruxolitinib	501–502	3. Anticancer and immunomodulating drugs	Cytotoxics	
salicylates	532	3. Anticancer and immunomodulating drugs	Other immunomodulating drugs	
salmeterol	947–950	12. Respratory drugs	Bronchodilators	Beta-2 agonists
sapropterin	968	13. Metabolic drugs		
saquinavir	873, 876–879, 881, 882, 888–890, 892–895, 899–902, 904, 905	10. Drugs to treat infections	Protease inhibitors	
saxagliptin	631, 632	5. Antidiabetic drugs	Dipeptidyl peptidase-4 (DDP-4) inhibitors (gliptins)	
sedative	943	12. Respratory drugs	Antihistamines	
selective serotonin reuptake inhibitors	245–259	2. Drugs acting on the central nervous system	Antidepressants	
selegiline	344–346, 350, 351	2. Drugs acting on the central nervous system	Anti-Parkinson's drugs	Dopaminergics
semaxanib	502	3. Anticancer and immunomodulating drugs	Cytotoxics	
sertindole	356, 357, 361, 362	2. Drugs acting on the central nervous system	Antipsychotics	

(*Continued*)

Drug (primary)	Page	Part of the Book	Category	Subcategory (drug groups only)
sertraline	246, 248, 249, 253–257	2. Drugs acting on the central nervous system	Antidepressants	Selective serotonin reuptake inhibitors
sevelamer	1015	17. Miscellaneous	Miscellaneous pharmaceuticals	
sevoflurane	736	9. Anesthetic drugs	Anesthetics—General	
SGLT2 inhibitors	652–665	5. Antidiabetic drugs	Sulfonylureas	
sibutramine	337–338	2. Drugs acting on the central nervous system	Antiobesity drugs	
sildenafil	986–988	15. Drugs used to treat the urinary system	Drugs used for urinary retention	phosphodiesterase type 5 inhibitors
silodosin	66	1. Drugs acting on the cardiovascular system	Antihypertensives and heart failure drugs	Alpha-blockers
simvastatin	188–190	1. Drugs acting on the cardiovascular system	Lipid-lowering drugs	Statins
sirolimus	584–587	3. Anticancer and immunomodulating drugs	Other immunomodulating drugs	
sitagliptin	631, 632	5. Antidiabetic drugs	Dipeptidyl peptidase-4 (DDP-4) inhibitors (gliptins)	
sodium bicarbonate	989	15. Drugs used to treat the urinary system	Drugs used for urinary retention	urinary alkalinization
sodium oxybate	374	2. Drugs acting on the central nervous system	Anxiolytics and hypnotics	
sodium phenylbutyrate	968	13. Metabolic drugs		
solifenacin	341, 342	2. Drugs acting on the central nervous system	Anti-Parkinson's drugs	Antimuscarinics
somatropin	679	6. Other endocrine drugs	Somatropin	
sorafenib	502–504	3. Anticancer and immunomodulating drugs	Cytotoxics	
sotalol	109–110	1. Drugs acting on the cardiovascular system	Antiplatelet drugs	
spironolactone	171	1. Drugs acting on the cardiovascular system	Diuretics	
St. John's wort	248–255	2. Drugs acting on the central nervous system	Antidepressants	
statins	188–196, 1067	1. Drugs acting on the cardiovascular system	Lipid-lowering drugs	

(*Continued*)

Drug (primary)	Page	Part of the Book	Category	Subcategory (drug groups only)
		18. Over-the-counter/online drugs and remedies	Drugs for prevention of heart disease	
stavudine	851–854, 860, 861	10. Drugs to treat infections	Antivirals	
streptomycin	756	10. Drugs to treat infections	Antibiotics	
strontium ranelate	679	6. Other endocrine drugs	Steroid replacement therapy	
sucralfate	936–937	11. Drugs acting on the gastrointestinal tract		
sufentanil	712	7. Analgesics	Opioids	
sulfadiazine	785	10. Drugs to treat infections	Antibiotics	
sulfamethoxazole	786	10. Drugs to treat infections	Antibiotics	
sulfasalazine	531	3. Anticancer and immunomodulating drugs	Other immunomodulating drugs	
sulfinpyrazone	724–725	8. Musculoskeletal drugs	Antigout drugs	
sulfonamides	785–790	10. Drugs to treat infections	Antibiotics	
sulfonylureas	655	5. Antidiabetic drugs	Sulfonylureas	
sulpiride	354, 356, 364	2. Drugs acting on the central nervous system	Antipsychotics	
sumatriptan	330	2. Drugs acting on the central nervous system	Antimigraine drugs	
sunitinib	504–506	3. Anticancer and immunomodulating drugs	Cytotoxics	
suxamethonium	748–750	9. Anesthetic drugs	Muscle relaxants—Depolarizing	
sympathomimetics	207–216	1. Drugs acting on the cardiovascular system	Sympathomimetics	
tacrolimus	587–592	3. Anticancer and immunomodulating drugs	Other immunomodulating drugs	
tadalafil	985, 987, 988	15. Drugs used to treat the urinary system	Drugs used for urinary retention	Phosphodiesterase type 5 inhibitors
tamoxifen	524–530	3. Anticancer and immunomodulating drugs	Hormones and hormone antagonists	
tamsulosin	63, 66	1. Drugs acting on the cardiovascular system	Antihypertensives and heart failure drugs	Alpha-blockers

(*Continued*)

Drug (primary)	Page	Part of the Book	Category	Subcategory (drug groups only)
tegafur	439, 441, 442	3. Anticancer and immunomodulating drugs	Cytotoxics	
teicoplanin	802	10. Drugs to treat infections	Other antibiotics	
telithromycin	761, 763–765	10. Drugs to treat infections	Antibiotics	
telmisartan	69	1. Drugs acting on the cardiovascular system	Antihypertensives and heart failure drugs	Angiotensin II receptor antagonists
temazepam	366, 368	2. Drugs acting on the central nervous system	Anxiolytics and hypnotics	Benzodiazepines
temoporfin	506	3. Anticancer and immunomodulating drugs	Cytotoxics	
temozolomide	507	3. Anticancer and immunomodulating drugs	Cytotoxics	
temsirolimus	507	3. Anticancer and immunomodulating drugs	Cytotoxics	
tenofovir	850, 853, 855–857, 859, 861	10. Drugs to treat infections	Antivirals	
terbinafine	820	10. Drugs to treat infections	Antifungal drugs	Azoles
terbutaline	946	12. Respratory drugs	Bronchodilators	Beta-2 agonists
terfenadine	940–944	12. Respratory drugs	Antihistamines	
testosterone	679–680	6. Other endocrine drugs	Testosterone	
tetrabenazine	391	2. Drugs acting on the central nervous system	Parasympathomimetics	
tetracyclines	790–793, 1021	17. Miscellaneous	Miscellaneous pharmaceuticals	Minerals and vitamins
		10. Drugs to treat infections	Antibiotics	
thalidomide	593–594	3. Anticancer and immunomodulating drugs	Other immunomodulating drugs	
theophylline	950–959	12. Respratory drugs	Bronchodilators	Nonselective beta-agonists
thiazides	174–179	1. Drugs acting on the cardiovascular system	Diuretics	
thiazolidinediones	137	1. Drugs acting on the cardiovascular system	Calcium channel blockers	
thiopentone	295, 736, 740	2. Drugs acting on the central nervous system	Antiepileptics	Barbiturates
		9. Anesthetic drugs	Anesthetics—General	

(Continued)

Drug (primary)	Page	Part of the Book	Category	Subcategory (drug groups only)
thioridazine	363, 364	2. Drugs acting on the central nervous system	Antipsychotics	
thiotepa	508	3. Anticancer and immunomodulating drugs	Cytotoxics	
thrombolytics	616–617	4. Anticoagulants	thrombolytics	
thymoxamine	201	1. Drugs acting on the cardiovascular system	Peripheral vasodilators	
thyroid hormones	680–685	6. Other endocrine drugs	Thyroid hormones and iodine	
tibolone	982	14. Obstetrics and gynecology	Alprostadil	
ticagrelor	106–108	1. Drugs acting on the cardiovascular system	Antiplatelet drugs	
timolol	111, 115, 116, 120	1. Drugs acting on the cardiovascular system	Beta-blockers	
tinidazole	834	10. Drugs to treat infections	Other antiprotozoals	
tioguanine	508	3. Anticancer and immunomodulating drugs	Cytotoxics	
tipranavir	873, 875, 889, 895, 897, 899, 900, 905, 906	10. Drugs to treat infections	Protease inhibitors	
tizanidine	731–733	8. Musculoskeletal drugs	Skeletal muscle relaxants	
tocilizumab	595	3. Anticancer and immunomodulating drugs	Other immunomodulating drugs	
tofacitinib	509	3. Anticancer and immunomodulating drugs	Cytotoxics	
tofisopam	366	2. Drugs acting on the central nervous system	Anxiolytics and hypnotics	Benzodiazepines
tolbutamide	657, 658, 665–672	5. Antidiabetic drugs	Sulfonylureas Thiazolidinediones (glitazones)	
tolcapone	345, 349	2. Drugs acting on the central nervous system	Anti-Parkinson's drugs	Dopaminergics
tolterodine	340, 341	2. Drugs acting on the central nervous system	Anti-Parkinson's drugs	Antimuscarinics
tolvaptan	685	6. Other endocrine drugs	Tolvaptan	

(Continued)

Drug (primary)	Page	Part of the Book	Category	Subcategory (drug groups only)
topiramate	321–322	2. Drugs acting on the central nervous system	Antiepileptics	
topotecan	509	3. Anticancer and immunomodulating drugs	Cytotoxics	
trabectedin	510	3. Anticancer and immunomodulating drugs	Cytotoxics	
tramadol	701, 704–706, 708, 709, 712	7. Analgesics	Opioids	
tranexamic acid	1015	17. Miscellaneous	Miscellaneous pharmaceuticals	
tranylcypromine	227	2. Drugs acting on the central nervous system	Antidepressants	Monoamine oxidase inhibitors
trastuzumab	511	3. Anticancer and immunomodulating drugs	Cytotoxics	
trazodone	273, 277, 275	2. Drugs acting on the central nervous system	Antidepressants	Tricyclic antidepressants
treosulfan	512	3. Anticancer and immunomodulating drugs	Cytotoxics	
tretamine	512	3. Anticancer and immunomodulating drugs	Cytotoxics	
triazolam	366, 369	2. Drugs acting on the central nervous system	Anxiolytics and hypnotics	Benzodiazepines
trientine	968, 1023	13. Metabolic drugs 17. Miscellaneous	Miscellaneous pharmaceuticals	
trilostane	685	6. Other endocrine drugs	Trilostane	
trimethoprim	786, 789	10. Drugs to treat infections	Antibiotics	
trimipramine	274	2. Drugs acting on the central nervous system	Antidepressants	Tricyclic antidepressants
tripotassium dicitratobismuthate	937	11. Drugs acting on the gastrointestinal tract		
triptans	330, 331	2. Drugs acting on the central nervous system	Antimigraine drugs	
tropisetron	285, 286	2. Drugs acting on the central nervous system	Antiemetics	5-HT3 antagonists

(*Continued*)

Drug (primary)	Page	Part of the Book	Category	Subcategory (drug groups only)
trospium	342	2. Drugs acting on the central nervous system	Anti-Parkinson's drugs	Antimuscarinics
tryptophan	278–279	2. Drugs acting on the central nervous system	Antidepressants	
ulipristal	982	14. Obstetrics and gynecology	Alprostadil	
ursodeoxycholic acid	916	11. Drugs acting on the gastrointestinal tract	Antidiarrheals	
valdecoxib	698	7. Analgesics	Nonsteroidal anti-inflammatory drugs (NSAIDS)	
valproate	323–325	2. Drugs acting on the central nervous system	Antiepileptics	
valproic acid	1023	17. Miscellaneous	Miscellaneous pharmaceuticals	Antiepileptics
valrubicin	512	3. Anticancer and immunomodulating drugs	Cytotoxics	
valspodar	595	3. Anticancer and immunomodulating drugs	Other immunomodulating drugs	
vancomycin	803	10. Drugs to treat infections	Other antibiotics	
vandetanib	512–514	3. Anticancer and immunomodulating drugs	Cytotoxics	
vardenafil	987, 988	15. Drugs used to treat the urinary system	Drugs used for urinary retention	Phosphodiesterase type 5 inhibitors
vasodilator anti-hypertensives	83–92	1. Drugs acting on the cardiovascular system	Antihypertensives and heart failure drugs	
vecuronium	753, 754	9. Anesthetic drugs	Muscle relaxants—Nondepolarizings	
vemurafenib	514–517	3. Anticancer and immunomodulating drugs	Cytotoxics	
venlafaxine	255, 259–264	2. Drugs acting on the central nervous system	Antidepressants	Selective serotonin reuptake inhibitors Serotonin norepinephrine reuptake inhibitors
verapamil	128–140, 142, 144–150	1. Drugs acting on the cardiovascular system	Calcium channel blockers	
vigabatrin	325	2. Drugs acting on the central nervous system	Antiepileptics	

(*Continued*)

Drug (primary)	Page	Part of the Book	Category	Subcategory (drug groups only)
vinblastine	517, 518, 520, 522	3. Anticancer and immunomodulating drugs	Cytotoxics	
vinca alkaloids	517–519, 522, 523	3. Anticancer and immunomodulating drugs	Cytotoxics	
vincristine	517–520, 522	3. Anticancer and immunomodulating drugs	Cytotoxics	
vindesine	520	3. Anticancer and immunomodulating drugs	Cytotoxics	
vinflunine	517, 519–522	3. Anticancer and immunomodulating drugs	Cytotoxics	
vitamin A	1019	17. Miscellaneous	Miscellaneous pharmaceuticals	Minerals and vitamins
vitamin B12	1019	17. Miscellaneous	Miscellaneous pharmaceuticals	Minerals and vitamins
vitamin B3 (niacin)	1019	17. Miscellaneous	Miscellaneous pharmaceuticals	Minerals and vitamins
vitamin B6	1019	17. Miscellaneous	Miscellaneous pharmaceuticals	Minerals and vitamins
vitamin C	1019	17. Miscellaneous	Miscellaneous pharmaceuticals	Minerals and vitamins
vitamin D	1020	17. Miscellaneous	Miscellaneous pharmaceuticals	Minerals and vitamins
vitamin E	1020	17. Miscellaneous	Miscellaneous pharmaceuticals	Minerals and vitamins
voriconazole	805–811, 813–815	10. Drugs to treat infections	Antifungal drugs	Azoles
vorinostat	523	3. Anticancer and immunomodulating drugs	Cytotoxics	
warfarin	1021	17. Miscellaneous	Miscellaneous pharmaceuticals	Anticoagulants
zafirlukast	944–945	12. Respratory drugs	asthma prophylaxis	Leukotriene receptor antagonists
zalcitabine	858, 862	10. Drugs to treat infections	Antivirals	
zaleplon	375	2. Drugs acting on the central nervous system	Anxiolytics and hypnotics	
zidovudine	850–857, 859, 861, 1023	17. Miscellaneous	Miscellaneous pharmaceuticals	Antivirals
		10. Drugs to treat infections	Antivirals	
zoledronic acid	674	6. Other endocrine drugs	Bisphosphonates	
zolmitriptan	328, 330, 332, 333	2. Drugs acting on the central nervous system	Antimigraine drugs	

(Continued)

Drug (primary)	Page	Part of the Book	Category	Subcategory (drug groups only)
zolpidem	375	2. Drugs acting on the central nervous system	Anxiolytics and hypnotics	
zonisamide	325	2. Drugs acting on the central nervous system	Antiepileptics	
zopiclone	375	2. Drugs acting on the central nervous system	Anxiolytics and hypnotics	
zuclopenthixol	356, 363	2. Drugs acting on the central nervous system	Antipsychotics	

Introduction

Simon F.J. Clarke and Lakshman Delgoda Karalliedde

Despite continuing concerns and efforts to minimize the occurrence of ADIs, several obstacles to progress have emerged. When prescribing, a fundamental necessity is to consider all aspects of the pharmacological properties of the drug along with the disease state of the individual to whom the drug is prescribed. We are aware of the large (about sixfold) interpatient variation in the magnitude of interacting drugs that may occur. These variations are greater in patients taking particular drugs or having particular disease states. Thus, there are several classifications of high-risk drugs and high-risk patients.[1–5]

In addition, rates of drug-related problems (DRPs) vary with patients managed in different specialties. For example, 29% of neurology patients demonstrated at least one DRP while 80% DRPs were seen in a large study of 827 patients hospitalized in departments of internal medical and rheumatology.[6]

Patient groups reported to be at increased risk of ADIs are as follows:

1. Patients following transplants.
2. Disease states in older patients.[4]
3. Long-term care patients/elderly often require opioids that have been inadequately studied in special population groups, causing difficulties in predicting response.[7,8]
4. Patients with impaired renal function.
5. Patients with impaired hepatic function.
6. Neonates/children and those who are pregnant or breast feeding.
7. Long-standing or chronic diseases with a significant inflammatory component.
8. Obese patients.
9. Emergency Department (ED) patients taking three or more medications, and patients over the age of 50 years on two or more medications.[1]
10. Immigrant populations' continuing to use traditional medicines used in their countries of origin or birth.[8]

Horn and Hansten emphasized the necessity for a good general knowledge of common mechanisms, various pathways for drug elimination, common inhibitors and inducers of drug elimination, and an understanding of drug interaction (DI) risk management that may not be available in the computerized DI alert system.[9]

The computer/IT is invaluable at highlighting drug–drug interactions (DDIs), but it does not replace the knowledge and thinking of the prescriber essential for meaningful and practical interpretation of interaction alerts and rational and safe use of medicines for individual patients.[10] Duquet emphasized the need for vigilance while discussing interactions of nonsteroidal anti-inflammatory drugs (NSAIDs), as these potentially serious interactions will not be identified by computer systems.[11]

This second edition, in addition to providing an updated list of interactions, has added brief synopses on vulnerable population groups with reference to the pharmacokinetics that are known to occur in these groups, as suggested by Horn and Hansten, along with the influences of polymorphisms and ethnicity.

DDI alerting is considered an important tool for clinical decisions.[12] We commend the rapid expansion of electronically generated alerts aimed at minimizing medication errors (e.g., clinical decision support systems [CDSS], drug-interaction alert systems [DIAS]-JAVA language) and those that attempt to enhance the impact by including laboratory data.

Observations of Koplan et al. states that "as electronic health records (EHRs) become widely adopted, alerts and reminders can improve medication safety. Excessive alerts may irritate or overwhelm clinicians, thereby reducing their effectiveness." Overriding of alerts is a serious concern.[13–16]

The primary intent of this edition is to make the information clinically relevant—i.e., viewing DIs through the eyes of a busy prescriber who has to make decisions about the choice of a drug for a particular patient (individualized therapy) within the time frame of a consultation that may vary from 5 minutes to an hour in specialties, institutions, and countries in varying stages of technical development. This alternative would be accessible and available globally to all socioeconomic groups of prescribers, and by providing a "need-to-know" facility that is essentially patient related. It is hoped that the risk of "over-alerting" or "alert fatigue" would be minimized.

There would be lists of high-risk drugs and high-risk population groups, and cross-referencing would enable prescribers to assess risks/benefits of combinations of medications in nearly all population groups. We intend to reduce the margins for errors in prescribing to vulnerable population groups.

REFERENCES

1. Goldberg RM, Mabee J, Chan L, Wong S. Drug–drug and drug–disease interactions in the ED: Analysis of a high-risk population. *The American Journal of Emergency Medicine* 1996;14(5):447–450.
2. Institute for Safe Medication Practices. Results of ISMP survey on high-alert medications: Differences between nursing, pharmacy, and risk/quality/safety perspectives, Horsham, PA, 2012. www.ismp.org/Newsletters.
3. Saedder EA et al. Identifying high-risk medication: A systematic literature review. *European Journal of Clinical Pharmacology* 2014;70:637–645.
4. American Geriatrics Society 2015 Beers Criteria Update Expert Panel. American Geriatrics Society 2015 updated beers criteria for potentially inappropriate medication use in older adults. *Journal of the American Geriatrics Society* 2015;63(11):2227–2246.
5. Woods DJ. *New Zealand College of Pharmacists: Introduction to Drug Interactions.* www.psnz.org.nz/public/cop/college_information/affilaited/nzcp/drug interactions course/drug_int.aspx.
6. Chan DC et al. Drug-related problems (DRPs) identified from geriatric medication safety review clinics. *Archives of Gerontology and Geriatrics* 2012;54:168–174.
7. FDA February 2012. Guidance for Industry. E7 supported the requirement of studies in special populations: Geriatrics. Center for Drug Evaluation and Research (CDER), Center for Biologics Evaluation and Research (CBER), Silver Spring, MD, February 2012.
8. Tom L. Management of drug–drug interactions: Considerations for special populations—Focus on opioid use in the elderly and long term care. *American Journal of Managed Care* 2011;17:S293–S298. Published Online: September 20, 2011.
9. Horn JR, Hansten PD. How to address a drug interaction alert. *Pharmacy Times*. Published Online: August 17, 2010.
10. Ohno-Machado L. Health surveillance using the internet and other sources of information. *Journal of the American Medical Informatics Association* 2013 May–Jun;20(3):403.
11. Duquet N. Managing drug interactions at the pharmacy counter. The case of NSAIDs. *Journal de Pharmacie de Belgique* 2012;3:16–22.
12. Fritz D et al. Comparative evaluation of three clinical decision support systems: Prospective screening for medication errors in 100 medical inpatients. *European Journal of Clinical Pharmacology* 2012;68:1209–1219.
13. Isaac T et al. Overrides of medication alerts in ambulatory care. *Archives of Internal Medicine* 2009; 169:305–311.
14. Yeh ML et al. Physicians' responses to computerized drug–drug interaction alerts for outpatients. *Computer Methods and Programs in Biomedicine* 2013;111:17–25.
15. Isaac T et al. Overrides of medication alerts in ambulatory care. *Archives of Internal Medicine* 2009; 169:305–311.
16. Mille F et al. Analysis of overridden alerts in a drug–drug interaction detection system. *International Journal for Quality in Health Care* 2008;20:400–405.

Drug Metabolism and Elimination

Lakshman Delgoda Karalliedde, Simon F.J. Clarke, and Ursula Collignon

Metabolization of drugs serves to inactivate them and increase their solubility, thereby increasing their elimination via the kidneys. Much of the metabolism occurs in the liver primarily through the cytochrome P450 family (CYP) of enzymes located in the hepatic endoplasmic reticulum, but it may also occur through non-CYP enzyme systems, such as glucuronosyl- and sulfo-transferases. Some drug metabolizing enzymes (DME) are present in the gut wall and other extrahepatic tissues.

METABOLISM AND DRUG INTERACTIONS

Many metabolic routes of elimination can be inhibited or induced by concomitant drug treatment. Metabolic DDIs can cause substantial increases or decreases in blood and tissue concentrations of a drug or metabolites and influence the extent to which toxic or active metabolites are formed. These large changes in exposure alter the safety and efficacy profile of a drug and its active metabolites.

PHASES OF METABOLISM AND ELIMINATION

There are three phases of metabolism and elimination of xenobiotics:

- Phase I—Mainly oxidation
- Phase II—Mainly conjugation
- Phase III—Transport and elimination

Many phase I and II enzymes and phase III transporters are inducible and are the site of numerous DIs. There is also considerable variation in their activity, which is determined genetically and may be modified by environmental factors (see "Individual Variability of Adverse Drug Interactions" section).

Phase I

Cytochrome P450 Enzymes

These enzymes metabolize ~95% of the available drugs, making them more water soluble for elimination from the body. Usually phase I metabolism produces pharmacologically inactive metabolites; however, occasionally they are pharmacologically active or potentially toxic.

The classification of cytochromes has been undertaken by the Human Cytochrome P450 Allele Nomenclature Committee (drnelson.utmem.edu/Cytochrome450.html):

- Enzymes that share at least 40 amino acid sequences are included in families—these are designated with an Arabic numeral.
- Those that share 55% or more sequences are included in the same subfamily—these are designated with a capital letter.
- Enzymes sharing 97% amino acid sequences are individual enzymes designated by a number, for example, CYP3A4 = CYP (cytochrome P450) 3 (family) A (subfamily) 4 (individual enzyme).
- There are 18 families and 44 subfamilies of CYP enzymes.

Humans possess 57 CYP genes that could be functionally grouped into three main categories:

1. Fifteen are involved in drug metabolism.
2. Twenty-seven metabolize endogenous compounds such as bile acids, eicosanoids, and vitamins.
3. Fifteen have an unknown function.

The drug interaction database of the University of Washington (www.druginteractioninfo.org) reported that enzymes from subfamilies CYP1A, CYP2A, CYP2B, CYP2C, CYP2D, CYP2E, and CYP3A metabolize the majority of drugs in use.

Individual CYP enzymes can metabolize multiple substrates, while different drugs can either increase (inducers) or decrease (inhibitors) their activity; changes to the degree of activity of metabolizing enzymes are a significant mechanism of DDIs. The U.S. FDA (www.fda.gov) classifies inhibitors and inducers of CYP enzymes according to how much of an effect there is on the concentration or clearance of substrates by the affected enzyme.

Inhibitors

Degree of Inhibition	Increase in AUC of Substrate	Decrease in Clearance of Substrate
Strong	≥5-fold	>80%
Moderate	≥2-fold, <5-fold	50%–80%
Weak	≥1.25-fold, <2-fold	20%–50%

Inducers

Degree of Induction	Decrease in AUC of Substrate
Strong	≥80%
Moderate	50%–80%
Weak	20%–50%

Phase II

This is carried out by different groups of enzymes that are subdivided into families (according to similarities in amino acid sequences) and to subfamilies referred to as isoenzymes or isoforms. The isoforms are expressed in nearly all tissues and have broad and overlapping substrate specificity. These enzymes produce metabolites that are more polar, larger in molecular weight, and charged at physiological pH to enable easier excretion into urine or bile by transport proteins. Most conjugates are inactive and nontoxic, although there are a few exceptions.

The enzymes involved are

- UDP-glucuronyltransferases (UGT)
- Sulfonyl transferases (SULT)
- Glutathione S-transferases (GST)
- Methyl transferases (MTs)
- *n*-Actyltransferases (NAT)
- Acyl CoA ligase/*N*-acyltransferases

Glucuronidation is the most common reaction (35%) followed by sulfation (20%), GST reactions (15%), and NATs (10%).

Phase II metabolites often cannot exit cells through passive diffusion, requiring ATP-mediated transporters to cross cellular barriers.

Glucuronyl Transferases (UGTs)

There are 19 human UGTs. UGT1 and UGT2 are involved in the glucuronidation of drugs, possessing the largest capacity of phase II enzymes. Approximately 15 human UGTs expressed in the liver and the gastrointestinal (GI) tract have been identified, with nearly 350 individual compounds including 87% of commonly found medications substrates. UGTs also transform endogenous substrates such as bilirubin, bile acids, steroids, and glycolipids. Unlike the cytochromes that have their active sites facing the cytosol, active sites of UGTs face the luminal side of the endoplasmic reticulum where glucuronidation takes place.

Glucuronidation usually results in inactive metabolites. An important exception is the formation of morphine-6-glucurionide, which is 600 times more potent than morphine. Glucuronidation is a reversible process, as enzymes such as beta glucuronidases in the intestine are able to convert the conjugates back to the parent drug.

Expression: Mainly liver, but also skin, intestine, kidney, and brain.

Clinical Relevance

1. DIs involving glucuronidation are less frequent and result in less toxicity than those for CYP450s as UGTs have higher substrate K_m values, and metabolism occurs via multiple UGTs. V_{max} is the maximal speed of activity, i.e., conversion of substate to product, of the enzyme, measured as the rate at infinite substrate concentration. K_m is the concentration of substrate required to produce 50% of the V_{max} value. It is measured in units of concentration (generally M).
2. Lamotrigine coadministration with valproic acid increases the risk of skin rashes associated with lamotrigine attributed to valproic acid inhibiting glucuronidation of lamotrigine. The elimination half-life of lamotrigine monotherapy is 25–30 hours and is more than doubled, to 60 hours, when combined with valproic acid.
3. Factors affecting drug glucuronidation include
   a. Age
   b. Cigarette smoking
   c. Diet
   d. Disease states
   e. Ethnicity
   f. Genetic factors
   g. Hormonal factors
   h. Interaction with other drugs

Sulfotransferases (SULTs)

- There are four members in the SULT family.
- SULT1 and SULT2 play the most important role in drug metabolism.
- Sulfonation occurs more rapidly than glucuronidation; however, it is a saturable process due to lower liver content.
- Following saturation glucuronidation provides an alternative metabolic pathway.
- The cytosolic, and not the membrane-bound, form is involved in drug metabolism.

Expression: Liver, kidney, lung, skin, breast, GI tract (highest levels in small intestine), and brain.

Glutathione-S-Transferase (GST)

- GSTs may be cytosolic or membrane bound with a vital role in cell defence.
- GST inactivates reactive, toxic substances by catalyzing the conjugation of glutathione (GSH) to them. These substances may be formed by normal cellular metabolism or may enter the cell from outside, such as in drugs.
- Conjugation with GSH produces less reactive or damaging products that are more easily excreted, either by transport proteins into the bile or following conversion to *N*-acetylcysteine conjugates for excretion in the urine. However, some GSH conjugates may be *more* reactive than parent compounds.

GSTs are subdivided into classes according to amino acid groupings, e.g., alpha, mu, and pi. Additional classes have been identified in animals that do not have major roles in drug metabolism, e.g., sigma GSTs (function as prostaglandin synthases). The soluble glutathione transferases can be divided into the phi, tau, theta, zeta, and lambda classes. The theta and zeta GSTs have counterparts in animals, whereas the other classes are plant specific.

Methyltransferases

There are nearly 100 methyltransferases. Those involved in drug metabolism are

- Catechol methyltransferase (COMT)
- Cytosolic thiol methyltransferase (TMT)
- Thiopurine methyltransferase (TPMT)
- Nicotinamide *N*-methyltransferase (NNMT)

Expression: COMT is found in the highest concentrations in the liver and kidney and also in the brain, the lung, and erythrocytes.

Clinical Significance

Methyltranferases are the basis for theoretical interactions between NSAIDs and thiopurines. TPMT is a biotransformation phase II enzyme responsible for the metabolic inactivation of thiopurine drugs. Naproxen, tolfenamic acid, and mefenamic acid inhibited human TPMT in vitro, although in vivo evidence is lacking.

N-Acetyltransferases (NATs)

- Two distinct phenotypes of acetylation were identified: "rapid acetylators" and "slow acetylators." The phenotypes were later attributed to differences in the enzymatic activities of NAT1 and NAT2. Two human forms NAT1 and NAT2 are expressed from separate genes.
- In general, there is a three- to sixfold difference in the metabolic elimination between rapid and slow acetylators.
- NAT2 catalyzes the acetylation of aromatic amines and hydrazines.

Expression: NAT1 is widely distributed in most tissues. NAT2 is found in liver and gut.

Clinical Relevance

1. Because NAT2 metabolizes carcinogenic arylamines, NAT2 polymorphisms are associated with an increased susceptibility to cancers caused by industrial chemicals (α- and β-naphthylamine and benzidine).
2. Persons with a poor acetylator phenotype have increased risks of lung, bladder, and gastric cancers if exposed to carcinogenic arylamines for a long period of time.

3. Poor metabolizers (PMs) treated with isoniazid are at higher risk of peripheral neuropathy and liver disorders due to ↑ blood levels of isoniazid (↑ risk of isoniazid induced hepatitis).
4. When rifampicin and doxycycline are coadministered, rifampin levels are higher and doxycyciline levels are lower in rapid metabolizers compared to slow acetylators.
5. Risk of isoniazid-induced hepatotoxicity—no correlation with slow acetylators.

Amino Acid Conjugation

This is not a major metabolic pathway; it is essentially a detoxification pathway. An exception is with valproic acid when valproic acyl thioester, considered responsible at least in part for hepatotoxicity, is formed instead of the amino acid conjugate when the process becomes saturated due probably to the depletion of mitochondrial CoA with valproic acid.

The enzymes that catalyze amino acid conjugation (acyl CoA ligase and *N*-acetyl transferase) are located in hepatic mitochondria. Amino acid conjugates are easily eliminated in the urine. Glycine conjugation is easily saturated and is compensated by glucuronidation.

Clinical Relevance

1. Approximately 75% of a dose of aspirin conjugates with glycine.
2. Benzoic acid—a food preservative (used to treat hyperammonemia)—conjugates only with glycine.

Phase III

Metabolites from phase I and phase II metabolism are substrates for phase III metabolism.

Membrane Transporters

Membrane transporters exist for endogenous substrates; drugs and many environmental toxicants "hitchhike" onto these transporters, enabling entry or exit from cells. In contrast to ion channels that essentially exist in a closed state, these pumps may be open or closed. Transporters move their substrates either along or against a concentration gradient. All metabolizing enzymes are intracellular. Uptake of drugs from the extracellular space across the plasma membrane is a prerequisite for subsequent metabolism; transporters are involved in the uptake (influx) and exit (efflux) of drugs into and out of cells.

Transporters are involved in the absorption, distribution, and elimination of drugs and can affect the safety profile of a drug by altering its concentration or that of its metabolites in the blood or at the target organs. The renal excretion of drugs is due to a combination of three processes: glomerular filtration, renal tubule secretion, and renal tubular reabsorption. Transport proteins are involved in the last two processes. Inhibition of transporters is not necessarily associated with increase in toxicity. Cidofovir, which causes nephrotoxicity, is rendered relatively innocuous by probenecid due to inhibition of organic anion transporters (OAT) in the kidney, blocking the uptake of cidofovir into renal tubular cell and preventing nephrotoxicity. Inhibition of renal tubular secretion by OAT with probenecid was used clinically to extend the activity of cephalosporins and penicillin (during World War II when penicillin was in short supply).

Most membrane transporters are oligospecific (i.e., specialized for translocation of specific compounds) although there are a number of polyspecific transporters that accept compounds of different sizes and molecular structures.

Transporters can either serve as drug targets or as drug delivery systems. Recently exploited drug targets include

- Glucose transporters (SLC5 family)
- Neurotransmitter transporters (SLC6 family)

- Intestinal bile acid transporters (SLC10 family)
- Cation–chloride cotransporters (SLC12 family)

Classification

Nearly 400 transporters have been identified in humans and most are grouped into two superfamilies: ATP-binding cassette (ABC) and solute carrier (SLC).

ABC transporters

- ABC transporters are active transporters, using energy (ATP hydrolysis) to transport against steep concentration gradients and act as barriers to drug absorption in intestine and kidney.
- Active transporters (or cotransporters) couple the movement of one type of ion or molecule against its concentration gradient, to the movement of another ion or molecule down its concentration gradient.

SLC transporters

- SLC transporters are passive transporters and mitochondrial and vesicular transporters.
- Passive transporters transport substances down a concentration gradient.
- When the transported and the cotransported molecule or ion move in the same direction across a membrane, the transporter is called a *symporter*; when they move in opposite directions, the transporter is called an *antiporter* (or exchanger).

The number of substrates, inducers, and inhibitors of transport proteins is prohibitively large for this text. A number of online resources listing them are available, such as

- U.S. Food and Drug Administration. Available at: http://www.fda.gov/Drugs/DevelopmentApprovalProcess/DevelopmentResources/DrugInteractionsLabeling/ucm093664.htm
- *Pharmacology Weekly*. Available at: http://www.pharmacologyweekly.com/content/pages/drug-reference-table-cyp-p450-ugt-enzymes-transporters-or

ABC Transporters

P-Glycoprotein (Pgp)

Pgp has a wide range of roles protecting the body from toxins:

- It prevents the uptake of toxic drugs and food components from the gut into the body.
- It protects vital structures (e.g., brain, CSF, testis, and fetus) against toxins that enter the body.
- It limits the cellular uptake of drugs from the blood into the brain and from the intestinal lumen into epithelial cells.
- It mediates the export of phase II products of conjugation that cannot otherwise diffuse through cell membranes; in particular, it removes endogenous and xenobiotic compounds from hepatocytes into sinusoidal blood.
- It has a greater impact on limiting cellular uptake of drugs from blood circulation into the brain and placenta and from intestinal lumen into epithelial cells, than on enhancing excretion of drugs in the liver and kidney to the adjacent luminal spaces.

Expression:

Pgp is found in a wide range of organs and tissues:

- Intestinal enterocytes
- Kidney—proximal tubule

- Hepatocyte canalicules
- Blood–brain barrier
- Placenta
- Testes
- Endothelia
- Tumor cells
- Membranes of intracellular compartments (Golgi, endosome, multivesicular bodies, endoplasmic reticulum, peroxisome, and mitochondria)

Activity of Pgp varies widely between different tissues and between individuals:

- Expression in the liver is sevenfold lower than in the intestine.
- In the intestine, expression is highest in the jejunum, less in the ileum, and lowest in the colon.
- Highest expression levels are found in the placenta, liver, lung (alveolar type II pneumocytes), adrenal glands, and fetal tissues.
- Differential expression of Pgp in male and female with males expressing twofold higher amounts of Pgp than females.

Clinical implications:

1. Pgp plays a central role in bioavailability of oral drugs; some substrate drugs such as paclitaxel have to be given intravenously due to poor oral bioavailability. The MDR1 gene encoding Pgp is polymorphic. A change known as C3435T correlates with its intestinal expression. Those homozygous for the T allele have substantially lower Pgp expression in the GI tract compared with C-allele homozygotes, leading to genetic differences in the bioavailability of certain drugs (typically enhancing absorption). There is significant ethnic variation in the frequency of the different alleles: 83% of West Africans and 61% of African Americans are C-homozygous, compared with only 26% of whites.
   a. The increased frequency of the C/C genotype in blacks lowers bioavailability of certain highly active antiretroviral therapy (HAART) components.
   b. Valproate and carbamazepine are transported by Pgp—there is an increased risk of drug resistance in Iranian female epileptic patients with the ABCB1-1236CC genotype.
2. ABCC4 and ABCC5 transport cyclic nucleotides, and nucleotide analogues contribute to resistance against base and nucleoside analogues used in the treatment of cancer and viral disease. Pgp is able to cause the highest resistance to bulky amphipathic drugs—paclitaxel, anthracyclines, and vinca alkaloids—and it contributes to multidrug resistance (MDR) in cancer cells.
3. Pgp function decreases in the elderly resulting in an increased risk of drug toxicity not only due to enhanced intestinal absorption but also increased CNS side effects of drugs that cross the blood–brain barrier.
4. The potential risk of Pgp-mediated DIs might be underestimated by monitoring only the plasma concentration. Pgp inhibition has greater impact on tissue distribution of drugs in brain and placenta than on plasma concentration.
5. The three major categories of Pgp interaction are as follows:
   a. *Competitive inhibition*—the inhibitor binds to the same site on Pgp as the substrate
   b. *Noncompetitive inhibition*—the inhibitor binds to a different site than the substrate on Pgp
   c. Cooperative stimulation—Pgp is thought to have two separate binding sites that act cooperatively to increase the activity of Pgp.
6. Rifampicin increases intestinal Pgp content 3.5-fold; this reduces oral bioavailability of digoxin resulting in a lower digoxin level. Conversely, macrolides inhibit Pgp, resulting in an increased digoxin level due to increased intestinal absorption and reduced renal excretion.
7. The interaction between cyclosporin (a substrate of CYP3A4 and Pgp) and rifampicin (an inducer of CYP3A4 and Pgp) leads to decreased cyclosporin levels due to a combination of reduced Pgp-mediated bioavailability and increased CYP3A4-mediated metabolism.

Multidrug Resistance–Associated Proteins (MRP)

This large family of transporters, which are widely expressed throughout the body, are associated with transport of drugs both into and out of the body.

- *MRP 1*: Secretes drugs into the body, rather than moving them out of body; its role in DIs is uncertain.
- *MRP2*: Plays a key role in biliary elimination of glucuronide and sulfate conjugates and of divalent bile acids; it is also responsible for the excretion of GSH from liver into bile, maintaining a steep concentration gradient of GSH between blood (100 μmol/L) and bile (10–15 mmol/L), drawing water into bile to transport neutral drugs (e.g., vinblastine) out of cells. Mutation of its genes is associated with increased risk of diclofenac-associated hepatotoxicity due to intracellular accumulation of reactive metabolites. Its role in DIs is not clear.
- *MRP3*: Performs defence-related functions and contributes to the excretion of toxic anions. Its role in DIs is not clear.
- *MRP4*: Plays an important role in protecting hepatocytes. It actively transports PGE_1 and PGE_2.
- *MRP5*: Participates in hepatic drug transport. It is also widely expressed in the brain. Both MRP4 and MRP 5 have been proposed to reduce brain penetration of thiopurine nucleobase analogues of 6 mercaptopurine and 6 thioguanine (used widely for remission of acute lymphoblastic leukemia [ALL] in pediatric patients). Animal models showed that efflux of 6 MP from the brain was inhibited by OATs and or MRP inhibitors such as benzylpenicillin, cimetidine, and sulfinpyrazone.

Bile Salt Export Pump (BSEP) (ABCB11)

BSEP is located exclusively in the canalicular membrane of hepatocytes in humans and primarily governs biliary excretion of bile acids. A decrease in BSEP function may lead to reduced bile acid secretion. Inhibition of BSEP is associated with drug-induced intrahepatic cholestasis. Its role in DIs is not known.

SLC Transporters

The Human Genome Organisation (HUGO) Nomenclature Committee Database (http://www.gene.ucl.ac.uk/nomenclature/) provides a list of transporter families of the SLC gene series that encode passive transporters, ion-coupled transporters, and exchangers. There are 43 families of SLC transporters (families of SLC are comprised of transporters having at least 20%–25% of identical amino acid sequences).

The human SLC superfamily transports a broad spectrum of substrates such as nutrients, toxins, and prescription drugs. Passive transporters (or facilitated transporters) permit passage of drugs and other solutes (e.g., glucose, amino acids, and urea) across membranes down their electrochemical gradients. Among the SLC superfamily members, OATPs play a prominent role in transporting endogenous substances and xenobiotics, including numerous drugs across plasma membranes. Many genes in the SLC superfamily are involved in pediatric inherited disorders and other human diseases.

Organic Anion Transporting Polypeptides

Organic anion transporting polypeptides (OATPs) transport a wide range of endogenous substances (e.g., bile salts, hormones) and drugs (e.g., statins, ACE inhibitors, angiotensin receptor blockers, antibiotics, antihistaminics, antihypertensives, and anticancer drugs). Most OATPs are expressed in multiple tissues except OATP1B1 and OATP1B3, which are considered to be exclusively hepatic in expression.

Polymorphisms influence expression, localization, and transport kinetics, e.g., mutations of OATP1B1 cause decreased hepatic uptake of drugs, increasing their plasma concentrations.

Coadministration of a second drug that is also a substrate of the same transporter decreases hepatic uptake and increases plasma concentrations contributing to transporter-mediated DIs.

There are eleven OATPs in humans. They are classified according to shared amino acids (Hagenbuch and Meier, 2004):

- Proteins with more than 40% identity belong to the same family.
- Proteins with more than 60% identity belong to the same subfamily.

OATPs form six families (OATP1–OATP6) and thirteen subfamilies (e.g., OATP1A, OATP1B, OATP1C). There are numerous examples of OATP-mediated interactions, which include

- Reduced renal clearance and prolonged half-life of penicillin, methotrexate, and ACE inhibitors with probenecid
- Reduced renal clearance with an increased toxicity of methotrexate by penicillins
- Reduced renal clearance of furosemide by probenecid
- Increased plasma levels and toxicity of digoxin by amiodarone due to inhibition of OATPs and MDR1
- Reduced plasma concentrations of fexofenadine by fruit juices (grapefruit, orange juice)

Organic Cation Transporters (OCTs)

These are "polyspecific" transporters belonging to the SLC22 family. They accept drugs of different sizes and molecular structures and often display variations in affinity and turnover.

Approximately 40% of orally administered drugs are cations or weak bases at physiological pH; cation transporters are important determinants of drug PK. They are able to translocate organic cations across the plasma membrane in either direction—i.e., cation influx and cation efflux.

They consist of OCT1, OCTN1, OCTN2, OCT6, and the proton/cation antiporters MATE1, MATE2-K, and MATE2-B. OCT1, OCT2, and OCT3 translocate a range of organic cations and are inhibited by a number of compounds that are not transported.

Expression: Intestine, liver, kidney, and other tissues.

Clinical Features

- Polymorphisms—genetic variations in *SLC22A1* gene were associated with the altered pharmacokinetics of metformin increasing the risk of lactic acidosis.
- Coadministration of metformin with cimetidine, bisoprolol, carvedilol, metoprolol, or propranolol decreased the renal elimination of metformin (reduced OCT2-mediated uptake of metformin from blood into renal tubular cells).
- Imatinib, nilotinib, gefitinib, and erlotinib (tyrosine kinase inhibitors) inhibit MATE1- and MATE2-mediated metformin transport.
- Altered expression of OCT6 (SLC51A and SLC51B mutations) is found in cholestasis, primary biliary cirrhosis, and pediatric biliary atresia.
- Transporters in platelets—platelets represent a pharmacokinetic microcompartment where the interplay between uptake and elimination transporters determines intracellular drug concentrations. Platelets function as "long-haul truckers" for a variety of drugs and biologically active substances (e.g., serotonin). ABC and SLCs are present in platelets. Following coronary artery bypass graft surgery, platelets exhibit increased amounts of MRP4 resulting in active extrusion of aspirin from platelet cytosol with reduced COX-1 inhibition (suboptimal platelet inhibition-aspirin resistance). In the liver, uptake of statins is mediated by OATP transporters—mainly OATP1B1. OATP2B1 in platelets transports atorvastatin and rosuvastatin as high-affinity substrates.

REFERENCE

Hagenbuch B, Meier PJ. Organic anion transporting polypeptides of the OATP/SLC21 family:phylogenetic classification as OATO/SLCO superfamily, new nomenclature and molecular/functional properties. Pflugers Arch 2004;447:653–665.

Individual Variability of Adverse Drug Interactions

Simon F.J. Clarke, Lakshman Delgoda Karalliedde, Ursula Collignon, and Seneka Abeyratne

INTRODUCTION

The overall benefit of a drug therapy is determined by the balance between efficacy of the drug and the adverse drug reactions. Large randomized controlled trials are usually used to test the efficacy of drug treatments, yet they cannot predict the effect in individual patients or in different populations.

DDIs depend on the concentrations of affected drugs at different sites throughout the body. Drug concentrations are determined by their absorption, distribution, metabolism, and elimination, and all of these processes are subject to a number of influences including genetic, environmental, and (patho-)physiological states.

Drug Factors

DDIs may be beneficial but become adverse if the concentration of an affected drug becomes either too high (increased side effects or even toxic effects) or too low (loss of efficacy). Interactions involving drugs with a narrow therapeutic index are more likely to be associated with clinically significant adverse interactions.

Physiological Factors

Age, sex, disease states, pregnancy, exercise, starvation, and circadian rhythm contribute significantly to individual variations of the PK and PD properties of administered drugs.

Environmental Factors

Dietary constituents and tobacco and alcohol use are all known to induce or inhibit cytochrome P450s, other DMEs, and drug transporters. Environmental factors may also interact with drug targets to produce antagonism or synergy with drugs to alter drug therapeutic effects or toxicity.

Genetic Factors

The activity of the metabolizing and transport enzymes is determined genetically. Genetic polymorphisms can have a profound impact on drug disposition, drug efficacy, and drug safety. Depending on the drug, genetic factors have been suggested to account for 20%–95% of the variability in drug disposition and clinical effects observed not only between individuals but also between ethnic groups.[1]

Genetic polymorphisms of DMEs and transporters permanently change the structure of a target protein, altering the function and the rate and kinetic constants of metabolizing enzymes. Daily doses of warfarin vary 20- to 30-fold from patient to patient because of individual variations in its metabolism.

The remainder of this section is devoted to the genetic factors involved in DIs.

ROLE OF POLYMORPHISMS OF METABOLIZING ENZYMES, TRANSPORTERS, AND OF ETHNICITY IN ADVERSE DRUG INTERACTIONS

Since the 1950s, pharmacogenetic studies have systematically identified allelic variants at genes that influence drug response, including those of both DMEs and drug targets. Polymorphisms in DMEs can lead to acute toxic responses and unwanted DDIs or to therapeutic failure from augmented drug metabolism. The development of the complete human genome sequence has enabled the identification of the impact of variations of the human genome sequence, not only on the pathogenesis of diseases but also on the response to drug therapy.

An understanding of the variations of metabolizing enzymes and transporters can help to predict likely variations of concentrations in the blood and at target organs that may predispose to ADIs. Variations are predominantly genetically determined as polymorphisms influence the activity of the metabolizing and transport enzymes.

Genetic variations provide a molecular basis for ethnic differences in DMEs (e.g., CYP2C9, 2C19, 2D6, and 3A4), drug transporters (e.g., P glycoprotein), drug receptors (adrenoceptors), and other functionally important proteins (eNOS and G proteins).

Polymorphisms

More than 90% of human genes contain at least one single nucleotide polymorphism (SNP), and nearly every human gene is marked by a sequence variation.

- >14 million SNPs have been identified in the human genome.
- >60,000 SNPs are located in the coding regions of the genes.
- Most SNPs seem to have no apparent effect on gene function while others have a profound impact.
- Identification of a single SNP may not be sufficient to relate the variation of a target protein to a disease or a drug response.

Genetic polymorphisms are estimated to influence 20%–25% of all drug therapies. Genetic variations affect the amount and activity of metabolizing enzymes and transporters that determine the concentrations of drug in the blood and at target organs; they also affect the sensitivity of the target organs.

Genetic polymorphisms have been discovered in virtually all the major classes of DMEs, including the members of the important cytochrome P450 superfamily. As of March 2015, the Human Cytochrome P450 (*CYP*) Allele Nomenclature Database (www.cypallelles.ki.se) reported the number of alleles for the following CYPs:

- CYP1A2—41
- CYP2C8—16
- CYP2C9—67
- CYP2C19—48
- CYP2D6—154
- CYP3A4—46

As can be seen, CYP2D6 is a highly polymorphic enzyme and is responsible for more than 200-fold variations in the metabolism of nearly 100 drugs. Most of the known variant alleles are inactive or have decreased activity.

Simplistically, the presence of alleles with varying metabolizing activity within a cytochrome subfamily provides a basis for classification that guides clinicians to the probable blood levels following administration of a substrate drug. The following table shows the classification of phenotypes that is widely used for cytochrome 450 enzymes.

Alleles	Phenotype	Effect on Substrates	Examples of Effects
Nonfunctional variant	PMs	*Prodrug* • Slow metabolism • Poor efficacy • Greater risk of therapeutic failure • Accumulation of prodrug may increase the risk of associated side effects *Active drug* • Slow inactivation • Good efficacy • Rapid effect • Increased blood levels of active drug may be associated with increased risk of toxicity • Often required in lower doses	CYP2D6 PMs do not show DDIs predicted from in vitro studies. CYP2D6 PMs may cause interactions at alternative competing metabolic pathways Recommended dose for several antidepressants: 70%–80% of dose for EMs[2]
Low frequency of active alleles, e.g., CYP2D6*17 allele has approximately 20% activity of the wild type.	Intermediate metabolizers (IMs)	*Prodrug* • Metabolism slower than expected with risk of therapeutic failure • *Active drug* • Slower inactivation of active drug • May provide adequate efficacy in some but increased blood levels • Risk of toxic effects of active drug • May require lower doses in vulnerable populations, e.g., aged, infancy, some disease states	Under normal conditions of use, individuals most likely to display DDIs are those who are IMs with compromised drug metabolizing capacity or those who have inherited CYP2D6 alleles (such as CYP2D6*9, CYP2D6*10, or CYP2D6*17) with reduced or altered affinity for CYP2D6 substrates. Frequencies of the alleles with increased potential for DDIs vary widely between different ethnic groups Recommended dose for several antidepressants-80%–90% of dose for EMs[2]
Normal enzyme activity	Extensive metabolizers (EMs)	*Extensive Metabolizers* Extensive metabolizers have two normally functioning alleles for a particular enzyme	Expected response to standard dose medication.
Increased enzyme activity	Ultrarapid metabolizers (UMs)	*Active drug* • Fast inactivation of active drug • Poor drug efficacy • Risk of therapeutic failure • Higher doses often required	Ultrarapid metabolizers (UMs) with wide interethnic differences in prevalence do not exhibit expected DDIs due to a sufficiently large functional reserve of CYP2D6 activity, probably requiring much higher (and potentially toxic) doses of inhibitor to elicit an interaction. Recommended dose for several antidepressants-100%–130% of dose for EMs[2]

However, the situation is more complex, as is usually the case in pharmacology!

- The metabolism of drugs is usually the result of the expression of multiple genes and the distribution of genetic phenotypes is complex (e.g., they may be bimodal, multimodal, or broad without an apparent antimode). For drug responses that reflect the combined effects of multiple genes (i.e., polygenic inheritance), the phenotypic distribution of polygenic traits and their impact on drug therapy can be complex and obscure.

- Drugs are often metabolized by different pathways using different enzymes that may have different levels of activity. For example:
  - A strong CYP2D6 inhibitor (e.g., fluoxetine) will increase the plasma levels of a CYP2D6 substrate (e.g., atomoxetine) in subjects who are extensive metabolizers (EMs).
  - Conversely, the inhibitor will have a minimal effect in subjects who are poor metabolizers (PMs), as they have no active enzyme to inhibit.
  - In some instances, inhibition has a greater effect in PMs than EMs.
  - When a drug is metabolized by a minor pathway (nonpolymorphic enzyme) and a major pathway (polymorphic enzyme), inhibition of the minor pathway will usually have minimal effect on plasma concentrations in EMs.
  - The minor pathway plays a greater role in the clearance of the drug in PMs of the major pathway; in this circumstance, the inhibition of the minor pathway in PMs of the major pathway may have a significant effect on drug clearance and resulting drug concentrations.

Ethnicity

There is increasing evidence that genetic differences between different ethnic populations influence pharmacokinetics and pharmacodynamics and should be taken into account by prescribers. Significant interethnic differences exist in the frequency of variant alleles that express the activity of metabolizing and transport enzymes. Genetic polymorphisms often vary more than 10-fold between populations. For example

- The frequency of CYP2D6 PMs is much higher in populations of Western Caucasian origin (5%–10%) than in Far East and Asian ethnic groups (0%–2%).[3–5]
- The frequency of PMs of CYP2C19 is lower in Western Caucasians (2%–4%) compared to East Asians (about 15%–25%), reaching as high as 60%–70% in Vanuatu and other Pacific islands.[6,7]

Clinically significant interethnic differences in drug metabolism are more likely to occur when the drug is only metabolized by a single pathway. In addition, drugs most likely to exhibit ethnic differences in their pharmacokinetics are those that undergo significant gut metabolism/transport and/or hepatic first-pass metabolism, are highly bound to plasma proteins, or have hepatic metabolism as a major route of elimination. As important are variations in structure and function of targets-receptors of drug action, as they do produce ethnic differences in responses to drug classes such as antipsychotics, tricyclic antidepressants, and adrenergics.

Environmental influences add to genetic variations to produce interethnic or intergeographic differences in drug response. The definition of ethnicity encompassing both genetic and environmental factors is different from that of race. Self-identification of race may be challenging.

With increasing global migration and admixing of different ethnic populations within a community, prediction of DDI attributable to ethnicity would be most challenging. Geographical differences in the pattern of drug usage complicate interethnic differences in DIs.

Specific Examples

1. Ethnic differences in responses to cardiovascular drugs have been recognized since the 1980s. The Fourth Report of the Joint National Committee (JNC-IV) on the Detection, Evaluation, and Treatment of High Blood Pressure (1988) was the first to recommend consideration of race/ethnicity in the selection of antihypertensive therapy, and the three subsequent sets of JNC guidelines have contained similar recommendations. FDA and similar regulatory authorities subsequently recommended that the choice of medications for certain disease states such as hypertensive heart disease should take ethnicity into account. Distinction would be to the three major continental populations

from which the human population mainly derives (namely, European, African, and Asian ancestry), i.e., ethnic groups who may have similar ancestral origins and who share certain social or cultural practices.[8] For example, Caucasians (those of European origin) responded better to β-blockers and ACE inhibitors, while blacks of African ancestry responded better to diuretics.[9]

2. A study in Singapore revealed differences in warfarin requirements between different ethnic groups within the country.[10] Warfarin maintenance requirements of Indians (5.9 mg) was nearly twice that of Chinese (3.5 mg) and Malays (3.6 mg); the difference persisted after adjusting for body weight (Indians required 0.089 mg/kg body weight daily, Chinese 0.058 mg/kg/day, and Malays 0.059 mg/kg/day). In the absence of genetic information, race was an important predictor of warfarin dosage in the Singapore population.
3. The FDA, the European Medicines Agency (EMA), the Pharmaceuticals and Medical Devices Agency (PMDA) in Japan, and other regulatory agencies have enforced the availability of pharmacogenetic information (e.g., in FDA-approved labels) for more than 100 drugs (e.g., atorvastatin, carvedilol, clopidogrel, and hydralazine).

Awareness of the molecular basis underlying ethnic differences in drug metabolism, transport, and response will enable prescribers to consider this important variable while prescribing and expanding the acumen in predicting or managing DDIs.

EXAMPLES OF POLYMORPHISMS AND ETHNIC VARIABILITY IN DIFFERENT ENZYMES

Cytochromes P 450 Enzymes

CYP3A4

- Forty percent of total CYP is expressed in liver and intestines.
- Environmental and genetic factors influence CYP3A activity.

Polymorphisms:

- CYP3A adult phenotype four- to sixfold interindividual variation with 46 CYP3A4 variant proteins described
- Proteins with ↓ activity (*6,*17,*20)

Ethnic variations:

- CYP3A4*1B is absent in Chinese and Japanese (and present in Tanzanian healthy volunteers).
- CYP3A4-mediated demethylation more in Caucasians compared to Chinese.
- CYP3A4*2 frequency ~2.5%.
- Variant alleles of no functional significance in 45% African Americans.
- ↑ Frequencies of *CYP3A4*16* and *-*18* in Asian populations.
- High frequencies of *CYP3A4*2* and *-*7* in white people.

Clinical relevance:

- Interindividual variations of content and activity of these enzymes responsible for metabolism of nearly 140 frequently prescribed drugs diminishes the consistency of blood concentrations that would occur following metabolism.
- The impact of coadministered inhibitors and inducers would result in varying blood and primary drug concentrations at target organs among individuals and between ethnic groups.
- Nifedipine-Cl_s: 77% higher in Caucasians than Asian Indians. AUC threefold ↑ in Asian Indians compared to Caucasians.

- Alprazolam—Caucasians possess CYP3A4*1B with modest activity compared to wild type—frequency is 3.5%–11% in whites and Hispanics.
- Role in cyclophosphamide pharmacokinetics.

CYP 2B6

- Represents about 1%–6% of the total P450 *content* in the human liver
- Metabolizes nearly 35 drugs

Polymorphism:

- The CYP2B6*6 allele causes both ↑ and ↓ activity of CYP2B6.
- There is large interethnic differences in the distribution of alleles.
- Molecular basis for altered activity CYP2B6*18 is not clarified.
- Rare CYP2B6*28 allele is considered to be a genetic basis for some diseases, e.g., stomach, breast, and prostatic neoplasms.
- Homozygous combinations CYP2B6*6, CYP2B6*16, and CYP2B6*18 exhibit ↓ metabolism of CYP2B6 substrates (efavirenz). Efavirenz AUC is significantly different for CYP2B6 516G NT (Q172H) genotypes (more common in Africans).

Ethnic variations:

- CYP2B6*6—frequency in populations (20%–30%), rather common.
- CYP2B6*16 and CYP2B6*18 common in black subjects (7%–9%).
- The CYP2B6*4 allele possibly causes ↑ V_{max} of substrate drugs in vitro and in vivo and interindividual variability in CYP2B6 metabolic activity in vitro

Relevance:

- Efavirenz
  - The CYP2B6*4 allele ↑ V_{max} values → anti-HIV treatment is more effective.
  - CYP2B6 516T genotype individuals in combination with CYP2D6*6 allele → ↑ plasma levels.
  - The CYP2B6*6 allele causes both ↑ and ↓ activity of CYP 2B6.

CYP2C8

- CYP2C8 oxidizes arachidonic acid to vasoactive derivatives.
- Hepatic enzyme expressed at ↓ levels than CYP2C9 but ↑ than CYP2C19.

Polymorphisms:

- Gene relatively highly conserved.
- No important functional variants or null alleles in populations.
- Both CYP2C9 and CYP2C8 contribute to arachidonic acid oxidation. CYP2C8*3/CYP2C9*2 haplotypes decrease arachidonic acid oxidation. Recently, two CYP2C8 haplotypes have been identified: one associated with ↓ and the other with ↑ activity using both paclitaxel and repaglinide as substrates.
- High activity by the CYP2C8*1B allele.
- CYP2C8*1B binds nuclear factors.
- Altered CYP2C8 activity contributed to cerivastatin toxicity.
- Significant ↓ in arachidonic acid metabolism with CYP2C8*3/CYP2C9*2 haplotype compared with wild type.

Ethnicity:

- CYP2C8*2 mainly in Africans.
- CYP2C8 *3 and CYP2C8*4 mainly in Caucasians.
- Rare CYP2C8*5 plays a role in interindividual variability.

CYP2C9

- Mainly expressed in liver; contributes to ~20% of hepatic CYP activity. Metabolizes 10% of all drugs.
- Warfarin CYP 2C9 is the main enzyme for rate-limiting metabolism and has the largest impact on determining dose.
- Metabolizes the endogenous substrates arachidonic acid and linolenic acid.

Polymorphisms

- Clinically highly significant.
- Differences in substrate specificity among 3 CYP2C9 enzymes: CYP2C9.1, CYP2C9.2, and CYP2C9.3.
- Substrate affinity of CYP2C9.2 varies compared to wild type.
- CYP2C9*3 allele has stronger PK effects than CYP2C9*2 for most substrates but significant ↓ catalytic activity, 10% of intrinsic clearance of wild type for most CYP2C9 substrates.

Ethnicity:

- Concentrations of substrate drugs of CYP2C9 would be higher in whites.
- CYP2C9*3 is associated with ↓ warfarin requirements in Malays (9%) and Indians (18%), but does not solely account for lower warfarin requirements.
- CYP2C9*2 variant present in 10% of Caucasians.
- CYP2C9*2 and CYP2C9*3 variants absent or rare (0.4%) in Southeast Asians.
- Less than 2% of Southeast Asians are heterozygous for CYP2C9*3, none homozygous. Partly responsible are environmental factors.
- 0.5%–3% are homozygotes for CYP2C9*2 variant in black populations.
- In a study of three ethnic groups in Malaysia, CYP2C9*2 was not detected in Malays and Chinese but was present in Indians. Frequency of CYP2C9*3 was highest in Indians followed by Malays and the Chinese.
- Frequency of CYP2C9*3 reported to be higher in Caucasians (6%–10%), compared to Asians.
- As important are allele variations between communities within a country. In Pakistan, those of Baluchi origin (12 million), CYP2C9*3 alleles were more frequent compared to those of Sindhi origin (30 million) in whom the CYP2C9*2 was more frequent.

Clinical relevance:

- CYP2C9*1 metabolizes warfarin normally.
- CYP2C9*2 and CYP2C9*3, enzymes with ↓ activity (PMs): CYP2C9*2 reduces warfarin metabolism by 30% and CYP2C9*3 reduces warfarin metabolism by 90%.
- Compared with homozygous carriers of CYP2C9*1, homozygotes for CYP2C9*3 need 3.3-fold lower mean doses of warfarin to achieve the same INR.CYP2C9*2 carriers, and heterozygotes require doses in between.
- Patients with polymorphisms in CYP2C9 and VKORC1 often experience severe over-anticoagulation.
- CYP2C9*2 and CYP2C9*3 genotypes have ↑ rate of major bleeding complications during initiation of therapy with warfarin and acenocoumarol.

CYP2C19

- Metabolizes S-mephenytoin, diazepam, omeprazole, and other drugs.
- S-mephenytoin hydroxylation, catalyzed by CYP2C19, is genetically determined.
- CYP2C19 phenotype affects pharmacokinetics of moclobemide, amitriptyline, clomipramine, sertraline, and citalopram.

Polymorphisms:

- More than 20 polymorphisms of *CYP2C19* have been reported.
- Phenotype affects pharmacokinetics of moclobemide, amitriptyline, clomipramine, sertraline, and citalopram.
- CYP2C19 preferentially metabolizes the S-form of citalopram (mediates antidepressant effect) to a demethylated metabolite with ↓ plasma concentration and potency. AUC of citalopram and S-citalopram (escitalopram) significantly ↑ in PMs (frequency of PMs in Western Caucasians 2%–4%) compared with EMs.
- Patients on escitalopram therapy exhibited 42% lower plasma concentrations than those homozygous for CYP2C19*1, with a necessity of dose adjustment for those carrying CYP2C19*7.
- The CYP2C19*17 allele strongly associated with ↑ CYP2C19 activity in vivo; 42% ↓ plasma concentrations than those homozygous for CYP2C19*17.
- Dose adjustment for those carrying CYP2C19*17.

Ethnicity:

- The ethnic variation in CYP2C19*2: major factor for interethnic differences in PK of widely prescribed substrate drugs.
- 15%–25% of Chinese, Japanese, and Koreans are PMs compared with 2%–4% in Caucasians.
- 7% Africans are EMs compared with 5% in Caucasians.
- 20%–30% Caucasians are UMs.
- CYP2C19 deficient in 5% of Caucasians, 20% of Japanese.
- PM carrying two defective CYP2C19 genes—5% in Caucasian and African populations, 20% in Asians.
- Frequency of CYP2C19*2 allele is 15%.

Clinical relevance:

Clopidogrel

- Undergoes two sequential P450-mediated oxidations (formation of 2-oxo by CYP2C19, -1A2, and -2B6, followed by formation of active thiol metabolite by CYP3A4, -2B6, -2C19, and -2C9) to generate the active metabolite.
- Contributions by CYP2C19 and -3A4 are more important than by other P450s for bioactivation of clopidogrel. Formation of active metabolite via CYP2C19, 1A2, and 2B6.
- CYP2C19*2 polymorphism accounts for ~12% of variable responses.
- ↓ in CYP2C19 function → ↓ formation of clopidogrel's active metabolite → ↓ inhibition of platelet function.
- 30% of Caucasians and Africans carry one or two defective CYP2C19 alleles; they are not expected to respond to clopidrogel.
- The FDA issued a black box warning stating that "recommended doses of clopidogrel form less of metabolites and thus produce a smaller effect on platelet function in patients who are CYP2C19 PMs."

Cyclophosphamide

- *CYP2C19*2 and CYP2C19*3—responsible for majority of PM alleles.
- Inactive CYP2C19* allele significantly ↓ cyclophosphamide elimination.

- No functional significance of CYP3A4 variant alleles (minor haplotypes CYP3A7*2, CYP3A7_39256A, and CYP3A5*1).
- CYP2C19*17 allele strongly associated with ↑ CYP2C19 activity in vivo.
- Treatment in homozygous CYP2C19*2 patients significantly ↓ risk of developing premature ovarian failure.
- Homozygous CYP2C19*2 subjects ↑ probability of poor renal response.

Proton pump inhibitors

- *Omeprazole, Pantoprazole*: CYP2C19 metabolic capacity correlates inversely with exposure to omeprazole and clinical effects.
- Intragastric pH is
  - 4.5 for the PM subjects
  - 3.3 for the heterozygous EM subjects
  - 2.1 for the EM subjects
- Single dose (20 mg) of omeprazole: AUC is ↑ among PM subjects, ↓ among EM subjects, and in between in heterozygous EMs.

CYP2D6

- Only functional enzyme in human CYP2D family.
- Only P450 enzyme that cannot be induced.
- Protein content of CYP2D6 ↑ during the course of aging.
- Responsible for the metabolism of approximately 20%–25% of all marketed drugs.

Content:

- Expressed in liver (2.5% of total CYP), GI, brain, and lung.
- CYP2D6-mediated drug metabolism is ↑ in pregnancy.
- Confirmed existence of protein and mRNA at all stages of human growth: fetus, newborn, child, and adult.
- Therefore, activity of substrate drugs may ↑ slowly from neonate to young adult.
- CYP2D6 drug elimination obscured if renal clearance is significant in drug elimination.

Polymorphisms:

- Most clinically relevant of polymorphic genes in drug metabolism.
- Individual variation, mainly result from genetic variations; more than 150 variant alleles with over 63 different functional CYP2D6 gene variants described.
- Polymorphism significantly affects metabolism of 50% of substrate drugs.
- SNP is probably the most common variation associated with CYP2D6 polymorphism.
- Compared to *1, other functional alleles have moderate activity.
  - Theoretically, UMs carry at least three functional alleles (CYP2D6*1 (wild-type), *2,*9, *10, and *17) with increased enzyme activity.
  - Allele frequency of CYP2D6*2 is 28% in majority of UMs.
- EMs have two functional alleles (*1, *2, *9, *10, *17)
- IMs have one functional allele (frequently *2, *9, *10).
- The EM and UM phenotypes overlap more than PM and EM phenotypes.
- PMs (frequency is 51%–70%) have two of the following nonfunctional alleles: *3, *4, *5, *6, *7, *8, *14, *18, *21, and *44.

Ethnicity:

- The CYP2D6 alleles are subject to important inter-ethnic differences.
- UM phenotype has a higher prevalence worldwide than PMs.

- Caucasian liver microsomes ↑ CYP2D6 activity compared to Japanese.
- Hydroxylation of debrisoquine ↓ in Chinese compared to whites.
- Mean clearance of desipramine ↓ in Chinese compared to whites.
- UM phenotype has CYP2D6*1 wild-type.
- CYP2D6*1 frequency may reach 40%.
- CYP2D6*35, CYP2D6*2—UMs in North Africa and Oceania (20%).
- ↑ UM phenotype in Mozabite population in Algeria.
- Allele frequency of CYP2D6*2 is
  - 28% in North Africa
  - 40% in Ethiopians
  - 34% in Zimbabweans.
  - 17% in Tanzania
  - 2%–5% in other African populations
- UM alleles vary in frequency:
  - >25% black Americans compared with 0.2% in white Americans
  - ~10% in Northern Spain compared with 1%–2% in Sweden, very rare in Germans, and absent in British

Relevance:

- UM phenotype causes more adverse drug reactions due to ↑ levels of drug metabolites (UMs produce 10- to 30-fold ↑ amounts of metabolites). UM phenotype is a factor for lack of response to antidepressants and decreased levels of several CYP2D6 substrate drugs.

Codeine

- Case of infant death caused by breast-feeding mother of UM phenotype taking high doses of codeine-formation of morphine at levels lethal to the infant).
- The clearance of codeine via O-demethylation was higher in white American EMs than Chinese EMs. Chinese had a significantly lower ability to O-demethylate codeine compared to Japanese and Koreans.

Psychiatric drugs

- The clinical use of psychiatric drugs, many of which are metabolized by CYP2D6, illustrates the practicality of using CYP2D6 genotyping for dose selection in individual patients.
- Individual patients carrying CYP2D6*3, -*4, -*5, or -*6 variants should be given reduced doses of antidepressants to avoid or reduce drug side effects. In this scenario, the metabolism of the drugs is the major factor affecting drug response and safety, and genetic variations are well established. For this reason, psychiatrists at the Mayo Clinic have begun to request that the CYP2D6 genotype information be made available before psychiatric drug therapy is begun.

Tamoxifen

- Tamoxifen is metabolized by CYP2D6 to key metabolites 4-hydroxytamoxifen and endoxifen (about 100 times greater affinity for estrogen receptor).
- PMs (CYP2D6*4 is the most common null allele contributing to PM phenotype) are not able to activate tamoxifen with a risk of treatment failure.
- ↑ Incidence of moderate or severe hot flashes in patients with one or no *4 alleles (20%) compared with homozygotes of the *4 allele (0%).
- CYP2D6*4 homozygotes—shorter relapse-free time and worse disease-free survival with CYP2D6*4/*4 genotype (PM) compared with either one or no *4 alleles.

Clozapine

- Compared to Caucasians, Asian patients require ↓ dose for comparable clinical efficacy.

CYP2E1

- CYP2E1 accounts for 7% of total CYP content in liver.
- Most active member of 2E subfamily.
- Key role in pathogenesis of alcoholic liver disease.
- Metabolizes chloroxazone, ethanol, and paracetamol (acetaminophen).
- Activity affected by alcohol, drugs (isoniazid), organic solvents (e.g., carbon tetrachloride), and disease states (e.g., diabetes, ketonemia, and obesity).
- Key role in biodegradation of environmental carcinogens.
- Metabolizing activity is genetically determined. CYP2E1 mediates production of hepatotoxic hydrazine metabolite of isoniazid.
- Polymorphisms influence hepatotoxicity.
- ↑ Ethanol elimination rates among smokers.

GLUCURONYL TRANSFERASES (UGTs)

Polymorphisms:

- The major isoforms of these membrane-bound proteins are UGT1A1, UGT1A4, UGTT1A9, and UGT2B7 metabolizing 87% of the commonly used drugs.
- *UGT1A1* is highly polymorphic; more than 100 *UGT1A1* polymorphisms have been identified. The *UGT1A1*28* polymorphisms result in considerable reduction of UGT1A1 expression (~30%–80%) and reduced glucuronidation of SN-38.

Ethnicity:

- The frequency of *UGT1A1*6* polymorphism is high among Japanese and Chinese but low (<1%) in Caucasians.

Clinical relevance:

- The high frequency of the *UGT1A1*6* variant allele may contribute to the high incidence of neonatal hyperbilirubinemia in Asian populations, consistent with a major role of UGT1A1 in the glucuronidation of bilirubin.
- Irinotecan is metabolized in the liver to SN-38, which is inactivated via glucuronidation by UGT1A1 (and other UGTs to a lesser extent) and by secretion into the bile through ABCC2 (possibly other transporters as well). The majority of SN-38 glucuronide (SN-38G) in the intestine is reconverted to SN-38 by β-glucuronidase.
- Polymorphisms of *ABCC2* seem to influence the incidence of irinotecan-related diarrhea. The haplotype *ABCC2*2* associated with ↓ Cl of irinotecan from blood—↓ hepatobiliary secretion of SN-38 glucuronide through ABCC2, which ↓ exposure of intestinal epithelial cells to SN-38.
- A significant reduction of severe diarrhea was noted in patients who carry the *ABCC2*2* allele but not the *UGT1A1*28* allele (odds ratio of 0.15). This reduction was not observed in patients who carry at least one allele of *UGT1A1*28*.
- Patients homozygous or heterozygous for the *UGT1A1*28* allele have elevated levels of SN-38 as a result of reduced glucuronidation of SN-38 and accumulation of the active metabolite to a high level.

They are susceptible to bone marrow and gastrointestinal side effects of SN-38 when normal doses of irinotecan are used. FDA has recommended genotyping of patients for the *UGT1A1*28* polymorphism and dose-adjusting accordingly before irinotecan treatment.

SULFOTRANSFERASES (SULTs)

- Polymorphisms of SULT1A1 have been attributed to carcinogenicity due to the activation of endogenous substrates. Patients homozygous for SULT1A1*2 have an increased risk for cancers of the lung and breast.
- Polymorphism has not been associated with any DIs.

GLUTATHIONE-S-TRANSFERASE (GST)

- Polymorphisms are found within each class.
- The greatest impact of GST polymorphism on drug metabolism are due to mutations of classes μ and Θ, where genes encoding GSTM1*0 and GSTT1*0 are referred to as null alleles as genes encoding GSTM and GSTT are absent.
- GSTA1 gene polymorphism alters busulfan conjugation.
- Glutathione S-transferase P1 has an important role in cisplatin and carboplatin metabolism in ovarian cancer cells. Intertumor differences in GSTP1 expression may therefore influence response to platinum-based chemotherapy in ovarian cancer patients.

METHYLTRANSFERASES

- Polymorphic COMT is both cytosolic and membrane bound and requires Mg^{2+} for catalytic activity.
- Persons with defective *TPMT* alleles may have ↑ levels of cytotoxic thiopurine nucleotides → risk of severe hematological toxicity by parent drugs unless ↓ drug dose used.
- TPMT polymorphisms (18 mutant alleles identified): TPMT*2, TPMT*3A, and TPMT*3C have intermediate (frequency approximately 11%) or poor (frequency approximately 0.3%) enzyme activity.
- When persons who were homozygous for low levels of TPMT activity or for no activity ($TPMT^L$/$TPMT^L$) received standard doses of thiopurines, they had greatly elevated concentrations of active metabolites, 6-thioguanine nucleotides, and a greatly increased risk of life-threatening, drug-induced myelosuppression.
- As a result, a phenotypic test for the level of TPMT activity in red cells and, subsequently, DNA-based tests were among the first pharmacogenetic tests to be used in clinical practice.

N-ACETYLTRANSFERASES (NATs)

- Polymorphisms of NAT2 have been extensively studied: more than 20 variants of NAT-2 have been determined. People are categorized into fast, intermediate, and slow acetylators:
  - *Fast acetylators:* 98% of fast acetylators have wild-type allele *NAT-2*4*.
  - *Intermediate acetylators:* These are associated with *NAT2*5*, *NAT2*6A*, and *NAT2*7B*.
  - *Slow acetylators:* Major variants are *NAT2*5A (or B)*, *NAT2*6A*, and *NAT2*7A*.
- Slow acetylator phenotypes are present in up to 90% of some Arab populations, 40%–60% of whites, and 5%–25% of East Asians.

MEMBRANE TRANSPORTERS

- Some transporters showed extreme variability in expression (e.g., SLC13A1, SLC16A8, SLC16A14, ABCC13, and ABCA12), and these contribute to interindividual differences in the metabolism of endogenous and exogenous compounds.

REFERENCES

1. Weinshilboum R. Inheritance and drug response. *New England Journal of Medicine* 2003;348:529–537.
2. Kirchheimer J et al. CYP2D6 and CYP2C19 genotype based dose recommendations for antidepressants: A first step towards subpopulation-specificdoses. *Acta Psychiatrica Scandinavica* 2001;104:173–192.
3. Bradford LD. CYP2D6 allele frequency in European Caucasians, Asians, Africans and their descendants. *Pharmacogenomics* 2002;3:229–243.
4. Mizutani T. PM frequencies of major CYPs in Asians and Caucasians. *Drug Metabolism Reviews* 2003;35:99–106.
5. Ozawa S et al. Ethnic differences in genetic polymorphisms of CYP2D6, CYP2C19, CYP3As and MDR1/ABCB1. *Drug Metabolism and Pharmacokinetics* 2004;19:83–95.
6. Kaneko A et al. High and variable frequencies of CYP2C19 mutations: Medical consequences of poor drug metabolism in Vanuatu and other Pacific islands. *Pharmacogenetics* 1999;9:581–590.
7. Xie HG et al. Molecular basis of ethnic differences in drug disposition and response. *Annual Review of Pharmacology and Toxicology* 2001;41:815–850.
8. Johnson JA. Ethnic differences in cardiovascular drug response. *Potential Contribution of Pharmacogenetics Circulation* 2008;118:1383–1393.
9. Veterans Administration Cooperative Study Group on Antihypertensive Agents. Comparison of propranolol and hydrochlorothiazide for the initial treatment of hypertension, II: Results of long-term therapy. *JAMA* 1982;248:2004–2011.
10. Lee SC et al. Interethnic variability of warfarin maintenance requirement is explained by *VKORC1* genotype in an Asian population. *Clinical Pharmacology & Therapeutics* 2006;79:197–205.

OTHER SOURCES OF INFORMATION

Belle DJ, Singh H. Genetic factors in drug metabolism. *American Family Physician* 2008;77:1553–1560.

Brunham LR et al. Pharmacogenomic diversity in Singaporean populations and Europeans. *Pharmacogenomics Journal* 2014;14:555–563.

Constable S et al. Pharmacogenetics in clinical practice: Considerations for testing. *Expert Review of Molecular Diagnostics* 2006;6:193–205.

Efstratios K et al. Beta-adrenergic receptor polymorphisms: A basis for pharmacogenetics. *WJCD* 2013;6.

Jedlitschky G et al. Transport of glutathione, glucuronate and sulphate conjugates by the MRP gene encoded conjugate export pump. *Cancer Research* 1996;56:988–994.

Johnson JA. Predictability of the effects of race or ethnicity on pharmacokinetics of drugs. *International Journal of Clinical Pharmacology and Therapeutics* 2000;38:53–60. 12.

Lazarou J et al. Incidence of adverse drug reactions in hospitalized patients: A meta-analysis of prospective studies. *JAMA* 2006;279:1200–1205.

Qiang M et al. Pharmacogenetics, pharmacogenomics, and individualized medicine. *Pharmacological Reviews* 2011;63:437–459.

Shah RR. Pharmacogenetics in drug regulation: Promise, potential and pitfalls. *Philosophical Transcations of the Royal Society* 2005;360;1460.

Shah RR. Drug development and use in the elderly: Search for the right dose and dosing regimen. *British Journal of Clinical Pharmacology* 2004;58:452–469.

Spear BB et al. Clinical application of pharmacogenetics. *Trends in Molecular Medicine* 2001;7:201–220.

Wilkinson GR. Drug metabolism and variability among patients in drug response. *New England Journal of Medicine* 2005;352:2211–2221.

Yang L et al. Gene expression variability in human hepatic drug metabolizing enzymes and transporters. *PLOS ONE* April 23, 2013.

Yiping L et al. Individual differences in the pharmacokinetics of clozapine in healthy Chinese adults. *Bulletin of Clinical Psychopharmacology* 2012;22.

FURTHER SUGGESTED READING

There are a number of online resources listing the substrates, inhibitors, and inducers of metabolizing enzymes and transport proteins, such as

U.S. Food and Drug Administration. Available at: http://www.fda.gov/Drugs/DevelopmentApprovalProcess/DevelopmentResources/DrugInteractionsLabeling/ucm093664.htm

Pharmacology Weekly. Available at: http://www.pharmacologyweekly.com/content/pages/drug-reference-table-cyp-p450-ugt-enzymes-transporters-or

Pathological States That Are Associated with Increased Risk of Adverse Drug Interactions

Lakshman Delgoda Karalliedde, Simon F.J. Clarke, Ursula Collignon, Janaka Karalliedde, Niroshini Manthri Giles, Chulananda Goonasekera, and H.M.U. Amila Jayasinghe

As with polymorphisms and ethnicity, there are several physiological states and pathological diseases associated with changes in absorption, distribution, metabolism, and excretion and with altered response of target organs, e.g., receptors.

This section highlights the conditions associated with changes in PK and PD that may increase the risk of ADIs; understanding these factors is needed to promote safer prescribing.

- Liver disease
- Kidney disease
- Cardiovascular disease
- Obesity
- Malnutrition
- Inflammation/infection

LIVER DISEASE

The highest concentration of most cytochrome P450s responsible for drug metabolism is in the liver and activity of these enzymes may be reduced in liver disease. In particular, CYP2C19 is more sensitive to liver disease than other cytochromes while phase II enzymes are least affected by liver disease.

Causes

Types of liver diseases that can affect drug metabolism include

- Steatosis (fatty liver disease) and steatohepatitis—alcoholic and nonalcoholic
- Hepatitis—infectious and noninfectious
- Cirrhosis and primary biliary cirrhosis
- Hepatocellular carcinoma

Severity of liver disease, rather than a specific disease state, correlates with the extent of altered P450 metabolism.

Pathopharmacology

The class of drug determines which drugs are most affected by liver disease:

- Class I drugs (high solubility, high permeability)—pharmacokinetics are determined by enzymatic metabolism.
- Class II drugs (high permeability, low solubility)—both enzymes and transporters are important.
- Class III drugs (high solubility, low permeability)—transporters are more important.

Class I drugs are most affected by liver disease, class II are moderately affected and class III least affected (although their clearance may be altered by renal insufficiency, which often coexists with hepatic failure).

Pathological factors that influence pharmacokinetics in the presence of liver failure are summarized in Table P.1.

Drug dosing in patients with liver disease is complex; for example, hepatic metabolism of antibiotics such as fluoroquinolones and flucloxacillin is hampered by liver failure, though a reduction of at least 90% of the metabolic capacity of liver has to occur to substantially affect drug clearance. It requires an assessment of the severity of the disease, PK of drugs, and hemodynamic changes to the gut and liver. Unfortunately, common biochemical markers of hepatic function do not directly relate to drug clearance.

Assessment of Severity of Liver Disease

This is best obtained from the history of the disease as per variables such as alcohol consumption, illicit drug use, toxic industrial exposure, and use of medications (supplements such as iron, vitamin A, and herbal remedies). Family history of diseases (e.g., alpha-1 antitrypsin deficiency, iron storage diseases, porphyrias, and diabetes mellitus) alerts the possibility of liver impairment.

Clinical signs such as jaundice, spider naevi, palmar erythema, ascites, abdominal distention, hepatomegaly, splenomegaly, caput medusae, and encephalopathy also aid in assessing severity of liver disease.

The Child-Turcotte-Pugh score and the MELD (Model for End-Stage Liver Disease) scores are used to assess progression of liver disease. However, they cannot be used directly to calculate dose adjustments; there is no substitute for careful monitoring of the effects of changes in doses!

Clinical implications:

- Drugs with a wide therapeutic index and limited hepatic elimination (<20%) are minimally affected by liver disease.
- Drugs with a wide therapeutic range that undergo extensive hepatic metabolism should be used with caution. Dosing interval should be increased or the total dose reduced (e.g., carvedilol).
- Drugs with a narrow therapeutic index require dose adjustments (reduce by up to 50%) and frequent monitoring (at <48 h).
- The oral bioavailability of drugs with a relatively high hepatic extraction ratio may increase to reach toxic concentrations in patients with chronic liver disease; reduced doses should be given.
- The unbound fraction of drugs with low hepatic extraction and high degree of protein binding (>90%) may be significantly increased in patients with chronic liver disease. PK evaluation should be based on unbound blood/plasma concentrations, and dosage adjustment may be necessary even though total blood/plasma concentrations are within the normal range. Methods are available for simultaneous determination of total and free drug plasma concentrations (Nilsson et al., 2001).
- The elimination of drugs that are partly excreted in unchanged form by the kidneys may be impaired in patients with hepatorenal syndrome. Be aware that estimates of creatinine clearance significantly overestimate glomerular filtration rate (GFR) in these patients. Reduced doses should be given.

Liver Transplantation

Liver transplantation may not resolve altered metabolism in recipients immediately. Post–liver transplant (PLT) patients have fluid, electrolyte, and nutritional abnormalities and biliary tract dysfunction. Likely alterations in PK in PLT patients are shown in Table P.2.

Table P.1 Factors Predisposing to Interactions in Liver Disease

Ageing-Related Changes	**Effect**
Absorption	
Increased gastric pH Delayed gastric emptying	Delayed absorption of oral drugs. Note that although the extent of absorption may be unaffected, there is an increase in time to achieve C_{max}
Portal-systemic shunting Lower liver mass	Decreases presystemic elimination (i.e., first-pass effect) of high extraction drugs (e.g., propranolol, labetalol, lidocaine, salicylamide, meperidine, pentazocine, nicardipine) following oral administration
Distribution	
Increased body third space (ascites and edema)	The V_d of hydrophilic drugs (e.g., digoxin) ↑ in patients with edema and/or ascites—requiring higher loading doses and possibly reduced hepatic perfusion
Reduced serum albumin	V_d of highly protein-bound drugs (>90%) are likely to ↑ in patients with hypoalbuminemia or ascites. Increased free-fraction of highly protein-bound acidic drugs
Increased α 1-acid glycoprotein	Decreased free-fraction of basic drugs (e.g., propranolol, morphine, oxazepam, vancomycin)
Metabolism	
Reduced hepatic blood flow and overall liver mass.	Less effective first-pass metabolism and phase I metabolism
Fibrotic liver disease—cirrhosis	↓ CYP1A2, CYP2E1, CYP2C19, and CYP3A4 levels CYP2D6 unaffected
Nonalcoholic fatty liver disease	Microsomal CYP1A2, CYP2D6, and CYP2E1, and CYP3A4 activity reduced—correlated with disease progression. May be mediated by increased TNFα and IL-1β Microsomal CYP2A6, CYP2B6, and CYP2C9 mRNA expression increased—again correlated with disease progression. May be mediated by increased levels of lipid peroxidation products (resulting from oxidative stress)
Hepatic dysfunction caused by • Infection (associated with cholestasis or hepatocellular injury) • Ischemic hepatitis (shock liver through hypoperfusion) • Hemolysis • Direct damage from hepatotoxic pharmaceuticals—is reflected by ↑ liver enzymes, bilirubin, and ammonia, or ↓ synthesis of coagulant factors	Significantly increased levels of CYP2A6 CYP3A4 unaffected by cholestasis but may be decreased with hepatocellular injury
Primary biliary cirrhosis, alcoholic steatohepatitis, and cirrhotic patients	Reduced CYP1A2 and CYP3A4 activity. Significantly increased levels of CYP2A6
Excretion	
Reduced renal blood flow—seen in moderate to severe liver disease	• Impaired renal elimination of water-soluble drugs and metabolites especially in hepatorenal syndrome • Risk of ↑ toxicity of known nephrotoxic drugs (aminoglycosides, NSAIDs) following interactions that ↑ their plasma levels
Reduced biliary excretion	In cholestatic jaundice—drugs and their active metabolites that are dependent on biliary excretion for clearance will have impaired elimination. Further impairment is likely if the compound is excreted as a glucuronide and is subject to enterohepatic circulation
Transporters	
Efflux (Pgp) and influx (OATP) affected in cholestatic states	See "Transporters" section

Table P.2 Factors Predisposing to Interactions Following Liver Transplant

Post-Liver Transplantation–Related Changes	Effect
Absorption	PLT—oral absorption of lipophilic drugs (e.g., cyclosporine) may be dramatically improved.
Protein binding	Compared to patients with chronic liver disease, protein binding of salicylic acid and diazepam is greater because of the removal of endogenous binding proteins. The concentration of α 1-acid glycoprotein increases and remains elevated after a month resulting in lower free concentrations of drugs binding to this protein (e.g., lidocaine).
Hepatic clearance	Altered metabolism observed in the immediate posttransplant period may occur due to preservation injury, initially decreased hepatic blood flow, and induction or inhibition of enzymes by immunosuppressants. First-pass metabolism is altered in the transition to normal hepatic function. Biliary dysfunction results in high concentrations of cyclosporin metabolites in the blood. Cytochrome P450 activity is initially depressed and recovers over the first few months. The mRNA gene expression for CYP3A4, 3A5, 2E1 (often in first month), and 1A2 increases significantly over time. Substrate drugs of CYP2E1 may require dose adjustments. Donor gene polymorphisms are more important than recipient gene polymorphisms. No reports of altered phase II metabolism. Renal elimination of conjugates and metabolites of acetaminophen is often impaired.
High extraction vs. low extraction drugs	For low extraction drugs—influence of changes in plasma protein binding and intrinsic hepatic clearance result in an increase in both free and total steady-state drug concentrations. Examples: propranolol + 300% (CYP2D6); erythromycin, propoxyphene + 100% (CYP3A4); dihydrocodeine + 70% (CYP2D6); oxprenolol + 100% (CYP2D6).

REFERENCES AND SOURCES OF INFORMATION

Bedogni G et al. Prevalence of and risk factors for nonalcoholic fatty liver disease: The Dionysos nutrition and liver study. *Hepatology* 2005;42:44–52.

Craig DF et al. Hepatic cytochrome P450 enzyme alterations in humans with progressive stages of nonalcoholic fatty liver disease. *Drug Metabolism and Disposition* 2009;37:2087–2094.

Huang HL et al. Metabolic syndrome is related to nonalcoholic steatohepatitis in severely obese subjects. *Obesity Surgery* 2007;17:1457–1463.

Kock K, Brouwer KL. A perspective on efflux transport proteins in the liver. *Clinical Pharmacology & Therapeutics* 2012;92:599–612.

Malinchoc M et al. A model to predict poor survival in patients undergoing transjugularintrahepatic portosystemic shunts. *Hepatology* 2000;31:864–871.

Nilsson LB et al. Simultaneous determination of total and free drug plasma concentrations combined with batch-wise pH-adjustment for the free concentration determinations. *Journal of Pharmaceutical and Biomedical Analysis* 2001;24:921–927.

Park GR. Molecular mechanisms of drug metabolism in the critically ill. *British Journal of Anaesthesia* 1996;77:32–49.

Pelkonen O et al. Inhibition and induction of human cytochrome P450 enzymes: Current status. *Archives of Toxicology* 2008;82:667–715.

Perianez-Parraga L et al. Drug dosage recommendations in patients with chronic liver disease. *Revista espanola de enfermedades digestivas* 2012;104:165–184.

Prescott LF et al. Drug metabolism in liver disease. *Journal of Clinical Pathology—Supplement (Royal College of Pathologists)* 1975;9:62–65.

Tsunedomi R et al. Patterns of expression of cytochrome P450 genes in progression of hepatitis C virus-associated hepatocellular carcinoma. *International Journal of Oncology* 2005;27:661–667.

Verbeeck RK. Pharmacokinetics and dosage adjustment in patients with hepatic dysfunction. *European Journal of Clinical Pharmacology* 2008;64:1147–1161.

Villeneuve JP, Pichette V. Cytochrome P450 and liver diseases. *Current Drug Metabolism* 2004;5:273–282.

Yang LQ et al. Different alterations of cytochrome P450 3A4 isoform and its gene expression in livers of patients with chronic liver diseases. *World Journal of Anesthesiology* 2003;9:359–363.

RENAL FAILURE

Acute and or chronic renal failure alters absorption, distribution, metabolism, and elimination of drugs. This would lead to increases in free concentrations of drugs which, in turn, make ADIs more likely.

- Decreased renal elimination of drugs is expected in renal failure.
- Renal insufficiency significantly decreases both phase I and phase II reactions possibly due to the inhibitory effects of uremic toxins on metabolizing enzymes.
- Similarly, the actions of transporters can also be inhibited.

One large study (Marquito et al., 2014) looked at the pharmacological profile of 1651 prescriptions issued to 850 patients with chronic kidney disease:

- 1364 potential DIs were identified (82.6%).
- 5 (0.4%) interactions were due to coadministration of drugs that were known to be contraindicated.
- Severe DIs included dual blockade of the renin-angiotensin system (RAS) (22% of severe DDIs) and prescriptions of RAS inhibitor with a xanthine oxidase inhibitor (allopurinol).
- The probability of occurrence of a DI increased 2.5-fold for each drug added to a prescription.

Another study looked into the prevalence of DIs in CKD patients by analyzing 205 prescriptions. A total of 474 combinations with potential for interactions were detected, with a mean of 2.7 interactions per prescription. The probability of occurrence of DDI increased 4.7-fold in patients with stage 5 CKD when compared to individuals with CKD stages 1 and 2. Severe DIs involving cardiovascular medications were seen in 19.6% of the cases.

The FDA recommends PK studies in renal patients for drugs with a narrow therapeutic index that are cleared predominantly by nonrenal mechanisms (http://www.fda.gov/downloads/Drugs/GuidanceComplianceRegulatoryInformation/Guidances/UCM204959.pdf). This should include at least one abbreviated PK study in end-stage renal disease (ESRD) patients.

Pathological factors that influence pharmacokinetics in the presence of renal failure are summarized in Table P.3.

Clinical relevance:

Renal failure has been shown to increase plasma concentrations of

- Nimodipine (CYP3A4 alkylation)—87%
- Verapamil (CYP3A4 demethylation)—34%
- Metotclopramide (CYP2D6) deakylation/sulfation—66%
- Desmethyldiazepam (CYP2C9 hydroxylation)—50%
- Warfarin CYP2C9 hydroxylation—50%

In humans, renal failure is associated with a decrease in nonrenal clearance of some drugs:

- Captopril 50%
- Morphine 40%
- Procainamide 60%
- Imipenem 58%

Table P.3 Factors Predisposing to Interactions in Kidney Disease

Renal Impairment–Related Changes	Effect
Absorption	
Increased gastric pH (associated with therapy of phosphate binders, antacids, H_2-receptor antagonists, and PPI in these patients)	Delayed absorption of oral drugs. Note that although the extent of absorption may be unaffected, there is an increase in time to achieve C_{max}
Delayed gastric emptying	
Distribution	
Fluid retention	Increased V_d of hydrophilic drugs (e.g., pravastatin, fluvastatin, morphine, codeine); may cause decreased serum concentrations
Increased adipose tissue and muscle wasting	Reduced V_d with increased serum concentrations
Hypoalbuminemia (nephrotic syndrome)	Increases free drug fraction of acidic drugs highly bound to albumin (penicillins, cephalosporins, phenytoin, furosemide, salicylates)
Increased α 1-acid glycoprotein	Decreased free-fraction of basic drugs (e.g., propranolol, morphine, oxazepam, vancomycin)
Altered tissue binding in stage 5 CKD	V_d is reduced by 50% causing increases in digoxin plasma concentrations
Accumulation of metabolites, toxins (e.g., uremic toxins) and endogenous substances	Competitively bind with drugs increasing plasma concentrations of several drugs (e.g., digoxin, warfarin, phenytoin, valproic acid, dihydropyridine calcium channel blockers, NSAIDs). Reduced activity of drug transporters: decreases Pgp ~ 65%, OATP ~ 83%, ABCB1 ~ 41%, MRP2 ~ 61%, and MRP3 protein ~ 35%
Metabolism	
Uremic toxins that inhibit metabolizing enzymes include indoxyl sulfate (IS) and 3-carboxy-4-methyl-5-propyl-2-furan-propanoic acid (CMPF)	Decrease of hepatic and intestinal P450 metabolism by 40%–85% (particularly CYP2C9, 2C11, 2C19, 2D6, 3A2, and 3A4). Note: • Activity is not significantly improved in dialyzed ESRD patients • Animal models of ARF and CRF have shown reduced CYP activity *but with a retained susceptibility to induction* Phase II reactions (e.g., glucuronidation and acetylation) are also inhibited: • Zidovudine—AUC doubled (glucuronidation via UGT2B7) • Morphine glucuronidation via UGT2B7 reduced 40% • TPMT* sulfoxidation of captopril decrease of –50% • NAT-2 acetylation of procainamide decrease of –60% • Dehydropeptidase of imipenem decrease of –58%
Increased levels of parathyroid hormone	Downregulation of CYP3A2 and CYP2C11 protein expression by approximately 60%, an effect reversed by the adsorption of serum using anti-PTH antibodies
Excretion	
About one-third of medications used clinically are eliminated by the kidneys.	
Reduced glomerular filtration	Decreased GFR results in prolonged free drug elimination half-life
Reduced secretion by active transport	E.g., ampicillin, furosemide, penicillin G, dopamine, trimethoprim
Reduced passive reabsorption	E.g., aspirin, lithium. The rate of renal elimination is dependent on GFR, renal tubular secretion, and reabsorption
Accumulation of renally excreted active metabolites	Dosage adjustments may be necessary for certain medications in order to prevent toxicity from active metabolites

- Nimodipine 87%
- Verapamil 54%
- Metoclopramide 66%
- Desmethyldiazepam 63%
- Warfarin 50%

SOURCES OF INFORMATION

Bowman L, Luppa J. Principles of drug dosing in renal impairment. In: Cheng S et al., Eds., *Nephrology. The Washington Manual*, 3rd edn. Philadelphia, PA: Wolters Kluwer, 2012, Chapter 27.

Dreisbach AW, Lertora JJL. The effect of chronic renal failure on drug metabolism and transport. *Expert Opinion on Drug Metabolism & Toxicology* 2008;4:1065–1074.

Marquito AB et al. Summary of physiological and pharmacologic effects of CRF on drug metabolism and transport. *Jornal Brasileiro de Nefrologia* 2014;36 São Paulo Jan./Mar.

Sun H et al. Effects of renal failure on drug transport and metabolism. *Pharmacology & Therapeutics* 2006; 109:1–11.

CARDIOVASCULAR DISEASE

Patients with heart failure are at particular risk of ADIs:

- They have reduced physiological reserve so only minor degrees of change in drug action can cause symptoms.
- They are often taking multiple medications (a patient with heart failure takes on average 10 drugs).
- These "high-risk" patients often require "high-risk" medications, thus the margin for error either due to dosage or as a consequence of ADIs would have serious implications.
- A large number of cardiovascular medications, including β-blockers, calcium channel blockers, and angiotensin receptor antagonists, are metabolized to a significant extent by CYP enzymes.

Heart failure is associated with a number of alterations to metabolizing and transport proteins:

- Failing hearts expressed CYP11B1 and 11B2 (not detected in the normal human heart). Increased cardiac CYP11B2 mRNA was associated with increased myocardial fibrosis and the severity of left ventricular dysfunction in patients with heart failure.
- Upregulation in CYP2J2, 1B1, 2E1, 4A10, and 2F2 gene expression was reported in the failing heart.
- Studies have shown that increased circulating levels of TNF-alpha and IL-6 in patients with congestive heart failure were inversely proportional to CYP2C19 and CYP1A2 activity.[1]
- A recent study demonstrated a selective disease-dependent regulation of the high-affinity carnitine transporter, OCTN2, in patients with dilated cardiomyopathy, whereas the other OCT(N)s were unaffected.
- Cardiac cytokine release may affect OCTN2 expression during cardiomyopathy associated with inflammation.

Genetic polymorphisms of DMEs are commonly associated with heart failure and hypertension. A study in Japanese subjects reported that CYP2C9 wild-type carriers had lower systolic blood pressure after losartan (which is metabolized to the active metabolite EXP3174) therapy than PMs.

REFERENCE

1. Frye RF et al. Plasma levels of TNF-alpha and IL-6 are inversely related to cytochrome P 450 dependent drug metabolism in patients with congestive heart failure. *Journal of Cardiac Failure* 2002;8:315–319.

OBESITY

Obesity is the presence of excess amounts of body fat. Currently over 30% of the world's population is overweight, and this figure increases to over 65% for adults in the United States.

Different criteria are used to define obesity:

- Body mass index (BMI)
- Waist circumference
- In children
  - Weight >95th centile
  - Body fat percentage above 25% in boys and above 32% in girls
  - Body weight at least 20% higher than the healthy weight range for a child or adolescent of that height

Obesity may affect all four aspects of pharmacokinetics (Table P.4). Though clinicians tend to "under-dose" these individuals, the risk of toxicity is increased, necessitating therapeutic drug monitoring (TDM).

Clinical implications:

There is no dosing parameter (e.g., total body water [TBW], BSA) that can optimally control for body weight for drugs even of the same class. Note that dosage adjustments may not be as simple as doubling an antibiotic dose because a patient is morbidly obese. *Once again, there is no substitute for careful titration of drug doses with close monitoring of effects and use of TDM when available!*

The principles of safer prescribing include the following:

- Be aware that recommended doses are based on pharmacokinetic data obtained from normal weight individuals; obese individuals may require higher dosing.
- Be aware that comorbidity in the obese may affect the function of organs involved in drug elimination (kidney, liver).
- Dose lipid-soluble drugs on actual body weight (remifentanil is an exception).
- Dose water-soluble drugs on ideal body weight (IBW) or lean body weight (LBW).
- Specific guidelines exist for dosing different drugs:
  - The American Society of Clinical Oncology recommends that full weight-based chemotherapy doses be used in the treatment of obese patients with cancer.
  - Guidelines for dosing of drugs used during anesthesia of the obese are available—induction doses of propofol should be calculated using IBW while maintenance dosage should be using TBW or IBW+ (0.4 × excess weight); for midazolam, TBW should be used for initial dose and IBW in continuous dosage.

PK Changes following Bariatric Surgery

The increase in demand for bariatric surgery has been exponential (~180,000 surgeries performed annually in the United States). Procedures vary, e.g.,

- Restrictive (gastric banding, gastroplasty)
- Restrictive with limitation of digestive capacity (sleeve gastrectomy)

Table P.4 Factors Predisposing to Interactions in Obese Patients

Obesity-Related Changes	Effect
Absorption	
Data on the effects of drug absorption and obesity is limited	
Increased body surface area (BSA) and increased cardiac output with increased gut perfusion	Possibility of increased absorption of oral medications (increased gastric emptying); however, not shown to result in increased bioavailability
Distribution	
Increased ratio of adipose tissue to lean body mass	Increased V_d for lipid soluble drugs (this tends to be positively correlated with an increased half-life) Increased accumulation of lipophilic drugs in fat stores, reducing C_{max}
Altered protein binding	Plasma protein binding affinity may change in obesity without changes in protein concentrations Acidic drugs primarily bound by albumin (e.g., thiopental, phenytoin)—no clinically relevant differences were found Basic drugs binding to R1-acid glycoprotein (AAG) and those binding to lipoproteins vary in the obese. Studies do not provide conclusive results: • Significant ↑s in AAG concentrations lower free fractions of propranolol due to ↑ binding • However, some studies show that decreased AAG levels produce no change in plasma free-fractions of triazolam and verapamil, drugs principally bound to AAG
Metabolism	
Obesity probably affects different pathways by different mechanisms to varying degrees	Increased activity of CYP1A, CYP2B, CYP2E, CYP3A, and CYP4A in obese rats Consistent increases in CYP2E1 activity in obese humans Phase II conjugation pathways (glucuronidation and sulfation) may be affected to varying degrees: glucuronidation might ↑ significantly, sulfation to a lesser degree, with acetylation pathways relatively unaffected
Elimination	
There is conflicting evidence about the effect of obesity on overall renal function; however, there is some evidence that obesity is associated with ↑ tubular secretion and ↓ tubular reabsorption	Variable effect on elimination; note calculated and measured creatinine clearance correlate poorly in obesity
Coexisting disease may cause additional changes to renal function (e.g., diabetic and hypertensive nephropathy)	

- Restrictive/malabsorptive (gastric bypass)
- Purely malabsorptive (biliopancreatic diversion, jejunoileal bypass-jib)

Those associated with intestinal diversion interfere with absorption of drugs due to alterations in intestinal pH and nearly all oral agents are maximally absorbed in the small intestine. The most commonly performed procedure is Roux-en-Y gastric bypass. PK changes that occur post bariatric surgery include the following.

- Increasing gastric pH should
  - Increase the solubility of more basic drugs (become less ionized)
  - Decrease the solubility of more acidic drugs (more ionized)

    - Reduce disintegration of solid dosage forms of some medications. Substantial reductions may occur, which may require an increase in administered dose
- Reduced gastric motility that reduces gastric mixing, which is essential for drug disintegration: drugs with slow dissolution properties (sustained release or enteric coated preparations) more likely to exhibit ↓ absorption.
- Bypass of the proximal small intestine reduces bioavailability of some drugs:
    - Limited mixing of highly lipophilic drugs with bile acids
    - Increased relative influence of Pgp (expression of Pgp increases from proximal to the distal small intestine)
- Note that most of these effects tend to reduce blood levels of drugs that would cause therapeutic failure rather than a DDI. However, an ADI could occur if the level of a drug that induces metabolism of another drug is reduced (resulting in an increased concentration of the second drug); also, many baratric procedures are eventually reversed, which may lead to an increase in the concentration of some drugs.

SOURCES OF INFORMATION

Blouin R, Warren G. Pharmacokinetic considerations in obesity. *Journal of Pharmaceutical Sciences* 1999;88:No. 1.

De Baerdemaeker Luc EC et al. Pharmacokinetics in obese patients. *Continuing Education in Anaesthesia, Critical Care & Pain* 2004;4:152–155.

Green B, Duffull SB. What is the best size descriptor to use for pharmacokinetic studies in the obese? *British Journal of Clinical Pharmacology* 2004 Aug;58:119–133.

Hanley MJ et al. Effect of obesity on the pharmacokinetics of drugs in humans. *Clinical Pharmacokinetics* 2010;49(2):71–87.

Padwal R et al. A systematic review of drug absorption following bariatric surgery and its theoretical implications. *Obesity Reviews* 2010;11:41–50.

Shane P et al. Obesity and resistance to cancer chemotherapy: Interacting roles of inflammation and metabolic dysregulation. *Clinical Pharmacology & Therapeutics* 2014;96:458–463.

Velissaris D et al. Pharmacokinetic changes and dosing modification of aminoglycosides in critically ill obese patients: A literature review. *Journal of Clinical Medicine Research* 2014;6:227–233.

MALNUTRITION

Protein-energy malnutrition (PEM) affects a high proportion of infants and pre-children, particularly in developing countries (African, Asian, Latin American, and Caribbean regions). The clinical spectrum ranges from underweight, marasmus, and marasmic-kwashiorkor to kwashiorkor. The elderly in these regions are also highly vulnerable to PEM. Approximately 70% of the world's malnourished children live in Asia. Close to 11 million children (under 5 years of age) in developing countries die every year from illness. PEM directly or indirectly accounts for about half of these deaths. The World Health Organization (WHO) estimates that by 2015, the prevalence of PEM worldwide will be 17.6%—with the vast majority in people living in developing countries in southern Asia and sub-Saharan Africa. An additional 29% will have stunted growth due to poor nutrition.

Disease-related malnutrition costs in excess of £13 billion per annum in the United Kingdom based on annual malnutrition prevalence figures and associated costs of both health and social care. At any point of time, more than 3 million people in the United Kingdom are at risk of malnutrition with nearly 93% living in the community. It affects more than

- 1/3 of people recently admitted to care homes
- 1/2 of adults admitted to hospital

- ~1/5 of clients on admission to mental care units
- Up to 1/5 of patients attending hospital outpatients departments
- 1/10 of people attending GP practices

Those at increased risk are patients with COPD and malignant disease; patients who are elderly, frail, and immobile; and patients who are depressed and/or demented (excluding those with social issues).

A useful measure of malnourishment is the BMI—see Appendix J. Having a BMI less than 18.5 could suggest you are at a high risk of being malnourished, although you may also be considered at risk if your BMI is between 18.5 and 20.

Pharmacokinetics in Malnutrition

Severely malnourished children enter a physiologic state known as reductive adaptation. This energy-conserving process causes heart, kidney, and metabolic function to decline 25% from normal.

Malnutrition causes unpredictable changes to the free concentrations of drugs that contribute significantly to ADIs; these are summarized in Table P.5.

Table P.5 Factors Predisposing to Interactions in Malnourished Patients

Malnutrition-Related Changes	Effect
Absorption	
Diarrhea and vomiting are common Decrease in GI transit time Reduced blood flow to the GI tract. Intestinal malabsorption (associated with villous atrophy of the jejunal mucosa)	Reduced bioavailability of oral drugs: e.g., carbamazepine, chloroquine, sulphadiazine, chloramphenicol, and HAART drugs
Distribution	
TBW is increased in proportion to the degree of malnutrition	Increases V_d of water soluble drugs
Increase in extracellular fluid (ECF)	
Reduction in adipose mass and lean body mass (in marasmus, marasmic-kwashiorkor)	Alters the apparent V_d of drugs
	Distribution into adipose tissue of lipid-soluble drugs is reduced in PEM, increasing the concentration of lipid-soluble drugs at the target tissues—prolonging drug actions
Plasma albumin and fractions of glycoproteins for drug binding are decreased	Increased plasma free-drug fractions of highly protein-bound drugs with possible risk of increased drug toxicity.
Metabolism	
Hepatomegaly occurs with normal liver function tests but impaired hepatic drug metabolism	60%–80% suppression of hepatic microsomal CYP 1A2 and CYP2C11 levels
	40%–50% decrease in CYP2E1 and CYP3A1/2 levels
	Bilirubin-uridyldiphosphate (UDP) activities reported to be decreased
	Total levels of all involved in microsomal drug metabolism—significantly reduced in malnourished animals
Elimination	
GFR and renal blood flow diminished particularly in dehydration; *often blood urea nitrogen and creatinine are normal*	Impact relevant for drugs primarily excreted by the kidneys, e.g., methotrexate has a prolonged elimination of half-life. Relative weight, and not BSA or body weight, to be used for drug dosing

Clinical relevance:

1. There is often a need to reduce drug dosage due to ↓ in hepatic microsomal CYP levels.
2. ↑ V_d of water-soluble drugs resulting in lower peak blood concentrations.
3. Reduction in adipose mass and lean body mass ↑ concentration of lipid-soluble drugs at target organs.
4. Gross edema (greater than 30% of body weight) and shock may reduce bioavailability of intramuscular (I.M.) drugs.
5. Plasma albumin and fractions of glycoproteins for drug binding are decreased, resulting in substantial increases in plasma-free drug fractions of highly protein-bound drugs with possible risk of increased drug toxicity.

SOURCES OF INFORMATION

Heikens GT. How can we improve the care of severely malnourished children in Africa? *PLoS Medicine* 2007;4:e45.

Heikens GT et al. Case management of HIV-infected severely malnourished children: Challenges in the area of highest prevalence. *Lancet* 2008;371:1305–1307.

Musoke PM et al. Growth, immune and viral responses in HIV infected African children receiving highly active antiretroviral therapy: A prospective cohort study. *BMC Pediatrics* 2010;10:56.

Muller O, Krawinkel M. Malnutrition and health in developing countries. *CMAJ* 2005 Aug 2;173:279–286.

Malnutrition Universal Screening Tool (MUST); British Association of Parenteral and Enteral Nutrition (BAPEN). Available at: www.bapen.org.uk.

Man CJE, Startton RJ. Calculating the cost of disease related malnutrition in the UK in 2007 (public expenditure only) in: Combating malnutrition: Recommendations for action: Report from the Advisory Group on malnutrition led by BAPEN 2009.

Naidoo R et al. The influence of nutritional status on the response to HAART in HIV-infected children in South Africa. *Pediatric Infectious Disease Journal* 2010;29:511–513.

Nijs KA et al. Effect of family style mealtimes on quality of life, physical performance, and body weight of nursing home residents: Cluster randomised controlled trial. *BMJ* 2006;332:1180–1184.

Oshikoya KA, Senbanjo IO. Pathophysiological changes that affect drug disposition in protein-energy malnourished children. *Nutrition & Metabolism* 2009;6:50.

Prendergast A et al. Hospitalization for severe malnutrition among HIV-infected children starting antiretroviral therapy. *AIDS* 2011;25:951–956.

Rasheed S, Woods RT. Malnutrition and quality of life in older people: A systematic review and meta-analysis. *Ageing Research Reviews* 2012;12:561–566.

Russell CA, Elia M. Malnutrition in the UK: Where does it begin? *Proceedings of the Nutrition Society* 2010;69:465–469.

INFLAMMATORY DISEASES AND INFECTIONS

Several studies have shown that drug metabolism and transport is disrupted during infection primarily due to reductions in gene expression of associated enzymes and transporters. Inflammatory processes affect metabolism, distribution, and elimination of certain drugs.

- Changes in expression, activity of drug transporters, and metabolizing enzymes in liver and intestinal epithelial cells affect bioavailability.
- Altered levels of cytochromes P450 and drug transporters (such as Pgp) following inflammation in brain, intestine, and placenta influence drug therapy in diverse clinical settings. Drugs predominantly affected are those totally dependent on P450 or Pgp or on both pathways for disposition, particularly when administered to individuals with some impairment due to the presence of poor

metabolizing alleles. In these scenarios, repeated or continuous drug administration often may exceed the metabolizing capacity of the body resulting in higher free-drug concentrations, frequent occurrences of toxic manifestations, and an increased risk for DDIs.

Gram-Positive Infections

- Patients suffering from gram-positive bactereamia (e.g., *Pseudomonas* or *Staphylococcus* infections) have increases in V_d, thus dilution of antimicrobial agents in plasma and ECF may occur, requiring careful/frequent monitoring of the dosage regimen.
- Gram-positive bacterial component: lipoteichoic acid downregulates gene expression of several phase I and phase II DMEs in mice.
- *Streptococcus pneumonia* decreases benzocaine (antipyrine) clearance.

Gram-Negative Infections

- Lipopolysaccharides (LPS) endotoxins downregulate expression and activity of key hepatic, intestinal, and renal DMEs in several animal species, dependent on the route of administration.
- Recent data from the U.S. National Healthcare Safety Network indicate that gram-negative bacteria are responsible for more than 30% of hospital-acquired infections.
- In intensive care units (ICUs) in the United States, gram-negative bacteria account for about 70% of these infections.
- LPS injections in animals and humans altered PK parameters (↑ C_{max}), (↑ AUC) (↓ clearance) of several medications such as cisplatin, benzocaine (antipyrine), theophylline, hexobarbital, gentamicin, and vancomycin.

Viral Infections

- Often stimulate the immune system, releasing various inflammatory mediators from the immune cells.
- ↓ Levels of hepatic CYP1A2 detected in children with upper respiratory tract viral infections.
- Evidence for downregulation of renal CYP2E1 and hepatic CYP3A2 and CYP2C11 expression and activity, and induction of CYP4A protein expression.
- HIV-infected patients on HAART consisting of numerous drugs are reported to have caused both induction and suppression of drug transporters.

Inflammation

Metabolism

- Hepatic and intestinal cytochrome P450 enzymes are downregulated by proinflammatory cytokines (e.g., TNFα, IL-1β, IL-2, and IL-6), vasoactive amines (histamine), and peptides (bradykinin).
- Oxidative stress may also play a role in the downregulation of CYP enzymes (CYP3A11, 1A1, and 2E1).

Distribution

- Changes during both a local CNS and a systemic inflammatory response attributed to the loss in expression of the Pgp drug transporter protein within the blood–brain barrier. This allows levels of drugs that are normally transported out of the brain by Pgp to increase and cause CNS toxicity. Pgp drug efflux transporter is a major component of the blood–brain drug permeability barrier limiting the accumulation of several drugs in the CNS. Reduction in Pgp function may increase the risk for harmful DIs or toxicity produced by CNS-acting drugs, such as morphine and its biologically active metabolites.

Elimination

- Physiological functions, such as the GFR and Na^+ excretion are altered as is the blood flow to major excretory organs (liver, kidney), leading to decreased drug clearance.

Pharmacodynamics

- Several studies have shown that inflammation does not affect the PD of drugs though there have been suggestions of altered receptor-functioning or receptor-ligand binding. Increased permeability of imipenem is likely to cause seizures (less frequent or absent with penicillin).

1. Clinical significance is greater for drugs with a low therapeutic index. The 1980 influenza epidemic in Seattle resulted in several young children receiving daily theophylline as prophylactic treatment for asthma being admitted with severe drug toxicity (convulsions, cardiac conduction anomalies). Inflammatory mediators produced in response to virus caused a dramatic loss in CYP1A2-mediated metabolism of theophylline, resulting in significant toxicity.
2. Efficacy of prodrugs is reduced (activated by P450).

PK Alterations in Critical Illness

Absorption

- Shock reduces regional blood flow and motility-delayed gastric emptying and ↓ absorption.
- Vasopressors restoring arterial blood pressure will not normalize flow to increase absorption due to differing effects on flow to organs, e.g., splanchnic blood flow.
- Shock or use of vasopressors decreases skin blood flow ↓ s.c. absorption.
- Intravenous drug administration is usually recommended during critical illness.

Volume of Distribution (V_d)

- Sepsis, shock, burn injury, pancreatitis, and alterations in plasma protein-binding influence V_d.
- Sepsis and particularly septic shock is characterized by vasodilatation and ↑ vascular permeability leading to capillary leak syndrome. This shifts fluid from the intravascular compartment to the interstitial space leading to edema.
- This third-spacing phenomenon is enhanced by oncotic pressure caused by plasma proteins moving through the capillary leak.

Protein Binding

- Hypoalbuminemia is frequent during critical illness.
- >40% of patients admitted to ICUs have a serum albumin concentration of ≤25 g/dL at baseline.
- Protein binding is clinically relevant when the antimicrobial agent is highly protein bound (>85%–90%) and predominantly cleared by glomerular filtration, e.g., ertapenem, daptomycin, ceftriaxone, and teicoplanin. Hypoalbuminemia necessitates shorter dosing interval.

Drug Metabolism

- Cytochrome P450 enzyme system in the liver is dependent on blood flow and/or the hepatic extraction ratio of the drug for optimal enzymatic activity.
- Critical illness affects plasma protein concentration, hepatic enzymatic activity, and blood flow. Further, drugs used in critically ill patients may either induce or inhibit the activity of isoenzymes, including cytochrome P450s.

Elimination

- Critical illness may ↑ or ↓ renal clearance.
- ↑ Renal clearance occurs during sepsis, burn injury, or use of inotropic agents.
- Acute kidney injury will ↓ clearance.

Other Considerations

- Approximately 40%–50% of critically ill patients develop an infection during their stay in the ICU.
- In 100 surgical ICU patients with gram-negative sepsis, V_d and serum concentrations of aminoglycosides were investigated. V_d was ↑ by 36%–70%, necessitating larger loading dosages to achieve desirable target concentrations. Clinicians must be aware that PK of hydrophilic antimicrobials may be affected by the presence of sepsis due to limited tissue distribution usually to the ECF—dilution occurs whenever intravascular fluids escape into tissues. Almost all of these agents are normally cleared by the renal route. Changes in renal function in septic patients may ↑ or ↓ elimination rates. Lipophilic antimicrobials are less affected by the pathophysiology of sepsis as these are distributed within cells, and dilution does not take place from the ECF. Furthermore, most are cleared through the liver, whose function is often less significantly compromised during sepsis.

SOURCES OF INFORMATION

Blot S et al. Does contemporary vancomycin dosing achieve therapeutic targets in a heterogeneous clinical cohort of critically ill patients? Data from the multinational DALI Study. *Critical Care* 2014;18:R99.

Blot SI, Pea F, Lipman J. The effect of pathophysiology on pharmacokinetics in the critically ill patient—Concepts appraised by the example of antimicrobial agents. *Advanced Drug Delivery Reviews* 2014;77:11.

Cha R et al. Antimicrobial pharmacokinetics and pharmacodynamics in the treatment of nosocomial gram-negative infections. *Advances in Pharmacoepidemiology and Drug Safety* 2012. doi:ID4172/2167-1052 S1-005.

Taccone FS et al. Insufficient beta-lactam concentrations in the early phase of severe sepsis and septic shock. *Critical Care* 2010;14:R126.

Special Populations at Higher Risk of Adverse Drug Interactions

Andrea Corsonello, Giuseppe Maltese, Chulananda Goonasekera, and Niroshini Manthri Giles

Specific patient populations are at particular risk of ADIs for a variety of reasons:

- Different physiological reserves
- Differing activities of metabolizing and transport proteins
- Different patterns of pathology requiring different treatments

This section focuses on the following groups:

- The elderly
- Children
- Pregnancy

THE ELDERLY

Aging affects all aspects of the passage of a drug through the body—absorption, distribution, metabolism, and excretion (PK), and the effect of a drug at the target structures (PD). In the wealthier countries, as a whole, life expectancy is increasing due to the availability of a greater number of medications, including over-the-counter (OTC) and herbal and other traditional medicines. But as the elderly consume more and more drugs, it is likely that the incidence of ADIs in this group will rise proportionately.

In a study of 1601 elderly outpatients living in six European countries, 46% of patients had at least one potential clinically significant DDI, and 10% of these interactions were regarded as high severity. Davies and colleagues found that 25% and 11% of patients in elderly psychiatric wards had potential clinically relevant DDIs involving cytochromes 2D6 and 3A4, respectively. Hanlon and colleagues found that 6% of elderly inpatients had a DDI with a detectable adverse outcome and that 20% of these patients had an actual drug–disease interaction. Australian researchers reported that actual drug–disease interactions were two to three times more frequent than actual DDIs.

Adverse drug events that affect the elderly include the following:

- Polypharmacy is more common, making DDIs more likely.
- It is estimated that 20% of Medicare beneficiaries have five or more chronic conditions and 50% receive five or more medications.
- The average U.S. nursing home resident uses seven to eight different medications each month, and about one-third of residents have monthly drug regimens of nine or more medications.
- Polypharmacy (precise minimum number of medications used to define "polypharmacy" ranges from 5 to 10) increased from 14% in older women in 1998 to 49% in 2006.
- Prevalence of DDIs in older patients ranges from 35% to 60% and approaches 100% in patients taking eight or more medications.
- Physiological reserve is reduced, which makes DDIs more likely to be clinically significant, e.g., drug-induced orthostatic reactions (frequency of 5%–33%) with an increased risk of syncope (~11% are drug-induced).
- 90% loss of blood vessel distensibility from 20 to 80 years, increased intimal thickness, and endothelial dysfunction/loss of myocytes.
- Baroreflex-mediated heart rate response to hypotensive stimuli.
- Relative dehydration.
- Altered pharmacokinetics and pharmacodynamics (see Table P.6).

Table P.6 Factors Predisposing to Interactions in the Aged

Physiological Change(s)	Effect	Some Drugs Affected
Absorption		
↓ Esophagus peristalsis	↓ Rate of absorption—lower peak concentration delayed time to peak	Indomethacin, prazosin, digoxin
↓ Rate of gastric emptying	↑ Time in contact with gastric mucosa with ↑ ulcerogenic effect	NSAIDs, bisphosphonates
↓ Splanchnic blood flow	Slower absorption of drugs dependent on carrier-mediated transport mechanisms—lower peak concentration; delayed time to peak	Calcium, iron, vitamins, gabapentin, some nucleoside drugs
↓ Absorption surface	↓ Intestinal absorption, slower absorption of drugs dependent on carrier-mediated transport mechanisms	Calcium, iron, vitamins, gabapentin, some nucleoside drugs, vitamin B12
Reduction in liver volume Decreased liver blood flow	↓ First-pass metabolism; bioavailability may ↑ drugs with extensive first pass metabolism	↑ Bioavailability: • Propranolol • Labetalol
Distribution		
TBW content ↓ by 10%–15% until the age of 80	1. ↓ V_d of hydrophilic drugs—↑ C_{max} of water-soluble drugs (need for lower initial doses) 2. ↑ Adverse effects of diuretics. Diuretics ↑ risk of hypovolemia, hypokalemia (more in females > 65 years), hyponatremia, prerenal azotemia with thiazides in combination with loop diuretics	1. Aspirin, tubocurarine, edrophonium, famotidine, lithium, ethanol. 2. ↑ Adverse effects and ADIs with diuretics. ↓ Renal clearance of loop and thiazide diuretics—↑ plasma levels and systemic toxicity, ↓ diuretic and natriuretic effect
↑ Total body fat tends to occur (from 18% to 36% in men and from 33% to 45% in women)	↑ V_d for lipophilic drugs (more in men than in women). Results in ↑ half-life, ↑ time to reach steady-state serum concentrations with repeated drug doses	Amiodarone, diazepam, teicoplanin, and verapamil
Metabolism		
↓ In liver size in old age (25%–35% of endoplasmic reticulum is ↓, hepatic extracellular space ↑).	Metabolic clearance of some drugs ↓ by 20%–40%, irrespective of which CYP enzyme is involved. Age-dependent reduction	Antipyrine and theophylline
↓ Of liver blood flow by about 40%, ↓ bile flow	Drugs exhibiting high extraction display an age-related ↓ in metabolic clearance	Amitriptyline, imipramine, lidocaine, morphine, pethidine, propranolol, verapamil
Age-related ↓ (20%) in activity of CYP2D6	↑ C_{max} of 1. CVS drugs—hypotension, bradycardia. 2. TCAs—↑ antimuscarinic effects 3. Phenothiazines—CNS depression, falls	1. Increased effect of inhibitors (e.g., amiodarone) 2. ↑ Therapeutic effect of substrates (e.g., metoprolol, amitriptyline, diphenhydramine)
Phase II enzymes seem to be unchanged		

(*Continued*)

Table P.6 (*Continued*) Factors Predisposing to Interactions in the Aged

Physiological Change(s)	Effect	Some Drugs Affected
Elimination		
After the age of 40, there is a progressive development of glomerulosclerosis 1. ↓ Functioning glomeruli. GFR ↓ by 25%–50% between 20 and 90 2. Tubular secretion ↓ in proportion to loss of glomeruli 3. ↓ Renal blood flow (by ~1% per year)—due to ↑ angiotensin-II and endothelin levels, ↓ prostaglandin concentrations	Decline of total clearance is to be expected for all drugs predominantly eliminated by the kidneys. Renal elimination of most drugs—closely correlated with endogenous creatinine clearance	↑ Blood levels of several drugs, e.g., ↑ C_{max} of amantadine, digoxin (↑ risk of digoxin toxicity), methotrexate (↓ renal excretion and tubular secretion). ↓ Tubular secretion of cotrimoxazole, ciprofloxacin. ↑ Effects of anti-hypertensive drugs, diuretics, risk of bleeding with anticoagulants, GI irritation with NSAIDs
Pharmacodynamics		
Downregulated β-adrenoceptors; ↓ sensitivity of the myocardium to catecholamines	↓ Antihypertensive effect of β-blockers may be related to the lower renin levels in the elderly.	β-blockers
↓ Number of dopaminergic neurons and dopamine D2 receptors	Leads to extrapyramidal symptoms when a certain threshold of neuronal loss is reached	
↓ Number of cholinergic neurons	More sensitive to CNS effects of sedating antihistamines. Dizziness, sedation, risk of falls, dementia in those with ↓ cognitive function, delirium, hallucinations	First-generation antihistamines cross the BBB easily
↓ Number of muscarinic receptors.	Acute confusion, delerium, disorientation, hallucinations, delusion, and impaired memory. Peripheral antimuscarinic effects—constipation, blurred vision, dry mouth, urinary hesitancy/retention, acute glaucoma	Oxybutynin, amitryptiline, paroxetine, diphenhydramine, procyclidine, trixehyphenidyl
↓ Number of receptors involved in cognitive functions	May impede intellectual functions and motor coordination	Psychotropic drugs, anticonvulsants, centrally acting antihypertensives

- Decline in renal, hepatic, and cerebral blood flow.
- Nutritional disorders are more common (see "Malnutrition" section).

Clinical implications:

- Patients admitted with toxic effects of digoxin were 12 times more likely to have been prescribed clarithromycin in the week before admission.
- Patients on ACE inhibitors admitted with hyperkalemia were 20 times more likely to have been given a potassium-sparing diuretic in the previous week.
- Hospitalization for hypoglycemia was six times more likely in patients receiving cotrimaxazole with glyburide.
- ↑ The risk of serotonin syndrome in older adults is attributed by some to the increased risk of suicide in this age group-.
- Use of probenecid to boost beta-lactams concentrations should be avoided in older patients and in those with renal dysfunction or a history of seizure due to increased risk of antibiotic-induced convulsions.

- A retrospective study over 4 years in 17,661 veterans (>65 years of age) receiving warfarin in Australia revealed an incidence rate of bleeding-related hospitalizations per 100 person-years of
  - 4.1—no interacting medicines
  - 6.8—clopidogrel
  - 8.9—low-dose aspirin
  - 14.0—SSRIs
  - 16.6—tramadol
  - 17.9—amiodarone
  - 27.7—macrolides
  - 32.2—NSAIDs
- Other studies revealed an increased risk with doxycycline, amoxicillin and clavulanic acid, norfloxacin, trimethoprim, and cotrimoxazole. Enhanced warfarin response has been reported with almost every class of antibacterials.

Minimizing ADIs

- Prior to prescribing, make a complete clinical assessment of probable PK and PD alterations along with the list of current medications, including OTC's and herbals/traditional medicines.
- "Start low and go slow" with medications.
- Be aware of "unusual" presentation of ADIs in the elderly.
- Consider reducing dosages rather than changing medications unless safer alternatives are available.
- Give time for patients to stabilize.
- Monitor physiological parameters and drug levels. Advise patients/carers to report unusual symptoms (giving examples) and seek immediate medical attention.
- Consider multidisciplinary approach to drug therapy with nurses and pharmacists.

SOURCES OF INFORMATION

Baxter K. *Stockey's Drug Interactions*, 8th edn. London, U.K.: Pharmaceutical Press, 2008.

Bjorkman IK et al. Pharmaceutical Care Of The Elderly In Europe Research (PEER)Group. Drug–drug interactions in the elderly. *Annals of Pharmacotherapy* 2002;36:1675–1681.

Budnitz DS et al. Medication use leading to emergency department visits for adverse drug events in older adults. *Annals of Internal Medicine* 2007;147:755.

Crotty M et al. Does the addition of a pharmacist transition coordinator improveevidence-based medication management and health outcomes in older adults moving from the hospital to a long-term care facility? Results of a randomized, controlled trial. *American Journal of Geriatric Pharmacotherapy* 2004;2:257–264.

Davies SJ et al. Potential for drug interactions involving cytochromes P450 2D6 and 3A4 on general adult psychiatric and functional elderly psychiatric wards. *British Journal of Clinical Pharmacology* 2004;57:464–472.

Field TS et al. Risk factors for adverse drug events among nursing home residents. *Archives of Internal Medicine* 2001;161:1629.

Fox C et al. Anticholinergic medication use and cognitive impairment in the older population: The medical research council cognitive function and ageing study. *Journal of the American Geriatrics Society* 2011;59:1477.

Hanlon JT et al. Inappropriate medication use among frail elderly inpatients. *Annals of Pharmacotherapy* 2004;38:9–14.53.

Juurlink DN et al. Drug–drug interactions among elderly patients hospitalized for drugtoxicity. *JAMA* 2003;289:1652–1658.

Kinirons MT, O'Mahony MS. Drug metabolism and ageing. *British Journal of Clinical Pharmacology* May 2004;57(5):540–554.

Lane CJ et al. Potentially inappropriate prescribing in Ontario community-dwelling older adults and nursing home residents. *Journal of the American Geriatrics Society* 2004;52:861.

Pringle KE et al. Potential for alcohol and prescription drug interactions in older people. *Journal of the American Geriatrics Society* 2005;53:1930–1936.

Rochon PA et al. The challenge of managing drug interactions in elderly people. *Lancet* 2007;370:185.

Shi S, Morike K, Klotz U. The clinical implications of ageing for rational drug therapy. *European Journal of Clinical Pharmacology* 2008;64:183–199.

Turnheim K. When drug therapy gets old: Pharmacokinetics and pharmacodynamics in the elderly. *Experimental Gerontology* 2003;38:843–853.

Vitry AI et al. Major bleeding risk associated with warfarin and co-medications in the elderly population. *Pharmacoepidemiology and Drug Safety* 2011;20:1057–1063.

INFANCY AND CHILDHOOD

Drug Absorption

Oral Route

In the neonatal period, both passive and active transport become fully mature by approximately 4 months of age.

- Intragastric pH is relatively elevated (>4) due to ↓ basal acid output and ↓ total volume of gastric secretions leading to ↓ bioavailability of weak acids (e.g., phenobarbital), so ↑ oral doses are needed to achieve therapeutic plasma levels.
- Marked ↑ in gastric emptying during the first week of life. Absorption rates of most drugs are slower in neonates and young infants than older children.
- Age-associated changes in splanchnic blood flow during the first 2–3 weeks of life influence absorption rates by altering the concentration gradient across the intestinal mucosa.

Percutaneous Route

- ↑ Percutaneous absorption during infancy—thinner stratum corneum in preterm neonates and ↑ cutaneous perfusion and hydration of the epidermis (relative to adults). Although skin thickness is similar in infants and adults, the extent of perfusion and hydration diminishes from infancy to adulthood.
- Ratio of total body surface area to body mass in infants and young children greater than in adults. Relative systemic exposure of infants and children to topically applied drugs (e.g., corticosteroids, antihistamines, antiseptics) may ↑ risk of toxic effects.

Intramuscular Route

- ↓ Skeletal-muscle blood flow and inefficient muscular contractions (↓ drug dispersion) likely to result in a ↓ in the rate of absorption of drugs administered I.M. in neonates. However, this effect may be offset by the relatively greater density of skeletal-muscle capillaries in infants than in older children. I.M. absorption of specific agents (e.g., amikacin and cephalothin) is more efficient in neonates and infants than in older children.

Drug Distribution

- ↓ Plasma levels of drugs (particularly hydrophilic drugs) following administration in a weight-based manner. In the first 6 months of life, there is markedly expanded TBW and extracellular water (expressed as a % of total body weight compared with older infants and adults). Relatively ↑ ECF extracellular and TBW spaces in neonates and young infants compared with adults along with adipose stores having a ↑ ratio of water to lipid. The influence of age on V_d is not readily apparent for lipophilic drugs that are primarily distributed in tissue.
- Changes in the composition and amount of circulating plasma proteins such as albumin and a1-acid glycoprotein may influence the distribution of highly bound drugs.
  - Reduces the quantity of total plasma proteins (including albumin) in neonate and young infant, increases free-fraction of drug.
  - Fetal albumin has ↓ binding affinity for weak acids and ↑ in endogenous substances (e.g., bilirubin and free fatty acids) capable of displacing a drug from albumin binding sites during the neonatal period contribute to the ↑ free fractions of highly protein-bound drugs in neonates.
  - Variability in regional blood flow, organ perfusion, permeability of cell membranes, changes in acid–base balance, and cardiac output associated with development and disease also influence drug binding and distribution.

Transporters

- Pgp expression and localization in the CNS from neonates born at 23–42 weeks of gestational age suggests a pattern of localization similar to that in adults late in gestation and at term. However, the level of expression ↓ compared to adults. Passive diffusion of drugs into the CNS is age dependent. For example, progressive ↑ in the ratios of brain phenobarbital to plasma phenobarbital from 28 to 39 weeks of gestational age; ↑ transport of phenobarbital into the brain suggests changes in blood flow and pore density rather than pore size.

Metabolism

- Activity of cytochrome P450 isoforms and UGT isoform are very low during the first 2 months of life. Delayed maturation of drug-metabolizing enzyme may result in marked toxicity of drugs in the very young.
  - CYP2E1 activity surges after birth.
  - CYP2D6 becomes detectable soon thereafter.
  - CYP3A4 and CYP2C (CYP2C9 and CYP2C19) appear during the first week of life.
  - CYP1A2 is the last hepatic CYP to appear (1–3 months of life).
- Function of hepatic CYP3A4 and CYP3A5 ↑ during the first 3 months of life. Carbamazepine clearance is dependent on CYP3A4; activity in children is higher than in adults, necessitating higher weight-adjusted doses to achieve therapeutic plasma levels.
- The half-life of phenytoin (dependent on CYP2C9 and, to a lesser extent, CYP2C19) is prolonged (to approximately 75 hours) in preterm infants, but ↓ approximately to 20 hours in term infants during the first week of life and to ~8 hours after the second week of life. Concentration-dependent metabolism does not appear until ~10 days of age, demonstrating the developmental acquisition of CYP2C9 activity. Phenytoin dosages reflect CYP2C9 activity with values of 14 mg/kg per day in infants decreasing to 8 mg/kg per day in adolescents.
- Glucuronidation of acetaminophen (substrate for UGT1A6-lesser extent, UGT1A9) is less in newborns and young children compared with adolescents and adults.
- Glucuronidation by UGT2B7 of morphine is detected in premature infants as young as 24 weeks of gestational age. Clearance of morphine is positively correlated with postconceptional age and quadruples between 27 and 40 weeks postconceptional age, necessitating a corresponding ↑ in dose of morphine for effective analgesia.

Excretion

- Maturation of renal function beginning during fetal organogenesis is complete by early childhood. ↑ in GFR relies on normal nephrogenesis, beginning at 9 weeks of gestation and complete by 36 weeks of gestation, followed by postnatal changes in renal and intrarenal blood flow.
- The GFR is approximately 2–4 mL/min/1.73 m^2 in term neonates (0.6–0.8 mL/min/1.73 m^2 in preterm neonates). GFR increases rapidly during the first 2 weeks of life and then increases more steadily. Adult values are reached at 8–12 months of age.
- Tubular secretion is immature at birth reaching adult capacity during the first year of life.
    - Ceftazidime and famotidine excreted primarily by the glomeruli show correlations between plasma drug clearance and maturational changes in renal function.
    - Tobramycin is eliminated predominantly by glomerular filtration, necessitating dosing intervals of 36–48 hours in preterm newborns and of 24 hours in term newborns.
    - Failure to adjust aminoglycoside dosing regimens can result in the exposure of infants to potentially toxic serum levels of these drugs.
    - Drugs that are primarily eliminated by the kidney need individualized treatment regimens in an age-appropriate manner associated with maturational changes in kidney function.

Clinical implications:

- Current age-specific drug doses are based on probable effects of ontogenesis on drug disposition. However, these equations, though providing ranges of doses for drugs, are of no benefit regarding the frequency of administration as they do not consider drug clearance or the role of pharmacodynamics on dosing.
- Some drugs are known to adversely affect organ maturation that would influence PK; examples include isotretinoin, valproic acid, and carbamazepine.
- When fentanyl is used for sedation in neonates, the plasma concentrations required for satisfactory sedation steadily escalate, possibly indicating the rapid development of tolerance to the sedating effects of fentanyl.

SOURCES OF INFORMATION

Adams D et al. Complementary and alternative medicine use by pediatric specialty outpatients. *Pediatrics* 2013;131:225–232.

Agunod M et al. Correlative study of hydrochloric acid, pepsin and intrinsic factor secretion in newborns and infants. *American Journal of Digestive Disease* 1969;14:400–414.

Arnold JH et al. Changes in the pharmacodynamic response to fentanyl in neonates during continuous infusion. *The Journal of Pediatrics* 1991;119:639–643.

Fisher DM et al. Pharmacokinetics and pharmacodynamics of d-tubocurarine in infants, children, and adults. *Anesthesiology* 1982;57.

Sumpter A, Anderson BJ. *Current Anesthesiology Reports* 2013;3:27–36. Published online: December 12, 2012.

PREGNANCY

Many physiological changes occur during pregnancy that modulate drug pharmacokinetics. The fundamental pharmacokinetic parameters regulating drug absorption, distribution, metabolism, and excretion cannot be assumed to be constant, and change over the course of the pregnancy. Therefore constant monitoring of drug efficacy is required.

Cardiovascular Changes

During the first trimester, cardiac output begins to increase, due to a combination of higher heart rate and stroke volume, and it eventually plateaus at 30%–50% of that found in nonpregnant individuals. Cardiac output remains high throughout pregnancy and is accompanied by changes to peripheral resistance. Initially, peripheral resistance decreases, causing a period of hypotension that peaks around 20–24 weeks. Then blood pressure starts to rise and approaches prepregnancy levels. Total blood volume increases by 30%–40% (1500–1800 mL), while extravascular volume increases during the second and third trimesters. As a result of these blood pressure changes, patients who are being treated for cardiovascular disorders, such as hypertension, have to be carefully monitored throughout pregnancy.

Renal Changes

Starting at 6–8 weeks, and increasing until week 32, maternal blood volume increases by 50%. Sodium and water are retained to give hypervolemia, which may protect the mother from blood loss at the time of birth. As a result of this higher blood volume, hydrophilic drugs (those with a low V_d), which predominantly partition into plasma, have lower-than-predicted plasma concentrations in pregnant patients. Thus hydrophilic drugs require higher initial and maintenance doses. However, the increases in blood volume are not accompanied by increases in serum albumin. Therefore, effective albumin concentration in blood falls. This can have a major effect on drugs that are predominantly bound by serum albumin, with drugs that are highly bound in nonpregnant patients having a much higher active drug fraction than in pregnant patients. This phenomenon is known to affect the activity of digoxin, midazolam, and phenytoin.

During the third trimester, renal blood flow increases by 30%–50% and GFR by approximately 50%. This increases drug clearance rates, which can have a dramatic effect on drug half-life. For example, the clearance rate of lithium is doubled during the third trimester. Thus, renally excreted drugs would have a much higher rate of excretion during this period. Pregnancy is a condition well known to induce hyperdynamic changes, and the GFR increases by up to 1/3 during early pregnancy compared with the prepregnant value.

Respiratory Changes

Increased hormone levels during pregnancy lead to increased vascularization and edema of the upper respiratory tract. This is especially important for pregnant women who suffer from asthma, as they are considered to be at higher risk during pregnancy. Theoretically, such changes in the pulmonary physiology may affect the absorption rates for inhaled medications, such as beta agonists and steroids used for asthma treatment. There have been few clinical studies of drug uptake in pregnant women, but clinical guidelines recommend frequent monitoring of lung function and adjustment of asthma medication as required.

Metabolic Changes

Changes to hormone levels also result in changes in the expression of phase I and phase II enzymes involved in drug metabolism. Increases in activity have been reported for CYP2A6, CYP2D6, CYP2C9, CYP3A4, and UGT1A4, while CYP1A2 and CYP2C19 decrease in activity. These changes in drug pharmacokinetics can be modeled and drug dose adjusted accordingly if the underlying pharmacokinetic parameters are well established (see Xia et al., 2013).

Medications affected (thereby requiring dose adjustments/close monitoring of drug efficacy) include

- Amoxicillin
- Midazolam
- Phenytoin
- Indinavir
- Glyburide
- Tacrolimus
- Digoxin
- Metformin

In all of these cases, doses need to be increased due to increased clearance/decreased whole blood levels.

SOURCES OF INFORMATION

Alomar MJ, Strauch CC. A prospective evaluation of antihypertensive medications safety and efficacy in United Arab Emirates private hospitals. *American Journal of Pharmacology and Toxicology* 2010;5:89–94.

Costantine MM. Physiologic and pharmacokinetic changes in pregnancy. *Frontiers of Pharmacology* 2014; 5:1–5.

Hebert MF. Pregnancy on pharmacokinetics of medications. *Population Therapeutics and Clinical Pharmacology* 2013;20:e350–e357.

Jeong H. Altered drug metabolism during pregnancy: Hormonal regulation of drug-metabolizing enzymes. *Expert Opinion on Drug Metabolism and Toxicology* 2010;6:689–699.

Maselli DJ, Adams SG, Peters JI, Levine SM. Management of asthma during pregnancy. *Therapeutic Advances in Respiratory Disease* 2013;7:87–100.

Pacheco L et al. Physiological changes during pregnancy. In Mattison DR, Ed. *Clincal Pharmacology during Pregnancy*. San Diego, CA: Academic Press, 2013, pp. 5–14.

Xia B et al. Simplified PBPK modeling approach for prediction of pharmacokinetics of four primarily renally excreted and CYP3A metabolized compounds during pregnancy. *AAPS Journal* 2013;15:1012–1024.

Specific Clinical Problems

Simon F.J. Clarke, Lakshman Delgoda Karalliedde, and Ursula Collignon

Although ADIs can cause a whole range of clinical problems, there are a small number of conditions that are particularly serious. This section will give an overview of three problems:

1. Hyper/hypokalemia
2. QT prolongation and Torsades de Pointes ventricular tachycardia
3. Serotonin syndrome

DISTURBANCES IN SERUM POTASSIUM

Hypo- and hyperkalemia are often asymptomatic and increase the risk of cardiac arrhythmias. They often occur as the result of ADIs and are usually predictable and preventable. Therefore, it is vitally important to monitor serum potassium levels in all patients who take medications that may cause hypo- or hyperkalemia. An ECG will also be required, especially if serum K^+ levels are above normal.

Hyperkalemia

Hyperkalemia (serum potassium >5.5 mmol/L) is rare in healthy individuals. Levels >7 mmol/L indicate a medical emergency, as cardiac arrest may occur.

Elderly patients on many medicines are at greatest risk for DDIs. One study reports at least 7.8% of admissions of elderly people for hyperkalemia were predictable and therefore preventable ADIs.[1] Strategies for reducing the risk of hyperkalemia DDIs must consider both patient (e.g., those on K^+ increasing drugs, CKD, diabetes) and physician risk factors (e.g., lack of K^+ monitoring, use of alternative drugs with less effect on K^+).

Prescribers adhere poorly to hyperkalemia DDI alerts even in patients with risk factors for clinically significant interactions. Display of relevant laboratory data in the alerts did not improve adherence in the outpatient setting.[2] Clinical decision support systems[3] have been proposed with specific alerts, e.g., triggering for monitoring where a combination of potassium sparing diuretics and potassium supplements is prescribed and monitoring has been discontinued early. Use of such systems is currently limited and requires significant investment and further research is necessary to determine optimal strategies for conveying patient-specific DDI risk. Patient-oriented services provided by clinical pharmacists, including drug history taking and medicines reconciliation, drug therapy monitoring, and patient education, will reduce the frequency of DDIs.

Life-threatening and fatal hyperkalemia has been reported with combinations of ACEI and potassium-sparing diuretics or dual blockage of the RAS. In the United Kingdom, the MHRA now advises against coadministration of medicines from two classes of RAS blocking drugs.[4]

Specific care should also be taken in patients treated with ACEI, ARB, or diuretics who are coprescribed an NSAID for the first time; consider monitoring K^+ and creatinine every 24 hours especially in those with known CKD or diabetes. One study reports ACEI combined with spironolactone was the most common major preventable DDI, representing 20.0% of all preventable DDIs on admission and 25.6% on discharge.

Hypotension should also be avoided due to the risk of further deterioration of renal function and reduction of K^+ excretion.

Symptoms of hyperkalemia, if they occur, are often nonspecific, such as fatigue, weakness, paresthesia, and palpitations. Symptoms suggestive of hyperkalemia require immediate medical attention, as it can occur quickly. In one study, all patients who died of hyperkalemia had normal K^+ levels within 36 h prior to death. Drugs are implicated in the development of hyperkalemia in as many as 75% of cases.

Immediate management of hyperkalemia:

1. Check ECG—changes that may be seen are
   - Peaked T waves
   - Long PR interval
   - Broad P waves progressing to loss of P waves
   - Broad QRS
   - Second- and third-degree heart block
   - "Sine-wave" ECG
2. Discontinue K^+ sparing or K^+ containing medicines
3. Review other sources of K^+ intake, e.g., foods (low-salt/no-salt), supplements, and feeds.
4. Consider likelihood of digoxin toxicity.
5. Check for acidosis that can contribute to hyperkalemia.
6. Strategies to reduce K^+ levels:
   - If $K^+ \geq 7$ mmol/L and no ECG changes, start soluble insulin infusion (5 units in 50 mL of glucose 20%) over 15 min.
   - If $K^+ \geq 6.5$ mmol/L, give insulin as above or calcium resonium 15 g QDS plus a laxative depending on clinical situation.
   - If $K^+ < 6.5$ mmol/L, give oral treatment as above and ensure appropriate monitoring.
   - If there are any ECG changes, irrespective of the degree of hyperkalemia, give 10 mL of calcium chloride 10% over 3 min and start insulin infusion as above. Repeat calcium gluconate every 10 min until ECG normalizes.
   - If $K^+ \geq 5.5$ mmol/L and digoxin toxicity is suspected, avoid IV calcium; review with specialist toxicology team if possible and arrange for DigiFab administration.

Other treatment options:

- Nebulized salbutamol also increases K^+ excretion; it can be used while other therapies are being set up.
- Emergency dialysis may be required for hyperkalemia unresponsive to treatment.

Hypokalemia

Symptoms of hypokalemia include palpitations, skeletal muscle weakness, or cramping (including abdominal cramps), paresthesia, constipation, nausea or vomiting, polyuria, polydipsia, delirium, hallucinations, and depression.

U.S. studies show that ~20% of hospitalized patients are hypokalemic (a value of less than 3.6 mmol of potassium/L), but this is only clinically significant in 4%–5%.[5]

Immediate management of hypokalemia:

1. Check ECG—changes that may be seen are
   - Broad, tall P waves
   - Long PR interval
   - ST depression ± T wave flattening
   - U waves
   - Increased frequency of ectopic beats
   - Supraventricular tachycardias
   - Ventricular tachycardias
2. Consider likelihood of digoxin toxicity.

3. Establish IV access; assess if central access is required.
4. If $K^+ < 2.5$ mmol/L, give 40 mmol K^+, centrally as a concentrated solution (e.g., 20 mmol/100 mL) over 10–20 minutes or peripherally as a dilute solution (e.g., 40 mmol/1000 mL). Usual maximum peripheral rate is 10 mmol/h, but can be given over 10–20 minutes in an emergency.
5. If K^+ between 2.5–3.5 and ECG changes, give 20 mmol as above.
6. If K^+ between 2.5–3.5 and no ECG changes, supplement PO, 16 mmol TDS for 2–3 days.
7. Check magnesium levels and replace if necessary. Parenteral replacement is 20 mmol in 250 mL sodium chloride 0.9% over 4 h.

REFERENCES

1. Juurlink DN et al. Drug-drug interactions among elderly patients hospitalized for drug toxicity. *JAMA* 2003;289:1652–1658.
2. Fokter N et al. Potential drug–drug interactions and admissions due to drug–drug interactions in patients treated in medical departments. *Wiener klinische Wochenschrift* 2010;122:81–88.
3. Kawamoto K et al. Improving clinical practice using clinical decision support systems: A systematic review of trials to identify features critical to success. *BMJ* 2005;330:765.
4. Medicines and Healthcare Regulatory Authority (MHRA). Available at: https://www.gov.uk/drug-safety-update/combination-use-of-medicines-from-different-classes-of-renin-angiotensin-system-blocking-agents-risk-of-hyperkalaemia-hypotension-and-impaired-renal-function-new-warnings#combination-use-review (accessed February 4, 2015).
5. Gennari FJ. Hypokalemia. *New England Journal of Medicine* 1998;339:451–458.

FURTHER READING

Duke JD et al. Adherence to drug-drug interaction alerts in high-risk patients: A trial of context-enhancing alerting. *Journal of the American Medical Informatics Association* 2013;20:494–498.

Eschmann E et al. Patient and physician risk factors for hyperkalaemia in potassium increasing drug–drug interactions. *EJCP* 2014;70:215–223.

Horn JR, Hansten PD. Hyperkalemia due to drug interactions. Drug interactions: Insights and observations. *Pharmacy Times* January 2004.

Horn JR, Hansten PD. Hyperkalemia from drug interactions: New data. *Pharmacy Times* Published Online: Friday, July 11, 2014.

Uijtendaal EV et al. Serum potassium influencing interacting drugs: Risk-modifying strategies also needed at discontinuation. *Annals of Pharmacotherapy* 2012;46:176–182.

QT INTERVAL PROLONGATION AND TORSADES DE POINTES VENTRICULAR TACHYCARDIA

Introduction

QT prolongation is a common reason for withdrawal or restriction of use of drugs; it may cause polymorphic or Torsades de Pointes (TdP) ventricular tachycardia, which in turn may degenerate into ventricular fibrillation. It is an adverse effect of many different drugs and it continues to be a major concern due to unpredictability of its frequency of occurrence, individual variability, and risk of syncope and sudden death.

QT Interval

QT interval represents the measured interval between the beginnings of the QRS complex to the end of the T wave.

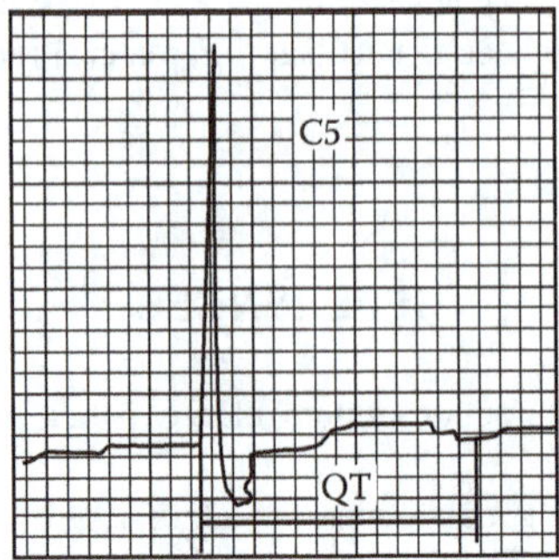

This includes both depolarization and repolarization of the ventricles, although the largest component is ventricular repolarization. Multiple ion currents contribute to normal repolarization. The most important clinically and pharmacologically are the inward rectifier potassium channels that open to allow potassium to enter the cell and return the myocyte membrane to its resting state. There are two main subtypes that are encoded by the potassium voltage-gated channel (KCN) family of genes:

1. The rapid delayed rectifier (I_{Kr}) potassium channel
   a. *KCNH2* gene (also known as *hERG*) regulates its structure.
   b. *KCNE2* gene codes for a molecule that regulates the activity of the channel.
2. The slow delayed rectifier (I_{Ks}) potassium channel
   a. *KCNQ1* gene regulates its structure.
   b. *KCNE1* gene codes for a molecule that regulates the activity of the channel.

The different ion channels provide a degree of "repolarization reserve"; this reserve is significantly reduced if channels are rendered less effective by genetic polymorphisms or disease states (such as heart failure or myocardial ischemia).

Factors Effecting QT Interval

Heart Rate

Heart rate is an important variable affecting the QT interval, and "rate-corrected" QT interval (QT_c) enables comparison of QT values at different heart rates. The Bazett formula is commonly used: $QT_c = QT/\sqrt{(RR\ interval)}$. There is no consensus about normal QT_c intervals; however, it is commonly thought that QT_c interval > 440–470 ms (males) and > 470–480 ms (females) are considered to be abnormal.

Disease States

The QT_c increases ~20 ms at night due to changes in autonomic tone that are more likely in disease states such as diabetes.

Treatment of congestive heart failure, renal impairment, and hypertension may cause electrolyte imbalances, which may result in prolonged QT syndrome.

Long QT syndrome (LQTS) may occur as a result of mutations in the genes encoding the potassium and sodium channels. At present, mutations of six genes associated with congenital long-QT syndrome have been identified:

1. *KCNH2*
2. *KCNE2*
3. *KCNQ1*
4. *KCNE1*
5. *SCN5A*—regulates the structure of a Na^+ channel
6. *ANK2*—regulates the position of K^+, Na^+, Ca^{2+} channels in the cardiac cell membrane

Gender and Ethnicity

More recently, the effect of gender and race on QT have been investigated:

1. One study observed that the baseline QT_c was about 10% longer in women than in men.
2. In a study of 2686 healthy middle-aged individuals, black men had a shorter QT_c length than white men.
3. Mansi et al. investigated ECG patterns (PR, QRS, and QT) in healthy individuals from six different ethnic groups (Saudi, Indian, Jordanian, Filipino, Sri Lankan, and Caucasian) living in the Middle East. No significant differences in ECG parameters were found among the male members of these groups, whereas the ECG patterns differed significantly among women; the P-wave axis in the Caucasian women and the QRS duration in the Jordanian women were significantly greater than those of the other populations, but there were no differences in QT_c.
4. A multiethnic cohort study of rural Hawaiians showed that significant differences in the prevalence of prolonged QT_c persisted after controlling for known metabolic and biochemical covariates related to the QT interval length.

These data support the hypothesis that genetic background is an important factor that contributes to ethnic disparities in cardiac electrophysiology.

The National Heart, Lung, and Blood Institute Family Heart Study on heritability of the QT interval duration found a major genetic effect accounting for 11% of the variation in QT interval duration and multiple other effects accounting for another 34%. Similarly, Newton-Cheh et al. found 35% heritability of QT interval duration. The evidence suggests that QT interval duration is a heritable trait although numerous other factors play an important role.

Torsades de Pointes

TdP is a type of ventricular tachycardia where the amplitude of the QRS varies. Torsades de Pointes translates to "twisting of the points" and is so named because the QRS complexes look like they are rotating around the isoelectric axis.

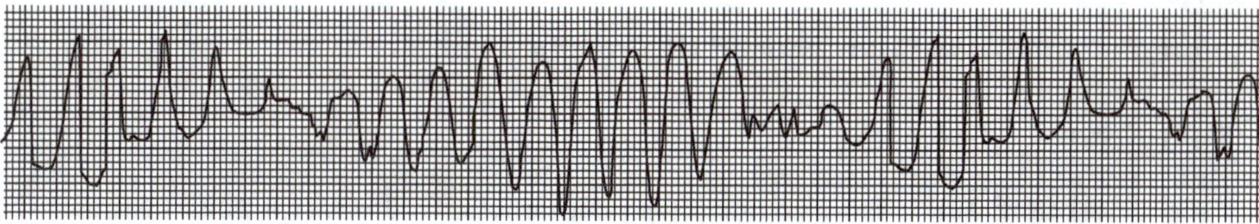

Risk of TdP differs in persons with similar QT prolongation as TdP does not increase in parallel with the increase in QT interval. This is because prolonged QT primes the heart for TdP but initiation of the arrhythmia requires a trigger, which involves a different mechanism.

Mechanisms

Two mechanisms are implicated in the development of TdP:

- After-depolarization—the trigger
- Reentry—maintains the arrhythmia

Alterations in repolarization prolong the action potential, which increases Ca^{2+} entry during the plateau phase. This triggers a transient inward current via Na^+/Ca^{2+} exchange that opens nonselective cation channels in the cell membranes that can cause early depolarizing currents. If these occur on a T wave (R-on-T phenomenon), an arrhythmia can be initiated.

When a depolarizing current meets an area of repolarization, a unidirectional block occurs, which is a prerequisite for the development of a reentry circuit. Homogeneity between repolarization in different cardiac cells (epicardial, mid-myocardial and endocardial myocytes and Purkinje fibers) provides this situation.

The risk for TdP increases as the QT_c interval increases. Each 10-ms increase in QT_c contributes approximately a 5%–7% *exponential* increase in risk for TdP; therefore, a patient with a QT_c of 540 ms has a 63%–97% higher risk of developing TdP than a patient with a QT_c of 440 ms. However, there is no threshold of QT_c prolongation at which TdP is certain to occur. Data from congenital LQTS studies indicate that a $QT_c > 500$ ms is associated with a two- to threefold higher risk for TdP and it is likely that there is a similar risk with drug-induced TdP.

Drugs That Prolong the QT Interval

Introduction

Drug-induced prolongation of repolarization as an antiarrhythmic mechanism was first described 35 years ago (Vaughan Williams class III action). Drug-induced long-QT syndrome (dLQTS) is associated with a risk of TdP. Withdrawal of the causative drugs results in the normalization of the QT interval after a washout period. Some drugs known to cause increased QT interval are listed in "QT Interval Prolongation and Torsades De Pointes Ventricular Tachycardia" section.

The overall incidence of drug-induced TdP is not known. Exposure of 1% of the population to a TdP genic drug doubles the risk ratio for sudden cardiac death and may account for about 10 deaths/million/year. Drugs vary in the degree by which they alter the QT interval and the heart rate particularly in patients with concurrent disease such as infections. Some cardiac drugs (sotalol, dofetilide, ibutilide) prolong the interval by more than 50 ms at prescribed doses. Noncardiac drugs may cause TdP causing a mean increase of 5–10 ms in some patients. Prolongation of the QT interval to longer than 500 ms during drug therapy requires immediate consideration of risks and benefits of that therapy, replacement with other drugs, and elimination of rectifiable risk factors.

Factors That Influence Drug-Induced QT Prolongation

Pharmacological Factors

The incidence of TdP is more common with antiarrhythmic drugs (1%–10%) that have QT prolonging action than nonantiarrhythmic QT prolongers (0.001% for cisapride). Amiodarone is the exception to this rule; although chronic administration of amiodarone markedly prolongs the QT interval, it is very rarely associated with TdP because it also inhibits the late sodium currents that trigger TdP.

Potassium channel blockade is likely to be a dose–response effect; anything that increases dose of QT prolonging drugs will increase the effect on the QT interval. This includes

- Administration of an excessive dose.
- Rapid IV infusion—e.g., TdP can occur with rapid IV boluses of both erythromycin and ondansetron.
- Inhibition of metabolism of a QT prolonger by a food or another drug usually mediated by the cytochrome P450 (CYP) family, e.g., elevation of cisapride concentrations when used in combination with simvastatin—both metabolized by CYP3A4.
- Alterations in drug transporters (influx and efflux) by coadministered drugs.

Interestingly, quinidine is an exception to the direct dose–response rule. TdP is more likely occur at lower doses; it is a potent I_{Kr} blocker, so at low concentrations, it prolongs action potenti whereas at higher concentrations, its Na^+ channel–blocking properties inhibit initiation of TdP.

Drug metabolites may also contribute to the clinical effects of the drug. For example, terfe dine is an I_{Kr} blocker but it is nearly completely biotransformed by the CYP3A enzyme system to noncardioactive fexofenadine before entering the systemic circulation. Although the QT prolo ing effect of terfenadine is minimal in healthy people exposed to normal doses (~6 ms), in patie with heart failure (a setting of reduced repolarization reserve), terfenadine-induced QT inter prolongation is greater. Similarly, when CYP3A is inhibited (e.g., coadministration of erythromy or ketoconazole) or overwhelmed (because of an overdose), or when its activity is reduced by d ease (cirrhosis), the concentration of unmetabolized terfenadine entering the systemic circulati increases markedly, resulting in a greater prolongation of the QT interval.

Coadministration of drugs that prolong the QT interval has an additive effect with a theoreti increased risk of TdP. Although, as previously stated, QT prolongation does not necessarily lead TdP, the potential life-threatening risk of TdP and the current difficulty in predicting which indiv uals will develop TdP means that coadministration of QT prolongers should be generally avoide

Disease States

A number of conditions increase the QT interval, which may add to the effect of QT prolonge others increase sensitivity of the I_{Kr} current to drug-blocking effects.

- Hypokalemia or hypomagnesemia.
- Preexisting cardiac disease reduces repolarization reserve.
- Bradycardia (the QT interval is greater at lower heart rates), e.g., after recent conversion from atrial fibrillation, therapy using cardiac glycosides, beta-blockers, or calcium channel blockers.
- Hepatic and renal disease—these may reduce metabolism and excretion of QT prolonging drugs; e.g., *N*-acetylprocainamide (NAPA), an active metabolite of procainamide, is renally excreted so there is a risk of TdP in patients with renal dysfunction. Other drugs that may be affected are sotalol and dofelitide (both significantly excreted unchanged by the kidneys).
- Thyroid disease.

Genetics

Potassium and Sodium Ion Channels

Clinical phenotype of dLQTS resembles that of congenital long-QT syndrome (cLQT and "latent" genetic factors probably underlie susceptibility of a subject to dLQTS and Td However, although dLQTS subjects had genetic backgrounds similar to cLQTS subjec functional changes associated with mutations identified in dLQTS were different from tho in cLQTS. Variants in ion channel genes have been identified in up to 15% of patients wi drug-induced TdP (Yang); in the Japanese population, polymorphisms have been identified ıe ıtients with drug-associated TdP. The current estimate is that LQTS mutation car-ıt in 1 of 1000–3000 individuals.

ymorphisms in ion channel genes have been shown to be associated with dLQTS:

'reliminary studies indicate that polymorphism (D85N) is more common (7%) among ith drug-associated TdP than among controls (2%–4%). Mutations have been implicated mias induced by cisapride and dofetilide. A variant has been identified in 22%–28% of ubjects (Horie M and Shimizu W, personal communication, December 2001).

ıERG): The majority of drugs associated with QT prolongation bind particularly to I_{Kr} hannels.

:o olymorphism of the *KCNE2* gene is present in 1.6% of the population (Sesti) and is associ-

ls drug-induced TdP with quinidine and sulfamethoxazole/trimethoprim.

1akita et al. reported that a group of patients with a subclinical mutation in the sodium

ı- subunit gene (SCN5A) may be prone to drug-induced arrhythmia. A mutant *SCN5A* chan-

ıe ıP) was reported in an elderly woman who had cisapride-induced TdP. Ethnically specific

ʒ- lymorphisms in these genes contribute to the length of the QT interval, both in the resting

ts n the context of drug-induced changes, and these might account for ethnic differences in

al :ed QT_c prolongation or arrhythmia.

n ete penetrance, family members with near-normal QT intervals may carry the same

ʒ- ciated with LQTS that cause QT-interval prolongation and an increased risk of sud-

n eir relatives. At present, 5%–10% of persons in whom TdP develops on exposure to olonging drugs harbor mutations associated with the long-QT syndrome and can be

ıl ıaving a subclinical form of the congenital syndrome.

o

l- *'sm and Transport*

lymorphisms determine the level of activity of drug-metabolizing enzymes, notably *:YP3A4*. Genotyping of *CYP2D6* is currently available to individualize the dosage of ; poor drug metabolization (seen in 5%–10% of Caucasians and African Americans) ıotentially dangerous levels of substrate drugs.

ʒ; iants of *CYP3A4* appear to be less relevant on their own. However, care should n the presence of other factors such as increased age, or ingestion of strong ıitors (such as grapefruit juice, some macrolide antibiotics, azole antifungals, and

ıolymorphisms will determine the activity of drug transporters (efflux and influx) fluence blood levels of substrate drugs. QT prolongers that are eliminated by a single isposition are likely to pose a greater risk.

of polymorphisms varies between different populations. Several studies have inves-lifferences in dLQTS and TdP:

ıbjects were less sensitive to quinidine-induced QT prolongation than Caucasian subjects, :end was particularly true for females (Shin). QT_c values of Caucasians were higher than :oreans at the same quinidine concentration. Gender and ethnicity are significant covari-

), ıinidine-induced QT_c prolongation. These results suggest that Koreans may be less vulner-

P. inidine-induced fatal arrhythmia than Caucasians.

s, et al. found a heterozygous polymorphism in the sodium channel gene *SCN5A* among

e mericans that increased the risk for drug-induced TdP. The polymorphism was present in

h patients with proarrhythmic episodes but in only 13% of control subjects.

n

3. Ackerman et al.[1] reported that the spectra and frequencies of potassium channel variants differed among four different ethnic populations including black, white, Asian, and Hispanic; black populations appeared to have a wider spectrum and higher frequency of potassium channel variants than any other ethnic population. This group also reported the first determination of the prevalence and spectrum of cardiac sodium channel variants in a range of different ethnic groups.[2]
4. Available data suggest that white Caucasians may be more susceptible than Asians to QT interval prolongation by hERG-regulated channel blockers.
5. The Japanese authority has received only a small fraction of the reports of drug-induced TdP received by the Western authorities from their corresponding regions. The International Conference on Harmonisation of Technical Requirements for Registration of Pharmaceuticals for Human Use (ICH E14) recommends that genotyping patients who experience marked prolongation of QT_c interval or TdP while on drug therapy should be considered.

Gender

Women have longer QT intervals and a greater propensity for drug-induced TdP due to differences in the densities of I_{Kr} and I_{K1} currents. Also, female sex is a risk factor for drug-induced TdP (~70% of TdP cases are attributed to lower levels of testosterone, which shortens the QT interval). Sex hormones may affect either the autonomic nervous system or the expression or activity of cardiac ion channels that contribute to gender-related differences in cardiac repolarization and possibly to greater susceptibility to TdP in women.

Clinical implications:

It is particularly important to balance the risks and benefits when prescribing drugs with QT prolonging action. The following principles should be applied:

1. *Is there an alternative, equally effective drug available that does not increase the QT interval?*
2. *Avoid QT prolongers in the following circumstances:*
   - When the patient is already taking a QT blocker
   - In patients with a past history of unexplained syncope or known long QT syndrome or a family history of sudden unexplained death

   If there is absolutely no alternative, coadministration should be undertaken under close supervision of a specialist (usually a cardiologist).
   - An ECG should be taken before starting treatment and at regular intervals after starting therapy or changing doses (at least weekly until stable).
   - If initiating therapy in hospital, the patient must have continuous cardiac monitoring.
3. *Caution should be exercised when there is a risk of poor metabolism or excretion of QT prolonging drugs or in situations that may increase their sensitivity:*
   - Hepatic disease
   - Renal dysfunction
   - Anorexia nervosa, protein-sparing diets, starvation, excessive fasting (Panagiotis Korantzopoulos, M.D. Konstantinos Siogas, M.D.G. Hatzikosta General Hospital of Ioannina, 45001 Ioannina, Greece pkor@oneway.gr)
   - Coadministration with a drug that inhibits its metabolism
   - Hypokalemia—e.g., gastroenteritis or the addition of a diuretic

   In these cases, the following are recommended:
   - It is prudent to start treatment at the lowest dose and gradually titrate the dose up.
   - In established hepatic/renal dysfunction, consider halving the dose.
   - An ECG should be taken before starting treatment and at regular intervals after starting therapy or changing doses (at least weekly until stable).
   - If initiating therapy in hospital, the patient must have continuous cardiac monitoring.

- Consider alternative therapy if QT_c exceeds 500 ms or it increases by >60 ms compared with the predrug baseline value.

4. *In all cases, patients should be warned to report promptly any symptoms such as new palpitations and near-syncope or syncope (even without palpitations).*

Management of prolonged QT and Torsades de Pointes

1. Assess and manage the patient using the standard A-B-C-D-E approach. Call for expert help.
2. Monitoring—ECG, SpO_2, NIBP as a minimum. $ETCO_2$ is required if the patient needs to be sedated.
3. Correct known aggravating factors:
   - Stop the QT prolonger.
   - Treat bradyarrhythmias.
   - Correct electrolyte abnormalities.
4. In the hemodynamically stable patient, magnesium sulfate 2 g infused over 20–30 minutes is the first-line agent irrespective of the serum magnesium level. This should be repeated if TdP persists.
5. In the unstable patient or where magnesium is ineffective, the patient will require synchronized DC cardioversion under sedation.

REFERENCES

1. Ackerman MJ et al. Ethnic differences in cardiac potassium channel variants: Implications for genetic susceptibility to sudden cardiac death and genetic testing for congenital long QT syndrome. *Journal of Molecular and Cellular Cardiology* 2004;37:79–89.
2. Ackerman MJ et al. Spectrum and prevalence of cardiac sodium channel variants among black, white, Asian, and Hispanic individuals: Implications for arrhythmogenic susceptibility and Brugada/long QT syndrome genetic testing. *Heart Rhythm* 2004;1:600–607.

FURTHER READING

Drew BJ et al. Prevention of Torsade de Pointes in hospital settings. A scientific statement from the American Heart Association and the American College of Cardiology Foundation. *Circulation* 2010;121:1047–1060.

ICH Guideline E14. The clinical evaluation of QT/QTc interval prolongation and proarrhythmic potential for non-antiarrhythmic drugs. 2005. http://www.ich.org/fileadmin/Public_Web_Site/ICH_Products/Guidelines/Efficacy/E14/E14_Guideline.pdf.

Makita M et al. Drug-induced long-QT syndrome associated with a subclinical *SCN5A* mutation. *Circulation* 2002;106; 1269–1274.

Mansi IA and Nash IS. Ethnic differences in electrocardiographic intervals and axes. *Journal of Electrocardiology* 2001;34:303–307.

Nachimuthu S et al. Drug-induced QT interval prolongation: Mechanisms and clinical management. *Therapeutic Advances in Drug Safety* 2012;3:241–253.

Newton-Cheh C et al. QT interval is a heritable quantitative trait with evidence of linkage to chromosome 3 in a genome-wide linkage analysis: The Framingham Heart Study. *Heart Rhythm* 2005;2:277–284.

Ritter JM. Drug-induced long QT syndrome and drug development. *British Journal of Clinical Pharmacology* 2008;66:341–344.

Ritter JM. Cardiac safety, drug-induced QT prolongation and torsade de pointes (TdP). *British Journal of Clinical Pharmacology* 2012;73:331–334.

Sesti F et al. A common polymorphism associated with antibiotic-induced cardiac arrhythmia. *Proceedings of the National Academy of Sciences* 2000;97:10613–10618.

Shin JG et al. Possible interethnic differences in quinidine-induced QT prolongation between healthy Caucasian and Korean subjects. *British Journal of Clinical Pharmacology* 2007;63;206–215.

Splawski I et al. Variant of SCN5A sodium channel implicated in risk of cardiac arrhythmia. *Science* 2002;297;1333–1336.

Yang P et al. Allelic variants in long-QT disease genes in patients with drug-associated Torsades de Pointes. *Circulation* 2002;105:1943–1948.

SEROTONIN SYNDROME

Serotonin, or 5-hydroxytryptamine (5HT), is a neurotransmitter found in the central and peripheral nervous system. Serotonin modulates a wide range of activities including mood, cognitive function, induction of sleep, appetite, sexual activity, pain perception, motor function, and temperature regulation. Fourteen types of serotonin receptors have been identified.

Serotonin syndrome is a constellation of signs and symptoms of excessive serotonin activity that progresses from mild side effects through to life-threatening toxicity, with increasing intrasynaptic serotonin levels. The increased serotonin levels cause hyperstimulation of the brain stem and spinal cord (possibly to a greater degree) $5HT_{1A}$ and $5HT_2$ receptors. Data from the 2012 Annual Report of the American Association of Poison Control Centers" National Poison Data System (AAPCC-NPDS) showed 2.3 million total toxic exposures and 2576 fatalities in 2012. SSRIs were involved in 47,115 of those exposures and 89 (3%) of deaths.

Causes

Overdose of serotonergic drugs is an important cause as is ADIs resulting in serotonin toxicity following coadministration of two serotonergic drugs.

The range of drugs with the potential to cause the syndrome includes

- Antidepressants (SSRIs, TCAs, SNRIs, MAOIs)
- Analgesics (opioids—pethidine, tramadol, methadone, fentanyl, dextromethorphan, dextropropoxyphene, pentazocine, oxycodone)
- Anticonvulsants (carbamazepine, valproate)
- Migraine therapies (triptans and ergot derivatives)
- Anxiolytics (buspirone)
- Antismoking aids (bupropion)
- Herbal products (St. John's wort)
- The diagnostic dye-methylthioninium chloride (methylene blue)—has reversible MAOI activity and could cause the syndrome
- Amphetamines, including its derived recreational drugs, and appetite suppressants
- Lithium

Most severe interactions occurs when monoamine oxidase inhibitors (MAOIs) are taken in combination with selective serotonin reuptake inhibitors (SSRIs), tricyclic antidepressants, or venlafaxine (a serotonin norepinephrine reuptake inhibitor). MAOIs prevent the breakdown of serotonin while SSRIs prevent reuptake of serotonin, increasing the levels at the receptors.

Clinical Features

Onset of symptoms occurs within 6 hours in 60% of patients after beginning concurrent therapy or a change of dose and resolves within 24 hours of stopping the serotonergic drug(s).

Clinical features are due to a combination of manifestations of altered mental status and neuromuscular hyperactivity.

These symptoms may not be present together in all patients. In severe life-threatening cases, hyperthermia, rhabdomyolysis, renal failure, and disseminated intravascular coagulopathy occur.

Biochemical changes include metabolic acidosis, hyperkalemia, elevated creatine kinase and transaminase activity, and renal impairment with myoglobinuria.

Management

Most important is to recognize this rare but serious condition!

This section provides an overview of management options; early involvement of clinicians experienced in emergency and critical care medicine and toxicology is mandatory.

Discontinue serotonergic medication.

Mild Cases

- Administer IV fluids. Antipyretics are not indicated, as the mechanism for temperature alteration is centrally mediated.
- Administer activated charcoal if a potentially lethal amount or combination of proserotonergic agents has been ingested and if the presentation is within 1–2 hours.
- Treat neuromuscular abnormalities with benzodiazepines.

Severe Cases

- Airway/breathing
  - All patients should be treated as above in an intensive care unit, with the addition of airway protection and ventilation if needed.
  - Paralysis and mechanical ventilation may also be necessary to avoid worsening muscle rigidity and increasing hyperthermia in any patient with a temperature higher than 41°C.
- Circulation
  - Hypotensives—e.g., nitroprusside, esmolol
- Disability
  - Anticonvulsants—lorazepam, diazepam, midazolam
- Specific therapies
  - 5 HT antagonists may be considered, such as cyproheptadine
  - Caution in hyperthermic patients, because cyproheptadine has anticholinergic properties and theoretically can worsen hyperthermia

Editors

Lakshman Delgoda Karalliedde, DA, FRCA, is honorary visiting professor, anesthesiology, Faculty of Medicine, Peradeniya, Sri Lanka. He was formerly honorary visiting professor in pharmacology, Faculty of Medicine, Peradeniya; visiting senior lecturer, Department of Public Health Sciences, King's College, London; consultant medical toxicologist, Health Protection Agency, United Kingdom; and senior lecturer and honorary consultant in anesthetics, Guy's and St Thomas Hospitals, London, United Kingdom. He is a recipient of a BMA book award (2011).

Simon F.J. Clarke, MbChB, DA, FRCSEd, FCEM, is consultant emergency physician, Frimley Health Foundation Trust (GSTFT), Frimley Park Hospital, Surrey, United Kingdom. Dr. Clarke undertook training in anesthesiology, primary care, and surgery before settling on a career in emergency medicine. He developed an interest in clinical toxicology in 2001 and worked at the Guys Poisons Unit, Chemical Incident Response Unit (London) and Health Protection Agency, Centre of Radiation, Chemical and Environmental Hazards (London) for 10 years. He has taught on the master's course, Toxicology for Public Health at Kings College London, worked on the Department of Health's (UK) Decontamination Optimization Working Group, and is a member of the All Party Parliamentary Carbon Monoxide Group. He has also presented to the MASH (mass casualties from chemical incidents) project for the European Union. He has published on chemical incident response and carbon monoxide epidemiology and has contributed to books on emergency medicine, management of opioid overdose, and clinical toxicology.

Ursula Gotel (nee Collignon) is the highly specialist pharmacist for Emergency Medicine at Guy's and St Thomas' NHS Foundation Trust, London, United Kingdom. She has worked as a clinical pharmacist in emergency medicine for over 10 years, likes challenges, enjoys changes, and innovates, particularly in the development and role of pharmacy/pharmacists in urgent and emergency care (UEC). Ursula is part of NHS London's UEC clinical leadership group, HEE pharmacy development group, and the national CEM/NPIS antidote guideline development group. She is coeditor of *Adverse Drug Interactions* (first edition, 2009, CRC Press, Boca Raton, Florida).

Ursula is the GHP regional representative for London & Eastern and a Unite accredited workplace representative. She is an Agenda for Change evaluator and was directly involved locally as an early implementer site. Recently, she has been involved in the consultation and change to 7-day services at GSTFT. She is part of staff side on the Trust Pay Group and ensures members' voices are heard and staff are effectively represented.

Janaka Karalliedde, MBChB, MRCP, PhD, is a Senior Lecturer in the Cardiovascular Division, Faculty of Life Science & Medicine, King's College London and Consultant Physician in Diabetes and Endocrinology at Guy's and St Thomas Hospital London. He graduated with a distinction in medicine from the University of London in 1998 and obtained his Membership of the Royal College of Physicians in 2001. He was awarded UK Medical Research Council Clinical Research Training Fellowship and PhD by the University of London for research on the pathophysiology and treatment of cardiovascular disease and renal disease in diabetes. He has published widely in the subject of diabetic nephropathy and cardiovascular disease and has been awarded research grants from the UK Medical Research Council, Diabetes UK, European Foundation for the Study of Diabetes, National Institute for Health Research, and the International Diabetes Federation. Dr Karalliedde is an active clinician and teacher with specialist interest in diabetic renal disease and vascular complications.

Coordinating Editor

Seneka Abeyratne earned his MS from Cornell University, Ithaca, New York. He has undertaken international consulting assignments for the Asian Development Bank (Manila) in public health and associated fields, provided technical and editorial assistance to policy documents, and is currently working on a dictionary of medicines and drugs.

Contributors

Rebecca Chanda
Pharmacy Department
St Thomas' Hospital
Guy's and St Thomas' NHS Foundation Trust
London, United Kingdom

Andrea Corsonello
Unit of Geriatric Pharmacoepidemiology
Italian National Research Center in Aging
Research Hospital of Cosenza
Cosenza, Italy

K.M.H.K. Ganegedara
Faculty of Medicine
University of Peradeniya
Peradeniya, Sri Lanka

Gregory Ian Giles
Department of Pharmacology & Toxicology
University of Otago
Dunedin, New Zealand

Niroshini Manthri Giles
Department of Pharmacology & Toxicology
University of Otago
Dunedin, New Zealand

Chulananda Goonasekera
Department of Anaesthesia
King's College Hospital
London, United Kingdom

H.M.U. Amila Jayasinghe
Department of Anaesthesia
Teaching Hospital
Peradeniya, Sri Lanka

Giuseppe Maltese
School of Medicine
King's College London
London, United Kingdom

Ruwan Parakramawansha
Department of Pharmacology
Faculty of Medicine
University of Peradeniya
Peradeniya, Sri Lanka

Vasanthi Pinto
Faculty of Medicine
University of Peradeniya
Peradeniya, Sri Lanka

Yohan P. Samarasinghe
Department of Medicine
Frimley Health NHS Foundation Trust
Frimley Park Hospital
Surrey, United Kingdom

Ming Ming Teh
Department of Endocrinology
Singapore General Hospital
and
Yong Loo Lin School of Medicine
National University of Singapore
and
DUKE-NUS Graduate School of Medicine
National University of Singapore
Singapore

E. Queenie Veerasingham
General Hospital
Avissawella, Sri Lanka

Winglam Yeung
Department of Pharmacy
Frimley Hospital NHS Foundation Trust
Surrey, United Kingdom

Patrick Yong
Frimley Park Hospital Foundation Trust
Camberley, United Kingdom

PART 1

Drugs Acting on the Cardiovascular System

Simon F.J. Clarke

1. ANTIARRHYTHMICS
2. ANTIHYPERTENSIVES AND HEART FAILURE DRUGS
   - ACE INHIBITORS
   - ADRENERGIC NEURONE BLOCKERS
   - ALISKIREN
   - ALPHA-BLOCKERS
   - ANGIOTENSIN II RECEPTOR ANTAGONISTS
   - CENTRALLY ACTING ANTIHYPERTENSIVES
   - 5-HT2 RECEPTOR AGONISTS—KETANSERIN
   - VASODILATOR ANTIHYPERTENSIVES
3. ANTIPLATELET DRUGS
4. BETA-BLOCKERS
5. CALCIUM CHANNEL BLOCKERS
6. CARDIAC GLYCOSIDES
7. DIURETICS
8. IVABRADINE
9. LIPID-LOWERING DRUGS
10. NITRATES
11. PERIPHERAL VASODILATORS
12. POTASSIUM CHANNEL ACTIVATORS—For example, NICORANDIL
13. RANOLAZINE
14. SELECTIVE PHOSPHODIESTERASE INHIBITORS
15. SYMPATHOMIMETICS

Primary Drug	Secondary Drug	Effect	Mechanism	Precautions
ANTIARRHYTHMICS				
ADENOSINE				
ADENOSINE	ANESTHETICS—LOCAL	↑ Myocardial depression	Additive effect; local anesthetics and adenosine are myocardial depressants	Monitor PR, BP, and ECG closely
ADENOSINE	ANTIARRHYTHMICS	Risk of bradycardia and ↓ BP	Additive myocardial depression	Monitor PR, BP, and ECG closely
ADENOSINE	ANTIPLATELET AGENTS—DIPYRIDAMOLE	↑ Effect of adenosine; ↓ doses needed to terminate supraventricular tachycardias; case report of profound bradycardia when adenosine infusion was given for myocardial stress testing	Dipyridamole inhibits adenosine uptake into cells	↓ Bolus doses of adenosine by up to fourfold when administering it for treating supraventricular tachycardias. Some recommend avoiding adenosine for patients taking dipyridamole. Advise patients to stop dipyridamole for 24 h before using adenosine infusions
ADENOSINE	ANTIPSYCHOTICS	Risk of ventricular arrhythmias, particularly torsades de pointes, with phenothiazines and pimozide. There is also a theoretical risk of QT prolongation with the atypical antipsychotics	All of these drugs prolong the QT interval	Avoid coadministration of phenothiazines, amisulpride, pimozide, or sertindole with adenosine. Monitor the ECG closely when adenosine is coadministered with atypical antipsychotics
ADENOSINE	BRONCHODILATORS—THEOPHYLLINE	↓ Efficacy of adenosine	Theophylline and other xanthines are adenosine receptor antagonists	Watch for poor response to adenosine; higher doses may be required
AJMALINE				
AJMALINE	**DRUGS THAT PROLONG THE QT INTERVAL**			
AJMALINE	1. ANTIARRHYTHMICS—amiodarone, azimilide, cibenzoline, disopyramide, dofetilide, dronedarone, ibutilide, procainamide, propafenone, quinidine	Risk of ventricular arrhythmias, particularly torsades de pointes	Additive effect; these drugs prolong the QT interval	Avoid coadministration

(*Continued*)

Primary Drug	Secondary Drug	Effect	Mechanism	Precautions
ANTIARRHYTHMICS				
	2. ANTIBIOTICS—macrolides (especially azithromycin, clarithromycin, parenteral erythromycin, telithromycin), quinolones (especially moxifloxacin), quinupristin/dalfopristin 3. ANTICANCER AND IMMUNOMODULATING DRUGS—arsenic trioxide, bosutinib, crizotinib, dasatinib, eribulin, fingolimod, lapatinib, nilotinib, pazopanib, sunitinib, vandetanib, vemurafenib 4. ANTIDEPRESSANTS—TCAs, venlafaxine 5. ANTIEMETICS—ondansetron 6. ANTIFUNGALS—fluconazole, posaconazole, voriconazole 7. ANTIHISTAMINES—terfenadine, hydroxyzine, mizolastine 8. ANTIHYPERTENSIVES—ketanserin 9. ANTIMALARIALS—artemether with lumefantrine, chloroquine, halofantrine, hydroxychloroquine, mefloquine, quinine 10. ANTIPROTOZOALS—pentamidine isethionate 11. ANTIPSYCHOTICS—atypicals, phenothiazines, pimozide 12. ANTIVIRALS—boceprevir, rilpivirine, telaprevir 13. BETA-BLOCKERS—sotalol 14. BRONCHODILATORS—parenteral bronchodilators 15. CNS STIMULANTS—atomoxetine 16. RANOLAZINE			
AJMALINE	ANTIEPILEPTICS—PHENOBARBITAL	↓ Ajmaline levels	Unknown	Monitor PR, BP, ECG closely; watch for poor response to ajmaline

(*Continued*)

Primary Drug	Secondary Drug	Effect	Mechanism	Precautions
ANTIARRHYTHMICS				
AMIODARONE				
Amiodarone has a long half-life and therefore, interactions may persist for weeks after stopping therapy				
AMIODARONE	**DRUGS THAT PROLONG THE QT INTERVAL**			
AMIODARONE	1. ANTIARRHYTHMICS—ajmaline, azimilide, cibenzoline, disopyramide, dofetilide, dronedarone, ibutilide, procainamide, propafenone, quinidine 2. ANTIBIOTICS—macrolides (especially azithromycin, clarithromycin, parenteral erythromycin, telithromycin), quinolones (especially moxifloxacin), quinupristin/dalfopristin 3. ANTICANCER AND IMMUNOMODULATING DRUGS—arsenic trioxide, bosutinib, crizotinib, dasatinib, eribulin, fingolimod, lapatinib, nilotinib, pazopanib, sunitinib, vandetanib, vemurafenib 4. ANTIDEPRESSANTS—TCAs, venlafaxine 5. ANTIEMETICS—ondansetron 6. ANTIFUNGALS—fluconazole, posaconazole, voriconazole 7. ANTIHISTAMINES—terfenadine, hydroxyzine, mizolastine 8. ANTIHYPERTENSIVES—ketanserin 9. ANTIMALARIALS—artemether with lumefantrine, chloroquine, halofantrine, hydroxychloroquine, mefloquine, quinine 10. ANTIPROTOZOALS—pentamidine isethionate 11. ANTIPSYCHOTICS—atypicals, phenothiazines, pimozide 12. ANTIVIRALS—boceprevir, rilpivirine, telaprevir 13. BETA-BLOCKERS—sotalol	Risk of ventricular arrhythmias, particularly torsades de pointes	Additive effect; these drugs prolong the QT interval	Avoid coadministration

(*Continued*)

Primary Drug	Secondary Drug	Effect	Mechanism	Precautions
ANTIARRHYTHMICS				
	14. BRONCHODILATORS—parenteral bronchodilators 15. CNS STIMULANTS—atomoxetine 16. RANOLAZINE			
AMIODARONE	AGALSIDASE	↓ Clinical effect of agalsidase beta	Uncertain	Avoid coadministration
AMIODARONE	ANALGESICS—FENTANYL	Profound bradycardia, sinus arrest, and hypotension have reported	Exact mechanism is uncertain	Coadministration of fentanyl and amiodarone should be avoided wherever possible Fentanyl should not be used as an adjunct to sedation or analgesic in any patient who may reasonably be foreseen as requiring amiodarone. Fentanyl should never be administered following amiodarone administration
AMIODARONE	ANESTHETICS—GENERAL	Amiodarone may ↑ the myocardial depressant effects of inhalational anesthetics	Additive effect	Monitor PR, BP, and ECG closely
AMIODARONE	ANESTHETICS—LOCAL	Risk of ↓ BP	Additive myocardial depression	Particular care should be taken to avoid inadvertent intravenous administration during bupivacaine infiltration; monitor PR, BP, and ECG during epidural administration of bupivacaine
AMIODARONE	ANTIARRHYTHMICS			
AMIODARONE	ANTIARRHYTHMICS	Risk of bradycardia and ↓ BP	Additive myocardial depression	Monitor PR and BP closely
AMIODARONE	FLECAINIDE	↑ Plasma levels of flecainide	Amiodarone is a potent inhibitor of the CYP2D6-mediated metabolism of flecainide	↓ The dose of flecainide (by up to 50%)

(Continued)

		arrhythmias		
AMIODARONE	RIFAMPICIN	↓ Levels of amiodarone	Uncertain, but rifampicin is a known enzyme inducer and therefore may ↑ metabolism of amiodarone	Watch for a poor response to amiodarone
AMIODARONE	**ANTICANCER AND IMMUNOMODULATING DRUGS**			
AMIODARONE	AFATINIB	Possible increase in afatinib levels	P-glycoprotein inhibition	Manufacturer recommends staggered dosing 6–12 h apart or dose reduction
AMIODARONE	CICLOSPORIN	Ciclosporin levels may be ↑ by amiodarone; risk of nephrotoxicity	Uncertain; ciclosporin is metabolized by CYP3A4, which is markedly inhibited by amiodarone. Amiodarone also interferes with renal elimination of ciclosporin and inhibits intestinal Pgp, which may ↑ the bioavailability of ciclosporin	Monitor renal function closely; consider reducing the dose of ciclosporin when coadministering amiodarone
AMIODARONE	CORTICOSTEROIDS	Risk of arrhythmias	Cardiac toxicity directly related to hypokalemia	Monitor potassium levels every 4–6 weeks until stable, then at least annually
AMIODARONE	CYCLOPHOSPHAMIDE	Increased risk of pulmonary toxicity	Possible additive effect	Be aware of potential for increased pulmonary toxicity
AMIODARONE	CYTOTOXICS	↑ Risk of photosensitivity reactions	Attributed to additive effects	Avoid exposure of skin and eyes to direct sunlight for 30 days after porfimer therapy
AMIODARONE	SIROLIMUS, TACROLIMUS	Increased sirolimus and tacrolimus levels	CYP3A4 inhibition	Monitor closely
AMIODARONE	THALIDOMIDE	Possible increased risk of peripheral neuropathy	Additive	Manufacturer advises caution

(Continued)

DRUGS ACTING ON THE CARDIOVASCULAR SYSTEM ANTIARRHYTHMICS

Primary Drug	Secondary Drug	Effect	Mechanism	Precautions
ANTIARRHYTHMICS				
AMIODARONE	**ANTICOAGULANTS—ORAL**			
AMIODARONE	DABIGATRAN	↑ Dabigatran levels	Inhibition of Pgp	Reduce dose of dabigatran to 150 mg/day (75 mg in renal failure)
AMIODARONE	WARFARIN	Cases of bleeding within 4 weeks of starting amiodarone in patients previously stabilized on warfarin. The effect was seen to last up to 16 weeks after stopping amiodarone	Amiodarone inhibits CYP2C9- and CYP3A4-mediated metabolism of warfarin	↓ The dose of anticoagulant by 30%–50% and monitor INR closely for at least the first month of starting amiodarone and for 4 months after stopping amiodarone. If the INR suddenly ↑ after being initially stabilized, check TSH level
AMIODARONE	**ANTIDEPRESSANTS**			
AMIODARONE	LITHIUM	1. Rare risk of ventricular arrythmias, particularly torsades de pointes 2. Risk of hypothyroidism	1. Additive effect; lithium rarely causes QT prolongation 2. Additive effect; both drugs can cause hypothyroidism	1. Manufacturer of amiodarone recommends avoiding coadministration 2. If coadministration is thought to be necessary, watch for symptoms/signs of hypothyroidism; check TFTs every 3–6 months
AMIODARONE	SSRIs—SERTRALINE	Sertraline may ↑ amiodarone levels	Sertraline may inhibit CYP3A4-mediated metabolism of amiodarone	Watch for amiodarone toxicity; for those taking high doses of amiodarone, consider using an alternative SSRI with a lower affinity for CYP3A4
AMIODARONE	ANTIEPILEPTICS—PHENYTOIN	Phenytoin levels may be ↑ by amiodarone; conversely, amiodarone levels may be ↓ by phenytoin	Uncertain; amiodarone inhibits CYP2C9, which plays a role in phenytoin metabolism, while phenytoin is a known hepatic enzyme inducer. Also, amiodarone inhibits intestinal Pgp, which may ↑ the bioavailability of phenytoin	↓ Phenytoin dose by 25%–30% and monitor levels; watch for amiodarone toxicity. Note that phenytoin and amiodarone share similar features of toxicity, such as arrhythmias and ataxia

(*Continued*)

Primary Drug	Secondary Drug	Effect	Mechanism	Precautions
ANTIARRHYTHMICS				
AMIODARONE	ANTIHYPERTENSIVES AND HEART FAILURE DRUGS—ALISKIREN	Aliskiren levels ↑ by amiodarone	Amiodarone is a moderate Pgp inhibitor	Monitor BP and serum potassium at least weekly until stable
AMIODARONE	ANTIOBESITY DRUGS—ORLISTAT	Possible ↓ amiodarone levels	↓ Absorption of amiodarone	Watch for poor response to amiodarone
AMIODARONE	**ANTIVIRALS**			
AMIODARONE	ANTIVIRAL DRUGS—COBICISTAT	Theoretical risk of ↑ levels of amiodarone	Cobicistat inhibits CYP3A4	Monitor ECG closely
AMIODARONE	PROTEASE INHIBITORS	Amiodarone levels may be ↑ by protease inhibitors	Uncertain, but postulated to be due to ↓ metabolism of amiodarone	Watch closely for amiodarone toxicity; for those taking high doses of amiodarone, consider reducing the dose when starting protease inhibitor anti-HIV therapy
AMIODARONE	BETA-BLOCKERS	Risk of bradycardia (occasionally severe), ↓ BP and heart failure. Also, ↑ plasma levels of metoprolol	Additive negative inotropic and chronotropic effects. In addition, high-dose amiodarone is associated with ↑ plasma levels of metoprolol due to inhibition of CYP2D6	For patients on beta-blockers, monitor BP closely when loading with amiodarone
AMIODARONE	BRONCHODILATORS—THEOPHYLLINE	Theophylline levels may be ↑ by amiodarone (single case report of theophylline levels doubling)	Uncertain; amiodarone probably inhibits the metabolism of theophylline	Watch for theophylline toxicity; monitor levels regularly until stable
AMIODARONE	CALCIUM CHANNEL BLOCKERS	Risk of bradycardia, AV block, and ↓ BP when amiodarone is coadministered with diltiazem or verapamil	Additive negative inotropic and chronotropic effect. Also, amiodarone inhibits intestinal Pgp, which ↑ the bioavailability of diltiazem and verapamil	Monitor PR, BP, and ECG closely; watch for heart failure

(*Continued*)

Primary Drug	Secondary Drug	Effect	Mechanism	Precautions
ANTIARRHYTHMICS				
AMIODARONE	**CARDIAC GLYCOSIDES**			
AMIODARONE	DIGOXIN	Amiodarone may ↑ plasma levels of digoxin (in some cases up to fourfold)	Uncertain; thought to be due to inhibition of Pgp-mediated renal clearance of digoxin. Amiodarone is also known to inhibit intestinal Pgp, which may ↑ the bioavailability of digoxin	↓ Digoxin dose by one-third to one-half when starting amiodarone. Monitor digoxin levels; watch for digoxin toxicity, especially for ↓ weeks after initiating or adjusting amiodarone therapy
AMIODARONE	DIGITOXIN	Reports of digitoxin toxicity in two patients on digitoxin after starting amiodarone	Uncertain; thought to be due to inhibition of Pgp-mediated renal clearance of digoxin	Watch for digitoxin toxicity
AMIODARONE	**DIURETICS**			
AMIODARONE	CARBONIC ANHYDRASE ANTAGONISTS, LOOP DIURETICS, THIAZIDES	Risk of arrhythmias	Cardiac toxicity directly related to hypokalemia	Monitor potassium levels every 4–6 weeks until stable, then at least annually
AMIODARONE	POTASSIUM-SPARING DIURETICS	Risk of ↑ levels of eplerenone with amiodarone; risk of hyperkalemia directly related to serum levels	Potassium channel blockers inhibit CYP3A4-mediated metabolism of eplerenone	Restrict dose of eplerenone to 25 mg/day. Monitor serum potassium concentrations closely; watch for hyperkalemia
AMIODARONE	DRUG DEPENDENCE THERAPIES—BUPROPION	↑ Plasma concentrations of amiodarone, with risk of toxic effects	Bupropion and its metabolite hydroxybupropion inhibit CYP2D6	Initiate therapy of these drugs at the lowest effective dose
AMIODARONE	GRAPEFRUIT JUICE	Possibly ↓ effect of amiodarone. Torsade de pointes reported with high volumes of GFJ	Inhibition of CYP3A4-mediated metabolism of amiodarone to its active metabolite	Warn patients to avoid GFJ; if amiodarone becomes less effective, ask the patient about GFJ ingestion

(*Continued*)

Primary Drug	Secondary Drug	Effect	Mechanism	Precautions
ANTIARRHYTHMICS				
AMIODARONE	H2 RECEPTOR BLOCKERS	Cimetidine may ↑ amiodarone levels	Uncertain	Monitor PR and BP at least weekly until stable. Warn patients to report symptoms of hypotension (light-headedness, dizziness on standing, etc.). Consider alternative acid suppression therapy
AMIODARONE	IVABRADINE	Risk of arrhythmias	Additive effect	Monitor ECG closely
AMIODARONE	LAXATIVES—STIMULANT	Risk of arrhythmias	Cardiac toxicity directly related to hypokalemia	Manufacturers recommend using alternative laxatives
AMIODARONE	**LIPID-LOWERING DRUGS**			
AMIODARONE	ANION EXCHANGE RESINS	Cholestyramine ↓ amiodarone levels	Cholestyramine binds amiodarone, reducing its absorption and interrupting its enterohepatic circulation	Avoid coadministration
AMIODARONE	STATINS—SIMVASTATIN, ATORVASTATIN	↑ Risk of myopathy with high doses (>40 mg daily) of simvastatin	Amiodarone inhibits CYP3A4-mediated metabolism of these statins. It inhibits intestinal Pgp, which may ↑ the bioavailability of statins	Avoid >20 mg daily doses of simvastatin in patients taking amiodarone; if higher doses are required, switch to an alternative statin
AMIODARONE	OXYGEN	Risk of pulmonary toxicity (adult respiratory distress syndrome) in patients on amiodarone who were ventilated with 100% oxygen during surgery	Uncertain	Manufacturers recommend that, for patients on amiodarone undergoing surgery, the lowest possible oxygen concentrations to achieve adequate oxygenation should be given
AMIODARONE	PIRFENIDONE	↑ Pirfenidone levels	Inhibition of metabolism of pirfenidone	Manufacturer recommends avoiding coadministration
AMIODARONE	THYROID HORMONES	Risk of either under- or overtreatment of thyroid function	Amiodarone contains iodine and has been reported to cause both hyperthyroidism and hypothyroidism	Monitor triiodothyronine, thyroxine, and TSH levels at least 6 months

(*Continued*)

Primary Drug	Secondary Drug	Effect	Mechanism	Precautions
ANTIARRHYTHMICS				
AMIODARONE	URINARY ALKALINIZERS—AMMONIUM CHLORIDE, SODIUM BICARBONATE	Urinary alkalinization ↑ amiodarone levels	Amiodarone excretion ↓ in the presence of an alkaline urine; amiodarone exists in predominantly a nonionic form, which is more readily reabsorbed from the renal tubules	Monitor PR and BP closely
AZIMILIDE				
AZIMILIDE	**DRUGS THAT PROLONG THE QT INTERVAL**			
AZIMILIDE	1. ANTIARRHYTHMICS—ajmaline, amiodarone, cibenzoline, disopyramide, dofetilide, dronedarone, ibutilide, procainamide, propafenone, quinidine 2. ANTIBIOTICS—macrolides (especially azithromycin, clarithromycin, parenteral erythromycin, telithromycin), quinolones (especially moxifloxacin), quinupristin/dalfopristin 3. ANTICANCER AND IMMUNOMODULATING DRUGS—arsenic trioxide, bosutinib, crizotinib, dasatinib, eribulin, fingolimod, lapatinib, nilotinib, pazopanib, sunitinib, vandetanib, vemurafenib 4. ANTIDEPRESSANTS—TCAs, venlafaxine 5. ANTIEMETICS—ondansetron 6. ANTIFUNGALS—fluconazole, posaconazole, voriconazole 7. ANTIHISTAMINES—terfenadine, hydroxyzine, mizolastine 8. ANTIHYPERTENSIVES—ketanserin 9. ANTIMALARIALS—artemether with lumefantrine, chloroquine, halofantrine, hydroxychloroquine, mefloquine, quinine	Risk of ventricular arrhythmias, particularly torsades de pointes	Additive effect; these drugs prolong the QT interval	Avoid coadministration

(*Continued*)

Primary Drug	Secondary Drug	Effect	Mechanism	Precautions
ANTIARRHYTHMICS				
	10. ANTIPROTOZOALS—pentamidine isethionate 11. ANTIPSYCHOTICS—atypicals, phenothiazines, pimozide 12. ANTIVIRALS—boceprevir, rilpivirine, telaprevir 13. BETA-BLOCKERS—sotalol 14. BRONCHODILATORS—parenteral bronchodilators 15. CNS STIMULANTS—atomoxetine 16. RANOLAZINE			
CIBENZOLINE				
CIBENZOLINE	**DRUGS THAT PROLONG THE QT INTERVAL**			
CIBENZOLINE	1. ANTIARRHYTHMICS—ajmaline, amiodarone, azimilide, disopyramide, dofetilide, dronedarone, ibutilide, procainamide, propafenone, quinidine 2. ANTIBIOTICS—macrolides (especially azithromycin, clarithromycin, parenteral erythromycin, telithromycin), quinolones (especially moxifloxacin), quinupristin/dalfopristin 3. ANTICANCER AND IMMUNOMODULATING DRUGS—arsenic trioxide, bosutinib, crizotinib, dasatinib, eribulin, fingolimod, lapatinib, nilotinib, pazopanib, sunitinib, vandetanib, vemurafenib 4. ANTIDEPRESSANTS—TCAs, venlafaxine 5. ANTIEMETICS—ondansetron 6. ANTIFUNGALS—fluconazole, posaconazole, voriconazole 7. ANTIHISTAMINES—terfenadine, hydroxyzine, mizolastine	Risk of ventricular arrhythmias, particularly torsades de pointes	Additive effect; these drugs prolong the QT interval	Avoid coadministration

(Continued)

Primary Drug	Secondary Drug	Effect	Mechanism	Precautions
ANTIARRHYTHMICS				
	8. ANTIHYPERTENSIVES—ketanserin 9. ANTIMALARIALS—artemether with lumefantrine, chloroquine, halofantrine, hydroxychloroquine, mefloquine, quinine 10. ANTIPROTOZOALS—pentamidine isethionate 11. ANTIPSYCHOTICS—atypicals, phenothiazines, pimozide 12. ANTIVIRALS—boceprevir, rilpivirine, telaprevir 13. BETA-BLOCKERS—sotalol 14. BRONCHODILATORS—parenteral bronchodilators 15. CNS STIMULANTS—atomoxetine 16. RANOLAZINE			
DISOPYRAMIDE				
DISOPYRAMIDE	**DRUGS THAT PROLONG THE QT INTERVAL**			
DISOPYRAMIDE	1. ANTIARRHYTHMICS—ajmaline, amiodarone, azimilide, cibenzoline, dofetilide, dronedarone, ibutilide, procainamide, propafenone, quinidine 2. ANTIBIOTICS—macrolides (especially azithromycin, clarithromycin, parenteral erythromycin, telithromycin), quinolones (especially moxifloxacin), quinupristin/dalfopristin 3. ANTICANCER AND IMMUNOMODULATING DRUGS—arsenic trioxide, bosutinib, crizotinib, dasatinib, eribulin, fingolimod, lapatinib, nilotinib, pazopanib, sunitinib, vandetanib, vemurafenib 4. ANTIDEPRESSANTS—TCAs, venlafaxine 5. ANTIEMETICS—ondansetron 6. ANTIFUNGALS—fluconazole, posaconazole, voriconazole	Risk of ventricular arrhythmias, particularly torsades de pointes	Additive effect; these drugs prolong the QT interval	Avoid coadministration

(*Continued*)

Primary Drug	Secondary Drug	Effect	Mechanism	Precautions
ANTIARRHYTHMICS				
	7. ANTIHISTAMINES—terfenadine, hydroxyzine, mizolastine 8. ANTIHYPERTENSIVES—ketanserin 9. ANTIMALARIALS—artemether with lumefantrine, chloroquine, halofantrine, hydroxychloroquine, mefloquine, quinine 10. ANTIPROTOZOALS—pentamidine isethionate 11. ANTIPSYCHOTICS—atypicals, phenothiazines, pimozide 12. ANTIVIRALS—boceprevir, rilpivirine, telaprevir 13. BETA-blockers—sotalol 14. BRONCHODILATORS—parenteral bronchodilators 15. CNS STIMULANTS—atomoxetine 16. RANOLAZINE			
DISOPYRAMIDE	**DRUGS WITH ANTIMUSCARINIC EFFECTS**			
DISOPYRAMIDE	1. ANALGESICS—nefopam 2. ANTIARRHYTHMICS—propafenone 3. ANTI DEPRESSANTS—TCAs 4. ANTIEMETICS—cyclizine 5. ANTIHISTAMINES—chlorphenamine, cyprohep tadine, hydroxyzine 6. ANTIMUSCARINICS—atropine, benztropine, cyclopentolate, dicycloverine, flavoxate, homatropine, hyoscine, orphenadrine, oxybutynin, procyclidines, propantheline, tolterodine, trihexyphenidyl, tropicamide 7. ANTI-PARKINSON'S DRUGS—DOPAMINERGICS 8. ANTIPSYCHOTICS—phenolthiazines, clozapine, pimozide 9. MUSCLE RELAXANTS—baclofen 10. NITRATES—isosorbide dinitrate	↑ Risk of antimuscarinic side effects. *NB ↓ efficacy of sublingual nitrate tablets*	Additive effect; both drugs cause antimuscarinic side effects. *Antimuscarinic effects ↓ salivary production, which ↓ dissolution of the tablet*	Warn patient of this additive effect. *Consider changing the formulation to a sublingual nitrate spray*

(Continued)

Primary Drug	Secondary Drug	Effect	Mechanism	Precautions
ANTIARRHYTHMICS				
DISOPYRAMIDE	ANESTHETICS—LOCAL	Risk of ↓ BP	Additive myocardial depression	Particular care should be taken to avoid inadvertent intravenous administration during bupivacaine infiltration; monitor PR, BP, and ECG during epidural administration of bupivacaine
DISOPYRAMIDE	ANALGESICS	Disopyramide may slow the onset of action of intermittent dose paracetamol	These drugs have anticholinergic effects that include delayed gastric emptying. This will delay absorption	Warn patients that the action of paracetamol may be delayed. This will not be the case when paracetamol is taken regularly
DISOPYRAMIDE	ANTIARRHYTHMICS	Risk of bradycardia and ↓ BP	Additive effects; antiarrhythmics are myocardial depressants	Monitor PR, BP, and ECG closely
DISOPYRAMIDE	ANTIBIOTICS—RIFAMPICIN	Disopyramide levels are ↓ by rifampicin	Rifampicin induces hepatic metabolism of disopyramide	Watch for poor response to disopyramide; check serum levels if necessary
DISOPYRAMIDE	ANTICANCER AND IMMUNOMODULATING DRUGS—CORTICOSTEROIDS	Risk of hypokalemia	Additive effect	Monitor potassium levels closely
DISOPYRAMIDE	ANTIDIABETIC DRUGS	↑ Risk of hypoglycemic episodes, particularly in patients with impaired renal function. Hypoglycemic attacks may occur even when plasma levels of disopyramide are within the normal range (attacks occurring with plasma disopyramide levels of 1–4 ng/mL)	Disopyramide and its metabolite mono-isopropyl disopyramide ↑ secretion of insulin (considered to be due to inhibition of potassium-ATP channels). Suggestion that disopyramide causes an impairment of the counterregulatory (homeostatic) mechanisms that follow hypoglycemia	In patients receiving antidiabetic drugs, start with the lowest dose of disopyramide if there is no alternative. Measure creatinine clearance. If creatinine clearance is 40 mL/min or less, the dose of disopyramide should not exceed 100 mg and should be administered once daily if creatinine clearance is less than 15 mL/min ➢ ***For signs and symptoms of hypoglycemia, see Clinical Features of Some Adverse Drug Interactions, Hypoglycemia***

(*Continued*)

Primary Drug	Secondary Drug	Effect	Mechanism	Precautions
ANTIARRHYTHMICS				
DISOPYRAMIDE	ANTIEPILEPTICS—BARBITURATES, PHENYTOIN	Disopyramide levels are ↓ by phenobarbital, primidone, and phenytoin	Induction of hepatic metabolism	Monitor PR and BP weekly until stable
DISOPYRAMIDE	**ANTIVIRALS**			
DISOPYRAMIDE	ANTIVIRAL DRUGS—COBICISTAT	Theoretical risk of ↑ levels of disopyramide	Cobicistat inhibits CYP3A4	Monitor ECG closely
DISOPYRAMIDE	PROTEASE INHIBITORS	Disopyramide levels may be ↑ by protease inhibitors, possible ↑ side effects	Inhibition of CYP3A4-mediated metabolism of disopyramide	Avoid coadministration with saquinavir. Watch closely for disopyramide toxicity and cardiac and neurological side effects
DISOPYRAMIDE	BETA-BLOCKERS	Risk of bradycardia (occasionally severe), ↓ BP, and heart failure	Additive negative inotropic and chronotropic effects	Monitor PR, BP, and ECG at least weekly until stable; watch for development of heart failure
DISOPYRAMIDE	CALCIUM CHANNEL BLOCKERS	Risk of myocardial depression and asystole when disopyramide is coadministered with verapamil, particularly in the presence of heart failure	Disopyramide is a myocardial depressant like verapamil and can cause ventricular tachycardia, ventricular fibrillation, or torsades de pointes	Avoid coadministering verapamil with disopyramide if possible. If single-agent therapy is ineffective, monitor PR, BP, and ECG closely; watch for heart failure
DISOPYRAMIDE	DIURETICS—CARBONIC ANHYDRASE INHIBITORS, LOOP DIURETICS, THIAZIDES	Risk of hypokalemia	Additive effect	Monitor potassium levels closely
DISOPYRAMIDE	GRAPEFRUIT JUICE	Possibly ↓ effect of disopyramide	Likely to be due to inhibited CYP3A4-mediated metabolism of disopyramide	Monitor ECG and side effects more closely
DISOPYRAMIDE	IVABRADINE	Risk of arrhythmias	Additive effect	Monitor ECG closely

(*Continued*)

DRUGS ACTING ON THE CARDIOVASCULAR SYSTEM ANTIARRHYTHMICS Disopyramide

DRUGS ACTING ON THE CARDIOVASCULAR SYSTEM ANTIARRHYTHMICS Dofetilide

Primary Drug	Secondary Drug	Effect	Mechanism	Precautions
ANTIARRHYTHMICS				
DOFETILIDE				
DOFETILIDE	**DRUGS THAT PROLONG THE QT INTERVAL**			
DOFETILIDE	1. ANTIARRHYTHMICS—ajmaline, amiodarone, azimilide, cibenzoline, disopyramide, dronedarone, ibutilide, procainamide, propafenone, quinidine 2. ANTIBIOTICS—macrolides (especially azithromycin, clarithromycin, parenteral erythromycin, telithromycin), quinolones (especially moxifloxacin), quinupristin/dalfopristin 3. ANTICANCER AND IMMUNOMODULATING DRUGS—arsenic trioxide, bosutinib, crizotinib, dasatinib, eribulin, fingolimod, lapatinib, nilotinib, pazopanib, sunitinib, vandetanib, vemurafenib 4. ANTIDEPRESSANTS—TCAs, venlafaxine 5. ANTIEMETICS—ondansetron 6. ANTIFUNGALS—fluconazole, posaconazole, voriconazole 7. ANTIHISTAMINES—terfenadine, hydroxyzine, mizolastine 8. ANTIHYPERTENSIVES—ketanserin 9. ANTIMALARIALS—artemether with lumefantrine, chloroquine, halofantrine, hydroxychloroquine, mefloquine, quinine 10. ANTIPROTOZOALS—pentamidine isethionate 11. ANTIPSYCHOTICS—atypicals, phenothiazines, pimozide 12. ANTIVIRALS—boceprevir, rilpivirine, telaprevir 13. BETA-BLOCKERS—sotalol	Risk of ventricular arrhythmias, particularly torsades de pointes	Additive effect; these drugs prolong the QT interval	Avoid coadministration

(*Continued*)

Primary Drug	Secondary Drug	Effect	Mechanism	Precautions
ANTIARRHYTHMICS				
	14. BRONCHODILATORS—parenteral bronchodilators 15. CNS STIMULANTS—atomoxetine 16. RANOLAZINE			
DOFETILIDE	ANTIBIOTICS—TRIMETHOPRIM	↑ Dofetilide levels with risk of ↑ QT prolongation	Trimethoprim reduces renal excretion of dofetilide	Avoid coadministration
DOFETILIDE	ANTICANCER AND OTHER IMMUNOMODULATING DRUGS—MEGESTROL	↑ Dofetilide levels with risk of ↑ QT prolongation	Megestrol reduces renal excretion of dofetilide	Avoid coadministration
DOFETILIDE	ANTIEMETICS—PROCHLORPERAZINE	↑ Dofetilide levels with risk of ↑ QT prolongation	Prochlorperazine reduces renal excretion of dofetilide	Avoid coadministration
DOFETILIDE	ANTIFUNGALS—KETOCONAZOLE	↑ Dofetilide levels with risk of ↑ QT prolongation	Ketoconazole inhibits CYP3A4-mediated metabolism; it also inhibits renal excretion of dofetilide	Avoid coadministration
DOFETILIDE	**ANTIVIRALS**			
DOFETILIDE	DOLUTEGRAVIR	Possible ↑ plasma concentration of dofetilide, risk of toxicity	Inhibition of transport via OCT2	Avoid coadministration
DOFETILIDE	PROTEASE INHIBITORS	Risk of ↑ dofetilide levels with risk of ↑ QT prolongation	PIs inhibit CYP3A4-mediated metabolism of dofetilide	Avoid coadministration
DOFETILIDE	CALCIUM CHANNEL BLOCKERS—DILTIAZEM, VERAPAMIL	Risk of ↑ dofetilide levels with risk of ↑ QT prolongation	Diltiazem and verapamil inhibits CYP3A4-mediated metabolism of dofetilide	Avoid coadministration
DOFETILIDE	DIURETICS—HYDROCHLOROTHIAZIDE	↑ Dofetilide levels with risk of ↑ QT prolongation	Unknown	Avoid coadministration
DOFETILIDE	GRAPEFRUIT JUICE	Risk of ↑ dofetilide levels with risk of ↑ QT prolongation	Grapefruit juice inhibits CYP3A4-mediated metabolism of dofetilide	Avoid coadministration

(Continued)

Primary Drug	Secondary Drug	Effect	Mechanism	Precautions
ANTIARRHYTHMICS				
DOFETILIDE	H2-RECEPTOR BLOCKERS—CIMETIDINE	↑ Dofetilide levels with risk of ↑ QT prolongation	Cimetidineinhibits CYP3A4-mediated metabolism; it also inhibits renal excretion of dofetilide	Avoid coadministration
DRONEDARONE				
DRONEDARONE	**DRUGS THAT PROLONG THE QT INTERVAL**			
DRONEDARONE	1. ANTIARRHYTHMICS—ajmaline, amiodarone, azimilide, cibenzoline, disopyramide, dofetilide, ibutilide, procainamide, propafenone, quinidine 2. ANTIBIOTICS—macrolides (especially azithromycin, clarithromycin, parenteral erythromycin, telithromycin), quinolones (especially moxifloxacin), quinupristin/dalfopristin 3. ANTICANCER AND IMMUNOMODULATING DRUGS—arsenic trioxide, bosutinib, crizotinib, dasatinib, eribulin, fingolimod, lapatinib, nilotinib, pazopanib, sunitinib, vandetanib, vemurafenib, vemurafenib 4. ANTIDEPRESSANTS—TCAs, venlafaxine 5. ANTIEMETICS—ondansetron 6. ANTIFUNGALS—fluconazole, posaconazole, voriconazole 7. ANTIHISTAMINES—terfenadine, hydroxyzine, mizolastine 8. ANTIHYPERTENSIVES—ketanserin 9. ANTIMALARIALS—artemether with lumefantrine, chloroquine, halofantrine, hydroxychloroquine, mefloquine, quinine 10. ANTIPROTOZOALS—pentamidine isethionate 11. ANTIPSYCHOTICS—atypicals, phenothiazines, pimozide	Risk of ventricular arrhythmias, particularly torsades de pointes	Additive effect; these drugs prolong the QT interval	Avoid coadministration

(Continued)

Primary Drug	Secondary Drug	Effect	Mechanism	Precautions
ANTIARRHYTHMICS				
	12. ANTIVIRALS—boceprevir, rilpivirine, telaprevir 13. BETA-BLOCKERS—sotalol 14. BRONCHODILATORS—parenteral bronchodilators 15. CNS STIMULANTS—atomoxetine 16. RANOLAZINE			
DRONEDARONE	ANTIBIOTICS—RIFAMPICIN	Risk of ↓ levels of dronedarone	Rifampicin increases CYP3A4-mediated metabolism of dronedarone	Watch for poor response to dronedarone
DRONEDARONE	**ANTICANCER AND IMMUNOMODULATING DRUGS**			
DRONEDARONE	BOSUTINIB	Increased bosutinib levels	CYP3A inhibition	Manufacturer advises to avoid concurrent use. If not possible, interruption of therapy or dose reduction should be considered
DRONEDARONE	EVEROLIMUS	Predicted increase in everolimus levels	CYP3A4 inhibition P-glycoprotein inhibition	Monitor closely with concurrent use
DRONEDARONE	SIROLIMUS AND TACROLIMUS	↑ Plasma levels of sirolimus and possibly tacrolimus	Dronedarone inhibits CYP3A4-mediated metabolism of sirolimus and tacrolimus	Monitor blood sirolimus and tacrolimus levels closely
DRONEDARONE	TEMSIROLIMUS	Predicted increase in temsirolimus levels	CYP3A4 inhibition P-glycoprotein inhibition	Monitor closely with concurrent use
DRONEDARONE	**ANTICOAGULANTS—ORAL**			
DRONEDARONE	DABIGATRAN	↑ Dabigatran levels	Possible inhibition of Pgp. Coadministration increases dabigatran exposure by 70%–140%; when dronedarone administered 2 h after dabigatran, exposure increased only 30%–60%	Reduce dose of dabigatran to 150 mg/day (75 mg in renal failure)

(Continued)

Primary Drug	Secondary Drug	Effect	Mechanism	Precautions
ANTIARRHYTHMICS				
DRONEDARONE	RIVAROXABAN	No information on specific effect with rivaroxaban	No specific information relating to mechanism	Manufacturer of rivaroxaban advises to avoid concomitant use with dronedarone
DRONEDARONE	WARFARIN	Case reports of ↑ INR when dronedarone given with warfarin	Likely inhibition of metabolism of warfarin	Monitor INRs closely until stable in patients on warfarin when starting and stopping dronedarone
DRONEDARONE	**ANTIDEPRESSANTS**			
DRONEDARONE	SSRIs	Risk of ↑ plasma levels of SSRIs	Dronedarone inhibits CYP2D6-metabolism SSRIs	Warn patients to report about symptoms of SSRI toxicity, e.g., GI effects and anorexia. Reduce dose accordingly
DRONEDARONE	ST. JOHN'S WORT	Risk of ↓ levels of dronedarone	St. John's wort induces the hepatic metabolism of dronedarone	Watch for poor response to dronedarone
DRONEDARONE	ANTIEPILEPTICS—BARBITURATES, CARBAMAZEPINE, PHENYTOIN	Risk of ↓ levels of dronedarone	These antiepileptics induce the hepatic metabolism of dronedarone	Monitor PR and BP weekly until stable
DRONEDARONE	**ANTIVIRALS**			
DRONEDARONE	COBICISTAT	Theoretical risk of ↑ levels of dronedarone	Cobicistat inhibits CYP3A4	Monitor ECG closely
DRONEDARONE	MARAVIROC	Possible ↑ plasma levels dronedarone	Inhibition of metabolism via CYP3A	Avoid coadministration
DRONEDARONE	RITONAVIR	Marked ↑ levels of dronedarone	Ritonavir strongly inhibits CYP3A4-mediated metabolism of dronedarone	Manufacturer of dronedarone recommends avoiding coadministration
DRONEDARONE	BETA-BLOCKERS	Risk of bradycardia (occasionally severe), ↓ BP and heart failure. Also, ↑ plasma levels of metoprolol and propranolol	Additive negative inotropic and chronotropic effects. In addition, dronedarone inhibits CYP2D6-metabolism of metoprolol and propranolol	Monitor PR, BP, and ECG closely; watch for development of heart failure. Watch for propranolol and metoprolol toxicity; ↓ doses accordingly

(*Continued*)

Primary Drug	Secondary Drug	Effect	Mechanism	Precautions
ANTIARRHYTHMICS				
DRONEDARONE	**CALCIUM CHANNEL BLOCKERS**			
DRONEDARONE	DIHYDROPYRIDINES	↑ Levels of nifedipine and possibly other dihydropyridines	Dronedarone inhibits their metabolism	Monitor BP closely
DRONEDARONE	DILTIAZEM, VERAPAMIL	Risk of excessive bradycardia	Additive effect on slowing AV conduction	Monitor PR and BP closely. Cardiac monitoring is essential when giving calcium channel blockers parenterally (which should be administered slowly)
DRONEDARONE	CARDIAC GLYCOSIDES—DIGOXIN	Risk of excessive bradycardia and myocardial depression	Additive effect. In addition, dronedarone inhibits Pgp	Monitor PR and BP closely. Use lowest doses of these drugs and titrate carefully. Monitor digoxin levels
DRONEDARONE	GRAPEFRUIT JUICE	↑ Levels of dronedarone	Grapefruit juice inhibits CYP3A4-mediated metabolism of dronedarone	Warn patient to avoid GFJ while taking dronedarone
DRONEDARONE	LIPID-LOWERING DRUGS—STATINS	↑ Plasma levels of atorvastatin and simvastatin	Dronedarone inhibits CYP3A4-mediated metabolism of these statins	Titrate these statins slowly—warn the patient to look for signs of myopathy. Alternatively, consider an alternative statin
FLECAINIDE				
FLECAINIDE	AMMONIUM CHLORIDE	Urinary acidification ↓ flecainide levels	Flecainide excretion is ↑ in the presence of an acidic urine; flecainide exists in predominantly ionic form, which is less readily reabsorbed from the renal tubules	Watch for a poor response to flecainide

(Continued)

Primary Drug	Secondary Drug	Effect	Mechanism	Precautions
ANTIARRHYTHMICS				
FLECAINIDE	ANESTHETICS—LOCAL	Risk of ↓ BP	Additive myocardial depression	Particular care should be taken to avoid inadvertent intravenous administration during bupivacaine infiltration; monitor PR, BP, and ECG during epidural administration of bupivacaine
FLECAINIDE	**ANALGESICS**			
FLECAINIDE	NSAIDs	Parecoxib may ↑ flecainide levels	Parecoxib weakly inhibits CYP2D6-mediated metabolism of flecainide	Monitor PR and BP closely. If possible, use only short courses of NSAID
FLECAINIDE	OPIOIDS	Methadone and tramadol may ↑ flecainide levels	Methadone and tramadol inhibit CYP2D6-mediated metabolism of flecainide	Monitor PR and BP closely
FLECAINIDE	**ANTIARRHYTHMICS**			
FLECAINIDE	ANTIARRHYTHMICS	Risk of bradycardia and ↓ BP	Additive myocardial depression	Monitor PR and BP closely; watch for flecainide toxicity
FLECAINIDE	AMIODARONE	↑ Plasma levels of flecainide	Amiodarone is a potent inhibitor of CYP2D6-mediated metabolism of flecainide	↓ The dose of flecainide (by up to 50%)
FLECAINIDE	**ANTICANCER AND IMMUNOMODULATING DRUGS**			
FLECAINIDE	CORTICOSTEROIDS	Risk of arrhythmias	Cardiac toxicity is directly related to hypokalemia	Monitor potassium levels closely; watch for hypokalemia
FLECAINIDE	IMATINIB	Imatinib may cause an ↑ in plasma concentrations of flecainide with a risk of toxic effects, e.g., visual disturbances, dyspnea, liver dysfunction	Imatinib is a potent inhibitor of CYP2D6 isoenzymes, which metabolize flecainide	Monitor for clinical efficacy and toxicity of flecainide. Monitor liver function and BP, and do FBCs if toxicity is suspected

(*Continued*)

Primary Drug	Secondary Drug	Effect	Mechanism	Precautions
ANTIARRHYTHMICS				
FLECAINIDE	**ANTIDEPRESSANTS**			
FLECAINIDE	DULOXETINE	Duloxetine may ↑ flecainide levels	Duloxetine moderately inhibits CYP2D6, which metabolizes flecainide	Monitor PR and BP at least weekly until stable
FLECAINIDE	SSRIs	SSRIs may ↑ flecainide levels	SSRIs inhibit CYP2D6-mediated metabolism of flecainide	Monitor PR and BP closely; watch for flecainide toxicity ECG prior to treatment and repeated until stable
FLECAINIDE	TCAs	Risk of arrhythmias	Additive effect; both drugs may be proarrhythmogenic. In addition, amitriptyline and clomipramine may inhibit CYP2D6-mediated metabolism of flecainide	Monitor PR, BP, and ECG closely; watch for flecainide toxicity
FLECAINIDE	ANTIEMETICS—5-HT3-ANTAGONISTS	Risk of arrhythmias	Additive effect	Manufacturers recommend avoiding coadministration of flecainide with ondansetron. Caution with other 5-HT3-antagonists; monitor ECG closely
FLECAINIDE	ANTIFUNGALS—TERBINAFINE	↑ Flecainide levels	Inhibition of CYP2D6 mediated metabolism	Monitor PR and BP closely until stable
FLECAINIDE	ANTIHISTAMINES—TERFENADINE, HYDROXYZINE, MIZOLASTINE	Risk of arrhythmias	Additive effect	Avoid coadministration
FLECAINIDE	**ANTIMALARIALS**			
FLECAINIDE	ARTEMETHER/LUMEFANTRINE	Risk of arrhythmias	Additive effect	Avoid coadministration
FLECAINIDE	QUININE	Quinine may ↑ flecainide levels	Quinine inhibits CYP2D6-mediated metabolism of flecainide	The effect seems to be slight, but watch for flecainide toxicity; monitor PR and BP closely
FLECAINIDE	ANTIOBESITY—LORCASERIN	↑ Blood concentrations of flecainide	Inhibition of CYP2D6-mediated metabolism	Monitor PR, BP, and ECG closely until stable

(Continued)

Primary Drug	Secondary Drug	Effect	Mechanism	Precautions
ANTIARRHYTHMICS				
FLECAINIDE	ANTIPSYCHOTICS—PHENOTHIAZINES, AMISULPRIDE, CLOZAPINE, PIMOZIDE, SERTINDOLE	Risk of arrhythmias	Additive effect. Also, haloperidol and thioridazine inhibit CYP2D6-mediated metabolism of flecainide	Avoid coadministration
FLECAINIDE	**ANTIVIRALS**			
FLECAINIDE	COBICISTAT	Theoretical risk of ↑ levels of flecainide	Cobicistat inhibits CYP3A4	Monitor ECG closely
FLECAINIDE	PROTEASE INHIBITORS	Fosamprenavir, ritonavir and possibly saquinavir and tipranavir with ritonavir ↑ flecainide levels, with risk of ventricular arrhythmias	Uncertain; possibly inhibition of CYP3A4- and CYP2D6-mediated metabolism of flecainide	Manufacturers recommend avoiding coadministration of flecainide with amprenavir, ritonavir, and saquinavir
FLECAINIDE	BETA-BLOCKERS	Risk of bradycardia (occasionally severe), ↓ BP and heart failure. Note, a single case report has described bradycardia when timolol eye drops were given to a patient on flecainide	Additive negative inotropic and chronotropic effects	Monitor PR, BP, and ECG closely; watch for development of heart failure
FLECAINIDE	CALCIUM CHANNEL BLOCKERS	Risk of heart block and ↓ BP when flecainide is coadministered with verapamil. A single case of asystole has been reported	Additive negative inotropic and chronotropic effect	Monitor PR, BP, and ECG at least weekly until stable; watch for heart failure
FLECAINIDE	**DIURETICS**			
FLECAINIDE	CARBONIC ANHYDRASE INHIBITORS	Risk of ↑ myocardial depression. In addition, flecainide excretion is reduced in an alkaline urine	Cardiac toxicity is directly related to hypokalemia. Flecainide is in an ionized form in an alkaline environment, which is more readily reabsorbed from the renal tubule	Monitor potassium levels closely

(*Continued*)

Primary Drug	Secondary Drug	Effect	Mechanism	Precautions
ANTIARRHYTHMICS				
FLECAINIDE	LOOP DIURETICS, THIAZIDES	Risk of arrhythmias	Cardiac toxicity is directly related to hypokalemia	Monitor potassium levels closely; watch for hypokalemia
FLECAINIDE	DRUG DEPENDENCE THERAPIES—BUPROPION	↑ Levels of flecainide	Bupropion may inhibit CYP2D6-mediated metabolism of flecainide	Monitor PR and BP closely; start flecainide at the lowest dose for patients taking bupropion
FLECAINIDE	H2 RECEPTOR BLOCKERS	Cimetidine may ↑ flecainide levels	Cimetidine inhibits CYP2D6-mediated metabolism of flecainide. Ranitidine is a much weaker CYP2D6 inhibitor	Monitor PR and BP at least weekly until stable. Warn patients to report symptoms of hypotension (light-headedness, dizziness on standing, etc.). Consider alternative acid suppression therapy
FLECAINIDE	MIRABEGRON	↑ Flecainide and propafenone levels	Mirabegron inhibits CYP2D6. These drugs have a narrow therapeutic index	Manufacturer advises caution in coadministration. Warn patients to report symptoms such as dizziness, chest pain, or palpitations
FLECAINIDE	RANOLAZINE	Possible ↑ flecainide levels	Inhibition of CYP2D6 mediated metabolism of flecainide	Monitor PR and BP closely
FLECAINIDE	SODIUM BICARBONATE	Urinary alkalinization ↑ flecainide levels	Flecainide excretion is ↓ in the presence of an alkaline urine; flecainide exists in predominantly nonionic form, which is more readily reabsorbed from the renal tubules	Monitor PR and BP closely
FLECAINIDE	TOBACCO SMOKE	Flecainide levels lower in smokers	Uncertain; postulated that hepatic metabolism ↑ by a component of tobacco smoke	Watch for poor response to flecainide and ↑ the dose accordingly (studies have suggested that smokers need up to 20% higher doses)

(Continued)

Primary Drug	Secondary Drug	Effect	Mechanism	Precautions
ANTIARRHYTHMICS				
IBUTILIDE				
IBUTILIDE	**DRUGS THAT PROLONG THE QT INTERVAL**			
IBUTILIDE	1. ANTIARRHYTHMICS—ajmaline, amiodarone, azimilide, cibenzoline, disopyramide, dofetilide, dronedarone, procainamide, propafenone, quinidine 2. ANTIBIOTICS—macrolides (especially azithromycin, clarithromycin, parenteral erythromycin, telithromycin), quinolones (especially moxifloxacin), quinupristin/dalfopristin 3. ANTICANCER AND IMMUNOMODULATING DRUGS—arsenic trioxide, bosutinib, crizotinib, dasatinib, eribulin, fingolimod, lapatinib, nilotinib, pazopanib, sunitinib, vandetanib, vemurafenib 4. ANTIDEPRESSANTS—TCAs, venlafaxine 5. ANTIEMETICS—ondansetron 6. ANTIFUNGALS—fluconazole, posaconazole, voriconazole 7. ANTIHISTAMINES—terfenadine, hydroxyzine, mizolastine 8. ANTIHYPERTENSIVES—ketanserin 9. ANTIMALARIALS—artemether with lumefantrine, chloroquine, halofantrine, hydroxychloroquine, mefloquine, quinine 10. ANTIPROTOZOALS—pentamidine isethionate 11. ANTIPSYCHOTICS—atypicals, phenothiazines, pimozide 12. ANTIVIRALS—boceprevir, rilpivirine, telaprevir	Risk of ventricular arrhythmias, particularly torsades de pointes	Additive effect; these drugs prolong the QT interval	Avoid coadministration

(Continued)

Primary Drug	Secondary Drug	Effect	Mechanism	Precautions
ANTIARRHYTHMICS				
	13. BETA-BLOCKERS—sotalol 14. BRONCHODILATORS—parenteral bronchodilators 15. CNS STIMULANTS—atomoxetine 16. RANOLAZINE			
MEXILETINE				
MEXILETINE	**ANESTHETICS—LOCAL**			
MEXILETINE	BUPIVACAINE, LEVOBUPIVACAINE	Risk of ↓ BP	Additive myocardial depression	Particular care should be taken to avoid inadvertent intravenous administration during bupivacaine infiltration; monitor PR, BP, and ECG during epidural administration of bupivacaine
MEXILETINE	LIDOCAINE	Mexiletine ↑ lidocaine levels (with cases of toxicity when lidocaine is given intravenously)	Mexiletine displaces lidocaine from its tissue-binding sites; it also seems to ↓ its clearance, but the exact mechanism is uncertain at present	Watch for the early symptoms and signs of lidocaine toxicity (perioral paresthesia, ↑ muscle tone)
MEXILETINE	ANALGESICS—OPIOIDS	1. Absorption of oral mexiletine is ↓ by coadministration with morphine or diamorphine 2. Methadone may ↑ mexiletine levels	1. Uncertain, but thought to be due to opioid-induced delay in gastric emptying 2. Methadone inhibits CYP2D6-mediated metabolism of mexiletine	1. Watch for a poor response to mexiletine; consider starting at a higher dose or using the intravenous route 2. Monitor PR, BP, and ECG closely; watch for mexiletine toxicity
MEXILETINE	**ANTIARRHYTHMICS**			
MEXILETINE	ANTIARRHYTHMICS	Risk of bradycardia and ↓ BP; however, mexiletine ↓ the QT prolongation of other antiarrhythmics, so it is often beneficial	Additive effect; antiarrhythmics are all myocardial depressants	Monitor PR, BP, and ECG closely

(*Continued*)

Primary Drug	Secondary Drug	Effect	Mechanism	Precautions
ANTIARRHYTHMICS				
MEXILETINE	PROPAFENONE	↑ Serum levels of mexiletine	Propafenone inhibits CYP2D6-mediated metabolism of mexiletine; no case reports of adverse clinical effects but is potential for proarrhythmias	Monitor ECG closely
MEXILETINE	ANTIBIOTICS	Rifampicin ↓ mexiletine levels	Uncertain; postulated that rifampicin ↑ mexiletine metabolism	Watch for poor response to mexiletine
MEXILETINE	ANTICANCER AND IMMUNOMODULATING DRUGS—imatinib	Imatinib may cause an ↑ in plasma concentrations of mexiletine and a risk of toxic effects, e.g., nausea, vomiting, constipation, taste disturbances, dizziness, and confusion	Imatinib is a potent inhibitor of CYP2D6 isoenzymes, which metabolize mexiletine	Mexiletine is used for life-threatening ventricular arrhythmias. Close monitoring of BP and ECG is mandatory, and watch for signs and symptoms of heart failure
MEXILETINE	**ANTIDEPRESSANTS**			
MEXILETINE	SSRIs	SSRIs may ↑ mexiletine levels	SSRIs inhibit CYP2D6-mediated metabolism of mexiletine	Monitor PR and BP closely; watch for mexiletine toxicity ECG prior to treatment and repeated until stable
MEXILETINE	TCAs	Risk of arrhythmias	Additive effect; both drugs may be proarrhythmogenic. In addition, amitriptyline and clomipramine may inhibit CYP2D6-mediated metabolism of mexiletine, while mexiletine inhibits CYP1A2-mediated metabolism of amitriptyline, clomipramine, and imipramine	Monitor PR, BP, and ECG closely

(Continued)

Primary Drug	Secondary Drug	Effect	Mechanism	Precautions
ANTIARRHYTHMICS				
MEXILETINE	ANTIEMETICS—5-HT3-ANTAGONISTS	Risk of arrhythmias with ondansetron	Additive effect	Manufacturers recommend avoiding coadministration. Also caution with tropisetron; monitor ECG closely
MEXILETINE	ANTIEPILEPTICS—PHENYTOIN	↓ Mexiletine levels	Induction of hepatic metabolism	Monitor PR and BP weekly until stable, and watch for ↑ BP
MEXILETINE	ANTIFUNGALS—TERBINAFINE	↑ Mexiletine levels	Inhibition of CYP2D6 mediated metabolism	Monitor PR and BP closely until stable
MEXILETINE	ANTIHISTAMINES—MIZOLASTINE	Risk of arrhythmias	Additive effect	Avoid coadministration
MEXILETINE	ANTIMALARIALS—QUININE	Quinine may ↑ mexiletine levels	Quinine inhibits CYP2D6-mediated metabolism of mexiletine	Monitor PR and BP closely
MEXILETINE	ANTIMUSCARINICS—ATROPINE	Delayed absorption of mexiletine	Anticholinergic effects delay gastric emptying and absorption	May slow the onset of action of the first dose of mexiletine, but this is not of clinical significance for regular dosing (atropine does not ↓ the total dose absorbed)
MEXILETINE	**ANTIVIRALS**			
MEXILETINE	COBICISTAT	Theoretical risk of ↑ levels of mexiletine	Cobicistat inhibits CYP2D6	Monitor ECG closely
MEXILETINE	RITONAVIR	Mexiletine levels may be ↑ by ritonavir	Inhibition of metabolism via CYP2D6, particularly in rapid metabolizers (90% of the population)	Monitor PR, BP, and ECG closely
MEXILETINE	BETA-BLOCKERS	Risk of bradycardia (occasionally severe), ↓ BP and heart failure	Additive negative inotropic and chronotropic effects. Also, mexiletine is known to inhibit CYP1A2-mediated metabolism of propranolol	Monitor PR, BP, and ECG closely; watch for development of heart failure

(Continued)

Primary Drug	Secondary Drug	Effect	Mechanism	Precautions
ANTIARRHYTHMICS				
MEXILETINE	BRONCHODILATORS—THEOPHYLLINE	Theophylline levels may be ↑ by mexiletine; cases of theophylline toxicity have been reported	Mexiletine inhibits CYP1A2-mediated metabolism of theophylline	↓ The theophylline dose (by up to 50%). Monitor theophylline levels and watch for toxicity
MEXILETINE	CNS STIMULANTS—MODAFINIL	May cause ↓ mexiletine levels if CYP1A2 is the predominant metabolic pathway and alternative metabolic pathways are either genetically deficient or affected	Modafinil is a moderate inducer of CYP1A2 in a concentration-dependent manner	Be aware
MEXILETINE	DIURETICS—CARBONIC ANHYDRASE INHIBITORS, LOOP DIURETICS, THIAZIDES	Effect of mexiletine ↓ by hypokalemia	Uncertain	Normalize potassium levels before starting mexiletine
MEXILETINE	H2 RECEPTOR BLOCKERS	Cimetidine may ↑ plasma concentrations of mexiletine	Cimetidine inhibits CYP2D6-mediated metabolism of mexiletine. Ranitidine is a much weaker CYP2D6 inhibitor	Monitor PR and BP at least weekly until stable. Warn patients to report symptoms of hypotension (light-headedness, dizziness on standing, etc.). Consider alternative acid-suppression therapy
MORACIZINE				
MORACIZINE	BRONCHODILATORS—THEOPHYLLINE	↓ Plasma concentrations of theophylline and risk of therapeutic failure	Due to induction of microsomal enzyme activity	May need to ↑ dose of theophylline by 25%
MORACIZINE	CALCIUM CHANNEL BLOCKERS	Coadministration is associated with ↑ bioavailability of moracizine and ↓ availability of diltiazem	Postulated that diltiazem inhibits metabolism of moracizine, while moracizine ↑ metabolism of diltiazem; the precise mechanism of interaction is uncertain at present	Monitor PR, BP, and ECG; adjust doses of each drug accordingly

(*Continued*)

Primary Drug	Secondary Drug	Effect	Mechanism	Precautions
ANTIARRHYTHMICS				
MORACIZINE	CARDIAC GLYCOSIDES—DIGOXIN	Case reports of heart block when moracizine is coadministered with digoxin	Uncertain at present	Monitor PR and ECG closely
PROCAINAMIDE				
PROCAINAMIDE	**DRUGS THAT PROLONG THE QT INTERVAL**			
PROCAINAMIDE	1. ANTIARRHYTHMICS—ajmaline, amiodarone, azimilide, cibenzoline, disopyramide, dofetilide, dronedarone, ibutilide, propafenone, quinidine 2. ANTIBIOTICS—macrolides (especially azithromycin, clarithromycin, parenteral erythromycin, telithromycin), quinolones (especially moxifloxacin), quinupristin/dalfopristin 3. ANTICANCER AND IMMUNOMODULATING DRUGS—arsenic trioxide, bosutinib, crizotinib, dasatinib, eribulin, fingolimod, lapatinib, nilotinib, pazopanib, sunitinib, vandetanib, vemurafenib 4. ANTIDEPRESSANTS—TCAs, venlafaxine 5. ANTIEMETICS—ondansetron 6. ANTIFUNGALS—fluconazole, posaconazole, voriconazole 7. ANTIHISTAMINES—terfenadine, hydroxyzine, mizolastine 8. ANTIHYPERTENSIVES—ketanserin 9. ANTIMALARIALS—artemether with lumefantrine, chloroquine, halofantrine, hydroxychloroquine, mefloquine, quinine 10. ANTIPROTOZOALS—pentamidine isethionate 11. ANTIPSYCHOTICS—atypicals, phenothiazines, pimozide	Risk of ventricular arrhythmias, particularly torsades de pointes	Additive effect; these drugs prolong the QT interval	Avoid coadministration

(*Continued*)

Primary Drug	Secondary Drug	Effect	Mechanism	Precautions
ANTIARRHYTHMICS				
	12. ANTIVIRALS—boceprevir, rilpivirine, telaprevir 13. BETA-BLOCKERS—sotalol 14. BRONCHODILATORS—parenteral bronchodilators 15. CNS STIMULANTS—atomoxetine 16. RANOLAZINE			
PROCAINAMIDE	**ANESTHETICS—LOCAL**			
PROCAINAMIDE	BUPIVICAINE, LEVOBUPIVACAINE	Risk of ↓ BP	Additive myocardial depression	Particular care should be taken to avoid inadvertent intravenous administration during bupivacaine infiltration; monitor PR, BP, and ECG during epidural administration of bupivacaine
PROCAINAMIDE	LIDOCAINE	Case report of neurotoxicity when intravenous lidocaine is administered with procainamide. No significant interaction is expected when lidocaine is used for local anesthetic infiltration	Likely to be an additive effect; both may cause neurotoxicity in overdose	Care should be taken when administering lidocaine as an infusion for patients taking procainamide
PROCAINAMIDE	ANALGESICS—OPIOIDS	Methadone may ↑ flecainide levels	Methadone inhibits CYP2D6-mediated metabolism of flecainide	Monitor PR and BP closely
PROCAINAMIDE	ANTIARRHYTHMICS	Risk of bradycardia and ↓ BP	Additive effect; antiarrhythmics are all myocardial depressants	Monitor PR, BP, and ECG closely
PROCAINAMIDE	ANTIBIOTICS—TRIMETHOPRIM	Procainamide levels are ↑ by trimethoprim	Trimethoprim is a potent inhibitor of organic cation transport in the kidney, and elimination of procainamide is impaired	Watch for signs of procainamide toxicity; ↓ the dose of procainamide, particularly in the elderly

(Continued)

Primary Drug	Secondary Drug	Effect	Mechanism	Precautions
ANTIARRHYTHMICS				
PROCAINAMIDE	ANTICANCER AND OTHER IMMUNOMODULATING DRUGS—CRIZOTINIB	Possible increased levels of OCT1 and OCT2 substrates	OCT1 and OCT2 inhibition	Clinical significance uncertain; be aware of possible interaction
PROCAINAMIDE	ANTIDEPRESSANTS—SSRIs	SSRIs may ↑ procainamide levels	SSRIs inhibit CYP2D6-mediated metabolism of procainamide	Monitor PR and BP closely; watch for procainamide toxicity and ECG prior to treatment and repeated until stable
PROCAINAMIDE	ANTIHYPERTENSIVES AND HEART FAILURE DRUGS—ACE INHIBITORS	Possible ↑ risk of leukopenia	Uncertain at present	Monitor FBC before starting treatment, 2-weekly for 3 months after initiation of therapy, then periodically thereafter
PROCAINAMIDE	BETA-BLOCKERS	Risk of bradycardia (occasionally severe), ↓ BP and heart failure	Additive negative inotropic and chronotropic effects	Monitor PR, BP, and ECG closely; watch for development of heart failure
PROCAINAMIDE	CARDIAC GLYCOSIDES—DIGITOXIN	Single case report of toxicity in a patient taking both digitoxin and procainamide	Uncertain at present	Watch for digitoxin toxicity
PROCAINAMIDE	H2 RECEPTOR BLOCKERS	Cimetidine may ↑ plasma concentrations of procainamide	Cimetidine is a potent inhibitor of organic cation transport in the kidney, and elimination of procainamide is impaired. Cimetidine also inhibits CYP2D6-mediated metabolism of procainamide. Ranitidine is a much weaker CYP2D6 inhibitor	Monitor PR and BP at least weekly until stable. Warn patients to report symptoms of hypotension (light-headedness, dizziness on standing, etc.). Consider alternative acid-suppression therapy
PROCAINAMIDE	MUSCLE RELAXANTS—DEPOLARIZING	Possibility of ↑ neuromuscular blockade	Uncertain; procainamide may ↓ plasma cholinesterase levels	Be aware of the possibility of a prolonged effect of suxamethonium when administered to patients taking procainamide

(*Continued*)

Primary Drug	Secondary Drug	Effect	Mechanism	Precautions
ANTIARRHYTHMICS				
PROPAFENONE				
PROPAFENONE	**DRUGS THAT PROLONG THE QT INTERVAL**			
PROPAFENONE	1. ANTIARRHYTHMICS—ajmaline, amiodarone, azimilide, cibenzoline, disopyramide, dofetilide, dronedarone, ibutilide, procainamide, quinidine 2. ANTIBIOTICS—macrolides (especially azithromycin, clarithromycin, parenteral erythromycin, telithromycin), quinolones (especially moxifloxacin), quinupristin/dalfopristin 3. ANTICANCER AND IMMUNOMODULATING DRUGS—arsenic trioxide, bosutinib, crizotinib, dasatinib, eribulin, fingolimod, lapatinib, nilotinib, pazopanib, sunitinib, vandetanib, vemurafenib 4. ANTIDEPRESSANTS—TCAs, venlafaxine 5. ANTIEMETICS—ondansetron 6. ANTIFUNGALS—fluconazole, posaconazole, voriconazole 7. ANTIHISTAMINES—terfenadine, hydroxyzine, mizolastine 8. ANTIHYPERTENSIVES—ketanserin 9. ANTIMALARIALS—artemether with lumefantrine, chloroquine, halofantrine, hydroxychloroquine, mefloquine, quinine 10. ANTIPROTOZOALS—pentamidine isethionate 11. ANTIPSYCHOTICS—atypicals, phenothiazines, pimozide 12. ANTIVIRALS—boceprevir, rilpivirine, telaprevir 13. BETA-BLOCKERS—sotalol 14. BRONCHODILATORS—parenteral bronchodilators 15. CNS STIMULANTS—atomoxetine 16. RANOLAZINE	Risk of ventricular arrhythmias, particularly torsades de pointes	Additive effect; these drugs prolong the QT interval	Avoid coadministration

(*Continued*)

Primary Drug	Secondary Drug	Effect	Mechanism	Precautions
ANTIARRHYTHMICS				
PROPAFENONE	**DRUGS WITH ANTIMUSCARINIC EFFECTS**			
PROPAFENONE	1. ANALGESICS—nefopam 2. ANTIARRHYTHMICS—disopyramide 3. ANTIDEPRESSANTS—TCAs 4. ANTIEMETICS—cyclizine 5. ANTIHISTAMINES—chlorphenamine, cyproheptadine, hydroxyzine 6. ANTIMUSCARINICS—atropine, benztropine, cyclopentolate, dicycloverine, flavoxate, homatropine, hyoscine, orphenadrine, oxybutynin, procyclidine, propantheline, tolterodine, trihexyphenidyl, tropicamide 7. ANTI-PARKINSON'S DRUGS—dopaminergics 8. ANTIPSYCHOTICS—phenothiazines, clozapine, pimozide 9. MUSCLE RELAXANTS—baclofen 10. NITRATES—isosorbide dinitrate	↑ Risk of antimuscarinic side effects. NB ↓ efficacy of sublingual nitrate tablets	Additive effect; both drugs cause antimuscarinic side effects. Antimuscarinic effects ↓ salivary production, which ↓ dissolution of the tablet	Warn patient of this additive effect. Consider changing the formulation to a sublingual nitrate spray
PROPAFENONE	ANESTHETICS—LOCAL	Risk of ↓ BP	Additive myocardial depression	Particular care should be taken to avoid inadvertent intravenous administration during bupivacaine infiltration; monitor PR, BP, and ECG during epidural administration of bupivacaine
PROPAFENONE	**ANALGESICS**			
PROPAFENONE	NSAIDs	Serum levels of propafenone may be ↑ by parecoxib	Parecoxib is a weak inhibitor of CYP2D6-mediated metabolism of propafenone	Monitor PR and BP closely. If possible, use only short courses of NSAID
PROPAFENONE	OPIOIDS	Methadone may ↑ propafenone levels	Methadone inhibits CYP2D6-mediated metabolism of propafenone	Monitor PR and BP closely

(Continued)

Primary Drug	Secondary Drug	Effect	Mechanism	Precautions
ANTIARRHYTHMICS				
PROPAFENONE	PARACETAMOL	Propafenone may slow the onset of action of intermittent-dose paracetamol	Anticholinergic effects delay gastric emptying and absorption	Warn patients that the action of paracetamol may be delayed. This will not be the case when paracetamol is taken regularly
PROPAFENONE	**ANTIARRHYTHMICS**			
PROPAFENONE	ANTIARRHYTHMICS	Risk of bradycardia and ↓ BP with all antiarrhythmics	Additive myocardial depression	Monitor PR and BP closely
PROPAFENONE	MEXILETINE	↑ Serum levels of mexiletine	Propafenone inhibits CYP2D6-mediated metabolism of mexiletine; no case reports of adverse clinical effects but is a potential for proarrhythmias	Monitor ECG closely
PROPAFENONE	**ANTIBIOTICS**			
PROPAFENONE	ERYTHROMYCIN	Erythromycin may ↑ propafenone levels	Erythromycin inhibits metabolism of propafenone	Monitor PR and BP at least weekly until stable. Warn patients to report symptoms of hypotension (light-headedness, dizziness on standing, etc.)
PROPAFENONE	RIFAMPICIN	Rifampicin may ↓ propafenone levels	Rifampicin may increase CYP3A4- and CYP1A2-mediated metabolism of propafenone	Watch for poor response to propafenone
PROPAFENONE	ANTICANCER AND IMMUNOMODULATING DRUGS—CICLOSPORIN	Possible ↑ ciclosporin levels	Uncertain	Watch for signs of ciclosporin toxicity
PROPAFENONE	ANTICOAGULANTS—ORAL	Warfarin levels may be ↑ by propafenone	Propafenone seems to inhibit warfarin metabolism	Monitor INR at least weekly until stable

(*Continued*)

Primary Drug	Secondary Drug	Effect	Mechanism	Precautions
ANTIARRHYTHMICS				
PROPAFENONE	**ANTIDEPRESSANTS**			
PROPAFENONE	SNRIs	Duloxetine may ↑ propafenone levels	Duloxetine moderately inhibits CYP2D6, which metabolizes propafenone	Monitor PR and BP closely
PROPAFENONE	SSRIs	Levels of both may be ↑	Both SSRIs and propafenone are substrates for and inhibitors of CYP2D6	Monitor PR and BP closely
PROPAFENONE	ANTIEPILEPTICS—BARBITURATES	↓ Serum levels of propafenone with barbiturates	Barbiturates stimulate hepatic metabolism of propafenone	Watch for poor response to propafenone
PROPAFENONE	**ANTIFUNGALS**			
PROPAFENONE	KETOCONAZOLE	Ketoconazole may ↑ propafenone levels	Ketoconazole inhibits metabolism of propafenone	Monitor PR and BP at least weekly until stable. Warn patients to report symptoms of hypotension (light-headedness, dizziness on standing, etc.)
PROPAFENONE	TERBINAFINE	↑ Propefenone levels	Inhibition of CYP2D6-mediated metabolism	Monitor PR and BP closely until stable
PROPAFENONE	**ANTIVIRALS**			
PROPAFENONE	COBICISTAT	Theoretical risk of ↑ levels of propafenone	Cobicistat inhibits CYP2D6	Monitor ECG closely
PROPAFENONE	PROTEASE INHIBITORS	Fosamprenavir, ritonavir, and possibly saquinavir and tipranavir/ritonavir ↑ propafenone levels, with risk of ventricular arrhythmias	Probably inhibition of CYP2D6	Manufacturers recommend avoiding coadministration of propafenone with fosamprenavir, ritonavir, saquinavir, or tipranavir

(*Continued*)

Primary Drug	Secondary Drug	Effect	Mechanism	Precautions
ANTIARRHYTHMICS				
PROPAFENONE	BETA-BLOCKERS	Risk of bradycardia (occasionally severe), ↓ BP and heart failure. Also, ↑ plasma levels of metoprolol and propranolol	Additive negative inotropic and chronotropic effects. In addition, propafenone inhibits CYP2D6-metabolism of metoprolol and propranolol	Monitor PR, BP, and ECG closely; watch for development of heart failure. Watch for propranolol and metoprolol toxicity; ↓ doses accordingly
PROPAFENONE	BRONCHODILATORS—THEOPHYLLINE	Cases of ↑ theophylline levels with toxicity when propafenone added	Uncertain at present	Watch for signs of theophylline toxicity
PROPAFENONE	CARDIAC GLYCOSIDES—DIGOXIN	Digoxin concentrations may be ↑ by propafenone	Uncertain at present	Watch for digoxin toxicity; check digoxin levels if indicated and ↓ digoxin dose as necessary (15%–75% suggested by studies)
PROPAFENONE	DRUG DEPENDENCE THERAPIES—BUPROPION	Bupropion may ↑ propafenone levels	Bupropion may inhibit CYP2D6-mediated metabolism of propafenone	Monitor PR and BP closely; start propafenone at the lowest dose for patients taking bupropion
PROPAFENONE	GRAPEFRUIT JUICE	Grapefruit juice may ↑ propafenone levels	Grapefruit juice inhibits CYP2D6-mediated metabolism of propafenone	Advice patient to avoid GFJ
PROPAFENONE	H2 RECEPTOR BLOCKERS	Cimetidine may ↑ propafenone levels	Cimetidine inhibits CYP2D6-mediated metabolism of propafenone. Ranitidine is a weak CYP2D6 inhibitor	Monitor PR and BP at least weekly until stable. Warn patients to report symptoms of hypotension (light-headedness, dizziness on standing, etc.). Consider alternative acid-suppression therapy
PROPAFENONE	MIRABEGRON	↑ Flecainide and propafenone levels	Mirabegron inhibits CYP2D6. These drugs have a narrow therapeutic index	Manufacturer advises caution in coadministration. Warn patients to report symptoms such as dizziness, chest pain, or palpitations

(*Continued*)

Primary Drug	Secondary Drug	Effect	Mechanism	Precautions
ANTIARRHYTHMICS				
PROPAFENONE	PARASYMPATHOMIMETICS	↓ Efficacy of neostigmine and pyridostigmine	Uncertain; propafenone has a degree of antinicotinic action that may oppose the action of parasympathomimetic therapy for myasthenia gravis	Watch for poor response to these parasympathomimetics and ↑ dose accordingly
PROPAFENONE	PIRFENIDONE	↑ Pirfenidone levels	Inhibition of metabolism of pirfenidone	Manufacturer recommends avoiding coadministration
PROPAFENONE	RANOLAZINE	Possible ↑ propafenone levels	Inhibition of CYP2D6-mediated metabolism of propafenone	Monitor PR and BP closely
QUINIDINE				
QUINIDINE	**DRUGS THAT PROLONG THE QT INTERVAL**			
QUINIDINE	1. ANTIARRHYTHMICS—ajmaline, amiodarone, azimilide, cibenzoline, disopyramide, dofetilide, dronedarone, ibutilide, procainamide, propafenone 2. ANTIBIOTICS—macrolides (especially azithromycin, clarithromycin, parenteral erythromycin, telithromycin), quinolones (especially moxifloxacin), quinupristin/dalfopristin 3. ANTICANCER AND IMMUNOMODULATING DRUGS—arsenic trioxide, bosutinib, crizotinib, dasatinib, eribulin, fingolimod, lapatinib, nilotinib, pazopanib, sunitinib, vandetanib, vemurafenib 4. ANTIDEPRESSANTS—TCAs, venlafaxine 5. ANTIEMETICS—ondansetron	Risk of ventricular arrhythmias, particularly torsades de pointes	Additive effect; these drugs prolong the QT interval	Avoid coadministration

(*Continued*)

Primary Drug	Secondary Drug	Effect	Mechanism	Precautions
ANTIARRHYTHMICS				
	6. ANTIFUNGALS—fluconazole, posaconazole, voriconazole 7. ANTIHISTAMINES—terfenadine, hydroxyzine, mizolastine 8. ANTIHYPERTENSIVES—ketanserin 9. ANTIMALARIALS—artemether with lumefantrine, chloroquine, halofantrine, hydroxychloroquine, mefloquine, quinine 10. ANTIPROTOZOALS—pentamidine isethionate 11. ANTIPSYCHOTICS—atypicals, phenothiazines, pimozide 12. ANTIVIRALS—boceprevir, rilpivirine, telaprevir 13. BETA-BLOCKERS—sotalol 14. BRONCHODILATORS—parenteral bronchodilators 15. CNS STIMULANTS—atomoxetine 16. RANOLAZINE			
QUINIDINE	**ANALGESICS—OPIOIDS**			
QUINIDINE	CODEINE	↓ Analgesic effect of codeine	Inhibition of CYP2D6-mediated conversion of codeine to its active metabolite	Be aware that codeine may be less effective in patients taking codeine; there is a theoretical risk that dihydrocodeine and hydrocodone may be similarly affected
QUINIDINE	FENTANYL, PETHIDINE, TRAMADOL	↑ Fentanyl, pethidine, and tramadol levels	Quinidine inhibits CYP2D6	Theoretical drug interaction; watch for excessive narcotization
QUINIDINE	ANTIBIOTICS—RIFAMPICIN	↓ Quinidine levels	Induction of CYP3A4 and 2D6-mediated metabolism	↑ Quinidine dose (may need to be more than doubled). Monitor PR, BP, and ECG closely
QUINIDINE	**ANTICANCER AND IMMUNOMODULATING DRUGS**			
QUINIDINE	AFATINIB	Possible increase in afatinib levels	P-glycoprotein inhibition	Manufacturer recommends staggered dosing 6–12 h apart or dose reduction

(*Continued*)

Primary Drug	Secondary Drug	Effect	Mechanism	Precautions
ANTIARRHYTHMICS				
QUINIDINE	DASATINIB	Increased levels of quinidine	CYP3A4 inhibition	Caution with CYP3A4 substrates with narrow therapeutic window
QUINIDINE	GEFITINIB	Increased levels of gefitinib	CYP2D6 inhibition	Monitor closely
QUINIDINE	PACLITAXEL	Injectable preparations may increase levels of each drug	Uncertain-interference with excretion via Pgp	Clinical relevance uncertain
QUINIDINE	TAMOXIFEN	Theoretical risk of reduced efficacy of tamoxifen with increased recurrence of breast cancer	↓ CYP2D6-mediated metabolism of tamoxifen to its active metabolite	Avoid coadministration
QUINIDINE	**ANTICOAGULANTS**			
QUINIDINE	APIXABAN	↑ Quinidine levels	Inhibition of CYP3A4-mediated metabolism	Avoid coadministration
QUINIDINE	DABIGATRAN	↑ Dabigatran levels	Inhibition of Pgp	Reduce dose of dabigatran to 150 mg/day (75 mg in renal failure)
QUINIDINE	ANTIDEPRESSANTS—FLUVOXAMINE	Theoretical risk of ↑ quinidine levels	Fluvoxamine inhibits CYP3A4-mediated metabolism	Monitor PR, BP, and ECG closely
QUINIDINE	ANTIEPILEPTICS—BARBITURATES, PHENYTOIN	↓ Quinidine levels	Induction of CYP3A4 and 2D6-mediated metabolism	Monitor for poor response to quinidine and ↑ doses accordingly
QUINIDINE	ANTIFUNGALS—ITRACONAZOLE, POSSIBLY KETOCONAZOLE	↑ Quinidine levels	Itraconazole inhibits CYP3A4-mediated metabolism	Monitor PR, BP, and ECG closely

(Continued)

Primary Drug	Secondary Drug	Effect	Mechanism	Precautions
ANTIARRHYTHMICS				
QUINIDINE	ANTIGOUT DRUGS—COLCHICINE	Colchicine levels ↑ by quinidine	Quinidine is a moderate Pgp inhibitor	Avoid coadministration in the presence of renal failure. In the presence of normal renal function, UK manufacturer recommends reducing dose and/or increasing dosing interval. U.S. manufacturer recommends more specific dosage adjustments: for treatment of gout stat dose of 0.6 mg not to be repeated for 3 days. For gout prophylaxis if the patient is taking 0.6 mg bd, ↓ dose to 0.3 mg od; if the patient is taking 0.6 mg od, ↓ dose to 0.3 mg alternate days
QUINIDINE	**ANTIHYPERTENSIVE AND HEART FAILURE DRUGS**			
QUINIDINE	ALISKIREN	Aliskiren levels ↑ by quinidine	Quinidine is a moderate Pgp inhibitor	Monitor BP and serum potassium at least weekly until stable
QUINIDINE	ALPHA-BLOCKERS—TAMSULOSIN	↑ Tamsulosin levels	Inhibition of CYP2D6-mediated metabolism	Monitor BP closely; warn patient to report symptoms of orthostatic hypotension
QUINIDINE	ANTIMALARIALS—MEFLOQUINE	Risk of seizures	Additive effect	Warn patients of the risk; patients should be advised to avoid driving while taking these drugs in combination
QUINIDINE	ANTIPLATELET AGENTS—TICAGRELOR	Risk of ↑ ticagrelor levels	Inhibition of Pgp	Manufacturer recommends avoid coadministration
QUINIDINE	**ANTIVIRAL DRUGS**			
QUINIDINE	COBICISTAT	Theoretical risk of ↑ levels of quinidine	Cobicistat inhibits CYP2D6	Monitor PR, BP, and ECG closely
QUINIDINE	NNRTIs—ETRAVIRINE	Risk of ↓ quinidine levels	Etravirine induces CYP3A4	Monitor PR, BP, and ECG closely

(Continued)

Primary Drug	Secondary Drug	Effect	Mechanism	Precautions
ANTIARRHYTHMICS				
QUINIDINE	PROTEASE INHIBITORS—INDINAVIR, NELFINAVIR, RITONAVIR, SAQUINAVIR	Possibly ↑ plasma levels of quinidine, risk of ventricular arrhythmias	Possible inhibition of metabolism via CYP3A	Avoid coadministration
QUINIDINE	BETA-BLOCKERS—METOPROLOL, PROPRANOLOL, TIMOLOL	Risk of ↑ levels of these beta-blockers (report of bradycardia with timolol eye drops)	Inhibition of CYP2D6-mediated metabolism	Monitor PR and BP closely on initiation of coadministration. Warn patients to report symptoms of orthostatic hypotension
QUINIDINE	CALCIUM CHANNEL BLOCKERS—VERAPAMIL	↑ Quinidine levels; reports of quinidine toxicity	Verapamil inhibits CYP3A4-mediated metabolism	Reduce quinidine dose; monitor PR, BP, and ECG closely
QUINIDINE	CARDIAC GLYCOSIDES	↑ Levels of digoxin and digitoxin	Quinidine is a moderate Pgp inhibitor	Halve the dose of cardiac glycoside (reduce more in the presence of renal failure)
QUINIDINE	DIURETICS—AMILORIDE	Possible reduced efficacy of quinidine	Unknown	Monitor PR, BP, and ECG closely
QUINIDINE	ELIGLUSTAT	↑ Eliglustat levels	Inhibition of CYP2D6-mediated metabolism	Reduce dose to 85 mg od
QUINIDINE	GRAPEFRUIT JUICE	Absorption of quinidine is delayed (e.g., from 1.6 to 3.3 h) by grapefruit juice in a dose-dependent manner	Possibly due to effects on intestinal CYP3A4	Be aware. Avoid concomitant use. Torsade de pointes reported with high volumes of GFJ
QUINIDINE	H2 RECEPTOR BLOCKERS—CIMETIDINE	↑ Quinidine levels	Cimetidine inhibits CYP3A4-mediated metabolism. It also reduces renal excretion	Reduce quinidine dose; monitor PR, BP, and ECG closely
QUINIDINE	MUSCLE RELAXANTS—DEPOLARIZING AND NONDEPOLARIZING	↑ Effect and duration of both depolarizing and nondepolarizing muscle relaxants	Uncertain	Be aware of possible prolonged neuromuscular blockade in patients taking quinidine
QUINIDINE	PARASYMPATHOMIMETICS—DONEPEZIL, GALANTAMINE	Theoretical risk of ↑ donepezil and galantamine levels	Inhibition of CYP2D6 mediated metabolism	Warn patient to watch for development of side effects of donepezil and galantamine

(Continued)

Primary Drug	Secondary Drug	Effect	Mechanism	Precautions
ANTIARRHYTHMICS				
QUINIDINE	URINARY ALKALINIZERS—AMMONIUM CHLORIDE, SODIUM BICARBONATE	Urinary alkalinization ↑ quinidine levels	Quinidine excretion ↓ in the presence of an alkaline urine; quinidine exists predominantly in a nonionic form, which is more readily reabsorbed from the renal tubules	Monitor PR and BP closely
SOTALOL—*see Beta-blockers later*				

Primary Drug	Secondary Drug	Effect	Mechanism	Precautions
ANTIHYPERTENSIVES AND HEART FAILURE DRUGS				
ACE INHIBITORS				
ACE INHIBITORS	ALBUMIN-CONTAINING SOLUTIONS	Acute ↓ BP following *rapid* infusion with captopril or enalapril	Uncertain at present	Use alternative colloids; monitor BP closely while on infusion
ACE INHIBITORS	ALCOHOL	1. Acute alcohol ingestion may ↑ hypotensive effects 2. Chronic moderate/heavy drinking ↓ hypotensive effect	1. Additive hypotensive effect 2. Chronic alcohol excess is associated with hypertension	Monitor BP closely as unpredictable responses can occur. Advise patients to drink only in moderation and avoid large variations in the amount of alcohol drunk
ACE INHIBITORS	ANESTHETICS—GENERAL	Risk of severe hypotensive episodes during induction of anesthesia	Most general anesthetics are myocardial depressants and vasodilators. Additive hypotensive effect	Monitor BP closely, especially during induction of anesthesia
ACE INHIBITORS	ANESTHETICS—LOCAL	Risk of profound ↓ BP with epidural bupivacaine in patients on captopril	Additive hypotensive effect; epidural bupivacaine causes vasodilatation in the lower limbs	Monitor BP closely. Ensure that the patient is preloaded with fluids

(*Continued*)

Primary Drug	Secondary Drug	Effect	Mechanism	Precautions
ANTIHYPERTENSIVES AND HEART FAILURE DRUGS				
ACE INHIBITORS	ANALGESICS—NSAIDs	1. ↓ Hypotensive effect 2. ↑ Risk of renal impairment 3. ↑ Risk of hyperkalemia	1. NSAIDs cause sodium and water retention and raise BP by inhibiting vasodilating renal prostaglandins 2. Additive effect 3. Additive effect	Benefits often outweigh risks for short-term NSAID use but particular caution in the elderly. For longer-term use, monitor BP, renal function, and serum potassium at least weekly until stable
ACE INHIBITORS	ANTACIDS	↓ Effect, particularly of captopril, fosinopril, and enalapril	↓ Absorption due to ↑ in gastric pH	Watch for poor response to ACE inhibitors
ACE INHIBITORS	ANTIARRHYTHMICS—PROCAINAMIDE	Possible ↑ risk of leukopenia	Uncertain at present	Monitor FBC before starting treatment, 2-weekly for 3 months after initiation of therapy, then periodically thereafter
ACE INHIBITORS	**ANTIBIOTICS**			
ACE INHIBITORS	RIFAMPICIN	↓ Plasma concentrations and efficacy of imidapril and enalapril	Uncertain. ↓ Production of active metabolites noted despite rifampicin being an enzyme inducer	Monitor BP at least weekly until stable
ACE INHIBITORS	TETRACYCLINES	↓ Plasma concentrations and efficacy of tetracyclines with quinapril. The absorption of tetracyclines may be reduced when taken concurrently with quinapril, due to the presence of magnesium carbonate as an excipient in quinapril's pharmaceutical formulation	Magnesium carbonate (found in a formulation of quinapril) chelates with tetracyclines in the gut to form a less soluble substance that ↓ absorption of tetracycline	For short-term antibiotic use, consider stopping quinapril for duration of the course. For long-term use, consider an alternative ACE inhibitor

(Continued)

Primary Drug	Secondary Drug	Effect	Mechanism	Precautions
ANTIHYPERTENSIVES AND HEART FAILURE DRUGS				
ACE INHIBITORS	TRIMETHOPRIM	Risk of hyperkalemia when trimethoprim is coadministered with ACE inhibitors *in the presence of renal failure*	Uncertain at present	Avoid concurrent use in the presence of severe renal failure
ACE INHIBITORS	**ANTICANCER AND IMMUNOMODULATING DRUGS**			
ACE INHIBITORS	AZATHIOPRINE	Risk of anemia with captopril and enalapril and leukopenia with captopril	The exact mechanism is uncertain. Azathioprine-induced impairment of hematopoiesis and ACE inhibitor-induced ↓ in erythropoietin may cause additive effects. Enalapril has been used to treat postrenal transplant erythrocytosis	Monitor blood counts regularly
ACE INHIBITORS	BORTEZOMIB	↑ Hypotensive effect	Additive hypotensive effect	Monitor BP at least weekly until stable, particularly on initiation of therapy
ACE INHIBITORS	EVEROLIMUS, (TELI)SIROLIMUS	Reports of angioedema	Uncertain—possibly additive effect (both can cause angioedema)	Warn patient to report facial swelling immediately
ACE INHIBITORS	CICLOSPORIN	↑ Risk of hyperkalemia and renal failure	Ciclosporin causes a dose-dependent ↑ in serum creatinine, urea, and potassium, especially in renal dysfunction	Monitor renal function and serum potassium weekly until stable, then at least every 3–6 months
ACE INHIBITORS	CORTICOSTEROIDS	↓ Hypotensive effect	Corticosteroids cause sodium and water retention leading to ↑ BP	Monitor BP at least weekly until stable

(*Continued*)

Primary Drug	Secondary Drug	Effect	Mechanism	Precautions
ANTIHYPERTENSIVES AND HEART FAILURE DRUGS				
ACE INHIBITORS	ESTRAMUSTINE	Possible increased risk of angioedema	Additive	Manufacturer recommends stopping treatment with estramustine if angioedema occurs
ACE INHIBITORS	INTERLEUKIN-2 (ALDESLEUKIN)	↑ Hypotensive effect	Additive hypotensive effect; may be used therapeutically. Aldesleukin causes ↓ vascular resistance and ↑ capillary permeability	Monitor BP at least weekly until stable. Warn patients to report symptoms of hypotension (light-headedness, dizziness on standing, etc.)
ACE INHIBITORS	PORFIMER	↑ Risk of photosensitivity reactions when porfimer is administered with enalapril	Attributed to additive effects	Avoid exposure of skin and eyes to direct sunlight for 30 days after porfimer therapy
ACE INHIBITORS	PROCARBAZINE	Hypotension	Additive	Monitor closely
ACE INHIBITORS	TEMSIROLIMUS	Possible increased risk of angioedema	Additive	Monitor closely
ACE INHIBITORS	ANTICOAGULANTS—PARENTERAL	↑ Risk of hyperkalemia with heparins	Heparin inhibits aldosterone secretion, causing hyperkalemia	Monitor potassium levels closely
ACE INHIBITORS	**ANTIDEPRESSANTS**			
ACE INHIBITORS—CAPTOPRIL ENALAPRIL, LISINOPRIL, RAMIPRIL, BENAZEPRIL	LITHIUM	↑ Lithium levels (up to 1/3) with risk of developing lithium toxicity	↓ Renal excretion (↑ lithium reabsorbtion by renal tubules)	Watch for lithium toxicity. Monitor lithium levels
ACE INHIBITORS	MAOIs	Possible ↑ hypotensive effect. MAOIs cause orthostatic hypotension	Additive hypotensive effect	Monitor BP at least weekly until stable. Warn patients to report about symptoms of hypotension (light-headedness, dizziness on standing, etc.)

(Continued)

Primary Drug	Secondary Drug	Effect	Mechanism	Precautions
ANTIHYPERTENSIVES AND HEART FAILURE DRUGS				
ACE INHIBITORS	TCAs	Risk of postural hypotension	Additive hypotensive effect	Monitor BP at least weekly until stable. Warn patients to report symptoms of hypotension (light-headedness, dizziness on standing, etc.)
ACE INHIBITORS	**ANTIDIABETIC DRUGS**			
ACE INHIBITORS	ANTIDIABETIC DRUGS	↑ Risk of hypoglycemic episodes	Mechanism uncertain. ACE inhibitors possibly ↑ insulin sensitivity and glucose utilization. Altered renal function may also be a factor. ACE inhibitors may ↑ bradykinin levels, which ↓ production of glucose by the liver. Hypoglycemia is reported as a side effect (rare) of ACE inhibitors. It is suggested that the occurrence of hypoglycemia is greater with captopril than enalapril. Captopril and enalapril are used in the treatment of diabetic nephropathy	Concurrent treatment need not be avoided and is often beneficial in type II diabetes. Watch for and warn patients about symptoms of hypoglycemia. Be aware that risk of hypoglycemia is greater in elderly people and people with poor glycemic control ➢ ***For signs and symptoms of hypoglycemia, see Clinical Features of Some Adverse Drug Interactions, Hypoglycemia***
ACE INHIBITORS—ENALAPRIL	DDP-4 INHIBITORS—SITAGLIPTIN	Hypotensive effects altered with sitagliptin	Mechanism unknown	Monitor blood pressure
LOVASTATIN	GLP-1 ANALOGUES	AUC and C_{max} reduced by 40% and 28%, respectively	Unknown mechanism	Monitor lipid levels
ACE INHIBITORS	**ANTIGOUT DRUGS**			
ALLOPURINOL	ANTIHYPERTENSIVES AND HEART FAILURE DRUGS—ACE INHIBITORS	Risk of serious hypersensitivity with captopril and enalapril. ↑ Risk of leukopenia	Uncertain. Both drugs can cause hypersensitivity reactions	Warn patient to look for clinical features of hypersensitivity and Stevens–Johnson syndrome

(Continued)

	Secondary Drug	Effect	Mechanism	Precautions
ANTIHYPERTENSIVES AND HEART FAILURE DRUGS				
ACE INHIBITORS	PROBENECID	↑ Plasma concentrations of captopril and enalapril; uncertain clinical significance	Renal excretion of captopril and enalapril ↓ by probenecid	Monitor BP closely
ACE INHIBITORS	**ANTIHYPERTENSIVES AND HEART FAILURE DRUGS**			
ACE INHIBITORS	ALISKIREN	Reports of hypotension with syncope or stroke, renal impairment, and hyperkalemia	Additive effect on renin-angiotensin system	1. Contraindicated in patients with diabetes mellitus or renal impairment (GFR < 60) 2. Other patients need close monitoring of renal function, serum potassium, and blood pressure
ACE INHIBITORS	ANTIHYPERTENSIVES AND HEART FAILURE DRUGS	↑ Hypotensive effect. Episodes of severe first dose ↓ BP when alpha-blockers are added to ACE inhibitors	Additive hypotensive effect; may be used therapeutically	Monitor BP at least weekly until stable, particularly on initiation of therapy. Consider starting therapy at night
ACE INHIBITORS—CAPTOPRIL	ANTIOBESITY—LORCASERIN	↑ Blood concentrations of captopril	Inhibition of CYP2D6-mediated metabolism	Monitor PR and BP closely until stable
ACE INHIBITORS	**ANTI-PARKINSON'S DRUGS**			
ACE INHIBITORS	LEVODOPA	↑ Hypotensive effect	Additive effect	Monitor BP at least weekly until stable. Warn patients to report symptoms of hypotension (light-headedness, dizziness on standing, etc.)
ACE INHIBITORS	PERGOLIDE	Possible ↑ hypotensive effect	Additive effect; a single case of severe ↓ BP with lisinopril and pergolide has been reported	Monitor BP at least weekly until stable. Warn patients to report about symptoms of hypotension (light-headedness, dizziness on standing, etc.)

(Continued)

Primary Drug	Secondary Drug	Effect	Mechanism	Precautions
ANTIHYPERTENSIVES AND HEART FAILURE DRUGS				
ACE INHIBITORS	ANTIPLATELET DRUGS—ASPIRIN	↑ Risk of renal impairment. ↓ Efficacy of captopril and enalapril with high-dose (>100 mg/day) aspirin	Aspirin and NSAIDs can cause elevation of BP. Prostaglandin inhibition leads to sodium and water retention and poor renal function in those with impaired renal blood flow	Monitor renal function every 3–6 months; watch for poor response to ACE inhibitors when >100 mg/day aspirin is given
ACE INHIBITORS	ANTIPSYCHOTICS	↑ Hypotensive effect	Dose-related ↓ BP (due to vasodilatation) is a side effect of most antipsychotics, particularly phenothiazines	Monitor BP closely, especially during initiation of treatment. Warn patients to report symptoms of hypotension (light-headedness, dizziness on standing, etc.)
ACE INHIBITORS	ANXIOLYTICS AND HYPNOTICS	↑ Hypotensive effect	Additive hypotensive effect	Monitor BP at least weekly until stable. Warn patients to report symptoms of hypotension (light-headedness, dizziness on standing, etc.)
ACE INHIBITORS	BETA-BLOCKERS	↑ Hypotensive effect	Additive hypotensive effect; may be used therapeutically	Monitor BP at least weekly until stable. Warn patients to report symptoms of hypotension (light-headedness, dizziness on standing, etc.)
ACE INHIBITORS	CALCIUM CHANNEL BLOCKERS	↑ Hypotensive effect	Additive hypotensive effect; may be used therapeutically	Monitor BP at least weekly until stable. Warn patients to report symptoms of hypotension (light-headedness, dizziness on standing, etc.)
ACE INHIBITORS	CARDIAC GLYCOSIDES—DIGOXIN	↑ Plasma concentrations of digoxin when captopril is coadministered in the presence of heart failure (class II or more severe) or renal insufficiency. No other ACE inhibitors seem to interact in the same way	Uncertain; postulated to be due to ↓ renal excretion of digoxin	Monitor digoxin levels; watch for digoxin toxicity

(Continued)

Primary Drug	Secondary Drug	Effect	Mechanism	Precautions
ANTIHYPERTENSIVES AND HEART FAILURE DRUGS				
ACE INHIBITORS	**DIURETICS**			
ACE INHIBITORS	LOOP DIURETICS	↑ Hypotensive effect. Risk of first-dose ↓ BP greater when ACE inhibitors are added to high-dose diuretics	Additive hypotensive effect; may be used therapeutically	Monitor BP at least weekly until stable. Warn patients to report about symptoms of hypotension (light-headedness, dizziness on standing, etc.). Benefits often outweigh risks
ACE INHIBITORS	POTASSIUM-SPARING DIURETICS, ALDOSTERONE ANTAGONISTS	↑ Risk of hyperkalemia	Additive retention of potassium	Monitor serum potassium every week until stable, then every 3–6 months
ACE INHIBITORS	THIAZIDES	↑ Hypotensive effect. Risk of first-dose ↓ BP greater when ACE inhibitors are added to high-dose diuretics	Additive hypotensive effect; may be used therapeutically	Monitor BP at least weekly until stable. Warn patients to report symptoms of hypotension (light-headedness, dizziness on standing, etc.). Benefits often outweigh risks
ACE INHIBITORS	EPOETIN	↓ Hematopoietic effects of epoetin ↓ Efficacy of ACE inhibitors	Angiotensin II is believed to be responsible for sustaining secretion of erythropoietin and for stimulating the bone marrow to produce erythrocytes. Epoetin has direct contractile effects on vessels (causing ↑ BP)	Watch for poor response to erythropoietin and to ACE inhibitors. These effects may be delayed, so monitor for the duration of coadministration
ACE INHIBITORS	GOLD (SODIUM AUROTHIOMALATE)	Cases of ↓ BP. May be delayed by several months	Additive vasodilating effects	Monitor BP at least weekly until stable. Warn patients to report symptoms of hypotension (light-headedness, dizziness on standing, etc.). If reaction occurs, consider changing to alternative gold formulation or stopping ACE inhibitor

(*Continued*)

Primary Drug	Secondary Drug	Effect	Mechanism	Precautions
ANTIHYPERTENSIVES AND HEART FAILURE DRUGS				
ACE INHIBITORS	INTERFERON ALFA	Risk of severe granulocytopenia	Possibly due to synergistic hematological toxicity	Monitor blood counts frequently; warn patients to report promptly any symptoms of infection
ACE INHIBITORS	MUSCLE RELAXANTS—SKELETAL	↑ Hypotensive effect with tizanidine and baclofen	Additive hypotensive effect	Monitor BP at least weekly until stable. Warn patients to report symptoms of hypotension (light-headedness, dizziness on standing, etc.)
ACE INHIBITORS	NITRATES	↑ Hypotensive effect	Additive hypotensive effect; may be used therapeutically	Monitor BP at least weekly until stable. Warn patients to report symptoms of hypotension (light-headedness, dizziness on standing, etc.)
ACE INHIBITORS	ESTROGENS	↓ Hypotensive effect	Estrogens cause sodium and fluid retention	Monitor BP at least weekly until stable; routine prescription of estrogens in patients with ↑ BP is not advisable
ACE INHIBITORS	ORLISTAT	↓ Hypotensive effect found with enalapril. Rare cases of marked hypertension	Uncertain at present	Monitor BP at least weekly until stable
ACE INHIBITORS	PERIPHERAL VASODILATORS—MOXISYLYTE (THYMOXAMINE)	↑ Hypotensive effect	Additive hypotensive effect	Monitor BP at least weekly until stable. Warn patients to report symptoms of hypotension (light-headedness, dizziness on standing, etc.)
ACE INHIBITORS	POTASSIUM	↑ Risk of hyperkalemia	Retention of potassium by ACE inhibitors and additional intake of potassium	Monitor serum potassium daily
ACE INHIBITORS	POTASSIUM CHANNEL ACTIVATORS	↑ Hypotensive effect	Additive effect	Monitor BP closely

(*Continued*)

Primary Drug	Secondary Drug	Effect	Mechanism	Precautions
ANTIHYPERTENSIVES AND HEART FAILURE DRUGS				
ACE INHIBITORS	PROGESTOGENS	↑ Risk of hyperkalemia	Drospirenone (component of some combined contraceptive pills) is a progestogen derived from spironolactone that can cause potassium retention	Monitor serum potassium weekly until stable, then every 6 months.
ACE INHIBITORS	PROSTAGLANDINS—ALPROSTADIL	↑ Hypotensive effect	Additive hypotensive effect	Monitor BP at least weekly until stable. Warn patients to report symptoms of hypotension (light-headedness, dizziness on standing, etc.)
ACE INHIBITORS	SYMPATHOMIMETICS	↓ Hypotensive effect. Note there is a risk of interactions even with topical sympathomimetics (eye and nose drops)	Adrenergic neurone blockers act mainly by preventing the release of norepinephrine. Sympathomimetics stimulate adrenergic receptors, which causes a rise in BP	Monitor BP at least weekly until stable
ADRENERGIC NEURONE BLOCKERS				
ADRENERGIC NEURONE BLOCKERS	ALCOHOL	1. Acute alcohol ingestion may ↑ hypotensive effects 2. Chronic moderate/heavy drinking ↓ hypotensive effect	1. Additive hypotensive effect 2. Chronic alcohol excess is associated with hypertension	Monitor BP closely as unpredictable responses can occur. Advise patients to drink only in moderation and avoid large variations in the amount of alcohol drunk
ADRENERGIC NEURONE BLOCKERS	ANESTHETICS—GENERAL	Risk of severe hypotensive episodes during induction of anesthesia	Most general anesthetics are myocardial depressants and vasodilators. Additive hypotensive effect	Monitor BP closely, especially during induction of anesthesia

(Continued)

Primary Drug	Secondary Drug	Effect	Mechanism	Precautions
ANTIHYPERTENSIVES AND HEART FAILURE DRUGS				
ADRENERGIC NEURONE BLOCKERS—GUANETHIDINE	ANESTHETICS—LOCAL	↓ Clinical efficacy of guanethidine when used in the treatment of complex regional pain syndrome-type I	The local anesthetic ↓ the reuptake of guanethidine	Be aware. Consider use of a local anesthetic that minimally inhibits reuptake, e.g., lidocaine, when possible
ADRENERGIC NEURONE BLOCKERS	ANALGESICS—NSAIDs	↓ Hypotensive effect reported with phenylbutazone. Theoretical risk of similar effect with other NSAIDs	NSAIDs cause sodium and water retention and raise BP by inhibiting vasodilating renal prostaglandins	Benefits often outweigh risks for short-term NSAID use but particular caution in the elderly. For longer-term use, monitor BP, renal function, and serum potassium at least weekly until stable
ADRENERGIC NEURONE BLOCKERS	**ANTICANCER AND IMMUNOMODULATING DRUGS**			
ADRENERGIC NEURONE BLOCKERS	BORTEZOMIB	↑ Hypotensive effect	Additive hypotensive effect	Monitor BP at least weekly until stable, particularly on initiation of therapy
ADRENERGIC NEURONE BLOCKERS	CORTICOSTEROIDS	↓ Hypotensive effect	Corticosteroids cause sodium and water retention leading to ↑ BP	Monitor BP at least weekly until stable
ADRENERGIC NEURONE BLOCKERS	INTERLEUKIN-2 (ALDESLEUKIN)	↑ Hypotensive effect	Additive hypotensive effect; may be used therapeutically. Aldesleukin causes ↓ vascular resistance and ↑ capillary permeability	Monitor BP at least weekly until stable. Warn patients to report symptoms of hypotension (light-headedness, dizziness on standing, etc.)
ADRENERGIC NEURONE BLOCKERS	PROCARBAZINE	Hypotension	Additive	Monitor closely

(*Continued*)

Primary Drug	Secondary Drug	Effect	Mechanism	Precautions
ANTIHYPERTENSIVES AND HEART FAILURE DRUGS				
ADRENERGIC NEURONE BLOCKERS	**ANTIDEPRESSANTS**			
ADRENERGIC NEURONE BLOCKERS	MAOIs	Possible ↑ hypotensive effect. MAOIs cause orthostatic hypotension	Additive hypotensive effect	Monitor BP at least weekly until stable. Warn patients to report symptoms of hypotension (light-headedness, dizziness on standing, etc.)
ADRENERGIC NEURONE BLOCKERS	MAOIs	Risk of adrenergic syndrome	Due to inhibition of MAOI, which breaks down sympathomimetics	Avoid concurrent use. Onset may be 6–24 h after ingestion
ADRENERGIC NEURONE BLOCKERS	TCAs	↓ Hypotensive effect. There is possibly less effect with maprotiline and mianserin	TCAs compete with adrenergic neurone blockers for reuptake to nerve terminals	Monitor BP at least weekly until stable
ADRENERGIC NEURONE BLOCKERS	ANTIDIABETIC DRUGS	↑ Hypoglycemic effect	Catecholamines are diabetogenic; guanethidine blocks the release of catecholamines from nerve endings	Monitor blood glucose closely
ADRENERGIC NEURONE BLOCKERS	**ANTIHYPERTENSIVES AND HEART FAILURE DRUGS**			
ADRENERGIC NEURONE BLOCKERS	ANTIHYPERTENSIVES AND HEART FAILURE DRUGS	↑ Hypotensive effect. Episodes of severe first dose	Additive hypotensive effect; may be used therapeutically	Monitor BP at least weekly until stable, particularly on initiation of therapy. Consider starting therapy at night
ADRENERGIC NEURONE BLOCKERS	VASODILATOR ANTIHYPERTENSIVES—MINOXIDIL	Risk of excessive hypotension	Additive effect	Manufacturer recommends stopping guanethidine before starting minoxidil. If this is not possible, minoxidil should be started in hospital with close monitoring of BP

(*Continued*)

Primary Drug	Secondary Drug	Effect	Mechanism	Precautions
ANTIHYPERTENSIVES AND HEART FAILURE DRUGS				
ADRENERGIC NEURONE BLOCKERS	ANTI-PARKINSON'S DRUGS—LEVODOPA	↑ Hypotensive effect	Additive effect	Monitor BP at least weekly until stable. Warn patients to report symptoms of hypotension (light-headedness, dizziness on standing, etc.)
ADRENERGIC NEURONE BLOCKERS	ANTIPLATELET DRUGS—ASPIRIN	↓ Hypotensive effect; not noted with low-dose aspirin	Aspirin may cause sodium retention and vasoconstriction at possibly both renal and endothelial sites	Monitor BP at least weekly until stable when high-dose aspirin is prescribed
ADERENERGIC NEURONE BLOCKERS	**ANTIPSYCHOTICS**			
ADERENERGIC NEURONE BLOCKERS	ANTIPSYCHOTICS	↑ Hypotensive effect	Dose-related ↓ BP (due to vasodilatation) is a side effect of most antipsychotics, particularly phenothiazines	Monitor BP closely, especially during initiation of treatment. Warn patients to report symptoms of hypotension (light-headedness, dizziness on standing, etc.)
ADRENERGIC NEURONE BLOCKERS	CHLORPROMAZINE	Variable effect: some cases of ↑ hypotensive effect; other cases where hypotensive effects ↓ by higher doses (>100 mg) of chlorpromazine	Additive hypotensive effect. Phenothiazines cause vasodilatation; however, chlorpromazine blocks uptake of guanethidine into adrenergic neurons	Monitor BP at least weekly until stable. Warn patients to report symptoms of hypotension (light-headedness, dizziness on standing, etc.)
ADRENERGIC NEURONE BLOCKERS	HALOPERIDOL	↓ Hypotensive effect	Haloperidol blocks the uptake of guanethidine into adrenergic neurones	Monitor BP at least weekly until stable
ADRENERGIC NEURONE BLOCKERS	ANXIOLYTICS AND HYPNOTICS	↑ Hypotensive effect	Additive hypotensive effect	Monitor BP at least weekly until stable. Warn patients to report symptoms of hypotension (light-headedness, dizziness on standing, etc.)

(*Continued*)

Primary Drug	Secondary Drug	Effect	Mechanism	Precautions
ANTIHYPERTENSIVES AND HEART FAILURE DRUGS				
ADRENERGIC NEURONE BLOCKERS	BETA-BLOCKERS	↑ Hypotensive effect	Additive hypotensive effect; may be used therapeutically	Monitor BP at least weekly until stable. Warn patients to report symptoms of hypotension (light-headedness, dizziness on standing, etc.)
ADRENERGIC NEURONE BLOCKERS	CALCIUM CHANNEL BLOCKERS	↑ Hypotensive effect	Additive hypotensive effect; may be used therapeutically	Monitor BP at least weekly until stable. Warn patients to report symptoms of hypotension (light-headedness, dizziness on standing, etc.)
ADRENERGIC NEURONE BLOCKERS	DIURETICS—LOOP	↑ Hypotensive effect	Additive hypotensive effect; may be used therapeutically	Monitor BP at least weekly until stable. Warn patients to report symptoms of hypotension (light-headedness, dizziness on standing, etc.). Benefits often outweigh risks
ADRENERGIC NEURONE BLOCKERS	MUSCLE RELAXANTS—SKELETAL	↑ Hypotensive effect with tizanidine and baclofen	Additive hypotensive effect	Monitor BP at least weekly until stable. Warn patients to report symptoms of hypotension (light-headedness, dizziness on standing, etc.)
ADRENERGIC NEURONE BLOCKERS	NITRATES	↑ Hypotensive effect	Additive hypotensive effect; may be used therapeutically	Monitor BP at least weekly until stable. Warn patients to report symptoms of hypotension (light-headedness, dizziness on standing, etc.)
ADRENERGIC NEURONE BLOCKERS	ESTROGENS	↓ Hypotensive effect	Estrogens cause sodium and fluid retention	Monitor BP at least weekly until stable; routine prescription of estrogens in patients with ↑ BP is not advisable
ADRENERGIC NEURONE BLOCKERS	PERIPHERAL VASODILATORS—MOXISYLYTE (THYMOXAMINE)	↑ Hypotensive effect	Additive hypotensive effect	Monitor BP at least weekly until stable. Warn patients to report symptoms of hypotension (light-headedness, dizziness on standing, etc.)

(Continued)

Primary Drug	Secondary Drug	Effect	Mechanism	Precautions
ANTIHYPERTENSIVES AND HEART FAILURE DRUGS				
ADRENERGIC NEURONE BLOCKERS	PIZOTIFEN	↓ Hypotensive effect	Pizotifen competes with adrenergic neurone blockers for reuptake to nerve terminals	Monitor BP at least weekly until stable
ADRENERGIC NEURONE BLOCKERS	POTASSIUM CHANNEL ACTIVATORS	↑ Hypotensive effect	Additive effect	Monitor BP closely
ADRENERGIC NEURONE BLOCKERS	PROSTAGLANDINS—ALPROSTADIL	↑ Hypotensive effect	Additive hypotensive effect	Monitor BP at least weekly until stable. Warn patients to report symptoms of hypotension (light-headedness, dizziness on standing, etc.)
ADRENERGIC NEURONE BLOCKERS	**SYMPATHOMIMETICS**			
ADRENERGIC NEURONE BLOCKERS	SYMPATHOMIMETICS	↓ Hypotensive effect. Note there is a risk of interactions even with topical sympathomimetics (eye and nose drops)	Adrenergic neuron blockers act mainly by preventing the release of norepinephrine. Sympathomimetics stimulate adrenergic receptors, which causes a rise in BP	Monitor BP at least weekly until stable
ADRENERGIC NEURONE BLOCKERS	SYMPATHOMIMETICS—DIRECT	For patients on guanethidine, ↑ pressor effects have been reported with the administration of norepinephrine and metaraminol, and a lower threshold for arrhythmias with norepinephrine. Prolonged mydriasis reported when eye drops are given to patients on guanethidine	Guanethidine blocks the release of norepinephrine from adrenergic neurones; this causes a hypersensitivity of the receptors that are normally stimulated by norepinephrine and leads to the ↑ response when they are stimulated by directly acting sympathomimetics	Start alpha- and beta-1 agonists at a lower dose; monitor BP and cardiac rhythm closely

(*Continued*)

Primary Drug	Secondary Drug	Effect	Mechanism	Precautions
ANTIHYPERTENSIVES AND HEART FAILURE DRUGS				
ALISKIREN				
ALISKIREN	ANALGESICS—NSAIDs	1. ↓ Hypotensive effect 2. ↑ Risk of renal impairment 3. ↑ Risk of hyperkalemia	1. NSAIDs cause sodium and water retention and raise BP by inhibiting vasodilating renal prostaglandins 2. Additive effect 3. Additive effect	Benefits often outweigh risks for short-term NSAID use but particular caution in the elderly. For longer-term use, monitor BP, renal function, and serum potassium at least weekly until stable
ALISKIREN	**ANTIARRHYTHMICS**			
ALISKIREN	AMIODARONE	Aliskiren levels ↑ by amiodarone	Amiodarone is a moderate Pgp inhibitor	Monitor BP and serum potassium at least weekly until stable
ALISKIREN	QUINIDINE	Aliskiren levels ↑ by quinidine	Quinidine is a moderate Pgp inhibitor	Monitor BP and serum potassium at least weekly until stable
ALISKIREN	**ANTIBIOTICS**			
ALISKIREN	ANTIBIOTICS—MACROLIDES	Aliskiren levels ↑ by macrolides.	Macrolides are moderate Pgp inhibitors	Monitor BP and serum potassium at least weekly until stable
ALISKIREN	ANTIBIOTICS—RIFAMPICIN	Likely to ↓ plasma concentrations of aliskiren	Rifampicin induces Pgp	Monitor BP weekly until stable
ALISKIREN	**ANTICANCER AND IMMUNOMODULATING DRUGS**			
ALISKIREN	BORTEZOMIB	↑ Hypotensive effect	Additive hypotensive effect	Monitor BP at least weekly until stable, particularly on initiation of therapy
ALISKIREN	CICLOSPORIN	Likely to ↑ plasma concentrations of aliskiren	Uncertain	Avoid coadministration
ALISKIREN	PROCARBAZINE	Hypotension	Additive	Monitor closely
ALISKIREN	VEMURAFENIB	Possible increased levels of P-glycoprotein substrates	Vemurafenib inhibits P-glycoprotein	Be aware. Clinical significance unknown
ALISKIREN	ANTICOAGULANTS—PARENTERAL	Risk of hyperkalemia with heparin	Additive effect	Monitor serum potassium closely

(*Continued*)

Primary Drug	Secondary Drug	Effect	Mechanism	Precautions
ANTIHYPERTENSIVES AND HEART FAILURE DRUGS				
ALISKIREN	ANTIDEPRESSANTS	Possible ↑ hypotensive effect. MAOIs cause orthostatic hypotension	Additive hypotensive effect	Monitor BP at least weekly until stable. Warn patients to report symptoms of hypotension (light-headedness, dizziness on standing, etc.)
ALISKIREN	**ANTIFUNGALS**			
ALISKIREN	ITRACONAZOLE	Aliskiren levels markedly ↑ by itraconazole	Itraconazole is a strong Pgp inhibitor	Avoid coadministration
ALISKIREN	KETOCONAZOLE	Aliskiren levels ↑ by ketoconazole	Ketoconazole is a moderate Pgp inhibitor	Monitor BP and serum potassium at least weekly until stable
ALISKIREN	**ANTIHYPERTENSIVES AND HEART FAILURE DRUGS**			
ALISKIREN	ACE INHIBITORS	Reports of hypotension with syncope or stroke, renal impairment, and hyperkalemia	Additive effect on renin-angiotensin system	1. Contraindicated in patients with diabetes mellitus or renal impairment (GFR < 60) 2. Other patients need close monitoring of renal function, serum potassium, and blood pressure
ALISKIREN	ANGIOTENSIN II RECEPTOR ANTAGONISTS	Reports of hypotension with syncope or stroke, renal impairment, and hyperkalemia	Additive effect on renin-angiotensin system	1. Contraindicated in patients with diabetes mellitus or renal impairment (GFR < 60) 2. Other patients need close monitoring of renal function, serum potassium, and blood pressure (weekly until stable)
ALISKIREN	BETA-BLOCKERS	↑ Hypotensive effect	Additive hypotensive effect; may be used therapeutically	Monitor BP at least weekly until stable. Warn patients to report symptoms of hypotension (light-headedness, dizziness on standing, etc.)
ALISKIREN	CALCIUM CHANNEL BLOCKERS—VERAPAMIL	Aliskiren levels ↑ by verapamil	Verapamil is a moderate Pgp inhibitor	Monitor BP and serum potassium at least weekly until stable

(*Continued*)

Primary Drug	Secondary Drug	Effect	Mechanism	Precautions
ANTIHYPERTENSIVES AND HEART FAILURE DRUGS				
ALISKIREN	**DIURETICS**			
ALISKIREN	LOOP DIURETICS	↓ Plasma levels of furosemide	Uncertain	Watch for poor response to furosemide
ALISKIREN	POTASSIUM-SPARING DIURETICS AND ALDOSTERONE ANTAGONISTS	Risk of hyperkalemia	Additive effect	Monitor serum potassium every week until stable, then every 3–6 months
ALISKIREN	FOOD—FRUIT JUICE AND HERBAL TEA	Risk of therapeutic failure	Inhibition of gastrointestinal Pgp	Manufacturers recommend patients taking aliskiren to avoid these drinks
ALISKIREN	GRAPEFRUIT JUICE	↓ Aliskiren levels	Possibly inhibition of enteric OATP-mediated uptake by GFJ could account for the reduced exposure	Monitor BP closely
ALISKIREN	POTASSIUM	Risk of hyperkalemia	Additive effect	Avoid coadministration
ALISKIREN	POTASSIUM CHANNEL ACTIVATORS	↑ Hypotensive effect	Additive effect	Monitor BP closely
ALPHA-BLOCKERS				
ALPHA-BLOCKERS	**ALCOHOL**			
ALPHA-BLOCKERS	ALCOHOL	1. Acute alcohol ingestion may ↑ hypotensive effects 2. Chronic moderate/heavy drinking ↓ hypotensive effect	1. Additive hypotensive effect 2. Chronic alcohol excess is associated with hypertension	Monitor BP closely as unpredictable responses can occur. Advise patients to drink only in moderation and avoid large variations in the amount of alcohol drunk
INDORAMIN	ALCOHOL	↑ Levels of both alcohol and indoramin occurs with concurrent use	Uncertain	Warn the patient about the risk of ↑ sedation
ALPHA-BLOCKERS	ANESTHETICS—GENERAL	Risk of severe hypotensive episodes during induction of anesthesia	Most general anesthetics are myocardial depressants and vasodilators. Additive hypotensive effect	Monitor BP closely, especially during induction of anesthesia

(Continued)

Primary Drug	Secondary Drug	Effect	Mechanism	Precautions
ANTIHYPERTENSIVES AND HEART FAILURE DRUGS				
ALPHA-BLOCKERS—TAMSULOSIN	QUINIDINE	↑ Tamsulosin levels	Inhibition of CYP2D6-mediated metabolism	Monitor BP closely; warn patient to report symptoms of orthostatic hypotension
ALPHA-BLOCKERS	ANTIBIOTICS-MACROLIDES	↑ Levels of alfuzosin, doxazosin, and possibly tamsulosin with clarithromycin and telithromycin	These drugs are strong inhibitors of CYP3A4-mediated metabolism of these drugs. Tamsulosin is also metabolized by CYP2D6	Monitor BP closely, especially during initiation of treatment. Warn patients to report symptoms of hypotension (light-headedness, dizziness on standing, etc.)
ALPHA-BLOCKERS	**ANTICANCER AND IMMUNOMODULATING DRUGS**			
ALPHA-BLOCKERS	BORTEZOMIB	↑ Hypotensive effect	Additive hypotensive effect	Monitor BP at least weekly until stable, particularly on initiation of therapy
ALPHA-BLOCKERS	CICLOSPORIN	1. Slight reduced GFR with prazosin in renal transplants 2. Predicted increase in silodosin levels	1. Uncertain 2. P-glycoprotein inhibition	1. Prazosin not ideal antihypertensive 2. Avoid concurrent use
ALPHA-BLOCKERS	CORTICOSTEROIDS	↓ Hypotensive effect	Corticosteroids cause sodium and water retention leading to ↑ BP	Monitor BP at least weekly until stable
ALPHA-BLOCKERS	INTERLEUKIN-2 (ALDESLEUKIN)	↑ Hypotensive effect	Additive hypotensive effect; may be used therapeutically. Aldesleukin causes ↓ vascular resistance and ↑ capillary permeability	Monitor BP at least weekly until stable. Warn patients to report symptoms of hypotension (light-headedness, dizziness on standing, etc.)
ALPHA-BLOCKERS	PROCARBAZINE	Hypotension	Additive	Monitor closely
ALPHA-BLOCKERS	THALIDOMIDE	Excessive bradycardia	Additive effect	Monitor BP and PR closely
ALPHA-BLOCKERS	ANTIDEPRESSANTS—MAOIs	Possible ↑ hypotensive effect. MAOIs cause orthostatic hypotension	Additive hypotensive effect	Monitor BP at least weekly until stable. Warn patients to report symptoms of hypotension (light-headedness, dizziness on standing, etc.)

(*Continued*)

Primary Drug	Secondary Drug	Effect	Mechanism	Precautions
ANTIHYPERTENSIVES AND HEART FAILURE DRUGS				
ALPHA-BLOCKERS	ANTIFUNGALS—AZOLES	↑ Levels of alfuzosin, doxazosin, and possibly tamsulosin with itraconazole, ketoconazole, and voriconazole	These drugs are strong inhibitors of CYP3A4-mediated metabolism of these drugs. Tamsulosin is also metabolized by CYP2D6	Monitor BP closely, especially during initiation of treatment. Warn patients to report symptoms of hypotension (light-headedness, dizziness on standing, etc.)
ALPHA-BLOCKERS	ANTIHYPERTENSIVES AND HEART FAILURE DRUGS	↑ Hypotensive effect. Risk of severe first dose ↓ BP when alpha-blockers are added to ACE inhibitors and angiotensin II receptor blockers	Additive hypotensive effect; may be used therapeutically	Monitor BP at least weekly until stable, particularly on initiation of therapy. Consider starting therapy at night
ALPHA-BLOCKERS	ANTI-PARKINSON'S DRUGS—APOMORPHINE	↑ Hypotensive effect	Not clear—effect seen with vasodilators but not other antihypertensives	Monitor BP closely, especially during initiation of treatment. Warn patients to report symptoms of hypotension (light-headedness, dizziness on standing, etc.)
ALPHA-BLOCKERS	ANTIPLATELET DRUGS—ASPIRIN	↓ Hypotensive effect; not noted with low-dose aspirin	Aspirin may cause sodium retention and vasoconstriction at possibly both renal and endothelial sites	Monitor BP at least weekly until stable when high-dose aspirin is prescribed
ALPHA-BLOCKERS	ANTIPSYCHOTICS	↑ Hypotensive effect	Dose-related ↓ BP (due to vasodilatation) is a side effect of most antipsychotics, particularly phenothiazines	Monitor BP closely, especially during initiation of treatment. Warn patients to report symptoms of hypotension (light-headedness, dizziness on standing, etc.)

(*Continued*)

Primary Drug	Secondary Drug	Effect	Mechanism	Precautions
ANTIHYPERTENSIVES AND HEART FAILURE DRUGS				
ALPHA-BLOCKERS	**ANTIVIRALS**			
ALPHA-BLOCKERS—ALFUZOSIN	COBICISTAT	↑ Plasma levels	Inhibition of metabolism via CYP3A	Avoid coadministration
ALPHA-BLOCKERS	PROTEASE INHIBITORS	↑ Levels of alfuzosin, doxazosin, and possibly tamsulosin with boceprevir and telaprevir	These drugs are strong inhibitors of CYP3A4-mediated metabolism of these drugs. Tamsulosin is also metabolized by CYP 2D6	Monitor BP closely, especially during initiation of treatment. Warn patients to report symptoms of hypotension (light-headedness, dizziness on standing, etc.)
ALPHA-BLOCKERS	ANXIOLYTICS AND HYPNOTICS	↑ Hypotensive effect	Additive hypotensive effect	Monitor BP at least weekly until stable. Warn patients to report symptoms of hypotension (light-headedness, dizziness on standing, etc.)
ALPHA-BLOCKERS	BETA-BLOCKERS	↑ Efficacy of alpha-blockers; ↑ risk of first-dose ↓ BP when alfuzosin, prazosin, or terazosin is started in patients already taking beta-blockers	Additive hypotensive effect; may be used therapeutically	Monitor BP at least weekly until stable. Warn patients to report symptoms of hypotension (light-headedness, dizziness on standing, etc.). Watch for first-dose ↓ BP
ALPHA-BLOCKERS	CALCIUM CHANNEL BLOCKERS	↑ Efficacy of alpha-blockers; ↑ risk of first-dose ↓ BP with alfuzosin, prazosin, and terazosin	Additive hypotensive effect; may be used therapeutically	Watch for first-dose ↓ BP when starting either drug when the patient is already established on the other; consider reducing the dose of the established drug and starting the new agent at the lowest dose and titrating up
ALPHA-BLOCKERS	CARDIAC GLYCOSIDES	Possibility of ↑ plasma concentrations of digoxin with prazosin; no cases of toxicity have been reported	Uncertain	Monitor digoxin levels

(*Continued*)

Primary Drug	Secondary Drug	Effect	Mechanism	Precautions
ANTIHYPERTENSIVES AND HEART FAILURE DRUGS				
ALPHA-BLOCKERS	**DIURETICS**			
ALPHA-BLOCKERS	LOOP DIURETICS	↑ Hypotensive effect	Additive hypotensive effect; may be used therapeutically	Monitor BP at least weekly until stable. Warn patients to report symptoms of hypotension (light-headedness, dizziness on standing, etc.). Benefits often outweigh risks. Patients with congestive cardiac failure on diuretics should be started on a low dose of alpha-blocker
ALPHA-BLOCKERS	THIAZIDES	↑ Hypotensive effect	Additive hypotensive effect; may be used therapeutically	Monitor BP at least weekly until stable. Warn patients to report symptoms of hypotension (light-headedness, dizziness on standing, etc.). Benefits often outweigh risks. Patients with congestive cardiac failure on diuretics should be started on a low dose of alpha-blocker
ALPHA-BLOCKERS—SILODOSIN, TAMSULOSIN	GRAPEFRUIT JUICE	↑ Silodosin and tamsulosin levels	Inhibition of metabolism (UGT2B7 and CYP3A4)	Avoid grapefruit juice while taking silodosin and tamsulosin
ALPHA-BLOCKERS	H2 RECEPTOR BLOCKERS	↓ Efficacy of tolazoline	Uncertain; possibly ↓ absorption	Watch for poor response to tolazoline
ALPHA-BLOCKERS	MUSCLE RELAXANTS—SKELETAL	↑ Hypotensive effect with tizanidine and baclofen	Additive hypotensive effect	Monitor BP at least weekly until stable. Warn patients to report symptoms of hypotension (light-headedness, dizziness on standing, etc.)
ALPHA-BLOCKERS	NITRATES	↑ Hypotensive effect	Additive hypotensive effect; may be used therapeutically	Monitor BP at least weekly until stable. Warn patients to report symptoms of hypotension (light-headedness, dizziness on standing, etc.)

(*Continued*)

Primary Drug	Secondary Drug	Effect	Mechanism	Precautions
ANTIHYPERTENSIVES AND HEART FAILURE DRUGS				
ALPHA-BLOCKERS	ESTROGENS	↓ Hypotensive effect	Estrogens cause sodium and fluid retention	Monitor BP at least weekly until stable; routine prescription of estrogens in patients with ↑ BP is not advisable
ALPHA-BLOCKERS	PERIPHERAL VASODILATORS—MOXISYLYTE (THYMOXAMINE)	↑ Hypotensive effect	Additive hypotensive effect	Monitor BP at least weekly until stable. Warn patients to report symptoms of hypotension (light-headedness, dizziness on standing, etc.)
ALPHA-BLOCKERS	PHOSPHODIESTERASE TYPE 5 INHIBITORS	Risk of marked ↓ BP	Additive hypotensive effect	Avoid coadministration if possible (manufacturers particularly mention tadalafil). If others must be administered with alpha blockers, warn patients about the clinical features of orthostatic hypotension
ALPHA-BLOCKERS	POTASSIUM CHANNEL ACTIVATORS	↑ Hypotensive effect	Additive effect	Monitor BP closely
ALPHA-BLOCKERS	PROSTAGLANDINS—ALPROSTADIL	↑ Hypotensive effect	Additive hypotensive effect	Monitor BP at least weekly until stable. Warn patients to report symptoms of hypotension (light-headedness, dizziness on standing, etc.)
ANGIOTENSIN II RECEPTOR ANTAGONISTS				
ANGIOTENSIN II RECEPTOR ANTAGONISTS	ALCOHOL	1. Acute alcohol ingestion may ↑ hypotensive effects 2. Chronic moderate/heavy drinking ↓ hypotensive effect	1. Additive hypotensive effect 2. Chronic alcohol excess is associated with hypertension	Monitor BP closely as unpredictable responses can occur. Advise patients to drink only in moderation and avoid large variations in the amount of alcohol drunk
ANGIOTENSIN II RECEPTOR ANTAGONISTS	ALISKIREN	Aliskiren levels possibly ↓ by irbesartan	Uncertain	Monitor BP at least weekly until stable
ANGIOTENSIN II RECEPTOR ANTAGONISTS	ANESTHETICS—GENERAL	Risk of severe hypotensive episodes during induction of anesthesia	Most general anesthetics are myocardial depressants and vasodilators. Additive hypotensive effect	Monitor BP closely, especially during induction of anesthesia

(*Continued*)

Primary Drug	Secondary Drug	Effect	Mechanism	Precautions
ANTIHYPERTENSIVES AND HEART FAILURE DRUGS				
ANGIOTENSIN II RECEPTOR ANTAGONISTS	ANALGESICS—NSAIDs	1. ↓ Hypotensive effect 2. ↑ Risk of renal impairment 3. ↑ Risk of hyperkalemia	1. NSAIDs cause sodium and water retention and raise BP by inhibiting vasodilating renal prostaglandins 2. Additive effect 3. Additive effect	Benefits often outweigh risks for short-term NSAID use but particular caution in the elderly. For longer-term use, monitor BP, renal function, and serum potassium at least weekly until stable
LOSARTAN	ANTIBIOTICS—RIFAMPICIN	↓ Antihypertensive effect of losartan	Rifampicin induces CYP2C9	Monitor BP at least weekly until stable
ANGIOTENSIN II RECEPTOR ANTAGONISTS	**ANTICANCER AND IMMUNOMODULATING DRUGS**			
ANGIOTENSIN II RECEPTOR ANTAGONISTS	BORTEZOMIB	↑ Hypotensive effect	Additive hypotensive effect	Monitor BP at least weekly until stable, particularly on initiation of therapy
ANGIOTENSIN II RECEPTOR ANTAGONISTS	CICLOSPORIN	↑ Risk of hyperkalemia and renal failure	Ciclosporin causes a dose-dependent ↑ in serum creatinine, urea, and potassium, especially in renal dysfunction	Monitor renal function and serum potassium weekly until stable, then at least every 3–6 months
ANGIOTENSIN II RECEPTOR ANTAGONISTS	CORTICOSTEROIDS	↓ Hypotensive effect	Corticosteroids cause sodium and water retention leading to ↑ BP	Monitor BP at least weekly until stable
ANGIOTENSIN II RECEPTOR ANTAGONISTS—LOSARTAN	EVEROLIMUS	Reports of angioedema	Uncertain—possibly additive effect (both can cause angioedema)	Warn patient to report facial swelling immediately
ANGIOTENSIN II RECEPTOR ANTAGONISTS—LOSARTAN	FLUOROURACIL	Inhibition of losartan to its active metabolite, E-3174	CYP2C9 inhibition	Clinical significance unclear

(*Continued*)

Primary Drug	Secondary Drug	Effect	Mechanism	Precautions
ANTIHYPERTENSIVES AND HEART FAILURE DRUGS				
ANGIOTENSIN II RECEPTOR ANTAGONISTS	INTERLEUKIN-2 (ALDESLEUKIN)	↑ Hypotensive effect	Additive hypotensive effect; may be used therapeutically. Aldesleukin causes ↓ vascular resistance and ↑ capillary permeability	Monitor BP at least weekly until stable. Warn patients to report symptoms of hypotension (light-headedness, dizziness on standing, etc.)
ANGIOTENSIN II RECEPTOR ANTAGONISTS	IMATINIB	↑ Plasma concentrations of losartan, irbesartan, and valsartan	Imatinib is a potent inhibitor of CYP2C9 isoenzymes, which metabolize these angiotensin II receptor blockers	Monitor for toxic effects of losartan, e.g., hypotension, hyperkalemia, diarrhea, cough, vertigo, and liver toxicity
TELMISARTAN	MYCOPHENOLATE	Reduced mycophenolic acid levels	Unknown	Consider monitoring mycophenolate levels
ANGIOTENSIN II RECEPTOR ANTAGONISTS	PROCARBAZINE	Hypotension	Additive	Monitor closely
ANGIOTENSIN II RECEPTOR ANTAGONISTS	TACROLIMUS	↑ Risk of hyperkalemia	Uncertain	Monitor serum potassium weekly until stable, then every 6 months
ANGIOTENSIN II RECEPTOR ANTAGONISTS	ANTICOAGULANTS—PARENTERAL	↑ Risk of hyperkalemia with heparins	Heparin inhibits aldosterone secretion, causing hyperkalemia	Monitor potassium levels closely
ANGIOTENSIN II RECEPTOR ANTAGONISTS	**ANTIDEPRESSANTS**			
ANGIOTENSIN II RECEPTOR ANTAGONISTS	LITHIUM	Risk of lithium toxicity	↓ Excretion of lithium possibly due to ↓ renal tubular reabsorption of sodium in proximal tubule	Watch for lithium toxicity; monitor lithium levels
ANGIOTENSIN II RECEPTOR ANTAGONISTS	MAOIs	Possible ↑ hypotensive effect. MAOIs cause orthostatic hypotension	Additive hypotensive effect	Monitor BP at least weekly until stable. Warn patients to report symptoms of hypotension (light-headedness, dizziness on standing, etc.)

(*Continued*)

Primary Drug	Secondary Drug	Effect	Mechanism	Precautions
ANTIHYPERTENSIVES AND HEART FAILURE DRUGS				
ANGIOTENSIN II RECEPTOR ANTAGONISTS—IRBESARTAN	ANTIDIABETIC DRUGS—SULFONYLUREAS	Possible ↑ hypotensive effect of irbesartan by tolbutamide	Tolbutamide competitively inhibits CYP2C9-mediated metabolism of irbesartan	Monitor BP at least weekly until stable. Warn patients to report symptoms of hypotension (light-headedness, dizziness on standing, etc.)
ANGIOTENSIN II RECEPTOR ANTAGONISTS	**ANTIHYPERTENSIVES AND HEART FAILURE DRUGS**			
ANGIOTENSIN II RECEPTOR ANTAGONISTS	ANTIHYPERTENSIVES AND HEART FAILURE DRUGS	↑ Hypotensive effect. Episodes of severe first-dose ↓ BP when alpha-blockers are added to angiotensin II receptor antagonists	Additive hypotensive effect; may be used therapeutically	Monitor BP at least weekly until stable, particularly on initiation of therapy. Consider starting therapy at night
ANGIOTENSIN II RECEPTOR ANTAGONISTS	ACE INHIBITORS	Risk of hyperkalemia	Additive retention of potassium	Monitor renal function and serum potassium every 4–6 weeks until stable and then at least annually
ANGIOTENSIN II RECEPTOR ANTAGONISTS	ALISKIREN	Reports of hypotension with syncope or stroke, renal impairment, and hyperkalemia	Additive effect on renin-angiotensin system	1. Contraindicated in patients with diabetes mellitus or renal impairment (GFR < 60) 2. Other patients need close monitoring of renal function, serum potassium, and blood pressure (weekly until stable)
ANGIOTENSIN II RECEPTOR ANTAGONISTS	ANTI-PARKINSON'S DRUGS—LEVODOPA	↑ Hypotensive effect	Additive effect	Monitor BP at least weekly until stable. Warn patients to report symptoms of hypotension (light-headedness, dizziness on standing, etc.)

(*Continued*)

Primary Drug	Secondary Drug	Effect	Mechanism	Precautions
ANTIHYPERTENSIVES AND HEART FAILURE DRUGS				
ANGIOTENSIN II RECEPTOR ANTAGONISTS	ANTIPLATELET DRUGS—ASPIRIN	Risk of renal impairment when olmesartan is administered with high-dose aspirin (>3 g daily). Effect not noted with low-dose aspirin	Additive effect on reducing glomerular filtration rate	Monitor renal function regularly until stable
ANGIOTENSIN II RECEPTOR ANTAGONISTS	ANTIPSYCHOTICS	↑ Hypotensive effect	Dose-related ↓ BP (due to vasodilatation) is a side effect of most antipsychotics, particularly phenothiazines	Monitor BP closely, especially during initiation of treatment. Warn patients to report symptoms of hypotension (light-headedness, dizziness on standing, etc.)
ANGIOTENSIN II RECEPTOR ANTAGONISTS	ANXIOLYTICS AND HYPNOTICS	↑ Hypotensive effect	Additive hypotensive effect	Monitor BP at least weekly until stable. Warn patients to report symptoms of hypotension (light-headedness, dizziness on standing, etc.)
ANGIOTENSIN II RECEPTOR ANTAGONISTS	BETA-BLOCKERS	↑ Hypotensive effect	Additive hypotensive effect; may be used therapeutically	Monitor BP at least weekly until stable. Warn patients to report symptoms of hypotension (light-headedness, dizziness on standing, etc.)
ANGIOTENSIN II RECEPTOR ANTAGONISTS	CALCIUM CHANNEL BLOCKERS	↑ Hypotensive effect	Additive hypotensive effect; may be used therapeutically	Monitor BP at least weekly until stable. Warn patients to report symptoms of hypotension (light-headedness, dizziness on standing, etc.)
ANGIOTENSIN II RECEPTOR ANTAGONISTS	CARDIAC GLYCOSIDES—DIGOXIN	Telmisartan may ↑ plasma levels of digoxin	Uncertain; telmisartan thought to ↑ the rate of absorption of digoxin	Watch for digoxin toxicity, monitor digoxin levels

(*Continued*)

Primary Drug	Secondary Drug	Effect	Mechanism	Precautions
ANTIHYPERTENSIVES AND HEART FAILURE DRUGS				
ANGIOTENSIN II RECEPTOR ANTAGONISTS	**DIURETICS**			
ANGIOTENSIN II RECEPTOR ANTAGONISTS	LOOP DIURETICS	↑ Hypotensive effect. Risk of first-dose ↓ BP greater when angiotensin II receptor antagonists are added to high-dose diuretics	Additive hypotensive effect; may be used therapeutically	Monitor BP at least weekly until stable. Warn patients to report symptoms of hypotension (light-headedness, dizziness on standing, etc.). Benefits often outweigh risks
ANGIOTENSIN II RECEPTOR ANTAGONISTS	POTASSIUM-SPARING DIURETICS, ALDOSTERONE ANTAGONISTS	↑ Risk of hyperkalemia	Additive retention of potassium	Monitor serum potassium every week until stable, then every 3–6 months
ANGIOTENSIN II RECEPTOR ANTAGONISTS	THIAZIDES	↑ Hypotensive effect	Additive hypotensive effect; may be used therapeutically	Monitor BP at least weekly until stable. Warn patients to report symptoms of hypotension (light-headedness, dizziness on standing, etc.). Benefits often outweigh risks
ANGIOTENSIN II RECEPTOR ANTAGONISTS	EPOETIN	↓ Efficacy of angiotensin II receptor antagonists and possible ↑ risk of hyperkalemia	Angiotensin II is believed to sustain the secretion of erythropoietin and to stimulate the bone marrow to produce erythrocytes. Epoetin has a direct contractile effect on vessels	Monitor BP at least weekly until stable. Monitor serum potassium every week until stable, then every 3–6 months
ANGIOTENSIN II RECEPTOR ANTAGONISTS	MUSCLE RELAXANTS—SKELETAL	↑ Hypotensive effect with tizanidine and baclofen	Additive hypotensive effect	Monitor BP at least weekly until stable. Warn patients to report symptoms of hypotension (light-headedness, dizziness on standing, etc.)
ANGIOTENSIN II RECEPTOR ANTAGONISTS	NITRATES	↑ Hypotensive effect	Additive hypotensive effect; may be used therapeutically	Monitor BP at least weekly until stable. Warn patients to report symptoms of hypotension (light-headedness, dizziness on standing, etc.)

(*Continued*)

Primary Drug	Secondary Drug	Effect	Mechanism	Precautions
ANTIHYPERTENSIVES AND HEART FAILURE DRUGS				
ANGIOTENSIN II RECEPTOR ANTAGONISTS	ESTROGENS	↓ Hypotensive effect	Estrogens cause sodium and fluid retention	Monitor BP at least weekly until stable; routine prescription of estrogens in patients with ↑ BP is not advisable
ANGIOTENSIN II RECEPTOR ANTAGONISTS	ORLISTAT	Cases of ↓ efficacy of losartan, rare cases of marked hypertension	Uncertain at present	Monitor BP at least weekly until stable
ANGIOTENSIN II RECEPTOR ANTAGONISTS	PERIPHERAL VASODILATORS—MOXISYLYTE (THYMOXAMINE)	↑ Hypotensive effect	Additive hypotensive effect	Monitor BP at least weekly until stable. Warn patients to report symptoms of hypotension (light-headedness, dizziness on standing, etc.)
ANGIOTENSIN II RECEPTOR ANTAGONISTS	POTASSIUM	↑ Risk of hyperkalemia	Retention of potassium by ACE inhibitors and additional intake of potassium	Monitor serum potassium daily
ANGIOTENSIN II RECEPTOR ANTAGONISTS	POTASSIUM CHANNEL ACTIVATORS	↑ Hypotensive effect	Additive effect	Monitor BP closely
ANGIOTENSIN II RECEPTOR ANTAGONISTS	PROGESTOGENS	↑ Risk of hyperkalemia	Drospirenone (component of some brands of combined contraceptive pill) is a progestogen derived from spironolactone that can cause potassium retention	Monitor serum potassium weekly until stable, then every 6 months
ANGIOTENSIN II RECEPTOR ANTAGONISTS	PROSTAGLANDINS—ALPROSTADIL	↑ Hypotensive effect	Additive hypotensive effect	Monitor BP at least weekly until stable. Warn patients to report symptoms of hypotension (light-headedness, dizziness on standing, etc.)

(*Continued*)

Primary Drug	Secondary Drug	Effect	Mechanism	Precautions
ANTIHYPERTENSIVES AND HEART FAILURE DRUGS				
CENTRALLY ACTING ANTIHYPERTENSIVES				
CENTRALLY ACTING ANTIHYPERTENSIVES	**ALCOHOL**			
CENTRALLY ACTING ANTIHYPERTENSIVES	ALCOHOL	1. Acute alcohol ingestion may ↑ hypotensive effects 2. Chronic moderate/heavy drinking ↓ hypotensive effect	1. Additive hypotensive effect 2. Chronic alcohol excess is associated with hypertension	Monitor BP closely as unpredictable responses can occur. Advise patients to drink only in moderation and avoid large variations in the amount of alcohol drunk
CENTRALLY ACTING ANTIHYPERTENSIVES—CLONIDINE AND MOXONIDINE	ALCOHOL	Clonidine and moxonidine may exacerbate the sedative effects of alcohol, particularly during initiation of therapy	Uncertain	Warn patients of this effect and advise them to avoid driving or operating machinery if they suffer from sedation
CENTRALLY ACTING ANTIHYPERTENSIVES	ANESTHETICS—GENERAL	Risk of severe hypotensive episodes during induction of anesthesia	Most general anesthetics are myocardial depressants and vasodilators. Additive hypotensive effect	Monitor BP closely, especially during induction of anesthesia
CENTRALLY ACTING ANTIHYPERTENSIVES	**ANTICANCER AND IMMUNOMODULATING DRUGS**			
CENTRALLY ACTING ANTIHYPERTENSIVES	BORTEZOMIB	↑ Hypotensive effect	Additive hypotensive effect	Monitor BP at least weekly until stable, particularly on initiation of therapy
CENTRALLY ACTING ANTIHYPERTENSIVES—CLONIDINE	CICLOSPORIN	Single case of increased ciclosporin levels	Uncertain	Be aware of interaction
CENTRALLY ACTING ANTIHYPERTENSIVES—CLONIDINE	CRIZOTINIB	Risk of excessive bradycardia	Additive	Caution with concurrent use

(*Continued*)

Primary Drug	Secondary Drug	Effect	Mechanism	Precautions
ANTIHYPERTENSIVES AND HEART FAILURE DRUGS				
CENTRALLY ACTING ANTIHYPERTENSIVES	CORTICOSTEROIDS	↓ Hypotensive effect	Corticosteroids cause sodium and water retention leading to ↑ BP	Monitor BP at least weekly until stable
CENTRALLY ACTING ANTIHYPERTENSIVES—CLONIDINE	HISTAMINE	Possible increased toxicity of histamine	Additive effect on lowering blood pressure	Avoid concurrent use
CENTRALLY ACTING ANTIHYPERTENSIVES	INTERLEUKINL-2 (ALDESLEUKIN)	↑ Hypotensive effect	Additive hypotensive effect; may be used therapeutically. Aldesleukin causes ↓ vascular resistance and ↑ capillary permeability	Monitor BP at least weekly until stable. Warn patients to report symptoms of hypotension (light-headedness, dizziness on standing, etc.)
CENTRALLY ACTING ANTIHYPERTENSIVES	PROCARBAZINE	Hypotension	Additive	Monitor closely
CENTRALLY ACTING ANTIHYPERTENSIVES	**ANTIDEPRESSANTS**			
METHYLDOPA	ANTIDEPRESSANTS	Methyldopa may ↓ the effect of antidepressants	Methyldopa can cause depression	Methyldopa should be avoided in patients with depression
CENTRALLY ACTING ANTIHYPERTENSIVES	LITHIUM	Case reports of lithium toxicity when coingested with methyldopa. It was noted that lithium levels were in the therapeutic range	Uncertain at present	Avoid coadministration if possible; if not, watch closely for clinical features of toxicity and do not rely on lithium levels
METHYLDOPA	MAOIs	Risk of adrenergic syndrome. Reports of an enhanced hypotensive effect and hallucinations with methyldopa, which may cause depression	Due to inhibition of MAOI, which breaks down sympathomimetics	Avoid concurrent use. Onset may be 6–24 h after ingestion

(Continued)

Primary Drug	Secondary Drug	Effect	Mechanism	Precautions
ANTIHYPERTENSIVES AND HEART FAILURE DRUGS				
CENTRALLY ACTING ANTIHYPERTENSIVES	TCAs	1. Possibly hypotensive effect of clonidine and moxonidine antagonized by TCAs (some cases of hypertensive crisis) 2. Conversely, clonidine and moxonidine may exacerbate the sedative effects of TCAs, particularly during initiation of therapy	Uncertain	1. Monitor BP at least weekly until stable 2. Warn patients of the risk of sedation and advise them to avoid driving or operating machinery if they suffer from sedation
CENTRALLY ACTING ANTIHYPERTENSIVES	**ANTIHYPERTENSIVES AND HEART FAILURE DRUGS**			
CENTRALLY ACTING ANTIHYPERTENSIVES	ANTIHYPERTENSIVES AND HEART FAILURE DRUGS	↑ Hypotensive effect. Episodes of severe first dose ↓ BP when alpha-blockers are added to ACE inhibitors	Additive hypotensive effect; may be used therapeutically	Monitor BP at least weekly until stable, particularly on initiation of therapy. Consider starting therapy at night
CENTRALLY ACTING ANTIHYPERTENSIVES	ACE INHIBITORS	Some evidence that when switching from clonidine to captopril, there may be a delayed onset of action of captopril	Sudden cessation of clonidine causes rebound of ↑ BP, and this may be the reason for the delay in onset of captopril	Monitor BP at least weekly until stable
CLONIDINE	ALPHA-BLOCKERS—PRAZOSIN	Small case series indicate that prazosin may ↓ the antihypertensive effect of clonidine	Uncertain at present	Monitor BP at least weekly until stable
CENTRALLY ACTING ANTIHYPERTENSIVES	**ANTI-PARKINSON'S DRUGS**			
CENTRALLY ACTING ANTIHYPERTENSIVES	AMANTADINE	↓ Efficacy of amantadine with methyldopa	Antagonism of antiparkinsonian effect; these drugs have extrapyramidal side effects	Use with caution; avoid in patients aged under 20 years

(Continued)

Primary Drug	Secondary Drug	Effect	Mechanism	Precautions
ANTIHYPERTENSIVES AND HEART FAILURE DRUGS				
CENTRALLY ACTING ANTIHYPERTENSIVES	LEVODOPA	↑ Hypotensive effect	Additive effect	Monitor BP at least weekly until stable. Warn patients to report symptoms of hypotension (light-headedness, dizziness on standing, etc.)
CLONIDINE	LEVODOPA	Clonidine may oppose the effect of levodopa/carbidopa	Uncertain at present	Watch for deterioration in control of symptoms of Parkinson's disease
METHYLDOPA	LEVODOPA	Methyldopa may ↓ levodopa requirements, although there are case reports of deteriorating dyskinesias in some patients	Uncertain at present	Levodopa needs may ↓; in cases of worsening Parkinson's control, use an alternative antihypertensive
CENTRALLY ACTING ANTIHYPERTENSIVES	ASPIRIN	↓ Hypotensive effect; not noted with low-dose aspirin	Aspirin may cause sodium retention and vasoconstriction at possibly both renal and endothelial sites	Monitor BP at least weekly until stable when high-dose aspirin is prescribed
CENTRALLY ACTING ANTIHYPERTENSIVES	**ANTIPSYCHOTICS**			
CENTRALLY ACTING ANTIHYPERTENSIVES	ANTIPSYCHOTICS	↑ Hypotensive effect	Dose-related ↓ BP (due to vasodilatation) is a side effect of most antipsychotics, particularly phenothiazines	Monitor BP closely, especially during initiation of treatment. Warn patients to report symptoms of hypotension (light-headedness, dizziness on standing, etc.)
METHYLDOPA	HALOPERIDOL	Case reports of sedation or confusion on initiating coadministration of haloperidol and methyldopa	Uncertain; possible additive effect	Watch for excess sedation when starting therapy

(*Continued*)

Primary Drug	Secondary Drug	Effect	Mechanism	Precautions
ANTIHYPERTENSIVES AND HEART FAILURE DRUGS				
CENTRALLY ACTING ANTIHYPERTENSIVES	**ANXIOLYTICS AND HYPNOTICS**			
CENTRALLY ACTING ANTIHYPERTENSIVES	ANXIOLYTICS AND HYPNOTICS	↑ Hypotensive effect	Additive hypotensive effect	Monitor BP at least weekly until stable. Warn patients to report symptoms of hypotension (light-headedness, dizziness on standing, etc.)
CENTRALLY ACTING ANTIHYPERTENSIVES	ANXIOLYTICS AND HYPNOTICS	Clonidine and moxonidine may exacerbate the sedative effects of BZDs, particularly during initiation of therapy	Uncertain	Warn patients of this effect and advise them to avoid driving or operating machinery if they suffer from sedation
CENTRALLY ACTING ANTIHYPERTENSIVES	**BETA-BLOCKERS**			
CENTRALLY ACTING ANTIHYPERTENSIVES	BETA-BLOCKERS	↑ Hypotensive effect	Additive hypotensive effect; may be used therapeutically	Monitor BP at least weekly until stable. Warn patients to report symptoms of hypotension (light-headedness, dizziness on standing, etc.)
CLONIDINE, MOXONIDINE	BETA-BLOCKERS	Risk of withdrawal ↑ BP (rebound ↑ BP) with clonidine and possibly moxonidine	Withdrawal of clonidine, and possibly moxonidine, is associated with ↑ circulating catecholamines; beta-blockers, especially noncardioselective ones, will allow the catecholamines to exert an unopposed alpha action (vasoconstriction)	Do not withdraw clonidine or moxonidine while a patient is taking beta-blockers. Withdraw beta-blockers several days before slowly withdrawing clonidine and moxonidine
CENTRALLY ACTING ANTIHYPERTENSIVES	BRONCHODILATORS—BETA-2 AGONISTS	Cases of ↓ BP when intravenous salbutamol is given with methyldopa	Uncertain at present	Monitor BP closely

(*Continued*)

Primary Drug	Secondary Drug	Effect	Mechanism	Precautions
ANTIHYPERTENSIVES AND HEART FAILURE DRUGS				
CENTRALLY ACTING ANTIHYPERTENSIVES	**CALCIUM CHANNEL BLOCKERS**			
CENTRALLY ACTING ANTIHYPERTENSIVES	CALCIUM CHANNEL BLOCKERS	↑ Hypotensive effect	Additive hypotensive effect; may be used therapeutically	Monitor BP at least weekly until stable. Warn patients to report symptoms of hypotension (light-headedness, dizziness on standing, etc.)
CENTRALLY ACTING ANTIHYPERTENSIVES	VERAPAMIL	Two cases of complete heart block when clonidine was added to a patient on verapamil	Additive effect; both drugs are known rarely to cause AV dysfunction	Monitor ECG closely when coadministering
CENTRALLY ACTING ANTIHYPERTENSIVES	**DIURETICS**			
CENTRALLY ACTING ANTIHYPERTENSIVES	LOOP DIURETICS	↑ Hypotensive effect	Additive hypotensive effect; may be used therapeutically	Monitor BP at least weekly until stable. Warn patients to report symptoms of hypotension (light-headedness, dizziness on standing, etc.). Benefits often outweigh risks
CENTRALLY ACTING ANTIHYPERTENSIVES	THIAZIDES	↑ Hypotensive effect	Additive hypotensive effect; may be used therapeutically	Monitor BP at least weekly until stable. Warn patients to report symptoms of hypotension (light-headedness, dizziness on standing, etc.). Benefits often outweigh risks
CENTRALLY ACTING ANTIHYPERTENSIVES	IRON COMPOUNDS	↓ Antihypertensive effect of methyldopa	Ferrous sulfate and possibly ferrous gluconate may chelate methyldopa in the intestine and ↓ its absorption	Monitor BP at least weekly until stable

(*Continued*)

Primary Drug	Secondary Drug	Effect	Mechanism	Precautions
ANTIHYPERTENSIVES AND HEART FAILURE DRUGS				
CENTRALLY ACTING ANTIHYPERTENSIVES	**MUSCLE RELAXANTS—SKELETAL**			
CENTRALLY ACTING ANTIHYPERTENSIVES	MUSCLE RELAXANTS—SKELETAL	↑ Hypotensive effect with tizanidine and baclofen	Additive hypotensive effect	Monitor BP at least weekly until stable. Warn patients to report symptoms of hypotension (light-headedness, dizziness on standing, etc.)
CLONIDINE	TIZANIDINE	Theoretical risk of marked hypotension	Additive effect—tizanidine is structurally related to clonidine	Manufacturers recommend avoiding coadministration
CENTRALLY ACTING ANTIHYPERTENSIVES	NITRATES	↑ Hypotensive effect	Additive hypotensive effect; may be used therapeutically	Monitor BP at least weekly until stable. Warn patients to report symptoms of hypotension (light-headedness, dizziness on standing, etc.)
CENTRALLY ACTING ANTIHYPERTENSIVES	ESTROGENS	↓ Hypotensive effect	Estrogens cause sodium and fluid retention	Monitor BP at least weekly until stable; routine prescription of estrogens in patients with ↑ BP is not advisable
CENTRALLY ACTING ANTIHYPERTENSIVES	PERIPHERAL VASODILATORS—MOXISYLYTE (THYMOXAMINE)	↑ Hypotensive effect	Additive hypotensive effect	Monitor BP at least weekly until stable. Warn patients to report symptoms of hypotension (light-headedness, dizziness on standing, etc.)
CENTRALLY ACTING ANTIHYPERTENSIVES	POTASSIUM CHANNEL ACTIVATORS	↑ Hypotensive effect	Additive effect	Monitor BP closely
CENTRALLY ACTING ANTIHYPERTENSIVES	PROSTAGLANDINS—ALPROSTADIL	↑ Hypotensive effect	Additive hypotensive effect	Monitor BP at least weekly until stable. Warn patients to report symptoms of hypotension (light-headedness, dizziness on standing, etc.)
CENTRALLY ACTING ANTIHYPERTENSIVES	SYMPATHOMIMETICS—DIRECT	Risk of ↑ BP when clonidine is given with epinephrine or norepinephrine	Additive effect; clonidine use associated with ↑ circulating catecholamines	Monitor BP at least weekly until stable

(*Continued*)

Primary Drug	Secondary Drug	Effect	Mechanism	Precautions
ANTIHYPERTENSIVES AND HEART FAILURE DRUGS				
CENTRALLY ACTING ANTIHYPERTENSIVES	SYMPATHOMIMETICS—INDIRECT	1. Indirect sympathomimetics may ↓ the hypotensive effect of methyldopa 2. Methyldopa may ↓ the mydriatic effect of ephedrine eye drops	1. Uncertain 2. Uncertain	1. Monitor BP at least weekly until stable 2. Watch for a poor response to ephedrine eye drops
5-HT2 RECEPTOR AGONISTS—KETANSERIN				
KETANSERIN	**DRUGS THAT PROLONG THE QT INTERVAL**			
KETANSERIN	1. ANTIARRHYTHMICS—ajmaline, amiodarone, azimilide, cibenzoline, disopyramide, dofetilide, dronedarone, ibutilide, procainamide, propafenone, quinidine 2. ANTIBIOTICS—macrolides (especially azithromycin, clarithromycin, parenteral erythromycin, telithromycin), quinolones (especially moxifloxacin), quinupristin/dalfopristin 3. ANTICANCER AND IMMUNOMODULATING DRUGS—arsenic trioxide, bosutinib, crizotinib, dasatinib, eribulin, fingolimod, lapatinib, nilotinib, pazopanib, sunitinib, vandetanib, vemurafenib 4. ANTIDEPRESSANTS—TCAs, venlafaxine 5. ANTIEMETICS—ondansetron 6. ANTIFUNGALS—fluconazole, posaconazole, voriconazole 7. ANTIHISTAMINES—terfenadine, hydroxyzine, mizolastine 8. ANTIMALARIALS—artemether with lumefantrine, chloroquine, halofantrine, hydroxychloroquine, mefloquine, quinine	Risk of ventricular arrhythmias, particularly torsades de pointes	Additive effect; these drugs prolong the QT interval	Avoid coadministration

(Continued)

Primary Drug	Secondary Drug	Effect	Mechanism	Precautions
ANTIHYPERTENSIVES AND HEART FAILURE DRUGS				
	9. ANTIPROTOZOALS—pentamidine isethionate 10. ANTIPSYCHOTICS—atypicals, phenothiazines, pimozide 11. ANTIVIRALS—boceprevir, rilpivirine, telaprevir 12. BETA-BLOCKERS—sotalol 13. BRONCHODILATORS—parenteral bronchodilators 14. CNS STIMULANTS—atomoxetine 15. RANOLAZINE			
KETANSERIN	ALCOHOL	1. Acute alcohol ingestion may ↑ hypotensive effects 2. Chronic moderate/heavy drinking ↓ hypotensive effect	1. Additive hypotensive effect 2. Chronic alcohol excess is associated with hypertension	Monitor BP closely as unpredictable responses can occur. Advise patients to drink only in moderation and avoid large variations in the amount of alcohol drunk
KETANSERIN	ANTICANCER AND IMMUNOMODULATING DRUGS—PROCARBAZINE	Hypotension	Additive	Monitor closely
KETANSERIN	BETA-BLOCKERS	Risk of first dose hypotension	Additive effect	Monitor BP closely; start at a low dose and titrate up to effect
KETANSERIN	CALCIUM CHANNEL BLOCKERS—NIFEDIPINE	Small number of cases of ectopic beats and VT	Unknown	Monitor PR, BP, and ECG closely
KETANSERIN	DIURETICS—LOOP, THIAZIDES	Risk of ventricular arrhythmias, particularly torsades de pointes	These drugs ↓ potassium levels, which ↑ the risk of QT prolongation	Avoid coadministration
KETANSERIN	MUSCLE RELAXANTS—SKELETAL—BACLOFEN	↑ Hypotensive effect with tizanidine and baclofen	Additive hypotensive effect	Monitor BP at least weekly until stable. Warn patients to report symptoms of hypotension (light-headedness, dizziness on standing, etc.)

(*Continued*)

Primary Drug	Secondary Drug	Effect	Mechanism	Precautions
ANTIHYPERTENSIVES AND HEART FAILURE DRUGS				
KETANSERIN	ESTROGENS	↓ Hypotensive effect	Estrogens cause sodium and fluid retention	Monitor BP at least weekly until stable; routine prescription of estrogens in patients with ↑ BP is not advisable
KETANSERIN	POTASSIUM CHANNEL ACTIVATORS	↑ Hypotensive effect	Additive effect	Monitor BP closely
VASODILATOR ANTIHYPERTENSIVES				
VASODILATOR ANTIHYPERTENSIVES	ALCOHOL	1. Acute alcohol ingestion may ↑ hypotensive effects 2. Chronic moderate/heavy drinking ↓ hypotensive effect	1. Additive hypotensive effect 2. Chronic alcohol excess is associated with hypertension	Monitor BP closely as unpredictable responses can occur. Advise patients to drink only in moderation and avoid large variations in the amount of alcohol drunk
VASODILATOR ANTIHYPERTENSIVES	ANESTHETICS—GENERAL	Risk of severe hypotensive episodes during induction of anesthesia	Most general anesthetics are myocardial depressants and vasodilators. Additive hypotensive effect	Monitor BP closely, especially during induction of anesthesia
VASODILATOR ANTIHYPERTENSIVES	ANALGESICS—NSAIDs	1. Etoricoxib may ↑ minoxidil levels 2. Indometacin opposes the hypotensive effect of IV hydralazine	1. Etoricoxib inhibits sulfotransferase activity 2. Unknown mechanism	1. Monitor BP closely 2. Monitor BP closely
VASODILATOR ANTIHYPERTENSIVES	**ANTIBIOTICS**			
VASODILATOR ANTIHYPERTENSIVES	MACROLIDES	Erythromycin and clarithromycin may ↑ levels of sildenafil, tadalafil, and vardenafil	Inhibition of CYP3A4 mediated metabolism of these phosphodiesterase inhibitors	Monitor BP closely
VASODILATOR ANTIHYPERTENSIVES	RIFAMPICIN	1. ↓ Bosentan levels 2. Theoretical risk of abnormal liver function	1. Induction of metabolism 2. Additive effect—both may adversely affect liver function	Manufacturer recommends avoiding coadministration

(Continued)

Primary Drug	Secondary Drug	Effect	Mechanism	Precautions
ANTIHYPERTENSIVES AND HEART FAILURE DRUGS				
VASODILATOR ANTIHYPERTENSIVES	**ANTICANCER AND IMMUNOMODULATING DRUGS**			
VASODILATOR ANTIHYPERTENSIVES—BOSENTAN	BOSUTINIB	Reduced bosutinib levels	CYP3A induction	Manufacturer advises avoid concurrent use. Dose increase unlikely to sufficiently compensate
VASODILATOR ANTIHYPERTENSIVES	BORTEZOMIB	↑ Hypotensive effect	Additive hypotensive effect	Monitor BP at least weekly until stable, particularly on initiation of therapy
VASODILATOR ANTIHYPERTENSIVES	CICLOSPORIN	1. Coadministration of bosentan and ciclosporin leads to ↑ bosentan and ↓ ciclosporin levels 2. Ciclosporin moderately ↑ ambrisentan levels 3. Risk of hypertrichosis when minoxidil given with ciclosporin	1. Additive effect; both drugs inhibit the bile sodium export pump, which is associated with hepatotoxicity 2. Uncertain 3. Additive effect	1. Avoid coadministration of bosentan and ciclosporin 2. Limit ambrisentan to 5 mg/day and monitor BP closely until stable 3. Warn patients of the potential interaction
VASODILATOR ANTIHYPERTENSIVES	CORTICOSTEROIDS	↓ Hypotensive effect	Corticosteroids cause sodium and water retention leading to ↑ BP	Monitor BP at least weekly until stable
VASODILATOR ANTIHYPERTENSIVES—DIAZOXIDE	CORTICOSTEROIDS	Risk of hyperglycemia when diazoxide is coadministered with corticosteroids	Additive effect; both drugs have a hyperglycemic effect	Monitor blood glucose closely, particularly with diabetes
VASODILATOR ANTIHYPERTENSIVES—BOSENTAN	DOCETAXEL	Predicted reduced docetaxel levels	CYP3A4 induction	Monitor closely Dose increase may be required

(*Continued*)

Primary Drug	Secondary Drug	Effect	Mechanism	Precautions
ANTIHYPERTENSIVES AND HEART FAILURE DRUGS				
VASODILATOR ANTIHYPERTENSIVES	INTERLEUKIN-2 (ALDESLEUKIN)	↑ Hypotensive effect	Additive hypotensive effect; may be used therapeutically. Aldesleukin causes ↓ vascular resistance and ↑ capillary permeability	Monitor BP at least weekly until stable. Warn patients to report symptoms of hypotension (light-headedness, dizziness on standing, etc.)
BOSENTAN	METHOTREXATE	Reduced efficacy with oral methotrexate Case of hepatotoxicity with subcutaneous methotrexate	Reduced efficacy due to bosentan displacing methotrexate from its protein-binding sites, reducing conversion to active metabolites Heptatoxocity due to additive effects	Interaction not firmly established Caution with concurrent use
AMBRISENTAN	PONATINIB	Predicted increased in levels of ambrisentan	P-glycoprotein inhibition	Be aware
VASODILATOR ANTIHYPERTENSIVES	PROCARBAZINE	Hypotension	Additive	Monitor closely
VASODILATOR ANTIHYPERTENSIVES	ANTICOAGULANTS—ORAL	1. Bosentan may ↓ warfarin levels 2. Iloprost and sitaxentan may ↑ warfarin levels	1. Uncertain; postulated that bosentan induces CYP3A4 and 2C9 2. Uncertain	Monitor INR closely
VASODILATOR ANTIHYPERTENSIVES	ANTICOAGULANTS—PARENTERAL	Possible ↑ risk of bleeding with iloprost	Anticoagulant effects of heparins ↑ by a mechanism that is uncertain at present	Monitor APTT closely
VASODILATOR ANTIHYPERTENSIVES	ANTIDEPRESSANTS—MAOIs	Possible ↑ hypotensive effect. MAOIs cause orthostatic hypotension	Additive hypotensive effect	Monitor BP at least weekly until stable. Warn patients to report symptoms of hypotension (light-headedness, dizziness on standing, etc.)

(*Continued*)

Primary Drug	Secondary Drug	Effect	Mechanism	Precautions
ANTIHYPERTENSIVES AND HEART FAILURE DRUGS				
VASODILATOR ANTIHYPERTENSIVES	**ANTIDIABETIC DRUGS**			
VASODILATOR ANTIHYPERTENSIVES—BOSENTAN	SULFONYLUREAS	1. Risk of hepatotoxicity when bosentan is given with glibenclamide 2. ↑ Risk of hypoglycemic episodes when bosentan is given with tolbutamide	1. Additive effect: both drugs inhibit the bile sodium export pump 2. Bosentan may inhibit CYP2C9-mediated metabolism of tolbutamide	1. Avoid coadministration of bosentan and glibenclamide 2. Monitor blood glucose levels closely. Warn patients about the signs and symptoms of hypoglycemia. ***For signs and symptoms of hypoglycemia, see Clinical Features of Some Adverse Drug Interactions, Hypoglycemia***
VASODILATOR ANTIHYPERTENSIVES—DIAZOXIDE	ANTIDIABETIC DRUGS	May ↑ antidiabetic requirements	Diazoxide causes hyperglycemia by inhibiting insulin release and probably by a catecholamine-induced extrahepatic effect. Used in the treatment of hypoglycemia due to insulinomas	Larger doses of antidiabetic are often required; need to monitor blood sugar until adequate control of blood sugar is achieved
VASODILATOR ANTIHYPERTENSIVES	ANTIEPILEPTICS	Coadministration of diazoxide and phenytoin ↓ phenytoin levels and possibly ↓ efficacy of diazoxide	Uncertain at present	Monitor phenytoin levels and BP closely
VASODILATOR ANTIHYPERTENSIVES	ANTIFUNGALS—AZOLES	↑ Bosentan levels	Azoles inhibit CYP3A4 and CYP2C9	Monitor BP at least weekly until stable, particularly on initiation of therapy
VASODILATOR ANTIHYPERTENSIVES	**VASODILATOR ANTIHYPERTENSIVES**			
VASODILATOR ANTIHYPERTENSIVES	ANTIHYPERTENSIVES AND HEART FAILURE DRUGS	↑ Hypotensive effect	Additive hypotensive effect; may be used therapeutically	Monitor BP at least weekly until stable, particularly on initiation of therapy. Consider starting therapy at night

(*Continued*)

Primary Drug	Secondary Drug	Effect	Mechanism	Precautions
ANTIHYPERTENSIVES AND HEART FAILURE DRUGS				
VASODILATOR ANTIHYPERTENSIVES—MINOXIDIL	ADRENERGIC NEURONE BLOCKERS	Risk of excessive hypotension	Additive effect	Manufacturer recommends stopping guanethidine before starting minoxidil. If this is not possible, minoxidil should be started in hospital with close monitoring of BP
VASODILATOR ANTIHYPERTENSIVES—DIAZOXIDE	VASODILATOR ANTIHYPERTENSIVES—HYDRALAZINE	Profound, refractory ↓ BP may occur when diazoxide is coadministered with hydralazine	Additive effect; uncertain why the effect is so refractory to treatment	Avoid coadministration
VASODILATOR ANTIHYPERTENSIVES	**ANTI-PARKINSON'S DRUGS**			
VASODILATOR ANTIHYPERTENSIVES	APOMORPHINE	Theoretical risk of ↑ hypotensive effect	Not clear—effect seen with vasodilators but not other antihypertensives	Monitor BP closely, especially during initiation of treatment. Warn patients to report symptoms of hypotension (light-headedness, dizziness on standing, etc.)
VASODILATOR ANTIHYPERTENSIVES	LEVODOPA	↑ Hypotensive effect	Additive effect	Monitor BP at least weekly until stable. Warn patients to report symptoms of hypotension (light-headedness, dizziness on standing, etc.)
VASODILATOR ANTIHYPERTENSIVES	**ANTIPLATELET AGENTS**			
VASODILATOR ANTIHYPERTENSIVES—ILOPROST	ANTIPLATELET AGENTS	↑ Risk of bleeding when antiplatelets are coadministered with iloprost	Additive effect—iloprost has antiplatelet activity	Closely monitor the effects; watch for signs of excess bleeding
VASODILATOR ANTIHYPERTENSIVES	ASPIRIN	1. ↓ Hypotensive effect; not noted with low-dose aspirin 2. ↑ Risk of bleeding when aspirin is coadministered with iloprost	1. Aspirin may cause sodium retention and vasoconstriction at possibly both renal and endothelial sites 2. Additive effect—iloprost has antiplatelet activity	1. Monitor BP at least weekly until stable when high-dose aspirin is prescribed 2. Closely monitor the effects; watch for signs of excess bleeding

(*Continued*)

Primary Drug	Secondary Drug	Effect	Mechanism	Precautions
ANTIHYPERTENSIVES AND HEART FAILURE DRUGS				
VASODILATOR ANTIHYPERTENSIVES—DIAZOXIDE	ANTIPSYCHOTICS—CHLORPROMAZINE	Risk of hyperglycemia when diazoxide is coadministered with chlorpromazine	Additive effect; both drugs have a hyperglycemic effect	Monitor blood glucose closely, particularly with diabetes
VASODILATOR ANTIHYPERTENSIVES	**ANTIVIRALS**			
VASODILATORS ANTIHYPERTENSIVES—BOSENTAN	COBICISTAT	1. Possible ↓ plasma levels of cobicistat, risk of treatment failure, and resistance 2. Possible ↓ plasma levels of medicines being boosted, e.g., protease inhibitor	Induction of metabolism via CYP3A	Combination not recommended
VASODILATORS ANTIHYPERTENSIVES—BOSENTAN	ELVITEGRAVIR	↓ Plasma levels of elvitegravir, risk of treatment failure, and resistance	Increased metabolism through induction of CYP3A	Coadministration not recommended
VASODILATORS ANTIHYPERTENSIVES—BOSENTAN	MARAVIROC	Possible ↓ plasma levels of maraviroc, risk of treatment failure, and resistance	Induction of metabolism via CYP3A	Coadministration not recommended
VASODILATORS ANTIHYPERTENSIVES	PROTEASE INHIBITORS	1. ↑ Adverse effects of bosentan, sildenafil, tadalafil, and vardenafil by boceprevir, lopinavir, ritonavir, and telaprevir 2. Risk of failure of telaprevir when given with bosentan	1. Inhibition of CYP3A4-mediated metabolism of bosentan 2. Bosentan induces CYP3A4-mediated metabolism of telaprevir	1. Monitor BP closely; warn patient to report adverse features of bosentan (edema, headache) 2. Monitor efficacy of telaprevir
VASODILATOR ANTIHYPERTENSIVES	NNRTIs	Risk of peripheral neuropathy when hydralazine is coadministered with didanosine, stavudine, or zalcitabine	Additive effect; both drugs can cause peripheral neuropathy	Warn patient to report early features of peripheral neuropathy; if it occurs, the NNRTI should be stopped

(Continued)

Primary Drug	Secondary Drug	Effect	Mechanism	Precautions
ANTIHYPERTENSIVES AND HEART FAILURE DRUGS				
VASODILATOR ANTIHYPERTENSIVES	ANXIOLYTICS AND HYPNOTICS	↑ Hypotensive effect	Additive hypotensive effect	Monitor BP at least weekly until stable. Warn patients to report symptoms of hypotension (light-headedness, dizziness on standing, etc.)
VASODILATOR ANTIHYPERTENSIVES	BETA-BLOCKERS	↑ Hypotensive effect	Additive hypotensive effect with diazoxide, hydralazine, minoxidil, and sodium nitroprusside; may be used therapeutically. In addition, hydralazine may ↑ the bioavailability of beta-blockers with a high first-pass metabolism (e.g., propranolol and metoprolol), possibly due to alterations in hepatic blood flow or inhibited hepatic metabolism	Monitor BP at least weekly until stable. Warn patients to report symptoms of hypotension (light-headedness, dizziness on standing, etc.)
VASODILATOR ANTIHYPERTENSIVES	CALCIUM CHANNEL BLOCKERS	↑ Hypotensive effect	Additive hypotensive effect; may be used therapeutically	Monitor BP at least weekly until stable. Warn patients to report symptoms of hypotension (light-headedness, dizziness on standing, etc.)
VASODILATOR ANTIHYPERTENSIVES	**DIURETICS**			
VASODILATOR ANTIHYPERTENSIVES	LOOP DIURETICS	↑ Hypotensive effect	Additive hypotensive effect; may be used therapeutically	Monitor BP at least weekly until stable. Warn patients to report symptoms of hypotension (light-headedness, dizziness on standing, etc.). Benefits often outweigh risks

(*Continued*)

Primary Drug	Secondary Drug	Effect	Mechanism	Precautions
ANTIHYPERTENSIVES AND HEART FAILURE DRUGS				
VASODILATOR ANTIHYPERTENSIVES	THIAZIDES	↑ Hypotensive effect	Additive hypotensive effect; may be used therapeutically	Monitor BP at least weekly until stable. Warn patients to report symptoms of hypotension (light-headedness, dizziness on standing, etc.). Benefits often outweigh risks
VASODILATOR ANTIHYPERTENSIVES—DIAZOXIDE	THIAZIDES	Risk of hyperglycemia when diazoxide is coadministered with thiazides	Additive effect; both drugs have a hyperglycemic effect	Monitor blood glucose closely, particularly with diabetes
VASODILATOR ANTIHYPERTENSIVES—BOSENTAN	IVACAFTOR	↓ Ivacaftor levels	Induction of CYP3A4-mediated metabolism of ivacaftor	Manufacturers advice against coadministration
VASODILATOR ANTIHYPERTENSIVES	LIPID-LOWERING DRUGS	Bosentan lowers simvastatin levels	Uncertain; bosentan moderately inhibits CYP3A4	Monitor lipid profile closely; look for poor response to simvastatin
VASODILATOR ANTIHYPERTENSIVES	MUSCLE RELAXANTS—SKELETAL	↑ Hypotensive effect with tizanidine and baclofen	Additive hypotensive effect	Monitor BP at least weekly until stable. Warn patients to report symptoms of hypotension (light-headedness, dizziness on standing, etc.)
VASODILATOR ANTIHYPERTENSIVES	NITRATES	↑ Hypotensive effect	Additive hypotensive effect; may be used therapeutically	Monitor BP at least weekly until stable. Warn patients to report symptoms of hypotension (light-headedness, dizziness on standing, etc.)
VASODILATOR ANTIHYPERTENSIVES	**ESTROGENS**			
VASODILATOR ANTIHYPERTENSIVES	ESTROGENS	↓ Hypotensive effect	Estrogens cause sodium and fluid retention	Monitor BP at least weekly until stable; routine prescription of estrogens in patients with ↑ BP is not advisable

(Continued)

Primary Drug	Secondary Drug	Effect	Mechanism	Precautions
ANTIHYPERTENSIVES AND HEART FAILURE DRUGS				
VASODILATOR ANTIHYPERTENSIVES—BOSENTAN	ESTROGENS	↓ Estrogen levels, which may lead to failure of contraception or poor response to treatment of menorrhagia	Possibly induction of metabolism of estrogens	1. <2 month course of bosentan: advise patients to use additional contraception for the period of intake and for 1 month after stopping coadministration with these drugs 2. For long-term use, consider alternative contraceptive methods
VASODILATOR ANTIHYPERTENSIVES—DIAZOXIDE	ESTROGENS	Risk of hyperglycemia when diazoxide is coadministered with combined oral contraceptives	Additive effect; both drugs have a hyperglycemic effect	Monitor blood glucose closely, particularly with diabetics
VASODILATOR ANTIHYPERTENSIVES	PERIPHERAL VASODILATORS—MOXISYLYTE (THYMOXAMINE)	↑ Hypotensive effect	Additive hypotensive effect	Monitor BP at least weekly until stable. Warn patients to report symptoms of hypotension (light-headedness, dizziness on standing, etc.)
VASODILATOR ANTIHYPERTENSIVES—BOSENTAN	PHOSPHODIESTERASE TYPE 5 INHIBITORS—SILDENAFIL	↓ Sildenafil levels	Probable induction of metabolism	Watch for poor response
VASODILATOR ANTIHYPERTENSIVES	POTASSIUM CHANNEL ACTIVATORS	↑ Hypotensive effect	Additive effect	Monitor BP closely
VASODILATOR ANTIHYPERTENSIVES—BOSENTAN	PROGESTOGENS	↓ Progesterone levels, which may lead to failure of contraception or poor response to treatment of menorrhagia	Possibly induction of metabolism of progestogens	1. <2 month course of bosentan: advise patients to use additional contraception for the period of intake and for 1 month after stopping coadministration with these drugs 2. For long-term use, consider alternative contraceptive methods
VASODILATOR ANTIHYPERTENSIVES	PROSTAGLANDINS—ALPROSTADIL	↑ Hypotensive effect	Additive hypotensive effect	Monitor BP at least weekly until stable. Warn patients to report symptoms of hypotension (light-headedness, dizziness on standing, etc.)

(*Continued*)

Primary Drug	Secondary Drug	Effect	Mechanism	Precautions
ANTIHYPERTENSIVES AND HEART FAILURE DRUGS				
VASODILATOR ANTIHYPERTENSIVES	SAPROPTERIN	↑ Hypotensive effect	Additive hypotensive effect	Monitor BP at least weekly until stable. Warn patients to report symptoms of hypotension (light-headedness, dizziness on standing, etc.)
VASODILATOR ANTIHYPERTENSIVES	SYMPATHOMIMETICS—DIRECT	Cases of ↑ tachycardia when epinephrine is given for perioperative ↓ BP in patients on hydralazine	Additive effect	Avoid coadministration

Primary Drug	Secondary Drug	Effect	Mechanism	Precautions
ANTIPLATELET DRUGS				
ASPIRIN				
ASPIRIN	ANESTHETICS—GENERAL	↓ Requirements of thiopentone when aspirin (1 g) used as premedication	Uncertain at present	Be aware of possible ↓ dose requirements for thiopentone
ASPIRIN	ANALGESICS—NSAIDs	1. Risk of gastrointestinal bleeding when aspirin, even low dose, is coadministered with NSAIDs 2. Ibuprofen ↓ antiplatelet effect of aspirin 3. Reduced cardioprotective effect of aspirin when taken with NSAIDs including COXIBs	1. Additive effect 2. Ibuprofen competitively inhibits binding of aspirin to platelets 3. Uncertain; possibly related to variable inhibition of cyclo-oxygenase 1 and 2 isoenzymes	1. Avoid coadministration; if essential to coprescribe, add a proton pump inhibitor 2. Avoid coadministration; if there is no alternative, low-dose aspirin (81 mg daily) should be taken 30 min before or 8 h after taking ibuprofen 3. Avoid coadministration
ASPIRIN	ANTACIDS	Antacids may reduce high-dose aspirin to subtherapeutic levels	Alkalinizing the urine increases aspirin loss in the urine	Monitor salicylate levels when high-dose aspirin therapy is used

(Continued)

Primary Drug	Secondary Drug	Effect	Mechanism	Precautions
ANTIPLATELET DRUGS				
ASPIRIN	**ANTICANCER AND IMMUNOMODULATING DRUGS**			
ASPIRIN	CORTICOSTEROIDS	Corticosteroids ↓ aspirin levels, and therefore, there is a risk of salicylate toxicity when withdrawing corticosteroids. Risk of gastric ulceration when aspirin is coadministered with corticosteroids	Uncertain	Watch for features of salicylate toxicity when withdrawing corticosteroids. Use aspirin in the lowest dose. Remember that corticosteroids may mask the features of peptic ulceration
ASPIRIN	DASATINIB	Increased risk of bleeding	Additive	Caution with concurrent use
ASPIRIN (ANALGESIC DOSES)	GOLD	Increased risk of aspirin induced hepatotoxicity compared to fenoprofen	Uncertain	Safer with fenoprofen
ASPIRIN	METHOTREXATE	Risk of methotrexate toxicity when coadministered with high-dose aspirin. There is a risk of toxic effects of methotrexate, e.g., liver cirrhosis, blood dyscrasias that may be fatal, pulmonary toxicity, and stomatitis. Hematopoietic suppression can occur abruptly. Other adverse effects include anorexia, dyspepsia, gastrointestinal ulceration and bleeding, and pulmonary edema	Aspirin ↓ plasma protein binding of methotrexate (a relatively minor contribution to the interaction) and the renal excretion of high doses of methotrexate. Salicylates compete with methotrexate for renal elimination	Check FBC, U&Es, and LFTs before starting treatment and repeat weekly until stabilized, then every 2–3 months. Patients should be advised to report symptoms such as sore throat, fever, or gastrointestinal discomfort immediately. Stop methotrexate and initiate supportive therapy if the white cell or platelet counts drop. Do not administer aspirin within 10 days of high-dose methotrexate treatment
ASPIRIN	PEMETREXED	Increased pemetrexed toxicity	Reduced renal clearance	Caution with concurrent use

(*Continued*)

Primary Drug	Secondary Drug	Effect	Mechanism	Precautions
ANTIPLATELET DRUGS				
ASPIRIN	**ANTICOAGULANTS**			
ASPIRIN	ANTICOAGULANTS	Risk of bleeding when high-dose aspirin is coadministered with anticoagulants; less risk with low-dose aspirin	Additive effect on the clotting mechanism; aspirin also irritates the gastric mucosa	Avoid coadministration of anticoagulants and high-dose aspirin. Patients on warfarin should be warned that many OTC and some herbal remedies contain aspirin
ASPIRIN	APIXABAN	↑ Risk of bleeding	Additive effect	Contraindicated unless benefits outweigh risks and no alternatives available
ASPIRIN	DABIGATRAN	↑ Risk of bleeding	Additive effect	Avoid coadministration
ASPIRIN	**ANTIDEPRESSANTS**			
ASPIRIN	SSRIs	Possible ↑ risk of bleeding with SSRIs	Uncertain. Possible additive effects including inhibition of serotonin release by platelets, SSRI-induced thrombocytopenia, and ↓ platelet aggregation	Avoid coadministration with high-dose aspirin
ASPIRIN	SNRIs	Possible ↑ risk of bleeding with SNRIs	Uncertain. Possible additive effects including inhibition of serotonin release by platelets, SNRI-induced thrombocytopenia, and ↓ platelet aggregation	Avoid coadministration with high-dose aspirin
ASPIRIN	ANTIDIABETIC DRUGS	Risk of hypoglycemia when high-dose aspirin (3.5–7.5 g/day) is given with antidiabetic agents	Additive effect; aspirin has a hypoglycemic effect	Avoid high-dose aspirin
ASPIRIN	ANTIEMETICS	↑ Aspirin levels with metoclopramide	↑ Absorption of aspirin	Watch for early features of salicylate toxicity

(Continued)

Primary Drug	Secondary Drug	Effect	Mechanism	Precautions
ANTIPLATELET DRUGS				
ASPIRIN	ANTIEPILEPTICS	Possible ↑ levels of phenytoin and valproate	Possibly ↑ unbound phenytoin or valproate fraction in the blood	Monitor phenytoin or valproate levels when coadministering high-dose aspirin
ASPIRIN	**ANTIGOUT DRUGS**			
ASPIRIN	PROBENICID	High doses of aspirin antagonize the effects of probenecid	Uncertain	Watch for poor response to probenecid
ASPIRIN	BENZBROMARONE	High doses of aspirin antagonize the effects of benzbromarone	Uncertain	Watch for poor response to benzbromarone
ASPIRIN	SULFINPYRAZONE	High-dose aspirin antagonizes the urate-lowering effect of sulfinpyrazone	Salicylates block sulfinpyrazone-induced inhibition of renal tubular reabsorption of urate	Avoid long-term coadministration of high-dose aspirin with sulfinpyrazone. Low-dose aspirin does not seem to have this effect
ASPIRIN	**ANTIHYPERTENSIVES AND HEART FAILURE DRUGS**			
ASPIRIN	ANTIHYPERTENSIVES AND HEART FAILURE DRUGS	↓ Antihypertensive effect with aspirin; effect not noted with low-dose aspirin	Aspirin may cause sodium retention and vasoconstriction at possibly both renal and endothelial sites	Monitor BP at least weekly until stable when high-dose is aspirin prescribed
ASPIRIN	ACE INHIBITORS	↑ Risk of renal impairment. ↓ efficacy of captopril and enalapril with high-dose (>100 mg/day) aspirin	Aspirin and NSAIDs can cause elevation of BP. Prostaglandin inhibition leads to sodium and water retention and poor renal function in those with impaired renal blood flow	Monitor renal function every 3–6 months, watch for poor response to ACE inhibitors when >100 mg/day aspirin is given
ASPIRIN	ANGIOTENSIN II RECEPTOR BLOCKERS	Risk of renal impairment when olmesartan is administered with high-dose (>3 g daily) aspirin. Effect not noted with low-dose aspirin	Additive effect on reducing glomerular filtration rate	Monitor renal function regularly until stable

(*Continued*)

Primary Drug	Secondary Drug	Effect	Mechanism	Precautions
ANTIPLATELET DRUGS				
ASPIRIN	VASODILATOR ANTIHYPERTENSIVES	1. ↓ Hypotensive effect; not noted with low-dose aspirin 2. ↑ Risk of bleeding when aspirin is coadministered with iloprost	1. Aspirin may cause sodium retention and vasoconstriction at possibly both renal and endothelial sites 2. Additive effect—iloprost has antiplatelet activity	1. Monitor BP at least weekly until stable when high-dose aspirin is prescribed 2. Closely monitor the effects; watch for signs of excess bleeding
ASPIRIN	ANTIOBESITY DRUGS—SIBUTRAMINE	Risk of bleeding	Additive effect; sibutramine may cause thrombocytopenia	Warn the patient to report any signs of ↑ bleeding
ASPIRIN	ANTIPLATELET AGENTS	Risk of bleeding when aspirin is coadministered with other antiplatelet agents. The addition of dipyridamole to low-dose aspirin does not seem to confer an ↑ risk of bleeding	Additive effect	Closely monitor effects; watch for signs of excess bleeding
ASPIRIN	ANXIOLYTICS AND HYPNOTICS	↓ Requirements of midazolam when aspirin (1 g) is coadministered	Uncertain at present	Be aware of possible ↓ dose requirements for midazolam
ASPIRIN	CALCIUM CHANNEL BLOCKERS	↓ Antihypertensive effect with aspirin; effect not noted with low-dose aspirin	Aspirin may cause sodium retention and vasoconstriction at possibly both renal and endothelial sites	Monitor BP at least weekly until stable when high-dose is aspirin prescribed
ASPIRIN	**DIURETICS**			
ASPIRIN	CARBONIC ANHYDRASE INHIBITORS	↑ Risk of salicylate toxicity with high-dose aspirin	Uncertain at present	Use low-dose aspirin

(*Continued*)

Primary Drug	Secondary Drug	Effect	Mechanism	Precautions
ANTIPLATELET DRUGS				
ASPIRIN	LOOP DIURETICS	1. Risk of renal failure when loop diuretics are given with high-dose aspirin 2. Risk of ototoxicty when bumetanide or furosemide is given with high-dose aspirin	1. Additive adverse effect on renal function 2. Additive effect; all are ototoxic	1. Monitor renal function closely; warn the patient to maintain good hydration 2. Monitor hearing regularly
ASPIRIN	POTASSIUM-SPARING DIURETICS	↓ Efficacy of spironolactone	Uncertain	Watch for poor response to spironolactone
ASPIRIN	DINOPROSTONE	Theoretical risk of ↓ efficacy of dinoprost; not confirmed in clinical studies	Antagonism of effect	UK manufacturers recommend stopping aspirin (in analgesic doses) before administering dinoprostone. U.S. manufacturer does not give this advice
ASPIRIN	DROTRECOGIN ALFA	↑ Risk of bleeding	Additive effect on clotting mechanism; drotrecogin alfa has antithrombotic and fibrinolytic effects	Careful risk–benefit analysis should be undertaken if drotrecogin alfa is given within 7 days of aspirin
ASPIRIN	LEUKOTRIENE ANTAGONISTS	↑ Levels of zafirlukast	Uncertain	Watch for early features of zafirlukast toxicity. Monitor FBC and liver function closely
ASPIRIN	MIFEPRISTONE	↓ Efficacy of mifepristone	Antiprostaglandin effect of aspirin antagonizes action of mifepristone	Avoid coadministration
ASPIRIN	NITRATES	↓ Antihypertensive effect with aspirin; effect not noted with low-dose aspirin	Aspirin may cause sodium retention and vasoconstriction at possibly both renal and endothelial sites	Monitor BP at least weekly until stable when high-dose aspirin is prescribed
ASPIRIN	PERIPHERAL VASODILATORS	Possible ↑ risk of bleeding with cilostazol. Low-dose aspirin (<80 mg) appears to be safe	Additive effect; cilostazol has antiplatelet activity	Warn the patient to report any signs of ↑ bleeding

(*Continued*)

Primary Drug	Secondary Drug	Effect	Mechanism	Precautions
ANTIPLATELET DRUGS				
ASPIRIN	THROMBOLYTICS	↑ Risk of intracerebral bleeding when streptokinase is coadministered with higher dose (300 mg) aspirin	Additive effect	Avoid coingestion when streptokinase is given for cerebral infarction; use low-dose aspirin when coadministered for myocardial infarction
CLOPIDOGREL				
CLOPIDOGREL	ANALGESICS—NSAIDs	1. Risk of gastrointestinal bleeding when clopidogrel is coadministered with NSAIDs 2. Case of intracerebral hemorrhage when clopidogrel given with celecoxib	1. NSAIDs may cause gastric mucosal irritation/ulceration; clopidogrel inhibits platelet aggregation 2. Uncertain; possible that celecoxib inhibits CYP2D6-mediated metabolism of clopidogrel	1. Warn patients to report immediately any gastrointestinal symptoms; use NSAIDs for as short a course as possible 2. Avoid coingestion of clopidogrel and celecoxib
CLOPIDOGREL	**ANTIBIOTICS**			
CLOPIDOGREL	CHLORAMPHENICOL, CIPROFLOXACIN	Theoretical risk of ↓ efficacy of clopidogrel	Inhibition of CYP2C19-mediated activation of clopidogrel	Avoid coadministration
CLOPIDOGREL	MACROLIDES—ERYTHROMYCIN	Theoretical risk of ↓ efficacy of clopidogrel	Inhibition of CYP3A4-mediated activation of clopidogrel	Assess risk:benefit of coadministration carefully
CLOPIDOGREL	RIFAMPICIN	Theoretical risk of bleeding	Rifampicin increases CYP3A4-mediated activation of clopidogrel. No clinical reports of bleeding	Warn patient to report abnormal bleeding immediately
CLOPIDOGREL	ANTICANCER AND OTHER IMMUNOMODULATING DRUGS—DASATINIB	Increased risk of bleeding	Additive	Caution with concurrent use

(Continued)

Primary Drug	Secondary Drug	Effect	Mechanism	Precautions
ANTIPLATELET DRUGS				
CLOPIDOGREL	ANTICOAGULANTS	Risk of bleeding when clopidogrel is coadministered with anticoagulants	Additive effect on different parts of the clotting mechanism	Closely monitor effects; watch for signs of excess bleeding
CLOPIDOGREL	DABIGATRAN	↑ Risk of bleeding	Additive effect	Avoid coadministration
CLOPIDOGREL	**ANTIDEPRESSANTS**			
CLOPIDOGREL	SSRIs	Possible ↑ risk of bleeding with SSRIs	Uncertain. Possible additive effects including inhibition of serotonin release by platelets, SSRI-induced thrombocytopenia, and ↓ platelet aggregation	Avoid coadministration
CLOPIDOGREL	SNRIs	Possible ↑ risk of bleeding with SNRIs	Uncertain. Possible additive effects including inhibition of serotonin release by platelets, SNRI-induced thrombocytopenia, and ↓ platelet aggregation	Avoid coadministration
CLOPIDOGREL	ST. JOHN'S WORT	Theoretical risk of bleeding	St. John's wort increases CYP3A4- and 2C19-mediated activation of clopidogrel. No clinical reports of bleeding	Warn patient to report abnormal bleeding immediately
CLOPIDOGREL	ANTIEPILEPTICS—CARBAMAZEPINE, OXCARBAZEPINE	Theoretical risk of ↓ efficacy of clopidogrel	Inhibition of CYP2C19-mediated activation of clopidogrel	Consider using an alternative antiepileptic
CLOPIDOGREL	ANTIFUNGALS—AZOLES	1. ↓ Efficacy of clopidogrel with fluconazole and voriconazole 2. Theoretical risk of ↓ efficacy of clopidogrel with ketoconazole	1. Inhibition of CYP2C19-mediated activation of clopidogrel 2. Inhibition of CYP3A4-mediated activation of clopidogrel	1. Avoid coadministration of clopidogrel with fluconazole or voriconazole 2. Assess risk:benefit of coadministration carefully

(*Continued*)

Primary Drug	Secondary Drug	Effect	Mechanism	Precautions
ANTIPLATELET DRUGS				
CLOPIDOGREL	ANTIHYPERTENSIVES AND HEART FAILURE DRUGS—VASODILATOR ANTIHYPERTENSIVES	↑ Risk of bleeding when clopidogrel is coadministered with iloprost	Additive effect—iloprost has antiplatelet activity	Closely monitor effects; watch for signs of excess bleeding
CLOPIDOGREL	ANTIPLATELET AGENTS	Risk of bleeding when clopidogrel is coadministered with other antiplatelet agents	Additive effect	Closely monitor effects; watch for signs of excess bleeding
CLOPIDOGREL	ANTIVIRALS—ETRAVIRINE	Possible ↓ efficacy of clopidogrel	Predicted inhibition of metabolism to clopidogrel's active metabolite	Combination not recommended
CLOPIDOGREL	CNS STIMULANTS—MODAFINIL	May cause moderate ↑ in plasma concentrations of these substrates	Modafinil is a reversible inhibitor of CYP2C19 when used in therapeutic doses	Be aware
CLOPIDROGEL	GRAPEFRUIT JUICE	↓ Peak plasma concentration (C_{max}) of the active metabolite of clopidogrel to 13% of the control, AUC from 0 to 3 h to 14% of the control	No significant effect on parent clopidogrel. GFJ markedly ↓ the platelet-inhibitory effect of clopidogrel	Concomitant use of grapefruit juice may impair the efficacy of clopidogrel. Use of GFJ is best avoided during clopidogrel therapy
CLOPIDOGREL	H2-RECEPTOR BLOCKERS—CIMETIDINE	Theoretical risk of ↓ efficacy of clopidogrel	Inhibition of CYP2C19-mediated activation of clopidogrel	Consider using an alternative H2-receptor blocker
CLOPIDOGREL	LIPID-LOWERING DRUGS	Atorvastatin and possibly simvastatin ↓ the antiplatelet effect of clopidogrel in a dose-dependent manner. The clinical significance of this effect is uncertain	Atorvastatin and simvastatin inhibit CYP3A4-mediated activation of clopidogrel	Use these statins at the lowest possible dose; otherwise, consider using an alternative statin

(Continued)

DRUGS ACTING ON THE CARDIOVASCULAR SYSTEM ANTIPLATELET DRUGS Dipyridamole

Primary Drug	Secondary Drug	Effect	Mechanism	Precautions
ANTIPLATELET DRUGS				
CLOPIDOGREL	PERIPHERAL VASODILATORS	Possible ↑ risk of bleeding with cilostazol	1. Additive effect; cilostazol has antiplatelet activity 2. Clopidogrel ↑ the levels of a metabolite of cilostazol that has high antiplatelet activity, by a mechanism that is uncertain at present	Warn the patient to report any signs of ↑ bleeding
CLOPIDOGREL	PROTON PUMP INHIBITORS—OMEPRAZOLE	↓ Efficacy of clopidogrel	Inhibition of CYP2C19-mediated activation of clopidogrel	Avoid coadministration. Use an alternative PPI
DIPYRIDAMOLE				
DIPYRIDAMOLE	ANTACIDS	Possible ↓ bioavailability of dipyridamole	Dipyridamole tablets require an acidic environment for adequate dissolution; ↑ in pH of the stomach impairs dissolution and therefore may ↓ absorption of the drug	↑ The dose of dipyridamole or consider using an alternative antiplatelet drug
DIPYRIDAMOLE	ANTIARRHYTHMICS—ADENOSINE	↑ Effect of adenosine; ↓ doses needed to terminate supraventricular tachycardias; case report of profound bradycardia when adenosine infusion was given for myocardial stress testing	Dipyridamole inhibits adenosine uptake into cells	↓ Bolus doses of adenosine by up to fourfold when administering it to treat supraventricular tachycardias. Some recommend avoiding adenosine for patients taking dipyridamole. Advise patients to stop dipyridamole for 24 h before using adenosine infusions

(Continued)

Primary Drug	Secondary Drug	Effect	Mechanism	Precautions
ANTIPLATELET DRUGS				
DIPYRIDAMOLE	**ANTICANCER AND IMMUNOMODULATING DRUGS**			
DIPYRIDAMOLE	CYTARABINE	Single report of increased cytarabine toxicity	Dipyridamole inhibits the nucleoside transporter that transports cytarabine extracellularly, resulting in increased intracellular concentration in hepatocytes	Significance unclear, consider interaction if unexpected toxicity
DIPYRIDAMOLE	DASATINIB	Increased risk of bleeding	Additive	Caution with concurrent use
DIPYRIDAMOLE	FLUDARABINE	Possible ↓ efficacy of fludarabine	Uncertain	Consider using an alternative antiplatelet drug
DIPYRIDAMOLE	ANTICOAGULANTS	Cases of mild bleeding when dipyridamole is added to anticoagulants	Antiplatelet effects of dipyridamole add to the anticoagulant effects	Warn patients to report early signs of bleeding
DIPYRIDAMOLE	**ANTIDEPRESSANTS**			
DIPYRIDAMOLE	SSRIs	Possible ↑ risk of bleeding with SSRIs	Uncertain. Possible additive effects including inhibition of serotonin release by platelets, SSRI-induced thrombocytopenia, and ↓ platelet aggregation	Avoid coadministration
DIPYRIDAMOLE	SNRIs	Possible ↑ risk of bleeding with SNRIs	Uncertain. Possible additive effects including inhibition of serotonin release by platelets, SSRI-induced thrombocytopenia, and ↓ platelet aggregation	Avoid coadministration

(Continued)

Primary Drug	Secondary Drug	Effect	Mechanism	Precautions
ANTIPLATELET DRUGS				
DIPYRIDAMOLE	ANTIPLATELET AGENTS	Risk of bleeding when dipyridamole is coadministered with other antiplatelet drugs. The addition of dipyridamole to low-dose aspirin does not seem to confer an ↑ risk of bleeding	Additive effect	Closely monitor effects; watch for signs of excess bleeding
DIPYRIDAMOLE	H2 RECEPTOR BLOCKERS	Possible ↓ bioavailability of dipyridamole	Dipyridamole tablets require an acidic environment for adequate dissolution; ↑ pH of the stomach impairs dissolution and may therefore ↓ absorption of drug	Use M/R prep of dipyridamole. Consider using an alternative antiplatelet drug or ≠ dose of dipyridamole tablets
DIPYRIDAMOLE	PERIPHERAL VASODILATORS	Possible ↑ risk of bleeding with cilostazol	Additive effect; cilostazol has antiplatelet activity	Warn the patient to report any signs of ↑ bleeding
DIPYRIDAMOLE	PROTON PUMP INHIBITORS	Possible ↓ bioavailability of dipyridamole	Dipyridamole tablets require an acidic environment for adequate dissolution; an ↑ in pH of the stomach impairs dissolution and therefore may ↓ absorption of the drug	Modified release preparations are not affected or ↑ dose of dipyridamole or consider using an alternative antiplatelet drug
DIPYRIDAMOLE	SYMPATHOMIMETICS—DOBUTAMINE	Case reports of marked hypotension when given together	Uncertain	Avoid coadministration
GLYCOPROTEIN IIb/IIIa INHIBITORS				
GLYCOPROTEIN IIb/IIIa INHIBITORS	ANTICOAGULANTS	Risk of bleeding when glycoprotein IIb/IIIa inhibitors are coadministered with anticoagulants	Additive effect on different parts of the clotting mechanism	Closely monitor APTT or INR as appropriate; watch for signs of excess bleeding

(*Continued*)

Primary Drug	Secondary Drug	Effect	Mechanism	Precautions
ANTIPLATELET DRUGS				
GLYCOPROTEIN IIb/IIIa INHIBITORS	DABIGATRAN	↑ Risk of bleeding	Additive effect	Avoid coadministration
GLYCOPROTEIN IIb/IIIa INHIBITORS	ANTICANCER AND OTHER IMMUNOMODULATING DRUGS—DASATINIB	Increased risk of bleeding	Additive	Caution with concurrent use
GLYCOPROTEIN IIb/IIIa INHIBITORS	**ANTIDEPRESSANTS**			
GLYCOPROTEIN IIb/IIIa INHIBITORS	SSRIs	Possible ↑ risk of bleeding with SSRIs	Uncertain. Possible additive effects including inhibition of serotonin release by platelets, SSRI-induced thrombocytopenia, and ↓ platelet aggregation	Avoid coadministration
GLYCOPROTEIN IIb/IIIa INHIBITORS	SNRIs	Possible ↑ risk of bleeding with SNRIs	Uncertain. Possible additive effects including inhibition of serotonin release by platelets, SNRI-induced thrombocytopenia, and ↓ platelet aggregation	Avoid coadministration
GLYCOPROTEIN IIb/IIIa INHIBITORS	ANTIHYPERTENSIVES AND HEART FAILURE DRUGS—VASODILATOR ANTIHYPERTENSIVES	↑ Risk of bleeding when eptifibatide or tirofiban is coadministered with iloprost	Additive effect—iloprost has antiplatelet activity	Closely monitor effects; watch for signs of excess bleeding
GLYCOPROTEIN IIb/IIIa INHIBITORS	ANTIPLATELET AGENTS	Risk of bleeding when glycoprotein IIb/IIIa inhibitors are coadministered with other antiplatelet agents	Additive effect	Closely monitor effects; watch for signs of excess bleeding
GLYCOPROTEIN IIb/IIIa INHIBITORS	PERIPHERAL VASODILATORS	Possible ↑ risk of bleeding with cilostazol	Additive effect; cilostazol has antiplatelet activity	Warn the patient to report any signs of ↑ bleeding

(Continued)

Primary Drug	Secondary Drug	Effect	Mechanism	Precautions
ANTIPLATELET DRUGS				
GLYCOPROTEIN IIb/IIIa INHIBITORS	THROMBOLYTICS	1. ↑ Risk of major hemorrhage when coadministered with alteplase 2. Possible ↑ risk of bleeding complications when streptokinase is coadministered with eptifibatide	1. Uncertain; other thrombolytics do not seem to interact 2. Additive effect	1. Avoid coadministration 2. Watch for bleeding complications. Risk–benefit analysis is needed before coadministering; this will involve the availability of alternative therapies such as primary angioplasty
PRASUGREL				
PRASUGREL	ANALGESICS—NSAIDs	↑ Risk of gastrointestinal bleeding	Pharmacodynamic additive effect on GI mucosal irritation and bleeding	Watch for features of gastrointestinal bleeding. Use gastroprotection if combination cannot be avoided
PRASUGREL	ANTICANCER AND OTHER IMMUNOMODULATING DRUGS—DASATINIB	Increased risk of bleeding	Additive	Caution with concurrent use
PRASUGREL	**ANTICOAGULANTS**			
PRASUGREL	ANTICOAGULANTS	Risk of bleeding when prasugrel is coadministered with anticoagulants	Additive effect on different parts of the clotting mechanism	Closely monitor effects; watch for signs of excess bleeding. Avoid coadministration with dabigatran
PRASUGREL	DABIGATRAN	↑ Risk of bleeding	Additive effect	Avoid coadministration
PRASUGREL	**ANTIDEPRESSANTS**			
PRASUGREL	SSRIs	Possible ↑ risk of bleeding with SSRIs	Uncertain. Possible additive effects including inhibition of serotonin release by platelets, SSRI-induced thrombocytopenia, and ↓ platelet aggregation	Avoid coadministration

(*Continued*)

Primary Drug	Secondary Drug	Effect	Mechanism	Precautions
ANTIPLATELET DRUGS				
PRASUGREL	SNRIs	Possible ↑ risk of bleeding with SNRIs	Uncertain. Possible additive effects including inhibition of serotonin release by platelets, SNRI-induced thrombocytopenia, and ↓ platelet aggregation	Avoid coadministration
PRASUGREL	ANTIHYPERTENSIVES AND HEART FAILURE DRUGS—ILOPROST	↑ Risk of bleeding when prasugrel is coadministered with iloprost	Additive effect—iloprost has antiplatelet activity	Closely monitor effects; watch for signs of excess bleeding
PRASUGREL	ANTIPLATELET AGENTS	Risk of bleeding when prasugrel is coadministered with other antiplatelet agents	Additive effect	Closely monitor effects; watch for signs of excess bleeding
PRASUGREL	ANTIVIRALS—COBICISTAT	↓ Activation of prasugrel, risk of treatment failure	Inhibition of metabolism to active metabolite via CYP3A4	Consider using clopidogrel as an alternative
PRASUGREL	PERIPHERAL VASODILATORS	Possible ↑ risk of bleeding with cilostazol	Additive effect; cilostazol has antiplatelet activity	Warn the patient to report any signs of ↑ bleeding
TICAGRELOR				
TICAGRELOR	NSAIDs	↑ Risk of gastrointestinal bleeding	Pharmacodynamic additive effect on GI mucosal irritation and bleeding	Watch for features of gastrointestinal bleeding. Use gastroprotection if combination cannot be avoided
TICAGRELOR	ANTIARRHYTHMICS—QUINIDINE	Risk of ↑ ticagrelor levels	Inhibition of Pgp	Manufacturer recommends to avoid coadministration
TICAGRELOR	**ANTIBIOTICS**			
TICAGRELOR	MACROLIDES	Marked ↑ ticagrelor levels by clarithromycin, erythromycin, and telithromycin	Inhibition of CYP3A4-mediated metabolism of ticagrelor	Manufacturer recommends to avoid coadministration

(*Continued*)

Primary Drug	Secondary Drug	Effect	Mechanism	Precautions
ANTIPLATELET DRUGS				
TICAGRELOR	RIFAMPICIN	↓ Ticagrelor levels	Induction of CYP3A4-mediated metabolism of ticagrelor	Manufacturer recommends to avoid coadministration
TICAGRELOR	**ANTICANCER AND IMMUNOMODULATING DRUGS—CICLOSPORIN**			
TICAGRELOR	CICLOSPORIN	Risk of ↑ ticagrelor levels	Inhibition of Pgp	Manufacturer recommends to avoid coadministration
TICAGRELOR	DASATINIB	Increased risk of bleeding	Additive	Caution with concurrent use
TICAGRELOR	**ANTICOAGULANTS**			
TICAGRELOR	ANTICOAGULANTS	Risk of bleeding when prasugrel is coadministered with anticoagulants	Additive effect on different parts of the clotting mechanism	Closely monitor effects; watch for signs of excess bleeding
TICAGRELOR	DABIGATRAN	↑ Risk of bleeding	Additive effect	Avoid coadministration
TICAGRELOR	**ANTIDEPRESSANTS**			
TICAGRELOR	SSRIs	Possible ↑ risk of bleeding with SSRIs	Uncertain. Possible additive effects including inhibition of serotonin release by platelets, SSRI-induced thrombocytopenia, and ↓ platelet aggregation	Avoid coadministration
TICAGRELOR	SNRIs	Possible ↑ risk of bleeding with SNRIs	Uncertain. Possible additive effects including inhibition of serotonin release by platelets, SNRI-induced thrombocytopenia, and ↓ platelet aggregation	Avoid coadministration
TICAGRELOR	ANTIEPILEPTICS—CARBAMAZEPINE, PHENOBARBITONE, PHENYTOIN, PRIMIDONE	↓ Ticagrelor levels	Induction of CYP3A4-mediated metabolism of ticagrelor	Manufacturer recommends to avoid coadministration

(*Continued*)

Primary Drug	Secondary Drug	Effect	Mechanism	Precautions
ANTIPLATELET DRUGS				
TICAGRELOR	ANTIFUNGALS—AZOLES	Marked ↑ ticagrelor levels with ketoconazole, fluconazole, itraconazole, posaconazole, and voriconazole	Inhibition of CYP3A4-mediated metabolism of ticagrelor	Manufacturer recommends to avoid coadministration
TICAGRELOR	ANTIPLATELET AGENTS	Risk of bleeding when prasugrel is coadministered with other antiplatelet agents	Additive effect	Closely monitor effects; watch for signs of excess bleeding
TICAGRELOR	**ANTIVIRALS**			
TICAGRELOR	COBICISTAT	↑ Risk of side effects	Inhibition of metabolism via CYP3A4	Consider using clopidogrel as an alternative
TICAGRELOR	PROTEASE INHIBITORS	Marked ↑ ticagrelor levels by boceprevir, ritonavir, saquinavir, and telaprevir	Inhibition of CYP3A4-mediated metabolism of ticagrelor	Manufacturer recommends to avoid coadministration
TICAGRELOR	CALCIUM CHANNEL BLOCKERS	Risk of ↑ ticagrelor levels with diltiazem and verapamil	Inhibition of CYP3A4 mediated metabolism of ticagrelor. Verapamil also inhibits Pgp	Manufacturer recommends to avoid coadministration
TICAGRELOR	CARDIAC GLYCOSIDES—DIGOXIN	Risk of ↑ digoxin levels	Inhibition of Pgp	Monitor PR and BP closely
TICAGRELOR	GRAPEFRUIT JUICE	↑ Ticagrelor levels	Inhibition of the first-pass metabolism of ticagrelor	Do not coadminsiter
TICAGRELOR	PERIPHERAL VASODILATORS	Possible ↑ risk of bleeding with cilostazol	Additive effect; cilostazol has antiplatelet activity	Warn the patient to report any signs of ↑ bleeding

DRUGS ACTING ON THE CARDIOVASCULAR SYSTEM BETA-BLOCKERS

Primary Drug	Secondary Drug	Effect	Mechanism	Precautions
BETA-BLOCKERS				
SOTALOL	**DRUGS THAT PROLONG THE QT INTERVAL**			
SOTALOL	1. ANTIARRHYTHMICS—ajmaline, amiodarone, azimilide, cibenzoline, disopyramide, dofetilide, dronedarone, ibutilide, procainamide, propafenone, quinidine 2. ANTIBIOTICS—macrolides (especially azithromycin, clarithromycin, parenteral erythromycin, telithromycin), quinolones (especially moxifloxacin), quinupristin/dalfopristin 3. ANTICANCER AND IMMUNOMODULATING DRUGS—arsenic trioxide, bosutinib, crizotinib, dasatinib, eribulin, fingolimod, lapatinib, nilotinib, pazopanib, sunitinib, vandetanib, vemurafenib 4. ANTIDEPRESSANTS—TCAs, venlafaxine 5. ANTIEMETICS—ondansetron 6. ANTIFUNGALS—fluconazole, posaconazole, voriconazole 7. ANTIHISTAMINES—terfenadine, hydroxyzine, mizolastine 8. ANTIHYPERTENSIVES—ketanserin 9. ANTIMALARIALS—artemether with lumefantrine, chloroquine, halofantrine, hydroxychloroquine, mefloquine, quinine 10. ANTIPROTOZOALS—pentamidine isethionate 11. ANTIPSYCHOTICS—atypicals, phenothiazines, pimozide 12. ANTIVIRALS—boceprevir, rilpivirine, telaprevir 13. BRONCHODILATORS—parenteral bronchodilators 14. CNS STIMULANTS—atomoxetine 15. RANOLAZINE	Risk of ventricular arrhythmias, particularly torsades de pointes	Additive effect; these drugs prolong the QT interval	Avoid coadministration

(Continued)

Primary Drug	Secondary Drug	Effect	Mechanism	Precautions
BETA-BLOCKERS				
SOTALOL	IVABRADINE	Risk of arrhythmias	Additive effect; ivabradine slows the sinus node	Monitor ECG closely
BETA-BLOCKERS	ALCOHOL	Acute alcohol ingestion may ↑ hypotensive effect. Chronic moderate/heavy drinking ↓ hypotensive effect	Additive hypotensive effect. Mechanism of opposite effect with chronic intake is uncertain	Monitor BP closely as unpredictable responses can occur. Advise patients to drink only in moderation and to avoid large variations in the amount of alcohol drunk
BETA-BLOCKERS	ANESTHETICS—GENERAL	Risk of severe hypotensive episodes during induction of anesthesia (including patients using timolol eye drops)	Most general anesthetics are myocardial depressants and vasodilators, so additive ↓ BP may occur	Monitor BP closely, especially during induction of anesthesia
BETA-BLOCKERS	**ANESTHETICS—LOCAL**			
➢ **Remember that ↑ BP can occur when epinephrine-containing local anesthetics are used in patients on beta-blockers**				
BETA-BLOCKERS	BUPIVACAINE	Risk of bupivacaine toxicity	Beta-blockers, particularly propranolol, inhibit hepatic microsomal metabolism of bupivacaine	Watch for bupivacaine toxicity—monitor ECG and BP
BETA-BLOCKERS	LIDOCAINE	1. Risk of bradycardia (occasionally severe), ↓ BP and heart failure with intravenous lidocaine 2. Risk of lidocaine toxicity due to ↑ plasma concentrations of lidocaine, particularly with propranolol and nadolol 3. ↑ Plasma concentrations of propranolol and possibly some other beta-blockers	1. Additive negative inotropic and chronotropic effects 2. Uncertain, but possibly a combination of beta-blocker-induced reduction in hepatic blood flow (due to ↓ cardiac output) and inhibition of metabolism of lidocaine 3. Attributed to inhibition of metabolism by lidocaine	1. Monitor PR, BP, and ECG closely; watch for development of heart failure when intravenous lidocaine is administered to patients on beta-blockers 2. Watch for lidocaine toxicity 3. Be aware. Regional anesthetics should be used cautiously in patients with bradycardia. Beta-blockers could cause dangerous hypertension due to stimulation of alpha-receptors if epinephrine is used with local anesthetic

(*Continued*)

DRUGS ACTING ON THE CARDIOVASCULAR SYSTEM BETA-BLOCKERS

Primary Drug	Secondary Drug	Effect	Mechanism	Precautions
BETA-BLOCKERS				
BETA-BLOCKERS	**ANALGESICS**			
BETA-BLOCKERS	NSAIDs—INDOMETACIN, PIROXICAM, POSSIBLY IBUPROFEN, NAPROXEN	↓ Hypotensive efficacy of beta-blockers. This effect is absent in other NSAIDs	Additive toxic effects on kidney, and sodium and water, retention by NSAIDs. NSAIDs can raise BP by inhibiting renal synthesis of vasodilating prostaglandins. It is uncertain why this effect is specific to these NSAIDs	Watch for ↓ response to beta-blockers
METOPROLOL	CELECOXIB, VALDECOXIB	Risk of ↑ hypotensive efficacy of metoprolol	Inhibition of CYP2D6-mediated metabolism of metoprolol	Monitor BP at least weekly until stable. Warn patients to report symptoms of hypotension (light-headedness, dizziness on standing, etc.)
BETA-BLOCKERS	OPIOIDS	1. Risk of ↑ plasma concentrations and effects of labetalol, metoprolol, and propranolol; ↑ systemic effects of timolol eye drops 2. ↑ Plasma concentrations of esmolol when morphine is added 3. ↑ Plasma concentrations of metoprolol and propranolol when dextro-propoxyphene is added	1. Methadone inhibits CYP2D6, which metabolizes these beta-blockers 2. Unknown 3. ↓ Hepatic clearance of metoprolol and propranolol	1. Monitor BP at least weekly until stable 2. Monitor BP closely 3. Monitor BP at least weekly until stable. Warn patients to report symptoms of hypotension (light-headedness, dizziness on standing, etc.)

(*Continued*)

Primary Drug	Secondary Drug	Effect	Mechanism	Precautions
BETA-BLOCKERS				
BETA-BLOCKERS	ANTACIDS CONTAINING MAGNESIUM AND ALUMINUM	↑ Bioavailability of metoprolol and ↓ bioavailability of atenolol, which may produce mild variation in response to metoprolol and atenolol	Variations in absorption of the respective beta-blockers	Clinical significance may be minimal but be aware; monitor BP at least weekly until stable when initiating antacid therapy. Warn patients to report symptoms of hypotension (light-headedness, dizziness on standing, etc.)
BETA-BLOCKERS	**ANTIARRHYTHMICS**			
BETA-BLOCKERS	AMIODARONE, DISOPYRAMIDE, DRONEDARONE, FLECAINIDE, MEXILETINE, PROCAINAMIDE, PROPAFENONE	Risk of bradycardia (occasionally severe), ↓ BP, and heart failure. A single case report has described bradycardia when timolol eye drops were given to a patient on flecainide. Also, propafenone and dronedarone ↑ plasma levels of propranolol and metoprolol	Additive negative inotropic and chronotropic effects. In addition: 1. High-dose amiodarone is associated with ↑ plasma levels of metoprolol due to inhibition of CYP2D 2. Dronedarone inhibits CYP2D6-metabolism of metoprolol and propranolol 3. Mexiletine is known to inhibit CYP1A2-mediated metabolism of propranolol 4. Propafenone inhibits CYP2D6-metabolism of propranolol	Monitor PR, BP, and ECG closely, especially when loading patients on beta-blockers with antiarrhythmics; watch for the development of heart failure. ↓ Doses of beta-blocker accordingly, especially when coadministering propafenone with metoprolol or propranolol
BETA-BLOCKERS—METOPROLOL, PROPRANOLOL, TIMOLOL	QUINIDINE	Risk of ↑ levels of these beta-blockers (report of bradycardia with timolol eye drops)	Inhibition of CYP2D6-mediated metabolism	Monitor PR and BP closely on initiation of coadministration. Warn patients to report symptoms of orthostatic hypotension

(Continued)

DRUGS ACTING ON THE CARDIOVASCULAR SYSTEM BETA-BLOCKERS

Primary Drug	Secondary Drug	Effect	Mechanism	Precautions
BETA-BLOCKERS				
BETA-BLOCKERS	**ANTIBIOTICS**			
BETA-BLOCKERS	AMPICILLIN	Plasma concentrations of atenolol are halved by 1 g doses of ampicillin (but not smaller doses)	Uncertain	Monitor BP closely during initiation of therapy with ampicillin
BETA-BLOCKERS	RIFAMPICIN	↓ Plasma concentrations and efficacy of bisoprolol, carvedilol, celiprolol, metoprolol, and propranolol	Rifampicin induces hepatic enzymes (e.g., CYP2C19), which ↑ metabolism of the beta-blockers; in addition, it may also ↑ Pgp expression	Monitor PR and BP; watch for poor response to beta-blockers
BETA-BLOCKERS	**ANTICANCER AND IMMUNOMODULATING DRUGS**			
BETA-BLOCKERS	BORTEZOMIB	↑ Hypotensive effect	Additive hypotensive effect	Monitor BP at least weekly until stable, particularly on initiation of therapy
ACEBUTOLOL, ATENOLOL, BETAXOLOL, BISOPROLOL, METOPROLOL, PROPRANOLOL	CICLOSPORIN	↑ Risk of hyperkalemia	Beta-blockers cause an efflux of potassium from cells, and side effect has been observed during ciclosporin therapy	➢ Monitor serum potassium levels during coadministration ***For signs and symptoms of hyperkalemia, see Clinical Features of Some Adverse Drug Interactions, Hyperkalemia***
CARVEDILOL	CICLOSPORIN	Possible ↑ in plasma concentrations of ciclosporin	Carvedilol is metabolized primarily by CYP2D6 and CYP2D9, with a minor contribution from CYP3A4	Usually a dose reduction (20%) of ciclosporin is required
BETA-BLOCKERS	CORTICOSTEROIDS	↓ Efficacy of beta-blockers	Mineralocorticoids cause ↑ BP as a result of sodium and water retention	Watch for poor response to beta-blockers
BETA-BLOCKERS	CRIZOTINIB	Risk of excessive bradycardia	Additive	Caution with concurrent use

(Continued)

Primary Drug	Secondary Drug	Effect	Mechanism	Precautions
BETA-BLOCKERS				
BETA-BLOCKERS	FINGOLIMOD	Possible increased risk of bradycardia	Additive	Monitor for bradycardia, ECG prior to starting fingolimod
BETA-BLOCKERS	INTERLEUKIN-2 (ALDESLEUKIN)	↑ Hypotensive effect	Additive hypotensive effect. Aldesleukin causes ↓ vascular resistance and ↑ capillary permeability	Monitor BP at least weekly until stable
BETA-BLOCKERS	IMATINIB	Imatinib may cause an ↑ in plasma concentrations of metoprolol, propranolol, and timolol, with a risk of toxic effects	Imatinib is a potent inhibitor of CYP2D6 isoenzymes, which metabolize beta-blockers	Monitor for clinical efficacy and toxicity of beta-adrenergic blockers
BETA-BLOCKERS	PASIREOTIDE	Risk of bradycardia	Additive effect	Monitor PR closely until stable
BETA-BLOCKERS—PROPRANOLOL	PIXANTRONE	Theoretical risk of increased drug levels	Pixantrone inhibits CYP1A2	Manufacturer advises to monitor closely
BETA-BLOCKERS	THALIDOMIDE	Excessive bradycardia	Additive effect	Monitor BP and PR closely
BETA-BLOCKERS	**ANTIDEPRESSANTS**			
BETA-BLOCKERS—PROPRANOLOL	LITHIUM	Report of episode of ↑ lithium levels in elderly patient after starting low-dose propranolol. However, propranolol is often used to treat lithium-induced tremor without problems	Mechanism uncertain at present, but propranolol seems to ↓ lithium clearance	Monitor lithium levels when starting propranolol therapy in elderly people. Warn patients to report dizziness and to measure pulse rate
BETA-BLOCKERS	MAOIs	↑ Hypotensive effect	Additive hypotensive effect. Postural ↓ BP is a common side effect of MAOIs	Monitor BP at least weekly until stable. Warn patients to report symptoms of hypotension (light-headedness, dizziness on standing, etc.)
BETA-BLOCKERS	SNRIs—VENLAFAXINE	↑ Plasma concentrations and efficacy of metoprolol, propranolol, and timolol	Venlafaxine inhibits CYP2D6-mediated metabolism of metoprolol, propranolol, and timolol	Monitor PR and BP at least weekly; watch for metoprolol toxicity (in particular, loss of its cardioselectivity) and propranolol toxicity

(Continued)

DRUGS ACTING ON THE CARDIOVASCULAR SYSTEM BETA-BLOCKERS

DRUGS ACTING ON THE CARDIOVASCULAR SYSTEM BETA-BLOCKERS

Primary Drug	Secondary Drug	Effect	Mechanism	Precautions
BETA-BLOCKERS				
METOPROLOL, PROPRANOLOL, AND TIMOLOL	SSRIs	↑ Plasma concentrations and efficacy of metoprolol, propranolol, and timolol	Fluvoxamine inhibits the CYP1A2-, 2C19-, and 2D6-mediated metabolism of propranolol and 2D6-mediated metabolism of metoprolol Fluoxetine inhibits CYP2C19- and 2D6-mediated metabolism of propranolol and timolol and 2D6-mediated metabolism of metoprolol Paroxetine, sertraline, and venlafaxine inhibit CYP2D6-mediated metabolism of metoprolol, propranolol. and timolol and can impair conduction through the AV node	Monitor PR and BP at least weekly. Warn patients to report symptoms of hypotension (light-headedness, dizziness on standing, etc.). Watch for propranolol toxicity and loss of metoprolol cardioselectivity
BETA-BLOCKERS	**TCAS AND RELATED ANTIDEPRESSANTS**			
BETA-BLOCKERS	AMITRIPTYLINE, CLOMIPRAMINE	Risk of ↑ levels of beta-blockers with amitriptyline and clomipramine	These TCAs inhibit CYP2D6-mediated metabolism of beta-blockers	Monitor BP at least weekly until stable. Warn patients to report symptoms of hypotension (light-headedness, dizziness on standing, etc.)
LABETALOL, PROPRANOLOL	IMIPRAMINE	↑ Imipramine levels with labetalol and propranolol	Uncertain at present. Postulated that imipramine metabolism ↓ due to competition at CYP2D6 and CYP2C8	Monitor plasma levels of imipramine when initiating beta-blocker therapy

(Continued)

Primary Drug	Secondary Drug	Effect	Mechanism	Precautions
BETA-BLOCKERS				
PROPRANOLOL	MAPROTILINE	Cases of ↑ plasma levels of maprotiline with propranolol	Uncertain at present. Postulated that maprotiline metabolism ↓ with alterations in hepatic blood flow	Monitor plasma levels of maprotiline when initiating beta-blocker therapy
BETA-BLOCKERS	**ANTIDIABETIC DRUGS**			
BETA-BLOCKERS	ANTIDIABETIC DRUGS	Beta-blockers may mask the symptoms and signs of hypoglycemia. They also ↓ insulin sensitivity; however, beta-blockers that also have vasodilating properties (carvedilol, celiprolol, labetalol, nebivolol) seem to ↑ sensitivity to insulin	Beta-blockers ↓ glucose tolerance and interfere with the metabolic and autonomic responses to hypoglycemia	➢ Warn patients about masking of signs of hypoglycemia. Vasodilating beta-blockers are preferred in patients with diabetes, and all beta-blockers should be avoided in those having frequent hypoglycemic attacks. Monitor capillary blood glucose levels closely, especially during initiation of therapy ***For signs and symptoms of hypoglycemia, see Clinical Features of Some Adverse Drug Interactions, Hypoglycemia***
PINDOLOL, PROPRANOLOL, OR TIMOLOL EYE DROPS	INSULIN	Hypoglycemia has occurred in patients on insulin with patients taking oral propranolol and pindolol, propranolol or timolol eye drops	These beta-blockers inhibit the rebound in blood glucose that occurs as a response to a fall in blood glucose levels	➢ Cardioselective beta-blockers are preferred, and all beta-blockers should be avoided in those having frequent hypoglycemic attacks. Monitor capillary blood glucose levels closely, especially during initiation of therapy ***For signs and symptoms of hypoglycemia, see Clinical Features of Some Adverse Drug Interactions, Hypoglycemia***

(*Continued*)

DRUGS ACTING ON THE CARDIOVASCULAR SYSTEM BETA-BLOCKERS

DRUGS ACTING ON THE CARDIOVASCULAR SYSTEM BETA-BLOCKERS

Primary Drug	Secondary Drug	Effect	Mechanism	Precautions
BETA-BLOCKERS				
BETA-BLOCKERS	ANTIDIARRHEALS—KAOLIN	Possibly ↓ levels of atenolol, propranolol and sotalol	↓ Absorption	Separate doses by at least 2 h
BETA-BLOCKERS	**ANTIEPILEPTICS**			
BETA-BLOCKERS	BARBITURATES	Regular barbiturate use may ↑ elimination of those beta-blockers metabolized by the liver (metoprolol, propranolol, timolol)	Barbiturates induce CYP1A2-, CYP2C9-, and CYP2C19-mediated metabolism of propranolol	Monitor BP at least weekly until stable and watch for ↑ BP
BETA-BLOCKERS	PHENYTOIN	↓ Levels of propranolol with risk of therapeutic failure	Induction of hepatic metabolism	Monitor PR and BP weekly until stable, and watch for ↑ BP
BETA-BLOCKERS	ANTIFUNGALS—TERBINAFINE	↑ Metoprolol and propanolol levels	Inhibition of CYP2D6 mediated metabolism	Monitor PR and BP closely until stable
BETA-BLOCKERS	ANTIGOUT DRUGS—SULFINPYRAZONE	Antihypertensive effects of oxprenolol ↓ by sulfinpyrazone	Unknown	Monitor PR and BP closely; consider starting an alternative beta-blocker
BETA-BLOCKERS	**ANTIHYPERTENSIVES AND HEART FAILURE DRUGS**			
BETA-BLOCKERS	ACE INHIBITORS, ADRENERGIC NEURONE BLOCKERS, ALISKIREN, ANGIOTENSIN II RECEPTOR ANTAGONISTS	↑ Hypotensive effect	Additive hypotensive effect; may be used therapeutically	Monitor BP at least weekly until stable. Warn patients to report symptoms of hypotension (light-headedness, dizziness on standing, etc.)
BETA-BLOCKERS	ALPHA-BLOCKERS	↑ Efficacy of alpha-blockers; ↑ risk of first-dose ↓ BP with alfuzosin, prazosin, and terazosin	Additive hypotensive effect; may be used therapeutically. Beta-blockers prevent the ability to mount a tachycardia in response to ↓ BP; this ↑ the risk of first-dose ↓ BP when starting alpha-blockers in patients already on beta-blockers	Monitor BP at least weekly until stable; watch for first-dose ↓ BP. Warn patients to report symptoms of hypotension (light-headedness, dizziness on standing, etc.)

(Continued)

Primary Drug	Secondary Drug	Effect	Mechanism	Precautions
BETA-BLOCKERS				
BETA-BLOCKERS	CENTRALLY ACTING ANTIHYPERTENSIVES	Risk of withdrawal ↑ BP (rebound ↑ BP) with clonidine and possibly moxonidine	Withdrawal of clonidine, and possibly moxonidine, is associated with ↑ circulating catecholamines; beta-blockers, especially noncardioselective ones, allow the catecholamines to exert an unopposed alpha-receptor action (vasoconstriction)	Do not withdraw clonidine or moxonidine while a patient is taking beta-blockers. Withdraw beta-blockers several days before slowly withdrawing clonidine and moxonidine
BETA-BLOCKERS	KETANSERIN	Risk of first-dose hypotension	Additive effect	Monitor BP closely; start at a low dose and titrate up to effect
BETA-BLOCKERS	VASODILATOR ANTIHYPERTENSIVES	↑ Hypotensive effect	Additive hypotensive effect with diazoxide, hydralazine, minoxidil, and sodium nitroprusside; may be used therapeutically. In addition, hydralazine may ↑ the bioavailability of beta-blockers with a high first-pass metabolism (e.g., propranolol and metoprolol), possibly due to alterations in hepatic blood flow or inhibited hepatic metabolism	Monitor BP at least weekly until stable. Warn patients to report symptoms of hypotension (light-headedness, dizziness on standing, etc.)
BETA-BLOCKERS	**ANTIMALARIALS**			
METOPROLOL	ARTEMETHER/LUMEFANTRINE	↑ Risk of toxicity	Uncertain	Avoid coadministration

(Continued)

DRUGS ACTING ON THE CARDIOVASCULAR SYSTEM BETA-BLOCKERS

DRUGS ACTING ON THE CARDIOVASCULAR SYSTEM BETA-BLOCKERS

Primary Drug	Secondary Drug	Effect	Mechanism	Precautions
BETA-BLOCKERS				
BETA-BLOCKERS	MEFLOQUINE	↑ Risk of bradycardia	Mefloquine can cause cardiac conduction disorders, e.g., bradycardia. Additive bradycardic effect. Single case report of cardiac arrest with coadministration of mefloquine and propranolol, possibly caused by QT prolongation	Monitor PR closely
BETA-BLOCKERS	QUININE	Risk of ↑ plasma concentrations and effects of labetalol, metoprolol, and propranolol; ↑ systemic effects of timolol eye drops	Quinine inhibits CYP2D6, which metabolizes these beta-blockers	Monitor BP at least weekly until stable
BETA-BLOCKERS—BETAXOLOL, CARVEDILOL	ANTIOBESITY—LORCASERIN	↑ Blood concentrations of betaxolol and carvedilol	Inhibition of CYP2D6-mediated metabolism	Monitor PR and BP closely until stable
BETA-BLOCKERS	ANTI-PARKINSON'S DRUGS—LEVODOPA	↑ Hypotensive effect	Additive hypotensive effect; however, overall, adding beta-blockers to levodopa can be beneficial (e.g., by reducing the risk of dopamine-mediated risk of arrhythmias)	Monitor BP at least weekly until stable
BETA-BLOCKERS	**ANTIPSYCHOTICS**			
BETA-BLOCKERS	ANTIPSYCHOTICS	↑ Hypotensive effect	Dose-related ↓ BP (due to vasodilatation) is a side effect of most antipsychotics, particularly the phenothiazines	Monitor BP at least weekly until stable, especially during initiation of treatment. Warn patients to report symptoms of hypotension (light-headedness, dizziness on standing, etc.)

(*Continued*)

Primary Drug	Secondary Drug	Effect	Mechanism	Precautions
BETA-BLOCKERS				
PROPRANOLOL, TIMOLOL	CHLORPROMAZINE, HALOPERIDOL	↑ Plasma concentrations and efficacy of both chlorpromazine and propranolol during coadministration	Propranolol and chlorpromazine mutually inhibit each other's hepatic metabolism. Haloperidol inhibits CYP2D6-mediated metabolism of propranolol and timolol	Watch for toxic effects of chlorpromazine and propranolol; ↓ doses accordingly
BETA-BLOCKERS	**ANTIVIRALS**			
BETA-BLOCKERS—METOPROLOL, TIMOLOL	COBICISTAT	Possible ↑ plasma levels	Inhibition of metabolism via CYP3A	Monitor more closely; if patient is already on the beta-blocker, a dose reduction may be required
BETA-BLOCKERS	PROTEASE INHIBITORS—RITONAVIR, TIPRANAVIR	↑ Adverse effects of carvedilol, metoprolol, propranolol, and timolol	Inhibition of CYP2D6-mediated metabolism of these beta-blockers and CYP2C19-mediated metabolism of propranolol	Use an alternative beta-blocker if possible; if not, monitor closely
BETA-BLOCKERS	**ANXIOLYTICS AND HYPNOTICS**			
BETA-BLOCKERS	ANXIOLYTICS AND HYPNOTICS	↑ Hypotensive effect	Additive hypotensive effect; anxiolytics and hypnotics can cause postural ↓ BP	Watch for ↓ BP. Monitor BP at least weekly until stable. Warn patients to report symptoms of hypotension (light-headedness, dizziness on standing, etc.)
BETA-BLOCKERS	DIAZEPAM	May occasionally cause ↑ sedation during metoprolol and propranolol therapy	Propranolol and metoprolol inhibit the metabolism of diazepam	Warn patients about ↑ sedation
BETA-BLOCKERS	POTASSIUM CHANNEL ACTIVATORS	↑ Hypotensive effect	Additive effect	Monitor BP closely
BETA-BLOCKERS	**BRONCHODILATORS**			
BETA-BLOCKERS	BETA-2 AGONISTS	Nonselective beta-blockers (e.g., propranolol) ↓ or prevent the bronchodilator effect of beta-2 agonists	Nonselective beta-blockers antagonize the effect of beta-2 agonists on bronchial smooth muscle	Avoid coadministration

(Continued)

DRUGS ACTING ON THE CARDIOVASCULAR SYSTEM BETA-BLOCKERS

Primary Drug	Secondary Drug	Effect	Mechanism	Precautions
BETA-BLOCKERS				
BETA-BLOCKERS	THEOPHYLLINE	↑ Plasma levels of theophylline with propranolol	Propranolol exerts a dose-dependent inhibitory effect on the metabolism of theophylline	Monitor theophylline levels during propranolol coadministration
BETA-BLOCKERS	**CALCIUM CHANNEL BLOCKERS**			
BETA-BLOCKERS	CALCIUM CHANNEL BLOCKERS	↑ Hypotensive effect, bradycardia, conduction defects, and heart failure	Additive hypotensive effect; may be used therapeutically	Monitor PR, BP, and ECG at least weekly until stable. Warn patients to report symptoms of hypotension (light-headedness, dizziness on standing, etc.)
BETA-BLOCKERS	DIHYDROPYRIDINES	Rare cases of severe ↓ BP and heart failures when nifedipine and nisoldipine are given to patients on beta-blockers	It is uncertain why this severe effect occurs	Monitor PR, BP, and ECG at least weekly until stable. Warn patients to report symptoms of hypotension (light-headedness, dizziness on standing, etc.)
BETA-BLOCKERS	DILTIAZEM	↑ Hypotensive and bradycardic effects: cases of severe bradycardia and AV block when both drugs are administered concurrently in the presence of pre-existing heart failure or conduction abnormalities	Additive effects on conduction; diltiazem causes bradycardia, sinoatrial block, and AV block. Also, diltiazem inhibits CYP1A2-mediated metabolism of propranolol	Monitor PR, BP, and ECG at least weekly until stable. Warn patients to report symptoms of hypotension (light-headedness, dizziness on standing, etc.)
BETA-BLOCKERS	VERAPAMIL	1. Risk of cardiac arrest when parenteral verapamil is given to patients on beta-blockers 2. Risk of bradycardias when both are given orally	Additive effect. Also, verapamil inhibits CYP1A2-mediated metabolism of propranolol	1. Do not administer intravenous verapamil to patients taking beta-blockers 2. Monitor ECG and BP carefully when both are given orally
BETA-BLOCKERS	**CARDIAC GLYCOSIDES**			
BETA-BLOCKERS	DIGOXIN	Risk of bradycardia and AV block	Additive bradycardia	Monitor PR, BP, and ECG closely

(*Continued*)

Primary Drug	Secondary Drug	Effect	Mechanism	Precautions
BETA-BLOCKERS				
CARVEDILOL	DIGOXIN	Carvedilol may ↑ digoxin plasma concentrations, particularly in children	↓ Pgp-mediated renal clearance of digoxin	↓ The dose of digoxin by 25%; watch for signs of digoxin toxicity and monitor digoxin levels
BETA-BLOCKERS	COCAINE	Risk of hypertensive crisis	Cocaine produces both alpha- and beta-adrenergic agonist effects; selective beta-blockade leads to unopposed alpha-agonism (vasoconstriction)	Avoid concurrent use
PROPRANOLOL	CNS STIMULANTS—MODAFINIL	Variable effect on propranolol levels	Modafinil is a reversible inhibitor of CYP2C19 when used in therapeutic doses, and a moderate inducer of CYP1A2 in a concentration-dependent manner	Be aware
BETA-BLOCKERS	DRUG DEPENDENCE THERAPIES—BUPROPION	↑ Plasma concentrations of metoprolol, propranolol, and timolol, with risk of toxic effects	Bupropion and its metabolite hydroxybupropion inhibit CYP2D6	Initiate therapy of these drugs at the lowest effective dose
BETA-BLOCKERS	DIURETICS	↑ Hypotensive effect	Additive hypotensive effect; may be used therapeutically	Monitor BP at least weekly until stable. Warn patients to report symptoms of hypotension (light-headedness, dizziness on standing, etc.)
BETA-BLOCKERS—METOPROLOL	ELIGLUSTAT	↑ Metoprolol levels	Inhibition of CYP2D6-mediated metabolism	Reduce dose of metoprolol; monitor PR and BP closely

(*Continued*)

DRUGS ACTING ON THE CARDIOVASCULAR SYSTEM BETA-BLOCKERS

Primary Drug	Secondary Drug	Effect	Mechanism	Precautions
BETA-BLOCKERS				
BETA-BLOCKERS	ERGOT DERIVATIVES	Three reported cases of arterial vasoconstriction and one of ↑ BP occurred when ergotamine or methysergide was added to propranolol or oxprenolol	Ergotamine can cause peripheral vasospasm, and absence of beta-adrenergic activity can ↑ the risk of vasoconstriction	Ergot derivatives and beta-blockers are often coadministered without trouble; however, monitor BP at least weekly until stable (watch for ↑ BP) and warn patients to stop the ergot derivative and seek medical attention if they develop cold, painful feet
PROPRANOLOL	5-HT1 AGONISTS—RIZATRIPTAN	Plasma levels of rizatriptan almost doubled during propranolol therapy	Propranolol inhibits the metabolism of rizatriptan	Initiate therapy with 5 mg rizatriptan and do not exceed 10 mg in 24 h. The manufacturers recommend separating doses by 2 h, although this has not been proved by the studies
BETA-BLOCKERS	GLUCAGON	↓ Hyperglycemic effect of glucagon	Uncertain	Monitor blood sugar closely
BETA-BLOCKERS	**H2 RECEPTOR BLOCKERS**			
BETA-BLOCKERS	CIMETIDINE	↑ Plasma concentrations and effects of labetalol, metoprolol, and propranolol; ↑ systemic effects of timolol eye drops	Cimetidine inhibits CYP2D6, which metabolizes these beta-blockers, and inhibits CYP1A2- and CYP2E1-mediated metabolism of propranolol. Ranitidine is a weaker inhibitor of CYP2D6	Monitor BP and PR, risk of worsening heart failure, monitor these patients more closely. Nebivolol and levels of other CYP2D6 substrates are likely to be increased
BETA-BLOCKERS	NIZATIDINE	↑ Bradycardia when nizatidine is added to atenolol. Other beta-blockers have not been studied	Uncertain	Monitor PR when administering nizatidine to patients on beta-blockers

(Continued)

Primary Drug	Secondary Drug	Effect	Mechanism	Precautions
BETA-BLOCKERS				
BETA-BLOCKERS	**MUSCLE RELAXANTS**			
BETA-BLOCKERS	NONDEPOLARIZING	1. Modest ↑ in efficacy of muscle relaxants, particularly with propranolol 2. Risk of ↓ BP with atracurium and alcuronium	1 and 2. Uncertain	1. Watch for prolonged muscular paralysis after muscle relaxants 2. Monitor BP at least weekly until stable
BETA-BLOCKERS	SKELETAL—BACLOFEN, TIZANIDINE	↑ Hypotensive effect with baclofen or tizanidine. Risk of bradycardia with tizanidine	Additive hypotensive effect. Tizanidine shows negative inotropic and chronotropic effects	Monitor BP at least weekly until stable. Warn patients to report symptoms of hypotension (light-headedness, dizziness on standing, etc.)
BETA-BLOCKERS	NITRATES	↑ Hypotensive effect	Additive hypotensive effect; may be used therapeutically	Monitor BP at least weekly until stable
BETA-BLOCKERS	ESTROGENS	↓ Hypotensive effect	Estrogens cause sodium and fluid retention	Monitor BP at least weekly until stable; routine prescription of estrogens in patients with ↑ BP is not advisable
BETA-BLOCKERS	ORLISTAT	Case report of severe ↑ BP when orlistat started on a patient on atenolol	Uncertain at present	Monitor BP at least weekly until stable
BETA-BLOCKERS	**PARASYMPATHOMIMETIC**			
BETA-BLOCKERS	NEOSTIGMINE, PYRIDOSTIGMINE	1. Cases of bradycardia and ↓ BP when neostigmine or physostigmine was given to reverse anesthesia 2. ↓ Effectiveness of neostigmine and pyridostigmine in myasthenia gravis	1. Neostigmine and pyridostigmine cause accumulation of ACh, which may cause additive bradycardia and ↓ BP 2. Beta-blockers are thought to have a depressant effect on the neuromuscular junction and thereby ↑ weakness	1. Monitor PR and BP closely when giving anticholinesterases to reverse anesthesia in patients on beta-blockers 2. Monitor the response to neostigmine and pyridostigmine when starting beta-blockers

(Continued)

DRUGS ACTING ON THE CARDIOVASCULAR SYSTEM BETA-BLOCKERS

DRUGS ACTING ON THE CARDIOVASCULAR SYSTEM BETA-BLOCKERS

Primary Drug	Secondary Drug	Effect	Mechanism	Precautions
BETA-BLOCKERS				
BETA-BLOCKERS	PILOCARPINE	↑ Risk of arrhythmias	Pilocarpine is a parasympathomimetic and can cause additive bradycardia	Monitor PR and ECG closely
BETA-BLOCKERS	PERIPHERAL VASODILATORS—MOXISYLYTE (THYMOXAMINE)	↑ Hypotensive effect	Additive hypotensive effect	Monitor BP at least weekly until stable
BETA-BLOCKERS	POTASSIUM CHANNEL ACTIVATORS	↑ Hypotensive effect	Additive effect	Monitor BP at least weekly until stable
BETA-BLOCKERS	PROSTAGLANDINS—ALPROSTADIL	↑ Hypotensive effect	Additive hypotensive effect	Monitor BP at least weekly until stable. Warn patients to report symptoms of hypotension (light-headedness, dizziness on standing, etc.)
BETA-BLOCKERS	PROTON PUMP INHIBITORS	Risk of ↑ plasma concentrations and effects of propranolol	Omeprazole inhibits CYP2D6- and CYP2C19-mediated metabolism of propranolol	Monitor BP at least weekly until stable
BETA-BLOCKERS	RANOLAZINE	↑ Metoprolol levels	Inhibition of CYP2D6 mediated metabolism of metoprolol	Monitor PR and BP closely
BETA-BLOCKERS	**SYMPATHOMIMETICS**			
BETA-BLOCKERS	SYMPATHOMIMETICS—INDIRECT	↓ Hypotensive efficacy of beta-blockers	The hypertensive effect of sympathomimetics opposes the hypotensive actions of beta-blockers	Monitor BP at least weekly until stable; watch for poor response to beta-blockers

(*Continued*)

Primary Drug	Secondary Drug	Effect	Mechanism	Precautions
BETA-BLOCKERS				
BETA-BLOCKERS	SYMPATHOMIMETICS—DIRECT	1. Severe ↑ BP and bradycardia with noncardioselective beta-blockers (including reports of severe ↑ BP in patients given infiltrations of local anesthetics containing epinephrine, and one case of a fatal reaction with phenylephrine eye drops) 2. Patients on beta-blockers may respond poorly to epinephrine when given to treat anaphylaxis	1. Unopposed alpha stimulation causes vasoconstriction, which results in a rise in BP. Beta-2 receptors, when stimulated, cause vasodilatation, which counteracts any alpha action; nonselective beta-blockers antagonize beta-2 receptors 2. Uncertain mechanism	1. Monitor BP at least weekly until stable. When using local anesthetics with epinephrine, use small volumes of low concentrations (such as 1 in 200,000 epinephrine); avoid high concentrations (e.g., 1 in 1,000 mixtures) 2. Look for failure of epinephrine therapy and consider using salbutamol, isoprenaline, or glucagon
BETA-BLOCKERS	X-RAY CONTRAST SOLUTIONS	Beta-blockers are associated with ↑ risk of anaphylactoid reactions to iodinated x-ray contrast materials	Uncertain, but postulated that beta-receptors have a role in suppressing the release of mediators of anaphylaxis	Consider using low-osmolality contrast media and pretreating with antihistamines and corticosteroids. Stopping beta-blockers a few days before the x-ray may reduce the risk: a risk–benefit assessment must therefore be made

Primary Drug	Secondary Drug	Effect	Mechanism	Precautions
CALCIUM CHANNEL BLOCKERS				
CALCIUM CHANNEL BLOCKERS	ALCOHOL	1. Acute alcohol ingestion may ↑ hypotensive effect. Chronic moderate/heavy drinking ↓ hypotensive effect 2. Verapamil may ↑ peak serum concentration and prolong the effects of alcohol	1. Additive hypotensive effect with acute alcohol excess. Chronic alcohol excess is associated with hypertension 2. Uncertain at present, but presumed to be due to an inhibition of hepatic metabolism of alcohol	1. Monitor BP closely as unpredictable responses can occur. Advise patients to drink only in moderation and avoid large variations in the amount of alcohol drunk 2. Warn the patient about the ill-effects of alcohol, particularly the risks of driving

(*Continued*)

DRUGS ACTING ON THE CARDIOVASCULAR SYSTEM CALCIUM CHANNEL BLOCKERS

DRUGS ACTING ON THE CARDIOVASCULAR SYSTEM CALCIUM CHANNEL BLOCKERS

Primary Drug	Secondary Drug	Effect	Mechanism	Precautions
CALCIUM CHANNEL BLOCKERS				
CALCIUM CHANNEL BLOCKERS	ANESTHETICS—GENERAL, INHALATIONAL	↑ Hypotensive effects of dihydropyridines, and hypotensive/bradycardic effects of diltiazem and verapamil	Additive hypotensive and negative inotropic effects. General anesthetics tend to be myocardial depressants and vasodilators; they also ↓ sinus automaticity and AV conduction	Monitor BP and ECG closely
CALCIUM CHANNEL BLOCKERS	ANESTHETICS—LOCAL	Case reports of severe ↓ BP when bupivacaine epidural was administered to patients on calcium channel blockers	Additive hypotensive effect; both bupivacaine and calcium channel blockers are cardiodepressant; in addition, epidural anesthesia causes sympathetic block in the lower limbs, which leads to vasodilatation and ↓ BP	Monitor BP closely. Preload intravenous fluids prior to the epidural
CALCIUM CHANNEL BLOCKERS	**ANALGESICS**			
CALCIUM CHANNEL BLOCKERS	NSAIDs	↓ Antihypertensive effect of calcium channel blockers	NSAIDs cause sodium retention and vasoconstriction at possibly both renal and endothelial sites	Monitor BP at least weekly until stable
CALCIUM CHANNEL BLOCKERS	OPIOIDS	Diltiazem prolongs the action of alfentanil	Diltiazem inhibits CYP3A4-mediated metabolism of alfentanil	Watch for the prolonged action of alfentanil in patients taking calcium channel blockers; case reports of delayed extubation in patients recovering from anesthetics involving large doses of alfentanil in patients on diltiazem

(*Continued*)

Primary Drug	Secondary Drug	Effect	Mechanism	Precautions
CALCIUM CHANNEL BLOCKERS				
CALCIUM CHANNEL BLOCKERS	**ANTIARRHYTHMICS**			
CALCIUM CHANNEL BLOCKERS	AMIODARONE	Risk of bradycardia, AV block, and ↓ BP when amiodarone is coadministered with diltiazem or verapamil	Additive negative inotropic and chronotropic effects. Also, amiodarone inhibits intestinal Pgp, which ↑ the bioavailability of diltiazem and verapamil	Monitor PR, BP, and ECG closely; watch for heart failure
CALCIUM CHANNEL BLOCKERS	DISOPYRAMIDE	Risk of myocardial depression and asystole when disopyramide is coadministered with verapamil, particularly in the presence of heart failure	Disopyramide is a myocardial depressant like verapamil and can cause ventricular tachycardia, ventricular fibrillation, or torsades de pointes	Avoid coadministering verapamil with disopyramide if possible. If single-agent therapy is ineffective, monitor PR, BP, and ECG closely; watch for heart failure
DIHYDROPYRIDINES	DRONEDARONE	↑ Levels of nifedipine and possibly other dihydropyridines	Dronedarone inhibits their metabolism	Monitor BP closely
DILTIAZEM, VERAPAMIL	DRONEDARONE	Risk of excessive bradycardia	Additive effect on slowing AV conduction	Monitor PR and BP closely. Cardiac monitoring is essential when giving calcium channel blockers pareterally (which should be administered slowly)
CALCIUM CHANNEL BLOCKERS—DILTIAZEM, VERAPAMIL	DOFETILIDE	Risk of ↑ dofetilide levels with risk of ↑ QT prolongation	Diltiazem and verapamil inhibits CYP3A4-mediated metabolism of dofetilide	Avoid coadministration
CALCIUM CHANNEL BLOCKERS	FLECAINIDE	Risk of heart block and ↓ BP when flecainide is coadministered with verapamil. A single case of asystole has been reported	Additive negative inotropic and chronotropic effects	Monitor PR, BP, and ECG at least weekly until stable; watch for heart failure

(Continued)

DRUGS ACTING ON THE CARDIOVASCULAR SYSTEM CALCIUM CHANNEL BLOCKERS

DRUGS ACTING ON THE CARDIOVASCULAR SYSTEM CALCIUM CHANNEL BLOCKERS

DRUGS ACTING ON THE CARDIOVASCULAR SYSTEM CALCIUM CHANNEL BLOCKERS

Primary Drug	Secondary Drug	Effect	Mechanism	Precautions
CALCIUM CHANNEL BLOCKERS				
CALCIUM CHANNEL BLOCKERS	MORACIZINE	Coadministration is associated with ↑ bioavailability of moracizine and ↓ availability of diltiazem	Postulated that diltiazem inhibits metabolism of moracizine, while moracizine ↑ metabolism of diltiazem; the precise mechanism of interaction is uncertain at present	Monitor PR, BP, and ECG; adjust the doses of each drug accordingly
CALCIUM CHANNEL BLOCKERS—VERAPAMIL	QUINIDINE	↑ Quinidine levels; reports of quinidine toxicity	Verapamil inhibits CYP3A4-mediated metabolism	Reduce quinidine dose; monitor PR, BP, and ECG closely
CALCIUM CHANNEL BLOCKERS	**ANTIBIOTICS**			
CALCIUM CHANNEL BLOCKERS	MACROLIDES	↑ Plasma concentrations of felodipine when coadministered with erythromycin; cases of adverse effects of verapamil (bradycardia and ↓ BP) with both erythromycin and clarithromycin	Erythromycin inhibits CYP3A4-mediated metabolism of felodipine and verapamil. Clarithromycin and erythromycin inhibit intestinal Pgp, which may ↑ the bioavailability of verapamil	Monitor PR and BP closely; watch for bradycardia and ↓ BP. Consider reducing the dose of calcium channel blocker during macrolide therapy
CALCIUM CHANNEL BLOCKERS	RIFAMPICIN	Plasma concentrations of calcium channel blockers may be ↓ by rifampicin	Rifampicin induces CYP3A4-mediated metabolism of calcium channel blockers. It also induces CYP2C9-mediated metabolism of verapamil and induces intestinal Pgp, which may ↓ the bioavailability of verapamil	Monitor BP closely; watch for ↓ effect of calcium channel blockers

(Continued)

Primary Drug	Secondary Drug	Effect	Mechanism	Precautions
CALCIUM CHANNEL BLOCKERS				
CALCIUM CHANNEL BLOCKERS	QUINUPRISTIN/DALFOPRISTIN	Plasma levels of nifedipine may be ↑ by quinupristin–dalfopristin	Quinupristin inhibits CYP3A4-mediated metabolism of calcium channel blockers	Monitor BP closely; watch for ↓ BP
CALCIUM CHANNEL BLOCKERS	**ANTICANCER AND IMMUNOMODULATING DRUGS**			
CALCIUM CHANNEL BLOCKERS—VERAPAMIL	AFATINIB	Possible increase in afatinib levels	P-glycoprotein inhibition	Manufacturer recommends staggered dosing 6–12 h apart or dose reduction
CALCIUM CHANNEL BLOCKERS	BORTEZOMIB	↑ Hypotensive effect	Additive hypotensive effect	Monitor BP at least weekly until stable, particularly on initiation of therapy
CALCIUM CHANNEL BLOCKERS—DILTIAZEM, MIBEFRADIL, VERAPAMIL	BOSUTINIB	↑ Bosutinib levels	CYP3A inhibition	Manufacturer advises to avoid concurrent use. If not possible, interruption of therapy or dose reduction should be considered
CALCIUM CHANNEL BLOCKERS	BUSULFAN	↑ Plasma concentrations of busulfan and ↑ risk of toxicity of busulfan such as veno-occlusive disease and pulmonary fibrosis, when coadministered with diltiazem, nifedipine, or verapamil	Due to inhibition of CYP3A4-mediated metabolism of busulfan by these calcium channel blockers. Busulfan clearance may be ↓ by 25%, and the AUC of busulfan may ↑ by 1500 μmol/L	Monitor clinically for veno-occlusive disease and pulmonary toxicity in transplant patients. Monitor busulfan blood levels as AUC of below 1500 μmol/L/min tends to prevent toxicity

(Continued)

DRUGS ACTING ON THE CARDIOVASCULAR SYSTEM CALCIUM CHANNEL BLOCKERS

Primary Drug	Secondary Drug	Effect	Mechanism	Precautions
CALCIUM CHANNEL BLOCKERS				
CALCIUM CHANNEL BLOCKERS	CICLOSPORIN	1. Plasma concentrations of ciclosporin are ↑ when coadministered with diltiazem, nicardipine, verapamil, and possibly amlodipine and nisoldipine. However, calcium channel blockers seem to protect renal function 2. Ciclosporin ↑ nifedipine levels	1. Uncertain; presumed to be due to impaired hepatic metabolism. Also, diltiazem and verapamil inhibit intestinal Pgp, which may ↑ the bioavailability of ciclosporin. Uncertain mechanism of renal protection 2. Uncertain effect of ciclosporin on nifedipine	1. Monitor ciclosporin levels and ↓ dose accordingly (possibly by up to 25%–50% with nicardipine) 2. Monitor BP closely and warn patients to watch for signs of nifedipine toxicity
CALCIUM CHANNEL BLOCKERS	CORTICOSTEROIDS	1. Antihypertensive effects of calcium channel blockers are antagonized by corticosteroids 2. ↑ Adrenal-suppressive effects of dexamethasone, methylprednisolone, and prednisolone when coadministered with diltiazem, nifedipine, or verapamil. This may ↑ the risk of infections and produce an inadequate response to stress scenarios	1. Mineralocorticoids cause sodium and water retention, which antagonizes the hypotensive effects of calcium channel blockers 2. Due to inhibition of metabolism of these corticosteroids	1. Monitor BP at least weekly until stable 2. Monitor cortisol levels and warn patients to report symptoms such as fever and sore throat
CALCIUM CHANNEL BLOCKERS—VERAPAMIL AND DILTIAZEM	CRIZOTINIB	Risk of excessive bradycardia	Additive	Caution with concurrent use
CALCIUM CHANNEL BLOCKERS—DILTIAZEM, FELODIPINE, NICARDIPINE, NIFEDIPINE, VERAPAMIL	DABRAFENIB	Possible reduced levels of CYP3A4/CYP2Cs/CYP2B6 substrates. Level of reduction may vary	Dabrafenib induces CYP3A4/CYP2Cs/ CYP2B6	Monitor closely or avoid concurrent use

(Continued)

Primary Drug	Secondary Drug	Effect	Mechanism	Precautions
CALCIUM CHANNEL BLOCKERS				
CALCIUM CHANNEL BLOCKERS—BEPRIDIL	DASATINIB	↑ Levels of bepridil	CYP3A4 inhibition	Caution with CYP3A4 substrates with narrow therapeutic window
CALCIUM CHANNEL BLOCKERS	DOXORUBICIN	↑ Serum concentrations and efficacy of doxorubicin when coadministered with verapamil, nicardipine, and possibly diltiazem and nifedipine; however, no cases of doxorubicin toxicity have been reported	Uncertain; however, verapamil is known to inhibit intestinal Pgp, which may ↑ the bioavailability of doxorubicin	Watch for symptoms/signs of toxicity (tachycardia, heart failure, and hand-foot syndrome)
CALCIUM CHANNEL BLOCKERS	EPIRUBICIN	Cases of ↑ bone marrow suppression when verapamil is added to epirubicin	Uncertain at present	Monitor FBC closely
CALCIUM CHANNEL BLOCKERS—VERAPAMIL	ERLOTINIB	Altered distribution or elimination of erlotinib	P-glycoprotein inhibition	Caution with concurrent use
CALCIUM CHANNEL BLOCKERS	ETOPOSIDE	↑ Serum concentrations and risk of toxicity when verapamil is given to patients on etoposide	Verapamil inhibits CYP3A4-mediated metabolism of etoposide	Watch for symptoms/signs of toxicity (nausea, vomiting, and bone marrow suppression) in patients taking calcium channel blockers
CALCIUM CHANNEL BLOCKERS—VERAPAMIL, DILTIAZEM	EVEROLIMUS	↑ Levels of everolimus and verapamil Predicted increased levels of everolimus with diltiazem	CYP3A4 and P-glycoprotein inhibition (verapamil) CYP3A4 inhibition (diltiazem)	Monitor closely with concurrent use Consider dose reduction of everolimus
CALCIUM CHANNEL BLOCKERS—DILTIAZEM, VERAPAMIL	FINGOLIMOD	Possible increased risk of bradycardia	Additive	Monitor for bradycardia, get ECG prior to starting fingolimod

(Continued)

DRUGS ACTING ON THE CARDIOVASCULAR SYSTEM CALCIUM CHANNEL BLOCKERS

DRUGS ACTING ON THE CARDIOVASCULAR SYSTEM CALCIUM CHANNEL BLOCKERS

Primary Drug	Secondary Drug	Effect	Mechanism	Precautions
CALCIUM CHANNEL BLOCKERS				
CALCIUM CHANNEL BLOCKERS	IFOSFAMIDE	↓ Plasma concentrations of 4-hydroxyifosfamide, the active metabolite of ifosfamide and risk of inadequate therapeutic response when it is coadministered with diltiazem, nifedipine, or verapamil	Due to inhibition of the isoenzymatic conversion to active metabolites by diltiazem	Monitor clinically the efficacy of ifosfamide and ↑ the dose accordingly
CALCIUM CHANNEL BLOCKERS	IMATINIB	↑ Plasma concentrations of imatinib when it is coadministered with diltiazem, nifedipine, or verapamil. ↑ Risk of toxicity (e.g., abdominal pain, constipation, and dyspnea) and of neurotoxicity (e.g., taste disturbances, dizziness, headache, paresthesias, and peripheral neuropathy)	Due to inhibition of hepatic metabolism of imatinib by the CYP3A4 isoenzymes by diltiazem	Monitor for clinical efficacy and for the signs of toxicity listed along with convulsions, confusion, and signs of edema (including pulmonary edema). Monitor electrolytes and liver function, and for cardiotoxicity
CALCIUM CHANNEL BLOCKERS	INTERLEUKIN-2 (ALDESLEUKIN)	↑ Hypotensive effect	Additive hypotensive effect. Aldesleukin causes ↓ vascular resistance and ↑ capillary permeability	Monitor BP at least weekly until stable. Warn patients to report symptoms of hypotension (light-headedness, dizziness on standing, etc.)
CALCIUM CHANNEL BLOCKERS	IRINOTECAN	Risk of ↑ serum concentrations of irinotecan with nifedipine. No cases of toxicity reported	Inhibition of hepatic microsomal enzymes but exact mechanism is uncertain at present	Watch for symptoms/signs of toxicity (especially diarrhea, an early manifestation of acute cholinergic syndrome)
CALCIUM CHANNEL BLOCKERS—DIHYDROPYRIDINES	LAPATINIB	Possible ↑ levels of dihydropyridine calcium channel blockers	CYP3A4 inhibition	Interactions related to case reports. General relevance uncertain. Monitor concurrent use
CALCIUM CHANNEL BLOCKERS—VERAPAMIL	LAPATINIB	↑ Lapatinib levels	P-glycoprotein inhibition	Caution with concurrent use

(*Continued*)

Primary Drug	Secondary Drug	Effect	Mechanism	Precautions
CALCIUM CHANNEL BLOCKERS				
CALCIUM CHANNEL BLOCKERS—VERAPAMIL	LENALIDOMIDE	Lenalidomide levels increased, ↑ risk of toxicity	Inhibition of P-glycoprotein	Monitor closely and adjust dose as necessary
CALCIUM CHANNEL BLOCKERS—VERAPAMIL	NILOTINIB	↑ Nilotinib levels	P-glycoprotein inhibition	Caution with concurrent use
CALCIUM CHANNEL BLOCKERS—R-VERAPAMIL (HIGH DOSE)	PACLITAXEL	↑ Paclitaxel levels, ↑ hematological toxicity	Inhibition of P-glycoprotein	Clinical relevance uncertain as R-verapamil is usually used for investigation purposes only
CALCIUM CHANNEL BLOCKERS—VERAPAMIL	PASIREOTIDE	1. Risk of bradycardia 2. ↑ Pasireotide levels	1. Additive effect 2. Inhibition of Pgp	1. Monitor PR closely until stable 2. Warn patient to report adverse effects of pasireotide
CALCIUM CHANNEL BLOCKERS	PORFIMER	↑ Risk of photosensitivity reactions with diltiazem	Attributed to additive effects	Avoid exposure of skin and eyes to direct sunlight for 30 days after porfimer therapy
CALCIUM CHANNEL BLOCKERS—DILTIAZEM, MIBEFRADIL	RUXOLITINIB	↑ Levels of ruxolitinib	CYP3A4 inhibition	Manufacturer advises dose reduction Monitor closely
CALCIUM CHANNEL BLOCKERS	SIROLIMUS	Plasma concentrations of sirolimus are ↑ when given with diltiazem. Plasma levels of both drugs are ↑ when verapamil and sirolimus are coadministered	Diltiazem and verapamil inhibit intestinal CYP3A4, which is the main site of sirolimus metabolism	Watch for side effects of sirolimus when it is coadministered with diltiazem or verapamil; monitor renal and hepatic function. Monitor PR and BP closely when sirolimus is given with verapamil
CALCIUM CHANNEL BLOCKERS	TACROLIMUS	Plasma concentrations of tacrolimus are ↑ when given with diltiazem, felodipine, or nifedipine; however, they appear to protect renal function	Uncertain, but presumed to be due to inhibition of CYP3A4-mediated tacrolimus metabolism	Watch for side effects of tacrolimus; monitor ECG, blood count, and renal and hepatic functions
CALCIUM CHANNEL BLOCKERS	THALIDOMIDE	Risk of bradycardia	Additive effect	Monitor BP and PR closely

(*Continued*)

DRUGS ACTING ON THE CARDIOVASCULAR SYSTEM CALCIUM CHANNEL BLOCKERS

Primary Drug	Secondary Drug	Effect	Mechanism	Precautions
CALCIUM CHANNEL BLOCKERS				
CALCIUM CHANNEL BLOCKERS	TOCILIZUMAB	↓ Levels	Tocilizumab reverses cytochrome P450 isoenzyme suppression by IL-6	Monitor closely and consider dose adjustment
CALCIUM CHANNEL BLOCKERS	TOREMIFENE	↑ Plasma concentrations of toremifene when coadministered with diltiazem, nifedipine, or verapamil	Due to inhibition of CYP3A4-mediated metabolism of toremifene	Clinical relevance is uncertain. Necessary to monitor for clinical toxicities
CALCIUM CHANNEL BLOCKERS	TRABECTIN	↑ Plasma concentrations of trabectin when coadministered with verapamil	Due to inhibition of Pgp	Warn patient to report features of toxicity (GI upset, headaches, and edema). Monitor FBC, U&Es, and LFTs closely
CALCIUM CHANNEL BLOCKERS	TRETINOIN	↓ Plasma tretinoin levels and risk of ↓ antitumor activity when it is coadministered with diltiazem, nifedipine, or verapamil	Due to induction of CYP3A4-mediated metabolism of tretinoin	Avoid coadministration if possible
CALCIUM CHANNEL BLOCKERS	ANTICOAGULANTS—DABIGATRAN	↑ Dabigatran levels	Inhibition of Pgp	Reduce dose: 1. VTE prophylaxis—150 mg od (taken at the same time as verapamil)—reduce further to 75 mg od in the presence of renal impairment 2. Stroke prophylaxis—110 mg bd
CALCIUM CHANNEL BLOCKERS	ANTIDEMENTIA DRUGS—DONEPEZIL, GALANTAMINE, RIVASTIGMINE	Risk of bradycardia	Additive effect	Monitor PR and BP closely until stable

(*Continued*)

Primary Drug	Secondary Drug	Effect	Mechanism	Precautions
CALCIUM CHANNEL BLOCKERS				
CALCIUM CHANNEL BLOCKERS	**ANTIDEPRESSANTS**			
CALCIUM CHANNEL BLOCKERS	LITHIUM	Small number of cases of neurotoxicity when coadministered with diltiazem or verapamil. Alterations in lithium levels (both ↑ and ↓) reported with verapamil and ↓ levels reported with nifedipine. These effects are variable	Uncertain, but thought to be due to an additive effect on neurotransmission	Monitor closely for side effects
CALCIUM CHANNEL BLOCKERS	MAOIs	↑ Antihypertensive effect of calcium channel blockers when coadministered with MAOIs	Additive hypotensive effects; postural ↓ BP is a side effect of MAOIs	Monitor BP at least weekly until stable. Warn patients to report symptoms of hypotension (light-headedness, dizziness on standing, etc.)
CALCIUM CHANNEL BLOCKERS	SSRIs	Reports of ↑ serum levels of nimodipine and episodes of adverse effects of nifedipine and verapamil (edema, flushing, and ↓ BP) attributed to ↑ levels when coadministered with fluoxetine	Fluoxetine inhibits CYP3A4-mediated metabolism of calcium channel blockers. It also inhibits intestinal Pgp, which may ↑ the bioavailability of verapamil. Nefazodone also inhibits CYP3A4	Monitor BP at least weekly until stable. Warn patients to report symptoms of hypotension (light-headedness, dizziness on standing, etc.). Consider reducing the dose of calcium channel blocker or using an alternative antidepressant
CALCIUM CHANNEL BLOCKERS	ST. JOHN'S WORT	St. John's wort is associated with ↓ verapamil levels	St. John's wort induces CYP3A4, which metabolizes calcium channel blockers, and induces intestinal Pgp, which may ↓ the bioavailability of verapamil	Monitor BP regularly for at least the first 2 weeks of initiating St. John's wort

(*Continued*)

DRUGS ACTING ON THE CARDIOVASCULAR SYSTEM CALCIUM CHANNEL BLOCKERS

DRUGS ACTING ON THE CARDIOVASCULAR SYSTEM CALCIUM CHANNEL BLOCKERS

Primary Drug	Secondary Drug	Effect	Mechanism	Precautions
CALCIUM CHANNEL BLOCKERS				
CALCIUM CHANNEL BLOCKERS	TCAs	↑ Plasma concentrations of TCAs when coadministered with diltiazem and verapamil. Reports of cardiotoxicity (first- and second-degree block) when imipramine is given with diltiazem or verapamil	Uncertain, but may be due to a combination of ↓ clearance of TCAs (both diltiazem and verapamil are known to inhibit CYP1A2, which has a role in the metabolism of amitriptyline, clomipramine, and imipramine) and ↑ intestinal absorption (diltiazem and verapamil inhibit intestinal Pgp, which may ↑ amitriptyline bioavailability)	Monitor ECG when commencing or altering treatment
CALCIUM CHANNEL BLOCKERS	**ANTIDIABETIC DRUGS**			
CALCIUM CHANNEL BLOCKERS	INSULIN	Single case reports of impaired glucose intolerance requiring ↑ insulin requirements with diltiazem and nifedipine	Uncertain at present	Evidence suggests that calcium channel blockers are safe in diabetics; monitor blood glucose levels when starting calcium channel blockers
CALCIUM CHANNEL BLOCKERS	SAXAGLIPTIN	Likely to ↑ plasma concentrations of saxagliptin and ↑ risk of hypoglycemic episodes with diltiazem and verapamil	Inhibition of CYP3A4-mediated metabolism of saxagliptin	➢ Watch for and warn patients about hypoglycemia ***For signs and symptoms of hypoglycemia, see Clinical Features of Some Adverse Drug Interactions, Hypoglycemia***
CALCIUM CHANNEL BLOCKERS—NIFEDIPINE THIAZOLIDINEDIONES	THIAZOLIDINEDIONES	↓ Levels of Nifedipine in the blood	Possibly related to metabolism using the same CYP3A4 pathway	Nifedipine dose may need to be increased

(Continued)

Primary Drug	Secondary Drug	Effect	Mechanism	Precautions
CALCIUM CHANNEL BLOCKERS				
CALCIUM CHANNEL BLOCKERS	**ANTIEPILEPTICS**			
CALCIUM CHANNEL BLOCKERS	BARBITURATES	↓ Plasma concentrations of felodipine, nifedipine, nimodipine, nisoldipine, and verapamil with phenobarbital	Phenobarbital induces CYP3A4, which metabolizes calcium channel blockers. It also induces intestinal Pgp, which may ↓ the bioavailability of verapamil	Monitor PR and BP closely; watch for ↑ BP
CALCIUM CHANNEL BLOCKERS	CARBAMAZEPINE	1. Diltiazem and verapamil ↑ plasma concentrations of carbamazepine (cases of toxicity) 2. ↓ Plasma concentrations of felodipine, nifedipine, and possibly nimodipine and nisoldipine	1. Diltiazem and verapamil inhibit CYP3A4-mediated metabolism of carbamazepine. They also inhibit intestinal Pgp, which may ↑ the bioavailability of carbamazepine 2. Carbamazepine, in turn, induces CYP3A4, which metabolizes calcium channel blockers	1. Monitor carbamazepine levels when initiating calcium channel blockers, particularly diltiazem and verapamil 2. Monitor PR and BP closely; watch for ↑ BP when starting carbamazepine in patients already on calcium channel blockers
CALCIUM CHANNEL BLOCKERS	PHENYTOIN	1. Phenytoin levels are ↑ by diltiazem and possibly nifedipine and isradipine 2. ↓ Plasma concentrations of diltiazem, felodipine, nisoldipine, verapamil, and possibly nimodipine	1. Postulated to be due to inhibition of CYP3A4-mediated metabolism of phenytoin. Diltiazem is also known to inhibit intestinal Pgp, which may ↑ the bioavailability of phenytoin 2. Phenytoin induces CYP3A4, which metabolizes calcium channel blockers	1. Monitor phenytoin levels when initiating calcium channel blockers, particularly diltiazem and verapamil 2. Monitor PR and BP closely; watch for ↑ BP when starting phenytoin in patients already on calcium channel blockers

(Continued)

DRUGS ACTING ON THE CARDIOVASCULAR SYSTEM CALCIUM CHANNEL BLOCKERS

DRUGS ACTING ON THE CARDIOVASCULAR SYSTEM CALCIUM CHANNEL BLOCKERS

Primary Drug	Secondary Drug	Effect	Mechanism	Precautions
CALCIUM CHANNEL BLOCKERS				
CALCIUM CHANNEL BLOCKERS	PRIMIDONE	↓ Plasma concentrations of calcium channel blockers	Primidone induces CYP3A4, which metabolizes calcium channel blockers	Monitor PR and BP closely; watch for ↑ BP
CALCIUM CHANNEL BLOCKERS	SODIUM VALPROATE	Nimodipine levels may be ↑ by valproate	Uncertain at present	Monitor BP at least weekly until stable. Warn patients to report symptoms of hypotension (light-headedness, dizziness on standing, etc.)
CALCIUM CHANNEL BLOCKERS	ANTIFUNGALS—AZOLES	Plasma concentrations of dihydropyridine calcium channel blockers are ↑ by fluconazole, itraconazole, and ketoconazole. Risk of ↑ verapamil levels with ketoconazole and itraconazole. Itraconazole and possibly posaconazole may ↑ diltiazem levels	The azoles are potent inhibitors of CYP3A4 isoenzymes, which metabolize calcium channel blockers. They also inhibit CYP2C9-mediated metabolism of verapamil. Ketoconazole and itraconazole both inhibit intestinal Pgp, which may ↑ the bioavailability of verapamil. Diltiazem is mainly a substrate of CYP3A5 and CYP3A5P1, which are inhibited by itraconazole. Around 75% of the metabolism of diltiazem occurs in the liver and the rest in the intestine. Diltiazem is a substrate of Pgp (also an inhibitor but unlikely to be significant at therapeutic doses), which is inhibited by itraconazole, resulting in ↑ bioavailability of diltiazem	Monitor PR, BP, and ECG, and warn patents to watch for symptoms/signs of heart failure

(*Continued*)

Primary Drug	Secondary Drug	Effect	Mechanism	Precautions
CALCIUM CHANNEL BLOCKERS				
CALCIUM CHANNEL BLOCKERS	**ANTIGOUT DRUGS**			
CALCIUM CHANNEL BLOCKERS	COLCHICINE	↑ Colchicine levels by diltiazem and verapamil—reports of toxicity	Combination of inhibition of CYP3A4 and Pgp	Reduce dose of colchicines—monitor FBC regularly and warn patients to report features of colchicines toxicity (GI upset, muscle aches, sore throat)
CALCIUM CHANNEL BLOCKERS	SULFINPYRAZONE	Serum concentrations pf verapamil are significantly ↓ when coadministered with sulfinpyrazone	Uncertain, but presumed to be due to ↑ hepatic metabolism	Monitor PR and BP at least weekly until stable. Watch for poor response to verapamil
CALCIUM CHANNEL BLOCKERS	**ANTIHYPERTENSIVES AND HEART FAILURE DRUGS**			
CALCIUM CHANNEL BLOCKERS	ANTIHYPERTENSIVES AND HEART FAILURE DRUGS	↑ Hypotensive effect	Additive hypotensive effect; may be used therapeutically	Monitor BP at least weekly until stable. Warn patients to report symptoms of hypotension (light-headedness, dizziness on standing, etc.)
VERAPAMIL	ALISKIREN	Aliskiren levels ↑ by verapamil	Verapamil is a moderate Pgp inhibitor	Monitor BP and serum potassium at least weekly until stable
CALCIUM CHANNEL BLOCKERS	ALPHA-BLOCKERS	↑ Efficacy of alpha-blockers; ↑ risk of first-dose ↓ BP with alfuzosin, prazosin, and terazosin	Additive hypotensive effect; may be used therapeutically	Watch for first-dose ↓ BP when starting either drug when the patient is already established on the other; consider reducing the dose of the established drug and starting the new agent at the lowest dose and titrating up
VERAPAMIL	CENTRALLY ACTING ANTIHYPERTENSIVES	Reports of two cases of complete heart block when clonidine was given to a patient on verapamil	Additive effect; both drugs are known to rarely cause AV dysfunction	Monitor ECG closely when coadministering
CALCIUM CHANNEL BLOCKERS—NIFEDIPINE	KETANSERIN	Small number of cases of ectopic beats and VT	Unknown	Monitor PR, BP, and ECG closely

(Continued)

DRUGS ACTING ON THE CARDIOVASCULAR SYSTEM CALCIUM CHANNEL BLOCKERS

DRUGS ACTING ON THE CARDIOVASCULAR SYSTEM CALCIUM CHANNEL BLOCKERS

Primary Drug	Secondary Drug	Effect	Mechanism	Precautions
CALCIUM CHANNEL BLOCKERS				
CALCIUM CHANNEL BLOCKERS	ANTIMALARIALS—MEFLOQUINE	Risk of bradycardia	Additive bradycardic effect; mefloquine can cause cardiac conduction disorders, e.g., bradycardia. Also a theoretical risk of QT prolongation with coadministration of mefloquine and calcium channel blockers	Monitor PR closely
VERAPAMIL	ANTIMUSCARINICS—DARIFENACIN	↑ Darifenacin levels	Inhibition of CYP3A4-mediated metabolism of darifenacin	Avoid coadministration (manufacturer's recommendation)
CALCIUM CHANNEL BLOCKERS	**ANTI-PARKINSON'S DRUGS**			
CALCIUM CHANNEL BLOCKERS	APOMORPHINE	Risk of ↑ hypotensive effect	Not clear—effect seen with vasodilators but not other antihypertensives	Monitor BP closely, especially during initiation of treatment. Warn patients to report symptoms of hypotension (light-headedness, dizziness on standing, etc.)
CALCIUM CHANNEL BLOCKERS	LEVODOPA	↑ Hypotensive effect	Additive hypotensive effect	Monitor BP at least weekly until stable. Warn patients to report symptoms of hypotension (light-headedness, dizziness on standing, etc.)
CALCIUM CHANNEL BLOCKERS	**ANTIPLATELET DRUGS**			
CALCIUM CHANNEL BLOCKERS	ASPIRIN	↓ Antihypertensive effect with aspirin; effect not noted with low-dose aspirin	Aspirin may cause sodium retention and vasoconstriction at possibly both renal and endothelial sites	Monitor BP closely when high-dose aspirin is prescribed

(Continued)

Primary Drug	Secondary Drug	Effect	Mechanism	Precautions
CALCIUM CHANNEL BLOCKERS				
CALCIUM CHANNEL BLOCKERS	TICAGRELOR	Risk of ↑ ticagrelor levels with diltiazem and verapamil	Inhibition of CYP3A4 mediated metabolism of ticagrelor. Verapamil also inhibits Pgp	Manufacturer recommends to avoid coadministration
CALCIUM CHANNEL BLOCKERS	**ANTIPSYCHOTICS**			
CALCIUM CHANNEL BLOCKERS	ANTIPSYCHOTICS	↑ Antihypertensive effect	Dose-related ↓ BP (due to vasodilatation) is a side effect of most antipsychotics, particularly phenothiazines	Monitor BP especially during initiation of treatment. Warn patients to report symptoms of hypotension (light-headedness, dizziness on standing, etc.)
CALCIUM CHANNEL BLOCKERS	CLOZAPINE	Plasma concentrations of clozapine may be ↑ by diltiazem and verapamil	Diltiazem and verapamil inhibit CYP1A2-mediated metabolism of clozapine	Watch about side effects of clozapine
CALCIUM CHANNEL BLOCKERS	SERTINDOLE	Plasma concentrations of sertindole are ↑ by diltiazem and verapamil	Diltiazem and verapamil inhibit CYP3A4-mediated metabolism of sertindole	Avoid coadministration; raised sertindole concentrations are associated with an ↑ risk of prolonged QT interval and therefore ventricular arrhythmias, particularly torsades de pointes
CALCIUM CHANNEL BLOCKERS	**ANTIVIRALS**			
CALCIUM CHANNEL BLOCKERS	COBICISTAT	Possible ↑ plasma levels	Inhibition of metabolism via CYP3A	Monitor more closely, dose reduction may be required
CALCIUM CHANNEL BLOCKERS—DILTIAZEM, VERAMAPIL	MARAVIROC	Possible ↑ plasma levels diltiazem	Inhibition of metabolism via CYP3A	Avoid coadministration
CALCIUM CHANNEL BLOCKERS	NONNUCLEOSIDE REVERSE TRANSCRIPTASE INHIBITORS	Theoretical risk of ↑ levels of diltiazem, verapamil, felodipine, nicardipine, nifedipine, and nisoldipine by efavirenz	Protease inhibitors inhibit CYP3A4-mediated metabolism of calcium channel blockers	Monitor PR, BP, and ECG closely; ↓ dose of calcium channel blocker if necessary

(*Continued*)

DRUGS ACTING ON THE CARDIOVASCULAR SYSTEM CALCIUM CHANNEL BLOCKERS

Primary Drug	Secondary Drug	Effect	Mechanism	Precautions
CALCIUM CHANNEL BLOCKERS				
CALCIUM CHANNEL BLOCKERS	PROTEASE INHIBITORS	↑ Levels of diltiazem, verapamil, felodipine, nicardipine, nifedipine, and nisoldipine by boceprevir, ritonavir, saquinavir, and telaprevir	Protease inhibitors inhibit CYP3A4-mediated metabolism of calcium channel blockers	Monitor PR, BP, and ECG closely; ↓ dose of calcium channel blocker if necessary (e.g., the manufacturers of diltiazem suggest starting at 50% of the standard dose and titrating to effect)
CALCIUM CHANNEL BLOCKERS	**ANXIOLYTICS AND HYPNOTICS**			
CALCIUM CHANNEL BLOCKERS	ANXIOLYTICS AND HYPNOTICS	↑ Hypotensive effect	Additive hypotensive effect; anxiolytics can cause postural ↓ BP	Monitor BP at least weekly until stable. Warn patients to report symptoms of hypotension (light-headedness, dizziness on standing, etc.). Consider reducing the dose of calcium channel blocker or using an alternative antidepressant
DILTIAZEM, VERAPAMIL	BENZODIAZEPINES	Plasma concentrations of midazolam and triazolam are ↑ by diltiazem and verapamil	Diltiazem and verapamil inhibit CYP3A4-mediated metabolism of midazolam and triazolam	↓ The dose of BZD by 50% in patients on calcium channel blockers; warn patients not to perform skilled tasks such as driving for at least 10 h after a dose of BZD
CALCIUM CHANNEL BLOCKERS	BUSPIRONE	Plasma concentrations of buspirone are ↑ by diltiazem and verapamil	Diltiazem and verapamil inhibit CYP3A4-mediated metabolism of buspirone	Start buspirone at a lower dose (2.5 mg twice daily suggested by the manufacturers) in patients on calcium channel blockers

(*Continued*)

Primary Drug	Secondary Drug	Effect	Mechanism	Precautions
CALCIUM CHANNEL BLOCKERS				
CALCIUM CHANNEL BLOCKERS	**BETA-BLOCKERS**			
CALCIUM CHANNEL BLOCKERS	BETA-BLOCKERS	↑ Hypotensive effect, bradycardia, conduction defects, and heart failure	Additive hypotensive effect; may be used therapeutically	Monitor PR, BP, and ECG at least weekly until stable. Warn patients to report symptoms of hypotension (light-headedness, dizziness on standing, etc.)
DIHYDROPYRIDINES	BETA-BLOCKERS	Rare cases of severe ↓ BP and heart failure when nifedipine and nisoldipine are given to patients on beta-blockers	Uncertain why this severe effect occurs	Monitor PR, BP, and ECG at least weekly until stable. Warn patients to report symptoms of hypotension (light-headedness, dizziness on standing, etc.)
DILTIAZEM	BETA-BLOCKERS	↑ Hypotensive and bradycardic effects: cases of severe bradycardia and AV block when both drugs are administered concurrently in the presence of pre-existing heart failure or conduction abnormalities	Additive effects on conduction; diltiazem causes bradycardia, sinoatrial block, and AV block. Also, diltiazem inhibits CYP1A2-mediated metabolism of propranolol	Monitor PR, BP, and ECG at least weekly until stable. Warn patients to report symptoms of hypotension (light-headedness, dizziness on standing, etc.)
VERAPAMIL	BETA-BLOCKERS	1. Risk of cardiac arrest when parenteral verapamil is given to patients on beta-blockers 2. Risk of bradycardias when both are given orally	Additive effect. Also, verapamil inhibits CYP1A2-mediated metabolism of propranolol	1. Do not administer intravenous verapamil to patients taking beta-blockers 2. Monitor ECG and BP carefully when both are given orally

(Continued)

DRUGS ACTING ON THE CARDIOVASCULAR SYSTEM CALCIUM CHANNEL BLOCKERS

DRUGS ACTING ON THE CARDIOVASCULAR SYSTEM CALCIUM CHANNEL BLOCKERS

DRUGS ACTING ON THE CARDIOVASCULAR SYSTEM CALCIUM CHANNEL BLOCKERS

Primary Drug	Secondary Drug	Effect	Mechanism	Precautions
CALCIUM CHANNEL BLOCKERS				
CALCIUM CHANNEL BLOCKERS	**BRONCHODILATORS**			
DILTIAZEM, VERAPAMIL	THEOPHYLLINE	↑ Theophylline levels with diltiazem and verapamil. Mostly not clinically significant, but two cases of theophylline toxicity with verapamil have been reported	Uncertain, but thought to be due to inhibition of CYP1A2-mediated metabolism of theophylline	Be aware of the small possibility of theophylline toxicity when commencing calcium channel blockers; check levels if any problems occur, and consider either reducing the dose of theophylline or using an alternative calcium channel blocker
NIFEDIPINE	THEOPHYLLINE	Clinically nonsignificant ↓ theophylline levels with nifedipine, but there are case reports of theophylline toxicity after starting nifedipine	Uncertain; probably due to alterations in either metabolism or volume of distribution of theophylline	Be aware of the small possibility of theophylline toxicity when commencing calcium channel blockers; check levels if any problems occur, and consider either reducing the dose of theophylline or using an alternative calcium channel blocker
CALCIUM CHANNEL BLOCKERS	CALCIUM CHANNEL BLOCKERS	Coadministration of nifedipine and diltiazem leads to ↑ plasma concentrations of both drugs	Uncertain, but presumed mutual inhibition of CYP3A isoform-mediated metabolism	Monitor PR, BP, and ECG at least weekly until stable. Warn patients to report symptoms of hypotension (light-headedness, dizziness on standing, etc.)
CALCIUM CHANNEL BLOCKERS	**CARDIAC GLYCOSIDES**			
VERAPAMIL	DIGOXIN	1. Verapamil causes an ↑ in serum digoxin levels, and there have been case reports of significant toxicity 2. ↑ AV block when digoxin is coadministered with verapamil	1. Verapamil seems to inhibit Pgp-mediated renal and biliary clearances of digoxin. Inhibition of intestinal Pgp would also ↑ the bioavailability of digoxin. 2. Additive effect	1. It is recommended to ↓ digoxin doses by 33%–50% when starting verapamil; monitor digoxin levels and watch for symptoms/signs of toxicity 2. Monitor ECG closely when coadministering digoxin and verapamil, especially when verapamil is being given parenterally

(Continued)

Primary Drug	Secondary Drug	Effect	Mechanism	Precautions
CALCIUM CHANNEL BLOCKERS				
CALCIUM CHANNEL BLOCKERS	DIGOXIN	Possible ↑ plasma concentrations of digoxin with diltiazem, felodipine, lacidipine, lercanidipine, nicardipine, nifedipine, and nisoldipine	These calcium channel blockers are thought to ↓ renal excretion of digoxin	Monitor digoxin levels carefully
CALCIUM CHANNEL BLOCKERS	DIGITOXIN	Plasma concentrations of digitoxin may be ↑ by diltiazem and verapamil	Uncertain at present	Watch for digitoxin toxicity
VERAPAMIL	CNS STIMULANTS—MODAFINIL	May cause ↓ verapamil levels if CYP1A2 is the predominant metabolic pathway and alternative metabolic pathways are either genetically deficient or affected	Modafinil is a moderate inducer of CYP1A2 in a concentration-dependent manner	Be aware
CALCIUM CHANNEL BLOCKERS	**DIURETICS**			
CALCIUM CHANNEL BLOCKERS	DIURETICS	↑ Hypotensive effect	Additive hypotensive effect; may be used therapeutically	Monitor BP at least weekly until stable. Warn patients to report symptoms of hypotension (light-headedness, dizziness on standing, etc.)
CALCIUM CHANNEL BLOCKERS	POTASSIUM-SPARING DIURETICS	↑ Serum concentrations of eplerenone when given with diltiazem and verapamil	Calcium channel blockers inhibit CYP3A4-mediated metabolism of eplerenone	Restrict dose of eplerenone to 25 mg/day. Monitor serum potassium concentrations closely; watch for hyperkalemia
CALCIUM CHANNEL BLOCKERS	DUTASTERIDE	Plasma concentrations of dutasteride may ↑ when coadministered with diltiazem or verapamil	Uncertain, but postulated that it may be due to inhibition of CYP3A4-mediated metabolism of dutasteride	Watch for side effects of dutasteride

(Continued)

DRUGS ACTING ON THE CARDIOVASCULAR SYSTEM CALCIUM CHANNEL BLOCKERS

DRUGS ACTING ON THE CARDIOVASCULAR SYSTEM CALCIUM CHANNEL BLOCKERS

Primary Drug	Secondary Drug	Effect	Mechanism	Precautions
CALCIUM CHANNEL BLOCKERS				
DILTIAZEM, VERAPAMIL	ELIGLUSTAT	↑ Eliglustat levels	Inhibition of CYP3A4-mediated metabolism	Reduce dose to 85 mg od in extensive metabolizers. Avoid coadministration in intermediate and poor metabolizers
CALCIUM CHANNEL BLOCKERS	FINASTERIDE	Plasma concentrations of dutasteride may ↑ when coadministered with diltiazem or verapamil	Uncertain, but postulated that it may be due to inhibition of CYP3A4-mediated metabolism of dutasteride	Watch for side effects of dutasteride
DILTIAZEM, NIFEDIPINE, VERAPAMIL	5-HT1 AGONISTS—ALMOTRIPTAN, ELETRIPTAN	↑ Plasma concentrations of almotriptan and risk of toxic effects of almotriptan, e.g., flushing, sensations of tingling, heat, heaviness, pressure, or tightness of any part of the body, including the throat and chest, dizziness	Almotriptan is metabolized mainly by CYP3A4 isoenzymes. Most CYP isoenzymes are inhibited by diltiazem to varying degrees, and since there is an alternative pathway of metabolism by MAO-A, toxicity responses vary between individuals	CSM has advised that if chest tightness or pressure is intense, then triptan should be discontinued immediately and the patient need to be investigated for ischemic heart disease by measuring cardiac enzymes and doing an ECG. Avoid concomitant use in patients with coronary artery disease and in those with severe or uncontrolled hypertension
CALCIUM CHANNEL BLOCKERS	GRAPEFRUIT JUICE	↑ Bioavailability of felodipine and nisoldipine (with reports of adverse effects), and ↑ bioavailability of isradipine, lacidipine, lercanidipine, nicardipine, nifedipine, nimodipine, and verapamil (without reported adverse clinical effects)	Postulated that flavonoids in grapefruit juice (and possibly Seville oranges and limes) inhibit intestinal (but not hepatic) CYP3A4. They also inhibit intestinal Pgp, which may ↑ the bioavailability of verapamil	Avoid concurrent use of felodipine and nisoldipine and grapefruit juice

(Continued)

Primary Drug	Secondary Drug	Effect	Mechanism	Precautions
CALCIUM CHANNEL BLOCKERS				
CALCIUM CHANNEL BLOCKERS	**H2 RECEPTOR BLOCKERS**			
CALCIUM CHANNEL BLOCKERS	CIMETIDINE, RANITIDINE	↑ Levels of calcium channel blockers, especially diltiazem, nifedipine, and isradipine, particularly with cimetidine	Inhibition of CYP3A isoform-mediated metabolism, cimetidine being the most potent inhibitor	Monitor BP and HR closely; be aware of possibility of significant ↓ BP. Consider ↓ dose of diltiazem, nifedipine, and isradipine by up to 50%
CALCIUM CHANNEL BLOCKERS	FAMOTIDINE	Reports of heart failure and ↓ BP when famotidine is given with nifedipine	Additive negative inotropic effects	Caution when coadministering famotidine with calcium channel blockers, especially in elderly people
CALCIUM CHANNEL BLOCKERS	IVABRADINE	↑ Levels with diltiazem and verapamil	Reduced CYP3A4-mediated metabolism of ivabradine	Avoid coadministration
CALCIUM CHANNEL BLOCKERS	**LIPID-LOWERING DRUGS**			
CALCIUM CHANNEL BLOCKERS	ANION EXCHANGE RESINS	Colestipol ↓ diltiazem levels	Colestipol binds diltiazem in the intestine	Monitor for poor response to diltiazem. Separating doses of diltiazem and colestipol does not seem to ↓ this interaction
CALCIUM CHANNEL BLOCKERS—DIHYDROPYRIDINES	STATINS	Slight ↑ plasma levels of simvastatin and possible atorvastatin with amlodipine. Clinical relevance not clear	Uncertain	Manufacturer advises restricting dose of simvastatin to 20 mg when coadministered with amlodipine
CALCIUM CHANNEL BLOCKERS—DILTIAZEM, VERAPAMIL	STATINS	↑ Plasma levels of atorvastatin, lovastatin, and simvastatin; case reports of myopathy when atorvastatin and simvastatin are coadministered with diltiazem or verapamil	Inhibition of CYP3A4-mediated metabolism of statins	Watch for side effects of statins. Monitor lipid profile closely. The lowest effective dose should be used; manufacturers recommend: 1. Simvastatin 20 mg with verapamil or diltiazem 2. Lovastatin 20 mg with verapamil

(*Continued*)

DRUGS ACTING ON THE CARDIOVASCULAR SYSTEM CALCIUM CHANNEL BLOCKERS

DRUGS ACTING ON THE CARDIOVASCULAR SYSTEM CALCIUM CHANNEL BLOCKERS

Primary Drug	Secondary Drug	Effect	Mechanism	Precautions
CALCIUM CHANNEL BLOCKERS				
CALCIUM CHANNEL BLOCKERS	MAGNESIUM (PARENTERAL)	Cases of profound muscular weakness when nifedipine is given with parenteral magnesium	Both drugs inhibit calcium influx across cell membranes, and magnesium promotes movement of calcium into the sarcoplasmic reticulum; this results in muscular paralysis	Do not administer calcium channel blockers during parenteral magnesium therapy
CALCIUM CHANNEL BLOCKERS—DILTIAZEM, VERAPAMIL	NITISINONE	Possible ↑ nitisinone levels	Inhibition of CYP3A4-mediated metabolism	Monitor carefully
CALCIUM CHANNEL BLOCKERS	**MUSCLE RELAXANTS**			
CALCIUM CHANNEL BLOCKERS	DEPOLARIZING	↑ Effect of suxamethonium with parenteral, but not oral, calcium channel blockers	Uncertain; postulated that ACh release at the synapse is calcium dependent; ↓ calcium concentrations at the nerve ending may ↓ ACh release, which in turn prolongs the nerve blockade	Monitor nerve blockade carefully, particularly during short procedures
CALCIUM CHANNEL BLOCKERS	NONDEPOLARIZING	↑ Effect of nondepolarizing muscle relaxants with parenteral calcium channel blockers; the effect is less certain with oral therapy. In two cohort studies, vecuronium requirements were halved in patients on diltiazem. Nimodipine does not seem to share this interaction	Uncertain; postulated that ACh release at the synapse is calcium dependent; ↓ calcium concentrations at the nerve ending may ↓ ACh release, which in turn prolongs the nerve blockade	Monitor nerve blockade carefully in patients on calcium channel blockers, particularly near to the end of surgery, when muscle relaxation may be prolonged and difficult to reverse

(Continued)

Primary Drug	Secondary Drug	Effect	Mechanism	Precautions
CALCIUM CHANNEL BLOCKERS				
CALCIUM CHANNEL BLOCKERS	**SKELETAL**			
CALCIUM CHANNEL BLOCKERS	BACLOFEN AND TIZANIDINE	↑ Hypotensive effect with baclofen of tizanidine. Risk of bradycardia with tizanidine	Additive hypotensive effect. Tizanidine has a negative inotropic and chronotropic effects	Monitor BP at least weekly until stable. Warn patients to report symptoms of hypotension (light-headedness, dizziness on standing, etc.)
CALCIUM CHANNEL BLOCKERS	DANTROLENE	Risk of arrhythmias when diltiazem is given with intravenous dantrolene. Risk of ↓ BP, myocardial depression, and hyperkalemia when verapamil is given with intravenous dantrolene	Uncertain at present	Extreme caution must be exercised when administering parenteral dantrolene to patients on diltiazem or verapamil. Monitor BP and cardiac rhythm closely; watch for hyperkalemia
CALCIUM CHANNEL BLOCKERS	NITRATES	↑ Hypotensive effect	Additive effect	Monitor BP at least weekly until stable. Warn patients to report symptoms of hypotension (light-headedness, dizziness on standing, etc.)
CALCIUM CHANNEL BLOCKERS	ESTROGENS	↓ Hypotensive effect	Estrogens cause sodium and fluid retention	Monitor BP at least weekly until stable; routine prescription of estrogens in patients with ↑ BP is not advisable
CALCIUM CHANNEL BLOCKERS	ORLISTAT	Case report of ↑ BP when orlistat was started for a patient on amlodipine	Uncertain at present	Monitor BP at least weekly until stable
CALCIUM CHANNEL BLOCKERS	**PERIPHERAL VASODILATORS**			
CALCIUM CHANNEL BLOCKERS	CILOSTAZOL	↑ Plasma concentrations and efficacy of cilostazol with diltiazem, verapamil, and nifedipine	These calcium channel blockers inhibit CYP3A4-mediated metabolism of cilostazol	Avoid coadministration

(*Continued*)

Primary Drug	Secondary Drug	Effect	Mechanism	Precautions
CALCIUM CHANNEL BLOCKERS				
CALCIUM CHANNEL BLOCKERS	MOXISYLYTE (THYMOXAMINE)	↑ Hypotensive effect	Additive hypotensive effect	Monitor BP at least weekly until stable. Warn patients to report symptoms of hypotension (light-headedness, dizziness on standing, etc.)
CALCIUM CHANNEL BLOCKERS	PHOSPHODIESTERASE TYPE 5 INHIBITORS	↑ Hypotensive action particularly with sildenafil and vardenafil	Additive effect; phosphodiesterase type 5 inhibitors cause vasodilation	Warn patients of the small risk of postural ↓ BP
CALCIUM CHANNEL BLOCKERS	POTASSIUM CHANNEL ACTIVATORS	↑ Hypotensive effect	Additive effect	Monitor BP closely
CALCIUM CHANNEL BLOCKERS	PROSTAGLANDINS—ALPROSTADIL	↑ Hypotensive effect	Additive hypotensive effect	Monitor BP at least weekly until stable. Warn patients to report symptoms of hypotension (light-headedness, dizziness on standing, etc.)
CALCIUM CHANNEL BLOCKERS—DILTIAZEM, VERAPAMIL	RANOLAZINE	↑ Ranolazine levels	Inhibition of CYP3A4-mediated metabolism of ranolazine	May be used therapeutically. Reduce dose of ranolazine
CALCIUM CHANNEL BLOCKERS	X-RAY CONTRAST SOLUTIONS	↑ Hypotensive effect when intravenous ionic contrast solutions are given to patients on calcium channel blockers	Additive hypotensive effect	Consider using a nonionic x-ray contrast solution for patients on calcium channel blockers

Primary Drug	Secondary Drug	Effect	Mechanism	Precautions
CARDIAC GLYCOSIDES				
DIGITOXIN				
DIGITOXIN	**ANTIARRHYTHMICS**			
DIGITOXIN	AMIODARONE	Reports of digitoxin toxicity in two patients after starting amiodarone	Uncertain; thought to be due to inhibition of Pgp-mediated renal clearance of digoxin	Watch for digitoxin toxicity

(Continued)

Primary Drug	Secondary Drug	Effect	Mechanism	Precautions
CARDIAC GLYCOSIDES				
DIGITOXIN	PROCAINAMIDE	Single case report of toxicity in a patient taking both digitoxin and procainamide	Uncertain at present	Watch for digitoxin toxicity
DIGITOXIN	QUINIDINE	↑ Levels of digitoxin	Quinidine is a moderate Pgp inhibitor	Halve the dose of cardiac glycoside (reduce more in the presence of renal failure)
DIGITOXIN	ANTIBIOTICS—RIFAMPICIN	Plasma concentrations of digitoxin may be halved by rifampicin	Due to ↑ hepatic metabolism	Watch for poor response to digitoxin
DIGITOXIN	ANTIEPILEPTICS—BARBITURATES, PHENYTOIN	Plasma concentrations of digitoxin may be ↓ (by up to half by barbiturates)	Possibly ↑ hepatic metabolism	Watch for poor response to digitoxin
DIGITOXIN	CALCIUM CHANNEL BLOCKERS	Plasma concentrations of digitoxin may be ↑ by diltiazem and verapamil	Uncertain at present	Watch for digitoxin toxicity
DIGITOXIN	DIURETICS—SPIRONOLACTONE	Conflicting results from volunteer studies; some showed ↑ (up to one-third) in the half-life of digitoxin, others a ↓ (up to one-fifth)	Uncertain at present	Watch for either digitoxin toxicity or a poor response, particularly for the first month after starting spironolactone
DIGITOXIN	LIPID-REGULATING DRUGS—ANION EXCHANGE RESINS	Both colestipol and cholestyramine may ↓ digitoxin levels	Both colestipol and cholestyramine are ion exchange resins that bind bile sodiums and prevent reabsorption in the intestine; this breaks the enterohepatic cycle of digitoxin	Colestipol and cholestyramine should be given at least 1.5 h after digitoxin

(*Continued*)

Primary Drug	Secondary Drug	Effect	Mechanism	Precautions
CARDIAC GLYCOSIDES				
DIGOXIN				
DIGOXIN	AMINOSALICYLATES	Sulfasalazine may ↓ digoxin levels. The manufacturers of balsalazide also warn against the possibility of this interaction in spite of a lack of case reports	Uncertain at present	Watch for poor response to digoxin; check levels if there are signs of ↓ effect
DIGOXIN	**ANALGESICS**			
DIGOXIN	NSAIDs	Diclofenac, indometacin, and possibly fenbufen, ibuprofen, and tiaprofenic acid ↑ plasma concentrations of digoxin and ↑ risk of precipitating cardiac failure and renal dysfunction	Uncertain; postulated that NSAID-induced renal impairment plays as role; however, since all NSAIDs have this effect, it is not understood why only certain NSAIDs actually influence digoxin levels	Monitor renal function closely. Monitor digoxin levels; watch for digoxin toxicity
DIGOXIN	OPIOIDS	↑ Concentrations of digoxin may occur with tramadol	Uncertain at present	Watch for digoxin toxicity; check levels and ↓ the dose of digoxin as necessary
DIGOXIN	ANTACIDS	Plasma concentrations of digoxin may be ↓ by antacids	Uncertain; probably ↓ absorption of digoxin	Watch for poor response to digoxin
DIGOXIN	**ANTIARRHYTHMICS**			
DIGOXIN	AMIODARONE	Amiodarone may ↑ plasma levels of digoxin (in some cases up to fourfold)	Uncertain; thought to be due to inhibition of Pgp-mediated renal clearance of digoxin. Amiodarone is also known to inhibit intestinal Pgp, which may ↑ the bioavailability of digoxin	↓ Digoxin dose by one-third to one-half when starting amiodarone. Monitor digoxin levels; watch for digoxin toxicity, especially for ↓ weeks after initiating or adjusting amiodarone therapy

(*Continued*)

Primary Drug	Secondary Drug	Effect	Mechanism	Precautions
CARDIAC GLYCOSIDES				
DIGOXIN	DRONEDARONE	Risk of excessive bradycardia and myocardial depression	Additive effect. In addition, dronedarone inhibits Pgp	Monitor PR and BP closely. Use lowest doses of these drugs and titrate carefully. Monitor digoxin levels
DIGOXIN	MORICIZINE	Case reports of heart block when moracizine is coadministered with digoxin	Uncertain at present	Monitor PR and ECG closely
DIGOXIN	PROPAFENONE	Digoxin concentrations may be ↑ by propafenone	Uncertain at present	Watch for digoxin toxicity; check digoxin levels if indicated and ↓ digoxin dose as necessary (15%–70% is suggested by studies)
DIGOXIN	QUINIDINE	↑ Levels of digoxin	Quinidine is a moderate Pgp inhibitor	Halve the dose of cardiac glycoside (reduce more in the presence of renal failure)
DIGOXIN	**ANTIBIOTICS**			
DIGOXIN	AMINOGLYCOSIDES	1. Gentamicin may ↑ plasma concentrations of digoxin 2. Neomycin may ↓ plasma concentrations of digoxin	1. Uncertain; postulated to be due to impaired renal clearance of digoxin 2. Neomycin ↓ absorption of digoxin; this may be offset in some patients by ↓ intestinal bacterial breakdown of digoxin	1. Monitor digoxin levels; watch for ↑ levels, particularly with diabetes and in the presence of renal insufficiency 2. Monitor digoxin levels; watch for poor response to digoxin
DIGOXIN	MACROLIDES	Digoxin concentrations may be ↑ by macrolides	Uncertain; postulated that macrolides inhibit Pgp in both the intestine (↑ bioavailability) and kidney (↓ clearance). It is possible that alterations in intestinal flora may also have a role	Monitor digoxin levels; watch for digoxin toxicity

(Continued)

Primary Drug	Secondary Drug	Effect	Mechanism	Precautions
CARDIAC GLYCOSIDES				
DIGOXIN	RIFAMPICIN	Plasma concentrations of digoxin may be ↓ by rifampicin	Rifampicin seems to induce Pgp-mediated excretion of digoxin in the kidneys	Watch for a ↓ response to digoxin, check plasma levels, and ↑ the dose as necessary
DIGOXIN	TRIMETHOPRIM, COTRIMOXAZOLE	Trimethoprim may ↑ plasma concentrations of digoxin, particularly in elderly people	Uncertain; postulated that trimethoprim ↓ renal clearance of digoxin	Monitor digoxin levels; watch for digoxin toxicity
DIGOXIN	**ANTICANCER AND IMMUNOMODULATING DRUGS**			
DIGOXIN	AMINOSALICYLATES	Sulfasalazine may ↓ digoxin levels. The manufacturers of balsalazide also warn against the possibility of this interaction in spite of a lack of case reports	Uncertain at present	Watch for poor response to digoxin; check levels if there are signs of ↓ effect
DIGOXIN	CICLOSPORIN	↑ Plasma digoxin levels, with risk of toxicity. Digoxin may ↑ ciclosporin bioavailability (by 15%–20%)	Attributed to inhibition of intestinal Pgp and renal Pgp, which ↑ bioavailability and ↑ renal elimination. Digoxin ↑ bioavailability of ciclosporin is due to substrate competition for Pgp	Watch for digoxin toxicity. Monitor plasma digoxin and ciclosporin levels
DIGOXIN	CORTICOSTEROIDS	Risk of digoxin toxicity due to hypokalemia	Corticosteroids may cause hypokalemia	Monitor potassium levels closely. Monitor digoxin levels; watch for digoxin toxicity
DIGOXIN	CRIZOTINIB	1. Possible ↑ levels of P-glycoprotein substrates 2. Risk of excessive bradycardia	1. Crizotinib inhibits P-glycoprotein 2. Additive	Monitor closely

(Continued)

Primary Drug	Secondary Drug	Effect	Mechanism	Precautions
CARDIAC GLYCOSIDES				
DIGOXIN	CYTOTOXICS	Cytotoxics may ↓ levels of digoxin (by up to 50%) when digoxin is given in tablet form	Cytotoxic-induced damage to the mucosa of the intestine may ↓ absorption; this does not seem to be a problem with liquid or liquid-containing capsule formulations	Watch for poor response to digoxin; check levels if there are signs of ↓ effect, and consider swapping to liquid digoxin or liquid-containing capsules
DIGOXIN	DABRAFENIB	Possible ↓ levels of CYP3A4/CYP2Cs/CYP2B6 substrates. Level of reduction may vary	Dabrafenib induces CYP3A4/CYP2Cs/CYP2B6	Monitor closely or avoid concurrent use
DIGOXIN	INTERFERON GAMMA	↑ Plasma concentrations of digoxin may occur with interferon gamma	Interferon gamma ↓ Pgp-mediated renal and biliary excretion of digoxin	Monitor digoxin levels; watch for digoxin toxicity
DIGOXIN	LAPATINIB	↑ Levels of digoxin	P-glycoprotein inhibition	Monitor closely, measure digoxin levels and consider dose reduction with digoxin
DIGOXIN	NILOTINIB	↑ Levels of digoxin	P-glycoprotein inhibition	Monitor closely, measure digoxin levels and consider dose reduction with digoxin
DIGOXIN	PENICILLAMINE	Plasma concentrations of digoxin may be ↓ by penicillamine	Uncertain at present	Watch for poor response to digoxin
DIGOXIN	REGORAFENIB	Possible ↑ levels of digoxin	P-glycoprotein inhibition	Monitor PR and BP closely
DIGOXIN	RUXOLITINIB	Predicted ↑ in P-glycoprotein or BCRP substrate levels	P-glycoprotein/BCRP inhibition	Monitor closely. Separate administration of drugs
DIGOXIN	TACROLIMUS	Digoxin toxicity (pharmacodynamic)	Possibly due to tacrolimus-induced hyperkalemia and hypomagnesemia	Watch for digoxin toxicity. Monitor potassium and magnesium levels
DIGOXIN	THALIDOMIDE	Excessive bradycardia	Additive effect	Monitor BP and PR closely

(Continued)

DRUGS ACTING ON THE CARDIOVASCULAR SYSTEM CARDIAC GLYCOSIDES

Primary Drug	Secondary Drug	Effect	Mechanism	Precautions
CARDIAC GLYCOSIDES				
DIGOXIN	VEMURAFENIB	Possible ↑ levels of P-glycoprotein substrates	Vemurafenib inhibits P-glycoprotein	Clinical significance unknown
DIGOXIN	**ANTIDEPRESSANTS**			
DIGOXIN	ST. JOHN'S WORT	Plasma concentrations of digoxin seem to be ↓ by St. John's wort	St. John's wort seems to ↓ Pgp-mediated intestinal absorption of digoxin	Watch for a ↓ response to digoxin
DIGOXIN	SSRIs	Theoretical risk of ↑ digoxin levels	Inhibition of Pgp by sertraline and paroxetine observed *in vitro*; unlikely of major clinical significance	Be aware
DIGOXIN	TRAZODONE	Reports of two cases of ↑ plasma concentrations of digoxin after starting trazodone	Uncertain at present	Watch for digoxin toxicity; check levels and ↓ the dose of digoxin as necessary
DIGOXIN	**ANTIDIABETIC DRUGS**			
DIGOXIN	ACARBOSE	Acarbose may ↓ plasma levels of digoxin	Uncertain; possibly ↓ absorption of digoxin	Monitor digoxin levels; watch for ↓ levels
DIGOXIN	SITAGLIPTIN	Possibly ↑ levels of digoxin	Uncertain at present	Monitor digoxin levels; watch for ↑ levels
DIGOXIN	ANTIDIARRHEALS—KAOLIN	Possibly ↓ levels of digoxin	↓ Absorption	Separate doses by at least 2 h
DIGOXIN	ANTIEPILEPTICS			
DIGOXIN	PHENYTOIN	Phenytoin may ↓ plasma levels of digoxin	Uncertain at present	Watch for poor response to digoxin; check levels if there are signs of ↓ effect
DIGOXIN	TOPIRAMATE	Small ↓ in peak plasma levels of digoxin	Oral clearance of digoxin was slightly increased	Watch for a decreased response to digoxin therapy. Increase digoxin therapy if symptoms and signs of cardiac failure or arrhythmia persist

(*Continued*)

Primary Drug	Secondary Drug	Effect	Mechanism	Precautions
CARDIAC GLYCOSIDES				
DIGOXIN	**ANTIFUNGALS**			
DIGOXIN	AMPHOTERICIN	Risk of digoxin ↑ by toxicity due to hypokalemia	Amphotericin may cause hypokalemia	Monitor potassium levels closely. Monitor digoxin levels; watch for digoxin toxicity
DIGOXIN	AZOLES	Itraconazole and possibly ketoconazole and posaconazole may cause ↑ plasma levels of digoxin; cases reported of digoxin toxicity	These azoles inhibit Pgp-mediated renal clearance and ↑ intestinal absorption of digoxin	Monitor digoxin levels; watch for digoxin toxicity
DIGOXIN	ANTIGOUTS—COLCHICINE	↑ Risk of myopathy	Possible competition for Pgp	Ask patients to report signs of myopathy
DIGOXIN	**ANTIHYPERTENSIVES AND HEART FAILURE DRUGS**			
DIGOXIN	ACE INHIBITORS	↑ Plasma concentrations of digoxin when captopril is coadministered in the presence of heart failure (class II or more severe) or renal insufficiency. No other ACE inhibitors seem to interact in the same way	Uncertain; postulated to be due to ↓ renal excretion of digoxin	Monitor digoxin levels; watch for digoxin toxicity
DIGOXIN	ALPHA-BLOCKERS	Possibility of ↑ plasma concentrations of digoxin with prazosin; no cases of toxicity have been reported	Uncertain	Monitor digoxin levels
DIGOXIN	ANGIOTENSIN II RECEPTOR ANTAGONISTS	Telmisartan may ↑ plasma levels of digoxin	Uncertain; telmisartan thought to ↑ rate of absorption of digoxin	Monitor digoxin levels; watch for digoxin toxicity
DIGOXIN	**ANTIMALARIALS**			
DIGOXIN	CHLOROQUINE, HYDROXYCHLOROQUINE	Chloroquine may ↑ plasma concentrations of digoxin	Uncertain at present	Monitor digoxin levels; watch for digoxin toxicity

(*Continued*)

Primary Drug	Secondary Drug	Effect	Mechanism	Precautions
CARDIAC GLYCOSIDES				
DIGOXIN	MEFLOQUINE	Risk of bradycardia	Uncertain; probably additive effect; mefloquine can cause AV block	Monitor PR and ECG closely
DIGOXIN	QUININE	Plasma concentrations of digoxin may ↑ when coadministered with quinine	Uncertain, but seems to be due to ↓ nonrenal (possibly biliary) excretion of digoxin	Monitor digoxin levels; watch for digoxin toxicity
DIGOXIN	ANTIMUSCARINICS—PROPANTHELINE	↑ Digoxin levels (30%–40%) but only with slow-release formulations	Slowed gut transit time allows more digoxin to be absorbed	Use alternative formulation of digoxin
DIGOXIN	ANTIPLATELETS—TICAGRELOR	Risk of ↑ digoxin levels	Inhibition of Pgp	Monitor PR and BP closely
DIGOXIN	**ANTIVIRALS**			
DIGOXIN	COBICISTAT	↑ Peak plasma levels	Inhibition of transport via Pgp and metabolism via CYP3A	Start with lowest dose, increase slowly and monitor levels
DIGOXIN	NONNUCLEOSIDE REVERSE TRANSCRIPTASE INHIBITORS	Plasma digoxin concentrations may be ↑ by etravirine and rilpivirine	Uncertain; probably due to inhibition of Pgp-mediated renal excretion of digoxin and ↑ intestinal absorption	Monitor digoxin levels; watch for digoxin toxicity
DIGOXIN	PROTEASE INHIBITORS—RITONAVIR BOOSTED PROTEASE INHIBITORS, INDINAVIR, RITONAVIR, SAQUINAVIR, TAPRANAVIR	1. Plasma digoxin concentrations may be ↑ 2. ↑ or ↓ by tipranavir/ritonavir	1. Inhibition of Pgp-mediated renal excretion of digoxin and ↑ intestinal absorption 2. Initial inhibition of Pgp and then induction of Pgp	If already on digoxin, reduce digoxin dose by half and monitor digoxin levels; watch for digoxin toxicity
DIGOXIN	ANXIOLYTICS AND HYPNOTICS	Alprazolam and possibly diazepam may ↑ digoxin levels, particularly in people above 65	Uncertain at present	Monitor digoxin levels; watch for digoxin toxicity

(*Continued*)

Primary Drug	Secondary Drug	Effect	Mechanism	Precautions
CARDIAC GLYCOSIDES				
DIGOXIN	**BETA-BLOCKERS**			
DIGOXIN	BETA-BLOCKERS	Risk of bradycardia and AV block	Additive bradycardia	Monitor PR, BP, and ECG at least weekly until stable
DIGOXIN	CARVEDILOL	Carvedilol may ↑ digoxin plasma concentrations, particularly in children	↓ Pgp-mediated renal clearance of digoxin	↓ The dose of digoxin by 25%; watch for signs of digoxin toxicity and monitor digoxin levels
DIGOXIN	BRONCHODILATORS—BETA-2 AGONISTS	1. Hypokalemia may exacerbate digoxin toxicity 2. Salbutamol may ↓ digoxin levels (by 16%–22%) after 10 days of concurrent therapy	1. Beta-2 agonists may cause hypokalemia 2. Uncertain	1. Monitor potassium levels closely 2. Clinical significance is uncertain. Useful to monitor digoxin levels if there is a clinical indication of ↓ response to digoxin
DIGOXIN	CALCIUM	Risk of cardiac arrhythmias with large intravenous doses of calcium	Uncertain; it is known that calcium levels directly correlate with the action of digoxin; therefore, high levels, even if transient, may ↑ the chance of toxicity	It is recommended that parenteral administration of calcium should be avoided in patients taking digoxin. If this is not possible, administer calcium slowly and in small aliquots
DIGOXIN	**CALCIUM CHANNEL BLOCKERS**			
DIGOXIN	VERAPAMIL	1. Verapamil causes an ↑ in serum digoxin levels, and there have been case reports of significant toxicity 2. ↑ AV block when digoxin is coadministered with verapamil	1. Verapamil seems to inhibit Pgp-mediated renal and biliary clearance of digoxin. Inhibition of intestinal Pgp would also ↑ the bioavailability of digoxin 2. Additive effect	1. It is recommended to ↓ digoxin doses by 33%–50% when starting verapamil; monitor digoxin levels and watch for symptoms/signs of toxicity 2. Monitor ECG closely when coadministering digoxin and verapamil, especially when verapamil is being given parenterally

(Continued)

DRUGS ACTING ON THE CARDIOVASCULAR SYSTEM CARDIAC GLYCOSIDES

Primary Drug	Secondary Drug	Effect	Mechanism	Precautions
CARDIAC GLYCOSIDES				
DIGOXIN	DILTIAZEM, NIFEDIPINE, FELODIPINE, LACIDIPINE, LERCANIDIPINE, NICARDIPINE, NISOLDIPINE	Possible ↑ plasma concentrations of digoxin	These calcium channel blockers are thought to ↓ the renal excretion of digoxin	Monitor digoxin levels carefully
DIGOXIN	**DIURETICS**			
DIGOXIN	CARBONIC ANHYDRASE INHIBITORS, LOOP DIURETICS, THIAZIDES	Risk of digoxin toxicity ↑ due to hypokalemia	Uncertain	Monitor potassium levels closely. Monitor digoxin levels; watch for digoxin toxicity
DIGOXIN	POTASSIUM-SPARING DIURETICS AND ALDOSTERONE ANTAGONISTS	Spironolactone may ↑ plasma concentrations of digoxin	Uncertain; spironolactone possibly ↓ the volume of distribution of digoxin	Monitor digoxin levels; watch for digoxin toxicity
DIGOXIN	ELIGLUSTAT	↑ Digoxin levels	Inhibition of Pgp	Reduce dose of digoxin by 30%. Monitor digoxin levels
DIGOXIN	GRAPEFRUIT JUICE	Possible ↑ efficacy and ↑ adverse effects	Possibly via altered absorption	Most patients have been unaffected; consider if unexpected bradycardia or heart block with digoxin
DIGOXIN	HERBAL MEDICINES	1. Bufalin, danshen, and ginseng interfere with some of the assays for digoxin 2. Liquorice may ↑ the risk of digoxin toxicity 3. Many herbal medicines contain digoxin-like compounds, e.g., black cohosh root, cayenne pepper	1. Bufalin cross-reacts with the antibody used in some digoxin assays. The mechanism of interaction of danshen and ginseng is uncertain at present 2. Liquorice causes electrolyte imbalances, which may precipitate digoxin toxicity	Ask about Chinese herbal remedies in patients taking digoxin; inform the laboratory when monitoring digoxin levels. Watch for symptoms/signs of toxicity in patients taking liquorice-containing remedies
DIGOXIN	IVACAFTOR	Plasma digoxin concentrations may be ↑ by ivacaftor	Uncertain; probably due to inhibition of Pgp-mediated renal excretion of digoxin and ↑ intestinal absorption	Monitor digoxin levels; watch for digoxin toxicity

(*Continued*)

Primary Drug	Secondary Drug	Effect	Mechanism	Precautions
CARDIAC GLYCOSIDES				
DIGOXIN	**LIPID-LOWERING DRUGS**			
DIGOXIN	ANION EXCHANGE RESINS	Colestipol and cholestyramine both may ↓ digoxin levels	Both colestipol and cholestyramine are ion exchange resins that bind bile sodiums and prevent reabsorption in the intestine; this breaks the enterohepatic cycle of digoxin	Colestipol and cholestyramine should be given at least 1.5 h after digoxin
DIGOXIN	STATINS	High-dose (80 mg) atorvastatin may ↑ digoxin levels	Atorvastatin inhibits intestinal Pgp, which ↑ absorption of digoxin	Watch for digoxin toxicity
DIGOXIN	MIRABEGRON	↑ Digoxin levels	Mirabegron inhibits Pgp	Monitor digoxin levels
DIGOXIN	**MUSCLE RELAXANTS**			
DIGOXIN	DEPOLARIZING	Risk of ventricular arrhythmias when suxamethonium is given to patients taking digoxin	Uncertain; postulated that the mechanism involves rapid efflux of potassium from the cells	Use caution and monitor ECG closely if suxamethonium needs to be used in patients taking digoxin
DIGOXIN	NONDEPOLARIZING	Case reports of ST segment/T wave changes and sinus/atrial tachycardia when pancuronium given to patients on digoxin	Uncertain	Avoid pancuronium in patients taking digoxin
DIGOXIN	SKELETAL	Risk of bradycardia when tizanidine given with digoxin	Tizanidine has a negative inotropic effect	Monitor PR closely
DIGOXIN	PARASYMPATHOMIMETICS—EDROPHONIUM	Risk of bradycardia	Additive AV block	Avoid coadministration

(Continued)

Primary Drug	Secondary Drug	Effect	Mechanism	Precautions
CARDIAC GLYCOSIDES				
DIGOXIN	PROTON PUMP INHIBITORS	Plasma concentrations of digoxin are possibly ↑ by proton pump inhibitors	Small ↑ in bioavailability possible via ↑ intragastric pH or altered intestinal Pgp transport	Be aware; may not be clinically significant unless it is a poor CYP2C19 metabolizer or high-dose digoxin. Different proton pump inhibitors may interact differently—monitor if changing therapy or doses
DIGOXIN	RANOLAZINE	↑ Digoxin levels	Inhibition of Pgp	Monitor digoxin levels closely until stable
DIGOXIN	SUCRALFATE	Plasma concentrations of digoxin may be ↓ by sucralfate	Uncertain; possibly sucralfate binds with digoxin and ↓ its absorption	Watch for poor response to digoxin
DIGOXIN	VITAMIN D	Theoretical risk of cardiac arrhythmias if hypercalcemia occurs due to vitamin D therapy	Uncertain; it is known that calcium levels directly correlate with the action of digoxin; therefore, high levels, even if transient, may ↑ the chance of toxicity	Monitor serum calcium levels closely

Primary Drug	Secondary Drug	Effect	Mechanism	Precautions
DIURETICS				
CARBONIC ANHYDRASE INHIBITORS—ACETAZOLAMIDE				
CARBONIC ANHYDRASE INHIBITORS	**ANTIARRHYTHMICS**			
CARBONIC ANHYDRASE INHIBITORS	AMIODARONE, FLECAINIDE	Risk of ↑ myocardial depression. In addition, flecainide excretion is reduced in an alkaline urine	Cardiac toxicity directly related to hypokalemia. Flecainide is in an ionized form in an alkaline environment, which is more readily reabsorbed from the renal tubule	Monitor potassium levels closely

(Continued)

Primary Drug	Secondary Drug	Effect	Mechanism	Precautions
DIURETICS				
CARBONIC ANHYDRASE INHIBITORS	DISOPYRAMIDE	Risk of hypokalemia	Additive effect	Monitor potassium levels closely
CARBONIC ANHYDRASE INHIBITORS	MEXILETINE	Effect of mexiletine ↓ by hypokalemia	Uncertain	Normalize potassium levels before starting mexiletine
CARBONIC ANHYDRASE INHIBITORS	ANTIBIOTICS—METHENAMINE	↓ Efficacy of methenamine	Methenamine is only effective at a low pH; raising the urinary pH ↓ its effects	Avoid coadministration
CARBONIC ANHYDRASE INHIBITORS	ANTICANCER AND OTHER IMMUNOMODULATING DRUGS—CICLOSPORIN	Reports of rapid ↑ in ciclosporin levels	Uncertain	Monitor ciclosporin dose closely—consider reducing dose of ciclosporin and titrating to blood levels
CARBONIC ANHYDRASE INHIBITORS	ANTIDEMENTIA DRUGS—MEMANTINE	Possibly ↑ memantine levels	↓ Renal excretion: clearance of memantine was reduced by about 80% under alkaline urine conditions at pH 8	Watch for early features of memantine toxicity
CARBONIC ANHYDRASE INHIBITORS	ANTIDEPRESSANTS—LITHIUM	↓ Plasma concentrations of lithium, with risk of inadequate therapeutic effect	↑ Renal elimination of lithium	Monitor clinically and by measuring blood lithium levels to ensure adequate therapeutic efficacy
CARBONIC ANHYDRASE INHIBITORS	ANTIEPILEPTICS—BARBITURATES, PHENYTOIN	Risk of osteomalacia	Barbiturates and phenytoin have a small risk of causing osteomalacia; this may be ↑ by acetazolamide-induced urinary excretion of calcium	Be aware
CARBONIC ANHYDRASE INHIBITORS	ANTIPLATELET AGENTS—ASPIRIN	↑ Risk of salicylate toxicity with high-dose aspirin	Uncertain at present	Use low-dose aspirin

(Continued)

DRUGS ACTING ON THE CARDIOVASCULAR SYSTEM DIURETICS Loop diuretics

Primary Drug	Secondary Drug	Effect	Mechanism	Precautions
DIURETICS				
CARBONIC ANHYDRASE INHIBITORS	BETA-BLOCKERS—SOTALOL	↑ Risk of ventricular arrhythmias, particularly torsades de pointes, caused by sotalol	Hypokalemia, a side effect of these diuretics, predisposes to arrhythmias during sotalol therapy	Normalize potassium levels before starting sotalol in patients already taking these diuretics. When starting these diuretics in patients already taking sotalol, monitor potassium levels every 4–6 weeks until stable
CARBONIC ANHYDRASE INHIBITORS	BRONCHODILATORS—BETA-2 AGONISTS, THEOPHYLLINE	Risk of hypokalemia	Additive effects	Monitor blood potassium levels prior to concomitant administration and during therapy. Administer potassium supplements to prevent hypokalemia
CARBONIC ANHYDRASE INHIBITORS	CARDIAC GLYCOSIDES	Risk of digoxin toxicity ↑ by acetazolamide due to hypokalemia	Uncertain	Monitor potassium levels closely. Watch for digoxin toxicity and check levels
LOOP DIURETICS				
LOOP DIURETICS	ANESTHETICS—GENERAL	↑ Hypotensive effect	Additive hypotensive effect	Monitor BP closely, especially during induction of anesthesia
LOOP DIURETICS	ANALGESICS			
LOOP DIURETICS	NSAIDs	1. Reduced efficacy of diuretics 2. ↑ Risk of nephrotoxicity	1. NSAIDs cause sodium and water retention 2. Additive effect	Monitor BP and U&Es closely
LOOP DIURETICS	OPIODS	Opioids may enhance the orthostatic hypotensive effect of diuretics	Additive hypotensive effect	Warn about dizziness when standing up suddenly and other symptoms of orthostatic hypotension
LOOP DIURETICS	**ANTIARRHYTHMICS**			
LOOP DIURETICS	AMIODARONE, FLECAINIDE	Risk of arrhythmias	Cardiac toxicity directly related to hypokalemia	Monitor potassium levels every 4–6 weeks until stable, then at least annually

(*Continued*)

Primary Drug	Secondary Drug	Effect	Mechanism	Precautions
DIURETICS				
LOOP DIURETICS	DISOPYRAMIDE	Risk of hypokalemia	Additive effect	Monitor potassium levels closely
LOOP DIURETICS	MEXILETINE	Effect of mexiletine ↓ by hypokalemia	Uncertain	Normalize potassium levels before starting mexiletine
LOOP DIURETICS	**ANTIBIOTICS**			
LOOP DIURETICS	AMINOGLYCOSIDES	↑ Risk of ototoxicity and nephrotoxicity as a result of concomitant use of furosemide or bumetanide and gentamicin	Additive effect	If used concurrently, patients should be monitored for any hearing impairment. Monitor U&Es closely
LOOP DIURETICS	COLISTIN	↑ Risk of ototoxicity and possible deafness as a result of concomitant use of furosemide and colistin	Additive effect	If used concurrently, patients should be monitored for any hearing impairment
LOOP DIURETICS	TETRACYCLINES	Possible risk of renal toxicity	Additive effect	Some recommend avoiding coadministration; others advise monitoring renal function closely. Doxycycline is likely to be less of a problem
LOOP DIURETICS	VANCOMYCIN	Risk of renal toxicity	Additive effect	Monitor renal function closely
LOOP DIURETICS	**ANTICANCER AND IMMUNOMODULATING DRUGS**			
LOOP DIURETICS	BORTEZOMIB	↑ Hypotensive effect	Additive hypotensive effect	Monitor BP at least weekly until stable, particularly on initiation of therapy
LOOP DIURETICS	CISPLATIN	Theoretical risk of auditory toxic effects with cisplatin	Loop diuretics cause tinnitus and deafness as side effects. Additive toxic effects on auditory system likely	Monitor hearing—test auditory function regularly, particularly if patients report symptoms such as tinnitus or impaired hearing
LOOP DIURETICS	CICLOSPORIN	Risk of nephrotoxicity	Additive effect	Monitor renal function weekly
LOOP DIURETICS	CORTICOSTEROIDS	Risk of hypokalemia	Additive effect	Monitor serum potassium weekly until stable

(Continued)

Primary Drug	Secondary Drug	Effect	Mechanism	Precautions
DIURETICS				
LOOP DIURETICS	INTERLEUKIN 2 (ALDESLEUKIN)	↑ Hypotensive effect	Additive hypotensive effect	Monitor BP at least weekly until stable. Warn patients to report symptoms of hypotension (light-headedness, dizziness on standing, etc.)
LOOP DIURETICS	PORFIMER	↑ Risk of photosensitivity reactions when porfimer is coadministered with bumetanide or furosemide	Attributed to additive effects	Avoid exposure of skin and eyes to direct sunlight for 30 days after porfimer therapy
LOOP DIURETICS	PEMETREXED	↑ Pemetrexed toxicity	Reduced renal clearance	Caution with concurrent use
LOOP DIURETICS	**ANTIDEPRESSANTS**			
LOOP DIURETICS	LITHIUM	↑ Plasma concentrations of lithium, with risk of toxic effects	↓ Renal excretion of lithium	Monitor clinically and by measuring blood lithium levels for lithium toxicity. Loop diuretics are safer than thiazides
LOOP DIURETICS	REBOXETINE	Risk of hypokalemia	Additive effect	Monitor potassium levels closely
LOOP DIURETICS	SSRIs	Hyponatremia associated with SSRI use, with the incidence varying from 0.5% to 32%	Hyponatremia developed within the first few weeks of treatment and resolved within 2 weeks after therapy was discontinued. Mechanism secondary to development of SIADH (inappropriate secretion of ADH)	Risk factors include older age, female gender, low body weight, and lower baseline serum sodium
LOOP DIURETICS	**ANTIDIABETICS**			
LOOP DIURETICS	SGLT2 INHIBITORS	Potential for intravascular depletion and hypotension	Osmotic (natriuresis) effects of both classes of drug enhance diuresis	Manufacturer does not recommend use in combination with loop diuretics

(*Continued*)

Primary Drug	Secondary Drug	Effect	Mechanism	Precautions
DIURETICS				
LOOP DIURETICS	**ANTIEPILEPTICS**			
LOOP DIURETICS	CARBAMAZEPINE	Risk of hyponatremia	Additive effect	Monitor serum sodium closely
LOOP DIURETICS	PHENYTOIN	↓ Efficacy of furosemide	Uncertain	Be aware; watch for poor response to furosemide
LOOP DIURETICS	ANTIFUNGALS—AMPHOTERICIN	Risk of hypokalemia	Additive effect	Monitor potassium closely
LOOP DIURETICS	**ANTIHYPERTENSIVES AND HEART FAILURE DRUGS**			
LOOP DIURETICS	ANTIHYPERTENSIVES AND HEART FAILURE DRUGS	↑ Hypotensive effect; Risk of first-dose ↓ BP greater when ACE inhibitors are added to high-dose diuretics	Additive hypotensive effect; may be used therapeutically	Monitor BP at least weekly until stable. Warn patients to report symptoms of hypotension (light-headedness, dizziness on standing, etc.). Benefits often outweigh risks. Patients with congestive cardiac failure on diuretics should be started on a low dose of alpha-blocker
LOOP DIURETICS	ALISKIREN	↓ Plasma levels of furosemide	Uncertain	Watch for poor response to furosemide
LOOP DIURETICS	KETANSERIN	Risk of ventricular arrhythmias, particularly torsades de pointes	These drugs ↓ potassium levels, which ↑ the risk of QT prolongation	Avoid coadministration
LOOP DIURETICS	ANTI-PARKINSON'S DRUGS—LEVODOPA	↑ Hypotensive effect	Additive effect	Monitor BP at least weekly until stable. Warn patients to report symptoms of hypotension (light-headedness, dizziness on standing, etc.)
LOOP DIURETICS	ASPIRIN	1. Risk of renal failure when loop diuretics given with high-dose aspirin 2. Risk of ototoxicty when bumetanide or furosemide given with high-dose aspirin	1. Additive adverse effect on renal function 2. Additive effect; all are ototoxic	1. Monitor renal function closely; warn the patient to maintain good hydration 2. Monitor hearing regularly

(Continued)

Primary Drug	Secondary Drug	Effect	Mechanism	Precautions
DIURETICS				
LOOP DIURETICS	ANTIPSYCHOTICS—ATYPICALS, PHENOTHIAZINES, PIMOZIDE	Risk of arrhythmias	Cardiac toxicity directly related to hypokalemia	Monitor potassium levels every 4–6 weeks until stable, then at least annually
LOOP DIURETICS	**BETA-BLOCKERS**			
LOOP DIURETICS	BETA-BLOCKERS	↑ Hypotensive effect	Additive hypotensive effect; may be used therapeutically	Monitor BP at least weekly until stable. Warn patients to report symptoms of hypotension (light-headedness, dizziness on standing, etc.)
LOOP DIURETICS	SOTALOL	↑ Risk of ventricular arrhythmias, particularly torsades de pointes	Hypokalemia, a side effect of these diuretics, and predisposes to arrhythmias during sotalol therapy	Normalize potassium levels before starting sotalol in patients already taking these diuretics. When starting these diuretics in patients already taking sotalol, monitor potassium levels every 4–6 weeks until stable
LOOP DIURETICS	BRONCHODILATORS—BETA-2 AGONISTS, THEOPHYLLINE	Risk of hypokalemia	Additive effects	Monitor blood potassium levels prior to concomitant administration and during therapy. Administer potassium supplements to prevent hypokalemia
LOOP DIURETICS	CALCIUM CHANNEL BLOCKERS	↑ Hypotensive effect	Additive hypotensive effect; may be used therapeutically	Monitor BP at least weekly until stable. Warn patients to report symptoms of hypotension (light-headedness, dizziness on standing, etc.)
LOOP DIURETICS	CARDIAC GLYCOSIDES	Risk of digoxin toxicity ↑ due to hypokalemia	Uncertain	Monitor potassium levels closely. Watch for digoxin toxicity and check levels
LOOP DIURETICS	CNS STIMULANTS—ATOMOXETINE	↑ Risk of arrhythmias with hypokalemia	These diuretics may cause hypokalemia	Monitor potassium levels closely

(*Continued*)

Primary Drug	Secondary Drug	Effect	Mechanism	Precautions
DIURETICS				
LOOP DIURETICS	LIPID-LOWERING DRUGS—COLESTIPOL, CHOLESTYRAMINE	Both colestipol and cholestyramine markedly ↓ levels of loop diuretics	Colestipol and cholestyramine bind diuretics in the intestine	Give the anion exchange resin 3 h after furosemide
LOOP DIURETICS	**MUSCLE RELAXANTS**			
LOOP DIURETICS	BACLOFEN, TIZANIDINE	↑ Hypotensive effect	Additive hypotensive effect	Monitor BP at least weekly until stable. Warn patients to report symptoms of hypotension (light-headedness, dizziness on standing, etc.)
LOOP DIURETICS	NONDEPOLARIZING—MIVACURIUM	↑ Neuromuscular block	Uncertain; multiple factors likely, including electrolyte disturbances and possible direct effect on muscle contractility	Monitor neuromuscular block and titrate doses of mivacurium
LOOP DIURETICS	NITRATES	↑ Hypotensive effect	Additive hypotensive effect	Monitor BP at least weekly until stable. Warn patients to report symptoms of hypotension (light-headedness, dizziness on standing, etc.)
LOOP DIURETICS	PERIPHERAL VASODILATORS—MOXISYLYTE (THYMOXAMINE)	↑ Hypotensive effect	Additive hypotensive effect	Monitor BP at least weekly until stable. Warn patients to report symptoms of hypotension (light-headedness, dizziness on standing, etc.)
LOOP DIURETICS	POTASSIUM CHANNEL ACTIVATORS	↑ Hypotensive effect	Additive hypotensive effect	Monitor BP at least weekly until stable. Warn patients to report symptoms of hypotension (light-headedness, dizziness on standing, etc.)
POTASSIUM-SPARING DIURETICS AND ALDOSTERONE ANTAGONISTS				
POTASSIUM-SPARING DIURETICS	ANESTHETICS—GENERAL	↑ Hypotensive effect	Additive hypotensive effect	Monitor BP closely, especially during induction of anesthesia

(Continued)

Primary Drug	Secondary Drug	Effect	Mechanism	Precautions
DIURETICS				
POTASSIUM-SPARING DIURETICS	ANALGESICS—NSAIDs	1. Risk of hyperkalemia with NSAIDs 2. Reports of acute renal failure when triamterene coadministered with indometacin	1. Renal insufficiency caused by NSAIDs can exacerbate potassium retention by these diuretics 2. Uncertain	1. Monitor renal function and potassium closely 2. Avoid coadministration of triamterene and indometacin
POTASSIUM-SPARING DIURETICS	**ANTIARRHYTHMICS**			
POTASSIUM-SPARING DIURETICS	AMIODARONE	Risk of ↑ levels of eplerenone with amiodarone; risk of hyperkalemia directly related to serum levels	Amiodarone inhibits CYP3A4-mediated metabolism of eplerenone	Restrict dose of eplerenone to 25 mg/day. Monitor serum potassium concentrations closely; watch for hyperkalemia
DIURETICS—AMILORIDE	QUINIDINE	Possible ↓ efficacy of quinidine	Unknown	Monitor PR, BP, and ECG closely
POTASSIUM-SPARING DIURETICS	**ANTIBIOTICS**			
POTASSIUM-SPARING DIURETICS	MACROLIDES—ERYTHROMYCIN	↑ Eplerenone results in an ↑ risk of hypotension and hyperkalemia	Eplerenone is primarily metabolized by CYP3A4; there are no active metabolites. Erythromycin moderately inhibits CYP3A4, leading to ↑ levels of eplerenone	Dosage should not exceed 25 mg daily
POTASSIUM-SPARING DIURETICS	RIFAMPICIN	↓ Eplerenone levels	Induction of metabolism	Avoid coadministration
POTASSIUM-SPARING DIURETICS	TRIMETHOPRIM	Risk of hyponatremia ± hyperkalemia when trimethoprim is coadministered with thiazides combined with eplerenone or triamterene	Additive effect	Monitor potassium levels closely

(Continued)

Primary Drug	Secondary Drug	Effect	Mechanism	Precautions
DIURETICS				
POTASSIUM-SPARING DIURETICS	**ANTICANCER AND IMMUNOMODULATING DRUGS**			
POTASSIUM-SPARING DIURETICS	CICLOSPORIN	↑ Risk of hyperkalemia	Additive effect	Avoid coadministration
POTASSIUM-SPARING—EPLERENONE	CORTICOSTEROIDS	↓ Antihypertensive effect	Corticosteroids cause fluid and sodium retention	Be aware of interaction
SPIRONOLACTONE	MITOTANE	Case report of reduced mitotane efficacy	Unknown	Avoid concurrent use
POTASSIUM-SPARING DIURETICS	TACROLIMUS	Risk of hyperkalemia	Additive effect	Monitor potassium levels closely
POTASSIUM-SPARING DIURETICS	**ANTIDEPRESSANTS**			
POTASSIUM-SPARING DIURETICS	LITHIUM	Spironolactone and eplerenone possibly ↑ plasma concentrations of lithium, with risk of toxic effects	↓ Renal excretion of lithium	Monitor clinically and by measuring blood lithium levels for lithium toxicity
POTASSIUM-SPARING DIURETICS	ST. JOHN'S WORT	↓ Eplerenone levels	Induction of metabolism	Avoid coadministration
POTASSIUM-SPARING DIURETICS	**ANTIDIABETIC DRUGS**			
AMILORIDE	METFORMIN	↑ Metformin levels and risk of lactic acidosis	Metformin is not metabolized in humans and is not protein bound. Competition for renal tubular excretion is the basis for ↑ activity or retention of metformin	Theoretical possibility. Requires reduction of metformin dose to be considered, or the avoidance of coadministration

(Continued)

Primary Drug	Secondary Drug	Effect	Mechanism	Precautions
DIURETICS				
POTASSIUM-SPARING DIURETICS	REPAGLINIDE	↓ Hypoglycemic effect	Antagonistic effect	Higher doses of repaglinide needed
POTASSIUM-SPARING DIURETICS	ANTIEPILEPTICS—BARBITURATES, CARBAMAZEPINE	↓ Eplerenone levels	Induction of hepatic metabolism	Be aware; watch for poor response to eplerenone
POTASSIUM-SPARING DIURETICS	ANTIFUNGALS—KETOCONAZOLE	↑ Eplerenone levels	Inhibition of metabolism	Avoid coadministration
POTASSIUM-SPARING DIURETICS	ANTIHYPERTENSIVES AND HEART FAILURE DRUGS—ACE INHIBITORS, ALISKIREN, ANGIOTENSIN II RECEPTOR ANTAGONISTS	↑ Risk of hyperkalemia	Additive retention of potassium	Monitor serum potassium every week until stable, then every 3–6 months
POTASSIUM-SPARING DIURETICS	ANTIPLATELET AGENTS—ASPIRIN	↓ Efficacy of spironolactone	Uncertain	Watch for poor response to spironolactone
POTASSIUM-SPARING DIURETICS	ANTIVIRALS—PROTEASE INHIBITORS	Possibly ↑ adverse effects of eplerenone with nelfinavir, ritonavir (with or without lopinavir), and saquinavir	Inhibition of CYP3A4-mediated metabolism of eplerenone	Avoid concomitant use
POTASSIUM-SPARING DIURETICS	CALCIUM CHANNEL BLOCKERS	↑ Serum concentrations of eplerenone when given with diltiazem and verapamil	Calcium channel blockers inhibit CYP3A4-mediated metabolism of eplerenone	Restrict dose of eplerenone to 25 mg/day. Monitor serum potassium concentrations closely; watch for hyperkalemia
POTASSIUM-SPARING DIURETICS	**CARDIAC GLYCOSIDES**			
POTASSIUM-SPARING DIURETICS	DIGITOXIN	Conflicting results from volunteer studies; some showed ↑ (up to one-third) in the half-life of digitoxin, others a ↓ (up to one-fifth)	Uncertain at present	Watch for either digitoxin toxicity or a poor response, particularly for the first month after starting spironolactone
POTASSIUM-SPARING DIURETICS	DIGOXIN	Spironolactone may ↑ plasma concentrations of digoxin	Uncertain; spironolactone possibly ↓ The volume of distribution of digoxin	Watch for digoxin toxicity; check levels

(Continued)

Primary Drug	Secondary Drug	Effect	Mechanism	Precautions
DIURETICS				
POTASSIUM-SPARING DIURETICS	POTASSIUM	Risk of hyperkalemia	Additive effect	Monitor potassium levels closely
POTASSIUM-SPARING DIURETICS	PROGESTOGENS	↑ Risk of hyperkalemia	Drospirenone (component of some brands of combined contraceptive pill) is a progestogen derived from spironolactone that can cause potassium retention	Monitor serum potassium weekly until stable, then every 6 months
POTASSIUM-SPARING DIURETICS	TRILOSTANE	Risk of hyperkalemia	Additive effect	Monitor potassium levels regularly during coadministration
THIAZIDES				
THIAZIDES	ALCOHOL	1. Acute alcohol ingestion may ↑ hypotensive effects 2. Chronic moderate/heavy drinking ↓ hypotensive effect	1. Additive hypotensive effect 2. Chronic alcohol excess is associated with hypertension	Monitor BP closely as unpredictable responses can occur. Advise patients to drink only in moderation and avoid large variations in the amount of alcohol drunk
THIAZIDES	ANESTHETICS—GENERAL	↑ Hypotensive effect	Additive hypotensive effect	Monitor BP closely, especially during induction of anesthesia
THIAZIDES	ANALGESICS—NSAIDs	1. Reduced efficacy of diuretics 2. ↑ Risk of nephrotoxicity	1. NSAIDs cause sodium and water retention 2. Additive effect	Monitor BP and U&Es closely
THIAZIDES	**ANTIARRHYTHMICS**			
THIAZIDES	AMIODARONE, FLECAINIDE	Risk of arrhythmias	Cardiac toxicity directly related to hypokalemia	Monitor potassium levels every 4–6 weeks until stable, then at least annually
THIAZIDES	DISOPYRAMIDE	Risk of hypokalemia	Additive effect	Monitor potassium levels closely
DOFETILIDE	DIURETICS—HYDROCHLOROTHIAZIDE	↑ Dofetilide levels with risk of ↑ QT prolongation	Unknown	Avoid coadministration

(*Continued*)

Primary Drug	Secondary Drug	Effect	Mechanism	Precautions
DIURETICS				
THIAZIDES	MEXILETINE	Effect of mexiletine ↓ by hypokalemia	Uncertain	Normalize potassium levels before starting mexiletine
THIAZIDES	**ANTIBIOTICS**			
THIAZIDES	TETRACYCLINES	Possible risk of renal toxicity	Additive effect	Some recommend avoiding coadministration; others advise monitoring renal function closely. Doxycycline likely to be less of a problem
THIAZIDES	TRIMETHOPRIM	Risk of hyponatremia ± hyperkalemia when trimethoprim is coadministered with thiazides combined with eplerenone or triamterene	Additive effect	Monitor potassium levels closely
THIAZIDES	**ANTICANCER AND IMMUNOMODULATING DRUGS**			
THIAZIDES	BORTEZOMIB	↑ Hypotensive effect	Additive hypotensive effect	Monitor BP at least weekly until stable, particularly on initiation of therapy
THIAZIDES	CICLOSPORIN	Risk of nephrotoxicity	Additive effect	Monitor renal function weekly
THIAZIDES	CORTICOSTEROIDS	Risk of hypokalemia	Additive effect	Monitor serum potassium weekly until stable
THIAZIDES	INTERLEUKIN 2 (ALDESLEUKIN)	↑ Hypotensive effect	Additive hypotensive effect	Monitor BP at least weekly until stable. Warn patients to report symptoms of hypotension (light-headedness, dizziness on standing, etc.)
THIAZIDES	PORFIMER	↑ Risk of photosensitivity reactions when porfimer is coadministered with hydrochlorothiazide	Attributed to additive effects	Avoid exposure of skin and eyes to direct sunlight for 30 days after porfimer therapy
THIAZIDES	TOREMIFENE	Risk of hypercalcemia	Additive effect	Monitor calcium levels closely. Warn patients about the symptoms of hypercalcemia

(*Continued*)

Primary Drug	Secondary Drug	Effect	Mechanism	Precautions
DIURETICS				
THIAZIDES	**ANTIDEPRESSANTS**			
THIAZIDES	LITHIUM	↑ Plasma concentrations of lithium, with risk of toxic effects	↓ Renal excretion of lithium	Monitor clinically and by measuring blood lithium levels for lithium toxicity. Loop diuretics are safer than thiazides
THIAZIDES	REBOXETINE	Risk of hypokalemia	Additive effect	Monitor potassium levels closely
THIAZIDES	SSRIs	Hyponatremia associated with SSRI use, with the incidence varying from 0.5% to 32%	Hyponatremia developed within the first few week of treatment and resolved within 2 weeks after therapy was discontinued. Mechanism secondary to development of SIADH (inappropriate secretion of ADH)	Risk factors include older age, female gender, low body weight, and lower baseline serum sodium
THIAZIDES	**ANTIDIABETIC DRUGS**			
THIAZIDES	SULFONYLUREAS	Hypoglycemic efficacy is ↓	Hyperglycemia due to antagonistic effect	Monitor blood glucose regularly until stable. Higher dose of oral antidiabetic agent often needed
THIAZIDES	CHLORPROPAMIDE	Risk of hyponatremia when chlorpropamide is given to a patient taking both potassium-sparing diuretics/aldosterone antagonists and thiazides	Additive effect; chlorpropamide enhances ADH secretion	Monitor serum sodium regularly
THIAZIDES	ANTIEPILEPTICS—CARBAMAZEPINE	Risk of hyponatremia	Additive effect	Monitor serum sodium closely
THIAZIDES	ANTIFUNGALS—AMPHOTERICIN	Risk of hypokalemia	Additive effect	Monitor potassium closely
THIAZIDES	ANTIGOUT DRUGS	Possible ↑ risk of severe allergic reactions when allopurinol is given with thiazides in the presence of renal impairment	Uncertain	Caution in coadministering allopurinol with thiazides in the presence of renal insufficiency

(Continued)

Primary Drug	Secondary Drug	Effect	Mechanism	Precautions
DIURETICS				
THIAZIDES	**ANTIHYPERTENSIVES AND HEART FAILURE DRUGS**			
THIAZIDES	ANTIHYPERTENSIVES AND HEART FAILURE DRUGS	↑ Hypotensive effect. Risk of first-dose ↓ BP greater when ACE inhibitors are added to high-dose diuretics	Additive hypotensive effect; may be used therapeutically	Monitor BP at least weekly until stable. Warn patients to report symptoms of hypotension (light-headedness, dizziness on standing, etc.). Benefits often outweigh risks. Patients with congestive cardiac failure on diuretics should be started on a low dose of alpha-blocker
THIAZIDES	KETANSERIN	Risk of ventricular arrhythmias, particularly torsades de pointes	These drugs ↓ potassium levels, which ↑ the risk of QT prolongation	Avoid coadministration
THIAZIDES	VASODILATOR ANTIHYPERTENSIVES—DIAZOXIDE	Risk of hyperglycemia when diazoxide is coadministered with thiazides	Additive effect; both drugs have a hyperglycemic effect	Monitor blood glucose closely, particularly with diabetes
THIAZIDES	ANTI-PARKINSON'S DRUGS—LEVODOPA	↑ Hypotensive effect	Additive effect	Monitor BP at least weekly until stable. Warn patients to report symptoms of hypotension (light-headedness, dizziness on standing, etc.)
THIAZIDES	ANTIPSYCHOTICS—ATYPICAL AGENTS, PHENOTHIAZINES, PIMOZIDE	Risk of arrhythmias	Cardiac toxicity directly related to hypokalemia	Monitor potassium levels every 4–6 weeks until stable, then at least annually
THIAZIDES	**BETA-BLOCKERS**			
THIAZIDES	BETA-BLOCKERS	↑ Hypotensive effect	Additive hypotensive effect; may be used therapeutically	Monitor BP at least weekly until stable. Warn patients to report symptoms of hypotension (light-headedness, dizziness on standing, etc.)

(*Continued*)

Primary Drug	Secondary Drug	Effect	Mechanism	Precautions
DIURETICS				
THIAZIDES	SOTALOL	↑ Risk of ventricular arrhythmias, particularly torsades de pointes, caused by sotalol	Hypokalemia a side effect of these diuretics, predisposes to arrhythmias during sotalol therapy	Normalize potassium levels before starting sotalol in patients already taking these diuretics. When starting these diuretics in patients already taking sotalol, monitor potassium levels every 4–6 weeks until stable
THIAZIDES	BRONCHODILATORS—BETA-2 AGONISTS, THEOPHYLLINE	Risk of hypokalemia	Additive effects	Monitor blood potassium levels prior to concomitant administration and during therapy. Administer potassium supplements to prevent hypokalemia
THIAZIDES	CALCIUM	Risk of hypercalcemia with high-dose calcium	↓ Renal excretion of calcium by thiazides	Monitor calcium levels closely
THIAZIDES	CALCIUM CHANNEL BLOCKERS	↑ Hypotensive effect	Additive hypotensive effect; may be used therapeutically	Monitor BP at least weekly until stable. Warn patients to report symptoms of hypotension (light-headedness, dizziness on standing, etc.)
THIAZIDES	CARDIAC GLYCOSIDES	Risk of digoxin toxicity ↑ due to hypokalemia	Uncertain	Monitor potassium levels closely. Watch for digoxin toxicity and check levels
THIAZIDES	CNS STIMULANTS—ATOMOXETINE	↑ Risk of arrhythmias with hypokalemia	These diuretics may cause hypokalemia	Monitor potassium levels closely
THIAZIDES	LIPID-LOWERING DRUGS—ANION EXCHANGE RESINS	Both colestipol and cholestyramine markedly ↓ levels of thiazides	Colestipol and cholestyramine bind diuretics in the intestine	Give the anion exchange resin 4–6 h after thiazides (although the effect of hydrochlorothiazide may still be ↓ by cholestyramine)
THIAZIDES	MUSCLE RELAXANTS—BACLOFEN, TIZANIDINE	↑ Hypotensive effect	Additive hypotensive effect	Monitor BP at least weekly until stable. Warn patients to report symptoms of hypotension (light-headedness, dizziness on standing, etc.)

(Continued)

Primary Drug	Secondary Drug	Effect	Mechanism	Precautions
DIURETICS				
THIAZIDES	NITRATES	↑ Hypotensive effect	Additive hypotensive effect	Monitor BP at least weekly until stable. Warn patients to report symptoms of hypotension (light-headedness, dizziness on standing, etc.)
THIAZIDES	ORLISTAT	Case of ↑ BP when orlistat is started for a patient on thiazides	Uncertain at present	Monitor BP at least weekly until stable
THIAZIDES	PERIPHERAL VASODILATORS—MOXISYLYTE (THYMOXAMINE)	↑ Hypotensive effect	Additive hypotensive effect	Monitor BP at least weekly until stable. Warn patients to report symptoms of hypotension (light-headedness, dizziness on standing, etc.)
THIAZIDES	POTASSIUM CHANNEL ACTIVATORS	↑ Hypotensive effect	Additive hypotensive effect	Monitor BP at least weekly until stable. Warn patients to report symptoms of hypotension (light-headedness, dizziness on standing, etc.)
THIAZIDES	VITAMIN D	Risk of hypercalcemia with vitamin D	↓ Renal excretion of calcium by thiazides	Monitor calcium levels closely

Primary Drug	Secondary Drug	Effect	Mechanism	Precautions
IVABRADINE				
IVABRADINE	ANTIARRHYTHMICS—AMIODARONE, DISOPYRAMIDE	Risk of arrhythmias	Additive effect	Monitor ECG closely
IVABRADINE	**ANTIBIOTICS**			
IVABRADINE	MACROLIDES	↑ Levels with erythromycin, clarithromycin, and telithromycin	Reduced CYP3A4-mediated metabolism of ivabradine	Avoid coadministration
IVABRADINE	RIFAMPICIN	↓ Levels of ivabradine	Increased CYP3A4-mediated metabolism of ivabradine	Monitor for reduced efficacy of ivabradine

(*Continued*)

Primary Drug	Secondary Drug	Effect	Mechanism	Precautions
IVABRADINE				
IVABRADINE	ANTIDEPRESSANTS—ST. JOHN'S WORT	↓ Levels of ivabradine	Increased CYP3A4-mediated metabolism of ivabradine	Monitor for reduced efficacy of ivabradine
IVABRADINE	ANTIEPILEPTICS—PHENOBARBITONE, PHENYTOIN	↓ Levels of ivabradine	Increased CYP3A4-mediated metabolism of ivabradine	Monitor for reduced efficacy of ivabradine
IVABRADINE	ANTIFUNGALS—AZOLES	↑ Levels with ketoconazole and possibly fluconazole and itraconazole	Reduced CYP3A4-mediated metabolism of ivabradine	Avoid coadministration
IVABRADINE	ANTIMALARIALS	Risk of arrhythmias with mefloquine	Additive effect	Monitor ECG closely
IVABRADINE	ANTIPROTOZOALS	Risk of arrhythmias with pentamidine	Additive effect	Monitor ECG closely
IVABRADINE	ANTIPSYCHOTICS	Risk of arrhythmias with pimozide and sertindole	Additive effect	Monitor ECG closely
IVABRADINE	ANTIVIRALS—PROTEASE INHIBITORS	↑ Levels with ritonavir	Reduced CYP3A4-mediated metabolism of ivabradine	Avoid coadministration
IVABRADINE	BETA-BLOCKERS—SOTALOL	Risk of arrhythmias	Additive effect; ivabradine slows the sinus node	Monitor ECG closely
IVABRADINE	CALCIUM CHANNEL BLOCKERS	↑ Levels with diltiazem and verapamil	Reduced CYP3A4-mediated metabolism of ivabradine	Avoid coadministration
IVABRADINE	GRAPEFRUIT JUICE	↑ Levels with grapefruit juice	Reduced CYP3A4-mediated metabolism of ivabradine	Avoid coadministration

DRUGS ACTING ON THE CARDIOVASCULAR SYSTEM IVABRADINE

Primary Drug	Secondary Drug	Effect	Mechanism	Precautions
LIPID-LOWERING DRUGS				
ANION EXCHANGE RESINS				
ANION EXCHANGE RESINS	**ANALGESICS**			
ANION EXCHANGE RESINS	NSAIDs	Cholestyramine ↓ absorption of NSAIDs	Cholestyramine binds NSAIDs in the intestine, reducing their absorption; it also binds those NSAIDs with a significant enterohepatic recirculation (meloxicam, piroxicam, sulindac, tenoxicam)	Give the NSAID 1 h before or 4–6 h after cholestyramine; however, meloxicam, piroxicam, sulindac, and tenoxicam should not be given with cholestyramine
ANION EXCHANGE RESINS	PARACETAMOL	Cholestyramine ↓ paracetamol by 60% when they are given together	Cholestyramine binds paracetamol in the intestine	Give cholestyramine and paracetamol at least 1 h apart
ANION EXCHANGE RESINS	ANTIARRHYTHMICS—AMIODARONE	Cholestyramine ↓ amiodarone levels	Cholestyramine binds amiodarone, reducing its absorption and interrupting its enterohepatic circulation	Avoid coadministration
ANION EXCHANGE RESINS	**ANTIBIOTICS**			
ANION EXCHANGE RESINS	TETRACYCLINE	↓ Levels of tetracycline and possible therapeutic failure	Tetracycline binds with colestipol and cholestyramine in the gut, therefore reducing its absorption	Dosing should be as separate as possible
ANION EXCHANGE RESINS	VANCOMYCIN (ORAL)	↓ Vancomycin levels	Inhibition of absorption	Separate doses as much as possible

(*Continued*)

Primary Drug	Secondary Drug	Effect	Mechanism	Precautions
LIPID-LOWERING DRUGS				
ANION EXCHANGE RESINS	**ANTICANCER AND IMMUNOMODULATING DRUGS**			
ANION EXCHANGE RESINS	CORTICOSTEROIDS	↓ Absorption of oral hydrocortisone and possibly budesonide and dexamethasone with cholestyramine and colestipol. Prednisolone is not affected	↓ Absorption	Give steroid 1 h before or 4–6 h after cholestyramine or colestipol
ANION EXCHANGE RESINS	LEFLUNOMIDE	↓ Levels of leflunomide	↓ Absorption	Avoid coadministration
ANION EXCHANGE RESINS	METHOTREXATE	Parenteral methotrexate levels may be ↓ by cholestyramine	Cholestyramine interrupts the enterohepatic circulation of methotrexate	Avoid coadministration
ANION EXCHANGE RESINS	MYCOPHENOLATE	↓ Plasma concentrations of mycophenolate by approximately 40%. Risk of therapeutic failure	Due to interruption of enterohepatic circulation because of binding of recirculating mycophenolate with cholestyramine in the intestine	Avoid coadministration
CHOLESTYRAMINE, CHOLESTAGEL	REGORAFENIB	Possible ↓ regorafenib levels	Formation of insoluble complexes with regorafenib reducing (re)absorption	Clinical significance unknown, but be aware of possible reduced efficacy of regorafenib. Consider separating doses
ANION EXCHANGE RESINS	ANTICOAGULANTS—ORAL	↓ Anticoagulant effect with cholestyramine	↓ Absorption of warfarin	Give warfarin 1 h before or 4–6 h after cholestyramine
ANION EXCHANGE RESINS	**ANTIDIABETIC DRUGS**			
ANION EXCHANGE RESINS	ACARBOSE	↑ Hypoglycemic effect of acarbose	Uncertain	Monitor blood glucose during and coadministration and after discontinuation of concurrent therapy

(*Continued*)

Primary Drug	Secondary Drug	Effect	Mechanism	Precautions
LIPID-LOWERING DRUGS				
ANION EXCHANGE RESINS	SULFONYLUREAS	1. Glipizide absorption may be ↓ by cholestyramine 2. Glibenclamide absorption may be ↓ by colesevelam	1. Cholestyramine interrupts the enterohepatic circulation of glipizide 2. Likely colesevelam binds glibenclamide in the stomach and small bowel	1. Avoid coadministration 2. Take glibenclamide 4 h before colesevelam
ANION EXCHANGE RESINS—COLESEVELAM	ANTIEPILEPTICS—PHENYTOIN	↓ Absorption of oral phenytoin	Possibly due to bonding	Administer phenytoin 4 h prior to colesevelam. Measure phenytoin concentrations and adjust the dose as required. Seizure diary is important
ANION EXCHANGE RESINS	ANTIMUSCARINICS—TROSPIUM	Risk of ↓ absorption of trospium	Colestipol and cholestyramine bind trospium in the intestine	Take trospium 1 h before or 4–6 h after colestipol or cholestyramine
ANION EXCHANGE RESINS	CALCIUM CHANNEL BLOCKERS	Colestipol ↓ diltiazem levels	Colestipol binds diltiazem in the intestine	Monitor for poor response to diltiazem. Separating doses of diltiazem and colestipol does not seem to ↓ this interaction.
ANION EXCHANGE RESINS	CARDIAC GLYCOSIDES	Colestipol and cholestyramine may ↓ digoxin and digitoxin levels	Both colestipol and cholestyramine are ion exchange resins that bind bile sodiums and prevent reabsorption in the intestine; this breaks the enterohepatic cycle of digoxin and digitoxin	Colestipol and cholestyramine should be given at least 1.5 h after digoxin and digitoxin
ANION EXCHANGE RESINS	DIURETICS	Both colestipol and cholestyramine markedly ↓ levels of loop diuretics and thiazides	Colestipol and cholestyramine bind diuretics in the intestine	Give the anion exchange resin 3 h after furosemide and 4–6 h after thiazides (although the effect of hydrochlorothiazide may still be ↓ by cholestyramine)
ANION EXCHANGE RESINS	IRON—ORAL	↓ Iron levels when iron is given orally with cholestyramine	↓ Absorption	Separate doses as much as possible—monitor FBC closely

(*Continued*)

Primary Drug	Secondary Drug	Effect	Mechanism	Precautions
LIPID-LOWERING DRUGS				
ANION EXCHANGE RESINS	**LIPID-LOWERING DRUGS**			
ANION EXCHANGE RESINS	EZETIMIBE	Cholestyramine ↓ the absorption of ezetimibe	Cholestyramine binds ezetimibe in the intestine	Giving ezetimibe 1 h before or 3–6 h after the anion exchange resin should minimize this effect
ANION EXCHANGE RESINS	FIBRATES	↓ Absorption of gemfibrozil and bezafibrate	Reduced absorption due to binding to anion exchange resins in the intestine	Manufacturer recommends separating doses by 2 h
ANION EXCHANGE RESINS	STATINS	Anion-binding resins ↓ the absorption of statins, but the overall lipid-lowering effect is not altered	Anion-binding resins bind statins in the intestine	Giving the statin 1 h before or 3–6 h after the anion exchange resin should minimize this effect
ANION EXCHANGE RESINS	ESTROGENS	Colesevelam probably ↓ absorption of combined oral contraceptives. Theoretical risk of contraceptive failure	Anion-binding resins bind oral contraceptives in the intestine	Giving the oral contraceptive 4 h before the anion exchange resin should minimize this effect
ANION EXCHANGE RESINS	PROGESTOGENS	Colesevelam probably ↓ absorption of combined oral contraceptives. Theoretical risk of contraceptive failure	Anion-binding resins bind oral contraceptives in the intestine	Giving the oral contraceptive 4 h before the anion exchange resin should minimize this effect
ANION EXCHANGE RESINS	RALOXIFENE	Raloxifene levels may be ↓ by cholestyramine	Cholestyramine interrupts the enterohepatic circulation of raloxifene	Avoid coadministration
ANION EXCHANGE RESINS	THYROID HORMONES	↓ Efficacy of thyroid hormones	↓ Absorption	Separate doses by at least 4–6 h. Monitor TFTs
ANION EXCHANGE RESINS	URSODEOXYCHOLIC ACID	Risk of ↓ absorption of ursodeoxycholic acid	Colestipol and cholestyramine bind ursodeoxycholic acid in the intestine	Take ursodeoxycholic acid 1 h before or 4–6 h after an anion exchange resin

(*Continued*)

Primary Drug	Secondary Drug	Effect	Mechanism	Precautions
LIPID-LOWERING DRUGS				
AVASIMIBE				
AVASIMIBE	RUXOLITINIB	↓ Levels of ruloxitinib	CYP3A4 induction	Monitor closely Titrate dose based on safety and efficacy
EZETIMIBE				
EZETIMIBE	ANTIBIOTICS—RIFAMPICIN	Possibly ↓ efficacy of ezetimibe	Uncertain	Monitor lipid profile closely
EZETIMIBE	**ANTICANCER AND IMMUNOMODULATING DRUGS**			
EZETIMIBE	CICLOSPORIN	↑ Levels of both drugs when ezetimibe is coadministered with ciclosporin	Uncertain	Watch for signs of ciclosporin toxicity
EZETIMIBE	TACROLIMUS	Possible slight ↑ in ezetimibe levels	P-glycoprotein inhibition	Unlikely to be of clinical significance
EZETIMIBE	**LIPID-LOWERING DRUGS**			
EZETIMIBE	ANION EXCHANGE RESINS	Cholestyramine ↓ the absorption of ezetimibe	Cholestyramine binds ezetimibe in the intestine	Giving ezetimibe 1 h before or 3–6 h after the anion exchange resin should minimize this effect
EZETIMIBE	LIPID-LOWERING DRUGS—FIBRATES	Risk of gallstones with fibrates	Uncertain	Stop coadministration if symptoms develop
FIBRATES				
FIBRATES	ANTACIDS	Gemfibrozil levels may be ↓ by antacids	Uncertain	Give gemfibrozil 1–2 h before the antacid
FIBRATES	ANTIBIOTICS—DAPTOMYCIN	Risk of myopathy	Additive effect	Avoid coadministration
FIBRATES	**ANTICANCER AND IMMUNOMODULATING DRUGS**			
GEMFIBROZIL	BEXAROTENE	Gemfibrozil may ↑ bexarotene levels	Uncertain at present	Avoid coadministration
FIBRATES	CICLOSPORIN	↑ Risk with renal failure	Uncertain at present	Monitor renal function closely

(Continued)

Primary Drug	Secondary Drug	Effect	Mechanism	Precautions
LIPID-LOWERING DRUGS				
GEMFIBROZIL	DABRAFENIB	Predicted ↑ dabrafenib levels	CYP2C8/CYP3A4 inhibition	Avoid concurrent use if possible. Caution if concurrent use necessary
GEMFIBROZIL	INTERFERON ALFA	Case reports of ↑ liver enzymes	Unknown	Monitor closely
GEMFIBROZIL	PACLITAXEL	Possible ↑ paclitaxel levels	CYP2C8 inhibition	Caution with concurrent use
FIBRATES	ANTICOAGULANTS—ORAL	↑ Efficacy of warfarin and phenindione	Uncertain; postulated that fibrates displace anticoagulants from their binding sites	Monitor INR closely
FIBRATES	**ANTIDIABETIC DRUGS**			
FIBRATES	SULFONYLUREAS—TOLBUTAMIDE	Fibrates may ↑ the efficacy of sulfonylureas	Uncertain; postulated that fibrates displace sulfonylureas from plasma proteins and ↓ their hepatic metabolism. In addition, fenofibrate may inhibit CYP2C9-mediated metabolism of tolbutamide	Monitor blood glucose levels closely
GEMFIBROZIL	REPAGLINIDE	Marked ↑ in repaglinide levels, with risk of severe hypoglycemia	Gemfibrozil is a relatively selective inhibitor of CYP2C8. Also drug transportation may have a role	Avoid coadministration. Bezafibrate and fenofibrate are suitable alternatives if a fibric acid derivative is required
GEMFIBROZIL	PIOGLITAZONE, ROSIGLITAZONE	↑ In blood levels of pioglitazone and rosiglitazone—often doubled	Gemfibrozil is a relatively selective inhibitor of CYP2C8	➢ Watch for hypoglycemic events and ↓ the dose of pioglitazone and rosiglitazone after repeated blood sugar measurements. Warn patients about hypoglycemia ***For signs and symptoms of hypoglycemia, see Clinical Features of Some Adverse Drug Interactions, Hypoglycemia***

(*Continued*)

Primary Drug	Secondary Drug	Effect	Mechanism	Precautions
LIPID-LOWERING DRUGS				
FIBRATES	ANTIEPILEPTICS	Gemfibrozil may ↑ carbamazepine levels	Uncertain at present	Watch for features of carbamazepine toxicity
FIBRATES	ANTIVIRALS—PROTEASE INHIBITORS	↓ Plasma levels gemfibrozil	Altered GI absorption	Monitor lipid profile closely
FIBRATES	**LIPID-LOWERING DRUGS**			
FIBRATES	ANION EXCHANGE RESINS	↓ Absorption of gemfibrozil and bezafibrate	Reduced absorption due to binding to anion exchange resins in the intestine	Manufacturer recommends separating doses by 2 h
FIBRATES	EZETIMIBE	Risk of gallstones with fibrates	Uncertain	Stop coadministration if symptoms develop
FIBRATES	STATINS	Gemfibrozil may ↑ atorvastatin, rosuvastatin, and simvastatin levels (risk of myopathy with simvastatin)	Uncertain	Avoid coadministration of simvastatin and gemfibrozil. When using other statins, warn patients to watch for the features of myopathy
LOMITAPIDE				
LOMITAPIDE	**ANTICANCER AND OTHER IMMUNOMODULATING DRUGS**			
LOMITAPIDE	LAPATINIB	Predicted increased levels of lapatinib	P-glycoprotein inhibition	Monitor closely with concurrent use
LOMITAPIDE	IMATINIB	Predicted increased levels of imatinib	P-glycoprotein inhibition	Monitor closely with concurrent use
LOMITAPIDE	NILOTINIB	Predicted increased levels of nilotinib	P-glycoprotein inhibition	Monitor closely with concurrent use
LOMITAPIDE	ELIGLUSTAT	↑ Eliglustat levels	Inhibition of CYP3A4-mediated metabolism	Avoid coadministration in poor metabolizers
LOMITAPIDE	NITISINONE	Possible ↑ nitisinone levels	Inhibition of CYP3A4-mediated metabolism	Monitor carefully
NICOTINIC ACID				
NICOTINIC ACID	LIPID-LOWERING DRUGS—STATINS	Slight risk of rhabdomyolysis	Uncertain at present	Monitor LFTs and CK closely; warn patients to report any features of rhabdomyolysis

(Continued)

Primary Drug	Secondary Drug	Effect	Mechanism	Precautions
LIPID-LOWERING DRUGS				
PROBUCOL				
PROBUCOL	ANTICANCER AND IMMUNOMODULATING DRUGS—CICLOSPORIN	Slight increase in ciclosporin levels	Unknown	Monitor concurrent use
STATINS				
STATINS	ANTACIDS	↓ Rosuvastatin levels	Likely reduced absorption. Unclear why other statins not similarly affected	Separate doses by at least 2 h
STATINS	**ANTIARRHYTHMICS**			
SIMVASTATIN, ATORVASTATIN	AMIODARONE	↑ Risk of myopathy with high doses (>40 mg daily) of simvastatin	Amiodarone inhibits CYP3A4-mediated metabolism of these statins. It inhibits intestinal Pgp, which may ↑ the bioavailability of statins	Avoid >20 mg daily doses of simvastatin in patients taking amiodarone; if higher doses are required, switch to an alternative statin
SIMVASTATIN, ATORVASTATIN	DRONEDARONE	↑ Plasma levels of atorvastatin and simvastatin	Dronedarone inhibits CYP3A4-mediated metabolism of these statins	Titrate these statins slowly—warn the patient to look for signs of myopathy. Alternatively consider an alternative statin
STATINS	**ANTIBIOTICS**			
STATINS	DAPTOMYCIN	Risk of myopathy	Additive effect	Avoid coadministration
STATINS	FUSIDIC ACID	Cases of rhabdomyolysis reported when fusidic acid was coadministered with atorvastatin or simvastatin	Uncertain at present	Monitor LFTs and CK closely; warn patients to report any features of rhabdomyolysis

(Continued)

Primary Drug	Secondary Drug	Effect	Mechanism	Precautions
LIPID-LOWERING DRUGS				
STATINS	MACROLIDES—CLARITHROMYCIN, ERYTHROMYCIN, TELITHROMYCIN	1. Marked ↑ levels of lovastatin and simvastatin 2. ↑ Levels of atorvastatin and pravastatin. Fluvastatin and rosuvastatin do not seem to interact	Inhibition of CYP3A4 mediated metabolism of statins (each to a different extent)	1. Avoid coadministration (temporarily stop the statin if the patient needs macrolide therapy) 2. Reduce dose of statin. Monitor lipid profile closely. Warn patients to report immediately muscle pain
STATINS	RIFAMPICIN	1. ↓ Atorvastatin and simvastatin efficacy when given at a separate time to rifampicin 2. Rifampicin has variable effects on fluvastatin levels	Uncertain	Administer atorvastatin and simvastatin at the same time as rifampicin. Monitor lipid profile closely; look for poor response
STATINS	**ANTICANCER AND IMMUNOMODULATING DRUGS**			
STATINS	BEXAROTENE	Levels of atorvastatin ↓ by bexarotene. Simvastatin and lovastatin may be affected	Possibly due to induction of CYP3A4	Atorvastatin dose increase may be necessary
STATINS—ATORVASTATIN, LOVASTATIN, ROSUVASTATIN, SIMVASTATIN	CICLOSPORIN	↑ Plasma concentrations of these statins, with risk of myopathy and rhabdomyolysis	Ciclosporin is a moderate inhibitor of CYP3A4, which metabolizes these statins	↓ Statins to lowest possible dose (do not give simvastatin in doses >10 mg). Monitor LFTs and CK closely; warn patients to report any features of rhabdomyolysis. This interaction does not occur with pravastatin
PRAVASTATIN	CRIZOTINIB	Possible ↑ levels of P-glycoprotein substrates	Crizotinib inhibits P-glycoprotein	Monitor closely
ATORVASTATIN, SIMVASTATIN	DABRAFENIB	Possible ↓ levels of CYP3A4/CYP2Cs/CYP2B6 substrates. Level of reduction may vary	Dabrafenib induces CYP3A4/CYP2Cs/CYP2B6	Monitor closely or avoid concurrent use

(Continued)

Primary Drug	Secondary Drug	Effect	Mechanism	Precautions
LIPID-LOWERING DRUGS				
STATINS	DASATINIB	Possible ↓ simvastatin levels	↑ Metabolism of simvastatin	Monitor lipid profile closely and adjust simvastatin dose accordingly when starting and stopping coadministration
SIMVASTATIN	ERLOTINIB	Single case of rhabdomyolysis	Unknown	Significance unknown
STATINS	IMATINIB	Imatinib may ↑ atorvastatin and simvastatin levels	Imatinib inhibits CYP3A4-mediated metabolism of simvastatin	Monitor LFTs, U&Es, and CK closely
STATINS	LENALIDOMIDE	↑ Risk of rhabdomyolysis	Additive	Monitor closely
SIMVASTATIN	PAZOPANIB	↑ ALT levels	Possibly due to inhibition of organic anion transporting polypeptide (OATP) 1B1	Monitor ALT and stop simvastatin if ALT increases
ROSUVASTATIN	PONATINIB	Predicted ↑ in levels of rosuvastatin	BCRP inhibition	Be aware
ROSUVASTATIN	RUXOLITINIB	Predicted ↑ in P-glycoprotein or BCRP substrate levels	P-glycoprotein/BCRP inhibition	Monitor closely Separate administration of drugs
STATINS	SIROLIMUS	Reports of rhabdomyolysis when sirolimus coadministered with simvastatin or fluvastatin	Uncertain	Warn patients to report immediately if there is any muscle pain
STATINS	TACROLIMUS	Single case report of rhabdomyolysis when simvastatin was added to tacrolimus	Uncertain at present	Monitor LFTs and CK closely; warn patients to report any features of rhabdomyolysis
STATINS	TOCILIZUMAB	↓ Levels of simvastatin. Other statins may be affected	Tocilizumab reverses cytochrome P450 isoenzyme suppression by IL-6	Monitor closely. Consider increasing statin dose

(Continued)

Primary Drug	Secondary Drug	Effect	Mechanism	Precautions
LIPID-LOWERING DRUGS				
STATINS	TRABECTEDIN	Possible ↑ risk of rhabdomyolysis	Additive	Caution with concurrent use
ROSUVASTATIN	VEMURAFENIB	Possible ↑ levels of BCRP substrates	Vemurafenib inhibits BCRP	Clinical significance unknown
STATINS	ANTICOAGULANTS—ORAL	Possible ↑ anticoagulant effect with fluvastatin and simvastatin	Uncertain; possibly due to inhibition of CYP2C9-mediated metabolism of warfarin	Monitor INR closely
STATINS	ANTIDEPRESSANTS—ST. JOHN'S WORT	St. John's wort may ↓ simvastatin levels	Uncertain at present	Monitor lipid profile closely; look for poor response to simvastatin
STATINS	**ANTIDIABETIC DRUGS**			
LOVASTATIN	GLP-1 ANALOGUES	AUC and C_{max} ↓ by 40% and 28%, respectively	Unknown mechanism	Monitor lipid levels
STATINS	NATEGLINIDE, REPAGLINIDE	↑ Incidence of adverse effects such as myalgia. There was an ↑ in maximum concentration of repaglinide by 25% with high variability	Uncertain. Statins are also substrates for CYP3A4, and competition for metabolism by the enzyme system may be a factor	Clinical significance is uncertain, but it is necessary to be aware of this. Warn patients about the adverse effects of statins and repaglinide
STATINS—ATORVASTATIN	THIAZOLIDINEDIONES	Decreased levels of both pioglitazone and atorvastatin in the blood	Possibly related to metabolism using the same CYP3A4 pathway	Consider increasing doses of both agents
STATINS	ANTIEPILEPTICS—PHENYTOIN	Reports of ↓ levels of atorvastatin and simvastatin	Induction of CYP3A4	Monitor lipid profile closely. If lipids increase, consider changing to another statin

(*Continued*)

Primary Drug	Secondary Drug	Effect	Mechanism	Precautions
LIPID-LOWERING DRUGS				
STATINS	ANTIFUNGALS	Azoles markedly ↑ atorvastatin, simvastatin (both with cases of myopathy reported), and possibly pravastatin. These effects are less likely with fluvastatin and rosuvastatin, although fluconazole may cause moderate rises in their levels	Itraconazole and ketoconazole inhibit CYP3A4-mediated metabolism of these statins; they also inhibit intestinal Pgp, which ↑ the bioavailability of statins; itraconazole may block the transport of atorvastatin due to inhibition of the OATP1B1 enzyme system. Some manufacturers suggest that the small ↑ in plasma levels of pravastatin may be due to ↑ absorption. Voriconazole is an inhibitor of CYP2C9. Fluconazole inhibits CYP2C9 and CYP3A4	Avoid coadministration of simvastatin and atorvastatin with azole antifungals. Care should be taken with coadministration of other statins and azoles. Although fluvastatin and rosuvastatin may be considered as alternatives, consider reducing the dose of statin and warn patients to report any features of rhabdomyolysis. Check LFTs and CK regularly
STATINS	ANTIGOUTS—COLCHICINE	↑ Risk of myopathy	Uncertain. Both drugs can cause myopathy	Ask patients to report signs of myopathy
STATINS	**ANTIHYPERTENSIVES AND HEART FAILURE DRUGS**			
STATINS	VASODILATOR ANTIHYPERTENSIVES	Bosentan lowers simvastatin levels	Uncertain; bosentan moderately inhibits CYP3A4	Monitor lipid profile closely; look for poor response to simvastatin
STATINS	ANTIPLATELET AGENTS—CLOPIDOGREL	Atorvastatin and possibly simvastatin ↓ the antiplatelet effect of clopidogrel in a dose-dependent manner	Atorvastatin and simvastatin inhibit CYP3A4-mediated activation of clopidogrel	Use these statins at the lowest possible dose; otherwise, consider using an alternative statin

(*Continued*)

Primary Drug	Secondary Drug	Effect	Mechanism	Precautions
LIPID-LOWERING DRUGS				
STATINS	**ANTIVIRALS**			
STATINS	COBICISTAT	↑ Plasma levels of simvastatin and lovastatin	Inhibition of metabolism via CYP3A	Avoid coadministration. Atorvastatin—combination not recommended, use with caution, start at lowest dose of statin, monitor closely for adverse effects. Pravastatin and rosuvastatin are suitable alternatives
STATINS	NNRTIs	1. ↓ Levels of atorvastatin, pravastatin, and simvastatin with efavirenz 2. Possible reduced (lovastatin, rosuvastatin, simvastatin) or increased levels (fluvastatin, rosuvastatin) with etravirine 3. ↓ Plasma levels of atorvastatin but ↑ levels of active metabolites with rilpivarine	1. Efavirenz induces CYP3A4 and intestinal Pgp, which may ↓ bioavailability of some statins (including atorvastatin) 2. Likely altered metabolism via CYP3A4 (lovastatin, rosuvastatin, simvastatin) and CYP2C9 (fluvastatin, rosuvastatin) 3. Possibly altered metabolism via CYP enzymes	Monitor lipid profile more closely, titrate doses as necessary. Atorvastatin can be used in combination without initial dose adjustment, including with rilpivirine. No interaction expected with pravastatin
STATINS	PROTEASE INHIBITORS—BOCEPREVIR, TELAPREVIR	Boceprevir and telaprevir ↑ levels of atorvastatin, lovastatin, and simvastatin	Inhibition of CYP3A4-mediated metabolism and possibly inhibition of OATP1B1	1. Manufacturer advised avoiding coadministration of telaprevir and atorvastatin 2. Other statins should be used at the lowest effective dose when coadministered with telaprevir or boceprevir. Monitor lipid profile closely. Warn patients to report immediately if there is any muscle pain

(*Continued*)

Primary Drug	Secondary Drug	Effect	Mechanism	Precautions
LIPID-LOWERING DRUGS				
STATINS	PROTEASE INHIBITORS—DARUNAVIR, FOSAMPRENAVIR, LOPINAVIR, RITONAVIR, SAQUINAVIR, TIPRANAVIR	1. Marked ↑ levels of lovastatin and simvastatin 2. ↑ Levels of atorvastatin, rosuvastatin, and possibly pravastatin	Inhibition of CYP3A4-mediated metabolism of statins (each to a different extent)	1. Avoid coadministration 2. Manufacturer advised the following maximum doses of atorvastatin: a. 10 mg with tipranivir b. 20 mg with lopinavir c. 40 mg with darunavir, fosamprenavir, ritonavir, saquinavir Manufacturers advised the following maximum doses of rosuvastatin: a. 5 mg with tipranavir b. 10 mg with other protease inhibitors Pravastatin should be used at the lowest effective dose. Monitor lipid profile closely. Warn patients to report immediately if there is any muscle pain
STATINS	**CALCIUM CHANNEL BLOCKERS**			
STATINS	DIHYDROPYRIDINES	Slight ↑ plasma levels of simvastatin and possibly atorvastatin with amlodipine. Clinical relevance not clear	Uncertain	Manufacturer advises restricting dose of simvastatin to 20 mg when coadministered with amlodipine
STATINS	DILTIAZEM, VERAPAMIL	↑ Plasma levels of atorvastatin, lovastatin, and simvastatin; case reports of myopathy when atorvastatin and simvastatin are coadministered with diltiazem or verapamil	Inhibition of CYP3A4-mediated metabolism of statins	Watch for side effects of statins. Monitor lipid profile closely. The lowest effective dose should be used; manufacturers recommend: 1. simvastatin 20 mg with verapamil or diltiazem 2. lovastatin 20 mg with verapamil
STATINS	CARDIAC GLYCOSIDES	High-dose (80 mg) atorvastatin may ↑ digoxin levels	Atorvastatin inhibits intestinal Pgp, which ↑ digoxin absorption	Watch for digoxin toxicity

(*Continued*)

Primary Drug	Secondary Drug	Effect	Mechanism	Precautions
LIPID-LOWERING DRUGS				
STATINS	CNS STIMULANTS—MODAFINIL	↓ Levels of atorvastatin and simvastatin	Induction of CYP3A4-mediated metabolism of these statins	Monitor lipid profile closely and consider increasing the dose of statin
STATINS	DANAZOL	↑ Levels of simvastatin and lovastatin. ↑ Risk of adverse effects such as myopathy	Inhibition of CYP3A4-mediated metabolism of simvastatin and lovastatin	Manufacturers advise avoiding coadministration of simvastatin and danazol. It would seem sensible to also avoid coadministration of danazol and lovastatin
STATINS	ELTROMBOPAG	↑ Levels of rosuvastatin; theoretical risk with other statins	Uncertain; possible inhibitor of OATP1B1 transporter	Manufacturer advises halving dose of rosuvastatin. It would seem sensible to use lowest effective dose of other statins; monitor lipid profile closely. Warn patients to report immediately when any muscle pains
STATINS	GRAPEFRUIT JUICE	↑ Levels of simvastatin; slight rise with atorvastatin. ↑ Risk of adverse effects such as myopathy	Constituent of grapefruit juice inhibits CYP3A4-mediated metabolism of simvastatin	Patients taking simvastatin and atorvastatin should avoid grapefruit juice
STATINS	**LIPID-LOWERING DRUGS**			
STATINS	ANION EXCHANGE RESINS	Anion-binding resins ↓ the absorption of statins, but the overall lipid-lowering effect is not altered	Anion-binding resins bind statins in the intestine	Giving the statin 1 h before or 3–6 h after the anion exchange resin should minimize this effect
STATINS	FIBRATES	Gemfibrozil may ↑ atorvastatin, rosuvastatin, and simvastatin levels, with risk of myopathy with simvastatin	Uncertain	Avoid coadministration of simvastatin and fibrates. When using other statins, warn patients to watch for the features of myopathy
STATINS	NICOTINIC ACID	Slight risk of rhabdomyolysis	Uncertain at present	Monitor LFTs and CK closely; warn patients to report any features of rhabdomyolysis

(*Continued*)

Primary Drug	Secondary Drug	Effect	Mechanism	Precautions
LIPID-LOWERING DRUGS				
STATINS	PROTON PUMP INHIBITORS	Possible ↑ efficacy and adverse effects of atorvastatin	Inhibition of Pgp, reducing first-pass clearance	Monitor closely
STATINS	RANOLAZINE	↑ Levels of simvastatin and possibly atorvastatin and lovastatin	Inhibition of CYP 3A4 mediated metabolism	Warn patients to report immediately when muscles pain

Primary Drug	Secondary Drug	Effect	Mechanism	Precautions
NITRATES				
NITRATES	**ADDITIVE HYPOTENSIVE EFFECT**			
NITRATES	1. ANESTHETICS—GENERAL 2. ANTICANCER AND IMMUNOMODULATING DRUGS—INTERLEUKIN-2 (ALDESLEUKIN) 3. ANTI DEPRESSANTS—MAOIs 4. ANTIHYPERTENSIVES AND HEART FAILURE DRUGS 5. ANTI PSYCHOTICS 6. ANXIOLYTICS AND HYPNOTICS 7. BETA-BLOCKERS 8. CALCIUM CHANNEL BLOCKERS 9. DIURETICS 10. MUSCLE RELAXANTS—BACLOFEN, TIZANIDINE 11. PERIPHERAL VASODILATORS—MOXISYLYTE (THYMOXAMINE) 12. PHOSPHODIESTERSASE TYPE V INHIBITORS 13. POTASSIUM CHANNEL ACTIVATORS	↑ Hypotensive effect	Additive hypotensive effect	Monitor BP at least weekly until stable. Warn patients to report symptoms of hypotension (lightheadedness, dizziness on standing, etc.). During anesthesia, monitor BP closely, especially during induction of anesthesia

(Continued)

DRUGS ACTING ON THE CARDIOVASCULAR SYSTEM NITRATES

DRUGS ACTING ON THE CARDIOVASCULAR SYSTEM NITRATES

Primary Drug	Secondary Drug	Effect	Mechanism	Precautions
NITRATES				
NITRATES	PHOSPHODIESTERASE TYPE 5 INHIBITORS	Risk of severe ↓ BP and precipitation of myocardial infarction	Additive effect	Avoid coadministration
NITRATES	**ADDITIVE ANTIMUSCARINIC EFFECTS**			
NITRATES	1. ANALGESICS—nefopam 2. ANTIARRHYTHMICS—disopyramide, propafenone 3. ANTIDEPRESSANTS—TCAs 4. ANTIEMETICS—cyclizine 5. ANTIHISTAMINES—chlorphenamine, cyproheptadine, hydroxyzine 6. ANTIMUSCARINICS—atropine, benztropine, cyclopentolate, dicycloverine, flavoxate, homatropine, hyoscine, orphenadrine, oxybutynin, procyclidine, propantheline, tolterodine, trihexyphenidyl, tropicamide 7. ANTI-PARKINSON'S DRUGS—dopaminergics 8. ANTIPSYCHOTICS—phenothiazines, clozapine, pimozide 9. MUSCLE RELAXANTS—baclofen	↑ Risk of antimuscarinic side effects. *NB ↓ efficacy of sublingual nitrate tablets*	Additive effect; both drugs cause antimuscarinic side effects. *Antimuscarinic effects ↓ salivary production, which ↓ dissolution of the tablet*	Warn patient of this additive effect. *Consider changing the formulation to a sublingual nitrate spray*
NITRATES	ALCOHOL	↑ Risk of postural ↓ BP when GTN taken with alcohol	Additive effect; both vasodilators	Warn the patient about the risk of feeling faint. Advise patients to drink only in moderation and to avoid binge drinking
NITRATES	ANALGESICS—NSAIDs	Hypotensive effects of hydralazine, minoxidil, and nitroprusside antagonized by NSAIDs	NSAIDs cause sodium and water retention in the kidney and can raise BP due to ↓ production of vasodilating renal prostaglandins	Monitor BP at least weekly until stable

(*Continued*)

Primary Drug	Secondary Drug	Effect	Mechanism	Precautions
NITRATES				
NITRATES	**ANTICANCER AND IMMUNOMODULATING DRUGS**			
NITRATES	BORTEZOMIB	↑ Hypotensive effect	Additive hypotensive effect	Monitor BP at least weekly until stable, particularly on initiation of therapy
NITRATES	CORTICOSTEROIDS	Antihypertensive effects of nitrates are antagonized by corticosteroids	Mineralocorticoids cause sodium and water retention	Monitor BP at least weekly until stable
NITRATES	PROCARBAZINE	Hypotension	Additive	Monitor closely
NITRATES	ANTICOAGULANTS—HEPARINS	Possible ↓ efficacy of heparin with GTN infusion	Uncertain	Monitor APTT closely
NITRATES	ANTIHYPERTENSIVES AND HEART FAILURE DRUGS	↑ Hypotensive effect	Additive hypotensive effect; may be used therapeutically	Monitor BP at least weekly until stable. Warn patients to report symptoms of hypotension (light-headedness, dizziness on standing, etc.)
NITRATES	ANTI-PARKINSON'S DRUGS—APOMORPHINE	Risk of ↑ hypotensive effect	Not clear—effect seen with vasodilators but not other antihypertensives	Monitor BP closely, especially during initiation of treatment. Warn patients to report symptoms of hypotension (light-headedness, dizziness on standing, etc.)
NITRATES	ANTIPLATELET AGENTS—ASPIRIN	↓ Antihypertensive effect with aspirin; effect not noted with low-dose aspirin	Aspirin may cause sodium retention and vasoconstriction at possibly both renal and endothelial sites	Monitor BP at least weekly until stable
NITRATES	DIURETICS	↑ Hypotensive effect	Additive hypotensive effect	Monitor BP at least weekly until stable. Warn patients to report symptoms of hypotension (light-headedness, dizziness on standing, etc.)

(Continued)

DRUGS ACTING ON THE CARDIOVASCULAR SYSTEM NITRATES

Primary Drug	Secondary Drug	Effect	Mechanism	Precautions
NITRATES				
NITRATES	ESTROGENS	↓ Antihypertensive effect of nitrates	Estrogens may cause fluid retention, and use of estrogens with hypertension needs to be closely monitored	Monitor BP at least weekly until stable; watch for poor response to nitrates
NITRATES	POTASSIUM CHANNEL ACTIVATORS	↑ Hypotensive effect	Additive effect	Monitor BP closely
NITRATES	PROSTAGLANDINS—ALPROSTADIL	↑ Risk of ↓ BP	Additive hypotensive effect	Monitor BP at least weekly until stable. Warn patients to report symptoms of hypotension (light-headedness, dizziness on standing, etc.)
NITRATES	SAPROPTERIN	↑ Hypotensive effect	Additive hypotensive effect	Monitor BP at least weekly until stable. Warn patients to report symptoms of hypotension (light-headedness, dizziness on standing, etc.)

Primary Drug	Secondary Drug	Effect	Mechanism	Precautions
PERIPHERAL VASODILATORS				
CILOSTAZOL				
CILOSTAZOL	ANAGRELIDE	Risk of adverse effects	Additive effect; anagrelide has phosphodiesterase inhibitory activity	Avoid coadministration
CILOSTAZOL	**ANTIBIOTICS**			
CILOSTAZOL	MACROLIDES	Cilostazol levels ↑ by erythromycin and possibly clarithromycin	Erythromycin and clarithromycin inhibit CYP3A4-mediated metabolism of cilostazol	Avoid coadministration
CILOSTAZOL	RIFAMPICIN	Theoretical risk of ↓ cilostazol levels	Induction of CYP3A4 by rifampicin	Monitor for evidence of poor response to cilostazol

(*Continued*)

Primary Drug	Secondary Drug	Effect	Mechanism	Precautions
PERIPHERAL VASODILATORS				
CILOSTAZOL	ANTIDEPRESSANTS—SSRIs	Fluoxetine, fluvoxamine, nefazodone, and sertraline ↑ cilostazol levels	Fluoxetine, fluvoxamine, and sertraline inhibit CYP3A4-mediated metabolism of cilostazol	Avoid coadministration
CILOSTAZOL	ANTIEPILEPTICS—CARBAMAZEPINE, PHENOBARBITAL, PHENYTOIN	Theoretical risk of ↓ cilostazol levels	Induction of CYP3A4 by these antiepileptics	Monitor for evidence of poor response to cilostazol
CILOSTAZOL	ANTIFUNGALS	Fluconazole, itraconazole, ketoconazole, and miconazole ↑ cilostazol levels	These azoles inhibit CYP3A4-mediated metabolism of cilostazol	Avoid coadministration
CILOSTAZOL	ANTIPLATELETS	Possible ↑ risk of bleeding. Low-dose aspirin (<80 mg) appears to be safe	1. Additive effect; cilostazol has antiplatelet activity 2. Clopidogrel ↑ the levels of a metabolite of cilostazol that has high antiplatelet activity, by an uncertain mechanism	Warn the patient to report any signs of ↑ bleeding
CILOSTAZOL	ANTIVIRALS—PROTEASE INHIBITORS	Amprenavir, indinavir, lopinavir, nelfinavir, ritonavir, and saquinavir ↑ cilostazol levels	These protease inhibitors inhibit CYP3A4-mediated metabolism of cilostazol	Reduce dose of cilostazol to 50 mg twice daily
CILOSTAZOL	ANXIOLYTICS AND HYPNOTICS	Midazolam ↑ cilostazol levels	Midazolam inhibits CYP3A4-mediated metabolism of cilostazol	Avoid coadministration
CILOSTAZOL	CALCIUM CHANNEL BLOCKERS	↑ Plasma concentrations and efficacy of cilostazol with diltiazem, verapamil, and nifedipine	These calcium channel blockers inhibit CYP3A4-mediated metabolism of cilostazol	Avoid coadministration
CILOSTAZOL	FOOD	Cilostazol levels are ↑ by taking it with a high-fat meal	Uncertain	Take cilostazol at least 30 min before or 2 h after a meal

(Continued)

DRUGS ACTING ON THE CARDIOVASCULAR SYSTEM PERIPHERAL VASODILATORS

Primary Drug	Secondary Drug	Effect	Mechanism	Precautions
PERIPHERAL VASODILATORS				
CILOSTAZOL	H2 RECEPTOR BLOCKERS	Cimetidine ↑ cilostazol levels	Cimetidine inhibits CYP3A4-mediated metabolism of cilostazol	Avoid coadministration
CILOSTAZOL	PROTON PUMP INHIBITORS	Cilostazol levels are ↑ by omeprazole and possibly lansoprazole	Omeprazole inhibits CYP2C19-mediated metabolism of cilostazol	Avoid concomitant use. U.S. manufacturer advises halving the dose of cilostazol
MOXISYLYTE (THYMOXAMINE)				
MOXISYLYTE	**ADDITIVE HYPOTENSIVE EFFECT**			
MOXISYLYTE	1. ANESTHETICS—GENERAL 2. ANTICANCER AND IMMUNOMODULATING DRUGS—INTERLEUKIN-2 (ALDESLEUKIN) 3. ANTIDEPRESSANTS—MAOIS 4. ANTIHYPERTENSIVES AND HEART FAILURE DRUGS 5. ANTIPSYCHOTICS 6. ANXIOLYTICS AND HYPNOTICS 7. BETA-BLOCKERS 8. CALCIUM CHANNEL BLOCKERS 9. DIURETICS 10. MUSCLE RELAXANTS—baclofen, tizanidine 11. NITRATES 12. POTASSIUM CHANNEL ACTIVATORS	↑ Hypotensive effect	Additive hypotensive effect	Monitor BP at least weekly until stable. Warn patients to report symptoms of hypotension (light-headedness, dizziness on standing, etc.). During anesthesia, monitor BP closely, especially during induction of anesthesia
MOXISYLYTE	PROSTAGLANDINS—ALPROSTADIL	Risk of priapism if intracavernous alprostadil is given with moxisylyte	Additive effect	Avoid coadministration
PENTOXIFYLLINE				
PENTOXIFYLLINE	ANALGESICS—NSAIDs	Risk of bleeding when pentoxifylline is given with ketorolac post surgery	Uncertain; possibly additive antiplatelet effect	Avoid coadministration of pentoxifylline and ketorolac

(*Continued*)

Primary Drug	Secondary Drug	Effect	Mechanism	Precautions
PERIPHERAL VASODILATORS				
PENTOXIFYLLINE	ANTIBIOTICS	Ciprofloxacin may ↑ pentoxifylline levels	Uncertain; likely to be due to inhibition of hepatic metabolism	Warn patients of the possibility of adverse effects of pentoxifylline
PENTOXIFYLLINE	ANTICOAGULANTS—ORAL	Case reports of major hemorrhage when pentoxifylline was given with acenocoumarol	Uncertain; possibly additive effect (pentoxifylline has an antiplatelet action)	Monitor INR closely
PENTOXIFYLLINE	BRONCHODILATORS—THEOPHYLLINE	Possibly ↑ theophylline levels	Uncertain; possibly competitive inhibition of theophylline metabolism (pentoxifylline is also a xanthine derivative)	Warn patients of the possibility of adverse effects of theophylline; monitor levels if necessary
PENTOXIFYLLINE	H2 RECEPTOR BLOCKERS	Cimetidine may ↑ pentoxifylline levels	Uncertain; likely to be due to inhibition of hepatic metabolism	Avoid coadministration

Primary Drug	Secondary Drug	Effect	Mechanism	Precautions
POTASSIUM CHANNEL ACTIVATORS—FOR EXAMPLE, NICORANDIL				
POTASSIUM CHANNEL ACTIVATORS	ALCOHOL	Acute alcohol ingestion may ↑ hypotensive effects. Chronic moderate/heavy drinking ↓ hypotensive effect	Additive hypotensive effect. Mechanism of opposite effect with chronic intake is uncertain	Monitor BP closely as unpredictable responses can occur. Advise patients to drink only in moderation and avoid large variations in the amount of alcohol drunk
POTASSIUM CHANNEL ACTIVATORS	ANESTHETICS—GENERAL	↑ Hypotensive effect	Additive effect	Monitor BP closely
POTASSIUM CHANNEL ACTIVATORS	**ANTICANCER AND IMMUNOMODULATING DRUGS**			
POTASSIUM CHANNEL ACTIVATORS	BORTEZOMIB	↑ Hypotensive effect	Additive hypotensive effect	Monitor BP at least weekly until stable, particularly on initiation of therapy

(Continued)

Primary Drug	Secondary Drug	Effect	Mechanism	Precautions
POTASSIUM CHANNEL ACTIVATORS—FOR EXAMPLE, NICORANDIL				
POTASSIUM CHANNEL ACTIVATORS	CORTICOSTEROIDS	Possible ↑ risk of gastric perforation	Uncertain	Monitor closely
POTASSIUM CHANNEL ACTIVATORS	INTERLEUKIN-2 (ALDESLEUKIN)	↑ Hypotensive effect	Additive effect	Monitor BP closely
POTASSIUM CHANNEL ACTIVATORS	ANTIDEPRESSANTS—MAOIs	↑ Hypotensive effect	Additive hypotensive effect. Postural ↓ BP is a common side effect of MAOIs	Monitor BP at least weekly until stable. Warn patients to report symptoms of hypotension (light-headedness, dizziness on standing, etc.)
POTASSIUM CHANNEL ACTIVATORS	ANTIHYPERTENSIVES AND HEART FAILURE DRUGS	↑ Hypotensive effect	Additive effect	Monitor BP closely
POTASSIUM CHANNEL ACTIVATORS	ANTIPSYCHOTICS	↑ Hypotensive effect	Additive effect	Monitor BP closely
POTASSIUM CHANNEL ACTIVATORS	ANXIOLYTICS AND HYPNOTICS	↑ Hypotensive effect	Additive effect	Monitor BP closely
POTASSIUM CHANNEL ACTIVATORS	BETA-BLOCKERS	↑ Hypotensive effect	Additive effect	Monitor BP closely
POTASSIUM CHANNEL ACTIVATORS	CALCIUM CHANNEL BLOCKERS	↑ Hypotensive effect	Additive effect	Monitor BP closely
POTASSIUM CHANNEL ACTIVATORS	DIURETICS	↑ Hypotensive effect	Additive effect	Monitor BP at least weekly until stable. Warn patients to report symptoms of hypotension (light-headedness, dizziness on standing, etc.)
POTASSIUM CHANNEL ACTIVATORS	MUSCLE RELAXANTS—BACLOFEN, TIZANIDINE	↑ Hypotensive effect	Additive effect	Monitor BP closely
POTASSIUM CHANNEL ACTIVATORS	NITRATES	↑ Hypotensive effect	Additive effect	Monitor BP closely

(*Continued*)

Primary Drug	Secondary Drug	Effect	Mechanism	Precautions
POTASSIUM CHANNEL ACTIVATORS—FOR EXAMPLE, NICORANDIL				
POTASSIUM CHANNEL ACTIVATORS	PERIPHERAL VASODILATORS—MOXISYLYTE (THYMOXAMINE)	↑ Hypotensive effect	Additive effect	Monitor BP at least weekly until stable. Warn patients to report symptoms of hypotension (light-headedness, dizziness on standing, etc.). During anesthesia, monitor BP closely, especially during induction of anesthesia
POTASSIUM CHANNEL ACTIVATORS	PHOSPHODIESTERASE TYPE 5 INHIBITORS	Risk of severe ↓ BP	Additive effect	Avoid coadministration

Primary Drug	Secondary Drug	Effect	Mechanism	Precautions
RANOLAZINE				
RANOLAZINE	**DRUGS THAT PROLONG THE QT INTERVAL**			
Ranolazine	1. ANTIARRHYTHMICS—ajmaline, amiodarone, azimilide, cibenzoline, disopyramide, dofetilide, dronedarone, ibutilide, procainamide, propafenone, quinidine 2. ANTIBIOTICS—macrolides (especially azithromycin, clarithromycin, parenteral erythromycin, telithromycin), quinolones (especially moxifloxacin), quinupristin/dalfopristin 3. ANTICANCER AND IMMUNOMODULATING DRUGS—arsenic trioxide, bosutinib, crizotinib, dasatinib, eribulin, fingolimod, lapatinib, nilotinib, pazopanib, sunitinib, vandetanib, vemurafenib 4. ANTIDEPRESSANTS—TCAs, venlafaxine	Risk of ventricular arrhythmias, particularly torsades de pointes	Additive effect; these drugs prolong the QT interval	Avoid coadministration

(Continued)

DRUGS ACTING ON THE CARDIOVASCULAR SYSTEM RANOLAZINE

Primary Drug	Secondary Drug	Effect	Mechanism	Precautions
RANOLAZINE				
	5. ANTIEMETICS—ondansetron 6. ANTIFUNGALS—fluconazole, posaconazole, voriconazole 7. ANTIHISTAMINES—terfenadine, hydroxyzine, mizolastine 8. ANTIHYPERTENSIVES—ketanserin 9. ANTIMALARIALS—artemether with lumefantrine, chloroquine, halofantrine, hydroxychloroquine, mefloquine, quinine 10. ANTIPROTOZOALS—pentamidine isethionate 11. ANTIPSYCHOTICS—atypicals, phenothiazines, pimozide 12. ANTIVIRALS—boceprevir, rilpivirine, telaprevir 13. BETA-BLOCKERS—sotalol 14. BRONCHODILATORS—parenteral bronchodilators 15. CNS STIMULANTS—atomoxetine			
RANOLAZINE	ANTIARRHYTHMICS—FLECAINIDE, PROPAFENONE	Possible ↑ flecainide and propafenone levels	Inhibition of CYP2D6-mediated metabolism of flecainide and propafenone	Monitor PR and BP closely
RANOLAZINE	ANTIBIOTICS—RIFAMPICIN	↓ Ranolazine levels with rifampicin	Induction of CYP 3A4-mediated metabolism of ranolazine	Manufacturer advises to avoid coadministration
RANOLAZINE	**ANTICANCER AND OTHER IMMUNOMODULATING DRUGS**			
RANOLAZINE	AFATINIB	Possible ↑ in afatinib levels	P-glycoprotein inhibition	Manufacturer recommends staggered dosing 6–12 h apart or dose reduction
RANOLAZINE	CICLOSPORIN	↑ Levels of both ciclosporin and ranolazine when coadministered	Mutual inhibition of Pgp	1. Watch for ciclosporin toxicity; ↓ dose as necessary and monitor levels if available 2. Monitor ECG carefully—titrate dose accordingly

(*Continued*)

Primary Drug	Secondary Drug	Effect	Mechanism	Precautions
RANOLAZINE				
RANOLAZINE	PONATINIB	Predicted ↑ in levels of ranolazine	P-glycoprotein inhibition	Be aware
RANOLAZINE	TACROLIMUS	↑ Tacrolimus levels	Possibly CYP3A4 and P-glycoprotein inhibition	Monitor tacrolimus levels closely
RANOLAZINE	ANTIDEPRESSANTS—ST. JOHN'S WORT	↓ Ranolazine levels with St. John's wort	Induction of CYP3A4-mediated metabolism of ranolazine	Manufacturer advises to avoid coadministration
RANOLAZINE	ANTIEPILEPTICS	↓ Ranolazine levels with carbamazepine, phenobarbitone, and phenytoin	Induction of CYP3A4-mediated metabolism of ranolazine	Manufacturer advises to avoid coadministration
RANOLAZINE	ANTIGOUT DRUGS—COLCHICINE	↑ Colchicine levels	Combination of inhibition of CYP3A4 and Pgp	Reduce dose of colchicine—monitor FBC regularly and warn patients to report features of colchicine toxicity (GI upset, muscle aches, sore throat)
RANOLAZINE	BETA-BLOCKERS	↑ Metoprolol levels	Inhibition of CYP2D6-mediated metabolism of metoprolol	Monitor PR and BP closely
RANOLAZINE	CALCIUM CHANNEL BLOCKERS—DILTIAZEM, VERAPAMIL	↑ Ranolazine levels	Inhibition of CYP3A4-mediated metabolism of ranolazine	May be used therapeutically. Reduce dose of ranolazine
RANOLAZINE	CARDIAC GLYCOSIDES—DIGOXIN	↑ Digoxin levels	Inhibition of Pgp	Monitor digoxin levels closely until stable
RANOLAZINE	ELIGLUSTAT	↑ Eliglustat levels	Inhibition of CYP3A4-mediated metabolism	Avoid coadministration in poor metabolizers
RANOLAZINE	LIPID LOWERING DRUGS	↑ Levels of simvastatin and possibly atorvastatin and lovastatin	Inhibition of CYP3A4 mediated metabolism	Warn patients to report immediately muscle pain
RANOLAZINE	NITISINONE	Possible ↑ nitisinone levels	Inhibition of CYP3A4-mediated metabolism	Monitor carefully

DRUGS ACTING ON THE CARDIOVASCULAR SYSTEM RANOLAZINE

DRUGS ACTING ON THE CARDIOVASCULAR SYSTEM SYMPATHOMIMETICS

Primary Drug	Secondary Drug	Effect	Mechanism	Precautions
SELECTIVE PHOSPHODIESTERASE INHIBITORS				
ENOXIMONE, MILRINONE	ANAGRELIDE	Risk of adverse effects	Additive effect; anagrelide has phosphodiesterase inhibitory activity	Avoid coadministration
ENOXIMONE	BRONCHODILATORS—THEOPHYLLINE	Theophylline may ↓ efficacy of enoximone	Possibly competitive inhibition of selective phosphodiesterases	Be aware; watch for poor response to enoximone

Primary Drug	Secondary Drug	Effect	Mechanism	Precautions
SYMPATHOMIMETICS				
SYMPATHOMIMETICS	**ANESTHETICS–GENERAL**			
DIRECT	ANESTHETICS–GENERAL	1. Risk of arrhythmias when inhalational anesthetics are coadministered with epinephrine or norepinephrine 2. Case report of marked ↑ BP when phenylephrine eye drops were given during general anesthesia	1. The arrhythmogenic threshold with injected epinephrine is lower with halothane than isoflurane or enflurane, which is attributed to sensitization to beta-adrenoceptor stimulation 2. Uncertain. Phenylephrine produces its effects by acting on alpha-adrenergic receptors; possible that these effects are enhanced	1. Use epinephrine in the smallest possible dose (when using 1:100,000 = 10 μg/mL infiltration to ↓ intraoperative bleeding, no more than 10 mL/10 min and less than 30 mL/h should be given). Prevent carbon dioxide retention during anesthesia as carbon dioxide increases sensitizing effect 2. Avoid use of phenylephrine eye drops during anesthesia
INDIRECT	ANESTHETICS—GENERAL	1. Risk of arrhythmias when inhalational anesthetics are coadministered with methylphenidate 2. Case report of ↓ sedative effect of midazolam and ketamine from methylphenidate	1. Uncertain; it is possible that inhalational anesthetics sensitize the myocardium to sympathetic stimulation 2. Uncertain at present	Avoid giving methylphenidate on the day of elective surgery

(Continued)

Primary Drug	Secondary Drug	Effect	Mechanism	Precautions
SYMPATHOMIMETICS				
INDIRECT	ANALGESICS	Dexamfetamine and methylphenidate ↑ the analgesic effects and ↓ the sedation of opioids when used for chronic pain	Uncertain; complex interaction between the sympathetic nervous system and the opioid receptors	Opioid requirements may be ↓ when patients also take indirect sympathomimetics
SYMPATHOMIMETICS	ANTACIDS—SODIUM BICARBONATE	Possibly ↑ ephedrine/pseudoephedrine levels	Alkalinizing urine ↓ excretion of these sympathomimetics	Watch for early features of toxicity
SYMPATHOMIMETICS	**ANTIBIOTICS**			
INDIRECT	FURAZOLIDINE	Risk of delayed onset ↑ BP	Metabolite of furazolidine has MAOI activity, which inhibits the breakdown of indirect sympathomimetics	Manufacturer advises against coadministration
SYMPATHOMIMETICS	LINEZOLID	Risk of ↑ BP when linezolid is coingested with either direct or indirect sympathomimetics	Linezolid causes accumulation of norepinephrine at the nerve ends; sympathomimetics stimulate the release of these ↑ reserves of norepinephrine, which in turn causes vasoconstriction and a rise in BP	Monitor BP closely; watch for ↑ BP. Warn patients taking linezolid not to take OTC remedies containing sympathomimetics
DIRECT	VANCOMYCIN	Vancomycin levels are ↓ by dobutamine or dopamine	Uncertain at present	Monitor vancomycin levels closely
SYMPATHOMIMETICS	**ANTICANCER AND IMMUNOMODULATING DRUGS**			
INDIRECT	CICLOSPORIN	Methylphenidate may ↑ ciclosporin levels	Uncertain at present	Watch for ciclosporin toxicity; ↓ levels as necessary and monitor levels if available

(Continued)

DRUGS ACTING ON THE CARDIOVASCULAR SYSTEM SYMPATHOMIMETICS

Primary Drug	Secondary Drug	Effect	Mechanism	Precautions
SYMPATHOMIMETICS				
INDIRECT	CORTICOSTEROIDS	Ephedrine may ↓ dexamethasone levels	Uncertain at present	Watch for poor response to dexamethasone; uncertain at present if other corticosteroids are similarly affected
SYMPATHOMIMETICS	PROCARBAZINE	Coadministration of ephedrine, metaraminol, methylphenidate, phenylephrine, or pseudoephedrine (including nasal and ophthalmic solutions) with procarbazine may cause a prolongation and ↑ intensity of the cardiac stimulant effects and effects on BP, which may lead to headache, arrhythmias, hypertensive, or hyperpyretic crisis	The metabolism of sympathomimetics is impaired due to an inhibition of MAO	It is recommended that sympathomimetics not be administered during and within 14 days of stopping procarbazine. Do not use any OTC nasal decongestants (sprays or oral preparations) or asthma relief agents without consulting the pharmacist/doctor
INDIRECT	ANTICOAGULANTS	Methylphenidate may ↑ efficacy of warfarin	Uncertain at present	Monitor INR closely
SYMPATHOMIMETICS	**ANTIDEPRESSANTS**			
DIRECT	MAOIs	Risk of adrenergic syndrome—see before. Unlikely to occur with moclobemide and selegiline. This is likely with some OTC medications, which may contain some of these sympathomimetics	Due to inhibition of MAOI, which breaks down sympathomimetics. Moclobemide is involved in the breakdown of serotonin, while selegiline is mainly involved in the breakdown of dopamine	Avoid concurrent use. Onset may be 6–24 h after ingestion. Do an ECG; measure electrolytes, FBC, CK, and coagulation profile. Before prescribing/dispensing, enquire about the use of MAOI antidepressants and related drugs such as linezolid

(*Continued*)

Primary Drug	Secondary Drug	Effect	Mechanism	Precautions
SYMPATHOMIMETICS				
INDIRECT	SSRIs	1. Case report of serotonin syndrome when dexamfetamine was coadministered with citalopram 2. Case reports of psychiatric disturbances when methylphenidate was given with sertraline and phenylpropanolamine coadministered with phenylpropanolamine	1. Uncertain; postulated that it is an additive effect of the inhibition of serotonin reuptake by citalopram with the release of serotonin by venlafaxine 2. Uncertain	1. Avoid coadministration of dexamfetamine and citalopram 2. Warn patients to watch for early signs such as anxiety
INDIRECT	TCAs	1. Methylphenidate ↑ TCA levels, which may improve their efficacy, but cases of toxicity with imipramine have been reported 2. TCAs possibly ↓ efficacy of indirect sympathomimetics	1. Uncertain; postulated to be due to inhibition of the hepatic metabolism of TCAs 2. Indirect sympathomimetics cause release of norepinephrine from the nerve endings; this is blocked by TCAs	1. Warn patients to watch for early signs of ↑ TCA efficacy such as drowsiness and dry mouth 2. Watch for poor response to indirect sympathomimetics
DIRECT	TCAs	↑ Efficacy of norepinephrine, epinephrine, or phenylephrine when coadministered with TCAs; risk of ↑ BP and tachyarrhythmias	TCAs block reuptake of norepinephrine into the nerve terminals, which prolongs its activity	Monitor PR, BP, and ECG closely; start inotropes at a lower dose. It would be advisable to monitor PR and BP even when using local anesthetics containing epinephrine, although there is no evidence of significant toxicity
INDIRECT	OTHER—VENLAFAXINE	Case report of serotonin syndrome when dexamfetamine was coadministered with venlafaxine	Uncertain; postulated to be an additive effect of the inhibition of serotonin reuptake by venlafaxine and the release of serotonin by venlafaxine	Avoid coadministration

(Continued)

DRUGS ACTING ON THE CARDIOVASCULAR SYSTEM SYMPATHOMIMETICS

Primary Drug	Secondary Drug	Effect	Mechanism	Precautions
SYMPATHOMIMETICS				
SYMPATHOMIMETICS—EPINEPHRINE	ANTIDIABETIC DRUGS	May ↑ antidiabetic therapy requirement	Epinephrine causes the release of glucose from the liver and is an important defence/homeostatic mechanism. Hyperglycemia may occur due to an antagonistic effect	Larger doses of antidiabetic therapy may be needed during the period of epinephrine use, which is usually in the short term or in emergency situations
SYMPATHOMIMETICS—DOPAMINE	ANTIEPILEPTICS—PHENYTOIN	Reports of severe hypotension when parenteral phenytoin is given to patients on dopamine	Uncertain; possibly additive effect (phenytoin can cause hypotension especially if given rapidly)	Use phenytoin with extreme caution; if needed, infuse it slowly
SYMPATHOMIMETICS	**ANTIHYPERTENSIVES AND HEART FAILURE DRUGS**			
SYMPATHOMIMETICS	ACE INHIBITORS, ADRENERGIC NEURON BLOCKERS	↓ Hypotensive effect. Note there is a risk of interactions even with topical sympathomimetics (eye and nose drops)	Adrenergic neurone blockers act mainly by preventing release of norepinephrine. Sympathomimetics ↑ cardiac output and/or cause vasoconstriction	Monitor BP at least weekly until stable
DIRECT	ADRENERGIC NEURON BLOCKERS	For patients on guanethidine 1. ↑ Pressor effects have been reported with the coadministration of norepinephrine or metaraminol 2. Lower threshold for arrhythmias with coadministration of norepinephrine 3. Prolonged mydriasis has been reported when eye drops were given to patients on guanethidine	Guanethidine blocks the release of norepinephrine from adrenergic neurones; this causes a hypersensitivity of the receptors that are normally stimulated by norepinephrine, and leads to the ↑ response when they are stimulated by directly acting sympathomimetics	Start alpha- and beta-1 agonists at a lower dose; monitor BP and cardiac rhythm closely

(*Continued*)

Primary Drug	Secondary Drug	Effect	Mechanism	Precautions
SYMPATHOMIMETICS				
DIRECT	CENTRALLY ACTING ANTIHYPERTENSIVES	Risk of ↑ BP when clonidine is given with epinephrine or norepinephrine	Additive effect; clonidine use is associated with ↑ circulating catecholamines	Monitor BP at least weekly until stable
INDIRECT	CENTRALLY ACTING ANTIHYPERTENSIVES	1. Indirect sympathomimetics may ↓ the hypotensive effect of methyldopa 2. Methyldopa may ↓ the mydriatic effect of ephedrine eye drops	1. Uncertain 2. Uncertain	Monitor BP at least weekly until stable; watch for poor response to methyldopa
DIRECT	VASODILATOR ANTIHYPERTENSIVES	Case reports of ↑ tachycardia when epinephrine was given for perioperative ↓ BP in patients on hydralazine	Additive effect	Avoid coadministration
SYMPATHOMIMETICS	ANTIMUSCARINICS—ATROPINE	Reports of hypertension when atropine was given to patients receiving 10% phenylephrine eye drops during eye surgery	Atropine abolishes the cholinergic response to phenylephrine-induced vasoconstriction	Use a lower concentration of phenylephrine
SYMPATHOMIMETICS—INCLUDING CENTRALLY ACTING APPETITE SUPPRESSANTS AND TOPICAL DECONGESTANTS	ANTIOBESITY DRUGS—SIBUTRAMINE	Risk of marked hypertension	Additive effect	Manufacturer advises against coadministration
SYMPATHOMIMETICS	**ANTI-PARKINSON'S DRUGS**			
INDIRECT	BROMOCRIPTINE	Case reports of severe, symptomatic ↑ BP when coadministered with indirect sympathomimetics	Likely additive effect; both can cause ↑ BP	Monitor BP closely; watch for ↑ BP

(Continued)

Primary Drug	Secondary Drug	Effect	Mechanism	Precautions
SYMPATHOMIMETICS				
INDIRECT	ENTACAPONE	Cases of severe, symptomatic ↑ BP when coadministered with indirect sympathomimetics	Likely additive effect; both can cause ↑ BP	Monitor BP closely; watch for ↑ BP
SYMPATHOMIMETICS	RASAGILINE	Risk of adrenergic syndrome—see before	Due to inhibition of MAOI, which breaks down sympathomimetics	Avoid concurrent use. Onset may be 6–24 h after ingestion. Do ECG; measure electrolytes, FBC, CK. and coagulation profile
DIRECT	SELEGILINE	Case report of ↑ hypertensive effect of dopamine when it was given to a patient already taking selegiline	Selegiline inhibits metabolism of dopamine	Titrate dopamine carefully
SYMPATHOMIMETICS—DOBUTAMINE	ANTIPLATELETS—DIPYRIDAMOLE	Case reports of marked hypotension when given together	Uncertain	Avoid coadministration
SYMPATHOMIMETICS	**ANTIPSYCHOTICS**			
SYMPATHOMIMETICS	ANTIPSYCHOTICS	Hypertensive effect of sympathomimetics is antagonized by antipsychotics	Dose-related ↓ BP (due to vasodilatation) is a side effect of most antipsychotics, particularly phenothiazines	Monitor BP closely
INDIRECT	ANTIPSYCHOTICS	1. Case reports of paralytic ileus with trifluoperazine and methylphenidate 2. Case report of acute dystonias with haloperidol and dexamfetamine 3. ↓ Efficacy of chlorpromazine when dexamfetamine was added	1. Additive anticholinergic effect 2. Uncertain; possibly due to ↑ dopamine release 3. Uncertain	1. Watch for signs of altered bowel habit 2. Warn patients of this rare interaction 3. Avoid coadministration

(*Continued*)

Primary Drug	Secondary Drug	Effect	Mechanism	Precautions
SYMPATHOMIMETICS				
SYMPATHOMIMETICS	ANTIVIRALS—PROTEASE INHIBITORS	1. Risk of serotonin syndrome when dexamfetamine is administered with ritonavir 2. Indinavir may ↑ phenylpropanolamine levels 3. Possibly ↑ plasma levels of amphetamine derivatives, e.g., methylphenidate with ritonavir or tipranavir	1. Protease inhibitors inhibit CYP2D6-mediated metabolism 2. Likely inhibition of phenylpropanolamine metabolism 3. Inhibition of metabolism via CYP2D6	1. Avoid coadministration 2. Monitor BP closely; watch for marked ↑ BP 3. Monitor therapeutic efficacy and adverse effects closely
SYMPATHOMIMETICS	**BETA-BLOCKERS**			
DIRECT	BETA-BLOCKERS	1. Severe ↑ BP and bradycardia with noncardioselective beta-blockers (including reports of severe ↑ BP in patients given infiltrations of local anesthetics containing epinephrine, and one case of a fatal reaction with phenylephrine eye drops) 2. Patients on beta-blockers may respond poorly to epinephrine when given to treat anaphylaxis	1. Unopposed alpha stimulation causes vasoconstriction, which results in a rise in BP. Beta-2 receptors, when stimulated, cause vasodilatation, which counteracts any alpha action; nonselective beta-blockers antagonize beta-2 receptors 2. Uncertain mechanism	1. Monitor BP at least weekly until stable. When using local anesthetics with epinephrine, use small volumes of low concentrations (such as 1 in 200,000 epinephrine); avoid high concentrations (e.g., 1 in 1,000 mixtures) 2. Look for failure of epinephrine therapy and consider using salbutamol, isoprenaline, or glucagon
INDIRECT	BETA-BLOCKERS	↓ Hypotensive efficacy of beta-blockers	The hypertensive effect of sympathomimetics opposes the hypotensive actions of beta-blockers	Monitor BP at least weekly until stable; watch for poor response to beta-blockers
SYMPATHOMIMETICS	BICARBONATE	Possibly ↑ ephedrine/pseudoephedrine levels	Alkalinizing urine ↓ the excretion of these sympathomimetics	Watch for early features of toxicity (tremor, insomnia, and tachycardia)

(*Continued*)

DRUGS ACTING ON THE CARDIOVASCULAR SYSTEM SYMPATHOMIMETICS

DRUGS ACTING ON THE CARDIOVASCULAR SYSTEM SYMPATHOMIMETICS

Primary Drug	Secondary Drug	Effect	Mechanism	Precautions
SYMPATHOMIMETICS				
SYMPATHOMIMETICS	**BRONCHODILATORS**			
INDIRECT	THEOPHYLLINE	↑ Incidence of side effects of theophylline (without a change in its serum concentrations) when coadministered with ephedrine	Uncertain	Warn patients to avoid OTC remedies containing ephedrine
DIRECT	THEOPHYLLINE	Case report of marked tachycardia when dobutamine was given to a patient already taking theophylline	Uncertain	Carefully titrate the dose of dobutamine in patients taking dobutamine
DIRECT	CALCIUM COMPOUNDS	Parenteral calcium administration may ↓ the positive inotropic effects of epinephrine and dobutamine	Uncertain; postulated that calcium modulates the signal transmission from the receptor	Monitor BP closely; watch for poor response to these inotropes
SYMPATHOMIMETICS	CNS STIMULANTS—MODAFINIL	May ↓ modafinil levels with dexamfetamine, methylphenidate	Due to delayed absorption	Be aware
SYMPATHOMIMETICS	DOXAPRAM	Risk of ↑ BP	Uncertain at present	Monitor BP closely
SYMPATHOMIMETICS	**DRUG DEPENDENCE THERAPIES**			
AMPHETAMINES	BUPROPION	1. ↑ Plasma concentrations of these substrates, with risk of toxic effects 2. ↑ Risk of seizures. This risk is marked in elderly people, patients with a history of seizures, those with an addiction to opiates/cocaine/stimulants, and those with diabetes treated with oral hypoglycemics or insulin	1. Bupropion and its metabolite hydroxybupropion inhibit CYP2D6 2. Bupropion is associated with a dose-related risk of seizures. These drugs that lower seizure threshold are individually epileptogenic. They have additive effects when combined	1. Initiate therapy with these drugs, particularly those with a narrow therapeutic index, at the lowest effective dose. Interaction is likely to be important with substrates for which CYP2D6 is considered the only metabolic pathway (e.g., amphetamines) 2. Extreme caution. The dose of bupropion should not exceed 450 mg/day (or 150 mg/day in those with severe hepatic cirrhosis)

(*Continued*)

Primary Drug	Secondary Drug	Effect	Mechanism	Precautions
SYMPATHOMIMETICS				
DEXAMFETAMINE, METHYLPHENIDATE	DISULFIRAM	Risk of psychosis	Additive effects; these drugs interfere with dopamine metabolism	Caution with coadministration. Warn patients and carers to watch for early features
SYMPATHOMIMETICS	**ERGOT DERIVATIVES**			
SYMPATHOMIMETICS	ERGOT DERIVATIVES	Risk of ergot toxicity when ergotamine is coadministered with sympathomimetics	Uncertain	Watch for early features of ergotamine toxicity (vertigo and gastrointestinal disturbance)
DIRECT	ERGOT DERIVATIVES	Case report of gangrene when dopamine was given to a patient on ergotamine	Thought to be due to additive vasoconstriction	Titrate dopamine carefully
SYMPATHOMIMETICS	H2 RECEPTOR BLOCKERS	↑ Efficacy and adverse effects of sympathomimetics	Unclear	↑ Hypertensive response; dose reduction may be required. Monitor ECG for tachycardias
SYMPATHOMIMETICS	OXYTOCICS	Risk of ↑ BP when oxytocin coadministered with ephedrine, metaraminol, norepinephrine, or pseudoephedrine	Additive vasoconstriction	Monitor PR, BP, and ECG closely; start inotropes at a lower dose
SYMPATHOMIMETICS	SYMPATHOMIMETICS	Risk of ↑ BP and tachycardia	Additive effect	May be used therapeutically in critical care medicine where invasive monitoring is used. Centrally acting appetite suppressants should not be coadministered with other sympatheticomimetics. Warn patients who are taking sympatheticomimetic medications not to use nasal decongestants

DRUGS ACTING ON THE CARDIOVASCULAR SYSTEM SYMPATHOMIMETICS

PART 2

Drugs Acting on the Central Nervous System

Lakshman Delgoda Karalliedde and Janaka Karalliedde

Primary Drug	Secondary Drug	Effect	Mechanism	Precautions
ANTIDEMENTIA DRUGS				
DONEPEZIL ➢ ***Drugs Used to Treat Neuromuscular Diseases and Movement Disorders, below***				
GALANTAMINE ➢ ***Drugs Used to Treat Neuromuscular Diseases and Movement Disorders, below***				
MEMANTINE				
MEMANTINE	ANESTHETICS—GENERAL—KETAMINE	↑ CNS side effects	Additive effects on NMDA receptors	Avoid coadministration
MEMANTINE	ANALGESICS—DEXTROMETHORPHAN	↑ CNS side effects	Additive effects on NMDA receptors	Avoid coadministration
MEMANTINE	ANTIEPILEPTICS—BARBITURATES	Possible ↓ Efficacy of primidone	Uncertain	Avoid coadministration
MEMANTINE	ANTIMUSCARINICS	Possible ↑ efficacy of antimuscarinics	Additive effect; memantine has weak antimuscarinic properties	Warn patients of this effect
MEMANTINE	ANTI-PARKINSON'S DRUGS—AMANTADINE	↑ CNS side effects	Additive effects on NMDA receptors	Manufacturers recommend avoiding coadministration of amantadine and memantine
MEMANTINE	DIURETICS—CARBONIC ANHYDRASE INHIBITORS	Possible ↑ memantine levels	↓ Renal excretion: clearance of memantine was reduced by about 80% under alkaline urine conditions at pH 8	Watch for early features of memantine toxicity
MEMANTINE	DOPAMINERGICS	Memantine augments the effect of dopaminergics	Memantine has some agonist activity at dopamine receptors	Be aware. May be used therapeutically
MEMANTINE	SODIUM BICARBONATE	Possible ↑ memantine levels	↓ Renal excretion	Watch for early features of memantine toxicity

(*Continued*)

Primary Drug	Secondary Drug	Effect	Mechanism	Precautions
ANTIDEMENTIA DRUGS				
RIVASTIGMINE ➢ ***Drugs Used to Treat Neuromuscular Diseases and Movement Disorders, below***				
LITHIUM				
LITHIUM	ANESTHETICS—GENERAL	1. Risk of hemodynamic instability and a range of arrhythmias 2. Decreased anesthetic requirements 3. Risk of lithium toxicity	1. Due to impaired renal excretion and interference with sodium and potassium levels 2. Sedative effect of lithium decreases anesthetic requirements 3. Sodium depletion decreases renal excretion of lithium and can lead to lithium toxicity	Discontinue lithium 72 h before surgery. The only reason not to stop lithium is minor surgery under local anesthesia. Lithium can be stopped abruptly, because no withdrawal symptoms occur To prevent significant renal absorption of lithium, administer sodium-based IV fluids during the perioperative period Lithium should be restarted, with monitoring of blood levels within 1 week. This is most important, because the psychiatric risk of recurrence or relapse is hazardous
LITHIUM	**ANALGESICS**			
LITHIUM	NSAIDs	NSAIDs may ↑ lithium levels; cases of toxicity have been reported; used to treat and prevent episodes of mania in manic depressive disorder that causes episodes of depression	Uncertain; NSAIDs possibly ↓ renal clearance of lithium	Avoid coadministration when possible. If not possible, monitor lithium levels closely; note blood concentrations of lithium may need to be measured for 4–7 days after an NSAID is either added or stopped
LITHIUM	OPIOIDS—DEXTROMETHORPHAN, PENTAZOCINE, TRAMADOL	Possible risk of serotonin syndrome	Additive effect of increased serotonin levels in brain	Be aware of the possibility of serotonin syndrome. Also need to monitor lithium levels with appropriate dose adjustments during coadministration ➢ ***For signs and symptoms of serotonin toxicity, see Clinical Features of Some Adverse Drug Interactions, Serotonin Toxicity and Serotonin Syndrome***

(*Continued*)

Primary Drug	Secondary Drug	Effect	Mechanism	Precautions
ANTIDEMENTIA DRUGS				
LITHIUM	ANTIARRHYTHMICS—AMIODARONE	1. Rare risk of ventricular arrythmias, particularly torsades de pointes 2. Risk of hypothyroidism	1. Additive effect; lithium rarely causes QT prolongation 2. Additive effect; both drugs can cause hypothyroidism	1. Manufacturers of amiodarone recommend avoiding coadministration. 2. If coadministration is thought to be necessary, watch for symptoms/signs of hypothyroidism; check TFTs every 3–6 months
LITHIUM	ANTIBIOTICS—METRONIDAZOLE	↑ Plasma concentrations of lithium with risk of toxicity	Uncertain	Monitor clinically and by measuring blood lithium levels for lithium toxicity
LITHIUM	ANTICANCER AND IMMUNOMODULATING DRUGS—CISPLATIN	Possible alteration in lithium levels	Unclear, possibly due to increased clearance due to cisplatin or hydration, or dilution	Monitor lithium levels closely
LITHIUM	**ANTIDEPRESSANTS**			
LITHIUM	MAOIs—PHENELZINE, TRANYLCYPROMINE	Possible risk of serotonin syndrome	Additive effect of increased serotonin levels in brain	Be aware of the possibility of serotonin syndrome. Also need to monitor lithium levels with appropriate dose adjustments during coadministration. ➢ ***For signs and symptoms of serotonin toxicity, see Clinical Features of Some Adverse Drug Interactions, Serotonin Toxicity and Serotonin Syndrome***
LITHIUM	SSRIs—FLUOXETINE, PAROXETINE, SERTRALINE	Lithium increases serotonin levels and the risk of serotonin syndrome. Excessive somnolence reported with fluvoxamine. Shivering, anxiety may occur. See symptoms of serotonin syndrome. There are reports of both ↑ and ↓ plasma concentrations of lithium, lithium toxicity	Lithium is a direct stimulant of 5-HT receptors, while SSRIs ↓ the reuptake of 5-HT; these are considered to ↑ the effects of serotonin in the brain. Seizures are a neurotoxic effect of lithium and could occur even with plasma lithium concentrations within the normal range. SSRIs and lithium may have additive effects to cause seizures	Be aware of the possibility of serotonin syndrome. Also need to monitor lithium levels with appropriate dose adjustments during coadministration. ➢ ***For signs and symptoms of serotonin toxicity, see Clinical Features of Some Adverse Drug Interactions, Serotonin Toxicity and Serotonin Syndrome***

(Continued)

Primary Drug	Secondary Drug	Effect	Mechanism	Precautions
ANTIDEMENTIA DRUGS				
LITHIUM	SNRIs—VENLAFAXINE	Possible risk of serotonin syndrome	Additive effect of increased serotonin levels in brain	Be aware of the possibility of serotonin syndrome. Also need to monitor lithium levels with appropriate dose adjustments during coadministration. ➢ ***For signs and symptoms of serotonin toxicity, see Clinical Features of Some Adverse Drug Interactions, Serotonin Toxicity and Serotonin Syndrome***
LITHIUM	TCAs—AMITRIPTYLINE, CLOMIPRAMINE, IMIPRAMINE, VENLAFAXINE	Possible risk of serotonin syndrome	Additive effect of increased serotonin levels in brain	Be aware of the possibility of serotonin syndrome. Also need to monitor lithium levels with appropriate dose adjustments during coadministration. ➢ ***For signs and symptoms of serotonin toxicity, see Clinical Features of Some Adverse Drug Interactions, Serotonin Toxicity and Serotonin Syndrome***
LITHIUM	ANTIEPILEPTICS—CARBAMAZEPINE, PHENYTOIN	↑ Risk of neurotoxicity	Uncertain; this may occur with normal lithium blood levels	Warn patients and carers to watch for drowsiness, ataxia, and tremor
LITHIUM	**ANTIHYPERTENSIVES AND HEART FAILURE DRUGS**			
LITHIUM	ACE INHIBITORS—CAPTOPRIL ENALAPRIL, LISINOPRIL, RAMIPRIL, BENAZAPRIL	↑ Lithium levels (up to 1/3) with risk of developing lithium toxicity	↓ Renal excretion (↑ lithium reabsorption by renal tubules)	Watch for lithium toxicity. Monitor lithium levels
LITHIUM	ANGIOTENSIN II RECEPTOR ANTAGONISTS	Risk of lithium toxicity	↓ Excretion of lithium possibly due to ↓ renal tubular reabsorption of sodium in the proximal tubule	Watch for lithium toxicity. Monitor lithium levels

(Continued)

Primary Drug	Secondary Drug	Effect	Mechanism	Precautions
ANTIDEMENTIA DRUGS				
LITHIUM	CENTRALLY ACTING ANTIHYPERTENSIVES	1. Methyldopa may reduce the effect of antidepressants 2. Case reports of lithium toxicity when coingested with methyldopa. It was noted that lithium levels were in the therapeutic range	1. Methyldopa can cause depression 2. Uncertain at present	1. Methyldopa should be avoided in patients with depression 2. Avoid coadministration if possible; if not, watch closely for clinical features of toxicity and do not rely on lithium levels
LITHIUM	**ANTIOBESITY DRUGS**			
LITHIUM	LORCASERIN	Risk of serotonin syndrome	Additive effect	Be aware of the possibility of serotonin syndrome. ➢ ***For signs and symptoms of serotonin toxicity, see Clinical Features of Some Adverse Drug Interactions, Serotonin Toxicity and Serotonin Syndrome***
LITHIUM	SIBUTRAMINE	Risk of serotonin syndrome	Additive effect	Manufacturer advises against coadministration
LITHIUM	**ANTIPSYCHOTICS**			
LITHIUM	CLOZAPINE, HALOPERIDOL, PHENOTHIAZINES, SULPIRIDE	1. ↑ Risk of extrapyramidal side effects and of neurotoxicity 2. Lithium might decrease effectiveness of phenothiazines (chlorpromazine, fluphenazine, trifluoperazine, thioridazine)	Uncertain	1. Watch for development of these symptoms (seizures, encephalopathy, pyrexia, extra-pyramidal symptoms) 2. Watch for deterioration in control of psychosis
LITHIUM	SERTINDOLE	↑ Risk of ventricular arrhythmias	Uncertain	Avoid concomitant use

(*Continued*)

Primary Drug	Secondary Drug	Effect	Mechanism	Precautions
ANTIDEMENTIA DRUGS				
LITHIUM	ANTIVIRALS—ACICLOVIR/ VALACICLOVIR	↑ Lithium levels with risk of toxicity	Possible ↓ renal excretion	Ensure adequate hydration, monitor lithium levels if intravenous aciclovir or >4 g/day valaciclovir required
LITHIUM	BETA-BLOCKERS—PROPANOLOL	Report of episode of ↑ lithium levels in an elderly patient after starting low-dose propanolol. However, propanolol is often used to treat lithium-induced tremor without problems	Mechanism uncertain at present, but propanolol seems to reduce lithium clearance	Monitor lithium levels when starting propanolol therapy in elderly patients. Warn patients to report dizziness and to measure pulse rate
LITHIUM	BRONCHODILATORS—METHYLXANTHINES (AMINOPHYLLINE, CAFFEINE, THEOPHYLLINE)	↓ Plasma levels of lithium, with risk of therapeutic failure	Theophylline ↑ renal clearance of lithium	May need to ↑ dose of lithium by 60%
LITHIUM	CALCIUM CHANNEL BLOCKERS	Small number of cases of neurotoxicity when coadministered with diltiazem or verapamil. Alterations in lithium levels (both ↑ and ↓) reported with verapamil and ↓ levels reported with nifedipine. These effects are variable	Uncertain, but thought to be due to additive effect on neurotransmission	Monitor closely for side effects
LITHIUM	**DIURETICS**			
LITHIUM	ACETAZOLAMIDE	↓ Plasma concentrations of lithium, with risk of inadequate therapeutic effect	↑ Renal elimination of lithium	Monitor clinically and by measuring blood lithium levels to ensure adequate therapeutic efficacy
LITHIUM	LOOP DIURETICS, POTASSIUM-SPARING DIURETICS, ALDOSTERONE ANTAGONISTS, THIAZIDES	Spironolactone and eplerenone possibly ↑ plasma concentrations of lithium, with risk of toxic effects	↓ Renal excretion of lithium	Monitor clinically and by measuring blood lithium levels for lithium toxicity. Loop diuretics are safer than thiazides

(*Continued*)

Primary Drug	Secondary Drug	Effect	Mechanism	Precautions
ANTIDEMENTIA DRUGS				
LITHIUM	**MUSCLE RELAXANTS**			
LITHIUM	NONDEPOLARIZING	Antagonism of effects of nondepolarizing muscle relaxants	Uncertain	Monitor intraoperative muscle relaxation closely; may need ↑ doses of muscle relaxants
LITHIUM	BACLOFEN	Enhancement of hyperkinesis associated with lithium	Uncertain	Consider alternative skeletal muscle relaxant
LITHIUM	PARASYMPATHOMIMETICS	↓ Efficacy of neostigmine and pyridostigmine	Uncertain	Watch for poor response to these parasympathomimetics and ↑ dose accordingly
LITHIUM	POTASSIUM IODIDE	Hypothyroidism	Uncertain	Be aware—monitor TFTs
LITHIUM	URINARY ALKALINIZERS—POTASSIUM ACETATE, POTASSIUM CITRATE, SODIUM BICARBONATE, AND SODIUM CITRATE	↓ Plasma concentrations of lithium with risk of lack of therapeutic effect	Due to ↑ renal excretion of lithium	Monitor clinically and by measuring blood lithium levels to ensure adequate therapeutic efficacy

Primary Drug	Secondary Drug	Effect	Mechanism	Precautions
ANTIDEPRESSANTS				
MONOAMINE OXIDASE INHIBITORS				
MAOIs ELEVATE THE LEVELS OF NOREPINEPHRINE, SEROTONIN, AND DOPAMINE BY INHIBITING AN ENZYME CALLED MONOAMINE OXIDASE				
MAOIs	ALCOHOL	Additive depression of CNS ranging from drowsiness to coma and respiratory depression	Synergistic depressant effects on CNS function	Necessary to warn patients, particularly regards activities that require attention, e.g., driving or using machinery and equipment that could cause self-harm

(*Continued*)

Primary Drug	Secondary Drug	Effect	Mechanism	Precautions
ANTIDEPRESSANTS				
MAOIs	ANESTHETICS—GENERAL	1. General anesthetics: • Reduced dose requirements of thiopentone • Risk of hypertensive crises with ketamine 2. Muscle relaxants: • Phenelzine prolongs the action of suxamethonium • Risk of hypertensive crises with pancuronium 3. Opioids: • Additive depression of CNS ranging from drowsiness to coma and respiratory depression • Risk of serotonin syndrome with dextromethorphan, pethidine, phenoperidine, or tramadol 4. Sympathomimetics: • Risk of adrenergic syndrome • Unlikely to occur with moclobemide and selegiline	1. General anesthetics: • MAOIs may cause a reduction in hepatic metabolism of barbiturates • Ketamine causes sympathetic stimulation • Benzodiazepines, inhalational anesthetic agents, anticholinergic drugs, and nonsteroidal anti-inflammatory drugs can be used safely in patients taking MAOIs 2. Muscle relaxants: • Phenelzine decreases plasma cholinesterase concentration • Pancuronium releases stored noradrenaline 3. Opioids: • Synergistic depressant effects on CNS function; in addition, MAOIs inhibit metabolism of opioids especially morphine • Additive effect: dextromethorphan, pethidine, phenoperidine, or tramadol inhibits serotonin reuptake 4. Sympathomimetics: • Due to inhibition of MAOI, which breaks down sympathomimetics • Moclobemide is involved in the breakdown of serotonin, while selegiline is mainly involved in the breakdown of dopamine	The decision to stop MAOIs therapy preoperatively for elective surgery should be made in advance on an individual basis after discussion among the anesthesiologist, psychiatric team, and patient. Although continuation of MAOIs carries risks, by careful anesthetic technique, these risks can be minimized and must be balanced against the risks of relapse and discontinuation syndrome If MAOIs are continued: 1. General anesthetics: • Be aware—reduce dose of thiopentone or use an alternative induction agent • Ketamine should be avoided as it causes sympathetic stimulation. Local anesthetics containing adrenaline should be used with caution 2. Muscle relaxants: • Be aware of the potential for prolonged relaxation of suxamethonium • Pancuronium should be avoided 3. Opioids: • Avoid coadministration of MAOIs with dextromethorphan, pethidine, phenoperidine, or tramadol for at least 2 weeks after cessation of MAOI • Other opioids are safe 4. Indirect-acting sympathomimetics are absolutely contraindicated with any MAOIs. Titrate doses of direct-acting sympathomimetics

(*Continued*)

Primary Drug	Secondary Drug	Effect	Mechanism	Precautions
ANTIDEPRESSANTS				
MAOIs	**ANALGESICS**			
MAOIs	NEFOPAM	Risk of arrhythmias	Additive effect; both drugs have sympathomimetic effects	Avoid coadministration
MAOIs	OPIOIDS	Additive depression of CNS ranging from drowsiness to coma and respiratory depression. Opioids may enhance the serotonergic effect of MAO inhibitors. This could result in serotonin syndrome	Synergistic depressant effects on CNS function	Necessary to warn patients, particularly regarding activities that require attention, e.g., driving or using machinery and equipment that could cause self-harm. Avoid use of fentanyl (and other anilidopiperidine opioids when possible) in patients who have used a monoamine oxidase inhibitor within the past 14 days due to reports of unpredictable but severe adverse effects
MAOIs	DEXTROMETHORPHAN, MORPHINE, PETHIDINE, PHENOPERIDINE, TRAMADOL	Two types of reactions are reported: 1. Risk of serotonin syndrome with dextromethorphan, pethidine, phenoperidine, or tramadol and MAOIs 2. Depressive—respiratory depression, hypotension, coma	Type I reactions are attributed to an inhibition of reuptake of serotonin; this is more common with pethidine, phenoperidine, dextromethorphan, and tramadol Type II reactions, attributed to MAOI inhibition of metabolism of opioids, are more common with morphine	Avoid coadministration; do not give dextromethorphan, pethidine, or tramadol for at least 2 weeks after cessation of MAOI
PHENELZINE	ANTIBIOTICS—ERYTHROMYCIN	Report of fainting and severe hypotension on initiation of erythromycin	Attributed to ↑ absorption of phenelzine due to rapid gastric emptying caused by erythromycin	Be aware
MAOIs	**ANTICANCER AND IMMUNOMODULATING DRUGS**			
MAOIs	HISTAMINE	Alter histamine metabolism	Altered histamine metabolism	Avoid concurrent use
MAOIs	PROCARBAZINE	Concurrent therapy ↑ risk of hypertensive crisis and severe seizures	Additive effect on inhibiting MAO	Concurrent treatment should not be started on an outpatient basis. Fourteen days should elapse before starting these medications after procarbazine treatment

(Continued)

DRUGS ACTING ON THE CENTRAL NERVOUS SYSTEM ANTIDEPRESSANTS Monoamine oxidase inhibitors

Primary Drug	Secondary Drug	Effect	Mechanism	Precautions
ANTIDEPRESSANTS				
MAOIs	THALIDOMIDE	Increased sedation	Additive	Caution with concurrent use
MAOIs	**ANTIDEPRESSANTS**			
MAOIs—PHENELZINE, TRANYLCYPROMINE	LITHIUM	Possible risk of serotonin syndrome	Additive effect of increased serotonin levels in brain	Be aware of the possibility of serotonin syndrome. Also need to monitor lithium levels with appropriate dose adjustments during coadministration ➢ ***For signs and symptoms of serotonin toxicity, see Clinical Features of Some Adverse Drug Interactions, Serotonin Toxicity and Serotonin Syndrome***
MAOIs	SSRIs	↑ Risk of serotonin syndrome ➢ ***For signs and symptoms of serotonin toxicity, see Clinical Features of Some Adverse Drug Interactions, Serotonin Toxicity and Serotonin Syndrome***	Additive inhibitory on serotonin reuptake	Avoid coadministration. MAOIs should not be started for at least 1 week after stopping SSRIs (2 weeks after sertraline, 5 weeks after fluoxetine). Conversely, SSRIs should not be started for at least 2 weeks after stopping MAOIs
MAOIs	TCAs—AMITRIPTYLINE, CLOMIPRAMINE, DESIPRAMINE, IMIPRAMINE, NORTRIPTYLINE	↑ Risk of stroke, hyperpyrexia, and convulsions. ↑ Plasma concentrations of TCAs, with risk of toxic effects. ↑ Risk of serotonin syndrome and of adrenergic syndrome with older MAOIs. Clomipramine may trigger acute confusion in Parkinson's disease when used with selegiline	TCAs are believed to also act by inhibiting the reuptake of serotonin and norepinephrine, increasing the risk of serotonin and adrenergic syndromes. The combination of TCAs and antidepressants can ↑ risk of seizures	Very hazardous interaction. Avoid concurrent use and consider the use of an alternative antidepressant. Be aware that seizures occur with overdose of TCAs just before cardiac arrest. See serotonergic syndrome in appendix

(*Continued*)

Primary Drug	Secondary Drug	Effect	Mechanism	Precautions
ANTIDEPRESSANTS				
MAOIs	**OTHER**			
MAOIs	SNRIs	Risk of severe hypertensive reactions and of serotonin syndrome ➢ ***For signs and symptoms of serotonin toxicity, see Clinical Features of Some Adverse Drug Interactions, Serotonin Toxicity and Serotonin syndrome***	Duloxetine inhibits the reuptake of both serotonin and norepinephrine. Due to impaired metabolism of these amines, there is an accumulation of serotonin and norepinephrine in the brain and at peripheral sites	Do not coadminister duloxetine and venlafaxine prior to 14 days after discontinuing an MAOI, and do not coadminister MAOI for 5 days after discontinuing duloxetine, 1 week after venlafaxine
MAOIs	MIRTAZAPINE	Risk of severe hypertensive reactions and of serotonin syndrome ➢ ***For signs and symptoms of serotonin toxicity, see Clinical Features of Some Adverse Drug Interactions, Serotonin Toxicity and Serotonin Syndrome***	Additive inhibition of both serotonin and norepinephrine reuptake	Avoid coadministration. MAOIs should not be started for at least 2 weeks after stopping mirtazapine (moclobemide can be started at least 1 week after stopping mirtazapine). Conversely, mirtazapine should not be started for at least 2 weeks after stopping MAOIs
MAOIs—INCLUDING LINEZOLID	REBOXETINE	Risk of severe hypertensive reactions	Additive inhibition of norepinephrine reuptake	Avoid coadministration. MAOIs should not be started for at least 1 week after stopping reboxetine. Conversely, reboxetine should not be started for at least 2 weeks after stopping MAOIs
MAOIs	TRYPTOPHAN	Risk of confusion and agitation	Tryptophan is a precursor to a number of neurotransmitters including serotonin. MAOIs inhibit the breakdown of neurotransmitters	Reduce dose of tryptophan
MAOIs	ANTIDIABETIC DRUGS—INSULIN, SULFONAMIDES	↑ Risk of hypoglycemic episodes	Monoamine oxidase inhibitors have an intrinsic hypoglycemic effect. MAOIs are considered to enhance the effect of hypoglycemic drugs	Watch for and warn patients about symptoms of hypoglycemia. ➢ ***For signs and symptoms of hypoglycemia, see Clinical Features of Some Adverse Drug Interactions, Hypoglycemia***

(Continued)

DRUGS ACTING ON THE CENTRAL NERVOUS SYSTEM ANTIDEPRESSANTS

Primary Drug	Secondary Drug	Effect	Mechanism	Precautions
ANTIDEPRESSANTS				
MAOIs	ANTIEPILEPTICS—BARBITURATES	1. ↑ Risk of seizures 2. Reports of prolonged hypnotic effects	1. MAOIs lower seizure threshold 2. Animal experiments showed that pretreatment with tranylcypromine prolonged amobarbital-induced hypnotic effects 2.5-fold. Inhibition of hepatic enzymes other than MAO has been proposed as an explanation for the exaggerated depressant effects associated with barbiturates and opioids	1. Care with coadministration. Watch for ↑ fit frequency; warn patients of this risk when starting these drugs, and take suitable precautions. Consider increasing the dose of antiepileptic 2. Be aware. Warn patients taking sleeping aids about activities requiring attention and co-ordination, e.g., driving or using machinery
MAOIs	**ANTIHYPERTENSIVES AND HEART FAILURE DRUGS**			
MAOIs	ANTIHYPERTENSIVES AND HEART FAILURE DRUGS	Possible ↑ hypotensive effect. MAOIs cause sudden drop in BP upon standing up (orthostatic hypotension)	Additive hypotensive effect	Monitor BP at least weekly until stable. Warn patients to report symptoms of hypotension (light-headedness, dizziness on standing, etc.)
MAOIs	ADRENERGIC NEURONE BLOCKERS—GUANETHIDINE, CENTRALLY ACTING ANTIHYPERTENSIVES—METHYLDOPA	Risk of adrenergic syndrome. Reports of an enhanced hypotensive effect and hallucinations with methyldopa, which may cause depression	Due to inhibition of MAOI, which breaks down sympathomimetics	Avoid concurrent use. Onset may be 6–24 h after ingestion
MAOIs	**ANTIHISTAMINES**			
MAOIs	ANTIHISTAMINES	↑ Occurrence of antimuscarinic effects such as blurred vision, confusion (in elderly patients), restlessness, and constipation	Additive antimuscarinic effects	Warn patients and carers, particularly those managing elderly patients. See anticholinergic risk scale in appendix
MAOIs	ANTIHISTAMINES—SEDATIVE	Additive depression of CNS ranging from drowsiness to coma and respiratory depression	Synergistic depressant effects on CNS function	Necessary to warn patients, particularly regarding activities that require attention, e.g., driving or using machinery and equipment that could cause self-harm

(*Continued*)

Primary Drug	Secondary Drug	Effect	Mechanism	Precautions
ANTIDEPRESSANTS				
MAOIs	ANTIMUSCARINICS	↑ Occurrence of antimuscarinic effects such as blurred vision, confusion (in elderly patients), restlessness, and constipation	Additive antimuscarinic effects	Warn patients and carers, particularly those managing elderly patients
MAOIs	**ANTIOBESITY DRUGS**			
MAOIs—INCLUDING LINEZOLID	LORCASERIN	Risk of serotonin syndrome	Additive effect	Be aware of the possibility of serotonin syndrome. ➢ ***For signs and symptoms of serotonin toxicity, see Clinical Features of Some Adverse Drug Interactions, Serotonin Toxicity and Serotonin Syndrome***
MAOIs	SIBUTRAMINE	Risk of serotonin syndrome	Additive effect	Manufacturer advises against coadministration. Do not start sibutramine for at least 2 weeks after stopping MAOIs
MAOIs	ANTI-PARKINSON'S DRUGS—DOPAMINERGICS—levodopa, selegiline, possibly rasagiline, entacapone, tolcapone	Risk of adrenergic syndrome—hypertension, hyperthermia, arrhythmias—and dopaminergic effects with selegiline	Levodopa and related drugs are precursors of dopamine. Levodopa is predominantly metabolized to dopamine, and a smaller proportion is converted to epinephrine and norepinephrine due to inhibition of MAOI, which breaks down dopamine and sympathomimetics	Avoid concurrent use. Onset may be 6–24 h after ingestion. Carbidopa and benserazide, which inhibit dopa decarboxylase that converts L-dopa to dopamine, is considered to minimize this interaction. However, MAOIs should not be used in patients with Parkinson's disease on treatment with levodopa. Imipramine and amitriptyline are considered safer by some clinicians
MAOIs	ANTIPSYCHOTICS	Additive depression of CNS ranging from drowsiness to coma and respiratory depression	Synergistic depressant effects on CNS function	Necessary to warn patients, particularly regarding activities that require attention, e.g., driving and using machinery and equipment that could cause self-harm

(*Continued*)

Primary Drug	Secondary Drug	Effect	Mechanism	Precautions
ANTIDEPRESSANTS				
MAOIs	**ANXIOLYTICS AND HYPNOTICS**			
MAOIs	BZDs	Additive depression of CNS ranging from drowsiness to coma and respiratory depression	Synergistic depressant effects on CNS function	Necessary to warn patients, particularly regarding activities that require attention, e.g., driving and using machinery and equipment that could cause self-harm
MAOIs	BUSPIRONE	Cases of hypertension	Uncertain	Monitor BP closely
MAOIs	CHLORAL HYDRATE	Case of fatal hyperpyrexia and cases of hypertension	Uncertain	Avoid coadministration
MAOIs	BETA-BLOCKERS	↑ Hypotensive effect	Additive hypotensive effect. Postural ↓ BP is a common side effect of MAOIs	Monitor BP at least weekly until stable. Warn patients to report symptoms of hypotension (light-headedness, dizziness on standing, etc.)
MAOIs	**BRONCHODILATORS**			
MAOIs	IPRATROPIUM, TIOTROPIUM	↑ Occurrence of antimuscarinic effects such as blurred vision, confusion (in elderly patients), restlessness, and constipation	Additive antimuscarinic effects	Warn patients and carers, particularly those managing elderly patients
MAOIs	BETA-2 AGONISTS	↑ Occurrence of headache, hypertensive episodes. Unlikely to occur with moclobemide and selegiline	Due to impaired metabolism of these sympathomimetic amines because of inhibition of MAO. Moclobemide is involved in the breakdown of serotonin, while selegiline is mainly involved in the breakdown of dopamine	Be aware. Monitor BP closely
MAOIs	CALCIUM CHANNEL BLOCKERS	↑ Antihypertensive effect of calcium channel blockers when coadministered with MAOIs	Additive hypotensive effects; postural ↓ BP is a side effect of MAOIs	Monitor BP at least weekly until stable. Warn patients to report symptoms of hypotension (light-headedness, dizziness on standing, etc.)

(Continued)

Primary Drug	Secondary Drug	Effect	Mechanism	Precautions
ANTIDEPRESSANTS				
MAOIs	**CNS STIMULANTS**			
MAOIs	ATOMOXETINE	Risk of severe hypertensive reactions	Additive inhibition of norepinephrine reuptake	Avoid coadministration. MAOIs should not be started for at least 2 weeks after stopping atomoxetine; conversely, atomoxetine should not be started for at least 2 weeks after stopping MAOI
MOCLOBEMIDE	MODAFINIL	May cause moderate ↑ plasma concentrations of these substrates	Modafinil is a reversible inhibitor of CYP2C19 when used in therapeutic doses	Be aware
PHENELZINE	DRUG DEPENDENCE THERAPIES—BUPROPION	↑ Acute toxicity of bupropion	Uncertain	Be aware
MAOIs	FOODS—TYRAMINE-CONTAINING—aged cheeses, aged pickles, smoked meats (e.g., salami), yeast extracts, beer (dark more than light, and tap more than bottles), red wine more than white wine, avocado, sauerkraut, marmite, banana peel, soy bean products, broad bean pods, foods containing msg	Risk of severe tyramine reactions—hypertension, occipital headaches, vomiting, palpitations, nausea, apprehension, chills, sweating. This reaction develops 20–60 min after ingestion of these foods	Tyramine has both direct and indirect sympathomimetic effects, and tyramine effects of foods may be potentiated by MAOIs 10–20-fold. A mild tyramine reaction occurs with 6 mg, moderate reaction with 10 mg, and severe reactions with 25 mg	Prompt treatment with phentolamine (0.5 mg intravenously) or nifedipine is effective, and death is rare (0.01%–0.02%). There is a recommendation that 25 mg tablet of chlorpromazine be given to patients on MAOIs to be taken if a tyramine reaction occurs
MAOIs	H2 RECEPTOR BLOCKERS—CIMETIDINE	↑ Plasma concentrations of moclobemide (by up to 40%)	Inhibition of metabolism	Reduce dose of moclobemide to one-half to one-third of original, then alter as required
MAOIs	**5-HT1 AGONISTS**			
MAOIs	RIZATRIPTAN, SUMATRIPTAN	↑ Plasma concentrations of rizatriptan and sumatriptan, with risk of toxic effects, e.g., flushing, sensations of tingling, heat, heaviness, pressure, or tightness of any part of body including the throat and chest, dizziness	These triptans are metabolized primarily by MAO-A	Avoid starting these triptans for at least 2 weeks after stopping MAOIs; conversely, avoid starting MAOIs for at least 2 weeks after stopping these triptans

(Continued)

Primary Drug	Secondary Drug	Effect	Mechanism	Precautions
ANTIDEPRESSANTS				
MOCLOBEMIDE	ZOLMITRIPTAN	Risk of agitation, confusion when zolmitriptan is coadministered with moclobemide	Uncertain	Watch for these effects and consider reducing the dose of zolmitriptan
MAOIs	**MUSCLE RELAXANTS**			
	BACLOFEN, TIZANIDINE	↑ Hypotensive effect	Additive hypotensive effect	Monitor BP at least weekly until stable. Warn patients to report symptoms of hypotension (light-headedness, dizziness on standing, etc.)
MAOIs	CYCLOBENZAPRINE	↑ Risk of serotonin syndrome and of adrenergic syndrome ➢ ***For signs and symptoms of serotonin toxicity, see Clinical Features of Some Adverse Drug Interactions, Serotonin Toxicity and Serotonin Syndrome***	Cyclobenzaprine is structurally similar to tricyclic antidepressants. TCAs are believed to act also by inhibiting the reuptake of serotonin and norepinephrine, increasing the risk of serotonin and adrenergic syndromes	Avoid coadministration
MAOIs	NONDEPOLARIZING—PANCURONIUM	Risk of severe hypertension	Pancuronium releases stored noradrenaline	Pancuronium should be avoided
MAOIs	NITRATES	↑ Hypotensive effect	Additive hypotensive effect. Postural ↓ BP is a common side effect of MAOIs	Monitor BP at least weekly until stable. Warn patients to report symptoms of hypotension (light-headedness, dizziness on standing, etc.)

(Continued)

Primary Drug	Secondary Drug	Effect	Mechanism	Precautions
ANTIDEPRESSANTS				
MAOIs	OTC MEDICATIONS—COUGH SYRUPS, SLEEP AIDS, MEDICINES FOR COLDS AND HAY FEVER, SOME PAIN RELIEVERS, SLIMMING AIDS, NASAL DECONGESTANTS	Due to the presence of sympathomimetics (amphetamines, ephedrine, ephedra, pseudoephedrine, phenylpropanolamine, etc., in nasal decongestants), opioids (pain relievers, e.g., codeine, dextromethorphan), fenfluramine (in slimming preparations), sedating antihistamines (promethazine, chlorpheniramine in hay fever and antiallergy preparations)	Patients on MAOIs cannot metabolize several of the active constituents of these OTC drugs	Mandatory that prior to dispensing these OTC medications, purchasers are questioned about the use of MAOIs
MAOIs	PERIPHERAL VASODILATORS—MOXISYLYTE	↑ Hypotensive effect	Additive hypotensive effect. Postural ↓ BP is a common side effect of MAOIs	Monitor BP at least weekly until stable. Warn patients to report symptoms of hypotension (light-headedness, dizziness on standing, etc.)
MAOIs	POTASSIUM CHANNEL ACTIVATORS	↑ Hypotensive effect	Additive hypotensive effect. Postural ↓ BP is a common side effect of MAOIs	Monitor BP at least weekly until stable. Warn patients to report symptoms of hypotension (light-headedness, dizziness on standing, etc.)
MOCLOBEMIDE	PROTON PUMP INHIBITORS—OMEPRAZOLE/ ESOMEPRAZOLE	Possible ↑ efficacy and adverse effects of both drugs	Inhibition of CYP2C19	Monitor more closely; effect only seen in extensive CYP2C19 metabolizers. Dose ↓ may be required
MAOIs	SYMPATHOMIMETICS	Risk of adrenergic syndrome. Unlikely to occur with moclobemide and selegiline. This is likely with some OTC medications, which may contain some of these sympathomimetics	Due to inhibition of MAOI, which breaks down sympathomimetics. Moclobemide is involved in the breakdown of serotonin, while selegiline is mainly involved in the breakdown of dopamine	Avoid concurrent use. Onset may be 6–24 h after ingestion. Do ECG, measure electrolytes, FBC, CK, and coagulation profile. Before prescribing/dispensing, enquire about use of MAOI antidepressants and related drugs such as linezolid

(*Continued*)

DRUGS ACTING ON THE CENTRAL NERVOUS SYSTEM ANTIDEPRESSANTS 235

Primary Drug	Secondary Drug	Effect	Mechanism	Precautions
ANTIDEPRESSANTS				
MAOIs	TETRABENAZINE	Risk of confusion and agitation	Uncertain; although tetrabenazine depletes norepinephrine, if it is started on a patient who is already taking MAOIs, it may stimulate the release of accumulated neurotransmitter. This would not be expected if a patient started MAOI while already taking tetrabenazine	Tetrabenazine may cause depression, so it should be used with caution in patients with depression. If necessary, consider using an alternative antidepressant or start an MAOI after tetrabenazine has been established
MIRTAZAPINE				
MIRTAZAPINE	ALCOHOL	↑ Sedation	Additive effect	Warn patients about this effect
MIRTAZAPINE	ANTICOAGULANTS—ORAL	↑ Anticoagulant effect of warfarin	Inhibition of metabolism of warfarin	Monitor INR at least weekly until stable
MIRTAZAPINE	ANTIDEPRESSANTS—MAOIs	Risk of severe hypertensive reactions and of serotonin syndrome. ➢ ***For signs and symptoms of serotonin toxicity, see Clinical Features of Some Adverse Drug Interactions, Serotonin Toxicity and Serotonin Syndrome***	Additive inhibition of both serotonin and norepinephrine reuptake	Avoid coadministration. MAOIs should not be started for at least 2 weeks after stopping mirtazapine (moclobemide can be started at least 1 week after stopping mirtazapine). Conversely, mirtazapine should not be started for at least 2 weeks after stopping MAOIs
MIRTAZAPINE	ANTIEPILEPTICS	↓ Mirtazapine levels with carbamazepine and phenytoin	Induction of metabolism of mirtazapine, possibly by CYP2D6	Watch for poor response to mirtazapine
MIRTAZAPINE	ANTIFUNGALS—KETOCONAZOLE	↑ Mirtazapine levels	Inhibition of metabolism via CYP1A2, CYP2D6, and CYP3A4	Consider alternative antifungals
MIRTAZAPINE	ANTIHYPERTENSIVES AND HEART FAILURE DRUGS—CENTRALLY ACTING ANTIHYPERTENSIVES—METHYLDOPA	Methyldopa may ↓ effect of antidepressants	Methyldopa can cause depression	Methyldopa should be avoided in patients with depression

(*Continued*)

Primary Drug	Secondary Drug	Effect	Mechanism	Precautions
ANTIDEPRESSANTS				
MIRTAZAPINE	**ANTIOBESITY DRUGS**			
MIRTAZAPINE	LORCASERIN	Risk of serotonin syndrome	Additive effect	Be aware of the possibility of serotonin syndrome. ➢ ***For signs and symptoms of serotonin toxicity, see Clinical Features of Some Adverse Drug Interactions, Serotonin Toxicity and Serotonin Syndrome***
MIRTAZAPINE	ANTIOBESITY DRUGS—SIBUTRAMINE	Risk of hypertension and agitation	Additive effect on norepinephrine transmission	Avoid coadministration
MIRTAZAPINE	ANXIOLYTICS AND HYPNOTICS	↑ Sedation	Additive effect	Warn patients about this effect
MIRTAZAPINE	H2 RECEPTOR BLOCKERS—CIMETIDINE	↑ Mirtazapine levels	Inhibition of metabolism via CYP1A2, CYP2D6, and CYPA4	Consider alternative acid suppression, e.g., H2 antagonist (proton pump inhibitors will interact in poor CYP2D6 metabolizers) or monitor more closely for side effects; ↓ dose as necessary
REBOXETINE				
Selective noradrenaline reuptake inhibitor (NaRI)				
REBOXETINE	ANALGESICS—TRAMADOL	Risk of ↑ reboxetine levels	Possibly inhibition of CYP3A4-mediated metabolism of reboxetine	Avoid coadministration
REBOXETINE	**ANTIBIOTICS**			
REBOXETINE	MACROLIDES	Risk of ↑ reboxetine levels	Possibly inhibition of CYP3A4-mediated metabolism of reboxetine	Avoid coadministration
REBOXETINE	LINEZOLID	Risk of severe hypertensive reactions	Additive inhibition of norepinephrine reuptake	Avoid coadministration. Linezolid should not be started for at least 1 week after stopping reboxetine. Conversely, reboxetine should not be started for at least 2 weeks after stopping linezolid

(Continued)

Primary Drug	Secondary Drug	Effect	Mechanism	Precautions
ANTIDEPRESSANTS				
REBOXETINE	RIFAMPICIN	Risk of ↓ reboxetine levels	Possibly induction of CYP3A4-mediated metabolism of reboxetine	May need to increase dose of reboxetine with close monitoring
REBOXETINE	**ANTIDEPRESSANTS**			
REBOXETINE	MAOIs	Risk of severe hypertensive reactions	Additive inhibition of norepinephrine reuptake	Avoid coadministration. MAOIs should not be started for at least 1 week after stopping reboxetine. Conversely, reboxetine should not be started for at least 2 weeks after stopping MAOIs
REBOXETINE	ST. JOHN'S WORT	Risk of ↓ reboxetine levels	Possibly induction of CYP3A4-mediated metabolism of reboxetine	May need to increase dose of reboxetine with close monitoring
REBOXETINE	SSRIs—FLUVOXAMINE	1. Risk of ↑ reboxetine levels 2. May ↑ fluvoxamine levels	1. Possibly inhibition of CYP3A4-mediated metabolism of reboxetine 2. Reboxetine is a selective norepinephrine reuptake inhibitor. Reboxetine inhibits metabolism of fluvoxamine	Avoid concurrent use (manufacturers' recommendation)
REBOXETINE	SSRIs—NEFAZODONE	Risk of ↑ reboxetine levels	Possibly inhibition of CYP3A4-mediated metabolism of reboxetine	Avoid coadministration
REBOXETINE	ANTIEPILEPTICS—CARBAMAZEPINE, PHENOBARBITOL, PHENYTOIN	Risk of ↓ reboxetine levels	Possibly induction of CYP3A4-mediated metabolism of reboxetine	May need to increase dose of reboxetine with close monitoring
REBOXETINE	ANTIFUNGALS—AZOLES	Risk of ↑ reboxetine levels	Possibly inhibition of CYP3A4-mediated metabolism of reboxetine	Avoid coadministration
REBOXETINE	ANTIHYPERTENSIVES AND HEART FAILURE DRUGS—CENTRALLY ACTING ANTIHYPERTENSIVES—METHYLDOPA	Methyldopa may ↓ effect of antidepressants	Methyldopa can cause depression	Methyldopa should be avoided in patients with depression

(Continued)

Primary Drug	Secondary Drug	Effect	Mechanism	Precautions
ANTIDEPRESSANTS				
REBOXETINE	ANTIMALARIALS—ARTEMETHER/LUMEFANTRINE	↑ Artemether/lumefantrine levels, with risk of toxicity, including arrhythmias	Uncertain	Avoid coadministration
REBOXETINE	ANTIMIGRAINE DRUGS—ERGOT DERIVATIVES	Risk of hypertension	Additive effect	Monitor BP closely
REBOXETINE	ANTIOBESITY DRUGS—SIBUTRAMINE	Risk of hypertension and agitation	Additive inhibition of norepinephrine reuptake	Avoid coadministration
REBOXETINE	ANTIVIRALS—COBICISTAT, PROTEASE INHIBITORS	Risk of ↑ reboxetine levels	Possibly inhibition of CYP3A4-mediated metabolism of reboxetine	Avoid coadministration
REBOXETINE	DIURETICS—LOOP, THIAZIDES	Risk of hypokalemia	Additive effect	Monitor potassium levels closely
ST. JOHN'S WORT				
ST. JOHNS WORT	ANTIARRHYTHMICS—DRONEDARONE	Risk of ↓ levels of dronedarone	St. John's wort induces the hepatic metabolism of dronedarone	Watch for poor response to dronedarone
ST. JOHN'S WORT	ANTIBIOTICS—TELITHROMYCIN	↓ Telithromycin levels	Due to induction of CYP3A4-mediated metabolism of telithromycin	Avoid coadministration for up to 2 weeks after stopping St. John's wort
ST. JOHN'S WORT	**ANTICANCER AND IMMUNOMODULATING DRUGS**			
ST. JOHN'S WORT	AFATINIB	Reduction in afatinib levels	P-glycoprotein induction	U.S. manufacturer recommends dose increase
ST. JOHN'S WORT	AXITINIB	Reduced axitinib levels	CYP3A4/5 induction	Manufacturer advises avoid concurrent use if possible. If concurrent use is necessary, dose adjustment is recommended
ST. JOHN'S WORT	BORTEZOMIB	Levels of bortezomib reduced	Possibly due to induction of CYP3A4	Avoid concomitant use
ST. JOHN'S WORT	BOSUTINIB	Reduced bosutinib levels	CYP3A induction	Manufacturer advises avoid concurrent use. Dose increase unlikely to sufficiently compensate
ST. JOHN'S WORT	CABAZITAXEL	Reduced cabazitaxel levels	CYP3A4 induction	Avoid coadministration
ST. JOHN'S WORT	CRIZOTINIB	Possible reduced crizotinib levels	CYP3A4 induction	Manufacturer advises to avoid concurrent use

(Continued)

Primary Drug	Secondary Drug	Effect	Mechanism	Precautions
ANTIDEPRESSANTS				
ST. JOHN'S WORT	DABRAFENIB	Predicted reduced dabrafenib levels	CYP2C8/CYP3A4 induction	Avoid concurrent use
ST. JOHN'S WORT	DASATINIB	↓ Dasatinib level; evidence for imatinib only but dasatinib is metabolized in a similar way	1. Dasatinib is a substrate and inhibitor of CYP3A4 2. St. John's wort ↑ metabolism of dasatinib by enzyme induction	Avoid concurrent use
ST. JOHN'S WORT	DOCETAXEL	Predicted reduced docetaxel levels	CYP3A4 induction	Monitor closely Dose increase may be required
ST. JOHN'S WORT	ERIBULIN	Possible reduced eribulin levels	CYP3A4 induction	Manufacturer recommends avoiding concurrent use
ST. JOHN'S WORT	EVEROLIMUS	Reduced everolimus levels	CYP3A4 induction	Avoid concurrent use Consider increasing dose of everolimus if concurrent use is necessary
ST. JOHN'S WORT	FINGOLIMOD	Fingolimod levels reduced	Induction of CYP3A4	Manufacturer advises to avoid concurrent use
ST. JOHN'S WORT	IFOSFAMIDE	↑ Rate of biotransformation to 4-hydroxyifosfamide, the active metabolite, but there is no change in AUC of 4-hydroxyifosfamide	Due to ↑ rate of metabolism and of clearance due to induction of CYP3A4 and CYP2D6	Be aware—but clinical significance may be minimal or none
ST. JOHN'S WORT	IMATINIB	↓ Imatinib levels	Due to induction of CYP3A4-mediated metabolism of imatinib	Avoid concurrent use
ST. JOHN'S WORT	IRINOTECAN	↓ Plasma concentrations of irinotecan and risk of ↓ therapeutic efficacy. The effects may last for 3 weeks after discontinuation of CYP-inducer therapy	Due to induction of CYP3A4-mediated metabolism of irinotecan	Avoid concomitant use whenever possible; if not, ↑ dose of irinotecan by 50%
ST. JOHN'S WORT	LAPATINIB	Reduced lapatinib levels	P-glycoprotein induction	Caution with concurrent use
ST. JOHN'S WORT	MITOTANE	Possible reduction in levels of St. John's wort	Mitotane has been shown to have an inductive effect on cytochrome 3A4	Mitotane dose should be adjusted to achieve a therapeutic plasma level of 14 to 20 mg/L. CNS toxicity has been associated with levels above 18–20 mg/L. Watch for poor response to St. John's Wort

(*Continued*)

Primary Drug	Secondary Drug	Effect	Mechanism	Precautions
ANTIDEPRESSANTS				
ST. JOHN'S WORT	NILOTINIB	↓ Nilotinib levels (though evidence for imatinib is stronger)	Induction of CYP3A4 metabolism of nilotinib by St. John's wort	Avoid concurrent use
ST. JOHN'S WORT	PACLITAXEL	↓ Plasma concentration of paclitaxel and ↓ efficacy of paclitaxel	Due to induction of hepatic metabolism of paclitaxel by the CYP isoenzymes	Monitor for clinical efficacy; need to ↑ dose if inadequate response is due to interaction
ST. JOHN'S WORT	PONATINIB	Possible reduced ponatinib levels	CYP3A4 induction	Avoid concurrent use if possible
ST. JOHN'S WORT	REGORAFENIB	Predicted reduced regorafenib levels	CYP3A4 induction	Manufacturer advises to avoid concurrent use
ST. JOHN'S WORT	RUXOLITINIB	Reduced levels of ruxolitinib	CYP3A4 induction	Monitor closely Titrate dose based on safety and efficacy
ST. JOHN'S WORT	TRABECTEDIN	Reduced trabectedin levels	CYP3A4 induction	Monitor closely
ST. JOHN'S WORT	VEMURAFENIB	Possible reduced levels of vemurafenib	CYP3A4 induction	Manufacturer recommends to avoid concurrent use
ST. JOHN'S WORT	VINCA ALKALOIDS—VINBLASTINE, VINCRISTINE, VINFLUNINE	↓ Plasma concentrations of vinblastine and vincristine, with risk of inadequate therapeutic response. Reports of AUC ↓ by 40%, elimination half-life ↓ by 35%, and clearance ↑ by 63% in patients with brain tumors taking vincristine	Due to induction of CYP3A4-mediated metabolism	Monitor for clinical efficacy, and ↑ dose of vinblastine and vincristine as clinically indicated; in the latter case, monitor clinically and radiologically for clinical efficacy in patients with brain tumors, and ↑ dose to obtain the desired response
ST. JOHN'S WORT	**HORMONES AND HORMONE ANTAGONIST**			
ST. JOHN'S WORT	TAMOXIFEN	↓ Plasma concentrations of tamoxifen and risk of inadequate therapeutic response	Due to induction of metabolism of tamoxifen by the CYP3A isoenzymes as a result of taking St. John's wort	Avoid concurrent use

(*Continued*)

Primary Drug	Secondary Drug	Effect	Mechanism	Precautions
ANTIDEPRESSANTS				
ST. JOHN'S WORT	**IMMUNOMODULATING DRUGS**			
ST. JOHN'S WORT	CICLOSPORIN	↓ Plasma concentrations of ciclosporin, with risk of transplant rejection	Due to induction of metabolism of ciclosporin by these drugs. The potency of induction varies. St. John's wort may produce its effects by an effect on Pgp	Avoid coadministration
ST. JOHN'S WORT	CORTICOSTEROIDS	↓ Plasma concentrations of corticosteroids and risk of poor or inadequate therapeutic response, which would be undesirable if used for, e.g., cerebral edema	Due to induction of the hepatic metabolism by the CYP3A4 isoenzymes	Monitor therapeutic response closely—clinically, with ophthalmoscopy and radiologically—and ↑ dose of corticosteroids for desired therapeutic effect
ST. JOHN'S WORT	TACROLIMUS	↓ Tacrolimus levels	Induction of CYP3A4-mediated metabolism of tacrolimus	Avoid coadministration
ST. JOHN'S WORT	ANTICOAGULANTS—ORAL			
ST. JOHN'S WORT	ANTICOAGULANTS—ORAL	↓ Warfarin levels	Induction of metabolism	Avoid coadministration
ST. JOHN'S WORT	APIXABAN	↓ Apixaban levels	Induction of CYP3A4-mediated metabolism and Pgp-mediated transport of apixaban	Avoid coadministration
ST. JOHN'S WORT	DABIGATRAN	↓ Dabigatran levels	Induction of Pgp	Manufacturers recommend avoiding coadministration
ST. JOHN'S WORT	RIVAROXABAN	↓ Rivaroxaban exposure	Induction of CYP3A4-mediated metabolism and Pgp-mediated efflux transport	Avoid coadministration
ST. JOHN'S WORT	**ANTIDEPRESSANTS**			
ST. JOHN'S WORT	REBOXETINE	Risk of ↓ reboxetine levels	Possibly induction of CYP3A4-mediated metabolism of reboxetine	May need to increase dose of reboxetine with close monitoring

(*Continued*)

Primary Drug	Secondary Drug	Effect	Mechanism	Precautions
ANTIDEPRESSANTS				
ST. JOHN'S WORT	SNRIs—DULOXETINE	↑ Risk of serotonin syndrome ➢ ***For signs and symptoms of serotonin toxicity, see Clinical Features of Some Adverse Drug Interactions, Serotonin Toxicity and Serotonin Syndrome***	Additive effect	Avoid coadministration
ST. JOHN'S WORT	SSRIs/TCA's/Triazolam	↑ Risk of serotonin syndrome ➢ ***For signs and symptoms of serotonin toxicity, see Clinical Features of Some Adverse Drug Interactions, Serotonin Toxicity and Serotonin Syndrome***	Additive effect	Caution with coadministration with TCAs or trazodone. Specialist advice should be sought and alternatives considered. Avoid coadministration of two SSRIs, and SSRIs with duloxetine or St. John's wort
ST. JOHN'S WORT	**ANTIDIABETIC DRUGS**			
ST. JOHN'S WORT	REPAGLINIDE	↓ Plasma concentrations of repaglinide likely	Due to inducing CYP3A4 isoenzymes, which metabolize repaglinide. However, the alternative pathway—CYP2C8—is unaffected by these inducers	Be aware and monitor for hyperglycemia. ➢ ***For signs and symptoms of hyperglycemia, see Clinical Features of Some Adverse Drug Interactions, Hyperglycemia***
ST. JOHN'S WORT	SULFONYLUREAS	↓ Hypoglycemic efficacy	↓ Plasma levels of sulfonylureas by induction of CYP-mediated metabolism	Watch for and warn patients about symptoms of hyperglycemia. ➢ ***For signs and symptoms of hyperglycemia, see Clinical Features of Some Adverse Drug Interactions, Hyperglycemia***
ST. JOHN'S WORT	**OTHER MEDICATIONS**			
ST. JOHN'S WORT	ANTIEMETICS—APREPITANT	↑ Aprepitant levels	Inhibition of CYP3A4-mediated metabolism of aprepitant	Avoid coadministration (manufacturers' recommendation)
ST. JOHN'S WORT	ANTIEPILEPTICS—BARBITURATES, CARBAMAZEPINE, PHENYTOIN LEVELS	↓ Antiepileptic levels	↑ Metabolism	Avoid coadministration

(*Continued*)

DRUGS ACTING ON THE CENTRAL NERVOUS SYSTEM ANTIDEPRESSANTS

Primary Drug	Secondary Drug	Effect	Mechanism	Precautions
ANTIDEPRESSANTS				
ST. JOHN'S WORT	ANTIMALARIALS—ARTEMETHER/LUMEFANTRINE	This antimalarial may cause dose-related dangerous arrhythmias	A substrate mainly of CYP3A4, which may be inhibited by St. John's wort	Manufacturers recommend to avoidance of antidepressants
ST. JOHN'S WORT	ANTIMIGRAINE DRUGS—TRIPTANS	↑ Risk of serotonin syndrome. ➢ ***For signs and symptoms of serotonin toxicity, see Clinical Features of Some Adverse Drug Interactions, Serotonin toxicity and Serotonin Syndrome***	Possibly additive effect	Avoid coadministration
ST. JOHN'S WORT	LORCASERIN	Risk of serotonin syndrome	Additive effect	Be aware of the possibility of serotonin syndrome. ➢ ***For signs and symptoms of serotonin toxicity, see Clinical Features of Some Adverse Drug Interactions, Serotonin Toxicity and Serotonin Syndrome***
ST. JOHN'S WORT	ANTIPLATELETS—CLOPIDOGREL	Theoretical risk of bleeding	St. John's wort increases CYP3A4- and 2C19-mediated activation of clopidogrel. No clinical reports of bleeding	Warn patient to report abnormal bleeding immediately
ST. JOHN'S WORT	**ANTIVIRALS**			
ST. JOHN'S WORT	COBICISTAT (Pharmacologic enhancer/booster)	↓ Plasma levels, risk of treatment failure, and resistance	Induction of cobicistat metabolism via CYP3A and CYP2D6 (minor)	Avoid coadministration
ST. JOHN'S WORT	DOLUTEGRAVIR	↓ Plasma levels, risk of treatment failure, and resistance	Induction of metabolism via CYP3A (all affected) and UGT1A1 (dolutegravir)	Avoid coadministration
ST. JOHN'S WORT	MARAVIROC	↓ Plasma levels, risk of treatment failure, and resistance	Induction of metabolism via CYP3A (all affected) and UGT1A1 (dolutegravir)	Avoid coadministration
ST. JOHN'S WORT	PROTEASE INHIBITORS	Markedly ↓ levels and efficacy of protease inhibitors by St. John's wort	Possibly ↑ CYP3A4-mediated metabolism of the protease inhibitors	Avoid coadministration

(*Continued*)

Primary Drug	Secondary Drug	Effect	Mechanism	Precautions
ANTIDEPRESSANTS				
ST. JOHN'S WORT	CALCIUM CHANNEL BLOCKERS	St. John's wort is associated with ↓ verapamil levels	St. John's wort induces CYP3A4, which metabolizes calcium channel blockers, and induces intestinal Pgp, which may ↓ bioavailability of verapamil	Monitor BP regularly for at least the first 2 weeks of initiating St. John's wort
ST. JOHN'S WORT	CARDIAC GLYCOSIDES—DIGOXIN	Plasma concentrations of digoxin seem to be ↓ by St. John's wort	St. John's wort seems to ↓ Pgp-mediated intestinal absorption of digoxin	Watch for ↓ response to digoxin
ST. JOHN'S WORT	CNS STIMULANTS—MODAFINIL	May ↓ modafinil levels	Induction of CYP3A4, which has a partial role in the metabolism of modafinil	Be aware
ST. JOHN'S WORT	DIURETICS—POTASSIUM-SPARING	↓ Eplerenone levels	Induction of metabolism	Avoid coadministration
ST. JOHN'S WORT	ELIGLUSTAT	↓ Eliglustat levels	Induction of CYP3A4-mediated metabolism	Avoid coadministration
ST. JOHN'S WORT	IVACAFTOR	↓ Ivacaftor levels	Induction of CYP3A4-mediated metabolism of ivacaftor	Manufacturers advice against coadministration
ST. JOHN'S WORT	IVABRADINE	↓ Levels of ivabradine	Increased CYP3A4 mediated metabolism of ivabradine	Monitor for reduced efficacy of ivabradine
ST. JOHN'S WORT	LIPID-LOWERING DRUGS—STATINS	St. John's wort may lower simvastatin levels	Uncertain at present	Monitor lipid profile closely; look for poor response to simvastatin
ST. JOHN'S WORT	MIFEPRISTONE	Theoretical risk of ↓ levels of mifepristone	Induction of CYP3A4-mediated metabolism of mifepristone	Watch for poor response to mifepristone
ST. JOHN'S WORT	NITISINONE	Possible ↓ nitisinone levels	Induction of CYP3A4-mediated metabolism	Avoid coadministration
ST. JOHN'S WORT	ESTROGENS	Marked ↓ contraceptive effect	Induction of metabolism of estrogens	Avoid coadministration

(Continued)

Primary Drug	Secondary Drug	Effect	Mechanism	Precautions
ANTIDEPRESSANTS				
ST. JOHN'S WORT	PROGESTOGENS	↓ Progesterone levels, which may lead to failure of contraception or a poor response to the treatment of menorrhagia	Possibly induction of metabolism of progestogens	Avoid coadministration
ST. JOHN'S WORT	RANOLAZINE	↓ RANOLAZINE levels with St. John's wort	Induction of CYP3A4-mediated metabolism of RANOLAZINE	Manufacturer advises to avoid coadministration
SELECTIVE SEROTONIN REUPTAKE INHIBITORS				
SSRIs	ALCOHOL	↑ Risk of sedation	Additive CNS depressant effects. Acute ingestion of alcohol inhibits CYP2D6 and CYP2C19, whereas chronic use induces CYP2E1 and CYP3A4	Be aware and caution against excessive alcohol intake
SSRIs	ANESTHETICS—GENERAL	No interactions with general anesthetics Note when considering balanced anesthesia, there is a risk of serotonin syndrome when dextromethorphan, pethidine, phenoperidine, or tramadol is used in patients taking SSRIs/SNRIs	Additive effect: these opioids inhibit serotonin uptake	SSRIs should be continued throughout the perioperative period to prevent discontinuation syndrome Avoid the use of dextromethorphan, pethidine, phenoperidine, or tramadol
FLUVOXAMINE	ANESTHETICS—LOCAL ROPIVACAINE	↑ Plasma concentrations and prolonged effects of ropivacaine—a local anesthetic related to bupivacaine but less potent and cardiotoxic. Adverse effects include nausea, vomiting, tachycardia, headache, and rigors	Fluvoxamine inhibits the metabolism of ropivacaine	Be aware of the possibility of prolonged effects and of toxicity. Take note of any numbness or tingling around the lips and mouth or slurring of speech after administration as they may be warning signs of more severe toxic effects such as seizures or loss of consciousness

(*Continued*)

Primary Drug	Secondary Drug	Effect	Mechanism	Precautions
ANTIDEPRESSANTS				
SSRIs	**ANALGESICS**			
SSRIs	OPIOIDS	1. Possible ↓ analgesic effect of codeine, and tramadol 2. ↑ Serotonin effects, including possible cases of serotonin syndrome, when opioids (oxycodone, pethidine, pentazocine, tramadol) are coadministered with SSRIs (fluoxetine, sertraline) 3. SSRIs may ↑ codeine, fentanyl, methadone, oxycodone, pethidine, and tramadol levels	1. Some SSRIs like paroxetine inhibit CYP2D6, which is required to produce the active form of codeine and tramadol 2. Additive effect; these opioids inhibit reuptake of serotonin 3. SSRIs inhibit CYP2D6-mediated metabolism of these opioids	1. Consider using an alternative opioid 2. Look for signs of ↑ serotonin activity, particularly on initiating therapy 3. Watch for excessive narcotization
SSRIs	NSAIDs	Slight ↑ risk of bleeding. SSRIs increase the risk of gastrointestinal adverse effects in first time users as compared with nonselective antidepressants	Unknown. SSRIs in combination with NSAIDs ↑ risk of gastrointestinal adverse effects: about 10 times higher than for SSRIs alone and about 4 times higher than the reported risk for NSAIDs alone	Warn patients to watch for early signs of bleeding. Combined use of SSRIs and NSAIDs strongly increases the risk of gastrointestinal adverse effects and should be avoided. The combination of nonselective antidepressants and NSAIDs does not have this effect
SSRIs	**ANTIARRHYTHMICS**			
SERTRALINE	AMIODARONE	Sertraline may ↑ amiodarone levels	Sertraline may inhibit CYP3A4-mediated metabolism of amiodarone	Watch for amiodarone toxicity; for those taking high doses of amiodarone, consider using an alternative SSRI with a lower affinity for CYP3A4
SSRIs	DRONEDARONE	Risk of ↑ plasma levels of SSRIs	Dronedarone inhibits CYP 2D6-metabolism SSRIs	Warn patients to report symptoms of SSRI toxicity, e.g., GI effects and anorexia. Reduce dose accordingly
SSRIs	FLECAINIDE, MEXILETINE, PROCAINAMIDE	SSRIs may ↑ levels of these antiarrhythmics	SSRIs inhibit CYP2D6-mediated metabolism	Monitor PR and BP closely; watch for toxicity. Get ECG prior to treatment and repeat this until stable

(*Continued*)

Primary Drug	Secondary Drug	Effect	Mechanism	Precautions
ANTIDEPRESSANTS				
SSRIs	PROPAFENONE	Levels of both may be ↑	Both SSRIs and propafenone are substrates for and inhibitors of CYP2D6	Monitor PR and BP closely
FLUVOXAMINE	QUINIDINE	Theoretical risk of ↑ quinidine levels	Fluvoxamine inhibits CYP3A4-mediated metabolism	Monitor PR, BP, and ECG closely
SSRIs	**ANTICANCER AND OTHER IMMUNOMODULATING DRUGS**			
SSRIs—NEFAZODONE	AXITINIB	Increased levels of axitinib	CYP3A4/5 inhibition	Manufacturer advises avoid concurrent use with strong CYP3A4/5 inhibitors if possible. If concurrent use is necessary, dose adjustment is recommended
FLUVOXAMINE	BENDAMUSTINE	Theoretical risk of increased bendamustine levels	CYP1A2 inhibition	Monitor closely
SSRIs—NEFAZODONE	BOSUTINIB	Increased bosutinib levels	CYP3A inhibition	Manufacturer advises to avoid concurrent use. If not possible, interruption of therapy or dose reduction should be considered
SSRIs—NEFAZODONE	CABAZITAXEL	Increased cabazitaxel levels	CYP3A4 inhibition	Avoid coadministration
SSRIs	CICLOSPORIN, TACROLIMUS	↑ Plasma concentrations of ciclosporin with risk of nephrotoxicity, myelosuppression, and neurotoxicity	Inhibition of CYP3A4-mediated metabolism of ciclosporin; these inhibitors vary in potency Potent—fluoxetine, nefazodone Moderate—fluvoxamine Weak—paroxetine, sertraline	Monitor plasma ciclosporin levels to prevent toxicity. Use SSRI with weak or no CYP3A4 inhibition
SSRIs—NEFAZODONE	DABRAFENIB	Predicted increased dabrafenib levels	CYP2C8/CYP3A4 inhibition	Avoid concurrent use if possible. Caution if concurrent use necessary
SSRIs—FLUVOXAMINE	ERLOTINIB	Increased levels of erlotinib	CYP1A2 inhibition	Caution with concurrent use. Consider dose reduction if toxicity occurs
SSRIs—FLUOXETINE, PAROXETINE	GEFITINIB	Increased levels of gefitinib	CYP2D6 inhibition	Monitor closely

(*Continued*)

Primary Drug	Secondary Drug	Effect	Mechanism	Precautions
ANTIDEPRESSANTS				
SERTRALINE	IMATINIB	↑ Plasma concentrations, with risk of toxic effects of sertraline	Imatinib is a potent inhibitor of CYP2C9 isoenzymes, which metabolize these drugs	Watch for the early toxic effects of these drugs. If necessary, consider using alternative drugs while the patient is being given imatinib
SSRIs—NEFAZODONE	PONATINIB	Possible increased ponatinib levels	CYP3A4 inhibition	Caution with concurrent use. Consider dose reduction
SSRIs—NEFAZODONE	PROCARBAZINE	↑ Risk of serotonin syndrome and CNS toxicity	Additive toxicity. Procarbazine has MAOI activity	Monitor BP closely and also CNS side effects. Because of the long half-life of fluoxetine and its active metabolites, at least 5 weeks should elapse between discontinuation of fluoxetine and initiation of therapy with procarbazine
SSRIs—NEFAZODONE	RUXOLITINIB	Increased levels of ruxolitinib	CYP3A4 inhibition	Manufacturer advises dose reduction Monitor closely
	TRABECTEDIN	Increased trabectedin levels	CYP3A4 inhibition	Avoid concurrent use with potent CP3A4 inhibitors if possible, monitor closely, and consider dose reduction
SSRIs—NEFAZODONE	VEMURAFENIB	Possible increased levels of vemurafenib	CYP3A4 inhibition	Manufacturers caution against concurrent use
SSRIs	**ANTICOAGULANTS**			
SSRIs	ANTICOAGULANTS—ORAL	Possible ↑ in anticoagulant effect with fluoxetine, fluvoxamine, paroxetine, and sertraline	Uncertain at present	Monitor INR at least weekly until stable
SSRIs	APIXABAN	↑ Effect of apixaban	Blockade of serotonin transfer to platelet causing ↓ platelet aggregation	Warn patient to report early evidence of bleeding
SSRIs	DABIGATRAN	↑ Effect of dabigatran	Blockade of serotonin transfer to platelet causing ↓ platelet aggregation	Warn patient to report early evidence of bleeding

(Continued)

Primary Drug	Secondary Drug	Effect	Mechanism	Precautions
ANTIDEPRESSANTS				
SSRIs	**ANTIDEPRESSANTS**			
SSRIs—FLUOXETINE, PAROXETINE, SERTRALINE	LITHIUM	Lithium increases serotonin levels and the risk of serotonin syndrome. Excessive somnolence reported with fluvoxamine. Shivering, anxiety may occur. See symptoms of serotonin syndrome. There are reports of both ↑ and ↓ plasma concentrations of lithium, lithium toxicity	Lithium is a direct stimulant of 5-HT receptors, while SSRIs ↓ reuptake of 5-HT; these are considered to ↑ effects of serotonin in the brain. Seizures are a neurotoxic effect of lithium and could occur even with plasma lithium concentrations within the normal range. SSRIs and lithium may have additive effects to cause seizures	Be aware of the possibility of serotonin syndrome. ➢ ***For signs and symptoms of serotonin toxicity, see Clinical Features of Some Adverse Drug Interactions, Serotonin Toxicity and Serotonin Syndrome.*** Also need to monitor lithium levels with appropriate dose adjustments during coadministration
SSRIs	MAOIs	↑ Risk of serotonin syndrome. ➢ ***For signs and symptoms of serotonin toxicity, see Clinical Features of Some Adverse Drug Interactions, Serotonin Toxicity and Serotonin Syndrome***	Additive inhibitory effects on serotonin reuptake	Avoid coadministration. MAOIs should not be started for at least 1 week after stopping SSRIs (2 weeks after sertraline, 5 weeks after fluoxetine). Conversely, SSRIs should not be started for at least 2 weeks after stopping MAOIs
SSRIs	ST. JOHN'S WORT SSRIs SNRIs—DULOXETINE TCAs TRAZODONE	↑ Risk of serotonin syndrome. ➢ ***For signs and symptoms of serotonin toxicity, see Clinical Features of Some Adverse Drug Interactions, Serotonin Toxicity and Serotonin Syndrome***	Additive effect. In addition, TCAs inhibit CYP2D6-mediated metabolism of SSRIs, increasing their levels	Caution with coadministration with TCAs or trazodone. Specialist advice should be sought and alternatives considered. Avoid coadministration of two SSRIs, and SSRIs with duloxetine or St. John's wort
FLUVOXAMINE	REBOXETINE	1. Risk of ↑ reboxetine levels 2. May ↑ fluvoxamine levels	1. Possibly inhibition of CYP3A4-mediated metabolism of reboxetine 2. Reboxetine is a selective norepinephrine reuptake inhibitor. Reboxetine inhibits metabolism of fluvoxamine	Avoid concurrent use (manufacturers' recommendation)
NEFAZODONE	REBOXETINE	Risk of ↑ reboxetine levels	Possibly inhibition of CYP3A4-mediated metabolism of reboxetine	Avoid coadministration

(*Continued*)

Primary Drug	Secondary Drug	Effect	Mechanism	Precautions
ANTIDEPRESSANTS				
SSRIs	TRYPTOPHAN	Risk of serotonin syndrome	Additive effect	Use with caution
SSRIs	ANTIDIABETIC DRUGS	Fluctuations in blood sugar are very likely, with both hypoglycemic and hyperglycemic events being reported in diabetics receiving hypoglycemic treatment. ↑ Plasma concentrations of sulfonylureas (e.g., tolbutamide) may occur	Brain serotonin and corticotropin-releasing hormone systems participate in the control of blood sugar levels. ↑ (usually acute) in brain serotonergic activity induces a hyperglycemic response. Fluvoxamine is a potent inhibitor and fluoxetine is a less potent inhibitor of CYP2C9, which metabolizes sulfonylureas	Both hyper- and hypoglycemic responses have been reported with SSRIs; there is a need to monitor blood glucose closely prior to, during, and after discontinuing SSRI treatment. ➢ ***For signs and symptoms of hypoglycemia, see Clinical Features of Some Adverse Drug Interactions, Hypoglycemia, Hyperglycemia***
FLUVOXAMINE	ANTIEMETICS—ONDANSETRON	Possible ↑ plasma concentrations of ondansetron	Fluvoxamine is potent inhibitor of CYP1A2, and fluoxetine, paroxetine, and sertraline are less potent inhibitors. Escitalopram and citalopram are not currently known to cause any inhibition	Warn patients to report ↑ in side effects of ondansetron
SSRIs	**ANTIEPILEPTICS**			
SSRIs	ANTIEPILEPTICS	↑ Risk of seizures	SSRIs lower seizure threshold	Risk of seizures is high; need to warn carers
PAROXETINE	BARBITURATES	↓ Paroxetine levels	Induction of hepatic metabolism	Be aware; watch for poor response to paroxetine
SSRIs	CARBAMAZEPINE	Risk of serotonin syndrome with carbamazepine	Carbamazepine ↑ serotonin concentrations in the brain	Avoid coadministration
SSRIs	PHENYTOIN	↑ Plasma concentrations of phenytoin	Phenytoin is a substrate of CYP2C9 and CYP2C19. Fluvoxamine and fluoxetine are known to inhibit CYP2C9/10/19. Paroxetine and sertraline cause less inhibition of CYP2C9/19	Monitor plasma phenytoin levels
SSRIs	**ANTIHISTAMINES**			
SSRIs	CYPROHEPTADINE	Antidepressant effect of SSRIs are possibly antagonized by cyproheptadine	Cyproheptadine is an antihistamine with antiserotonergic activity	Be aware

(Continued)

Primary Drug	Secondary Drug	Effect	Mechanism	Precautions
ANTIDEPRESSANTS				
SSRIs	TERFENADINE	Possibility of ↑ terfenadine levels with potential risk of dangerous arrhythmias	These drugs are metabolized mainly by CYP3A4. Fluvoxamine and fluoxetine are inhibitors of CYP3A4 but are relatively weak compared with ketoconazole, which is possibly 100 times more potent as an inhibitor	Avoid coadministration
SSRIs	**OTHER MEDICATIONS**			
SSRIs	ANTIHYPERTENSIVES AND HEART FAILURE DRUGS—METHYLDOPA	Methyldopa may ↓ effect of antidepressants	Methyldopa can cause depression	Methyldopa should be avoided in patients with depression
SSRIs	ANTIMALARIALS—ARTEMETHER/LUMEFANTRINE	This antimalarial may cause dose-related dangerous arrhythmias	A substrate, mainly of CYP3A4, which may be inhibited by high doses of fluvoxamine and to a lesser degree by fluoxetine and nefazodone	Manufacturers recommend avoiding coadministration
SSRIs	ANTIMIGRAINE DRUGS—5-HT1 AGONISTS	↑ Risk of serotonin syndrome. ➢ ***For signs and symptoms of serotonin toxicity, see Clinical Features of Some Adverse Drug Interactions, Serotonin Toxicity and Serotonin Syndrome*** A few cases of dyskinesias have been reported with fluoxetine	Triptans cause direct stimulation of 5-HT receptors, while SSRIs ↓ uptake of 5-HT, thus leading to ↑ serotonergic activity in the brain	The U.S. FDA (July 2006) issued a warning of possibility of occurrence of this life-threatening serotonin syndrome when SSRIs are used together with triptans. Advise patients to report immediately the onset of symptoms such as tremors, agitation, confusion, ↑ heart beat (palpitations), and fever, and either ↓ dose or discontinue SSRI
PAROXETINE	ANTIMUSCARINICS—DARIFENACIN, PROCYCLIDINE	↑ Levels of these antimuscarinics	Inhibition of metabolism	Watch for early features of toxicity

(*Continued*)

Primary Drug	Secondary Drug	Effect	Mechanism	Precautions
ANTIDEPRESSANTS				
SSRIs	**ANTIOBESITY DRUGS**			
SSRIs	LORCASERIN	Risk of serotonin syndrome	Additive effect	Be aware of the possibility of serotonin syndrome. ➢ ***For signs and symptoms of serotonin toxicity, see Clinical Features of Some Adverse Drug Interactions, Serotonin Toxicity and Serotonin Syndrome***
FLUOXETINE, FLUVOXAMINE	LORCASERIN	↑ Blood concentrations of these antidepressants	Inhibition of CYP2D6-mediated metabolism	Monitor PR and BP closely until stable
SSRIs	SIBUTRAMINE	Risk of serotonin syndrome	Additive effect	Manufacturer advises against coadministration
FLUVOXAMINE	ANTI-PARKINSON'S DRUGS—ROPINIROLE	↑ Ropinirole levels	Inhibition of CYP1A2-mediated metabolism to a greater extent by fluvoxamine compared to fluoxetine, paroxetine, and sertraline	Watch for early features of toxicity (nausea, drowsiness)
SSRIs	ANTI-PARKINSON'S DRUGS—SELEGILINE, RASAGILINE	Risk of severe hypertensive reactions and of serotonin syndrome. ➢ ***For signs and symptoms of serotonin toxicity, see Clinical Features of Some Adverse Drug Interactions, Serotonin Toxicity and Serotonin Syndrome***	Additive inhibitory effect on serotonin reuptake with SSRIs. There is an accumulation of serotonin in the brain and at peripheral sites. These dopaminergics are MAO-B inhibitors	Avoid coadministration. Rasagiline and selegiline should not be started for at least 2 weeks after stopping SSRIs (5 weeks after fluoxetine). Conversely, SSRIs should not be started for at least 2 weeks after stopping rasagiline and selegiline
SSRIs	**ANTIPLATELET AGENTS**			
SSRIs	ASPIRIN	Possible ↑ risk of bleeding with SSRIs	Uncertain. Possible additive effects including inhibition of serotonin release by platelets, SSRI-induced thrombocytopenia, and ↓ platelet aggregation	Avoid coadministration with high-dose aspirin
SSRIs	CLOPIDOGREL	Possible ↑ risk of bleeding with SSRIs	Uncertain. Possible additive effects including inhibition of serotonin release by platelets, SSRI-induced thrombocytopenia, and ↓ platelet aggregation	Avoid coadministration

(Continued)

Primary Drug	Secondary Drug	Effect	Mechanism	Precautions
ANTIDEPRESSANTS				
SSRIs	DIPYRIDAMOLE	Possible ↑ risk of bleeding with SSRIs	Uncertain. Possible additive effects including inhibition of serotonin release by platelets, SSRI-induced thrombocytopenia, and ↓ platelet aggregation	Avoid coadministration
SSRIs	GLYCOPROTEIN IIb/IIIa INHIBITORS	Possible ↑ risk of bleeding with SSRIs	Uncertain. Possible additive effects including inhibition of serotonin release by platelets, SSRI-induced thrombocytopenia, and ↓ platelet aggregation	Avoid coadministration
SSRIs	PRASUGREL	Possible ↑ risk of bleeding with SSRIs	Uncertain. Possible additive effects including inhibition of serotonin release by platelets, SSRI-induced thrombocytopenia, and ↓ platelet aggregation	Avoid coadministration
SSRIs	TICAGRELOR	Possible ↑ risk of bleeding with SSRIs	Uncertain. Possible additive effects including inhibition of serotonin release by platelets, SSRI-induced thrombocytopenia, and ↓ platelet aggregation	Avoid coadministration
SSRIs	**ANTIPSYCHOTICS**			
SSRIs	ARIPIPRAZOLE, CLOZAPINE, HALOPERIDOL, PERPHENAZINE, RISPERIDONE, SERTINDOLE, THIORIDAZINE	Possible ↑ plasma concentrations of these antipsychotics	Inhibition of CYP2D6-mediated metabolism of these drugs. The clinical significance of this depends upon whether alternative pathways of metabolism of these substrates are also inhibited by coadministered drugs. The risk is theoretically greater with clozapine, haloperidol, and olanzapine, because their CYP1A2-mediated metabolism is also inhibited by SSRIs	Warn patients to report ↑ side effects of these drugs, and consider reducing the dose of the antipsychotic
SERTRALINE	PIMOZIDE	↑ Plasma concentrations of these drugs and potential risk of dangerous arrhythmias	Sertraline inhibits metabolism of pimozide. Precise site of inhibition uncertain	Avoid coadministration

(Continued)

Primary Drug	Secondary Drug	Effect	Mechanism	Precautions
ANTIDEPRESSANTS				
SSRIs	**ANTIVIRALS**			
SSRIs	NNRTIs—EFAVIRENZ	Possible ↓ efficacy with sertraline	CYP2B6 contributes most to the demethylation of sertraline with lesser contributions from CYP2C19, CYP2C9, CYP3A4, and CYP2D6	Watch for therapeutic failure, and advise patients to report persistence or lack of improvement of symptoms of depression. ↑ Dose of sertraline as required, titrating to clinical response
SSRIs	PROTEASE INHIBITORS—RITONAVIR	↑ Adverse effects of fluoxetine, paroxetine, and sertraline when coadministered with ritonavir (with or without lopinavir). Cardiac and neurological events reported, including serotonin syndrome	Ritonavir is associated with the most significant interaction of the protease inhibitors due to potent inhibition of CYP3A, CYP2D6, CYP2C9, and CYP2C19 isoenzymes	Warn patients to watch for ↑ side effects of SSRIs, and consider reducing the dose of SSRI
SSRIs—PAROXETINE, SERTRALINE	DARUNAVIR/RITONAVIR	↓ Plasma levels of paroxetine and sertraline	Complex. Altered metabolism via CYP2D6 (paroxetine and sertraline) and CYP2C19 and 3A4 (sertraline)	Monitor more closely, may need ↑ dose of SSRI
SSRIs—PAROXETINE	FOSAMPRENAVIR/ RITONAVIR	↓ Plasma levels of paroxetine	Complex. Altered metabolism via CYP2D6	Warn patients to report altered treatment response for depression, watch for reduced efficacy as upward dose titration of paroxetine may be required
SSRIs	**ANXIOLYTICS AND HYPNOTICS**			
FLUOXETINE, FLUVOXAMINE, PAROXETINE	BZDs—ALPRAZOLAM, DIAZEPAM, MIDAZOLAM	↑ In plasma concentrations of these BZDs. Likely ↑ sedation and interference with psychomotor activity	Alprazolam, diazepam, and midazolam are subject to metabolism by CYP3A4. Fluvoxamine, fluoxetine, and possibly paroxetine are inhibitors of CYP3A4; sertraline is a weak inhibitor. SSRIs are relatively weak compared with ketoconazole, which is possibly 100 times more potent as an inhibitor	Warn patients about risks associated with activities that require alertness. Consider use of alternatives such as oxazepam, lorazepam, and temazepam, which are metabolized by glucuronidation. ➢ ***For signs and symptoms of CNS depression, see Clinical Features of Some Adverse Drug Interactions, Central Nervous System Depression***

(*Continued*)

DRUGS ACTING ON THE CENTRAL NERVOUS SYSTEM ANTIDEPRESSANTS

Primary Drug	Secondary Drug	Effect	Mechanism	Precautions
ANTIDEPRESSANTS				
SSRIs	CHLORAL HYDRATE	Case of excessive drowsiness	Uncertain; possibly additive effects, possibly displacement of chloral hydrate from protein binding sites	Warn patients to be aware of additional sedation
FLUOXETINE, PAROXETINE, SERTRALINE, VENLAFAXINE	ZOLPIDEM	Cases of agitation ± hallucinations	Uncertain	Avoid coadministration
SSRIs	**BETA-BLOCKERS**			
SSRIs	METOPROLOL, PROPRANOLOL, AND TIMOLOL	↑ Plasma concentrations and efficacy of metoprolol, propranolol, and timolol	Fluvoxamine inhibits the CYP1A2, 2C19, and 2D6-mediated metabolism of propranolol and 2D6-mediated metabolism of metoprolol Fluoxetine inhibits CYP2C19- and 2D6-mediated metabolism of propanolol and timolol and 2D6-mediated metabolism of metoprolol Paroxetine, sertraline, and venlafaxine inhibit CYP2D6-mediated metabolism of metoprolol, propanolol, and timolol and can impair conduction through the AV node	Monitor PR and BP at least weekly. Warn patients to report symptoms of hypotension (light-headedness, dizziness on standing, etc.). Watch for propanolol toxicity and loss of metoprolol cardioselectivity
FLUVOXAMINE	BRONCHODILATORS—THEOPHYLLINE	Possible ↑ plasma concentrations of theophylline	Fluvoxamine is potent inhibitor of CYP1A2, fluoxetine is less potent, and paroxetine and sertraline are weak inhibitors	Consider an alternative antidepressant, e.g., escitalopram and citalopram, which are not currently known to cause any inhibition
SSRIs	CALCIUM CHANNEL BLOCKERS	Reports of ↑ serum levels of nimodipine and episodes of adverse effects of nifedipine and verapamil (edema, flushing, ↓ BP) attributed to ↑ levels when coadministered with fluoxetine	Fluoxetine inhibits the CYP3A4-mediated metabolism of calcium channel blockers. It also inhibits intestinal Pgp, which may ↑ bioavailability of verapamil. Nefazodone also inhibits CYP3A4	Monitor BP at least weekly until stable. Warn patients to report symptoms of hypotension (light-headedness, dizziness on standing, etc.). Consider reducing the dose of calcium channel blocker or using an alternative antidepressant

(*Continued*)

Primary Drug	Secondary Drug	Effect	Mechanism	Precautions
ANTIDEPRESSANTS				
SSRIs	CARDIAC GLYCOSIDES—DIGOXIN	Theoretical risk of ↑ digoxin levels	Inhibition of Pgp by sertraline and paroxetine is observed in vitro, unlikely of major clinical significance	Be aware
SSRIs	**CNS STIMULANTS**			
SSRIs	ATOMOXETINE	↑ Plasma concentrations and risk of adverse effects (abdominal pain, vomiting, nausea, fatigue, irritability)	Atomoxetine is a selective norepinephrine reuptake inhibitor. ↑ Plasma concentrations due to inhibition of CYP2D6 by fluoxetine and paroxetine (potent), fluvoxamine and sertraline (less potent), and escitalopram and citalopram (weak)	Avoid coadministration. The interaction is usually severe with fluoxetine and paroxetine
FLUVOXAMINE	MODAFINIL	May cause ↓ imipramine levels if CYP1A2 is the predominant metabolic pathway and alternative metabolic pathways are either genetically deficient or affected	Modafinil is a moderate inducer of CYP1A2 in a concentration-dependent manner	Be aware
SSRIs	**DRUG DEPENDENCE THERAPIES**			
FLUOXETINE, FLUVOXAMINE, PAROXETINE, SERTRALINE	BUPROPION	↑ Plasma concentrations of bupropion and risk of adverse effects	Most SSRIs are inhibitors of CYP2D6-usually moderate. CYP2D6 is highly polymorphic and responses would vary. See Polymorphisms. Major pathway for Bupropion is via CYP2C8/9, inhibited weakly by fluoxetine, Fluvoxamine, paroxetine, and sertraline	Warn patients about adverse effects (dry mouth, taste disturbances, agitation, GI upset, insomnia), and use alternatives when possible
ESCITALOPRAM, FLUOXETINE, FLUVOXAMINE, PAROXETINE, SERTRALINE	BUPROPION	↑ Plasma concentrations of these SSRIs, with risk of toxic effects	Bupropion and its metabolite hydroxybupropion inhibit CYP2D6	Initiate therapy of these drugs at the lowest effective dose. Interaction is likely to be important with substrates for which CYP2D6 is considered the only metabolic pathway (e.g., paroxetine)

(Continued)

Primary Drug	Secondary Drug	Effect	Mechanism	Precautions
ANTIDEPRESSANTS				
SSRIs	DIURETICS	Hyponatremia associated with SSRI use, with the incidence varying from 0.5% to 32%	Hyponatremia developed within the first few week of treatment and resolved within 2 weeks after therapy was discontinued. Mechanism secondary to development of SIADH (inappropriate secretion of ADH)	Risk factors include older age, female gender, low body weight, and lower baseline serum sodium
SSRIs—FLUOXETINE, PAROXETINE	ELIGLUSTAT	↑ Eliglustat levels	Inhibition of CYP2D6-mediated metabolism	Reduce dose to 85 mg od
FLUVOXAMINE, NEFAZODONE	ELIGLUSTAT	↑ Eliglustat levels	Inhibition of CYP3A4-mediated metabolism	Nefazodone: reduce dose to 85 mg od in extensive metabolizers. Avoid coadministration in intermediate and poor metabolizers Fluvoxamine is a weak inhibitor of CYP3A4; it should be avoided in poor metabolizers
FLUVOXAMINE	FOOD—CHARGRILLED MEAT, BROCCOLI, CABBAGE, SPROUTS	↓ Plasma concentrations of fluvoxamine with loss of therapeutic efficacy	Fluvoxamine and fluoxetine are metabolized mainly by CYP1A2 isoenzymes, while the role of CYP1A2 in the metabolism of sertraline is probably not clinically significant	Monitor for lack of therapeutic effect. When inducers are withdrawn, monitor for fluvoxamine toxicity
FLUVOXAMINE, SERTRALINE	GRAPEFRUIT JUICE	Possibly ↑ efficacy and ↑ adverse effects	Possibly ↓ metabolism	Clinical significance unclear
SSRIs	H2 RECEPTOR BLOCKERS—CIMETIDINE	↑ Efficacy and adverse effects, e.g., nausea, diarrhea, dyspepsia, dizziness, sexual dysfunction	↑ Bioavailability	Use with caution, monitor for ↑ side effects. ↓ Dose may be necessary
SSRIs	MUSCLE RELAXANTS—CYCLOBENZAPRINE	↑ Risk of serotonin syndrome ➢ ***For signs and symptoms of serotonin toxicity, see Clinical Features of Some Adverse Drug Interactions, Serotonin Toxicity and Serotonin Syndrome***	Additive effect. Cyclobenzaprine is structurally similar to tricyclic antidepressants. TCAs block reuptake of serotonin	Caution with coadministration Specialist advice should be sought and alternatives considered

(*Continued*)

Primary Drug	Secondary Drug	Effect	Mechanism	Precautions
ANTIDEPRESSANTS				
SSRIs—FLUVOXAMINE, NEFAZODONE	NITISINONE	Possible ↑ nitisinone levels	Inhibition of CYP3A4-mediated metabolism	Monitor carefully
SSRIs	PARASYMPATHOMIMETICS—GALANTAMINE	↑ Galantamine levels	Inhibition of CYP2D6-mediated metabolism of galantamine Fluoxetine, paroxetine—potent Fluvoxamine, sertraline—less potent Escitalopram, citalopram—weak	Monitor PR and BP closely, watching for bradycardia and hypotension. Be aware that there is a theoretical risk with other SSRIs
SSRIs	PERIPHERAL VASODILATORS—CILOSTAZOL	Fluoxetine, fluvoxamine, and sertraline ↑ cilostazol levels	Fluoxetine, fluvoxamine, nefazodone, and sertraline inhibit CYP3A4-mediated metabolism of cilostazol	Avoid coadministration
SSRIs—CITALOPRAM/ESCITALOPRAM	OMEPRAZOLE/ESOMEPRAZOLE	↑ Plasma concentrations	Altered metabolism	Monitor more closely; ↓ dose may be required
FLUVOXAMINE	PROTON PUMP INHIBITORS—OMEPRAZOLE	1. ↓ Fluvoxamine levels with loss of therapeutic efficacy 2. ↑ Plasma concentration of proton pump inhibitor	1. Inhibition of CYP1A2-mediated metabolism by omeprazole 2. Fluvoxamine inhibits metabolism of proton pump inhibitors via CYP2C19	1. Monitor for lack of therapeutic effect of fluvoxamine. When omeprazole is withdrawn, monitor for fluvoxamine toxicity 2. Consider dose reduction of proton pump inhibitor
FLUVOXAMINE	PIRFENIDONE	↑ Pirfenidone levels	Inhibition of CYP1A2-mediated metabolism of pirfenidone	Manufacturer recommends avoiding coadministration
SSRIs	SYMPATHOMIMETICS	1. Case report of serotonin syndrome when dexamfetamine was coadministered with citalopram 2. Case reports of psychiatric disturbances when methylphenidate was given with sertraline, and phenylpropolamine was administered with fluoxetine was coadministered with phenylpropanolamine	1. Uncertain; postulated that there is an additive effect of inhibition of serotonin reuptake by citalopram 2. Generally considered that patients on SSRIs are more sensitive to sympathomimetics	1. Avoid coadministration of dexamfetamine and citalopram 2. Warn patients to watch for early signs such as anxiety 3. Be aware that phenylpropolamine is a constituent of several OTC medicines for nasal congestion

(*Continued*)

Primary Drug	Secondary Drug	Effect	Mechanism	Precautions
ANTIDEPRESSANTS				
FLUVOXAMINE	TOBACCO	↓ Plasma concentrations of fluvoxamine with loss of therapeutic efficacy	Fluvoxamine and fluoxetine are metabolized mainly by CYP1A2 isoenzymes, while the role of CYP1A2 in the metabolism of sertraline is probably not clinically significant	Monitor for lack of therapeutic effect. When inducers are withdrawn, monitor for fluvoxamine toxicity
SEROTONIN NOREPINEPHRINE REUPTAKE INHIBITORS—DULOXETINE, VENLAFAXINE				
VENLAFAXINE	**DRUGS THAT PROLONG THE QT INTERVAL**			
VENLAFAXINE	1. ANTIARRHYTHMICS—ajmaline, amiodarone, azimilide, cibenzoline, disopyramide, dofetilide, dronedarone, ibutilide, procainamide, propafenone, quinidine 2. ANTIBIOTICS—macrolides (especially azithromycin, clarithromycin, parenteral erythromycin, telithromycin), quinolones (especially moxifloxacin), quinupristin/dalfopristin 3. ANTICANCER AND IMMUNOMODULATING DRUGS—arsenic trioxide, bosutinib, crizotinib, dasatinib, eribulin, fingolimod, lapatinib, nilotinib, pazopanib, sunitinib, vandetanib, vemurafenib 4. ANTIDEPRESSANTS—TCAs 5. ANTIEMETICS—ondansetron	Risk of ventricular arrhythmias, particularly torsades de pointes	Additive effect; these drugs prolong the QT interval	Avoid coadministration

(*Continued*)

Primary Drug	Secondary Drug	Effect	Mechanism	Precautions
ANTIDEPRESSANTS				
	6. ANTIFUNGALS—fluconazole, posaconazole, voriconazole 7. ANTIHISTAMINES—terfenadine, hydroxyzine, mizolastine 8. ANTIHYPERTENSIVES—ketanserin 9. ANTIMALARIALS—artemether with lumefantrine, chloroquine, halofantrine, hydroxychloroquine, mefloquine, quinine 10. ANTIPROTOZOALS—pentamidine isothionate 11. ANTIPSYCHOTICS—atypicals, phenothiazines, pimozide 12. ANTIVIRALS—boceprevir, rilpivirine, telaprevir 13. BETA-BLOCKERS—sotalol 14. BRONCHODILATORS—parenteral bronchodilators 15. CNS STIMULANTS—atomoxetine 16. RANOLAZINE			
SNRIs	ANESTHETICS—GENERAL	No interactions with general anesthetics Note when considering balanced anesthesia, there is a risk of serotonin syndrome when dextromethorphan, pethidine, phenoperidine, or tramadol is used in patients taking SSRIs/SNRIs	Additive effect: these opioids inhibit serotonin uptake	SSRIs should be continued throughout the perioperative period to prevent discontinuation syndrome Avoid the use of dextromethorphan, pethidine, phenoperidine, or tramadol

(*Continued*)

Primary Drug	Secondary Drug	Effect	Mechanism	Precautions
ANTIDEPRESSANTS				
SNRIs	**ANALGESICS**			
VENLAFAXINE	NSAIDs	Slight ↑ risk of bleeding. SNRIs increase the risk of gastrointestinal adverse effects in first time users as compared with nonselective antidepressants	Attributed to ↓ serotonin content in platelets due to the SNRI causing ↓ platelet aggregation. SSRIs in combination with NSAIDs ↑ risk of gastrointestinal adverse effects: about 10 times higher than for SSRIs alone and about four times higher than the reported risk for NSAIDs alone	Warn patients to watch for early signs of bleeding. Combined use of SNRIs and NSAIDs strongly increases the risk of gastrointestinal adverse effects and should be avoided. The combination of nonselective antidepressants and NSAIDs does not have this effect. Acid suppressing drugs (e.g., PPIs) have some protective effect
DULOXETINE	OPIOIDS	↑ Serotonin effects, including possible cases of serotonin syndrome, when opioids (oxycodone, pethidine, pentazocine, tramadol) are given	Uncertain	Look for signs of ↑ serotonin activity, particularly on initiating therapy
DULOXETINE	ANTIARRHYTHMICS—FLECAINIDE, PROPAFENONE	Possibly ↑ flecainide and propafenone levels	Duloxetine moderately inhibits CYP2D6	Monitor PR and BP weekly until stable
DULOXETINE	ANTIBIOTICS—CIPROFLOXACIN	↑ Duloxetine levels with risk of side effects, e.g., arrhythmias	Inhibition of metabolism of duloxetine	Avoid coadministration
SNRIs	**ANTICOAGULANTS**			
SNRIs	APIXABAN	↑ Effect of dabigatran	Uncertain	Warn patient to report early evidence of bleeding
SNRIs	DABIGATRAN	↑ Effect of dabigatran	Uncertain	Warn patient to report early evidence of bleeding

(*Continued*)

Primary Drug	Secondary Drug	Effect	Mechanism	Precautions
ANTIDEPRESSANTS				
SNRIs	**ANTIDEPRESSANTS**			
VENLAFAXINE	LITHIUM	Possible risk of serotonin syndrome	Additive effect of increased serotonin levels in brain	Be aware of the possibility of serotonin syndrome. Also need to monitor lithium levels with appropriate dose adjustments during coadministration. ➢ ***For signs and symptoms of serotonin toxicity, see Clinical Features of Some Adverse Drug Interactions, Serotonin Toxicity and Serotonin Syndrome***
SNRIs	MAOIs	Risk of severe hypertensive reactions and of serotonin syndrome. ➢ ***For signs and symptoms of serotonin toxicity, see Clinical Features of Some Adverse Drug Interactions, Serotonin Toxicity and Serotonin Syndrome***	Duloxetine and venlafaxine inhibits the reuptake of both serotonin and norepinephrine. Due to impaired metabolism of these amines, there is an accumulation of serotonin and norepinephrine in the brain and at peripheral sites	Do not coadminister duloxetine and venlafaxine prior to 14 days after discontinuing an MAOI, and do not coadminister an MAOI for 5 days after discontinuing duloxetine and for 1 week after discontinuing venlafaxine.
DULOXETINE	ST. JOHN'S WORT, SSRIs, TCAs	↑ Risk of serotonin syndrome. ➢ ***For signs and symptoms of serotonin toxicity, see Clinical Features of Some Adverse Drug Interactions, Serotonin Toxicity and Serotonin Syndrome***	Additive effect	Avoid coadministration
SNRIs	ANTIHYPERTENSIVES AND HEART FAILURE DRUGS—CENTRALLY ACTING ANTIHYPERTENSIVES—METHYLDOPA	Methyldopa may ↑ effect of antidepressants	Methyldopa can cause depression	Methyldopa should be avoided in patients with depression
SNRIs	ANTIMALARIALS—ARTEMETHER/LUMEFANTRINE	↑ Artemether/lumefantrine levels with risk of toxicity, including arrhythmias	Venlafaxine inhibits CYP3A4, which is partly responsible for the metabolism of artemether	Avoid coadministration with venlafaxine and caution with duloxetine

(Continued)

Primary Drug	Secondary Drug	Effect	Mechanism	Precautions
ANTIDEPRESSANTS				
DULOXETINE	ANTIMIGRAINE DRUGS—5-HT1 AGONISTS	Possible ↑ risk of serotonin syndrome. ➢ ***For signs and symptoms of serotonin toxicity, see Clinical Features of Some Adverse Drug Interactions, Serotonin Toxicity and Serotonin Syndrome***	Triptans cause direct stimulation of 5-HT receptors, while SNRIs ↓ uptake of 5-HT, thus leading to ↑ serotonergic activity in the brain	The U.S. FDA (July 2006) warned of the possibility of life-threatening serotonin syndrome when SNRIs are used together with triptans (5-HT receptor agonists). Avoid concomitant use, or ↓ dose of SNRI
SNRIs	**ANTIOBESITY DRUGS**			
SNRIs	LORCASERIN	Risk of serotonin syndrome	Additive effect	Be aware of the possibility of serotonin syndrome. ➢ ***For signs and symptoms of serotonin toxicity, see Clinical Features of Some Adverse Drug Interactions, Serotonin Toxicity and Serotonin Syndrome***
DULOXETINE	LORCASERIN	↑ Blood concentrations of these antidepressants	Inhibition of CYP2D6-mediated metabolism	Monitor PR and BP closely until stable
SNRIs	SIBUTRAMINE	Risk of serotonin syndrome	Additive effect	Manufacturer advises against coadministration
VENLAFAXINE	ANTI-PARKINSON'S DRUGS—SELEGILINE, POSSIBLY RASAGILINE	Risk of severe hypertensive reactions and of serotonin syndrome ➢ ***For signs and symptoms of serotonin toxicity, see Clinical Features of Some Adverse Drug Interactions, Serotonin Toxicity and Serotonin Syndrome***	Venlafaxine inhibits the reuptake of both serotonin and norepinephrine. Due to impaired metabolism of these amines, there is an accumulation of serotonin and norepinephrine in the brain and at peripheral sites. These dopaminergics are MAO-B inhibitors	Do not start selegiline or rasagiline for at least 1 week after stopping venlafaxine; conversely, do not start venlafaxine for at least 2 weeks after stopping selegiline or rasagiline
SNRIs	**ANTIPLATELET AGENTS**			
SNRIs	ASPIRIN	Possible ↑ risk of bleeding	Uncertain. Possible additive effects including inhibition of serotonin release by platelets, SNRI-induced thrombocytopenia, and ↓ platelet aggregation	Avoid coadministration with high-dose aspirin

(*Continued*)

Primary Drug	Secondary Drug	Effect	Mechanism	Precautions
ANTIDEPRESSANTS				
SNRIs	CLOPIDOGREL	Possible ↑ risk of bleeding with SNRIs	Uncertain. Possible additive effects including inhibition of serotonin release by platelets, SNRI-induced thrombocytopenia, and ↓ platelet aggregation	Avoid coadministration
SNRIs	DIPYRIDAMOLE	Possible ↑ risk of bleeding with SNRIs	Uncertain. Possible additive effects including inhibition of serotonin release by platelets, SNRI-induced thrombocytopenia, and ↓ platelet aggregation	Avoid coadministration
SNRIs	CLOPIDOGREL	Possible ↑ risk of bleeding with SNRIs	Uncertain. Possible additive effects including inhibition of serotonin release by platelets, SNRI-induced thrombocytopenia, and ↓ platelet aggregation	Avoid coadministration
SNRIs	GLYCOPROTEIN IIB/IIIA INHIBITORS	Possible ↑ risk of bleeding with SNRIs	Uncertain. Possible additive effects including inhibition of serotonin release by platelets, SNRI-induced thrombocytopenia, and ↓ platelet aggregation	Avoid coadministration
SNRIs	PRASUGREL	Possible ↑ risk of bleeding with SNRIs	Uncertain. Possible additive effects including inhibition of serotonin release by platelets, SNRI-induced thrombocytopenia, and ↓ platelet aggregation	Avoid coadministration
SNRIs	TICAGRELOR	Possible ↑ risk of bleeding with SNRIs	Uncertain. Possible additive effects including inhibition of serotonin release by platelets, SNRI-induced thrombocytopenia, and ↓ platelet aggregation	Avoid coadministration
VENLAFAXINE	**ANTIPSYCHOTICS ➢ *also QT-prolonging drugs, above***			
VENLAFAXINE	HALOPERIDOL	↑ Haloperidol levels	Inhibited metabolism	Avoid coadministration

(Continued)

Primary Drug	Secondary Drug	Effect	Mechanism	Precautions
ANTIDEPRESSANTS				
VENLAFAXINE	BETA-BLOCKERS	↑ Plasma concentrations and efficacy of metoprolol, propranolol, and timolol	Venlafaxine inhibits CYP2D6-mediated metabolism of metoprolol, propanolol, and timolol	Monitor PR and BP at least weekly; watch for metoprolol toxicity (in particular, loss of its cardioselectivity) and propanolol toxicity
VENLAFAXINE	H2 RECEPTOR BLOCKERS—CIMETIDINE	↑ Efficacy and adverse effects	Inhibition of metabolism	Not thought to be clinically significant, but take care in elderly people and in patients with hepatic impairment
SNRIs	MUSCLE RELAXANTS—CYCLOBENZAPRINE	↑ Risk of serotonin syndrome ➢ ***For signs and symptoms of serotonin toxicity, see Clinical Features of Some Adverse Drug Interactions, Serotonin Toxicity and Serotonin Syndrome***	Additive effect. Cyclobenzaprine is structurally similar to tricyclic antidepressants. TCAs block reuptake of serotonin	Uncertain, postulated that there is an additive effect of inhibition of serotonin reuptake and of noradrenaline with increased release of serotonin
DESVENLAFAXINE	SYMPATHOMIMETICS—INDIRECT	Case of serotonin syndrome when dexamfetamine is coadministered	Uncertain; postulated that there is an additive effect of inhibition of serotonin reuptake and of noradrenaline with increased release of serotonin.	Avoid coadministration
TRICYCLIC AND TETRACYCLIC ANTIDEPRESSANTS				
TCAs	**DRUGS THAT PROLONG THE QT INTERVAL**			
TCAs	1. ANTIARRHYTHMICS—ajmaline, amiodarone, azimilide, cibenzoline, disopyramide, dofetilide, dronedarone, ibutilide, procainamide, propafenone, quinidine 2. ANTIBIOTICS—macrolides (especially azithromycin, clarithromycin, parenteral erythromycin, telithromycin), quinolones (especially moxifloxacin), quinupristin/dalfopristin	Risk of ventricular arrhythmias, particularly torsades de pointes	Additive effect; these drugs prolong the QT interval Also, amitriptyline, clomipramine, and desipramine levels may be ↑ by propafenone Amitriptyline and clomipramine may ↑ propafenone levels Propafenone and these TCAs inhibit CYP2D6-mediated metabolism of each other	Avoid coadministration

(Continued)

Primary Drug	Secondary Drug	Effect	Mechanism	Precautions
ANTIDEPRESSANTS				
	3. ANTICANCER AND IMMUNOMODULATING DRUGS—arsenic trioxide, bosutinib, crizotinib, dasatinib, eribulin, fingolimod, lapatinib, nilotinib, pazopanib, sunitinib, vandetanib, vemurafenib 4. ANTIDEPRESSANTS—venlafaxine 5. ANTIEMETICS—ondansetron 6. ANTIFUNGALS—fluconazole, posaconazole, voriconazole 7. ANTIHISTAMINES—terfenadine, hydroxyzine, mizolastine 8. ANTIHYPERTENSIVES—ketanserin 9. ANTIMALARIALS—artemether with lumefantrine, chloroquine, halofantrine,hydroxychloroquine, mefloquine, quinine 10. ANTIPROTOZOALS—pentamidine isothionate 11. ANTIPSYCHOTICS—atypicals, phenothiazines, pimozide 12. ANTIVIRALS—boceprevir, rilpivirine, telaprevir 13. BETA-BLOCKERS—sotalol 14. BRONCHODILATORS—parenteral bronchodilators 15. CNS STIMULANTS—atomoxetine 16. RANOLAZINE			

(*Continued*)

Primary Drug	Secondary Drug	Effect	Mechanism	Precautions
ANTIDEPRESSANTS				
TCAs	**DRUGS WITH ANTIMUSCARINIC EFFECTS**			
TCAs	1. ANALGESICS—nefopam 2. ANTIARRHYTHMICS—disopyramide, propafenone 3. ANTIEMETICS—cyclizine 4. ANTIHISTAMINES—chlorphenamine, cyproheptadine, hydroxyzine 5. ANTIMUSCARINICS—atropine, benzatropine, cyclopentolate, dicycloverine, flavoxate, homatropine, hyoscine, orphenadrine, oxybutynin, procyclidine, propantheline, tolterodine, trihexyphenidyl, tropicamide 6. ANTI-PARKINSON'S DRUGS—dopaminergics 7. ANTIPSYCHOTICS—phenothiazines, clozapine, pimozide 8. MUSCLE RELAXANTS—baclofen 9. NITRATES—isosorbide dinitrate	↑ Risk of antimuscarinic side effects. Also, possibly ↓ levodopa levels. *NB ↓ efficacy of sublingual nitrate tablets*	Additive effect. Delayed gastric emptying may cause more levodopa to be metabolized within the wall of the gastrointestinal tract. *Antimuscarinic effects ↓ saliva production, which ↓ dissolution of the tablet*	Warn patients of this additive effect. Consider increasing the dose of levodopa. *Consider changing the formulation to a sublingual nitrate spray*
TCAs	ALCOHOL	↑ Sedation	Additive effect	Warn patients about this effect

(*Continued*)

Primary Drug	Secondary Drug	Effect	Mechanism	Precautions
ANTIDEPRESSANTS				
TCAs	ANESTHETICS—GENERAL	Increased availability of neurotransmitters in the central nervous system can result in increased anesthetic requirements TCAs may result in increased response to intraoperatively administered anticholinergics, and those that cross the blood–brain barrier, such as atropine May cause postoperative confusion Exaggerated blood pressure responses following administration of indirect acting vasopressors such as ephedrine Chronic therapy depletes cardiac catecholamines, potentiating the cardiac depressant effects of anesthetic agents	Given chronically, TCAs decrease stores of noradrenergic catecholamines Cause changes on the ECG (changes in the T wave, widening of the QRS complex and prolongation of QT interval, bundle branch block or other conduction abnormalities, or PVCs) Predispose to ventricular arrhythmias Refractory hypotension may occur in higher doses Exaggerated responses to vasopressors due to increased availability of norepinephrine at the postsynaptic nervous system	The most important interaction between anesthetic agents and tricyclic antidepressant drugs is an exaggerated response to both indirect acting vasopressors and sympathetic stimulation Pancuronium, ketamine, meperidine, and epinephrine-containing solutions should be avoided Avoid use of vasopressors – necessary to maintain blood pressure with accurate replacement of blood or fluids During anesthesia and surgery, it is important to avoid stimulating the sympathetic nervous system. If hypotension occurs and vasopressors are needed, direct acting drugs such as phenylephrine are recommended. The dose should probably be decreased to minimize the likelihood of an exaggerated hypertensive response
TCAs	**ANALGESICS**			
TCAs	OPIOIDS	1. Risk of ↑ respiratory depression and sedation 2. ↑ Levels of morphine 3. Case reports of seizures when tramadol was coadministered with TCAs 4. TCAs may ↑ codeine, fentanyl, pethidine, and tramadol levels	1. Additive effect 2. Uncertain; likely ↑ bioavailability of morphine 3. Unknown 4. TCAs inhibit CYP2D6-mediated metabolism of these opioids	1. Warn patients of this effect. Titrate doses carefully 2. Warn patients of this effect. Titrate doses carefully 3. Consider an alternative opioid 4. Watch for excessive narcotization
TCAs	NEFOPAM	Risk of seizures with TCAs	Additive effect; both drugs lower the seizure threshold	Avoid coadministration

(*Continued*)

Primary Drug	Secondary Drug	Effect	Mechanism	Precautions
ANTIDEPRESSANTS				
TCAs	PARACETAMOL	TCAs may slow the onset of action of intermittent-dose paracetamol	Anticholinergic effects delay gastric emptying and absorption	Warn patients that the action of paracetamol may be delayed. This will not be the case when paracetamol is taken regularly
TCAs	ANTIARRHYTHMICS—FLECAINIDE, MEXILETINE	Risk of arrhythmias	Additive effect; both drugs may be proarrhythmogenic. In addition, amitriptyline and clomipramine may inhibit CYP2D6-mediated metabolism of flecainide and mexiletine, while mexiletine inhibits CYP1A2-mediated metabolism of amitriptyline, clomipramine, and imipramine	Monitor PR, BP, and ECG closely; watch for flecainide toxicity
TCAs	**ANTICANCER AND IMMUNOMODULATING DRUGS**			
TCAs	FLUOROURACIL, IMATINIB, LEFLUNOMIDE	Possible ↑ plasma concentrations of these cytotoxics	Inhibition of CYP2C9-mediated metabolism. The clinical significance of this depends upon whether alternative pathways of metabolism are also inhibited by coadministered drugs	Warn patients to report ↑ side effects and monitor blood count carefully
TCAs—AMITRIPTYLINE	PIXANTRONE	Theoretical risk of increased drug levels	Pixantrone inhibits CYP1A2	Manufacturer advises to monitor closely
TCAs	PROCARBAZINE	Interaction similar to tricyclics with conventional MAOIs	Procarbazine is weak MAO inhibitor	Avoid concurrent use
TCAs	THALIDOMIDE	Increased sedation	Additive	Caution with concurrent use
TCAs	VINBLASTINE	Possible ↑ plasma concentrations of vinblastine	Inhibition of CYP2D6-mediated metabolism of vinblastine. The clinical significance of this depends upon whether vinblastine's alternative pathways of metabolism are also inhibited by coadministered drugs	Warn patients to report ↑ side effects of vinblastine and monitor blood count carefully
TCAs	ANTICOAGULANTS—ORAL	Cases of both ↑ and ↓ effect of warfarin	Uncertain at present	Monitor INR at least weekly until stable

(*Continued*)

Primary Drug	Secondary Drug	Effect	Mechanism	Precautions
ANTIDEPRESSANTS				
TCAs	**ANTIDEPRESSANTS**			
TCAs—AMITRIPTYLINE, CLOMIPRAMINE, IMIPRAMINE	LITHIUM	Possible risk of serotonin syndrome	Additive effect of increased serotonin levels in brain	Be aware of the possibility of serotonin syndrome. Also need to monitor lithium levels with appropriate dose adjustments during coadministration. ➢ ***For signs and symptoms of serotonin toxicity, see Clinical Features of Some Adverse Drug Interactions, Serotonin Toxicity and Serotonin Syndrome***
TCAs—AMITRIPTYLINE, CLOMIPRAMINE, DESIPRAMINE, IMIPRAMINE, NORTRIPTYLINE	MAOIs	↑ Risk of stroke, hyperpyrexia, and convulsions. ↑ Plasma concentrations of TCAs, with risk of toxic effects. ↑ Risk of serotonin syndrome and of adrenergic syndrome with older MAOIs. Clomipramine may trigger acute confusion in Parkinson's disease when used with selegiline	TCAs are believed to act also by inhibiting the reuptake of serotonin and norepinephrine, increasing the risk of serotonin and adrenergic syndromes. A combination of TCAs and antidepressants can ↑ risk of seizures	Very hazardous interaction. Avoid concurrent use and consider use of alternative antidepressant. Be aware that seizures occur with overdose of TCAs just before cardiac arrest. See serotinergic syndrome in appendix SNRIs
TCAs	SSRIs, SNRIs—DULOXETINE VENLAFAXINE	↑ Risk of serotonin syndrome. ➢ ***For signs and symptoms of serotonin toxicity, see Clinical Features of Some Adverse Drug Interactions, Serotonin Toxicity and Serotonin Syndrome***	Additive effect. In addition, TCAs inhibit CYP2D6-mediated metabolism of SSRIs increasing their levels	Caution with coadministration. Specialist advice should be sought and alternatives considered
TCAs	HISTAMINE	Effects of histamine antagonized	Histamine blockade	Avoid concurrent use
TCAs	ANTIDIABETIC DRUGS	Likely to impair control of diabetes	TCAs may ↑ serum glucose levels by up to 150%, ↑ appetite (particularly carbohydrate craving) and ↓ metabolic rate	Be aware and monitor blood sugar weekly until stable. Generally considered safe unless diabetes is poorly controlled or is associated with significant cardiac or renal disease. Amitriptyline, imipramine, and citalopram are also used to treat painful diabetic neuropathy

(*Continued*)

Primary Drug	Secondary Drug	Effect	Mechanism	Precautions
ANTIDEPRESSANTS				
TCAs	ANTIEMETICS—ONDANSETRON, TROPISETRON	Possible ↑ plasma concentrations of these antiemetics	Inhibition of CYP2D6-mediated metabolism of these antiemetics. The clinical significance of this depends upon whether their alternative pathways of metabolism are also inhibited by coadministered drugs. The risk is theoretically higher with ondansetron, because TCAs also inhibit CYP1A2-mediated metabolism	Warn patients to report ↑ side effects of ondansetron and tropisetron
TCAs	**ANTIEPILEPTICS**			
TCAs	ANTIEPILEPTICS	Possible ↓ effect of antiepileptics	TCAs lower seizure threshold	Caution with coadministration. Consider an alternative antidepressant in patients on antiepileptics
MIANSERIN	BARBITURATES	↓ Mianserin levels	Induction of hepatic metabolism	Be aware and watch for signs of ↓ antidepressant effect of mianserin
MIANSERIN	CARBAMAZEPINE	1. ↑ Risk of bone marrow depression in patients on chemotherapy when used with TCAs 2. ↓ Plasma concentrations of mianserin	1. Additive effects 2. ↑ Metabolism of mianserin	1. Avoid concurrent use during chemotherapy 2. Be aware and watch for signs of ↓ antidepressant effect of mianserin
TCAs	PHENYTOIN	1. ↑ Risk of seizures 2. ↓ Levels of TCAs, with risk of therapeutic failure 3. Report of ↑ phenytoin levels with mianserin	1. TCAs drugs lower seizure threshold 2. Induction of hepatic metabolism 3. Inhibition of phenytoin metabolism	1. Care with coadministration 2. Watch for ↑ fit frequency; warn patient of this risk when starting these drugs and take suitable precautions. Consider increasing dose of antiepileptic 3. Monitor phenytoin levels when coadministered with mianserin
TCAs	VALPROATE	↑ Amitriptyline and nortriptyline levels	Uncertain	Be aware; watch for clinical features of ↑ levels of these TCAs (e.g., sedation, dry mouth)

(*Continued*)

Primary Drug	Secondary Drug	Effect	Mechanism	Precautions
ANTIDEPRESSANTS				
TCAs	ANTIFUNGALS—ITRACONAZOLE, KETOCONAZOLE, MICONAZOLE, GRISEOFULVIN	Possible ↑ plasma concentrations of TCAs	All TCAs are metabolized primarily by CYP2D6. Other pathways include CYP1A2 (e.g., amitriptyline, clomipramine, imipramine), CYP2C9, and CYP2C19 (e.g., clomipramine, imipramine). Ketoconazole and voriconazole are documented inhibitors of CYP2C19. Fluconazole and voriconazole are reported to inhibit CYP2C9	Warn patients to report ↑ side effects of TCAs such as dry mouth, blurred vision, and constipation, which may be an early sign of increasing TCA levels. In this case, consider reducing the dose of TCA
TCAs	**ANTIHYPERTENSIVES AND HEART FAILURE DRUGS**			
TCAs	ACE INHIBITORS	Risk of postural hypotension	Additive hypotensive effect	Monitor BP at least weekly until stable. Warn patients to report symptoms of hypotension (light-headedness, dizziness on standing, etc.)
MIANSERIN	ADRENERGIC NEURONE BLOCKERS	↓ Hypotensive effect. There is possibly less effect with maprotiline and mianserin	TCAs compete with adrenergic neurone blockers for reuptake to nerve terminals	Monitor BP at least weekly until stable
TCAs	CENTRALLY ACTING ANTIHYPERTENSIVES	1. Possibly hypotensive effect of clonidine and moxonidine antagonized by TCAs (some case reports of hypertensive crisis) 2. Conversely, clonidine and moxonidine may exacerbate the sedative effects of TCAs, particularly during initiation of therapy 3. Methyldopa may ↓ effect of antidepressants	1 and 2. Uncertain 3. Methyldopa can cause depression	1. Monitor BP at least weekly until stable 2. Warn patients of the risk of sedation and advise them to avoid driving or operating machinery if they suffer from sedation 3. Methyldopa should be avoided in patients with depression

(*Continued*)

Primary Drug	Secondary Drug	Effect	Mechanism	Precautions
ANTIDEPRESSANTS				
TCAs	ANTIMALARIALS—PROGUANIL	Possible ↑ plasma concentrations of proguanil	Inhibition of CYP2C19-mediated metabolism of proguanil. The clinical significance of this depends upon whether proguanil's alternative pathways of metabolism are also inhibited by coadministered drugs	Warn patient to report any evidence of excessive side effects such as change in bowel habit or stomatitis
TCAs	**ANTIOBESITY DRUGS**			
TCAs	LORCASERIN	Risk of serotonin syndrome	Additive effect	Be aware of the possibility of serotonin syndrome. ➢ ***For signs and symptoms of serotonin toxicity, see Clinical Features of Some Adverse Drug Interactions, Serotonin Toxicity and Serotonin Syndrome***
DESIPRAMINE, DOXEPIN	LORCASERIN	↑ Blood concentrations of these antidepressants	Inhibition of CYP2D6-mediated metabolism	Monitor PR and BP closely until stable
TCAs	ANTI-PARKINSON'S DRUGS—RASAGILINE, SELEGILINE	↑ Risk of stroke, hyperpyrexia, and convulsions. ↑ Plasma concentrations of TCAs, with risk of toxic effects. ↑ Risk of serotonin syndrome and of adrenergic syndrome. Clomipramine may trigger acute confusion in Parkinson's disease when used with selegiline	TCAs are believed to act also by inhibiting the reuptake of serotonin and norepinephrine, increasing the risk of serotonin and adrenergic syndromes. Serotonergic syndrome possibly less likely with TCAs compared to SSRIs	Very hazardous interaction. Avoid concurrent use and consider the use of an alternative antidepressant. Be aware that seizures occur with overdose of TCAs just before cardiac arrest
TCAs	**ANTIPSYCHOTICS ➢ *also QT-Prolonging Drugs***			
TCAs	HALOPERIDOL	Possible ↑ haloperidol levels	Inhibition of CYP2D6- and CYP1A2-mediated metabolism of thioridazine	Warn patients to report ↑ side effects of these drugs
TCAs	**ANTIVIRALS**			
TRAZODONE	COBICISTAT	Possible ↑ plasma levels	Inhibition of metabolism via CYP3A4 and 2D6	Dose adjustment may be required

(*Continued*)

Primary Drug	Secondary Drug	Effect	Mechanism	Precautions
ANTIDEPRESSANTS				
AMITRIPTYLINE	PROTEASE INHIBITORS	↑ Adverse effects when amitriptyline is coadministered with ritonavir (with or without lopinavir) and possibly atazanavir	Inhibition of CYP3A4-mediated metabolism. Note that SSRIs are metabolized by a number of enzymes, including CYP2C9, CYP2C19, CYP2D6 as well as CYP3A4; therefore, the effect of protease inhibitors is variable	Avoid coadministration with saquinavir. For other combinations, comma-monitor closely for adverse effects of TCAs
AMOXAPINE, CLOMIPRAMINE, DOXEPIN, IMIPRAMINE, NORTRIPTYLINE, TRIMIPRAMINE	PROTEASE INHIBITORS	Possibly ↑ adverse effects of amoxapine with atazanavir and ritonavir	Inhibition of CYP3A4-mediated metabolism of amoxapine, clomipramine, and doxepin; inhibition of CYP3A4-, CYP2D6,- and CYP2C9-mediated metabolism of imipramine; inhibition of CYP2D6-mediated metabolism of nortriptyline and trimipramine	Monitor closely
TCAs	**ANXIOLYTICS AND HYPNOTICS**			
TCAs	BZDs	Possible ↑ plasma concentrations of diazepam	Inhibition of CYP2C19-mediated metabolism of diazepam. The clinical significance of this depends upon whether diazepam's alternative pathways of metabolism are also inhibited by coadministered drugs	Watch for excessive sedation with diazepam
TCAs	SODIUM OXYBATE	Risk of CNS depression—coma, respiratory depression	Additive depression of CNS	Avoid coadministration
TCAs	**BETA-BLOCKERS**			
AMITRIPTYLINE, CLOMIPRAMINE	BETA-BLOCKERS	Risk of ↑ levels of beta-blockers with amitriptyline and clomipramine	These TCAs inhibit CYP2D6-mediated metabolism of beta-blockers	Monitor BP at least weekly until stable. Warn patients to report symptoms of hypotension (light-headedness, dizziness on standing, etc.)
IMIPRAMINE	LABETALOL, PROPANOLOL	↑ Imipramine with labetalol and propanolol	Uncertain at present. Postulated that imipramine metabolism ↓ by competition at CYP2D6 and CYP2C8	Monitor plasma levels of imipramine when initiating beta-blocker therapy

(*Continued*)

Primary Drug	Secondary Drug	Effect	Mechanism	Precautions
ANTIDEPRESSANTS				
MAPROTILINE	PROPANOLOL	Cases of ↑ plasma levels of maprotiline with propanolol	Uncertain at present. Postulated that maprotiline metabolism ↓ by alterations in hepatic blood flow	Monitor plasma levels of maprotiline when initiating beta-blocker therapy
TCAs	**BRONCHODILATORS**			
TCAs	THEOPHYLLINE	Possible ↑ plasma concentrations of theophylline	Inhibition of CYP1A2- and CYP2D6-mediated metabolism of theophylline. The clinical significance of this depends upon whether theophylline's alternative pathways of metabolism are also inhibited by coadministered drugs	Warn patients to report ↑ side effects of theophylline, and monitor PR and ECG carefully
TCAs	ZAFIRLUKAST	Possible ↑ plasma concentrations of zafirlukast	Inhibition of CYP2C9-mediated metabolism of zafirlukast. The clinical significance of this depends upon whether alternative pathways of metabolism are also inhibited by coadministered drugs	Warn patients to report ↑ side effects
TCAs	CALCIUM CHANNEL BLOCKERS	↑ Plasma concentrations of TCAs when coadministered with diltiazem and verapamil. Reports of cardiotoxicity (first- and second-degree block) when imipramine is given with diltiazem or verapamil	Uncertain but may be due to a combination of ↓ clearance of TCAs (both diltiazem and verapamil are known to inhibit CYP1A2, which has a role in the metabolism of amitriptyline, clomipramine, and imipramine) and ↑ intestinal absorption (diltiazem and verapamil inhibit intestinal Pgp, which may ↑ amitriptyline bioavailability)	Monitor ECG when commencing/ altering treatment
TRAZODONE	CARDIAC GLYCOSIDES—DIGOXIN	Two reported cases of ↑ plasma concentrations of digoxin after starting trazodone	Uncertain at present	Watch for digoxin toxicity; check levels and ↓ dose of digoxin as necessary

(*Continued*)

Primary Drug	Secondary Drug	Effect	Mechanism	Precautions
ANTIDEPRESSANTS				
TCAs	**CNS STIMULANTS**			
AMITRIPTYLINE	MODAFINIL	Variable effect on amitriptyline	Modafinil inhibits CYP2C9 and induces CYP1A2	Watch for both poor response and early features of toxicity of amitriptyline
CLOMIPRAMINE	MODAFINIL	Variable effect on clomipramine	CYP2C19 provides an ancillary pathway for the metabolism of clomipramine. Modafinil inhibits CYP2C19 reversibly at pharmacologically relevant concentrations. Modafinil also induces CYP1A2	Watch for both poor response and early features of toxicity of clomipramine
IMIPRAMINE	MODAFINIL	May cause ↓ imipramine levels if CYP1A2 is the predominant metabolic pathway and alternative metabolic pathways are either genetically deficient or affected	Modafinil is a moderate inducer of CYP1A2 in a concentration-dependent manner	Be aware
DESIPRAMINE	MODAFINIL	↑ Plasma concentrations of TCAs in a subset of the population (7%–10% of white people) who are deficient in CYP2D6	CYP2C19 provides an ancillary pathway for the metabolism of desipramine. Modafinil inhibits CYP2C19 reversibly at pharmacologically relevant concentrations	↓ In dose of TCAs is often necessary
TCAs	DRUG DEPENDENCE THERAPIES—BUPROPION	1. ↑ Risk of seizures. This risk is marked in elderly people, in patients with a history of seizures, addiction to opiates/cocaine/stimulants, and in diabetics treated with oral hypoglycemics or insulin 2. ↑ Plasma concentrations of amitriptyline, clomipramine, desipramine, doxepin, and imipramine, with risk of toxic effects	1. Bupropion is associated with a dose-related risk of seizures. TCAs lower the seizure threshold. Additive effects when combined 2. Bupropion and its metabolite hydroxybupropion inhibit CYP2D6	1. Extreme caution. The dose of bupropion should not exceed 450 mg/day (or 150 mg/day in those with severe hepatic cirrhosis) 2. Initiate therapy of these drugs at the lowest effective dose

(*Continued*)

Primary Drug	Secondary Drug	Effect	Mechanism	Precautions
ANTIDEPRESSANTS				
TCAs—AMITRIPTYLINE, IMIPRAMINE, NORTRIPTYLINE	ELIGLUSTAT	↑ Levels of these antidepressants	Inhibition of CYP2D6-mediated metabolism	Avoid coadministration
TCAs	H2 RECEPTOR BLOCKERS—CIMETIDINE	↑ Efficacy and adverse effects, e.g., dry mouth, urinary retention, blurred vision, constipation	↓ Metabolism	Use alternative acid suppression, e.g., famotidine or nizatidine or monitor more closely and ↓ dose. Rapid hydroxylators may be at ↑ risk
TCAs	MIRABEGRON	↑ TCA levels	Mirabegron inhibits CYP2D6. These drugs have a narrow therapeutic index	Manufacturer advises caution in coadministration. Warn patients to report symptoms such as drowsiness, dizziness, or palpitations
TCAs INCLUDING TRAZADONE	MUSCLE RELAXANTS—CYCLOBENZAPRINE	↑ Risk of serotonin syndrome and of adrenergic syndrome	Cyclobenzaprine is structurally similar to tricyclic antidepressants and may have an additive effect	Avoid coadministration
TCAs	NITRATES	1. ↑ Risk of antimuscarinic side effects when isosorbide dinitrate is coadministered with TCAs 2. ↓ Efficacy of sublingual nitrate tablets with TCAs	1. Additive effect; both of these drugs cause antimuscarinic side effects 2. Antimuscarinic effects ↓ saliva production, which ↓ dissolution of the tablet	1. Warn patients of this additive effect 2. Consider changing the formulation to a sublingual nitrate spray
TCAs	SUCRALFATE	Possible ↓ amitriptyline levels	↓ Absorption of amitriptyline	Watch for poor response to amitriptyline
TCAs	**SYMPATHOMIMETICS**			
TCAs	INDIRECT	1. Methylphenidate ↑ TCA levels, which may improve their efficacy, but cases of toxicity with imipramine reported 2. TCAs possibly ↓ efficacy of indirect sympathomimetics	1. Uncertain; postulated to be due to inhibition of hepatic metabolism of TCAs 2. Indirect sympathomimetics cause release of norepinephrine from nerve endings; this is blocked by TCAs	1. Warn patients to watch for early signs of ↑ TCA efficacy such as drowsiness and dry mouth 2. Watch for poor response to indirect sympathomimetics

(Continued)

Primary Drug	Secondary Drug	Effect	Mechanism	Precautions
ANTIDEPRESSANTS				
TCAs	DIRECT	↑ Efficacy of norepinephrine, epinephrine or phenylephrine when coadministered with TCAs; risk of ↑ BP and tachyarrhythmias	TCAs block reuptake of norepinephrine into the nerve terminals, which prolongs its activity	Monitor PR, BP, and ECG closely; start inotropes at a lower dose. It is advisable to monitor PR and BP even when using local anesthetics containing epinephrine, although there is no evidence of significant toxicity
TCAs	THYROID HORMONES	Possible ↑ antidepressant effect	Uncertain	May be beneficial, but there are cases of nausea and dizziness; warn patients to report these symptoms
TRYPTOPHAN				
TRYPTOPHAN	ANALGESICS—TRAMADOL	Risk of serotonin syndrome	Additive effect	Use with caution
TRYPTOPHAN	ANTICANCER AND IMMUNOMODULATING DRUGS—PROCARBAZINE	Risk of hyperreflexia, shivering, hyperventilation, hyperthermia, mania or hypomania, disorientation/confusion	Tryptophan is a precursor of a number of neurotransmitters, including serotonin. Procarbazine has MAOI activity, which inhibits the breakdown of neurotransmitters	Tryptophan should be started under specialist supervision. Recommended to start with low doses and titrate the dose upward with close monitoring of mental status and BP
TRYPTOPHAN	**ANTIDEPRESSANTS**			
TRYPTOPHAN	MAOIs	Risk of confusion and agitation	Tryptophan is a precursor of a number of neurotransmitters, including serotonin. MAOIs inhibit the breakdown of neurotransmitters	↓ Dose of tryptophan
TRYPTOPHAN	SSRIs	Risk of serotonin syndrome	Additive effect	Use with caution
TRYPTOPHAN	ANTIHYPERTENSIVES AND HEART FAILURE DRUGS—CENTRALLY ACTING ANTIHYPERTENSIVES—METHYLDOPA	Methyldopa may ↓ effect of antidepressants	Methyldopa can cause depression	Methyldopa should be avoided in patients with depression
TRYPTOPHAN	ANTIMALARIALS—ARTEMETHER/LUMEFANTRINE	↑ Artemether/lumefantrine levels, with risk of toxicity, including arrhythmias	Uncertain	Avoid coadministration

(*Continued*)

Primary Drug	Secondary Drug	Effect	Mechanism	Precautions
ANTIDEPRESSANTS				
TRYPTOPHAN	**ANTIOBESITY DRUGS**			
TRYPTOPHAN	LORCASERIN	Risk of serotonin syndrome	Additive effect	Be aware of the possibility of serotonin syndrome. ➢ ***For signs and symptoms of serotonin toxicity, see Clinical Features of Some Adverse Drug Interactions, Serotonin Toxicity and Serotonin Syndrome***
TRYPTOPHAN	SIBUTRAMINE	Risk of serotonin syndrome	Additive effect	Manufacturer advises against coadministration
TRYPTOPHAN	ANXIOLYTICS AND HYPNOTICS	Risk of sedation	Additive effect	Warn patient regarding risks when driving, using machinery, etc.

Primary Drug	Secondary Drug	Effect	Mechanism	Precautions
ANTIEMETICS				
APREPITANT				
APREPITANT	**ANTIBIOTICS**			
APREPITANT	MACROLIDES	↑ Aprepitant levels	Inhibition of CYP3A4-mediated metabolism of aprepitant	Use with caution; clinical significance unclear, so monitor closely
APREPITANT	RIFAMPICIN	↓ Aprepitant levels	Induction of CYP3A4-mediated metabolism of aprepitant	Watch for poor response to aprepitant
APREPITANT	ANTICANCER AND IMMUNOMODULATING DRUGS			
APREPITANT	BOSUTINIB	Increased bosutinib levels	CYP3A inhibition	Manufacturer advises avoid concurrent use. If not possible, interruption of therapy or dose reduction should be considered
APREPITANT	CORTICOSTEROIDS	↑ Dexamethasone and methylprednisolone levels	Inhibition of CYP3A4-mediated metabolism of these corticosteroids	Be aware

(*Continued*)

Primary Drug	Secondary Drug	Effect	Mechanism	Precautions
ANTIEMETICS				
APREPITANT	ERLOTINIB	Single case of increased erlotinib levels	Possibly CYP3A4 inhibition	Be aware of possible interaction
APREPITANT	EVEROLIMUS	Possible increased everolimus levels	CYP3A4 inhibition	Caution with concurrent use
APREPITANT	ANTICOAGULANTS—ORAL	Possible ↓ INR when aprepitant is added to warfarin	Aprepitant ↑ CYP2C9-mediated metabolism of warfarin	Monitor INR carefully for 2 weeks after completing each course of aprepitant
APREPITANT	ANTIDEPRESSANTS—ST. JOHN'S WORT	↑ Aprepitant levels	Inhibition of CYP3A4-mediated metabolism of aprepitant	Avoid coadministration (manufacturers' recommendation)
APREPITANT	ANTIDIABETIC DRUGS—TOLBUTAMIDE	↓ Tolbutamide levels	Aprepitant ↑ CYP2C9-mediated metabolism of tolbutamide	Monitor blood glucose closely
APREPITANT	ANTIEPILEPTICS—CARBAMAZEPINE, PHENOBARBITAL, PHENYTOIN	↓ Aprepitant levels	Induction of CYP3A4-mediated metabolism of aprepitant	Watch for poor response to aprepitant
APREPITANT	ANTIFUNGALS—KETOCONAZOLE	↑ Aprepitant levels	Inhibition of CYP3A4-mediated metabolism of aprepitant	Use with caution; clinical significance unclear; monitor closely
APREPITANT	ANTIPSYCHOTICS—PIMOZIDE	↑ Aprepitant levels	Inhibition of metabolism	Avoid coadministration (manufacturers' recommendation)
APREPITANT	ANTIVIRALS—PROTEASE INHIBITORS	↑ Aprepitant levels with nelfinavir and ritonavir (with or without lopinavir)	Inhibition of CYP3A4-mediated metabolism of aprepitant	Use with caution; clinical significance unclear; monitor closely
APREPITANT	ELIGLUSTAT	↑ Eliglustat levels	Inhibition of CYP3A4-mediated metabolism	Reduce dose to 85 mg od in extensive metabolizers. Avoid coadministration in intermediate and poor metabolizers
APREPITANT	NITISINONE	Possible ↑ nitisinone levels	Inhibition of CYP3A4-mediated metabolism	Monitor carefully
APREPITANT	ESTROGENS	↓ Estrogen levels with risk of contraceptive failure	Uncertain	Clinical significance uncertain. It would seem wise to advise patients to use an alternative form of contraception during and for 1 month after stopping coadministration with aprepitant

(*Continued*)

Primary Drug	Secondary Drug	Effect	Mechanism	Precautions
ANTIEMETICS				
APREPITANT	PROGESTOGENS	↓ Progestogen levels with risk of contraceptive failure	Uncertain	Advise patients to use an alternative form of contraception during and for 1 month after completing the course of aprepitant
ANTIHISTAMINES—CINNARIZINE, CYCLIZINE, PROMETHAZINE ➢ *Respiratory Drugs, Antihistamines*				
DOPAMINE RECEPTOR ANTAGONISTS—DOMPERIDONE, METOCLOPRAMIDE				
DOPAMINE RECEPTOR ANTAGONISTS	**ANALGESICS**			
DOMPERIDONE, METOCLOPRAMIDE	OPIOIDS	1. ↓ Efficacy of domperidone on gut motility by opioids 2. Metoclopramide ↑ speed of onset and effect of oral morphine	1. Antagonist effect 2. Uncertain; metoclopramide may promote the absorption of morphine by increasing gastric emptying	1. Caution with coadministration 2. Be aware that the effects of oral morphine are ↑
METOCLOPRAMIDE	NSAIDs	1. Metoclopramide speeds up the onset of action of tolfenamic acid 2. Metoclopramide ↓ efficacy of ketoprofen	Metoclopramide promotes gastric emptying. 1. Tolfenamic acid reaches its main site of absorption in the small intestine more rapidly 2. Ketoprofen has low solubility and has less time to dissolve in the stomach; therefore, less ketoprofen is absorbed	1. This interaction can be used beneficially to hasten the onset of analgesia 2. Take ketoprofen at least 2 h before metoclopramide
METOCLOPRAMIDE	**OTHER DRUGS**			
METOCLOPRAMIDE	CICLOSPORIN	Slight increase in ciclosporin levels	Increased ciclosporin absorption due to metoclopramide, increasing gastric emptying	Clinical significance uncertain
METOCLOPRAMIDE	EVEROLIMUS	Possible increased everolimus levels	CYP3A4 inhibition	Caution with concurrent use
METOCLOPRAMIDE	SIROLIMUS	Possible increased sirolimus levels	CYP3A4 inhibition	Caution with concurrent use
METOCLOPRAMIDE	TEMSIROLIMUS	Possible increased temsirolimus levels	CYP3A4 inhibition	Caution with concurrent use

(*Continued*)

Primary Drug	Secondary Drug	Effect	Mechanism	Precautions
ANTIEMETICS				
METOCLOPRAMIDE	ANTIMALARIALS—ATOVAQUONE	↓ Atovaquone levels	Uncertain	Avoid; consider an alternative antiemetic
DOMPERIDONE, METOCLOPRAMIDE	ANTIMUSCARINICS	↓ Efficacy of domperidone on gut motility by antimuscarinics	Some effects of metoclopramide are considered to be due to ↑ release of ACh and ↑ sensitivity of the cholinergic receptors to ACh. Antimuscarinics prevent the effects on muscarinic receptors	The gastrointestinal effects of metoclopramide will be impaired, while the antiemetic effects may not be. Thus, concurrent use with antimuscarinics is not advised because of effects on the gastrointestinal system
DOPAMINE RECEPTOR ANTAGONISTS	**ANTI-PARKINSON'S DRUGS**			
DOMPERIDONE, METOCLOPRAMIDE	AMANTADINE	↓ Efficacy of amantadine	Antagonism of anti-Parkinson's effect; these drugs have extrapyramidal side effects	Use with caution; avoid in patients <20 years
DOMPERIDONE, METOCLOPRAMIDE	BROMOCRIPTINE, CABERGOLINE	↓ Efficacy of bromocriptine and cabergoline for reducing prolactin levels	Domperidone and metoclopramide are associated with prolactin secretion	Use alternative antiemetics when bromocriptine and cabergoline are being used to treat prolactinomas. Domperidone has minimal central antidopaminergic effect and may therefore be used when bromocriptine and cabergoline are administered as treatments for Parkinson's disease
METOCLOPRAMIDE	DOPAMINERGICS	↓ Efficacy of dopaminergics	Metoclopramide is a centrally acting antidopaminergic	Use with caution; avoid in patients <20 years. Manufacturers recommend avoiding the coadministration of metoclopramide with ropinirole or rotigotine
METOCLOPRAMIDE	ANTIPLATELET AGENTS—ASPIRIN	↑ Aspirin levels with metoclopramide	↑ Absorption of aspirin	Watch for early features of salicylate toxicity
METOCLOPRAMIDE	ANTIPSYCHOTICS	↑ Risk of extrapyramidal effects	Additive effect	Consider using an alternative antiemetic

(*Continued*)

Primary Drug	Secondary Drug	Effect	Mechanism	Precautions
ANTIEMETICS				
METOCLOPRAMIDE	DRUG DEPENDENCE THERAPIES—BUPROPION	↑ Plasma concentrations of these substrates, with risk of toxic effects	Bupropion and its metabolite hydroxybupropion inhibit CYP2D6	Initiate therapy of these drugs at the lowest effective dose
METOCLOPRAMIDE	MUSCLE RELAXANTS—DANTROLENE	Possibly ↑ dantrolene levels	Uncertain	Be aware; monitor BP and LFTs closely
METOCLOPRAMIDE	SUXAMETHONIUM	Possible ↑ efficacy of suxamethonium	Uncertain; inhibition of pseudocholinesterase	Be aware and monitor effects of suxamethonium closely
METOCLOPRAMIDE	TETRABENAZINE	Risk of extrapyramidal symptoms	Additive effect	Avoid coadministration
5-HT3 ANTAGONISTS				
5-HT3 ANTAGONISTS	**DRUGS THAT PROLONG THE QT INTERVAL**			
5-HT3 ANTAGONISTS	1. ANTIARRHYTHMICS—ajmaline, amiodarone, azimilide, cibenzoline, disopyramide, dofetilide, dronedarone, ibutilide, procainamide, propafenone, quinidine 2. ANTIBIOTICS—macrolides (especially azithromycin, clarithromycin, parenteral erythromycin, telithromycin), quinolones (especially moxifloxacin), quinupristin/dalfopristin 3. ANTICANCER AND IMMUNOMODULATING DRUGS—arsenic trioxide, bosutinib, crizotinib, dasatinib, eribulin, fingolimod, lapatinib, nilotinib, pazopanib, sunitinib, vandetanib, vemurafenib 4. ANTIDEPRESSANTS—TCAs, venlafaxine 5. Antifungals—fluconazole, posaconazole, voriconazole	Risk of ventricular arrhythmias, particularly torsades de pointes	Additive effect; these drugs prolong the QT interval	Avoid coadministration

(*Continued*)

Primary Drug	Secondary Drug	Effect	Mechanism	Precautions
ANTIEMETICS				
	6. ANTIHISTAMINES—terfenadine, hydroxyzine, mizolastine 7. ANTIHYPERTENSIVES—ketanserin 8. ANTIMALARIALS—artemether with lumefantrine, chloroquine, halofantrine, hydroxychloroquine, mefloquine, quinine 9. ANTIPROTOZOALS—pentamidine isothionate 10. ANTIPSYCHOTICS—atypicals, phenothiazines, pimozide 11. ANTIVIRALS—boceprevir, rilpivirine, telaprevir 12. BETA-BLOCKERS—sotalol 13. BRONCHODILATORS—parenteral bronchodilators 14. CNS STIMULANTS—atomoxetine 15. RANOLAZINE			
ONDANSETRON	ANALGESICS—OPIOIDS	Ondansetron seems to ↓ analgesic effect of tramadol	Uncertain; tramadol exerts its analgesic properties via serotoninergic pathways in addition to stimulation of opioid receptors. Ondansetron is a serotonin receptor antagonist	Avoid coadministration. Although increasing tramadol restored the analgesic effect, it also caused a significant ↑ in vomiting that was poorly responsive to antiemetic
5-HT3-ANTAGONISTS	**ANTIARRHYTHMICS**			
5-HT3-ANTAGONISTS	FLECAINIDE	Risk of arrhythmias	Additive effect	Manufacturers recommend avoiding coadministration of flecainide with ondansetron. Caution with other 5-HT3-antagonists; monitor ECG closely

(*Continued*)

Primary Drug	Secondary Drug	Effect	Mechanism	Precautions
ANTIEMETICS				
5-HT3-ANTAGONISTS	MEXILETINE	Risk of arrhythmias with ondansetron	Additive effect	Manufacturers recommend avoiding coadministration. Also caution with tropisetron; monitor ECG closely
ONDANSETRON, TROPISETRON	ANTIBIOTICS—RIFAMPICIN	↓ Levels of these drugs	Induction of metabolism	Watch for poor response to ondansetron and tropisetron; consider using an alternative antiemetic
ONDANSETRON	ANTICANCER AND IMMUNOMODULATING DRUGS—PIXANTRONE	Theoretical risk of increased drug levels	Pixantrone inhibits CYP1A2	Manufacturer advises to monitor closely
5-HT3 ANTAGONISTS	**ANTIDEPRESSANTS**			
ONDANSETRON	FLUVOXAMINE	Possible ↑ plasma concentrations of ondansetron	Fluvoxamine is potent inhibitor of CYP1A2, and fluoxetine, paroxetine, and sertraline are less potent inhibitors. Escitalopram and citalopram are not currently known to cause any inhibition	Warn patients to report adverse effects of ondansetron (e.g., diarrhea, headache, fever, lightheadedness, dizziness, drowsiness, constipation, rash, blurred vision, and muscle spasm)
ONDANSETRON, TROPISETRON	TCAs	Possible ↑ plasma concentrations of these antiemetics	Inhibition of CYP2D6-mediated metabolism of these antiemetics. The clinical significance of this depends upon whether their alternative pathways of metabolism are also inhibited by coadministered drugs. The risk is theoretically higher with ondansetron, because TCAs also inhibit CYP1A2-mediated metabolism	Warn patients to report ↑ side effects of ondansetron and tropisetron
5-HT3 ANTAGONISTS	**ANTIEPILEPTICS**			
ONDANSETRON	CARBAMAZEPINE, PHENYTOIN	Reports of ↓ ondansetron levels	Induction of metabolism of ondansetron	Watch for poor response to ondansetron; care with other 5-HT3 antagonists

(*Continued*)

Primary Drug	Secondary Drug	Effect	Mechanism	Precautions
ANTIEMETICS				
TROPISETRON	PRIMIDONE	Reports of ↓ tropisetron levels	Induction of metabolism of tropisetron	Watch for poor response to ondansetron; care with other 5-HT3 antagonists
ONDANSETRON	CNS STIMULANTS—MODAFINIL	May cause ↓ ondansetron levels if CYP1A2 is the predominant metabolic pathway and alternative metabolic pathways are either genetically deficient or affected	Modafinil is moderate inducer of CYP1A2 in a concentration-dependent manner	Be aware
PHENOTHIAZINES—CHLORPROMAZINE, PERPHENAZINE, PROCHLORPERAZINE, TRIFLUOPERAZINE ➢ *Antipsychotics, below*				

Primary Drug	Secondary Drug	Effect	Mechanism	Precautions
ANTIEPILEPTICS				
BARBITURATES				
BARBITURATES	ALCOHOL	↑ Sedation	Additive sedative effect	Warn patients about this effect
BARBITURATES	ANESTHETICS—LOCAL—PROCAINE SOLUTIONS	Precipitation of drugs, which may not be immediately apparent	Pharmaceutical interaction	Do not mix in the same infusion or syringe
BARBITURATES	ANALGESICS—OPIOIDS	1. Barbiturates ↑ sedative effects of opioids 2. ↓ Efficacy of fentanyl and methadone	1. Additive sedative effect 2. ↑ Hepatic metabolism of fentanyl and methadone, and possibly an effect at the opioid receptor	1. Monitor respiratory rate and conscious levels 2. Be aware that the dose of fentanyl and methadone may need to be ↑
BARBITURATES	ANTIARRHYTHMICS—AMJALINE, DISOPYRAMIDE, DRONEDERONE, PROPAFENONE, QUINIDINE	↓ Levels of these drugs with risk of therapeutic failure	Induction of hepatic metabolism	Monitor for ↓ clinical efficacy and ↑ their dose as required

(Continued)

Primary Drug	Secondary Drug	Effect	Mechanism	Precautions
ANTIEPILEPTICS				
BARBITURATES	ANTIBIOTICS—CHLORAMPHENICOL, DOXYCYCLINE, METRONIDAZOLE, RIFAMPICIN, TELITHROMYCIN	↓ Levels of these drugs with risk of therapeutic failure	Induction of hepatic metabolism	1. Avoid coadministration of telithromycin for up to 2 weeks after stopping phenobarbital 2. With the other drugs, monitor for ↓ clinical efficacy and ↑ their dose as required
BARBITURATES	**ANTICANCER AND IMMUNOMODULATING DRUGS**			
BARBITURATES	AFATINIB	Reduction in afatinib levels	P-glycoprotein induction	U.S. manufacturer recommends dose increase
BARBITURATES	ANAKINRA	Possible reduced levels of phenytoin	Reversal of cytochrome P450 suppression by anakinra. Phenytoin has a narrow therapeutic index. The formation of CYP450 enzymes is suppressed by increased levels of cytokines (e.g., IL-1) during chronic inflammation. Thus, it may be expected that for an IL-1 receptor antagonist, such as anakinra, the formation of CYP450 enzymes could be normalized during treatment. This would be clinically relevant for CYP450 substrates with a narrow therapeutic index (e.g., warfarin and phenytoin)	Monitor closely, dose adjustment may be needed. Upon start or end of anakinra treatment in patients on these types of medicinal products, it may be relevant to consider therapeutic monitoring of the effect or concentration of these products and the individual dose of the medicinal product may need to be adjusted
BARBITURATES	AXITINIB	Reduced axitinib levels	CYP3A4/5 induction	Manufacturer advises to avoid concurrent use if possible. If concurrent use is necessary, dose adjustment is recommended
BARBITURATES	BORTEZOMIB	Levels of bortezomib possible reduced by phenobarbital	Possibly due to induction of CYP3A4	Avoid concomitant use
BARBITURATES	BOSUTINIB	Reduced bosutinib levels	CYP3A induction	Manufacturer advises to avoid concurrent use. Dose increase unlikely to sufficiently compensate
BARBITURATES	CABAZITAXEL	Reduced cabazitaxel levels	CYP3A4 induction	Avoid coadministration

(*Continued*)

Primary Drug	Secondary Drug	Effect	Mechanism	Precautions
ANTIEPILEPTICS				
BARBITURATES	CRIZOTINIB	Possible reduced crizotinib levels	CYP3A4 induction	Manufacturer advises to avoid concurrent use
BARBITURATES	CARMUSTINE, CICLOSPORIN, CORTICOSTEROIDS, DOXORUBICIN, ETOPOSIDE, IMATINIB, LOMUSTINE, PACLITAXEL, TACROLIMUS, TAMOXIFEN, TOREMIFENE, VINCA ALKALOIDS	↓ Levels of these drugs with risk of therapeutic failure	Induction of hepatic metabolism	1. Avoid coadministration of barbiturates with carmustine, etoposide, imatinib, lomustine, tacrolimus, tamoxifen; consider alternative nonenzyme-inducing antiepileptics 2. With the other drugs, monitor for ↓ clinical efficacy and ↑ their dose as required. Monitor ciclosporin levels
BARBITURATES	DABRAFENIB	Predicted reduced dabrafenib levels	CYP2C8/CYP3A4 induction	Avoid concurrent use
BARBITURATES	DOCETAXEL	Predicted reduced docetaxel levels	CYP3A4 induction	Monitor closely Dose increase may be required
BARBITURATES	ERLOTINIB	Reduced levels of erlotinib	CYP3A4 induction	Avoid concurrent use. If not possible, consider dose increase of erlotinib
BARBITURATES	EVEROLIMUS	Reduced everolimus levels	CYP3A4 induction	Avoid concurrent use Consider increasing dose of everolimus if concurrent use is necessary
BARBITURATES	FINGOLIMOD	Fingolimod levels reduced	Induction of CYP3A4	Uncertain
BARBITURATES	IFOSFAMIDE	↑ Rate of biotransformation to 4-hydroxyifosfamide, the active metabolite, but no change in AUC of 4-hydroxyifosfamide	Due to ↑ rate of metabolism and of clearance resulting from induction of CYP3A4 and CYP2D6	Be aware—clinical significance may be minimal or none
PHENOBARBITAL	METHOTREXATE	Increased clearance of methotrexate (as 24 h infusion), reduced efficacy in combination therapy for B-cell leukemia	Unknown	Clinical significance uncertain—further study needed

(Continued)

Primary Drug	Secondary Drug	Effect	Mechanism	Precautions
ANTIEPILEPTICS				
BARBITURATES	MITOTANE	Possible reduction in levels of barbiturates	Mitotane is a potent inducer of CYP enzymes	Be aware; watch for poor response to antiepileptic effect of barbiturates
BARBITURATES	PONATINIB	Possible reduced ponatinib levels	CYP3A4 induction	Avoid concurrent use if possible
BARBITURATES	PROCARBAZINE	↑ Risk of hypersensitivity reactions in patients with brain tumors	Strong correlation between therapeutic antiepileptic level and hypersensitivity reactions	Consider using nonenzyme-inducing agents
BARBITURATES	REGORAFENIB	Predicted reduced regorafenib levels	CYP3A4 induction	Manufacturer advises to avoid concurrent use
BARBITURATES	RUXOLITINIB	Reduced levels of ruloxitinib	CYP3A4 induction	Monitor closely Titrate dose based on safety and efficacy
BARBITURATES	SORAFENIB	Sorafenib levels reduced	CYP3A4 induction	Avoid concurrent use
BARBITURATES	TEMSIROLIMUS	Reduced temsirolimus levels	CYP3A4 induction	Avoid concurrent use. If not possible, consider temsirolimus dose increase
BARBITURATES	TRABECTEDIN	1. Reduced trabectedin levels 2. Reduced absorption of phenytoin	1. CYP3A4 induction 2. Trabectedin may damage gut mucosa, affecting absorption of phenytoin	1. Monitor closely 2. Monitor phenytoin levels
BARBITURATES	**ANTICOAGULANTS**			
BARBITURATES	ORAL	↓ Levels of these drugs with risk of therapeutic failure. The ↓ anticoagulant effect of warfarin reaches a maximum after 3 weeks and can last up to 6 weeks after stopping barbiturates	Induction of hepatic metabolism	Monitor INR carefully. Dose of anticoagulant may need to be ↑ by up to 60%
BARBITURATES	APIXABAN	↓ Apixaban levels	Induction of CYP3A4-mediated metabolism and Pgp-mediated transport of apixaban	Avoid coadministration
BARBITURATES	RIVAROXABAN	↓ Rivaroxaban exposure	Induction of CYP3A4-mediated metabolism and Pgp-mediated efflux transport	Avoid coadministration

(*Continued*)

Primary Drug	Secondary Drug	Effect	Mechanism	Precautions
ANTIEPILEPTICS				
BARBITURATES	ANTIDEMENTIA DRUGS—MEMANTINE	Possible ↓ efficacy of primidone	Uncertain	Avoid coadministration
BARBITURATES	**ANTIDEPRESSANTS**			
BARBITURATES	MAOIs	1. ↑ Risk of seizures 2. Reports of prolonged hypnotic effects with phenelzine	1. These drugs lower seizure threshold 2. Animal experiments showed that pretreatment with tranylcypromine prolonged amobarbital-induced hypnotic effects 2.5-fold. Inhibition of hepatic enzymes other than MAO has been proposed as an explanation for the exaggerated depressant effects associated with barbiturates and opioids	1. Care with coadministration. Watch for ↑ fit frequency; warn patient of this risk when starting these drugs and take suitable precautions. Consider increasing dose of antiepileptic 2. Be aware. Warn patients taking sleeping aids about activities requiring attention and co-ordination (e.g., driving or using machinery)
BARBITURATES	REBOXETINE	Risk of ↓ reboxetine levels	Possibly induction of CYP3A4-mediated metabolism of reboxetine	May need to increase dose of reboxetine with close monitoring
BARBITURATES	ST. JOHN'S WORT	↓ Barbiturate levels	↑ Metabolism	Avoid coadministration
BARBITURATES	SSRIs	1. ↑ Risk of seizures 2. ↓ Levels of paroxetine with risk of therapeutic failure	1. These drugs lower seizure threshold 2. Induction of hepatic metabolism	1. Care with coadministration. Watch for ↑ fit frequency; warn patient of this risk when starting these drugs and take suitable precautions. Consider increasing dose of antiepileptic 2. Monitor for ↓ clinical efficacy and ↑ their dose as required
BARBITURATES	TCAs	1. ↑ Risk of seizures 2. ↓ Levels of mianserin with risk of therapeutic failure	1. These drugs lower seizure threshold 2. Induction of hepatic metabolism	1. Care with coadministration. Watch for ↑ fit frequency; warn patient of this risk when starting these drugs and take suitable precautions. Consider increasing dose of antiepileptic 2. Monitor for ↓ clinical efficacy and ↑ their dose as required

(*Continued*)

Primary Drug	Secondary Drug	Effect	Mechanism	Precautions
ANTIEPILEPTICS				
BARBITURATES	ANTIDIABETIC DRUGS—REPAGLINIDE, SULFONYLUREAS	↓ Levels of these drugs with risk of therapeutic failure	Induction of hepatic metabolism	Monitor for ↓ clinical efficacy and ↑ their dose as required; monitor capillary blood glucose and warn patients about symptoms of hyperglycemia. ➢ ***For signs and symptoms of hyperglycemia, see Clinical Features of Some Adverse Drug Interactions, Hyperglycemia***
BARBITURATES	ANTIEMETICS—APREPITANT 5-HT3-ANTAGONISTS	↓ Levels of these drugs with risk of therapeutic failure. Dependent on the major metabolic pathways	Aprepitant is a substrate and moderate inhibitor of CYP3A4 and a mild inducer of CYP2C9	Monitor for ↓ clinical efficacy and ↑ their dose as required
BARBITURATES	**ANTIEPILEPTICS**			
BARBITURATES	CARBAMAZEPINE, LAMOTRIGINE, TIAGABINE, VALPROATE, ZONISAMIDE	↓ Levels of these antiepileptics	Induction of metabolism	Watch for poor response to these antiepileptics
BARBITURATES	PHENYTOIN	Variable effect on phenytoin levels. ↑ Phenobarbital levels	Phenobarbital induces metabolism of phenytoin but, at high levels, may competitively inhibit it. Uncertain why ↑ phenobarbital level occurs	Be aware and monitor levels. Watch for early features of phenytoin toxicity
BARBITURATES	**ANTIFUNGALS**			
BARBITURATES	**AZOLES**			
BARBITURATES	FLUCONAZOLE, ITRACONAZOLE, KETOCONAZOLE, VORICONAZOLE	↓ Azole levels with risk of therapeutic failure	Barbiturates induce CYP3A4, which metabolizes itraconazole and the active metabolite of itraconazole. Primidone is metabolized to phenobarbitone	Watch for inadequate therapeutic effects and ↑ dose of azole if effect is due to interaction
BARBITURATES	MICONAZOLE	↑ Phenobarbital levels	Inhibition of metabolism	Be aware; watch for early features of toxicity (e.g., ↑ sedation)

(*Continued*)

Primary Drug	Secondary Drug	Effect	Mechanism	Precautions
ANTIEPILEPTICS				
BARBITURATES	OTHER ANTIFUNGALS—GRISEOFULVIN	↓ Griseofulvin levels	↓ Absorption	Although the effect of ↓ plasma concentrations on therapeutic effect has not been established, concurrent use is preferably avoided
BARBITURATES	ANTIMALARIALS—CHLOROQUINE, MEFLOQUINE	↑ Risk of seizures	These drugs lower seizure threshold	Care with coadministration. Watch for ↑ fit frequency; warn patient of this risk when starting these drugs and take suitable precautions. Consider increasing dose of antiepileptic
BARBITURATES	ANTIMIGRAINE DRUGS—ALMOTRIPTAN, ELETRIPTAN	↓ Levels of these drugs with risk of therapeutic failure	Induction of hepatic metabolism	Monitor for ↓ clinical efficacy and ↑ their dose as required
BARBITURATES	ANTIPLATELET AGENTS—TICAGRELOR	↓ Ticagrelor levels	Induction of CYP 3A4-mediated metabolism of ticagrelor	Manufacturer recommends avoid coadministration
BARBITURATES	**ANTIPSYCHOTICS**			
BARBITURATES	ANTIPSYCHOTICS	↓ Efficacy of antiepileptics	Antipsychotics lower seizure threshold	Watch for ↑ fit frequency; warn patients of this risk when starting antipsychotics, and take suitable precautions. Consider increasing the dose of antiepileptic
BARBITURATES	ARPIPRAZOLE, CLOZAPINE, HALOPERIDOL, QUETIAPINE	↓ Levels of arpiprazole, haloperidol, clozapine, quetiapine	Induction of metabolism	Watch for poor response to these antipsychotics, and consider increasing the dose
BARBITURATES	**ANTIVIRALS**			
PHENOBARBITONE	COBICISTAT	1. Possible ↓ plasma levels of cobicistat, risk of treatment failure, and resistance 2. Possible ↓ plasma levels of medicines being boosted, e.g., protease inhibitor, risk of treatment failure, and resistance	Induction of metabolism via CYP3A and CYP2D6 (minor)	Avoid coadministration
PHENOBARBITONE	DOLUTEGRAVIR	Possible ↓ plasma levels of dolutegravir, risk of treatment failure, and resistance	Induction of UGT1A1 and CYP3A	Avoid coadministration

(*Continued*)

Primary Drug	Secondary Drug	Effect	Mechanism	Precautions
ANTIEPILEPTICS				
PHENOBARBITONE	MARAVIROC	Possible ↓ plasma levels of maraviroc, risk of treatment failure, and resistance	Induction of UGT1A1 and CYP3A	Avoid coadministration
PHENOBARBITONE	NNRTIs—EFAVIRENZ, ETRAVIRINE, RILPIVARINE	1. Possible ↑ or ↓ efficacy of antiepileptic with efavirenz 2. Possible ↓ plasma levels of etravirine and rilpivarine	Altered metabolism via CYP450	Monitor closely. Efavirenz: Monitor antiepileptic levels when starting, stopping, or changing treatment, and allow 2 weeks for phenytoin levels to accurately reflect dose changes. Etravirine: combination not recommended. Rilpivirine: avoid coadministration
PHENOBARBITAL	PROTEASE INHIBITORS	Possibly ↓ plasma levels of both protease inhibitors and phenobarbital	Increased metabolism of protease inhibitors mainly through induction of CYP3A4, and of phenobarbital through CYP2C9 and C19 induction	Use with caution. Monitor clinical outcomes closely including viral load and CD4 count, check phenobarbitone levels and monitor for side effects when initiating or changing treatment
BARBITURATES	**ANXIOLYTICS AND HYPNOTICS**			
BARBITURATES	BZDs—CLONAZEPAM	↓ Barbiturate levels	Induction of metabolism	Watch for poor response to barbiturates
BARBITURATES	SODIUM OXYBATE	Risk of CNS depression—coma, respiratory depression	Additive depression of CNS	Avoid coadministration. Caution even with relatively nonsedating antihistamines (cetirizine, desloratadine, fexofenadine, levocetirizine, loratadine, mizolastine) as they can impair performance of skilled tasks
BARBITURATES	**BETA-BLOCKERS**			
BARBITURATES	BETA-BLOCKERS	↑ Hypotensive effect	Additive hypotensive effect; anxiolytics and hypnotics can cause postural ↓ BP	Watch for ↓ BP; monitor BP at least weekly until stable. Warn patients to report symptoms of hypotension (light-headedness, dizziness on standing, etc.)
BARBITURATES	METOPROLOL, PROPANOLOL, TIMOLOL	↓ Levels of these drugs with risk of therapeutic failure	Induction of hepatic metabolism	Monitor PR and BP weekly until stable and watch for ↑ BP

(Continued)

Primary Drug	Secondary Drug	Effect	Mechanism	Precautions
ANTIEPILEPTICS				
BARBITURATES	BRONCHODILATORS—MONTELUKAST, THEOPHYLLINE	↓ Levels of these drugs with risk of therapeutic failure	Induction of hepatic metabolism	Monitor for ↓ clinical efficacy and ↑ their dose as required; may need to ↑ dose of theophylline by 25%
BARBITURATES	CALCIUM CHANNEL BLOCKERS—FELODIPINE, NIFEDIPINE, NIMODIPINE, NISOLDIPINE, VERAPAMIL	↓ Levels of these drugs with risk of therapeutic failure	Induction of hepatic metabolism	Monitor PR and BP weekly until stable and watch for ↑ BP
BARBITURATES	CARDIAC GLYCOSIDES—DIGITOXIN	↓ Levels of these drugs with risk of therapeutic failure	Induction of hepatic metabolism	Monitor PR and BP weekly until stable and watch for ↑ BP
BARBITURATES	CNS STIMULANTS—MODAFINIL	1. ↓ Plasma concentrations of modafinil with possibility of ↓ therapeutic effect 2. May cause moderate ↑ in plasma concentrations of phenobarbitone and primidone	1. Induction of CYP3A4, which has a partial role in the metabolism of modafinil 2. Modafinil is a reversible inhibitor of CYP2C19 when used in therapeutic doses	1 and 2. Be aware
BARBITURATES	**OTHER DRUGS**			
BARBITURATES	CARBONIC ANHYDRASE INHIBITORS	Risk of osteomalacia	Barbiturates have a small risk of causing osteomalacia; this may be ↑ by acetazolamide-induced urinary excretion of calcium	Be aware
BARBITURATES	EPLERENONE	↓ Levels of eplerenone risk of therapeutic failure	Induction of hepatic metabolism	Monitor for ↓ clinical efficacy and ↑ eplerenone dose as required
BARBITURATES	FOLIC ACID	↓ Levels of these antiepileptics	Uncertain; postulated that induction of CYP enzymes by these antiepileptics depletes folate reserves. Replacement of these reserves ↑ formation of CYP further, which ↑ metabolism of the antiepileptics	Watch for poor response to these antiepileptics and ↑ doses as necessary
BARBITURATES	GESTRINONE	↓ Levels of gestrinone with risk of therapeutic failure	Induction of hepatic metabolism	Monitor for ↓ clinical efficacy and ↑ gestrinone dose as required
BARBITURATES	IVABRADINE	↓ Levels of ivabradine	Increased CYP 3A4-mediated metabolism of ivabradine	Monitor for reduced efficacy of ivabradine

(Continued)

DRUGS ACTING ON THE CENTRAL NERVOUS SYSTEM ANTIEPILEPTICS Barbiturates

Primary Drug	Secondary Drug	Effect	Mechanism	Precautions
ANTIEPILEPTICS				
BARBITURATES	LOFEXIDINE	↑ Sedation	Additive effect	Warn patients of risk of excessive sedation
BARBITURATES	MIFEPRISTONE	Theoretical risk of ↓ levels of mifepristone	Induction of CYP3A4-mediated metabolism of mifepristone	Watch for poor response to mifepristone
BARBITURATES—THIOPENTONE	MUSCLE RELAXANTS—NONDEPOLARIZING—MIVACURIUM	Inactivation of mivacurium in the presence of an alkaline environment – pH > 8.5. In the presence of an alkaline solution, there is a risk that mivacurium may be inactivated and a free acid precipitated	Mivacurium injection is acidic (pH 3.5–5.5) and should not be mixed in the same syringe with highly alkaline solutions (e.g., some barbiturate solutions) or administered simultaneously through the same needle during i.v. infusion	Avoid mixing with alkaline solutions
BARBITURATES	NITISINONE	Possible ↓ nitisinone levels	Induction of CYP3A4-mediated metabolism	Avoid coadministration
BARBITURATES	ESTROGENS	↓ Levels of these drugs with risk of therapeutic failure	Induction of hepatic metabolism	Monitor for ↓ clinical efficacy and ↑ their dose as required; advise patients to use additional contraception for period of intake and for 1 month after stopping coadministration with these drugs
BARBITURATES	PERIPHERAL VASODILATORS—CILOSTAZOL	Theoretical risk of ↓ citolazol levels	Induction of CYP 3A4 by these antiepileptics	Monitor for evidence of poor response to cilostazol
BARBITURATES	PROGESTOGENS	↓ Levels of these drugs with risk of therapeutic failure	Induction of hepatic metabolism	Monitor for ↓ clinical efficacy and ↑ their dose as required; advise patients to use additional contraception for period of intake and for 1 month after stopping coadministration with these drugs
BARBITURATES	RANOLAZINE	↓ RANOLAZINE levels	Induction of CYP 3A4-mediated metabolism of RANOLAZINE	Manufacturer advises to avoid coadministration
BARBITURATES	THYROID HORMONES—LEVOTHYROXINE	↓ Levels of these drugs with risk of therapeutic failure	Induction of hepatic metabolism	Monitor TFTs regularly

(*Continued*)

Primary Drug	Secondary Drug	Effect	Mechanism	Precautions
ANTIEPILEPTICS				
BARBITURATES	TIBOLONE	↓ Tibolone levels	Induction of metabolism of tibolone	Watch for poor response to tibolone; consider increasing its dose
BARBITURATES	VITAMIN B6	↓ Plasma concentrations of these antiepileptics	Uncertain	Watch for poor response to these antiepileptics if large doses of vitamin B6 are given
CARBAMAZEPINE				
CARBAMAZEPINE	ANALGESICS—OPIOIDS	1. ↓ Efficacy of fentanyl and methadone 2. ↓ Tramadol levels	1. Additive sedative effect 2. Carbamazepine ↑ metabolism of tramadol 3. ↓ Carbamazepine levels	1. Monitor respiratory rate and conscious levels 2. Watch for poor effect of tramadol. Consider using an alternative opioid
CARBAMAZEPINE	ANTIARRHYTHMICS—DRONEDERONE, QUINIDINE	↓ Levels of these drugs with risk of therapeutic failure	Induction of hepatic metabolism	Monitor for ↓ clinical efficacy and ↑ their dose as required
CARBAMAZEPINE	**ANTIBIOTICS**			
CARBAMAZEPINE	DOXYCYCLINE	↓ Levels of doxycycline with risk of therapeutic failure	Induction of hepatic metabolism	Monitor for ↓ clinical efficacy and ↑ doxycycline dose as required
CARBAMAZEPINE	ISONIAZID	↑ Carbamazepine levels	Inhibition of metabolism	Monitor carbamazepine levels
CARBAMAZEPINE	MACROLIDES—CLARITHROMYCIN, ERYTHROMYCIN, TELITHROMYCIN,	1. ↑ Carbamazepine levels 2. ↓ Telithromycin levels	1. Inhibition of metabolism 2. Induction of hepatic metabolism	1. Monitor carbamazepine levels 2. Avoid coadministration of telithromycin for up to 2 weeks after stopping carbamazepine
CARBAMAZEPINE	RIFABUTIN	↓ Carbamazepine levels	Induction of metabolism	Monitor carbamazepine levels
CARBAMAZEPINE	**ANTICANCER AND IMMUNOMODULATING DRUGS**			
CARBAMAZEPINE	AFATINIB	Reduction in afatinib levels	P-glycoprotein induction	U.S. manufacturer recommends dose increase
CARBAMAZEPINE	ANAKINRA	Possible reduced levels of phenytoin	Reversal of cytochrome. P450 suppression by anakinra. Phenytoin has a narrow therapeutic index	Monitor closely, dose adjustment may be needed
CARBAMAZEPINE	AXITINIB	Reduced axitinib levels	CYP3A4/5 induction	Manufacturer advises to avoid concurrent use if possible. If concurrent use is necessary, dose adjustment is recommended

(Continued)

DRUGS ACTING ON THE CENTRAL NERVOUS SYSTEM ANTIEPILEPTICS Carbamazepine

Primary Drug	Secondary Drug	Effect	Mechanism	Precautions
ANTIEPILEPTICS				
CARBAMAZEPINE	BORTEZOMIB	Levels of bortezomib possible reduced by carbamazepine, phenobarbital, and phenytoin	Possibly due to induction of CYP3A4	Avoid concomitant use
CARBAMAZEPINE	BOSUTINIB	Reduced bosutinib levels	CYP3A induction	Manufacturer advises to avoid concurrent use. Dose increase unlikely to sufficiently compensate
CARBAMAZEPINE	CABAZITAXEL	Reduced cabazitaxel levels	CYP3A4 induction	Avoid coadministration
CARBAMAZEPINE	CICLOSPORIN, CORTICOSTEROIDS, IMATINIB, IRINOTECAN, PACLITAXEL, TAMOXIFEN, TOREMIFENE, VINCA ALKALOIDS	↓ Levels of these drugs with risk of therapeutic failure	Induction of hepatic metabolism	Avoid coadministration of carbamazepine with irinotecan (if not able to avoid, ↑ dose of irinotecan by 50%) or tamoxifen. With the other drugs, monitor for ↓ clinical efficacy and ↑ their dose as required. Monitor ciclosporin levels
CARBAMAZEPINE	CRIZOTINIB	Possible reduced crizotinib levels	CYP3A4 induction	Manufacturer advises to avoid concurrent use
CARBAMAZEPINE	DABRAFENIB	Predicted reduced dabrafenib levels	CYP2C8/CYP3A4 induction	Avoid concurrent use
CARBAMAZEPINE	DOCETAXEL	Predicted reduced docetaxel levels	CYP3A4 induction	Monitor closely Dose increase may be required
CARBAMAZEPINE	ERIBULIN	Possible reduced eribulin levels	CYP3A4 induction	Manufacturer recommends avoid concurrent use
CARBAMAZEPINE	ERLOTINIB	Reduced levels of erlotinib	CYP3A4 induction	Avoid concurrent use. If not possible, consider dose increase of erlotinib
CARBAMAZEPINE	ETOPOSIDE	Significantly ↓ plasma concentrations of etoposide (clearance may be >170%) and considerable risk of loss of therapeutic efficacy	Due to potent induction of the hepatic microsomal enzymes that metabolize etoposide	Do not coadminister. Consider use of alternative antiepileptics that do not induce hepatic microsomal enzymes, e.g., valproic acid
CARBAMAZEPINE	EVEROLIMUS	Reduced everolimus levels	CYP3A4 induction	Avoid concurrent use Consider increasing dose of everolimus if concurrent use is necessary

(Continued)

Primary Drug	Secondary Drug	Effect	Mechanism	Precautions
ANTIEPILEPTICS				
CARBAMAZEPINE	FINGOLIMOD	Fingolimod levels reduced	Induction of CYP3A4	Uncertain
CARBAMAZEPINE	LAPATINIB	Reduced lapatinib levels	CYP3A4 induction	Avoid concurrent use Consider dose increase if necessary
CARBAMAZEPINE	METHOTREXATE	Increased clearance of methotrexate (as 24 h infusion), reduced efficacy in combination therapy for B-cell leukemia	Unknown	Clinical significance uncertain—further study needed
CARBAMAZEPINE	MITOTANE	Possible reduction in levels of antiepileptics	Induction of CYP450	Be aware; watch for poor response to antiepileptics
CARBAMAZEPINE	PIXANTRONE	Theoretical risk of reduced pixantrone levels	Pixantrone excretion increased	Manufacturer advises caution
CARBAMAZEPINE	PLATINUM COMPOUNDS	↓ Plasma concentrations of antiepileptic, which ↑risk of seizures	Attributed to impaired absorption of antiepileptic	Monitor closely for seizure activity, and warn patient and carers. Need to adjust dosage using parameters such as blood levels to ensure therapeutic levels
CARBAMAZEPINE	PONATINIB	Possible reduced ponatinib levels	CYP3A4 induction	Avoid concurrent use if possible
CARBAMAZEPINE	PROCARBAZINE	↑ Risk of hypersensitivity reactions in patients with brain tumors	Strong correlation between therapeutic antiepileptic level and hypersensitivity reactions	Consider using nonenzyme-inducing agents
CARBAMAZEPINE	REGORAFENIB	Predicted reduced regorafenib levels	CYP3A4 induction	Manufacturer advises to avoid concurrent use
CARBAMAZEPINE	RUXOLINITIB	Reduced levels of ruxolinitib	CYP3A4 induction	Monitor closely Titrate dose based on safety and efficacy
CARBAMAZEPINE	SORAFENIB	Sorafenib levels reduced	CYP3A4 induction	Avoid concurrent use
CARBAMAZEPINE	TEMSIROLIMUS	Reduced temsirolimus levels	CYP3A4 induction	Avoid concurrent use. If not possible, consider temsirolimus dose increase

(Continued)

Primary Drug	Secondary Drug	Effect	Mechanism	Precautions
ANTIEPILEPTICS				
CARBAMAZEPINE	TRABECTEDIN	1. Reduced trabectedin levels 2. Reduced absorption of phenytoin	1. CYP3A4 induction 2. Trabectedin may damage gut mucosa, affecting absorption of phenytoin	1. Monitor closely
CARBAMAZEPINE	VEMURAFENIB	Possible reduced levels of vemurafenib	CYP3A4 induction	Manufacturer recommends to avoid concurrent use
CARBAMAZEPINE	**ANTICOAGULANTS**			
CARBAMAZEPINE	WARFARIN	↓ Levels of these drugs with risk of therapeutic failure	Induction of hepatic metabolism	Monitor INR at least weekly until stable
CARBAMAZEPINE	APIXABAN	↓ Apixaban levels	Induction of CYP3A4-mediated metabolism and Pgp-mediated transport of apixaban	Avoid coadministration
CARBAMAZEPINE	DABIGATRAN	↓ Dabigatran levels	Induction of Pgp	Manufacturers advise against coadministration
CARBAMAZEPINE	RIVAROXABAN	↓ Rivaroxaban exposure	Induction of CYP3A4-mediated metabolism and Pgp-mediated efflux transport	Avoid coadministration
CARBAMAZEPINE	**ANTIDEPRESSANTS**			
CARBAMAZEPINE	LITHIUM	↑ Risk of neurotoxicity	Uncertain; this may occur with normal lithium blood levels	Warn patient and carers to watch for drowsiness, ataxia, and tremor
CARBAMAZEPINE	MAOIs	↑ Risk of seizures	These drugs lower seizure threshold	Care with coadministration. Watch for ↑ fit frequency; warn patient of this risk when starting these drugs and take suitable precautions. Consider increasing dose of antiepileptic
CARBAMAZEPINE	MIRTAZAPINE	↓ Levels of mirtazapine with risk of therapeutic failure	Induction of hepatic metabolism	Monitor for ↓ clinical efficacy and ↑ their dose as required
CARBAMAZEPINE	REBOXETINE	Risk of ↓ reboxetine levels	Possibly induction of CYP3A4-mediated metabolism of reboxetine	May need to increase dose of reboxetine with close monitoring
CARBAMAZEPINE	ST. JOHN'S WORT	↓ Carbamazepine levels	Induction of metabolism	Avoid coadministration

(Continued)

Primary Drug	Secondary Drug	Effect	Mechanism	Precautions
ANTIEPILEPTICS				
CARBAMAZEPINE	SSRIs	1. ↑ Risk of seizures 2. Risk of serotonin syndrome with carbamazepine	1. These drugs lower seizure threshold 2. Carbamazepine ↑ serotonin concentrations in the brain	Avoid coadministration
CARBAMAZEPINE	TCAs	1. ↑ Risk of seizures 2. ↑ Risk of bone marrow depression in patients on chemotherapy when carbamazepine used with TCAs 3. ↓ Plasma concentrations of mianserin	1. These drugs lower seizure threshold 2. Additive effects 3. ↑ Metabolism of mianserin	1. Care with coadministration. Watch for ↑ fit frequency; warn patient of this risk when starting these drugs and take suitable precautions. Consider increasing dose of antiepileptic 2. Avoid concurrent use during chemotherapy 3. Be aware and watch for signs of ↓ antidepressant effect of mianserin
CARBAMAZEPINE	ANTIDIABETIC DRUGS—GLIPIZIDE, REPAGLINIDE	↓ Levels of these drugs with risk of therapeutic failure	Induction of hepatic metabolism	Monitor capillary blood glucose and warn patients about symptoms of hyperglycemia
CARBAMAZEPINE	ANTIEMETICS—APREPITANT, ONDANSETRON,	↓ Levels of these drugs with risk of therapeutic failure	Induction of hepatic metabolism	Monitor for ↓ clinical efficacy and ↑ their dose as required
CARBAMAZAPINE	**ANTIEPILEPTICS**			
CARBAMAZEPINE	1. ETHOSUXIMIDE 2. LAMOTRIGINE 3. TIAGABINE 4. TOPIRAMATE 5. VALPROATE 6. ZONISAMIDE	↓ Levels of these antiepileptics	Induction of metabolism	Watch for poor response to these antiepileptics
CARBAMAZEPINE	PHENYTOIN	Variable effect on phenytoin levels. ↓ Carbamazepine levels	Mutual induction of metabolism; uncertain why cases of ↑ phenytoin levels	Be aware and monitor levels. Watch for early features of phenytoin toxicity
CARBAMAZEPINE	ANTIFUNGALS—ITRACONAZOLE, KETOCONAZOLE, POSACONAZOLE, VORICONAZOLE, CASPOFUNGIN	1. ↓ Levels of these drugs with risk of therapeutic failure 2. Azoles also ↑ carbamazepine levels	1. Induction of hepatic metabolism 2. Inhibition of Pgp ↑ bioavailability of carbamazepine	Avoid coadministration of carbamazepine with azoles (consider using fluconazole). ↑ Dose of caspofungin to 70 mg daily

(Continued)

Primary Drug	Secondary Drug	Effect	Mechanism	Precautions
ANTIEPILEPTICS				
CARBAMAZEPINE	ANTIGOUT DRUGS—ALLOPURINOL	High-dose allopurinol (600 mg/day) may ↑ carbamazepine levels over a period of several weeks. 300 mg/day allopurinol does not seem to have this effect	Uncertain	Monitor carbamazepine levels in patients taking long-term, high-dose allopurinol
CARBAMAZEPINE	ANTIMALARIALS—CHLOROQUINE, MEFLOQUINE	↑ Risk of seizures	These drugs lower seizure threshold	Care with coadministration. Watch for ↑ fit frequency; warn patient of this risk when starting these drugs and take suitable precautions. Consider increasing dose of antiepileptic
CARBAMAZEPINE	ANTIMIGRAINE DRUGS—5-HT1 AGONISTS—ALMOTRIPTAN, ELETRIPTAN	Risk of serotonin syndrome with almotriptan and eletriptan	Additive effect—both triptans and carbamazepine stimulate 5-HT receptors, and carbamazepine also prevents reuptake of 5-HT	Be aware of the possibility of the occurrence of serotonin syndrome with 5-HT1 agonists
CARBAMAZEPINE	**ANTIPLATELET AGENTS**			
CARBAMAZEPINE, OXCARBAZEPINE	CLOPIDOGREL	Theoretical risk of ↓ efficacy of clopidogrel	Inhibition of CYP2C19-mediated activation of clopidogrel	Consider using an alternative antiepileptic
CARBAMAZEPINE	TICAGRELOR	↓ Ticagrelor levels	Induction of CYP3A4-mediated metabolism of ticagrelor	Manufacturer recommends avoid coadministration
CARBAMAZEPINE	ANTIPROTOZOALS—MEBENDAZOLE	↓ Levels of these drugs with risk of therapeutic failure	Induction of hepatic metabolism	Monitor for ↓ clinical efficacy and ↑ their dose as required
CARBAMAZEPINE	**ANTIPSYCHOTICS**			
CARBAMAZEPINE	ANTIPSYCHOTICS	↑ Risk of seizures	These drugs lower seizure threshold	Care with coadministration. Watch for ↑ fit frequency; warn patient of this risk when starting these drugs and take suitable precautions. Consider increasing dose of antiepileptic
CARBAMAZEPINE	ARPIPRAZOLE, CLOZAPINE, HALOPERIDOL, OLANZAPINE, QUETIAPINE, RISPERIDONE, SERTINDOLE	↓ Levels of arpiprazole, clozapine, haloperidol, olanzapine, quetiapine, risperidone, and sertindole	Induction of metabolism	Watch for poor response to these antipsychotics, and consider increasing the dose

(*Continued*)

Primary Drug	Secondary Drug	Effect	Mechanism	Precautions
ANTIEPILEPTICS				
CARBAMAZEPINE	**ANTIVIRALS**			
CARBAMAZEPINE	COBICISTAT	1. Possible ↓ plasma levels of cobicistat, risk of treatment failure, and resistance 2. Possible ↓ plasma levels of medicines being boosted, e.g., protease inhibitor, risk of treatment failure, and resistance	Induction of metabolism via CYP3A	Avoid coadministration
CARBAMAZEPINE	DOLUTEGRAVIR	Possible ↓ plasma levels of dolutegravir, risk of treatment failure, and resistance	Induction of UGT1A1 and CYP3A	Avoid coadministration
CARBAMAZEPINE	MARAVIROC	Possible ↓ plasma levels of dolutegravir, risk of treatment failure, and resistance	Induction of UGT1A1 and CYP3A	Avoid coadministration
CARBAMAZEPINE	NNRTIs	1. Possible ↓ efficacy of carbamazepine by etravirine and nevirapine 2. ↓ Plasma levels of efavirenz, possible ↓ efficacy of etravirine and efavirenz 3. Possible significant ↓ in plasma levels of rilpivirine, risk of antiviral therapeutic failure	1. ↑ Metabolism via CYP3A4 2. ↑ Metabolism via induction of CYP3A4 and CYP2B6 3. Uncertain	1. Monitor closely including carbamazepine levels and side effects when initiating or changing treatment 2. Combination with etravirine or efavirenz not recommended 3. Avoid coadministration
CARBAMAZEPINE	PROTEASE INHIBITORS	Possibly ↑ adverse effects of carbamazepine with protease inhibitors	Inhibition of CYP3A4-mediated metabolism of carbamazepine	Use with caution. Monitor carbamazepine levels and side effects when initiating or changing treatment
CARBAMAZEPINE	**ANXIOLYTICS AND HYPNOTICS**			
CARBAMAZEPINE	BZDs—CLONAZEPAM	↓ Carbamazepine levels	Induction of metabolism	Watch for poor response to carbamazepine
CARBAMAZEPINE	ZALEPLON, ZOLPIDEM, ZOPICLONE	↓ Levels of these drugs with risk of therapeutic failure	Induction of hepatic metabolism	Monitor for ↓ clinical efficacy and ↑ their dose as required

(*Continued*)

Primary Drug	Secondary Drug	Effect	Mechanism	Precautions
ANTIEPILEPTICS				
CARBAMAZEPINE	BRONCHODILATORS—THEOPHYLLINE	↓ Levels of these drugs with risk of therapeutic failure	Induction of hepatic metabolism	May need to ↑ dose of theophylline by 25%
CARBAMAZEPINE	**CALCIUM CHANNEL BLOCKERS**			
CARBAMAZEPINE	DILTIAZEM AND VERAPAMIL	Diltiazem and verapamil ↑ plasma concentrations of carbamazepine (have been cases of toxicity)	Diltiazem and verapamil inhibit CYP3A4-mediated metabolism of carbamazepine. They also inhibit intestinal Pgp, which may ↑ bioavailability of carbamazepine	Monitor carbamazepine levels when initiating calcium channel blockers, particularly diltiazem/verapamil
CARBAMAZEPINE	FELODIPINE, NIFEDIPINE, AND POSSIBLY NIMODIPINE AND NISOLDIPINE	↓ Levels of these drugs with risk of therapeutic failure	Induction of hepatic metabolism	Monitor PR and BP weekly until stable and watch for ↑
CARBAMAZEPINE	CNS STIMULANTS—MODAFINIL	↓ Plasma concentrations of modafinil, with possibility of ↓ therapeutic effect	Induction of CYP3A4, which has a partial role in the metabolism of modafinil	Be aware
CARBAMAZEPINE	DANAZOL	↑ Plasma concentrations of carbamazepine, with risk of toxic effects	Inhibition of carbamazepine metabolism	Watch for toxic effects of carbamazepine
CARBAMAZEPINE	**DIURETICS**			
CARBAMAZEPINE	EPLERENONE	↓ Levels of eplerenone with risk of therapeutic failure	Induction of hepatic metabolism	Avoid coadministration
CARBAMAZEPINE	LOOP, THIAZIDES	Risk of hyponatremia	Additive effect	Monitor serum sodium closely
CARBAMAZEPINE	GESTRINONE	↓ Levels of gestrinone with risk of therapeutic failure	Induction of hepatic metabolism	Monitor for ↓ clinical efficacy and ↑ gestrinone dose as required
CARBAMAZEPINE	GRAPEFRUIT JUICE	↑ Efficacy and ↑ adverse effects	Grapefruit juice irreversibly inhibits intestinal CYP3A4. Transport via Pgp and the MRP-2 efflux pumps is also inhibited	Monitor for ↑ side effects/toxicity and check carbamazepine levels. If levels or control of fits are variable, remove grapefruit juice and grapefruit from the diet

(*Continued*)

Primary Drug	Secondary Drug	Effect	Mechanism	Precautions
ANTIEPILEPTICS				
CARBAMAZEPINE	H2-RECEPTOR BLOCKERS—CIMETIDINE, FAMOTIDINE, RANITIDINE	↑ Plasma concentrations of carbamazepine and risk of adverse effects, including bone marrow depression and skin reactions	Transient inhibition of carbamazepine via CYP3A4, which may then be countered within a few days via autoinduction by carbamazepine	Cimetidine and carbamazpine—monitor for increased adverse effects though these should subside after about a week, rantidine appears not to interact with carbamazepine. Nizatidine appears not to interact with antiepileptics
CARBAMAZEPINE	IVACAFTOR	↓ Ivacaftor levels	Induction of CYP3A4-mediated metabolism of ivacaftor	Manufacturers advice against coadministration
CARBAMAZEPINE	LIPID-LOWERING DRUGS—FIBRATES	Gemfibrozil may ↑ carbamazepine levels	Uncertain at present	Watch for features of carbamazepine toxicity
CARBAMAZEPINE	MIFEPRISTONE	Theoretical risk of ↓ levels of mifepristone	Induction of CYP3A4-mediated metabolism of mifepristone	Watch for poor response to mifepristone
CARBAMAZEPINE	MUSCLE RELAXANTS	Resistance to neuromuscular blocking action may occur in patients who are taking regular carbamazepine or phenytoin. This results in a shorter duration of neuromuscular blockade	Unknown	Infusion rates of nondepolarizing muscle relaxants may need to be increased
CARBAMAZEPINE	NITISINONE	Possible ↓ nitisinone levels	Induction of CYP3A4-mediated metabolism	Avoid coadministration
CARBAMAZEPINE	ESTROGENS	↓ Levels of these drugs with risk of therapeutic failure	Induction of hepatic metabolism	Advise patients to use additional contraception for period of intake and for 1 month after stopping coadministration with these drugs
CARBAMAZEPINE	PROGESTOGENS	↓ Levels of these drugs with risk of therapeutic failure	Induction of hepatic metabolism	Advise patients to use additional contraception for period of intake and for 1 month after stopping coadministration with these drugs
CARBAMAZEPINE	PROTON PUMP INHIBITORS	Possible altered efficacy of carbamazepine	Unclear; possibly via ↓ clearance	Use with caution. Monitor carbamazepine levels when starting or stopping and use proton pump inhibitor regularly not PRN. Not reported with pantoprazole or rabeprazole

(*Continued*)

Primary Drug	Secondary Drug	Effect	Mechanism	Precautions
ANTIEPILEPTICS				
CARBAMAZEPINE	PERIPHERAL VASODILATORS—CILOSTAZOL	Theoretical risk of ↓ cilostazol levels	Induction of CYP3A4 by these antiepileptics	Monitor for evidence of poor response to cilostazol
CARBAMAZEPINE	RANOLAZINE	↓ RANOLAZINE levels	Induction of CYP3A4-mediated metabolism of RANOLAZINE	Manufacturer advises to avoid coadministration
CARBAMAZEPINE	ROFLUMILAST	↓ Efficacy of roflumilast	Induction of CYP3A4- and 1A2-mediated metabolism of roflumilast and its active metabolite	Monitor for poor response and increase dose as necessary
CARBAMAZEPINE	THYROID HORMONES—LEVOTHYROXINE	↓ Levels of these drugs with risk of therapeutic failure	Induction of hepatic metabolism	Monitor TFTs regularly
CARBAMAZEPINE	TIBOLONE	↓ Tibolone levels	Induction of metabolism of tibolone	Watch for poor response to tibolone; consider increasing its dose
ETHOSUXIMIDE				
ETHOSUXIMIDE	ANTIBIOTICS—ISONIAZID	Case of ↑ ethosuximide levels with toxicity	Inhibition of metabolism	Watch for early features of ethosuximide toxicity
ETHOSUXIMIDE	ANTIDEPRESSANTS—MAOIs, SSRIs, TCAs	↑ Risk of seizures	These drugs lower seizure threshold	Care with coadministration. Watch for ↑ fit frequency; warn patient of this risk when starting these drugs and take suitable precautions. Consider increasing dose of antiepileptic
ETHOSUXIMIDE	ANTIEPILEPTICS—PHENYTOIN	Cases of ↑ phenytoin levels	Uncertain	Watch for early features of phenytoin toxicity
ETHOSUXIMIDE	ANTIMALARIALS—CHLOROQUINE, MEFLOQUINE	↑ Risk of seizures	These drugs lower seizure threshold	Care with coadministration. Watch for ↑ fit frequency; warn patient of this risk when starting these drugs and take suitable precautions. Consider increasing dose of antiepileptic

(Continued)

Primary Drug	Secondary Drug	Effect	Mechanism	Precautions
ANTIEPILEPTICS				
ETHOSUXIMIDE	ANTIPSYCHOTICS	↑ Risk of seizures	These drugs lower seizure threshold	Care with coadministration. Watch for ↑ fit frequency; warn patient of this risk when starting these drugs and take suitable precautions. Consider increasing dose of antiepileptic
GABAPENTIN				
GABAPENTIN	ANTACIDS	↓ Gabapentin levels	↓ Absorption	Separate doses by at least 3 h
GABAPENTIN	ANALGESICS—MORPHINE	1. CNS depression 2. ↑ Analgesic effect	1. Pharmacodynamic additive CNS depression 2. Uncertain; partly due to ↑ plasma concentration of gabapentin due to ↓ gut mobility with morphine	Monitor for signs of CNS depression; titrate doses of gabapentin and/or morphine
GABAPENTIN	ANTIDEPRESSANTS—MAOIs, SSRIs, TCAs	↑ Risk of seizures	These drugs lower seizure threshold	Care with coadministration. Watch for ↑ fit frequency; warn patient of this risk when starting these drugs and take suitable precautions. Consider increasing dose of antiepileptic
GABAPENTIN	ANTIMALARIALS—CHLOROQUINE, MEFLOQUINE	↑ Risk of seizures	Antimalarials lower seizure threshold	Care with coadministration. Watch for ↑ fit frequency; warn patient of this risk when starting these drugs and take suitable precautions. Consider increasing dose of antiepileptic
GABAPENTIN	ANTIPSYCHOTICS	↑ Risk of seizures	These drugs lower seizure threshold	Care with coadministration. Watch for ↑ fit frequency; warn patient of this risk when starting these drugs and take suitable precautions. Consider increasing dose of antiepileptic

(Continued)

Primary Drug	Secondary Drug	Effect	Mechanism	Precautions
ANTIEPILEPTICS				
LAMOTRIGINE				
LAMOTRIGINE	ANTIBIOTICS—RIFAMPICIN	↓ Lamotrigine levels	↑ Metabolism	Monitor levels
LAMOTRIGINE	ANTIDEPRESSANTS—MAOIs, SSRIs, TCAs	↑ Risk of seizures	These drugs lower seizure threshold	Care with coadministration. Watch for ↑ fit frequency; warn patient of this risk when starting these drugs and take suitable precautions. Consider increasing dose of antiepileptic
LAMOTRIGINE	ANTIEPILEPTICS—CARBAMAZEPINE, OXCARBAZEPINE	1. Cases of ↑ levels of an active metabolite of carbamazepine with toxicity 2. Case of toxicity with oxcarbazepine	Uncertain	Be aware; watch for early features of toxicity of carbamazepine and oxcarbazepine
LAMOTRIGINE	ANTIMALARIALS—CHLOROQUINE, MEFLOQUINE	↑ Risk of seizures	These drugs lower seizure threshold	Care with coadministration. Watch for ↑ fit frequency; warn patient of this risk when starting these drugs and take suitable precautions. Consider increasing dose of antiepileptic
LAMOTRIGINE	ANTIPSYCHOTICS	↑ Risk of seizures	These drugs lower seizure threshold	Care with coadministration. Watch for ↑ fit frequency; warn patient of this risk when starting these drugs and take suitable precautions. Consider increasing dose of antiepileptic
LAMOTRIGINE	ANTIVIRALS—LOPINAVIR/RITONAVIR, RITONAVIR	↓ Plasma levels of lamotrigine	Increased glucuronidation of lamotrigine	Monitor more closely, take lamotrigine levels within 2 weeks of adjusting therapy. If lopinavir/ritonavir or ritoanvir is newly added, dose increase of antiepileptic may be required
LAMOTRIGINE	ESTROGENS	↓ Lamotrigine levels	↑ Metabolism	Monitor levels
LAMOTRIGINE	PROGESTOGENS	↓ Lamotrigine levels	↑ Metabolism	Monitor levels

(Continued)

Primary Drug	Secondary Drug	Effect	Mechanism	Precautions
ANTIEPILEPTICS				
OXCARBAZEPINE				
OXCARBAZEPINE	SORAFENIB	Sorafenib levels reduced	CYP3A4 induction	Avoid concurrent use
OXCARBAZEPINE	ANTIDEPRESSANTS—MAOIs, SSRIs, TCAs	↑ Risk of seizures	These drugs lower seizure threshold	Care with coadministration. Watch for ↑ fit frequency; warn patient of this risk when starting these drugs and take suitable precautions. Consider increasing dose of antiepileptic
OXCARBAZEPINE	**ANTIEPILEPTICS**			
OXCARBAZEPINE	1. BARBITURATES 2. PHENYTOIN	↑ Levels of these antiepileptics	Uncertain	Watch for early features of toxicity
OXCARBAZEPINE	CARBAMAZEPINE	Variable effect on carbamazepine levels	Uncertain	Be aware; monitor carbamazepine levels
OXCARBAZEPINE	ANTIMALARIALS—CHLOROQUINE, MEFLOQUINE	↑ Risk of seizures	These drugs lower seizure threshold	Care with coadministration. Watch for ↑ fit frequency; warn patient of this risk when starting these drugs and take suitable precautions. Consider increasing dose of antiepileptic
OXCARBAZEPINE	ANTIPLATELET AGENTS—CLOPIDOGREL	Theoretical risk of ↓ efficacy of clopidogrel	Inhibition of CYP2C19-mediated activation of clopidogrel	Consider using an alternative antiepileptic
OXCARBAZEPINE	ANTIPSYCHOTICS	↑ Risk of seizures	These drugs lower seizure threshold	Care with coadministration. Watch for ↑ fit frequency; warn patient of this risk when starting these drugs and take suitable precautions. Consider increasing dose of antiepileptic
OXCARBAZEPINE	**ANTIVIRALS**			
OXCARBAZEPINE	DOLUTEGRAVIR	Possible ↓ plasma levels of dolutegravir, risk of treatment failure, and resistance	Induction of UGT1A1 and CYP3A	Avoid coadministration
OXCARBAZEPINE	MARAVIROC	Possible ↓ plasma levels of dolutegravir, risk of treatment failure, and resistance	Induction of UGT1A1 and CYP3A	Avoid coadministration

(Continued)

Primary Drug	Secondary Drug	Effect	Mechanism	Precautions
ANTIEPILEPTICS				
OXCARBAZEPINE	ESTROGENS	Marked ↓ contraceptive effect	Induction of metabolism of estrogens	Advise patients to use additional contraception for period of intake and for 1 month after stopping coadministration
OXCARBAZEPINE	PROGESTOGENS	↓ Progesterone levels, which may lead to failure of contraception or poor response to treatment of menorrhagia	Possibly induction of metabolism of progestogens	Advise patients to use additional contraception for period of intake and for 1 month after stopping coadministration
PHENYTOIN/FOSPHENYTOIN				
PHENYTOIN	ACUTE AND CHRONIC ALCOHOL INGESTION	↑ Phenytoin levels	Uncertain	Warn patients regarding alcohol consumption
PHENYTOIN	ANESTHETICS—LOCAL—LIDOCAINE AND PROCAINE SOLUTIONS	Precipitation of drugs, which may not be immediately apparent	A pharmaceutical interaction	Do not mix in the same infusion or syringe
PHENYTOIN	**ANALGESICS**			
PHENYTOIN	NSAIDs—CELECOXIB, PARECOXIB	1. ↓ Levels of these drugs, with risk of therapeutic failure 2. Report of ↑ phenytoin levels with celecoxib	1. Induction of hepatic metabolism 2. Inhibition of CYP2C9-mediated metabolism of phenytoin by parecoxib	1. Monitor for ↓ clinical efficacy and ↑ their dose as required 2. Monitor phenytoin levels when coadministered with parecoxib
PHENYTOIN	OPIOIDS	1. ↓ Efficacy of fentanyl and methadone with carbamazepine, phenytoin 2. Risk of pethidine toxicity	1. ↑ Hepatic metabolism of fentanyl and methadone, and possibly an effect at the opioid receptor 2. Phenytoin induces metabolism of pethidine, which causes ↑ level of a neurotoxic metabolite	1. Be aware that the dose of fentanyl and methadone may need to be ↑ 2. Coadminister with caution; the effect may be ↓ by administering pethidine intravenously
PHENYTOIN	ANTACIDS	↓ Phenytoin levels	↓ Absorption	Separate doses by at least 3 h
PHENYTOIN	ANTIARRHYTHMICS—AMIODARONE, DISOPYRAMIDE, DRONEDERONE, MEXILETINE, QUINIDINE	1. ↓ Levels of these drugs, with risk of therapeutic failure 2. Phenytoin levels may be ↑ by amiodarone	1. Induction of hepatic metabolism 2. Uncertain; amiodarone inhibits CYP2C9, which plays a role in phenytoin metabolism and inhibits intestinal Pgp, which may ↑ bioavailability of phenytoin	1. Monitor PR and BP weekly until stable, and watch for ↑ BP 2. ↓ Phenytoin dose by 25%–30% and monitor levels; monitor phenytoin levels when coadministered with amiodarone

(*Continued*)

Primary Drug	Secondary Drug	Effect	Mechanism	Precautions
ANTIEPILEPTICS				
PHENYTOIN	**ANTIBIOTICS**			
PHENYTOIN	CHLORAMPHENICOL	↑ Phenytoin levels	Inhibited metabolism	Monitor phenytoin levels
PHENYTOIN	CIPROFLOXACIN	Variable effect on phenytoin levels	Unknown	Monitor phenytoin levels
PHENYTOIN	DOXYCYCLINE	↓ Levels of doxycycline with risk of therapeutic failure	Induction of hepatic metabolism	Monitor for ↓ clinical efficacy and ↑ doxycycline dose as required
PHENYTOIN	ISONIAZID	↑ Phenytoin levels	Inhibited metabolism	Monitor phenytoin levels
PHENYTOIN	METRONIDAZOLE	↑ Phenytoin levels	Inhibited metabolism	Monitor phenytoin levels
PHENYTOIN	MACROLIDES—CLARITHROMYCIN, ERYTHROMYCIN, TELITHROMYCIN	1. ↑ Phenytoin levels 2. ↓ Telithromycin levels	1. Inhibition of metabolism 2. Induction of hepatic metabolism	1. Monitor phenytoin levels 2. Avoid coadministration of telithromycin for up to 2 weeks after stopping phenytoin—erythromycin is unlikely to interact
PHENYTOIN	RIFAMPICIN, RIFABUTIN	↓ Phenytoin levels	Induced metabolism	Monitor phenytoin levels
PHENYTOIN	SULFONAMIDES, TRIMETHOPRIM	↑ Phenytoin levels	Inhibited metabolism	Monitor phenytoin levels
PHENYTOIN	**ANTICANCER AND IMMUNOMODULATING DRUGS**			
PHENYTOIN	ADALIMUMAB	Possible reduced levels of phenytoin	Reversal of cytochrome. P450 suppression by adalimumab. Phenytoin has a narrow therapeutic index	Monitor closely, dose adjustment may be needed
PHENYTOIN	AFATINIB	Reduction in afatinib levels	P-glycoprotein induction	U.S. manufacturer recommends dose increase
PHENYTOIN	ANAKINRA	Possible reduced levels of phenytoin	Reversal of cytochrome P450 suppression by anakinra. Phenytoin has a narrow therapeutic index	Monitor closely, dose adjustment may be needed
PHENYTOIN	AXITINIB	Reduced axitinib levels	CYP3A4/5 induction	Manufacturer advises to avoid concurrent use if possible. If concurrent use is necessary, dose adjustment is recommended

(Continued)

Primary Drug	Secondary Drug	Effect	Mechanism	Precautions
ANTIEPILEPTICS				
PHENYTOIN	BORTEZOMIB	Levels of bortezomib possibly reduced by carbamazepine, phenobarbital, and phenytoin	Possibly due to induction of CYP3A4	Avoid concomitant use
PHENYTOIN	BOSUTINIB	Reduced bosutinib levels	CYP3A induction	Manufacturer advises to avoid concurrent use. Dose increase unlikely to sufficiently compensate
PHENYTOIN	BUSULFAN, CICLOSPORIN, CORTICOSTEROIDS, ERLOTINIB, ETOPOSIDE, EXEMESTANE, IFOSFAMIDE, IRINOTECAN, PACLITAXEL, TACROLIMUS, TAMOXIFEN, TOPOTECAN, TOREMIFENE, VINCA ALKALOIDS	↓ Levels of these drugs, with risk of therapeutic failure	Induction of hepatic metabolism	1. Avoid coadministration of phenytoin with etoposide, irinotecan (if not able to avoid, ↑ dose of irinotecan by 50%), tacrolimus, and tamoxifen 2. ↑ Dose of erlotinib (manufacturer advises starting at 300 mg) 3. ↑ Dose of exemestane to 50 mg/day 4. With the other drugs, monitor for ↓ clinical efficacy and ↑ their dose as required. Monitor ciclosporin levels
PHENYTOIN	CABAZITAXEL	Reduced cabazitaxel levels	CYP3A4 induction	Avoid coadministration
PHENYTOIN	CRIZOTINIB	Possible reduced crizotinib levels	CYP3A4 induction	Manufacturer advises to avoid concurrent use
PHENYTOIN	DABRAFENIB	Predicted reduced dabrafenib levels	CYP2C8/CYP3A4 induction	Avoid concurrent use
PHENYTOIN	DOCETAXEL	Predicted reduced docetaxel levels	CYP3A4 induction	Monitor closely Dose increase may be required
PHENYTOIN	ERIBULIN	Possible reduced eribulin levels	CYP3A4 induction	Manufacturer recommends to avoid concurrent use
PHENYTOIN	ERLOTINIB	Reduced levels of erlotinib	CYP3A4 induction	Avoid concurrent use. If not possible, consider dose increase of erlotinib
PHENYTOIN	EVEROLIMUS	Reduced everolimus levels	CYP3A4 induction	Avoid concurrent use Consider increasing dose of everolimus if concurrent use is necessary

(*Continued*)

Primary Drug	Secondary Drug	Effect	Mechanism	Precautions
ANTIEPILEPTICS				
PHENYTOIN	FINGOLIMOD	Fingolimod levels reduced	Induction of CYP3A4	Uncertain
PHENYTOIN	FLUOROURACIL, CAPECITABINE, TEGAFUR	Increased risk of phenytoin toxicitiy	Flouuracil is classed as an irreversible inhibitor of enzymes. ↑ Phenytoin levels attributed to inhibition of CYP2C9	Avoid concurrent use If not possible, monitor phenytoin concentrations and adjust as necessary
PHENYTOIN	GEFITINIB	Gefitinib levels reduced	CYP3A4 induction	Avoid concurrent use. Consider dose increase if necessary
PHENYTOIN	GOLIMUMAB	Possible reduced levels of phenytoin	Induction of metabolism	Monitor closely, dose adjustment may be needed
FOSPHENYTOIN, PHENYTOIN	IMATINIB	1. ↓ Imatinib levels 2. ↑ Plasma concentrations, with risk of toxic effects of these drugs	1. Due to induction of CYP3A4-mediated metabolism of imatinib 2. Imatinib is a potent inhibitor of CYP2C9 isoenzymes, which metabolize these drugs	1. Monitor for clinical efficacy and adjust dose as required 2. Watch for the early toxic effects of these drugs. If necessary, consider using alternative drugs while the patient is being given imatinib
PHENYTOIN	INFLIXIMAB	Possible reduced levels of phenytoin	Reversal of cytochrome P450 suppression by adalimumab. Phenytoin has a narrow therapeutic index	Monitor closely, dose adjustment may be needed
PHENYTOIN	LEFLUNOMIDE	Possible increase in phenytoin toxicity	CYP2C9 inhibition by leflunomide metabolite	Monitor closely
PHENYTOIN	METHOTREXATE	1. Increased clearance of methotrexate (as 24 h infusion) reduced efficacy in combination therapy for B-cell leukemia 2. ↑ Plasma concentrations of phenytoin may occur and ↑ risk of toxic effects of phenytoin	High doses of methotrexate ↓ elimination of phenytoin	Monitor phenytoin levels and clinically watch for signs and symptoms of phenytoin toxicity, e.g., nausea, vomiting, insomnia, tremor, acne, hirsutism
PHENYTOIN	MITOTANE	Possible reduction in levels of antiepileptics	Induction of CYP450	Be aware; watch for poor response to antiepileptics

(Continued)

Primary Drug	Secondary Drug	Effect	Mechanism	Precautions
ANTIEPILEPTICS				
PHENYTOIN	PLATINUM COMPOUNDS	↓ Phenytoin levels with risk of seizures	Impaired absorption of antiepileptic	Monitor closely for seizure activity, and warn patients and carers. Need to adjust dosage using parameters such as blood levels to ensure therapeutic levels
PHENYTOIN	PONATINIB	Possible reduced ponatinib levels	CYP3A4 induction	Avoid concurrent use if possible
PHENYTOIN	PROCARBAZINE	↑ Risk of hypersensitivity reactions in patients with brain tumors	Strong correlation between therapeutic antiepileptic level and hypersensitivity reactions	Consider using nonenzyme-inducing agents
PHENYTOIN	REGORAFENIB	Predicted reduced regorafenib levels	CYP3A4 induction	Manufacturer advises to avoid concurrent use
PHENYTOIN	RUXOLITINIB	Reduced levels of ruloxitinib	CYP3A4 induction	Monitor closely Titrate dose based on safety and efficacy
PHENYTOIN	SIROLIMUS	Possible reduced sirolimus levels	CYP3A4 and P-glycoprotein induction	Monitor closely with concurrent use
PHENYTOIN	SORAFENIB	Sorafenib levels reduced	CYP3A4 induction	Avoid concurrent use
PHENYTOIN	TEMSIROLIMUS	Reduced temsirolimus levels	CYP3A4 induction	Avoid concurrent use. If not possible, consider temsirolimus dose increase
PHENYTOIN	THALIDOMIDE	Possible increased risk of peripheral neuropathy	Additive	Manufacturer advises caution
PHENYTOIN	TOCILIZUMAB	Reduced levels	Tocilizumab reverses cytochrome P450 isoenzyme suppression by IL-6	Monitor closely and consider dose adjustment
PHENYTOIN	**ANTICOAGULANTS**			
PHENYTOIN	WARFARIN	Initial ↑ in warfarin levels, then ↓ level with risk of therapeutic failure	Potential induction and inhibition of CYP2C9 by phenytoin—possibly leading to a biphasic interaction	Requires monitoring of INR at least three times a week until stable
PHENYTOIN	APIXABAN	↓ Apixaban levels	Induction of CYP3A4-mediated metabolism and Pgp-mediated transport of apixaban	Avoid coadministration

(*Continued*)

Primary Drug	Secondary Drug	Effect	Mechanism	Precautions
ANTIEPILEPTICS				
PHENYTOIN	DABIGATRAN	↓ Dabigatran levels	Induction of Pgp	Manufacturers advises against coadministration
PHENYTOIN	RIVAROXABAN	↓ Rivaroxaban exposure	Induction of CYP3A4-mediated metabolism and Pgp-mediated efflux transport	Avoid coadministration
PHENYTOIN	VEMURAFENIB	Possible reduced levels of vemurafenib	CYP3A4 induction	Manufacturer recommends to avoid concurrent use
PHENYTOIN	**ANTIDEPRESSANTS**			
PHENYTOIN	LITHIUM	↑ Risk of neurotoxicity	Uncertain; this may occur with normal lithium blood levels	Warn patients and carers to watch for drowsiness, ataxia, and tremor
PHENYTOIN	MAOIs	↑ Risk of seizures	These drugs lower seizure threshold	Care with coadministration. Watch for ↑ fit frequency; warn patient of this risk when starting these drugs and take suitable precautions. Consider increasing dose of antiepileptic
PHENYTOIN	MIRTAZAPINE	↓ Levels of these drugs, with risk of therapeutic failure	Induction of hepatic metabolism	Monitor for ↓ clinical efficacy and ↑ their dose as required
PHENYTOIN	REBOXETINE	Risk of ↓ reboxetine levels	Possibly induction of CYP3A4-mediated metabolism of reboxetine	May need to increase dose of reboxetine with close monitoring
PHENYTOIN	ST. JOHN'S WORT	↓ Phenytoin levels	Induction of metabolism	Avoid coadministration
PHENYTOIN	SSRIs	↑ Plasma concentrations of phenytoin	Phenytoin is a substrate of CYP2C9 and CYP2C19. Fluvoxamine and fluoxetine are known to inhibit CYP2C9/10/19. Paroxetine and sertraline cause less inhibition of CYP2C9/19	Monitor plasma phenytoin levels
PHENYTOIN	TCAs	1. ↑ Risk of seizures 2. ↓ Levels of TCAs, with risk of therapeutic failure 3. Report of ↑ phenytoin levels with mianserin	1. TCA drugs lower seizure threshold 2. Induction of hepatic metabolism. 3. Inhibition of phenytoin metabolism	1. Care with coadministration 2. Watch for ↑ fit frequency; warn patient of this risk when starting these drugs and take suitable precautions. Consider increasing dose of antiepileptic 3. Monitor phenytoin levels when coadministered with mianserin

(*Continued*)

Primary Drug	Secondary Drug	Effect	Mechanism	Precautions
ANTIEPILEPTICS				
PHENYTOIN	**ANTIDIABETIC DRUGS**			
PHENYTOIN	METFORMIN, SULFONYLUREAS	↓ Hypoglycemic efficacy	Hydantoins are considered to ↓ release of insulin	Monitor capillary blood glucose closely; higher doses of antidiabetic drugs needed
PHENYTOIN	REPAGLINIDE	↓ Levels of repaglinide with risk of therapeutic failure	Induction of hepatic metabolism	Monitor capillary blood glucose and warn patients about symptoms of hyperglycemia. ➢ ***For signs and symptoms of hyperglycemia, see Clinical Features of Some Adverse Drug Interactions, Hyperglycemia***
PHENYTOIN	ANTIEMETICS—APREPITANT, ONDANSETRON	↓ Levels of these drugs, with risk of therapeutic failure	Induction of hepatic metabolism	Monitor for ↓ clinical efficacy and ↑ their dose as required
PHENYTOIN	ANTIEPILEPTICS—LAMOTRIGINE, TIAGABINE, TOPIRAMATE, VALPROATE, ZONISAMIDE	↓ Levels of these antiepileptics. Topiramate sometimes ↑ phenytoin levels	Induction of metabolism. Uncertain why phenytoin alters topiramate levels	Watch for poor response to these antiepileptics
PHENYTOIN	ANTIFUNGALS—ITRACONAZOLE, KETOCONAZOLE, POSACONAZOLE, VORICONAZOLE, CASPOFUNGIN	↓ Levels of these drugs, with risk of therapeutic failure	Induction of hepatic metabolism	1. Avoid coadministration of phenytoin with these azoles (consider using fluconazole) 2. ↑ Dose of caspofungin to 70 mg daily
PHENYTOIN	ANTIGOUT DRUGS—ALLOPURINOL, SULFINPYRAZONE	Phenytoin levels may be ↑ in some patients	Uncertain for allopurinol. Possible displacement of phenytoin from its plasma protein-binding sites by sulfinpyrazone; inhibition of phenytoin metabolism by the liver	Monitor phenytoin levels
PHENYTOIN	**ANTIMALARIALS**			
PHENYTOIN	CHLOROQUINE, MEFLOQUINE	↑ Risk of seizures	These drugs lower seizure threshold	Care with coadministration. Watch for ↑ fit frequency; warn patient of this risk when starting these drugs and take suitable precautions. Consider increasing dose of antiepileptic

(*Continued*)

Primary Drug	Secondary Drug	Effect	Mechanism	Precautions
ANTIEPILEPTICS				
PHENYTOIN	PYRIMETHAMINE	1. ↓ Efficacy of phenytoin 2. ↑ Antifolate effect	1. Uncertain 2. Additive effect	1. Care with coadministration; ↑ dose of antiepileptic if ↑ incidence of fits 2. Monitor FBC closely; the effect may take a number of weeks to occur
PHENYTOIN	ANTIMIGRAINE DRUGS—5-HT1 AGONISTS—ALMOTRIPTAN, ELETRIPTAN	↓ Levels of these drugs, with risk of therapeutic failure	Induction of hepatic metabolism	Monitor for ↓ clinical efficacy and ↑ their dose as required
PHENYTOIN	ANTI-PARKINSON'S DRUGS—LEVODOPA	Possibly ↓ levodopa levels	Uncertain	Watch for poor response to levodopa and consider increasing its dose
PHENYTOIN	**ANTIPLATELET AGENTS**			
PHENYTOIN	ASPIRIN	Possible ↑ phenytoin levels	Possibly ↑ unbound phenytoin fraction in the blood	Monitor phenytoin levels when coadministering high-dose aspirin
PHENYTOIN	TICAGRELOR	↓ Ticagrelor levels	Induction of CYP3A4-mediated metabolism of ticagrelor	Manufacturer recommends to avoid coadministration
PHENYTOIN	**ANTIPROTOZOALS**			
PHENYTOIN	LEVAMISOLE	Possible ↑ phenytoin levels	Uncertain; case report of this interaction when levamisole and fluorouracil were coadministered with phenytoin	Monitor phenytoin levels and ↓ phenytoin dose as necessary
PHENYTOIN	MEBENDAZOLE	↓ Levels of these drugs, with risk of therapeutic failure	Induction of hepatic metabolism	Monitor for ↓ clinical efficacy and ↑ their dose as required
PHENYTOIN	**ANTIPSYCHOTICS**			
PHENYTOIN	ANTIPSYCHOTICS	↓ Efficacy of antiepileptics	Antipsychotics lower seizure threshold	Watch for ↑ fit frequency; warn patients of this risk when starting antipsychotics, and take suitable precautions. Consider increasing the dose of antiepileptic
PHENYTOIN	ANTIPSYCHOTICS	↓ Levels of arpiprazole, clozapine, quetiapine, sertindole	Induction of metabolism	Watch for poor response to these antipsychotics, and consider increasing the dose

(*Continued*)

Primary Drug	Secondary Drug	Effect	Mechanism	Precautions
ANTIEPILEPTICS				
PHENYTOIN	**ANTIVIRALS**			
PHENYTOIN	COBICISTAT	1. Possible ↓ plasma levels of cobicistat, risk of treatment failure, and resistance 2. Possible ↓ plasma levels of medicines being boosted, e.g., protease inhibitor, risk of treatment failure, and resistance	Induction of metabolism via CYP3A	Avoid coadministration
PHENYTOIN	DOLUTEGRAVIR	Possible ↓ plasma levels of dolutegravir, risk of treatment failure, and resistance	Induction of UGT1A1 and CYP3A	Avoid coadministration
PHENYTOIN	MARAVIROC	Possible ↓ plasma levels of dolutegravir, risk of treatment failure, and resistance	Induction of UGT1A1 and CYP3A	Avoid coadministration
PHENYTOIN,	NNRTIs—EFAVIRENZ, ETRAVIRINE, RILPIVARINE	1. Possible ↑ or ↓ efficacy of antiepileptic with efavirenz 2. Possible ↓ plasma levels of etravirine and rilpivarine	Altered metabolism via CYP450	Monitor closely. Efavirenz: monitor antiepileptic levels when starting, stopping, or changing treatment, and allow 2 weeks for phenytoin levels to accurately reflect dose changes. Etravirine: combination not recommended. Rilpivirine: avoid coadministration
PHENYTOIN	NRTIs—DIDANOSINE, STAVUDINE, ZIDOVUDINE	Possibly ↑ adverse effects (e.g., peripheral neuropathy) with didanosine, stavudine, and zidovudine	Additive effect	Monitor closely for peripheral neuropathy during prolonged combination
PHENYTOIN	PROTEASE INHIBITORS—INDINAVIR, NELFINAVIR, RITONAVIR WITH OR WITHOUT LOPINAVIR	Possibly ↓ efficacy of phenytoin, with a risk of fits when coadministered with indinavir, nelfinavir, and ritonavir (with or without lopinavir)	Uncertain; ↓ plasma levels of phenytoin	Use with caution. Monitor phenytoin levels weekly. Adjust doses at 7–10-day intervals. Maximum suggested dose adjustment each time is 25 mg
PHENYTOIN	ACICLOVIR/VALACICLOVIR	↓ Efficacy of phenytoin	Unclear	Warn patients and monitor seizure frequency

(Continued)

Primary Drug	Secondary Drug	Effect	Mechanism	Precautions
ANTIEPILEPTICS				
PHENYTOIN	**ANXIOLYTICS AND HYPNOTICS**			
PHENYTOIN	BZDs—CLONAZEPAM	↓ Phenytoin levels	Induction of metabolism	Watch for poor response to phenytoin
PHENYTOIN	ZALEPLON, ZOLPIDEM, ZOPICLONE	↓ Levels of these drugs, with risk of therapeutic failure	Induction of hepatic metabolism	Monitor for ↓ clinical efficacy and ↑ their dose as required
PHENYTOIN	BETA-BLOCKERS—PROPANOLOL	↓ Levels of propanolol with risk of therapeutic failure	Induction of hepatic metabolism	Monitor PR and BP weekly until stable, and watch for ↑ BP
PHENYTOIN	BRONCHODILATORS—THEOPHYLLINE	1. ↓ Levels of theophylline with risk of therapeutic failure 2. Phenytoin levels may be ↓ by theophylline	1. Induction of hepatic metabolism 2. Uncertain; theophylline ↓ absorption of phenytoin	1. Monitor for ↓ clinical efficacy and ↑ their dose as required. May need to ↑ dose of theophylline by 25% 2. Monitor phenytoin levels when coadministered with theophylline
PHENYTOIN	CALCIUM SALTS; OR ENTERAL FEEDING PRODUCTS (TUBE FEEDING)	↓ Phenytoin levels	↓ Absorption	Separate administration of phenytoin and enteral feeding products by at least 2 h
PHENYTOIN	CALCIUM CHANNEL BLOCKERS	1. Phenytoin levels are ↑ by diltiazem and possibly nifedipine and isradipine 2. ↓ Plasma concentrations of diltiazem, felodipine, nisoldipine, verapamil, and possibly nimodipine	1. Postulated to be due to inhibition of CYP3A4-mediated metabolism of phenytoin. Diltiazem is also known to inhibit intestinal Pgp, which may ↑ the bioavailability of phenytoin 2. Phenytoin induces CYP3A4, which metabolizes calcium channel blockers	1. Monitor phenytoin levels when initiating calcium channel blockers, particularly diltiazem and verapamil 2. Monitor PR and BP closely; watch for ↑ BP when starting phenytoin in patients already on calcium channel blockers
PHENYTOIN	CARDIAC GLYCOSIDES—DIGITOXIN, DIGOXIN	↓ Levels of these drugs, with risk of therapeutic failure	Induction of hepatic metabolism	Monitor PR and BP weekly until stable, and watch for ↑ BP
PHENYTOIN	CNS STIMULANTS—MODAFINIL	May ↓ modafinil levels	Induction of CYP3A4, which has a partial role in the metabolism of modafinil	Be aware
PHENYTOIN	**DIURETICS**			
PHENYTOIN	CARBONIC ANHYDRASE INHIBITORS	Risk of osteomalacia	Phenytoin is associated with a small risk of causing osteomalacia; this may be ↑ by acetazolamide-induced urinary excretion of calcium	Be aware

(*Continued*)

Primary Drug	Secondary Drug	Effect	Mechanism	Precautions
ANTIEPILEPTICS				
PHENYTOIN	LOOP DIURETICS—FUROSEMIDE	↓ Efficacy of furosemide	Uncertain	Be aware; watch for poor response to furosemide
PHENYTOIN	DRUG DEPENDENCE THERAPIES—DISULFIRAM	↑ Phenytoin levels	Inhibited metabolism	Monitor phenytoin levels closely
PHENYTOIN	FOLIC ACID	↓ Phenytoin levels	Uncertain; postulated that induction of CYP enzymes by these antiepileptics depletes folate reserves. Replacement of these reserves ↑ formation of CYP further, which ↑ metabolism of the antiepileptics	Watch for poor response to phenytoin and ↑ dose as necessary
PHENYTOIN	GESTRINONE	↓ Levels of gestrinone with risk of therapeutic failure	Induction of hepatic metabolism	Monitor for ↓ clinical efficacy and ↑ their dose as required
PHENYTOIN	H2 RECEPTOR BLOCKERS—CIMETIDINE, FAMOTIDINE, RANITIDINE	↑ Plasma concentrations of phenytoin, risk of adverse effects, including phenytoin toxicity, bone marrow depression, and skin reactions	Inhibition of phenytoin metabolism via CYP2C9 and CYP2C19	Avoid cimetidine and phenytoin, if there is no alternative. Use low-dose cimetidine <1.2 g/day regularly and monitor phenytoin levels closely. Famotidine or rantidine: monitor phenytoin levels more regularly when treatment is initiated. Nizatidine appears not to interact with antiepileptics
PHENYTOIN	IVACAFTOR	↓ Ivacaftor levels	Induction of CYP3A4-mediated metabolism of ivacaftor	Manufacturers advice against coadministration
PHENYTOIN	IVABRADINE	↓ Levels of ivabradine	Increased CYP3A4-mediated metabolism of ivabradine	Monitor for reduced efficacy of ivabradine
PHENYTOIN	**LIPID-LOWERING DRUGS**			
PHENYTOIN	COLESEVELAM	↓ Absorption of oral phenytoin	Possibly due to bonding	Administer phenytoin 4 h prior to colesevelam. Measure phenytoin concentrations and adjust the dose as required. Seizure diary is important
PHENYTOIN	STATINS	Reports of ↓ levels of atorvastatin and simvastatin	Induction of CYP3A4	Monitor lipid profile closely. If lipids increase, consider alternate statin

(*Continued*)

Primary Drug	Secondary Drug	Effect	Mechanism	Precautions
ANTIEPILEPTICS				
PHENYTOIN	MIFEPRISTONE	Theoretical risk of ↓ levels of mifepristone	Induction of CYP3A4-mediated metabolism of mifepristone	Watch for poor response to mifepristone
PHENYTOIN	MUSCLE RELAXANTS	Resistance to neuromuscular blocking action may occur in patients who are taking regular carbamazepine or phenytoin. This results in a shorter duration of neuromuscular blockade	Unknown	Infusion rates of nondepolarizing muscle relaxants may need to be increased
PHENYTOIN	NITISINONE	Possible ↓ nitisinone levels	Induction of CYP3A4-mediated metabolism	Avoid coadministration
PHENYTOIN	ESTROGENS	↓ Levels of these drugs, with risk of therapeutic failure	Induction of hepatic metabolism	Advise patients to use additional contraception for period of intake and for 1 month after stopping coadministration with these drugs
PHENYTOIN	PERIPHERAL VASODILATORS—CILOSTAZOL	Theoretical risk of ↓ cilostazol levels	Induction of CYP3A4 by these antiepileptics	Monitor for evidence of poor response to cilostazol
PHENYTOIN	PROGESTOGENS	↓ Levels of these drugs, with risk of therapeutic failure	Induction of hepatic metabolism	Advise patients to use additional contraception for period of intake and for 1 month after stopping coadministration with these drugs
PHENYTOIN	PROTON PUMP INHIBITORS—OMEPRAZOLE	Possible ↑ efficacy and adverse effects of phenytoin	Unclear; possible altered metabolism via CYP2C19	↓ Dose may be required. Use the proton pump inhibitor regularly, not PRN; monitor phenytoin levels when starting or stopping treatment. Patients have received omeprazole for 3 weeks without altered phenytoin levels. Effect not reported with pantoprazole or rabeprazole
PHENYTOIN	RANOLAZINE	↓ RANOLAZINE levels	Induction of CYP3A4-mediated metabolism of RANOLAZINE	Manufacturer advises to avoid coadministration
PHENYTOIN	ROFLUMILAST	↓ Efficacy of roflumilast	Induction of CYP3A4- and 1A2-mediated metabolism of roflumilast and its active metabolite	Monitor for poor response and increase dose as necessary

(*Continued*)

Primary Drug	Secondary Drug	Effect	Mechanism	Precautions
ANTIEPILEPTICS				
PHENYTOIN	SUCRALFATE	↓ Phenytoin levels	↓ Absorption of phenytoin	Give phenytoin at least 2 h after sucralfate
PHENYTOIN	SYMPATHOMIMETICS—DOPAMINE	Reports of severe hypotension when parenteral phenytoin is given to patients on dopamine	Uncertain; possibly additive effect (phenytoin can cause hypotension especially if given rapidly)	Use phenytoin with extreme caution; if needed, infuse it slowly
PHENYTOIN	TIBOLONE	↓ Tibolone levels	Induction of metabolism of tibolone	Watch for poor response to tibolone; consider ↑ its dose
PHENYTOIN	VASODILATOR ANTIHYPERTENSIVES	Coadministration of diazoxide and phenytoin ↓ phenytoin levels and possibly ↓ efficacy of diazoxide	Uncertain at present	Monitor phenytoin levels and BP closely
PHENYTOIN	VITAMIN B6	↓ Phenytoin levels	Uncertain	Watch for poor response to phenytoin if large doses of vitamin B6 are given
PHENYTOIN	VITAMIN D	↓ Efficacy of vitamin D	Uncertain	Be aware; consider increasing dose of vitamin D
TOPIRAMATE				
TOPIRAMATE	ALCOHOL	↑ Sedation	Additive sedative effect	Warn patients about this effect
TOPIRAMATE	ANTICANCER AND IMMUNOMODULATING DRUGS—IMATINIB	↑ Plasma concentrations, with risk of toxic effects of topiramate	Imatinib is a potent inhibitor of CYP2C9	Watch for the early toxic effects of topiramate. If necessary, consider using alternative drugs while the patient is being given imatinib
TOPIRAMATE	ANTIDEPRESSANTS—MAOIs, SSRIs, TCAs	↑ Risk of seizures	These drugs lower seizure threshold	Care with coadministration. Watch for ↑ fit frequency; warn patient of this risk when starting these drugs and take suitable precautions. Consider increasing dose of antiepileptic
TOPIRAMATE	ANTIDIABETIC DRUGS—METFORMIN	↑ Metformin levels	Unknown mechanism	Watch for and warn patients about hypoglycemia. ➢ ***For signs and symptoms of hypoglycemia, see Clinical Features of Some Adverse Drug Interactions, Hypoglycemia***

(*Continued*)

Primary Drug	Secondary Drug	Effect	Mechanism	Precautions
ANTIEPILEPTICS				
TOPIRAMATE	**ANTIEPILEPTICS**			
TOPIRAMATE	CARBAMAZEPINE, OXCARBAZEPINE	↓ Topiramate levels	Induction of metabolism of topiramate	Watch for poor response to these antiepileptics Watch for features of topiramate toxicity if coadministered carbamazepine or oxcarbazapine is discontinued
TOPIRAMATE	PHENYTOIN	Slight ↑ phenytoin levels and ↓ topiramate levels	Phenytoin induces metabolism of topiramate. Uncertain how topiramate affects phenytoin	Monitor phenytoin levels when topiramate is started or discontinued
TOPIRAMATE	ANTIMALARIALS—CHLOROQUINE, MEFLOQUINE	↑ Risk of seizures	These drugs lower seizure threshold	Care with coadministration. Watch for ↑ fit frequency; warn patient of this risk when starting these drugs and take suitable precautions. Consider increasing dose of antiepileptic
TOPIRAMATE	ANTIPSYCHOTICS	↑ Risk of seizures	These drugs lower seizure threshold	Care with coadministration. Watch for ↑ fit frequency; warn patient of this risk when starting these drugs and take suitable precautions. Consider increasing dose of antiepileptic
TOPIRAMATE	CARDIAC GLYCOSIDES—DIGOXIN	Small decrease in peak plasma levels of digoxin	Oral clearance of digoxin was slightly increased	Watch for a decreased response to digoxin therapy. Increase digoxin therapy if symptoms and signs of cardiac failure or arrhythmia persist
TOPIRAMATE	ESTROGENS	Marked ↓ contraceptive effect	Induction of metabolism of estrogens	Advise patients to use additional contraception for period of intake and for 1 month after stopping coadministration with topiramate
TOPIRAMATE	PROGESTOGENS	↓ Progesterone levels, which may lead to failure of contraception or poor response to treatment of menorrhagia	Possibly induction of metabolism of progestogens	Advise patients to use additional contraception for period of intake and for 1 month after stopping coadministration with topiramate

(Continued)

Primary Drug	Secondary Drug	Effect	Mechanism	Precautions
ANTIEPILEPTICS				
VALPROATE				
VALPROATE	**ANTIBIOTICS**			
VALPROATE	ERTAPENEM, MEROPENEM	↓ Valproate levels	Induced metabolism	Monitor levels
VALPROATE	ERYTHROMYCIN	↑ Valproate levels	Inhibited metabolism	Monitor levels
VALPROATE	**ANTICANCER AND IMMUNOMODULATING DRUGS**			
VALPROATE	DABRAFENIB	Possible reduced levels of CYP3A4/CYP2Cs/CYP2B6 substrates. Level of reduction may vary	Dabrafenib induces CYP3A4/CYP2Cs/CYP2B6	Monitor closely or avoid concurrent use
VALPROATE	PLATINUM COMPOUNDS	↓ Plasma concentrations of antiepileptic, which ↑ risk of seizures	Impaired absorption of valproate	Monitor for seizure activity closely, and warn patients and carers. Monitor valproate levels
VALPROATE	PROCARBAZINE	↑ Risk of hypersensitivity reactions in patients with brain tumors	Strong correlation between therapeutic antiepileptic level and hypersensitivity reactions	Consider using nonenzyme-inducing agents
VALPROATE	TEMOZOLOMIDE	Increased temozolomide levels	Unknown	Oral clearance reduced by 5%—significance unclear. Be aware
VALPROATE	**ANTIDEPRESSANTS**			
VALPROATE	MAOIs, SSRIs	↑ Risk of seizures	These drugs lower seizure threshold	Care with coadministration. Watch for ↑ fit frequency; warn patient of this risk when starting these drugs and take suitable precautions. Consider increasing dose of antiepileptic
VALPROATE	TCAs	1. ↑ Risk of seizures 2. ↑ Amitriptyline and nortriptyline levels	1. These drugs lower seizure threshold 2. Uncertain	1. Care with coadministration. Watch for ↑ fit frequency; warn patient of this risk when starting these drugs and take suitable precautions. Consider increasing dose of antiepileptic 2. Be aware; watch for clinical features of ↑ levels of these TCAs (e.g., sedation, dry mouth, etc.)

(*Continued*)

Primary Drug	Secondary Drug	Effect	Mechanism	Precautions
ANTIEPILEPTICS				
VALPROATE	ANTIDIABETIC DRUGS—ACARBOSE	Case of ↓ valproate levels	Uncertain	Monitor valproate levels
VALPROATE	**ANTIEPILEPTICS**			
VALPROATE	1. BARBITURATES—PHENOBARBITAL, PRIMIDONE 2. ?ETHOSUXIMIDE 3. LAMOTRIGINE	↑ Levels of these antiepileptics	Uncertain	Watch for early features of toxicity. Measure levels where possible
VALPROATE	PHENYTOIN	Variable effect on phenytoin levels	Uncertain	Be aware and monitor levels. Watch for early features of phenytoin toxicity
VALPROATE	ANTIMALARIALS—CHLOROQUINE, MEFLOQUINE	↑ Risk of seizures	These drugs lower seizure threshold	Care with coadministration. Watch for ↑ fit frequency; warn patient of this risk when starting these drugs and take suitable precautions. Consider increasing dose of antiepileptic
VALPROATE	ANTIPSYCHOTICS	↑ Risk of seizures	These drugs lower seizure threshold	Care with coadministration. Watch for ↑ fit frequency; warn patient of this risk when starting these drugs and take suitable precautions. Consider increasing dose of antiepileptic
VALPROATE	ANTIPLATELET AGENTS—ASPIRIN	Possible ↑ levels of valproate	Possibly ↑ unbound valproate fraction in the blood	Monitor or valproate levels when coadministering high-dose aspirin
VALPROATE	ANTIPSYCHOTICS—OLANZAPINE	Risk of bone marrow toxicity	Additive effect	Monitor FBC closely; warn patients to report sore throat, fever, etc.
VALPROATE	**ANTIVIRALS**			
VALPROATE	LOPINAVIR/RITONAVIR, RITONAVIR	1. Possible ↓ plasma levels of valproate 2. Possibly ↑ plasma levels of lopinavir	1. Increased glucuronidation of valproate 2. Uncertain	Use with caution, monitor more closely

(Continued)

DRUGS ACTING ON THE CENTRAL NERVOUS SYSTEM ANTIEPILEPTICS Zonisamide

Primary Drug	Secondary Drug	Effect	Mechanism	Precautions
ANTIEPILEPTICS				
VALPROATE	ZIDOVUDINE	↑ Zidovudine levels	Inhibition of metabolism	Watch for early features of toxicity of zidovudine
VALPROATE	CALCIUM CHANNEL BLOCKERS	Nimodipine levels may be ↑ by valproate	Uncertain at present	Monitor BP at least weekly until stable. Warn patients to report symptoms of hypotension (light-headedness, dizziness on standing, etc.)
VALPROATE	SODIUM PHENYLBUTYRATE	Possibly ↓ efficacy of sodium phenylbutyrate	These drugs are associated with ↑ ammonia levels	Avoid coadministration
VIGABATRIN				
VIGABATRIN	ANTIDEPRESSANTS—MAOIs, SSRIs, TCAs	↑ Risk of seizures	These drugs lower seizure threshold	Care with coadministration. Watch for ↑ fit frequency; warn patient of this risk when starting these drugs and take suitable precautions. Consider increasing dose of antiepileptic
VIGABATRIN	PHENYTOIN	Modest reduction in phenytoin levels may occur	Uncertain	Be aware
ZONISAMIDE				
ZONISAMIDE	ANTIEPILEPTICS—BARBITURATES, CARBAMAZEPINE, PHENYTOIN	↓ Levels of zonisamide likely	Induction of metabolism	Watch for poor response to zonisamide
ZONISAMIDE	CARBONIC ANHDRASE INHIBITORS—TOPIRAMATE, ACETAZOLAMIDE OR DICHLORPHENAMIDE	May increase the severity of metabolic acidosis and may also increase the risk of kidney stone formation	Additive effect of carbonic anhydrase enzyme inhibition	If zonisamide is given concomitantly with another carbonic anhydrase inhibitor, the patient should be monitored for the appearance or worsening of metabolic acidosis
ZONISAMIDE	Pgp SUBSTRATES—DIGOXIN, QUINIDINE	Theoretical potential for zonisamide to affect the pharmacokinetics of drugs which are Pgp substrates	Zonisamide is a weak inhibitor of Pgp (MDR1)	Caution is advised when starting or stopping zonisamide or changing the zonisamide dose in patients who are also receiving drugs which are Pgp substrates

Primary Drug	Secondary Drug	Effect	Mechanism	Precautions
ANTIMIGRAINE DRUGS				
ERGOT DERIVATIVES (INCLUDING METHYSERGIDE)				
ERGOT DERIVATIVES	ANESTHETICS—GENERAL—HALOTHANE	↓ Efficacy of ergometrine on the uterus	Uncertain	Use alternative form of anesthesia for surgery requiring use of ergotamine
ERGOT DERIVATIVES	**ANTIBIOTICS**			
ERGOT DERIVATIVES	MACROLIDES, QUINUPRISTIN/DALFOPRISTIN	↑ Ergotamine/methysergide levels with risk of toxicity	Inhibition of CYP3A4-mediated metabolism of the ergot derivatives	Avoid coadministration
ERGOT DERIVATIVES	TETRACYCLINES	Cases of ergotism with tetracyclines and ergotamine	Uncertain	Avoid coadministration. If absolutely necessary, advise patients to discontinue treatment immediately if numbness and tingling of the extremities are felt
ERGOTAMINE, DIHYDROERGOTAMINE	ANTICANCER AND IMMUNOMODULATING DRUGS—DASATINIB	Increased levels of these ergot alkaloids	CYP3A4 inhibition	Caution with CYP3A4 substrates with narrow therapeutic window
ERGOT DERIVATIVES	ANTIDEPRESSANTS—REBOXETINE	Risk of hypertension	Additive effect	Monitor BP closely
ERGOT DERIVATIVES	ANTIFUNGALS—VORICONAZOLE	↑ Ergotamine/methysergide levels with risk of toxicity	Inhibition of metabolism of the ergot derivatives	Avoid coadministration. If absolutely necessary, advise patients to discontinue treatment immediately if numbness and tingling of the extremities are felt
ERGOT ALKALOIDS—DIHYDROERGOTAMINE, ERGOTAMINE, ERGOMETRINE	COBICISTAT	↑ Plasma levels	Inhibition of metabolism via CYP3A	Avoid coadministration

(*Continued*)

Primary Drug	Secondary Drug	Effect	Mechanism	Precautions
ANTIMIGRAINE DRUGS				
ERGOTAMINE, METHYSERGIDE	ANTIMIGRAINE DRUGS—5-HT1 AGONISTS—TRIPTANS	↑ Risk of vasospasm: increased blood pressure, tachyarrhythmias, and abnormal ECG (PR & QTc prolongation, atrial flutter or fibrillation) and syncope	Additive effect	1. Do not administer ergotamine and almotriptan, rizatriptan, sumatriptan, or zolmitriptan within 6 h of each other 2. Do not administer methysergide and almotriptan, rizatriptan, sumatriptan, or zolmitriptan within 24 h of each other 3. Do not administer an ergot derivative and eletriptan or frovatriptan within 24 h of each other
DIHYDROERGOTAMINE	ANTIOBESITY DRUGS—SIBUTRAMINE	Risk of serotonin syndrome	Additive effect	Manufacturer advises against coadministration
ERGOT DERIVATIVES	**ANTIVIRALS**			
ERGOT DERIVATIVES	NNRTIs—EFAVIRENZ	↑ Ergotamine/methysergide levels, with risk of toxicity	↓ CYP3A4-mediated metabolism of ergot derivatives	Manufacturer contraindicates use within 24 h of an ergot alkaloid or methysergide and within 48 h of the CYP3A4 inhibitors
ERGOT DERIVATIVES	PROTEASE INHIBITORS	↑ Ergotamine/methysergide levels with risk of toxicity	↓ CYP3A4-mediated metabolism of ergot derivatives	Manufacturer contraindicates use within 24 h of an ergot alkaloid or methysergide and within 48 h of the CYP3A4 inhibitors
ERGOT DERIVATIVES	BETA-BLOCKERS	Three cases of arterial vasoconstriction and one of ↑ BP occurred when ergotamine or methysergide was added to propanolol or oxprenolol	Ergotamine can cause peripheral vasospasm, and absence of beta-adrenergic activity can ↑ risk of vasoconstriction	Ergot derivatives and beta-blockers are often coadministered without trouble; however, monitor BP at least weekly until stable (watch for ↑ BP) and warn patients to stop the ergot derivative and seek medical attention if they develop cold, painful feet
ERGOTAMINE	GRAPEFRUIT JUICE	Possibly ↑ efficacy and ↑ adverse effects, e.g., vasospasm, ergotism, peripheral vasoconstriction, gangrene	Possibly ↑ bioavailability by ↓ presystemic metabolism. Constituents of grapefruit juice irreversibly inhibit intestinal cytochrome CYP3A4	Monitor for ↑ side effects and stop intake of grapefruit preparations if side effects occur

(*Continued*)

Primary Drug	Secondary Drug	Effect	Mechanism	Precautions
ANTIMIGRAINE DRUGS				
ERGOT DERIVATIVES	H2 RECEPTOR BLOCKERS—CIMETIDINE	↑ Ergotamine/methysergide levels with risk of toxicity	Inhibition of metabolism via CYP3A4	Avoid coadministration
ERGOT DERIVATIVES	**SYMPATHOMIMETICS**			
ERGOT DERIVATIVES	SYMPATHOMIMETICS	Risk of ergot toxicity when ergotamine is coadministered with sympathomimetics. Case report of gangrene when dopamine was given to a patient on ergotamine	Thought to be due to additive vasoconstriction	Watch for early features of ergotamine toxicity (vertigo and gastrointestinal disturbance). Titrate dopamine carefully
5-HT1 AGONISTS—TRIPTANS				
TRIPTANS	**ANTIBIOTICS**			
ALMOTRIPTAN, ELETRIPTAN	MACROLIDES—CLARITHROMYCIN, ERYTHROMYCIN, TELITHROMYCIN	↑ Plasma concentrations of almotriptan and eletriptan, with risk of toxic effects, e.g., flushing, sensations of tingling, heat, heaviness, pressure, or tightness of any part of body including the throat and chest, dizziness	Almotriptan is metabolized mainly by CYP3A4 isoenzymes. Most CYP isoenzymes are inhibited by clarithromycin to varying degrees, and since there is an alternative pathway of metabolism by MAO-A, toxicity responses will vary between individuals	Avoid coadministration—do not use a triptan for at least 72 h after stopping a CYP3A4 inhibitor
ALMOTRIPTAN	RIFAMPICIN	Possible ↓ plasma concentrations of almotriptan, with risk of inadequate therapeutic efficacy	One of the major metabolizing enzymes of almotriptan—CYP3A4 isoenzymes—are induced by rifampicin. As there are alternative metabolic pathways, the effect may not be significant and can vary from individual to individual	Be aware of the possibility of ↓ response to triptan to be due to interaction
ZOLMITRIPTAN	QUINOLONES	Possible ↓ plasma concentrations of zolmitriptan, with risk of inadequate therapeutic efficacy	Possibly induced metabolism of zolmitriptan	Be aware of possibility of ↓ response to triptan to be due to interaction

(Continued)

Primary Drug	Secondary Drug	Effect	Mechanism	Precautions
ANTIMIGRAINE DRUGS				
ALMOTRIPTAN, ELETRIPTAN	**ANTICANCER AND IMMUNOMODULATING DRUGS**			
ALMOTRIPTAN, ELETRIPTAN	CYTOTOXICS—IMATINIB	↑ Plasma concentrations of almotriptan and risk of toxic effects of almotriptan, e.g., flushing, sensations of tingling, heat, heaviness, pressure, or tightness of any part of body including the throat and chest, dizziness	Almotriptan is metabolized mainly by CYP3A4 isoenzymes. Most CYP isoenzymes are inhibited by imatinib mesylate to varying degrees, and since there is an alternative pathway of metabolism by MAO-A, toxicity responses will vary between individuals sumitriptan is mainly metabolized by MAO	The CSM has advised, particularly for sumatriptan, that if chest tightness or pressure is intense, the triptan should be discontinued immediately and the patient is investigated for ischemic heart disease by measuring cardiac enzymes and doing an ECG. Avoid concomitant use in patients with coronary artery disease and in those with severe or uncontrolled hypertension
ALMOTRIPTAN, ELETRIPTAN	IMMUNOMODULATING DRUGS—CORTICOSTEROIDS—DEXAMETHASONE	Possible ↓ plasma concentrations of almotriptan and risk of inadequate therapeutic efficacy	One of the major metabolizing enzymes of almotriptan—CYP3A4 isoenzymes—are induced by corticosteroids. As there are alternative metabolic pathways, the effect may not be significant and can vary from individual to individual	Be aware of possibility of ↓ response to triptan, and consider ↑ dose if considered to be due to interaction
TRIPTANS	**ANTIDEPRESSANTS**			
TRIPTANS	SSRIs	↑ Risk of serotonin syndrome. ➢ ***For signs and symptoms of serotonin toxicity, see Clinical Features of Some Adverse Drug Interactions, Serotonin Toxicity and Serotonin Syndrome*** A few cases of dyskinesias have been reported with fluoxetine	Triptans cause direct stimulation of 5-HT receptors, while SSRIs ↓ uptake of 5-HT, thus leading to ↑ serotonergic activity in the brain	The U.S. FDA (July 2006) issued a warning of the possibility of this life-threatening serotonin syndrome when SSRIs are used together with triptans. Advise patients to report immediately the onset of symptoms such as tremors, agitation, confusion, ↑ heart beat (palpitations) and fever, and either ↓ dose or discontinue the SSRI

(*Continued*)

Primary Drug	Secondary Drug	Effect	Mechanism	Precautions
ANTIMIGRAINE DRUGS				
TRIPTANS	**MAOIs**			
RIZATRIPTAN, SUMATRIPTAN	MAOIs	↑ Plasma concentrations of rizatriptan and sumatriptan, with risk of toxic effects, e.g., flushing, sensations of tingling, heat, heaviness, pressure, or tightness of any part of body including the throat and chest, dizziness	These triptans are metabolized primarily by MAOI-A	Avoid starting these triptans for at least 2 weeks after stopping MAOIs; conversely, avoid starting MAOIs for at least 2 weeks after stopping these triptans
ZOLMITRIPTAN	MOCLOBEMIDE	Risk of agitation and confusion when zolmitriptan is coadministered with moclobemide	Uncertain	Watch for these effects and consider reducing the dose of zolmitriptan
TRIPTANS	DULOXETINE	Possible ↑ risk of serotonin syndrome. ➢ ***For signs and symptoms of serotonin toxicity, see Clinical Features of Some Adverse Drug Interactions, Serotonin Toxicity and Serotonin Syndrome***	Triptans cause direct stimulation of 5-HT receptors, while SSRIs ↓ uptake of 5-HT, thus leading to ↑ serotonergic activity in the brain	The U.S. FDA (July 2006) issued a warning of the possibility of this life-threatening serotonin syndrome when SSRIs are used together with triptans (5-HT receptor agonists). Avoid concomitant use or ↓ dose of the SSRI
TRIPTANS	ST. JOHN'S WORT	↑ Risk of serotonin syndrome. ➢ ***For signs and symptoms of serotonin toxicity, see Clinical Features of Some Adverse Drug Interactions, Serotonin Toxicity and Serotonin Syndrome***	Possibly additive effect	Avoid coadministration
TRIPTANS	**ANTIEPILEPTICS**			
ALMOTRIPTAN, ELETRIPTAN	CARBAMAZEPINE	Risk of serotonin syndrome with almotriptan and eletriptan	Additive effect—both triptans and carbamazepine stimulate 5-HT receptors, and carbamazepine also prevents reuptake of 5-HT	Be aware of the possibility of the occurrence of serotonin syndrome with 5-HT1 agonists

(*Continued*)

Primary Drug	Secondary Drug	Effect	Mechanism	Precautions
ANTIMIGRAINE DRUGS				
ALMOTRIPTAN, ELETRIPTAN	PHENOBARBITAL	Possible ↓ plasma concentrations of almotriptan and risk of inadequate therapeutic efficacy	One of the major metabolizing enzymes of almotriptan—CYP3A4 isoenzymes—is induced by azoles. As there are alternative metabolic pathways, the effect may not be significant and can vary from individual to individual	Be aware of possibility of ↓ response to triptan, and consider↑ dose if considered to be due to interaction
ALMOTRIPTAN, ELETRIPTAN	PHENYTOIN	↓ Levels of amlotriptan and eletriptan, with risk of therapeutic failure	Induction of hepatic metabolism	Monitor for ↓ clinical efficacy and ↑ their dose as required
TRIPTANS	ANTIFUNGALS—AZOLES	↑ Plasma concentrations of almotriptan and eletriptan, with risk of toxic effects, e.g., flushing, sensations of tingling, heat, heaviness, pressure, or tightness of any part of body including the throat and chest, dizziness	Almotriptan is metabolized mainly by CYP3A4 isoenzymes. Most CYP isoenzymes are inhibited by clarithromycin to varying degrees, and since there is an alternative pathway of metabolism by MAO-A, toxicity responses will vary between individuals	Manufacturer contraindicates use within 24 h of an ergot alkaloid or methysergide and within 48 h of the CYP3A4 inhibitors. Recommended that eletriptan should not be used for 72 h after use of a CYP3A4 inhibitor
TRIPTANS	ANTIMIGRAINE DRUGS—ERGOTAMINE, METHYSERGIDE	↑ Risk of vasospasm: increased blood pressure, tachyarrhythmias, and abnormal ECG (PR & QTc prolongation, atrial flutter or fibrillation) and syncope	Additive effect	1. Do not administer ergotamine and almotriptan, rizatriptan, sumatriptan, or zolmitriptan within 6 h of each other 2. Do not administer methysergide and almotriptan, rizatriptan, sumatriptan, or zolmitriptan within 24 h of each other 3. Do not administer an ergot derivative and eletriptan or frovatriptan within 24 h of each other
TRIPTANS	ANTIOBESITY DRUGS—LORCASERIN	Risk of serotonin syndrome	Additive effect	Be aware of the possibility of serotonin syndrome. ➢ ***For signs and symptoms of serotonin toxicity, see Clinical Features of Some Adverse Drug Interactions, Serotonin Toxicity and Serotonin Syndrome***

(*Continued*)

Primary Drug	Secondary Drug	Effect	Mechanism	Precautions
ANTIMIGRAINE DRUGS				
ALMOTRIPTAN, ELETRIPTAN	NONNUCLEOSIDE REVERSE TRANSCRIPTASE INHIBITORS—EFAVIRENZ	↑ Plasma concentrations of almotriptan and eletriptan, and risk of toxic effects, e.g., flushing, sensations of tingling, heat, heaviness, pressure, or tightness of any part of body including the throat and chest, dizziness	Almotriptan and eletriptan are metabolized by CYP3A4 isoenzymes, which may be inhibited by efavirenz. However, since there is an alternative pathway of metabolism by MAOA, the toxicity responses will vary between individuals	Manufacturer contraindicates use within 48 h of the CYP3A4 inhibitors. Recommended that eletriptan should not be used for 72 h after use of a CYP3A4 inhibitor
ALMOTRIPTAN, ELETRIPTAN	PROTEASE INHIBITORS—INDINAVIR, NELFINAVIR, RITONAVIR	Possibly ↑ adverse effects when almotriptan or eletriptan is coadministered with indinavir, ritonavir (with or without lopinavir), or nelfinavir	Inhibition of CYP3A4- and possibly CYP2D6-mediated metabolism of eletriptan, and CYP3A4-mediated metabolism of almotriptan	Manufacturer contraindicates use within 24 h of an ergot alkaloid or methysergide and within 48 h of the CYP3A4 inhibitors. Recommended that eletriptan should not be used for 72 h after use of a CYP3A4 inhibitor
RIZATRIPTAN	BETA-BLOCKERS—PROPRANOLOL	Plasma levels of rizatriptan almost doubled during propranolol therapy	Propanolol inhibits the metabolism of rizatriptan	Initiate therapy with 5 mg rizatriptan and do not exceed 10 mg in 24 h. The manufacturers recommend separating doses by 2 h, although this has not been proved by studies
ALMOTRIPTAN, ELETRIPTAN	CALCIUM CHANNEL BLOCKERS—DILTIAZEM, NIFEDIPINE, VERAPAMIL	↑ Plasma concentrations of almotriptan and risk of toxic effects of almotriptan, e.g., flushing, sensations of tingling, heat, heaviness, pressure, or tightness of any part of body including the throat and chest, dizziness	Almotriptan is metabolized mainly by CYP3A4 isoenzymes. Most CYP isoenzymes are inhibited by diltiazem to varying degrees, and since there is an alternative pathway of metabolism by MAO-A, toxicity responses vary between individuals	The CSM has advised that if chest tightness or pressure is intense, the triptan should be discontinued immediately and the patient is investigated for ischemic heart disease by measuring cardiac enzymes and doing an ECG. Avoid concomitant use in patients with coronary artery disease and in those with severe or uncontrolled hypertension
ZOLMITRIPTAN	CNS STIMULANTS—MODAFINIL	May cause ↓ zolmitriptan levels if CYP1A2 is the predominant metabolic pathway and alternative metabolic pathways are either genetically deficient or affected	Modafinil is a moderate inducer of CYP1A2 in a concentration-dependent manner	Be aware

(*Continued*)

DRUGS ACTING ON THE CENTRAL NERVOUS SYSTEM ANTIMIGRAINE DRUGS

Primary Drug	Secondary Drug	Effect	Mechanism	Precautions
ANTIMIGRAINE DRUGS				
TRIPTANS	ERGOT ALKALOIDS—ERGOTAMINE, METHYSERGIDE	↑ Risk of vasospasm	Additive effect	1. Do not administer ergotamine and almotriptan, rizatriptan, sumatriptan, or zolmitriptan within 6 h of each other 2. Do not administer methy-sergide and almotriptan, rizatriptan, sumatriptan, or zolmitriptan within 24 h of each other 3. Do not administer an ergot derivative and eletriptan or frovatriptan within 24 h of each other
ALMOTRIPTAN, ELETRIPTAN	GRAPEFRUIT JUICE	↑ Plasma concentrations of almotriptan and eletriptan, with risk of toxic effects, e.g., flushing, sensations of tingling, heat, heaviness, pressure, or tightness of any part of body including the throat and chest, dizziness	Almotriptan and eletriptan are metabolized mainly by CYP3A4 isoenzymes. Most CYP isoenzymes are inhibited by grapefruit juice to varying degrees, and since there is an alternative pathway of metabolism by MAO-A, toxicity responses will vary between individuals	The CSM has advised that if chest tightness or pressure is intense, the triptan should be discontinued immediately and the patient is investigated for ischemic heart disease by measuring cardiac enzymes and doing an ECG. Avoid concomitant use in patients with coronary artery disease and in those with severe or uncontrolled hypertension
ALMOTRIPTAN, ELETRIPTAN, ZOLMITRIPTAN	H2-RECEPTOR BLOCKERS—CIMETIDINE	↑ Efficacy and adverse effects of zolmitriptan, e.g., flushing, sensations of tingling, heat, heaviness, pressure, or tightness of any part of body including the throat and chest, dizziness	Inhibition of metabolism via CYP1A2	Consider alternative acid suppression, e.g., H2 antagonist or proton pump inhibitors (not omeprazole or lansoprazole), or monitor more closely and ↓ maximum dose of zolmitriptan to 5 mg/24 h
PIZOTIFEN				
PIZOTIFEN	ADRENERGIC NEURONE BLOCKERS	↓ Hypotensive effect	Pizotifen competes with adrenergic neuron blockers for reuptake to nerve terminals	Monitor BP at least weekly until stable

Primary Drug	Secondary Drug	Effect	Mechanism	Precautions
ANTIOBESITY DRUGS				
DIETHYLPROPION—*see Sympatheticomimetics—Indirect—CVS Section*				
LORCASERIN				
LORCASERIN	ANALGESICS—DEXTROMETHORPHAN, TRAMADOL	Risk of serotonin syndrome	Additive effect	Be aware of the possibility of serotonin syndrome. ➢ ***For signs and symptoms of serotonin toxicity, see Clinical Features of Some Adverse Drug Interactions, Serotonin Toxicity and Serotonin Syndrome***
LORCASERIN	ANTIARRHYTHMICS—FLECAINIDE	↑ Blood concentrations of flecainide	Inhibition of CYP2D6-mediated metabolism	Monitor PR, BP, and ECG closely until stable
LORCASERIN	ANTIBIOTICS—LINEZOLID	Risk of serotonin syndrome	Additive effect	Be aware of the possibility of serotonin syndrome. ➢ ***For signs and symptoms of serotonin toxicity, see Clinical Features of Some Adverse Drug Interactions, Serotonin Toxicity and Serotonin Syndrome***
LORCASERIN	ANTICANCER AND OTHER IMMUNOMODULATING DRUGS—DOXORUBICIN	↑ Blood concentrations of lorcaserin	Lorcaserin is a substrate of CYP3A4 and CYP2B6. Doxorubicin is an inhibitor of both these cytochrome enzymes	Monitor PR and BP closely until stable. Also monitor blood sugar and warn about muscle and joint pains. Report headaches and dizziness promptly
LORCASERIN	**ANTIDEPRESSANTS**			
LORCASERIN	LITHIUM, MIRTAZAPINE, MAOIs, ST. JOHN'S WORT, SSRIs, SNRIs, TCAs, TRYPTOPHAN	Risk of serotonin syndrome	Additive effect	Be aware of the possibility of serotonin syndrome. ➢ ***For signs and symptoms of serotonin toxicity, see Clinical Features of Some Adverse Drug Interactions, Serotonin Toxicity and Serotonin Syndrome***
LORCASERIN	DESIPRAMINE, DOXEPIN, DULOXETINE, FLUOXETINE, FLUVOXAMINE	↑ Blood concentrations of these antidepressants	Inhibition of CYP2D6-mediated metabolism	Monitor PR and BP closely until stable

(Continued)

Primary Drug	Secondary Drug	Effect	Mechanism	Precautions
ANTIOBESITY DRUGS				
LORCASERIN	ANTIHYPERTENSIVES AND HEART FAILURE DRUGS—CAPTOPRIL	↑ Blood concentrations of captopril	Inhibition of CYP2D6-mediated metabolism	Monitor PR and BP closely until stable
LORCASERIN	ANTIMIGRAINE DRUGS—TRIPTANS	Risk of serotonin syndrome	Additive effect	Be aware of the possibility of serotonin syndrome. ➢ ***For signs and symptoms of serotonin toxicity, see Clinical Features of Some Adverse Drug Interactions, Serotonin Toxicity and Serotonin Syndrome***
LORCASERIN	ANTI-PARKINSON'S DRUGS—RASAGILINE	Risk of serotonin syndrome	Additive effect	Be aware of the possibility of serotonin syndrome. ➢ ***For signs and symptoms of serotonin toxicity, see Clinical Features of Some Adverse Drug Interactions, Serotonin Toxicity and Serotonin Syndrome***
LORCASERIN	ANTIPSYCHOTICS—FLUPHENAZINE, HALOPERIDOL, ILOPERIDONE	↑ Blood concentrations of antipsychotics	Inhibition of CYP2D6-mediated metabolism	Monitor PR and BP closely until stable
LORCASERIN	BETA-BLOCKERS—BETAXOLOL, CARVEDILOL	↑ Blood concentrations of betaxol and carvedilol	Inhibition of CYP2D6-mediated metabolism	Monitor PR and BP closely until stable
LORCASERIN	ELIGLUSTAT	↑ Eliglustat levels	Inhibition of CYP2D6-mediated metabolism	Reduce dose to 85 mg od in extensive metabolizers. Avoid coadministration in intermediate and poor metabolizers
MAZINDOL—***see Sympatheticomimetics—Indirect—CVS Section***				
ORLISTAT				
ORLISTAT	ANTIARRHYTHMICS—AMIODARONE	Possible ↓ amiodarone levels	↓ Absorption of amiodarone	Watch for poor response to amiodarone
ORLISTAT	ANTICANCER DRUGS—CICLOSPORIN	↓ Plasma concentrations of ciclosporin and risk of transplant rejection	↓ Absorption of ciclosporin	Avoid coadministration

(Continued)

Primary Drug	Secondary Drug	Effect	Mechanism	Precautions
ANTIOBESITY DRUGS				
ORLISTAT	ANTICOAGULANTS—ORAL	↓ Anticoagulant effect	Probably ↓ absorption of coumarins	Monitor INR closely until stable
ORLISTAT	ANTIDIABETIC DRUGS—ACARBOSE, INSULIN, NATEGLINIDE, REPAGLINIDE, SULFONYLUREAS	Tendency for blood glucose levels to fluctuate	Antiobesity drugs change the dietary intake of carbohydrates and other foods, and the risk of such fluctuations is greater if there is a concurrent dietary regimen. A side effect of orlistat is hypoglycemia	These agents are used often in patients with type II diabetes who are on hypoglycemic therapy. Need to monitor blood sugars twice weekly until stable. Advise self-monitoring and warn about symptoms of hypoglycemia. Watch for and warn patients about symptoms of hypoglycemia. Avoid coadministration of acarbose and orlistat. ➢ ***For signs and symptoms of hypoglycemia, see Clinical Features of Some Adverse Drug Interactions, Hypoglycemia***
ORLISTAT	**ANTIHYPERTENSIVES AND HEART FAILURE DRUGS**			
ORLISTAT	ACE INHIBITORS	↓ Hypotensive effect found with enalapril. Rare cases of marked hypertension	Uncertain at present	Monitor BP at least weekly until stable
ORLISTAT	ANGIOTENSIN II RECEPTOR ANTAGONISTS	Cases of ↓ efficacy of losartan. Rare cases of marked hypertension	Uncertain at present	Monitor BP at least weekly until stable
ORLISTAT	BETA-BLOCKERS	Case of severe ↑ BP when orlistat is started in a patient on atenolol	Uncertain at present	Monitor BP at least weekly until stable
ORLISTAT	CALCIUM CHANNEL BLOCKERS	Case report of ↑ BP when orlistat was started in a patient on amlodipine	Uncertain at present	Monitor BP at least weekly until stable
ORLISTAT	DIURETICS—THIAZIDES	Case report of ↑ BP when orlistat was started in a patient on thiazides	Uncertain at present	Monitor BP at least weekly until stable
ORLISTAT	LAXATIVES	↑ Efficacy of laxatives	Additive effect; orlistat may cause soft stools	Start laxatives at low dose and titrate upward as needed

(Continued)

Primary Drug	Secondary Drug	Effect	Mechanism	Precautions
ANTIOBESITY DRUGS				
ORLISTAT	THYROID HORMONES	Possible risk of hypothyroidism	Uncertain	Monitor TFTs closely
ORLISTAT	VITAMINS—A, D, E, K, BETA-CAROTENE	↓ Absorption of the fat-soluble vitamins	Inhibition of pancreatic lipase by orlistat	Be aware that efficacy of these vitamins may be reduced, e.g., osteoporosis in postmenopausal women
PHENDIMETRAZINE—*see* ***Sympatheticomimetics—Indirect—CVS Section***				
PHENTERMINE—*see* ***Sympatheticomimetics—Indirect—CVS Section***				
RIMONABANT				
RIMONABANT	ANTICANCER AND IMMUNOMODULATING DRUGS—CICLOSPORIN	Slight increase in ciclosporin levels	Uncertain	Monitor ciclosporin levels closely
RIMONABANT	ANTIDIABETIC DRUGS—ACARBOSE, INSULIN, NATEGLINIDE, REPAGLINIDE, SULFONYLUREAS	Tendency for blood glucose levels to fluctuate	Antiobesity drugs change the dietary intake of carbohydrates and other foods, and the risk of such fluctuations is greater if there is a concurrent dietary regimen. A side effect of orlistat is hypoglycemia	These agents are used often in patients with type II diabetes who are on hypoglycemic therapy. Need to monitor blood sugars twice weekly until stable. Advise self-monitoring and warn about symptoms of hypoglycemia. Watch for and warn patients about symptoms of hypoglycemia. ➢ ***For signs and symptoms of hypoglycemia, see Clinical Features of Some Adverse Drug Interactions, Hypoglycemia***
RIMONABANT	ANTIFUNGALS—KETOCONAZOLE	↑ Rimonabant levels	Ketoconazole inhibits CYP3A4-mediated metabolism of rimonabant	Avoid coadministration
SIBUTRAMINE-WITHDRAWN FROM US AND BRITISH MARKETS IN 2010				
SIBUTRAMINE	**ANALGESICS**			
SIBUTRAMINE	NSAIDs	↑ Risk of bleeding	Additive effect	Avoid coadministration
SIBUTRAMINE	OPIOIDS—DEXTROMETHORPHAN, FENTANYL, PETHIDINE, PENTAZOCINE	Risk of serotonin syndrome	Additive effect	Manufacturer advises against coadministration

(*Continued*)

Primary Drug	Secondary Drug	Effect	Mechanism	Precautions
ANTIOBESITY DRUGS				
SIBUTRAMINE	ANTICOAGULANTS—HEPARINS	Possible ↑ risk of bleeding	Uncertain; possibly inhibiting platelet aggregation	Monitor APTT closely
SIBUTRAMINE	ANTIDEPRESSANTS—LITHIUM, MAOIs, SSRIs, SNRIs, TRYPTOPHAN	Risk of serotonin syndrome	Additive effect	Manufacturer advises against coadministration. Do not start sibutramine for at least 2 weeks after stopping MAOIs
SIBUTRAMINE	ANTIDIABETIC DRUGS—ACARBOSE, INSULIN, NATEGLINIDE, REPAGLINIDE, SULFONYL UREAS	Tendency for blood glucose levels to fluctuate	Antiobesity drugs change the dietary intake of carbohydrates and other foods, and the risk of such fluctuations is greater if there is a concurrent dietary regimen. A side effect of orlistat is hypoglycemia	These agents are used often in patients with type II diabetes who are on hypoglycemic therapy. Need to monitor blood sugars twice weekly until stable. Advise self-monitoring and warn about symptoms of hypoglycemia. Watch for and warn patients about symptoms of hypoglycemia. ➢ ***For signs and symptoms of hypoglycemia, see Clinical Features of Some Adverse Drug Interactions, Hypoglycemia***
SIBUTRAMINE	ANTIMIGRAINE DRUGS—DIHYDROERGOTAMINE	Risk of serotonin syndrome	Additive effect	Manufacturer advises against coadministration
SIBUTRAMINE	ANTIPLATELET AGENTS—ASPIRIN	Risk of bleeding	Additive effect; sibutramine may cause thrombocytopenia	Warn the patient to report any signs of ↑ bleeding
SIBUTRAMINE	SYMPATHOMIMETICS—including centrally acting appetite suppressants and topical decongestants	Risk of marked hypertension	Additive effect	Manufacturer advises against coadministration

Primary Drug	Secondary Drug	Effect	Mechanism	Precautions
ANTI-PARKINSON'S DRUGS				
AMANTADINE				
AMANTADINE	ANTIMUSCARINICS	↑ Risk of antimuscarinic side effects	Additive effect; both drugs cause antimuscarinic side effects	Warn patient of this additive effect

(Continued)

Primary Drug	Secondary Drug	Effect	Mechanism	Precautions
ANTI-PARKINSON'S DRUGS				
AMANTADINE	1. ANTIEMETICS—metoclopramide 2. ANTIPSYCHOTICS 3. CENTRALLY ACTING ANTIHYPERTENSIVES—methyldopa 4. TETRABENAZINE	↓ Efficacy of amantadine	Antagonism of anti-Parkinson's effect; these drugs have extrapyramidal side effects	Use with caution; avoid in patients <20 years
AMANTADINE	1. ANTI-PARKINSON'S DRUGS—dopaminergics 2. ANTIDEMENTIA DRUGS—memantine 3. DRUG DEPENDENCE THERAPIES—bupropion	↑ CNS side effects	Additive effects	Monitor more closely for confusion and gastrointestinal side effects. Initiate therapy with bupropion at the lowest dose and ↑ it gradually. Manufacturers recommend avoiding coadministration of amantadine and memantine
AMANTADINE	1. ANTIMALARIALS—quinine 2. ANTI-PARKINSON'S DRUGS—pramipexole	↑ Side effects	↓ Renal excretion	Monitor closely for confusion, disorientation, headache, dizziness, and nausea
ANTIMUSCARINICS				
ANTIMUSCARINICS	**ADDITIVE ANTICHOLINERGIC EFFECTS**			
ANTIMUSCARINICS	1. ANALGESICS—nefopam 2. ANTIARRHYTHMICS—disopyramide, propafenone 3. ANTIDEPRESSANTS—TCAs 4. ANTIEMETICS—cyclizine 5. ANTIHISTAMINES—chlorphenamine, cyproheptadine, hydroxyzine 6. ANTI-PARKINSON'S DRUGS—dopaminergics 7. ANTIPSYCHOTICS—phenothiazines, clozapine, pimozide 8. MUSCLE RELAXANTS—baclofen 9. NITRATES—isosorbide dinitrate	↑ Risk of antimuscarinic side effects. *NB ↓ efficacy of sublingual nitrate tablets*	Additive effect; both drugs cause antimuscarinic side effects. *Antimuscarinic effects ↓ saliva production, which ↓ dissolution of the tablet*	Warn patient of this additive effect. *Consider changing the formulation to a sublingual nitrate spray*

(*Continued*)

Primary Drug	Secondary Drug	Effect	Mechanism	Precautions
ANTI-PARKINSON'S DRUGS				
ATROPINE, GLYCOPYRRONIUM	ALCOHOL	↑ Sedation	Additive effect	Warn patients about this effect and advise them not to drink while taking these antimuscarinics
ANTIMUSCARINICS	ANALGESICS—PARACETAMOL	Atropine, benzatropine, orphenadrine, procyclidine, and trihexyphenidyl may slow the onset of action of intermittent-dose paracetamol	Anticholinergic effects delay gastric emptying and absorption	Warn patients that the action of paracetamol may be delayed. This will not be the case when paracetamol is taken regularly
ATROPINE	ANTIARRHYTHMICS—MEXILETINE	Delayed absorption of mexiletine	Anticholinergic effects delay gastric emptying and absorption	May slow the onset of action of the first dose of mexiletine, but is not of clinical significance for regular dosing (atropine does not ↓ total dose absorbed)
TOLTERODINE	ANTIBIOTICS—CLARITHROMYCIN, ERYTHROMYCIN	↑ Tolterodine levels	Inhibition of CYP3A4-mediated metabolism	Avoid coadministration (manufacturers' recommendation)
DARIFENACIN	ANTICANCER AND IMMUNOMODULATING DRUGS—CICLOSPORIN	↑ Levels of darifenacin	Ciclosporin inhibits Pgp and CYP3A4, which results in ↓ clearance of darifenacin	Avoid coadministration
ANTIMUSCARINICS	ANTIDEMENTIA DRUGS—MEMANTINE	Possible ↑ efficacy of antimuscarinics	Additive effect; memantine has weak antimuscarinic properties	Warn patients of this effect
ANTIMUSCARINICS	**ANTIDEPRESSANTS**			
DARIFENACIN, PROCYCLIDINE	PAROXETINE	↑ Levels of these antimuscarinics	Inhibition of metabolism	Watch for early features of toxicity
IPRATROPIUM, TIOTROPIUM	MAOIs	↑ Occurrence of antimuscarinic effects such as blurred vision, confusion (in elderly people), restlessness, and constipation	Additive antimuscarinic effects	Warn patients and carers, particularly those managing elderly patients

(Continued)

Primary Drug	Secondary Drug	Effect	Mechanism	Precautions
ANTI-PARKINSON'S DRUGS				
ANTIMUSCARINICS	ANTIEMETICS—DOMPERIDONE, METOCLOPRAMIDE	↓ Efficacy of domperidone on gut motility by antimuscarinics	Some effects of metoclopramide are considered to be due to ↑ release of ACh and ↑ sensitivity of the cholinergic receptors to ACh. Antimuscarinics prevent the effects on muscarinic receptors	The gastrointestinal effects of metoclopramide will be impaired, while the antiemetic effects may not be. Thus, concurrent use with antimuscarinics is not advised because of effects on the gastrointestinal system
ANTIMUSCARINICS	ANTIFUNGALS—ITRACONAZOLE, KETOCONAZOLE	1. ↓ Ketoconazole levels 2. ↑ Darifenacin, solifenacin, and tolterodine levels	1. ↓ Absorption 2. Inhibited metabolism	1. Watch for poor response to ketoconazole 2. Avoid coadministration of itraconazole, ketoconazole, and these antimuscarinics. The U.S. manufacturer of darifenacin recommends that its dose should not exceed 7.5 mg/day
ANTIMUSCARINICS	**ANTIVIRALS**			
DARIFENACIN	PROTEASE INHIBITORS	↑ Adverse effects with atazanavir and possibly with other protease inhibitors	Increased plasma levels as atazanavir reduced darifenacin metabolism via CYP3A4, 2D6 and PGP	Avoid coadministration
FESTERODINE	PROTEASE INHIBITORS—ATAZANAVIR, INDINAVIR, RITONAVIR, SAQUNAVIR	↑ Adverse effects	Increased plasma levels, reduces metabolism via CYP3A4 and 2D6	Limit maximum dose of festoterodine to 4 mg daily
MIRABEGRON	PROTEASE INHIBITORS—RITONAVIR	Possibly ↑ adverse effects	Combination of CYP3A4 inhibition and reduced renal elimination	Reduce dose if mild renal impairment, avoid if severe
SOLIFENACIN	PROTEASE INHIBITORS	↑ Adverse effects with nelfinavir and ritonavir (with or without lopinavir)	Inhibition of CYP3A4-mediated metabolism of solifenacin	Limit maximum dose of solifenacin to 5 mg daily
TOLTERODINE	PROTEASE INHIBITORS	Possibly ↑ adverse effects, including arrythmias, with protease inhibitors	Inhibition of CYP2D6- and 3A4-mediated metabolism of tolterodine	Avoid coadministration
ANTIMUSCARINICS	ANTI-PARKINSON'S—AMANTADINE	↑ Risk of antimuscarinic side effects	Additive effect; both drugs cause antimuscarinic side effects	Warn patients of this additive effect

(Continued)

Primary Drug	Secondary Drug	Effect	Mechanism	Precautions
ANTI-PARKINSON'S DRUGS				
IPRATROPIUM	BRONCHODILATORS—SALBUTAMOL	A few reports of acute angle closure glaucoma when nebulized ipratropium and salbutamol were coadministered	Ipratropium dilates the pupil, which ↓ drainage of aqueous humor, while salbutamol ↑ production of aqueous humor	Warn patients to prevent the solution to mist or enter the eye. Extreme caution in coadministering these bronchodilators by the nebulized route in patients with a history of acute closed-angle glaucoma
DARIFENACIN	CALCIUM CHANNEL BLOCKERS—VERAPAMIL	↑ Darifenacin levels	Inhibition of CYP3A4-mediated metabolism of darifenacin	Avoid coadministration (manufacturers' recommendation)
PROPANTHELINE	CARDIAC GLYCOSIDES—DIGOXIN	↑ Digoxin levels (30%–40%) but only with slow-release formulations	Slowed gut transit time allows more digoxin to be absorbed	Use alternative formulation of digoxin
ANTIMUSCARINICS—ARIFENACIN, FESOTERODINE, SOLIFENACIN	GRAPEFRUIT JUICE	↑ Levels of darifenacin and fesoterodine	Inhibition of metabolism	Avoid grapefruit juice while taking these antimuscarinics
TROSPIUM	LIPID LOWERING DRUGS—ANION EXCHANGE RESINS	Risk of ↓ absorption of trospium	Colestipol and colestyramine bind trospium in the intestine	Take trospium 1 h before or 4–6 h after colestipol or colestyramine
ANTIMUSCARINICS	PARASYMPATHOMIMETICS	↓ Efficacy of parasympathomimetics	Parasympathomimetics and antimuscarinics have opposing effects	Avoid coadministration where possible
ATROPINE	SYMPATHOMIMETICS	Reports of hypertension when atropine was given to patients receiving 10% phenylephrine eye drops during eye surgery	Atropine abolishes the cholinergic response to phenylephrine-induced vasoconstriction	Use a lower concentration of phenylephrine

(*Continued*)

DRUGS ACTING ON THE CENTRAL NERVOUS SYSTEM ANTI-PARKINSON'S DRUGS Dopaminergics

Primary Drug	Secondary Drug	Effect	Mechanism	Precautions
ANTI-PARKINSON'S DRUGS				
DOPAMINERGICS				
DOPAMINERGICS	**DRUGS WITH ANTIMUSCARINIC EFFECTS**			
DOPAMINERGICS	1. ANALGESICS—nefopam 2. ANTIARRHYTHMICS—disopyramide, propafenone 3. ANTIDEPRESSANTS—TCAs 4. ANTIEMETICS—cyclizine 5. ANTIHISTAMINES—chlorphenamine, cyproheptadine, hydroxyzine 6. ANTIMUSCARINICS—atropine, benzatropine, cyclopentolate, dicycloverine, flavoxate, homatropine, hyoscine, orphenadrine, oxybutynin, procyclidine, propantheline, tolterodine, trihexyphenidyl, tropicamide 7. ANTIPSYCHOTICS—phenothiazines, clozapine, pimozide 8. MUSCLE RELAXANTS—baclofen 9. NITRATES—isosorbide dinitrate	↑ Risk of antimuscarinic side effects. Also, possibly ↓ levodopa levels. *NB ↓ efficacy of sublingual nitrate tablets*	Additive effect. Delayed gastric emptying may cause more levodopa to be metabolized within the wall of the gastrointestinal tract. *Antimuscarinic effects ↓ saliva production, which ↓ dissolution of the tablet*	Warn patients of this additive effect. Consider increasing the dose of levodopa. *Consider changing the formulation to a sublingual nitrate spray*
LEVODOPA	ANESTHETICS—GENERAL—VOLATILE AGENTS	Possible risk of arrhythmias	Uncertain	Monitor EGC and BP closely. Consider using intravenous agents for maintenance of anesthesia
DOPAMINERGICS	**ANALGESICS**			
DOPAMINERGICS	NEFOPAM	↑ Anticholinergic effects	Additive effects	Warn patients about these effects

(*Continued*)

Primary Drug	Secondary Drug	Effect	Mechanism	Precautions
ANTI-PARKINSON'S DRUGS				
RASAGILINE, SELEGILINE	OPIOIDS—PETHIDINE, TRAMADOL	1. Risk of neurological toxicity when pethidine is coadministered with rasagiline 2. Risk of hyperpyrexia when pethidine and possibly tramadol is coadministered with selegiline.	Unknown	1. Avoid coadministration; do not use pethidine for at least 2 weeks after stopping rasagiline 2. Avoid coadministration
DOPAMINERGICS	PARACETAMOL	Amantadine, bromocriptine, levodopa, pergolide, pramipexole, and selegiline may slow the onset of action of intermittent-dose paracetamol	Anticholinergic effects delay gastric emptying and absorption	Warn patients that the action of paracetamol may be delayed. This will not be the case when paracetamol is taken regularly
DOPAMINERGICS	**ANTIBIOTICS**			
BROMOCRIPTINE, CABERGOLINE	ERYTHROMYCIN	↑ Bromocriptine and cabergoline levels	Inhibition of metabolism	Monitor BP closely and watch for early features of toxicity (nausea, headache, drowsiness)
ROPINIROLE	CIPROFLOXACIN	↑ Ropinirole levels	Inhibition of CYP1A2-mediated metabolism	Watch for early features of toxicity (nausea, drowsiness)
DOPAMINERGICS	**ANTICANCER AND IMMUNOMODULATING DRUGS**			
LEVODOPA	DACARBAZINE	Single report showed reduced effects of levodopa	Unknown	Be alert of the need
BROMOCRIPTINE	EVEROLIMUS	Possible increased everolimus levels	CYP3A4 inhibition	Caution with concurrent use
BROMOCRIPTINE	OCTREOTIDE	↑ Bromocriptine levels	Uncertain	Be aware
LEVODOPA	PENICILLAMINE	Possible increased levodopa levels	Uncertain	Parkinsonian symptoms may improve Monitor closely for increased levodopa side effects
BROMOCRIPTINE	PROCARBAZINE	May cause ↑ serum prolactin levels and interfere with the effects of bromocriptine	Uncertain	Watch for ↓ effect of bromocriptine

(Continued)

Primary Drug	Secondary Drug	Effect	Mechanism	Precautions
ANTI-PARKINSON'S DRUGS				
BROMOCRIPTINE	TEMSIROLIMUS	Possible increased temsirolimus levels	CYP3A4 inhibition	Caution with concurrent use
ENTACAPONE	ANTICOAGULANTS—ORAL	↑ Anticoagulant effect	Pharmacokinetic interaction with R-warfarin	Monitor INR at least weekly until stable
DOPAMINERGICS	ANTIDEMENTIA DRUGS—MEMANTINE	Memantine augments the effect of dopaminergics	Memantine has some agonist activity at dopamine receptors	Be aware. May be used therapeutically
DOPAMINERGICS	**ANTIDEPRESSANTS**			
LEVODOPA, SELEGILINE, POSSIBLY RASAGILINE, ENTACAPONE, TOLCAPONE	MAOIs	Risk of adrenergic syndrome—hypertension, hyperthermia, arrhythmias—and dopaminergic effects with selegiline; ↑ risk of serotonin syndrome and of adrenergic syndrome with older MAOIs	Levodopa and related drugs are precursors of dopamine. Levodopa is predominantly metabolized to dopamine, and a smaller proportion is converted to epinephrine and norepinephrine. Effects are due to inhibition of MAOI, which breaks down dopamine and sympathomimetics	Avoid concurrent use. Onset may be 6–24 h after ingestion. Carbidopa and benserazide, which inhibit dopa decarboxylase that converts L-dopa to dopamine, is considered to minimize this interaction. However, MAOIs should not be used in patients with Parkinson's disease on treatment with levodopa. Imipramine and amitriptyline are considered safer by some clinicians
RASAGILINE, SELEGILINE	SSRIs, VENLAFAXINE	Risk of severe hypertensive reactions and of serotonin syndrome. ➢ ***For signs and symptoms of serotonin toxicity, see Clinical Features of Some Adverse Drug Interactions, Serotonin Toxicity and Serotonin Syndrome***	Additive inhibitory effect on serotonin reuptake with SSRIs. Venlafaxine inhibits the reuptake of both serotonin and norepinephrine. Due to impaired metabolism of these amines, there is an accumulation of serotonin and norepinephrine in the brain and at peripheral sites. These dopaminergics are MAO-B inhibitors	Avoid coadministration. Rasagiline and selegiline should not be started for at least 2 weeks after stopping SSRIs (5 weeks after fluoxetine). Do not start selegiline or rasagiline for at least 1 week after stopping venlafaxine. Conversely, SSRIs and venlafaxine should not be started for at least 2 weeks after stopping rasagiline and selegiline

(*Continued*)

Primary Drug	Secondary Drug	Effect	Mechanism	Precautions
ANTI-PARKINSON'S DRUGS				
RASAGILINE, SELEGILINE	TCAs	↑ Risk of stroke, hyperpyrexia, and convulsions. ↑ Plasma concentrations of TCAs, with risk of toxic effects. Clomipramine may trigger acute confusion in Parkinson's disease when used with selegiline	TCAs are believed to also act by inhibiting the reuptake of serotonin and norepinephrine, increasing the risk of serotonin and adrenergic syndromes. The combination of TCAs and antidepressants can ↑ risk of seizures	Very hazardous interaction. Avoid concurrent use and consider the use of an alternative antidepressant. Be aware that seizures occur with overdose of TCAs just before cardiac arrest
ROPINIROLE	SSRI—FLUVOXAMINE	↑ Ropinirole levels	Inhibition of CYP1A2-mediated metabolism to a greater extent by fluvoxamine compared to fluoxetine, paroxetine, and sertraline	Watch for early features of toxicity (nausea, drowsiness)
RASAGILINE, SELEGILINE	ANTIDIABETIC DRUGS—INSULIN, SULFONYLUREAS	↑ Risk of hypoglycemic episodes	These drugs are MAO-B inhibitors. MAOIs have an intrinsic hypoglycemic effect and are considered to enhance the effect of hypoglycemic drugs	Watch for and warn patients about symptoms of hypoglycemia. ➢ ***For signs and symptoms of hypoglycemia, see Clinical Features of Some Adverse Drug Interactions, Hypoglycemia***
DOPAMINERGICS	**ANTIEMETICS**			
DOPAMINERGICS	METOCLOPRAMIDE	↓ Efficacy of dopaminergics	Metoclopramide is a centrally acting antidopaminergic	Use with caution, avoid in patients <20 years. Manufacturers recommend avoiding coadministration of metoclopramide with ropinirole or rotigotine
BROMOCRIPTINE, CABERGOLINE	DOMPERIDONE, METOCLOPRAMIDE	↓ Efficacy of bromocriptine and cabergoline at reducing prolactin levels	Domperidone and metoclopramide are associated with prolactin secretion	Use alternative antiemetics when bromocriptine and cabergoline are being used to treat prolactinomas. Domperidone has minimal central antidopaminergic effect and may therefore be used when bromocriptine and cabergoline are administered as treatments for Parkinson's disease

(Continued)

Primary Drug	Secondary Drug	Effect	Mechanism	Precautions
ANTI-PARKINSON'S DRUGS				
LEVODOPA	ANTIEPILEPTICS—PHENYTOIN	Possibly ↓ levodopa levels	Uncertain	Watch for poor response to levodopa and consider increasing its dose
DOPAMINERGICS	**ANTIHYPERTENSIVES AND HEART FAILURE DRUGS**			
APOMORPHINE	ALPHA-BLOCKERS	↑ Hypotensive effect	Not clear—effect seen with vasodilators but not other antihypertensives	Monitor BP closely, especially during initiation of treatment. Warn patients to report symptoms of hypotension (light-headedness, dizziness on standing, etc.)
APOMORPHINE	VASODILATOR ANTIHYPERTENSIVES	Theoretical risk of ↑ hypotensive effect	Not clear—effect seen with vasodilators but not other antihypertensives	Monitor BP closely, especially during initiation of treatment. Warn patients to report symptoms of hypotension (light-headedness, dizziness on standing, etc.)
LEVODOPA	ANTIHYPERTENSIVES AND HEART FAILURE DRUGS	↑ Hypotensive effect	Additive effect	Monitor BP at least weekly until stable. Warn patients to report symptoms of hypotension (light-headedness, dizziness on standing, etc.)
LEVODOPA	CENTRALLY ACTING ANTIHYPERTENSIVES	1. Clonidine may oppose the effect of levodopa/carbidopa 2. Methyldopa may ↓ levodopa requirements, although there are case reports of deteriorating dyskinesias in some patients	1. Uncertain at present 2. Uncertain at present	1. Watch for deterioration in control of symptoms of Parkinson's disease 2. Levodopa needs may ↓; in cases of worsening of Parkinson's control, use an alternative antihypertensive
PERGOLIDE	ACE INHIBITORS	Possible ↑ hypotensive effect	Additive effect; a single case of severe ↓ BP with lisinopril and pergolide has been reported	Monitor BP at least weekly until stable. Warn patients to report symptoms of hypotension (light-headedness, dizziness on standing, etc.)

(*Continued*)

Primary Drug	Secondary Drug	Effect	Mechanism	Precautions
ANTI-PARKINSON'S DRUGS				
RASAGILINE	ANTIOBESITY DRUGS—LORCASERIN	Risk of serotonin syndrome	Additive effect	Be aware of the possibility of serotonin syndrome. ➢ ***For signs and symptoms of serotonin toxicity, see Clinical Features of Some Adverse Drug Interactions, Serotonin Toxicity and Serotonin Syndrome***
DOPAMINERGICS	**ANTI-PARKINSON'S DRUGS**			
DOPAMINERGICS	AMANTADINE	↑ CNS side effects	Additive effects	Monitor more closely for confusion, gastrointestinal side effects. Initiate therapy with bupropion at the lowest dose and ↑ gradually. Manufacturers recommend avoiding coadministration of amantadine and memantine
PRAMIPEXOLE	AMANTADINE	↑ Side effects	↓ Renal excretion	Monitor closely for confusion, disorientation, headache, dizziness, and nausea
DOPAMINERGICS	ANTIPSYCHOTICS	↓ Efficacy of dopaminergics	Antipsychotics may cause extrapyramidal side effects, which oppose the effect of anti-Parkinson's drugs. The atypical antipsychotics cause less effect than the older drugs	Caution with coadministration; consider using atypical antipsychotics, and use antimuscarinic drugs if extrapyramidal symptoms occur. Manufacturers recommend avoiding coadministration of amisulpride with levodopa, and coadministration of antipsychotics with pramipexole, ropinirole, and rotigotine. Clozapine can be coadministered with Sinamet (Carbidiopa-Levodopa) and pergolide
LEVODOPA	ANXIOLYTICS AND HYPNOTICS—BZDs	Risk of ↓ effect of levodopa	Uncertain	Watch for poor response to levodopa and consider increasing its dose. If there is severe antagonism of effect, stop the BZD

(*Continued*)

Primary Drug	Secondary Drug	Effect	Mechanism	Precautions
ANTI-PARKINSON'S DRUGS				
LEVODOPA	BETA-BLOCKERS	↑ Hypotensive effect	Additive hypotensive effect; however, overall, adding beta-blockers to levodopa can be beneficial (e.g., by reducing the risk of a dopamine-mediated risk of arrhythmias)	Monitor BP at least weekly until stable
ANTI-PARKINSON'S DRUGS	**CALCIUM CHANNEL BLOCKERS**			
APOMORPHINE	CALCIUM CHANNEL BLOCKERS	Risk of ↑ hypotensive effect	Not clear—effect seen with vasodilators but not other antihypertensives; hypotension is a side effect of apomorphine	Monitor BP closely, especially during initiation of treatment. Warn patients to report symptoms of hypotension (light-headedness, dizziness on standing, etc.)
LEVODOPA	CALCIUM CHANNEL BLOCKERS	↑ Hypotensive effect	Additive hypotensive effect	Monitor BP at least weekly until stable. Warn patients to report symptoms of hypotension (light-headedness, dizziness on standing, etc.)
LEVODOPA	DIURETICS	↑ Hypotensive effect	Additive effect	Monitor BP at least weekly until stable. Warn patients to report symptoms of hypotension (light-headedness, dizziness on standing, etc.)
DOPAMINERGICS—ENTACAPONE, TOLCAPONE	DOPAMINERGICS—SELEGILINE	Possible risk of severe hypertensive reactions	Theoretical risk due to additive inhibitory effect on dopamine metabolism	Manufacturers recommend limiting the dose of selegiline to a maximum of 10 mg
LEVODOPA	DRUG DEPENDENCE THERAPIES—BUPROPION	↑ CNS side effects	Additive effects	Initiate therapy with bupropion at the lowest dose and ↑ gradually
PRAMIPEXOLE, ROPINIROLE	H2-RECEPTOR BLOCKER—CIMETIDINE	↑ Efficacy and adverse effects of pramipexole and possibly ropinirole	↓ Renal excretion of pramipexole by inhibition of cation transport system. Inhibition of CYP1A2-mediated metabolism of ropinirole	Monitor closely; ↓ dose of pramipexole may be required. Adjust dose of ropinirole as necessary or use alternative acid suppression, e.g., H2 antagonist proton pump inhibitor (not omeprazole or lansoprazole)

(*Continued*)

Primary Drug	Secondary Drug	Effect	Mechanism	Precautions
ANTI-PARKINSON'S DRUGS				
ENTACAPONE, LEVODOPA	IRON—ORAL	↓ Entacapone levels	Iron chelates with entacapone and levodopa, which ↓ their absorption	Separate doses as much as possible. Consider increasing the dose of anti-Parkinson's therapy
LEVODOPA	MUSCLE RELAXANTS—BACLOFEN	Reports of CNS agitation and ↓ efficacy of levodopa	Uncertain	Avoid coadministration
APOMORPHINE	NITRATES	Risk of ↑ hypotensive effect	Not clear—effect seen with vasodilators but not other antihypertensives	Monitor BP closely, especially during initiation of treatment. Warn patients to report symptoms of hypotension (light-headedness, dizziness on standing, etc.)
ROPINIROLE, SELEGILINE	ESTROGENS	↑ Levels of ropinirole and selegiline	Inhibition of metabolism (possibly *N*-demethylation)	Watch for early features of toxicity (nausea, drowsiness) when starting estrogens in a patient stabilized on these dopaminergics. Conversely, watch for poor response to them if estrogens are stopped
APOMORPHINE	PERIPHERAL VASODILATORS—MOXISYLYTE	↑ Hypotensive effect	Additive hypotensive effect	Monitor BP at least weekly until stable. Warn patients to report symptoms of hypotension (light-headedness, dizziness on standing, etc.)
SELEGILINE	PROGESTOGENS	↑ Selegiline levels	Inhibition of metabolism	Watch for early features of toxicity (nausea, drowsiness) when starting progestogens in a patient stabilized on these dopaminergics. Conversely, watch for poor response to them if progestogens are stopped
DOPAMINERGICS	**SYMPATHOMIMETICS**			
BROMOCRIPTINE, ENTACAPONE	INDIRECT	Cases of severe, symptomatic ↑ BP when coadministered with indirect sympathomimetics	Likely additive effect; both can cause ↑ BP	Monitor BP closely; watch for ↑ BP

(Continued)

DRUGS ACTING ON THE CENTRAL NERVOUS SYSTEM ANTIPSYCHOTICS

Primary Drug	Secondary Drug	Effect	Mechanism	Precautions
ANTI-PARKINSON'S DRUGS				
RASAGILINE	SYMPATHOMIMETICS	Risk of adrenergic syndrome	Due to inhibition of MAOI, which breaks down sympathomimetics	Avoid concurrent use. Onset may be 6–24 h after ingestion. Do ECG and measure electrolytes, FBC, CK, and coagulation profile
SELEGILINE	DOPAMINE	Case report of ↑ hypertensive effect of dopamine when it was given to a patient already taking selegiline	Selegiline inhibits metabolism of dopamine	Titrate dopamine carefully
LEVODOPA	VITAMIN B6	↓ Efficacy of levodopa (in the absence of a dopa decarboxylase inhibitor)	A derivative of vitamin B6 is a cofactor in the peripheral conversion of levodopa to dopamine, which ↓ the amount available for conversion in the CNS. Dopa decarboxylase inhibitors inhibit this peripheral reaction	Avoid coadministration of levodopa with vitamin B6; coadministration of vitamin B6 with co-beneldopa or co-careldopa is acceptable

Primary Drug	Secondary Drug	Effect	Mechanism	Precautions
ANTIPSYCHOTICS				
ANTIPSYCHOTICS	**DRUGS THAT PROLONG THE QT INTERVAL**			
ATYPICALS, PHENOTHIAZINE, PIMOZIDE	1. ANTIARRHYTHMICS—ajmaline, amiodarone, azimilide, cibenzoline, disopyramide, dofetilide, dronedarone, ibutilide, procainamide, propafenone, quinidine	Risk of ventricular arrhythmias, particularly torsades de pointes	Additive effect; these drugs prolong the QT interval Also, amitriptyline, clomipramine, and desipramine levels may be ↑ by propafenone Amitriptyline and clomipramine may ↑ propafenone levels Propafenone and these TCAs inhibit CYP2D6-mediated metabolism of each other	Avoid coadministration

(Continued)

Primary Drug	Secondary Drug	Effect	Mechanism	Precautions
ANTIPSYCHOTICS				
	2. ANTIBIOTICS—macrolides (especially azithromycin, clarithromycin, parenteral erythromycin, telithromycin), quinolones (especially moxifloxacin), quinupristin/dalfopristin 3. ANTICANCER AND IMMUNOMODULATING DRUGS—arsenic trioxide, bosutinib, crizotinib, dasatinib, eribulin, fingolimod, lapatinib, nilotinib, pazopanib, sunitinib, vandetanib, vemurafenib 4. ANTIDEPRESSANTS—TCAs, venlafaxine 5. ANTIEMETICS—ondansetron 6. ANTIFUNGALS—fluconazole, posaconazole, voriconazole 7. ANTIHISTAMINES—terfenadine, hydroxyzine, mizolastine 8. ANTIHYPERTENSIVES—ketanserin 9. ANTIMALARIALS—artemether with lumefantrine, chloroquine, halofantrine, hydroxychloroquine, mefloquine, quinine 10. ANTIPROTOZOALS—pentamidine isothionate 11. ANTIVIRALS—boceprevir, rilpivirine, telaprevir			

(*Continued*)

DRUGS ACTING ON THE CENTRAL NERVOUS SYSTEM ANTIPSYCHOTICS

Primary Drug	Secondary Drug	Effect	Mechanism	Precautions
ANTIPSYCHOTICS				
	12. BETA-BLOCKERS—sotalol 13. BRONCHODILATORS—parenteral bronchodilators 14. CNS STIMULANTS—atomoxetine 15. RANOLAZINE			
ANTIPSYCHOTICS	**DRUGS WITH ANTIMUSCARINIC EFFECTS**			
ANTIPSYCHOTICS—PHENOTHIAZINES, CLOZAPINE, PIMOZIDE	1. ANALGESICS—nefopam 2. ANTIARRHYTHMICS—disopyramide, propafenone 3. ANTIDEPRESSANTS—TCAs 4. ANTIEMETICS—cyclizine 5. ANTIHISTAMINES—chlorphenamine, cyproheptadine, hydroxyzine 6. ANTIMUSCARINICS—atropine, benzatropine, cyclopentolate, dicycloverine, flavoxate, homatropine, hyoscine, orphenadrine, oxybutynin, procyclidine, propantheline, tolterodine, trihexyphenidyl or tropicamide 7. ANTI-PSYCHOTICS—phenothiazines, clozapine, pimozide 8. MUSCLE RELAXANTS—baclofen 9. NITRATES—isosorbide dinitrate	↑ Risk of antimuscarinic side effects. Also, possibly ↓ levodopa levels. *NB ↓ efficacy of sublingual nitrate tablets*	Additive effect. Delayed gastric emptying may cause more levodopa to be metabolized within the wall of the gastrointestinal tract. *Antimuscarinic effects ↓ saliva production, which ↓ dissolution of the tablet*	Warn patients of this additive effect. Consider increasing the dose of levodopa. *Consider changing the formulation to a sublingual nitrate spray*
ANTIPSYCHOTICS	ALCOHOL	Risk of excessive sedation	Additive effect	Warn patients of this effect, and advise them to drink alcohol only in moderation
ANTIPSYCHOTICS	ANESTHETICS—GENERAL	Risk of hypotension	Additive effect	Monitor BP closely, especially during induction of anesthesia

(Continued)

Primary Drug	Secondary Drug	Effect	Mechanism	Precautions
ANTIPSYCHOTICS				
ANTIPSYCHOTICS	**ANALGESICS**			
ANTIPSYCHOTICS	NSAIDs	1. Reports of ↑ sedation when indometacin is added to haloperidol 2. Risk of agranulocytosis when azapropazone given with clozapine	1. Unknown 2. Likely additive effect	1. Avoid coadministration 2. Avoid coadministration
ANTIPSYCHOTICS	OPIOIDS	Risk of ↑ respiratory depression, sedation, and ↓ BP. This effect seems to be particularly marked with clozapine	Additive effects	Warn patients of these effects. Monitor BP closely. Titrate doses carefully
ANTIPSYCHOTICS	TRAMADOL	↑ Risk of fits	Additive effects	Consider using an alternative analgesic
PHENOTHIAZINES, SULPIRIDE	ANTACIDS	↓ Levels of these antipsychotics	↓ Absorption	Separate doses by 2 h (in the case of sulpiride, give sulpiride 2 h after but not before the antacid)
ANTIPSYCHOTICS	**ANTIARRHYTHMICS**			
ANTIPSYCHOTICS	ADENOSINE	Risk of ventricular arrhythmias, particularly torsades de pointes, with phenothiazines and pimozide. There is also a theoretical risk of QT prolongation with atypical antipsychotics	All of these drugs prolong the QT interval	Avoid coadministration of phenothiazines, amisulpride, pimozide, or sertindole with adenosine. Monitor the ECG closely when adenosine is coadministered with atypical antipsychotics
AMISULPRIDE, CLOZAPINE, PHENOTHIAZINES, PIMOZIDE, SERTINDOLE	FLECAINIDE	Risk of arrhythmias	Additive effect. Also, haloperidol and thioridazine inhibit CYP2D6-mediated metabolism of flecainide	Avoid coadministration
PROCHLOR-PERAZINE	DOFETILIDE	↑ Prolongation of action	Prochlorperazine reduces renal excretion of dofetilide	Avoid coadministration

(Continued)

DRUGS ACTING ON THE CENTRAL NERVOUS SYSTEM ANTIPSYCHOTICS

Primary Drug	Secondary Drug	Effect	Mechanism	Precautions
ANTIPSYCHOTICS				
ANTIPSYCHOTICS	**ANTIBIOTICS ➢ *QT-Prolonging Drugs, above***			
ARIPIPRAZOLE, CLOZAPINE, HALOPERIDOL	RIFABUTIN, RIFAMPICIN	↓ Levels of these antipsychotics	↑ Metabolism	Watch for poor response to these antipsychotics; consider increasing the dose
CLOZAPINE	CHLORAMPHENICOL, SULFONAMIDES	↑ Risk of bone marrow toxicity	Additive effect	Avoid coadministration
CLOZAPINE, OLANZAPINE	CIPROFLOXACIN	↑ Clozapine levels and possibly ↑ olanzapine levels	Ciprofloxacin inhibits CYP1A2; clozapine is primarily metabolized by CYP1A2, while olanzapine is partly metabolized by it	Watch for the early features of toxicity to these antipsychotics. ↓ In dose of clozapine and olanzapine may be required
CLOZAPINE	MACROLIDES—ERYTHROMYCIN	↑ Clozapine levels with risk of clozapine toxicity	Clozapine is metabolized by CYPIA2, which is moderately inhibited by erythromycin. Erythromycin is a potent inhibitor of CYP3A4, which has a minor role in the metabolism of clozapine. This may lead to ↓ clearance and therefore ↑ levels of clozapine	Cautious use advised
ANTIPSYCHOTICS	**ANTICANCER AND IMMUNOMODULATING DRUGS**			
CLOZAPINE	CYTOTOXICS	↑ Risk of bone marrow toxicity	Additive effect	Avoid coadministration
ANTIPSYCHOTICS—HALOPERIDOL	DABRAFENIB	Possible reduced levels of CYP3A4/CYP2Cs/CYP2B6 substrates. Level of reduction may vary	Dabrafenib induces CYP3A4/CYP2Cs/CYP2B6	Monitor closely or avoid concurrent use
ANTIPSYCHOTICS—PIMOZIDE	DASATINIB	Increased levels of pimozide	CYP3A4 inhibition	Caution with CYP3A4 substrates with narrow therapeutic window
ANTIPSYCHOTICS	HISTAMINE	Effects of histamine antagonized	Histamine blockade	Avoid concurrent use
CLOZAPINE, HALOPERIDOL, PERPHENAZINE, RISPERIDONE	IMATINIB	Imatinib may cause ↑ plasma concentrations of these drugs with a risk of toxic effects	Inhibition of CYP2D6-mediated metabolism of these drugs	Watch for early features of toxicity of these drugs

(*Continued*)

DRUGS ACTING ON THE CENTRAL NERVOUS SYSTEM ANTIPSYCHOTICS

Primary Drug	Secondary Drug	Effect	Mechanism	Precautions
ANTIPSYCHOTICS				
HALOPERIDOL, CLOZAPINE	PIXANTRONE	Theoretical risk of increased drug levels	Pixantrone inhibits CYP1A2	Manufacturer advises to monitor closely
CHLORPROMAZINE, FLUPHENAZINE	PORFIMER	↑ Risk of photosensitivity reactions	Attributed to additive effects	Avoid exposure of skin and eyes to direct sunlight for 30 days after porfimer therapy
CLOZAPINE	PROCARBAZINE, PENICILLAMINE	↑ Risk of bone marrow toxicity	Additive effect	Avoid coadministration
FLUPENTIXOL, PIMOZIDE, ZUCLOPENTHIXOL	PROCARBAZINE	Prolongation or greater intensity of sedative, hypotensive, and anticholinergic effects	Additive effect	Avoid coadministration
BROMOCRIPTINE	SIROLIMUS	Possible increased sirolimus levels	CYP3A4 inhibition	Caution with concurrent use
ANTIPSYCHOTICS	THALIDOMIDE	Increased sedation	Additive	Caution with concurrent use
ANTIPSYCHOTICS	**ANTIDEPRESSANTS**			
CLOZAPINE, HALOPERIDOL, PHENOTHIAZINE, SULPIRIDE	LITHIUM	1. ↑ Risk of extrapyramidal side effects and of neurotoxicity 2. Lithium might decrease effectiveness of phenothiazines (chlorpromazine, fluphenazine, trifluoperazine, thioridazine)	Uncertain	1. Watch for development of these symptoms (seizures, encephalopathy, pyrexia, extrapyramidal symptoms) 2. Watch for deterioration in control of psychosis
SERTINDOLE	LITHIUM	↑ Risk of ventricular arrhythmias	Uncertain	Avoid concomitant use
ANTIPSYCHOTICS	MAOIs	Additive depression of CNS ranging from drowsiness to coma and respiratory depression	Synergistic depressant effects on CNS function	Necessary to warn patients, particularly regarding activities that require attention, e.g., driving or using machinery and equipment that could cause self-harm

(*Continued*)

DRUGS ACTING ON THE CENTRAL NERVOUS SYSTEM ANTIPSYCHOTICS

DRUGS ACTING ON THE CENTRAL NERVOUS SYSTEM ANTIPSYCHOTICS

Primary Drug	Secondary Drug	Effect	Mechanism	Precautions
ANTIPSYCHOTICS				
ARIPIPRAZOLE, CLOZAPINE, HALOPERIDOL, PERPHENAZINE, RISPERIDONE, SERTINDOLE	SSRIs	Possible ↑ plasma concentrations of these antipsychotics	Inhibition of CYP2D6-mediated metabolism of these drugs. The clinical significance of this depends upon whether alternative pathways of metabolism of these substrates are also inhibited by coadministered drugs. The risk is theoretically greater with clozapine, haloperidol, and olanzapine, because their CYP1A2-mediated metabolism is also inhibited by SSRIs	Warn patients to report ↑ side effects of these drugs, and consider reducing the dose of the antipsychotic
PIMOZIDE	SERTRALINE	↑ Plasma concentrations of pimozide	Haloperidol is metabolized mainly by CYP3A4 and CYP2D6-TCAs inhibit CYP2D6	Warn patients to report early side effects of haloperidol (e.g., dizziness, tremors, palpitations). Particular care in the elderly. Be aware of CYP2D6 polymorphisms. See POLYMORPHISMS and ETHNICITY
HALOPERIDOL	TCAs	Possible ↑ haloperidol levels	Inhibition of CYP2D6- and CYP1A2-mediated metabolism of thioridazine	Warn patients to report ↑ side effects of these drugs
HALOPERIDOL	VENLAFAXINE	↑ Haloperidol levels	Inhibited metabolism	Avoid coadministration
ANTIPSYCHOTICS	**ANTIDIABETIC DRUGS**			
CLOZAPINE	ANTIDIABETIC DRUGS	May cause ↑ blood sugar and loss of control of blood sugar	Clozapine can cause resistance to the action of insulin	Watch for diabetes mellitus in patients on long-term clozapine treatment
OLANZAPINE, PHENOTHIAZINES	REPAGLINIDE	↓ Hypoglycemic effect	Antagonistic effect	Higher doses of repaglinide needed
PHENOTHIAZINES	METFORMIN	May ↑ blood sugar-lowering effect and risk of hypoglycemic episodes. Likely to occur with doses exceeding 100 mg/day	Phenothiazines such as chlorpromazine inhibit the release of epinephrine and ↑ risk of hypoglycemia. May inhibit the release of insulin	Chlorpromazine is nearly always used in the long term. Watch for and warn patients about symptoms of hypoglycemia. ➢ ***For signs and symptoms of hypoglycemia, see Clinical Features of Some Adverse Drug Interactions, Hypoglycemia***

(*Continued*)

Primary Drug	Secondary Drug	Effect	Mechanism	Precautions
ANTIPSYCHOTICS				
PHENOTHIAZINES	SULFONYLUREAS	May ↑ blood sugar-lowering effect and risk of hypoglycemic episodes. Likely to occur with doses exceeding 100 mg/day	Phenothiazines such as chlorpromazine inhibit the release of epinephrine and ↑ risk of hypoglycemia. May inhibit the release of insulin, which is the mechanism by which sulfonylureas act	Chlorpromazine is nearly always used in the long term. Watch for and warn patients about symptoms of hypoglycemia. ➢ ***For signs and symptoms of hypoglycemia, see Clinical Features of Some Adverse Drug Interactions, Hypoglycemia***
RISPERIDONE	NATEGLINIDE, REPAGLINIDE	↑ Risk of hypoglycemic episodes	Attributed to a synergistic effect	Watch for and warn patients about symptoms of hypoglycemia. ➢ ***For signs and symptoms of hypoglycemia, see Clinical Features of Some Adverse Drug Interactions, Hypoglycemia***
PIMOZIDE	ANTIEMETICS—APREPITANT	↑ Aprepitant levels	Inhibition of metabolism	Avoid coadministration (manufacturers' recommendation)
ANTIPSYCHOTICS	**ANTIEPILEPTICS**			
ANTIPSYCHOTICS	ANTIEPILEPTICS	↓ Efficacy of antiepileptics	Antipsychotics lower seizure threshold	Watch for ↑ fit frequency; warn patients of this risk when starting antipsychotics, and take suitable precautions. Consider increasing the dose of antiepileptic
ANTIPSYCHOTICS	BARBITURATES	↓ Levels of arpiprazole, haloperidol, clozapine, quetiapine	Induction of metabolism	Watch for poor response to these antipsychotics, and consider increasing the dose
CHLORPROMAZINE	PHENOBARBITAL	↓ Levels of both drugs	Induction of metabolism	Watch for poor response to these drugs, and consider increasing the dose
ANTIPSYCHOTICS	CARBAMAZEPINE	↓ Levels of arpiprazole, clozapine, haloperidol, olanzapine, quetiapine, risperidone, and sertindole	Induction of metabolism	Watch for poor response to these antipsychotics, and consider increasing the dose
ANTIPSYCHOTICS	PHENYTOIN	↓ Levels of arpiprazole, clozapine, quetiapine, sertindole	Induction of metabolism	Watch for poor response to these antipsychotics, and consider increasing the dose

(*Continued*)

DRUGS ACTING ON THE CENTRAL NERVOUS SYSTEM ANTIPSYCHOTICS

DRUGS ACTING ON THE CENTRAL NERVOUS SYSTEM ANTIPSYCHOTICS

Primary Drug	Secondary Drug	Effect	Mechanism	Precautions
ANTIPSYCHOTICS				
OLANZAPINE	VALPROATE	Risk of bone marrow toxicity	Additive effect	Monitor FBC closely; warn patients to report sore throat, fevers, etc.
ANTIPSYCHOTICS	**ANTIFUNGALS ≻ *QT-PROLONGING DRUGS, ABOVE***			
ARIPIPRAZOLE	ITRACONAZOLE, KETOCONAZOLE	↑ Aripiprazole levels	Inhibition of metabolism	↓ Dose of aripiprazole
ANTIPSYCHOTICS	**ANTIHYPERTENSIVES AND HEART FAILURE DRUGS**			
ANTIPSYCHOTICS	ANTIHYPERTENSIVES AND HEART FAILURE DRUGS	↑ Hypotensive effect	Dose-related ↓ BP (due to vasodilatation) is a side-effect of most antipsychotics, particularly phenothiazines	Monitor BP closely, especially during initiation of treatment. Warn patients to report symptoms of hypotension (light-headedness, dizziness on standing, etc.)
ANTIPSYCHOTICS	VASODILATOR ANTIHYPERTENSIVES	Risk of hyperglycemia when diazoxide is coadministered with chlorpromazine	Additive effect; both drugs have a hyperglycemic effect	Monitor blood glucose closely, particularly with diabetes
HALOPERIDOL	ADRENERGIC NEURONE BLOCKERS	↓ Hypotensive effect	Haloperidol blocks the uptake of guanethidine by adrenergic neurons	Monitor BP at least weekly until stable
HALOPERIDOL	CENTRALLY ACTING ANTIHYPERTENSIVES	Case reports of sedation or confusion on initiating coadministration of haloperidol and methyldopa	Uncertain; possible additive effect	Watch for excess sedation when starting therapy
PHENOTHIAZINES	ADRENERGIC NEURON BLOCKERS	Variable effect: some cases of ↑ hypotensive effect; other cases where hypotensive effects ↓ with higher doses (>100 mg) of chlorpromazine	Additive hypotensive effect. Phenothiazines cause vasodilatation; however, chlorpromazine blocks the uptake of guanethidine by adrenergic neurons	Monitor BP at least weekly until stable. Warn patients to report symptoms of hypotension (light-headedness, dizziness on standing, etc.)
ANTIPSYCHOTICS	**ANTIOBESITY DRUGS**			
ANTIPSYCHOTICS—FLUPHENAZINE, HALOPERIDOL, ILOPERIDONE	LORCASERIN	↑ Blood concentrations of lorcaserin	Inhibition of CYP2D6-mediated metabolism	Monitor PR and BP closely until stable

(Continued)

Primary Drug	Secondary Drug	Effect	Mechanism	Precautions
ANTIPSYCHOTICS				
ANTIPSYCHOTICS	ANTIOBESITY—SIBUTRAMINE	Risk of headache, agitation, fits	Additive effect	Avoid coadministration
ANTIPSYCHOTICS	**ANTI-PARKINSON'S DRUGS**			
ANTIPSYCHOTICS	AMANTADINE	↑ Extrapyramidal side effects	Additive effects	Use with caution, avoid in patients <20 years
ANTIPSYCHOTICS	DOPAMINERGICS	↓ Efficacy of dopaminergics	Antipsychotics may cause extrapyramidal side effects, which oppose the effect of anti-Parkinson's drugs. The atypical antipsychotics cause less effect than the older drugs	Caution with coadministration; consider using atypical antipsychotics, and use antimuscarinic drugs if extrapyramidal symptoms occur. Manufacturers recommend avoiding coadministration of amisulpride with levodopa, and coadministration of antipsychotics with pramipexole, ropinirole, and rotigotine. Clozapine can be coadministered with co-careldopa and pergolide
ANTIPSYCHOTICS	**ANTIPSYCHOTICS ➢ *QT-Prolonging Drugs, above***			
CLOZAPINE	DEPOT ANTIPSYCHOTICS	Risk of prolonged bone marrow suppression	Additive effects	Avoid coadministration
ANTIPSYCHOTICS	**ANTIVIRALS**			
PIMOZIDE	COBICISTAT	↑ Plasma levels	Inhibition of metabolism via CYP3A	Avoid coadministration
RISPERIDONE	COBICISTAT	Possible ↑ plasma levels	Inhibition of metabolism via CYP3A	Dose adjustment may be required
ARIPIPRAZOLE	NNRTIs	↓ Efficacy of aripiprazole	↑ CYP3A4-mediated metabolism of aripiprazole	Monitor patient closely, and ↑ dose of aripiprazole as necessary
PIMOZIDE	NNRTIs	Possible ↑ efficacy and ↑ adverse effects, e.g., ventricular arrhythmias of pimozide	↓ CYP3A4-mediated metabolism of pimozide	Avoid coadministration

(*Continued*)

DRUGS ACTING ON THE CENTRAL NERVOUS SYSTEM ANTIPSYCHOTICS

DRUGS ACTING ON THE CENTRAL NERVOUS SYSTEM ANTIPSYCHOTICS

Primary Drug	Secondary Drug	Effect	Mechanism	Precautions
ANTIPSYCHOTICS				
ARIPIPRAZOLE, HALOPERIDOL, CLOZAPINE, PIMOZIDE, RISPERIDONE, SERTINDOLE	PROTEASE INHIBITORS	Possibly ↑ levels of antipsychotic	Inhibition of CYP3A4- and/or CYP2D6-mediated metabolism	Avoid coadministration of clozapine with ritonavir, and pimozide or sertindole with protease inhibitors. Use other antipsychotics with caution as ↓ dose may be required; with risperidone, watch closely for extrapyramidal side effects and neuroepileptic malignant syndrome
OLANZAPINE	PROTEASE INHIBITORS	Possibly ↓ efficacy of olanzapine when coingested with ritonavir (with or without lopinavir)	Possibly ↑ metabolism via CYP1A2 and glucuronyl transferases	Monitor clinical response; ↑ dose as necessary
ANTIPSYCHOTICS	**ANXIOLYTICS AND HYPNOTICS**			
ANTIPSYCHOTICS	BZDs	Risk of excessive sedation. This effect seems to be particularly marked with clozapine	Additive effect	Warn patients and carers of this effect. Particular care should be exercised when parenteral doses are given, e.g., for emergency sedation
ANTIPSYCHOTICS	SODIUM OXYBATE	Risk CNS depression—coma, respiratory depression	Additive depression of CNS	Avoid coadministration
CHLORPROMAZINE	ZOLPIDEM, ZOPICLONE	Risk of sedation	Additive effect; uncertain why this occurs more with chlorpromazine	Warn patients of this effect
ANTIPSYCHOTICS	**BETA-BLOCKERS**			
ANTIPSYCHOTICS	BETA-BLOCKERS	↑ Hypotensive effect	Dose-related ↓ BP (due to vasodilatation) is a side-effect of most antipsychotics, particularly phenothiazines	Monitor BP at least weekly until stable, especially during initiation of treatment. Warn patients to report symptoms of hypotension (light-headedness, dizziness on standing, etc.)
CHLORPROMAZINE, HALOPERIDOL	PROPANOLOL, TIMOLOL	↑ Plasma concentrations and efficacy of both chlorpromazine and propranolol during coadministration	Propanolol and chlorpromazine mutually inhibit each other's hepatic metabolism. Haloperidol inhibits CYP2D6-mediated metabolism of propanolol and timolol	Watch for toxic effects of chlorpromazine and propranolol; ↓ doses accordingly

(*Continued*)

Primary Drug	Secondary Drug	Effect	Mechanism	Precautions
ANTIPSYCHOTICS				
CLOZAPINE	CAFFEINE	↑ Clozapine levels	Possibly ↑ metabolism via CYP1A2	Warn patients to avoid wide variations in caffeine intake once established on clozapine
ANTIPSYCHOTICS	**CALCIUM CHANNEL BLOCKERS**			
ANTIPSYCHOTICS	CALCIUM CHANNEL BLOCKERS	↑ Antihypertensive effect	Dose-related ↓ BP (due to vasodilatation) is a side-effect of most antipsychotics, particularly phenothiazines	Monitor BP, especially during initiation of treatment. Warn patients to report symptoms of hypotension (light-headedness, dizziness on standing, etc.)
CLOZAPINE	CALCIUM CHANNEL BLOCKERS	Plasma concentrations of clozapine may be ↑ by diltiazem and verapamil	Diltiazem and verapamil inhibit CYP1A2-mediated metabolism of clozapine	Watch for side effects of clozapine
SERTINDOLE	CALCIUM CHANNEL BLOCKERS	Plasma concentrations of sertindole are ↑ by diltiazem and verapamil	Diltiazem and verapamil inhibit CYP3A4-mediated metabolism of sertindole	Avoid coadministration; raised sertindole concentrations are associated with ↑ risk of prolonged QT interval and therefore ventricular arrhythmias, particularly torsades de pointes
CLOZAPINE, HALOPERIDOL, OLANZAPINE	CNS STIMULANTS—MODAFINIL	May cause ↓ plasma concentrations of these substrates if CYP1A2 is the predominant metabolic pathway and alternative metabolic pathways are either genetically deficient or affected	Modafinil is a moderate inducer of CYP1A2 in a concentration-dependent manner	Monitor efficacy of antipsychotics and consider ↑ of dose
PROCHLOR-PERAZINE	DEFEROXAMINE	Reports of coma when prochlorperazine is given with deferoxamine	Uncertain	Avoid coadministration
ATYPICALS, PHENOTHIAZINES PIMOZIDE	DIURETICS—LOOP AND THIAZIDES	Risk of arrhythmias	Cardiac toxicity directly related to hypokalemia	Monitor potassium levels every 4–6 weeks until stable, then at least annually

(*Continued*)

Primary Drug	Secondary Drug	Effect	Mechanism	Precautions
ANTIPSYCHOTICS				
ANTIPSYCHOTICS	**DRUG DEPENDENCE THERAPIES**			
ANTIPSYCHOTICS	BUPROPION	↑ Risk of seizures. This risk is marked in elderly people, in patients with a history of seizures, with addiction to opiates/cocaine/stimulants, and in diabetics treated with oral hypoglycemics or insulin	Bupropion is associated with a dose-related risk of seizures. These drugs, which lower seizure threshold, are individually epileptogenic. Additive effects occur when they are combined	Extreme caution. The dose of bupropion should not exceed 450 mg/day (or 150 mg/day in patients with severe hepatic cirrhosis)
CHLORPROMAZINE, PERPHENAZINE, RISPERIDONE	BUPROPION	↑ Plasma concentrations of these substrates with risk of toxic effects	Bupropion and its metabolite hydroxybupropion inhibit CYP2D6	Initiate therapy of these drugs at the lowest effective dose
CHLORPROMAZINE, CLOZAPINE, HALOPERIDOL, OLANZAPINE	BUPROPION	↑ Plasma concentrations of these drugs with risk of toxic/adverse effects	Smoking induces mainly CYP1A2 and CYP2E1. Thus, deinduction takes place following cessation of smoking	Be aware and watch for early features of toxicity. Consider reducing the dose
CHLORPROMAZINE, PERPHENAZINE	ELIGLUSTAT	↑ Levels of these antipsychotics	Inhibition of CYP2D6-mediated metabolism	Reduce doses of these antipsychotics; titrate to effect
ANTIPSYCHOTICS—PIMOZIDE	GRAPEFRUIT JUICE	Possibly ↑ efficacy and ↑ adverse effects	Not evaluated	Avoid concomitant use
ANTIPSYCHOTICS—ASENAPINE, CHLORPROMAZINE, CLOZAPINE, HALOPERIDOL, OLANZAPINE, PERPHENAZINE, RISPERIDONE, SERTINDOLE, THIORIDAZINE, ZUCLOPENTHIXOL	H2 RECEPTOR BLOCKERS—CIMETIDINE	Cimetidine is an inhibitor of CYP3A4 (sertindole, haloperidol, risperidone); CYP2D6 (chlorpromazine, risperidone, zuclopenthixol, thioridazine, perphenazine); and CYP1A2 (asenapine, clozapine, olanzapine, sertindole, haloperidol)	Due to inhibition of metabolism by cimetidine	Cimetidine is an inhibitor of CYP3A4 (sertindole, haloperidol, risperidone); CYP2D6 (chlorpromazine, risperidone, zuclopenthixol, thioridazine, perphenazine); and CYP1A2 (asenapine, clozapine, olanzapine, sertindole, haloperidol). Avoid concomitant use. Choose alternative acid suppression, nizatidine, famotidine, or rabeprazole that are likely not to interact significantly
ANTIPSYCHOTICS	IVABRADINE	Risk of arrhythmias with pimozide and sertindole	Additive effect	Monitor ECG closely

(Continued)

Primary Drug	Secondary Drug	Effect	Mechanism	Precautions
ANTIPSYCHOTICS				
THIORIDAZINE	MIRABEGRON	↑ Thioridazine levels	Mirabegron inhibits CYP2D6. These drugs have a narrow therapeutic index	Manufacturer advises caution in coadministration. Warn patients to report symptoms such as drowsiness or dizziness
ANTIPSYCHOTICS	**NITRATES**			
ANTIPSYCHOTICS	NITRATES	↑ Hypotensive effect	Additive hypotensive effect. Aldesleukin causes ↓ vascular resistance and ↑ capillary permeability	Monitor BP at least weekly until stable. Warn patients to report symptoms of hypotension (light-headedness, dizziness on standing, etc.)
ANTIPSYCHOTICS—PHENOTHIAZINE, CLOZAPINE, PIMOZIDE	NITRATES	1. ↑ Risk of antimuscarinic side effects when isosorbide dinitrate is coadministered with these drugs 2. ↓ Efficacy of sublingual nitrate tablets	1. Additive effect; both of these drugs cause antimuscarinic side effects. 2. Antimuscarinic effects ↓ saliva production, which ↓ dissolution of the tablet	1. Warn patient of these effects 2. Consider changing the formulation to a sublingual nitrate spray
ANTIPSYCHOTICS	POTASSIUM CHANNEL ACTIVATORS	↑ Hypotensive effect	Additive effect	Monitor BP closely
CLOZAPINE	PROTON PUMP INHIBITORS—OMEPRAZOLE	Possible ↓ efficacy of clozapine	↑ Metabolism via CYP1A2	Clinical significance unclear; monitor more closely
HALOPERIDOL	SODIUM PHENYLBUTYRATE	Possibly ↓ efficacy of sodium phenylbutyrate	These drugs are associated with ↑ ammonia levels	Avoid coadministration
CLOZAPINE	STRONTIUM RANELATE	Increased risk of bone marrow toxicity	Uncertain	Monitor FBC closely
SULPIRIDE	SUCRALFATE	↓ Sulpiride levels	↓ Absorption of sulpiride	Give sulpiride at least 2 h after sucralfate
ANTIPSYCHOTICS	**SYMPATHOMIMETICS**			
ANTIPSYCHOTICS	SYMPATHOMIMETICS	Hypertensive effect of sympathomimetics are antagonized by antipsychotics	Dose-related ↓ BP (due to vasodilatation) is a side effect of most antipsychotics, particularly phenothiazines	Monitor BP closely

(*Continued*)

DRUGS ACTING ON THE CENTRAL NERVOUS SYSTEM ANTIPSYCHOTICS
DRUGS ACTING ON THE CENTRAL NERVOUS SYSTEM ANTIPSYCHOTICS

Primary Drug	Secondary Drug	Effect	Mechanism	Precautions
ANTIPSYCHOTICS				
ANTIPSYCHOTICS	INDIRECT	1. Case reports paralytic ileus with trifluoperazine and methylphenidate 2. Case report of acute dystonias with haloperidol and dexamfetamine 3. ↓ Efficacy of chlorpromazine when dexamfetamine is added	1. Additive anticholinergic effect 2. Uncertain; possibly due to ↑ dopamine release 3. Uncertain	1. Watch for signs of altered bowel habit 2. Warn patients of this rare interaction 3. Avoid coadministration
ANTIPSYCHOTICS	TETRABENAZINE	Case report of extrapyramidal symptoms when tetrabenazine is given with chlorpromazine	Uncertain	Warn patients to report any extrapyramidal symptoms

Primary Drug	Secondary Drug	Effect	Mechanism	Precautions
ANXIOLYTICS AND HYPNOTICS				
ALL	CNS DEPRESSANTS—INCLUDING ALCOHOL	↑ Sedation	Additive effect	Warn patients to be aware of this added effect
ALL	DRUGS WITH HYPOTENSIVE EFFECTS	↑ Hypotensive effect	Additive hypotensive effect	Monitor BP at least weekly until stable. Warn patients to report symptoms of hypotension (light-headedness, dizziness on standing, etc.)
BARBITURATES ➢ *Antiepileptics, above*				
BENZODIAZEPINES				
BZDs	**ANALGESICS**			
BZDs	NSAIDs	Parenteral diclofenac may ↓ dose of midazolam needed to produce sedation	Unknown	Titrate the dose of midazolam carefully

(*Continued*)

Primary Drug	Secondary Drug	Effect	Mechanism	Precautions
ANXIOLYTICS AND HYPNOTICS				
BZDs	OPIOIDs	1. ↑ Sedation with BZDs 2. Respiratory depressant effect of morphine is antagonized by lorazepam	1. Additive effect; both drugs are sedatives 2. Uncertain	1. Closely monitor vital signs during coadministration 2. May be considered to be beneficial if the combination is used for sedation for painful procedures
BZDs	**ANTIBIOTICS**			
DIAZEPAM	ISONIAZID	↑ Diazepam levels	Inhibited metabolism	Watch for excessive sedation; consider reducing the dose of diazepam
MIDAZOLAM, TRIAZOLAM, POSSIBLY ALPRAZOLAM	MACROLIDES—ERYTHROMYCIN, CLARITHROMYCIN, TELITHROMYCIN	↑ BZD levels	Inhibition of CYP3A4-mediated metabolism	↓ Dose of BZD by 50%; warn patients not to perform skilled tasks such as driving for at least 10 h after the dose of BZD
MIDAZOLAM	QUINUPRISTIN/ DALFOPRISTIN	↑ Midazolam levels	Inhibited metabolism	Watch for excessive sedation; consider reducing the dose of midazolam
BZDs, NOT LORAZEPAM, OXAZEPAM, TEMAZEPAM	RIFAMPICIN	↓ BZD levels	Induction of CYP3A4-mediated metabolism	Watch for poor response to these BZDs; consider increasing the dose, e.g., diazepam or nitrazepam 2–3-fold
BZDs	**ANTICANCER AND IMMUNOMODULATING DRUGS**			
TOFISOPAM	BOSUTINIB	Increased bosutinib levels	CYP3A inhibition	Manufacturer advises avoid concurrent use. If not possible, interruption of therapy or dose reduction should be considered
ALPRAZOLAM, MIDAZOLAM, DIAZEPAM	CICLOSPORIN	Likely ↑ plasma concentrations and risk of ↑ sedation	These BZDs are metabolized primarily by CYP3A4, which is inhibited moderately by ciclosporin	Warn patients about ↑ sedation. Consider using alternative drugs, e.g., flurazepam. Warn about activities requiring attention. ➢ ***For signs and symptoms of CNS depression, see Clinical Features of Some Adverse Drug Interactions, Central Nervous SystemDepression***

(*Continued*)

Primary Drug	Secondary Drug	Effect	Mechanism	Precautions
ANXIOLYTICS AND HYPNOTICS				
MIDAZOLAM	CRIZOTINIB	Midazolam levels increased	CYP3A4 inhibition	Closer monitoring and possible dose reduction of midazolam with concurrent use
DIAZEPAM, MIDAZOLAM	DABRAFENIB	Possible reduced levels of CYP3A4/CYP2Cs/CYP2B6 substrates. Level of reduction may vary	Dabrafenib induces CYP3A4/CYP2Cs/CYP2B6	Monitor closely or avoid concurrent use
MIDAZOLAM	LAPATINIB	Midazolam levels slightly increased	CYP3A4 inhibition	Caution with concurrent use
MIDAZOLAM	NILOTINIB	Midazolam levels slightly increased	CYP3A4 inhibition	Caution with concurrent use
MIDAZOLAM	PAZOPANIB	Midazolam levels slightly increased	CYP3A4 inhibition	Caution with concurrent use
ANXIOLYTICS AND HYPNOTICS	THALIDOMIDE	Increased sedation	Additive	Caution with concurrent use
BZDs	**ANTIDEPRESSANTS**			
BZDs	MAOIs	Additive depression of CNS ranging from drowsiness to coma and respiratory depression	Synergistic depressant effects on CNS function	Necessary to warn patients, particularly regarding activities that require attention, e.g., driving or using machinery and equipment that could cause self-harm
BZDs	MIRTAZAPINE	↑ Sedation	Additive effect	Warn patients about this effect
BZDs	TCAs	Possible ↑ plasma concentrations of diazepam	Inhibition of CYP2C19-mediated metabolism of diazepam. The clinical significance of this depends upon whether diazepam's alternative pathways of metabolism are also inhibited by coadministered drugs	Watch for excessive sedation with diazepam

(*Continued*)

Primary Drug	Secondary Drug	Effect	Mechanism	Precautions
ANXIOLYTICS AND HYPNOTICS				
ALPRAZOLAM, DIAZEPAM, MIDAZOLAM	SSRIs—FLUOXETINE, FLUVOXAMINE, PAROXETINE	↑ In plasma concentrations of these BZDs. Likely ↑ sedation and interference with psychomotor activity	Alprazolam, diazepam, and midazolam are subject to metabolism by CYP3A4. Fluvoxamine, fluoxetine, and possibly paroxetine are inhibitors of CYP3A4; sertraline is a weak inhibitor	Warn patients about risks associated with activities that require alertness. Consider use of alternatives such as oxazepam, lorazepam, and temazepam, which are metabolized by glucuronidation. ➢ ***For signs and symptoms of CNS depression, see Clinical Features of Some Adverse Drug Interactions, Central Nervous System Depression***
ANXIOLYTICS AND HYPNOTICS	TRYPTOPHAN	Risk of sedation	Additive effect	Warn patient regarding risks when driving, using machinery, etc.
MIDAZOLAM	ANTIDIABETIC DRUGS—THIAZOLIDINEDIONES	Reduction in AUC of midazolam (syrup)	Possibly related to metabolism using the same CYP3A4 pathway	Midazolam dose may need compensatory increase when coadministered
CLONAZEPAM	ANTIEPILEPTICS—BARBITURATES, CARBAMAZEPINE, PHENYTOIN	↓ Levels of these antiepileptics	Induction of metabolism	Watch for poor response to these antiepileptics
ALPRAZOLAM, CHLORDIAZE-POXIDE, DIAZEPAM, LORAZEPAM, MIDAZOLAM, OXAZEPAM, TEMAZEPAM	ANTIFUNGALS—ITRACONAZOLE, KETOCONAZOLE, VORICONAZOLE	↑ Plasma concentrations of these BZDs with ↑ risk of adverse effects. These risks are greater following intravenous administration of midazolam compared with oral midazolam	Itraconazole and ketoconazole are potent inhibitors of phase I metabolism (oxidation and functionalization) of these BZDs by CYP3A4. In addition, the more significant ↑ in plasma concentrations following oral midazolam—15 times compared with 5 times following intravenous use—indicates that the inhibition of Pgp by ketoconazole is important following oral administration	Aim to avoid coadministration. If coadministration is necessary, always start with ↓ dose and monitor the effects closely. Consider the use of alternative BZDs, which predominantly undergo phase II metabolism by glucuronidation, e.g., flurazepam, quazepam. Fluconazole and posaconazole are unlikely to cause this interaction
NITRAZEPAM	ANTIGOUT—PROBENECID	Possibly ↑ nitrazepam levels	Possibly ↓ renal excretion of nitrazepam	Consider ↓ dose of nitrazepam Watch for excessive sedation

(*Continued*)

DRUGS ACTING ON THE CENTRAL NERVOUS SYSTEM ANXIOLYTICS AND HYPNOTICS Benzodiazepines

Primary Drug	Secondary Drug	Effect	Mechanism	Precautions
ANXIOLYTICS AND HYPNOTICS				
BZDs	ANTIHYPERTENSIVES AND HEART FAILURE DRUGS—CLONIDINE AND MOXONIDINE	Clonidine and moxonidine may exacerbate the sedative effects of BZDs, particularly during initiation of therapy	Uncertain	Warn patients of this effect and advise them to avoid driving or operating machinery if they suffer from sedation
BZDs	ANTI-PARKINSON'S DRUGS—LEVODOPA	Risk of ↓ effect of levodopa	Uncertain	Watch for poor response to levodopa and consider increasing its dose. If severe antagonism is the effect, stop BZD
BZDs	ANTIPLATELET AGENTS—ASPIRIN	↓ Requirements of midazolam when aspirin (1 g) is coadministered	Uncertain at present	Be aware of possible ↓ dose requirements for midazolam
BZDs	ANTIPSYCHOTICS	Risk of excessive sedation. This effect seems to be particularly marked with clozapine	Additive effect	Warn patients and carers of this effect. Particular care should be exercised when parenteral doses are given, e.g., for emergency sedation
BZDs	**ANTIVIRALS**			
MIDAZOLAM (PO), TRIAZOLAM (PO)	COBICISTAT	↑ Plasma levels	Inhibition of metabolism via CYP3A	Avoid coadministration. For other sedatives or hypnotics, monitor closely for increased sedation, dose reduction may be required
DIAZEPAM, MIDAZOLAM	NNRTIs—EFAVIRENZ	↑ Efficacy and ↑ adverse effects, e.g., prolonged sedation	↓ CYP3A4-mediated metabolism of diazepam and midazolam	1. Monitor more closely, especially sedation levels. May need ↓ dose of diazepam or alteration of timing of dose 2. Avoid coadministration with midazolam
BZDs	NUCLEOSIDE REVERSE TRANSCRIPTASE INHIBITORS—ZIDOVUDINE	↑ Adverse effects including ↑ Incidence of headaches when oxazepam is coadministered with zidovudine	Uncertain	Monitor closely

(*Continued*)

Primary Drug	Secondary Drug	Effect	Mechanism	Precautions
ANXIOLYTICS AND HYPNOTICS				
BZDs	PROTEASE INHIBITORS	↑ Adverse effects, e.g., prolonged sedation	Inhibition of CYP3A4-mediated metabolism of BZDs	Avoid coadministration of protease inhibitors and oral midazolam or triazolam, and alprazolam with indinavir. For IV midazolam consider a dose reduction and intensive monitoring, for other combinations, watch closely for ↑ sedation; ↓ dose of sedative as necessary. Some recommend considering substituting long-acting for shorter-acting BZDs with less active metabolites (e.g., lorazepam for diazepam) or less CYP3A4-dependent metabolism
BZDs	ANXIOLYTICS AND HYPNOTICS—SODIUM OXYBATE	Risk of CNS depression—coma, respiratory depression	Additive depression of CNS	Avoid coadministration. Caution even with relatively nonsedating antihistamines (cetirizine, desloratadine, fexofenadine, levocetirizine, loratadine, mizolastine) as they can impair the performance of skilled tasks
BZDs	**BETA-BLOCKERS**			
BZDs	BETA-BLOCKERS	↑ Hypotensive effect	Additive hypotensive effect; anxiolytics and hypnotics can cause postural ↓ BP	Watch for ↓ BP. Monitor BP at least weekly until stable. Warn patients to report symptoms of hypotension (light-headedness, dizziness on standing, etc.)
DIAZEPAM	BETA-BLOCKERS	May occasionally cause ↑ sedation during metoprolol and propranolol therapy	Propranolol and metoprolol inhibit the metabolism of diazepam	Warn patients about ↑ sedation
BZDs	BRONCHODILATORS—THEOPHYLLINE	↓ Therapeutic effect of BZDs	BZDs ↑ CNS concentrations of adenosine, a potent CNS depressant, while theophylline blocks adenosine receptors	Larger doses of diazepam are required to produce the desired therapeutic effects such as sedation. Discontinuation of theophylline without ↓ dose of BZD ↑ risk of sedation and of respiratory depression

(*Continued*)

Primary Drug	Secondary Drug	Effect	Mechanism	Precautions
ANXIOLYTICS AND HYPNOTICS				
BZDs	CALCIUM CHANNEL BLOCKERS—DILTIAZEM, VERAPAMIL	Plasma concentrations of midazolam and triazolam are ↑ by diltiazem and verapamil	Diltiazem and verapamil inhibit CYP3A4-mediated metabolism of midazolam and triazolam	↓ Dose of BZD by 50% in patients on calcium channel blockers; warn patients not to perform skilled tasks such as driving for at least 10 h after the dose of BZD
ALPRAZOLAM, DIAZEPAM	CARDIAC GLYCOSIDES—DIGOXIN	Alprazolam and possibly diazepam may ↑ digoxin levels, particularly in patients above 65	Uncertain at present; possibly ↓ renal excretion of digoxin	Monitor digoxin levels; watch for digoxin toxicity
BZDs	**CNS STIMULANTS**			
DIAZEPAM	MODAFINIL	May cause moderate ↑ plasma concentrations of diazepam	Modafinil is a reversible inhibitor of CYP2C19 when used in therapeutic doses	Be aware
TRIAZOLAM	MODAFINIL	May ↓ triazolam levels	Uncertain	Be aware
BZDs	**DRUG DEPENDENCE THERAPIES**			
BZDs	DISULFIRAM	↑ BZDs levels	Inhibited metabolism	Warn patients of risk of excessive sedation
BZDs	LOFEXIDINE	↑ Sedation	Additive effect	Warn patients of risk of excessive sedation
ALPRAZOLAM, DIAZEPAM, MIDAZOLAM—ORAL	GRAPEFRUIT JUICE	Possibly ↑ efficacy and ↑ adverse effects, e.g., sedation, CNS depression	Possibly ↑ bioavailability, ↓ presystemic metabolism. Constituents of grapefruit juice irreversibly inhibit intestinal CYP3A4. Transport via Pgp and MRP-2 efflux pumps is also inhibited	Avoid concomitant use. Be particularly vigilant in elderly patients or those with impaired liver function. Consider alternative, e.g., temazepam
BZDs (NOT LORAZEPAM OR TEMAZEPAM)	H2 RECEPTOR BLOCKERS—CIMETIDINE, RANITIDINE	↑ Efficacy and adverse effects of BZD, e.g., sedation	Cimetidine is an inhibitor of CYP3A4, CYP2D6, CYP2C19, and CYP1A2	Not clinically significant for most patients. Conflicting information for some BZDs. Monitor more closely, and ↓ dose if necessary
MIDAZOLAM	IVACAFTOR	Possible ↑ midazolam levels	Ivacaftor possibly inhibits CYP3A4-mediated metabolism of midazolam	Monitor levels of sedation closely

(*Continued*)

Primary Drug	Secondary Drug	Effect	Mechanism	Precautions
ANXIOLYTICS AND HYPNOTICS				
BZDs	**MUSCLE RELAXANTS**			
BZDs	BACLOFEN, TIZANIDINE	↑ Hypotensive effect	Additive hypotensive effect	Monitor BP at least weekly until stable. Warn patients to report symptoms of hypotension (light-headedness, dizziness on standing, etc.)
BZDs	BACLOFEN, METHOCARBAMOL, TIZANIDINE	↑ Sedation	Additive effect	Warn patients
BZDs	NITRATES	↑ Hypotensive effect	Additive hypotensive effect	Monitor BP at least weekly until stable. Warn patients to report symptoms of hypotension (light-headedness, dizziness on standing, etc.)
BZDs	ESTROGENS, PROGESTERONES	Reports of breakthrough bleeding when BZDs are coadministered with oral contraceptives	Uncertain	The clinical significance is uncertain. It would seem to be wise to advise patients to use an alternative form of contraception during and for 1 month after stopping BZDs
BZDs	**PERIPHERAL VASODILATORS**			
BZDs	CILOSTAZOL	Midazolam ↑ cilostazol levels	Midazolam inhibits CYP3A4-mediated metabolism of cilastazol	Avoid coadministration
BZDs	MOXISYLYTE	↑ Hypotensive effect	Additive hypotensive effect	Monitor BP at least weekly until stable. Warn patients to report symptoms of hypotension (light-headedness, dizziness on standing, etc.)
BZDs	POTASSIUM CHANNEL ACTIVATORS	↑ Hypotensive effect	Additive effect	Monitor BP closely
BZDs	PROTON PUMP INHIBITORS—OMEPRAZOLE/ESOMEPRAZOLE	↑ Efficacy and adverse effects, e.g., prolonged sedation	Inhibition of metabolism via CYP450 (some show competitive inhibition via CYP2C19)	Monitor for ↑ side effects, and ↓ dose as necessary. Likely to delay recovery after procedures for which BZDs have been used. Consider alternative proton pump inhibitor, e.g., lansoprazole or pantoprazole

(*Continued*)

Primary Drug	Secondary Drug	Effect	Mechanism	Precautions
ANXIOLYTICS AND HYPNOTICS				
BUSPIRONE				
BUSPIRONE	**ANTIBIOTICS**			
BUSPIRONE	MACROLIDES	↑ Buspirone levels	Inhibition of CYP3A4-mediated metabolism	Warn patients to be aware of additional sedation
BUSPIRONE	RIFAMPICIN	↓ Buspirone levels	Induction of CYP3A4-mediated metabolism	Watch for poor response to buspirone; consider increasing the dose
BUSPIRONE	ANTICANCER AND IMMUNOMODULATING DRUGS—PROCARBAZINE	Risk of elevation of blood pressure	Additive effect; buspirone acts at serotonin receptors; procarbazine inhibits the breakdown of sympathomimetics	Avoid concurrent use
BUSPIRONE	ANTIDEPRESSANTS—MAOIs	Cases of hypertension	Uncertain	Monitor BP closely
BUSPIRONE	ANTIFUNGALS—ITRACONAZOLE, KETOCONAZOLE	↑ Buspirone levels	Inhibition of CYP3A4-mediated metabolism	Warn patients to be aware of additional sedation
BUSPIRONE	**ANTIVIRALS**			
BUSPIRONE	COBICISTAT	Possible ↑ plasma levels of buspirone	Inhibition of metabolism via CYP3A	Use with caution, a reduced dose of buspirone may be required
BUSPIRONE	PROTEASE INHIBITORS	↑ Adverse effects, e.g., prolonged sedation	Inhibition of CYP3A4-mediated metabolism of buspirone	Warn patients of ↑ sedation and to avoid driving and using equipment that may cause self-harm
BUSPIRONE	ANXIOLYTICS AND HYPNOTICS—SODIUM OXYBATE	Risk of CNS depression—coma, respiratory depression	Additive depression of CNS	Avoid coadministration
BUSPIRONE	CALCIUM CHANNEL BLOCKERS	Plasma concentrations of buspirone are ↑ by diltiazem and verapamil	Diltiazem and verapamil inhibit CYP3A4-mediated metabolism of buspirone	Start buspirone at a lower dose (2.5 mg twice a day is suggested by the manufacturers) in patients on calcium channel blockers
BUSPIRONE—ORAL	GRAPEFRUIT JUICE	Possibly ↑ efficacy and ↑ adverse effects, e.g., sedation, CNS depression	Possibly ↑ bioavailability, ↓ presystemic metabolism. Constituents of grapefruit juice irreversibly inhibit intestinal CYP3A4. Transport via Pgp and MRP-2 efflux pumps is also inhibited	Avoid concomitant use. Be particularly vigilant in elderly patients or those with impaired liver function. Consider an alternative, e.g., temazepam

(Continued)

Primary Drug	Secondary Drug	Effect	Mechanism	Precautions
ANXIOLYTICS AND HYPNOTICS				
CHLORAL HYDRATE				
CHLORAL HYDRATE	**ANTIDEPRESSANTS**			
CHLORAL HYDRATE	MAOIs	Case report of fatal hyperpyrexia and cases of hypertension	Uncertain	Avoid coadministration
CHLORAL HYDRATE	SSRIs	Case of excessive drowsiness	Uncertain; possibly additive effects, possibly displacement of chloral hydrate from protein-binding sites	Warn patients to be aware of additional sedation
CHLORMETHIAZOLE				
CHLORMETHIAZOLE	H2 RECEPTOR BLOCKERS—CIMETIDINE	↑ Efficacy and adverse effects, e.g., sedation, "hangover" effect	Inhibition of metabolism by cimetidine	Monitor closely; ↓ dose may be required
MELATONIN				
MELATONIN	H2 RECEPTOR BLOCKERS—CIMETIDINE	↑ Plasma concentrations of melatonin	Inhibition of metabolism by cimetidine	Be aware
MEPROBAMATE				
MEPROBAMATE	ESTROGENS, PROGESTERONES	Reports of breakthrough bleeding when meprobamate is coadministered with oral contraceptives	Uncertain	The clinical significance is uncertain. It would seem to be wise to advise patients to use an alternative form of contraception during and for 1 month after stopping meprobamate
SODIUM OXYBATE				
SODIUM OXYBATE	1. ALCOHOL 2. ANALGESICS—opioids 3. ANTIDEPRESSANTS—TCAs 4. ANTIEPILEPTICS—barbiturates 5. ANTIHISTAMINES 6. ANTIPSYCHOTICS 7. ANXIOLYTICS AND HYPNOTICS—BZDs, buspirone	Risk of CNS depression—coma, respiratory depression	Additive depression of CNS	Avoid coadministration. Caution even with relatively nonsedating antihistamines (cetirizine, desloratadine, fexofenadine, levocetirizine, loratadine, mizolastine) as they can impair the performance of skilled tasks

(*Continued*)

Primary Drug	Secondary Drug	Effect	Mechanism	Precautions
ANXIOLYTICS AND HYPNOTICS				
ZALEPLON, ZOLPIDEM, ZOPICLONE				
ZALEPLON, ZOLPIDEM, ZOPICLONE	ANTIBIOTICS—RIFAMPICIN	↓ Levels of these hypnotics	Induction of CYP3A4-mediated metabolism	Watch for poor response to these agents
ZOLPIDEM	ANTICANCER AND IMMUNOMODULATING DRUGS—DABRAFENIB	↓ Zolpidem levels-though degree of reductions may vary	Dabrafenib induces CYP3A4/ CYP2Cs/CYP2B6	Monitor closely or avoid concurrent use
ZOLPIDEM	ANTIDEPRESSANTS—FLUOXETINE, PAROXETINE, SERTRALINE, VENLAFAXINE	Cases of agitation ± hallucinations	Uncertain	Avoid coadministration
ZALEPLON, ZOLPIDEM, ZOPICLONE	**ANTIEPILEPTICS**			
ZALEPLON, ZOLPIDEM, ZOPICLONE	CARBAMAZEPINE, RIFAMPICIN	↓ Levels of these hypnotics	Induction of CYP3A4-mediated metabolism	Watch for poor response to these agents
ZALEPLON, ZOLPIDEM, ZOPICLONE	PHENYTOIN	↓ Levels of these drugs, with risk of therapeutic failure	Induction of hepatic metabolism	Monitor for ↓ clinical efficacy and ↑ their dose as required
ZALEPLON, ZOLPIDEM, ZOPICLONE	ANTIFUNGALS—KETOCONAZOLE	↑ Zolpidem levels reported; likely to occur with zaleplon and zopiclone	Inhibition of CYP3A4 mediated metabolism by antifungals.	Warn patients of the risk of ↑ sedation
ZOLPIDEM, ZOPICLONE	ANTIPSYCHOTICS—CHLORPROMAZINE	Risk of sedation	Additive effect; uncertain why this occurs more with chlorpromazine	Warn patients of this effect
ZOLPIDEM	DRUG DEPENDENCE THERAPIES—BUPROPION	Cases of agitation ± hallucinations	Uncertain	Avoid coadministration
ZALEPLON	H2 RECEPTOR BLOCKERS—CIMETIDINE	↑ Plasma concentrations	Inhibition of metabolism	Monitor closely; ↓ dose may be required

Primary Drug	Secondary Drug	Effect	Mechanism	Precautions
CNS STIMULANTS				
ATOMOXETINE				
ATOMOXETINE	**DRUGS THAT PROLONG THE QT INTERVAL**			
ATOMOXETINE	1. ANTIARRHYTHMICS—ajmaline, amiodarone, azimilide, cibenzoline, disopyramide, dofetilide, dronedarone, ibutilide, procainamide, propafenone, quinidine 2. ANTIBIOTICS—macrolides (especially azithromycin, clarithromycin, parenteral erythromycin, telithromycin), quinolones (especially moxifloxacin), quinupristin/dalfopristin 3. ANTICANCER AND IMMUNOMODULATING DRUGS—arsenic trioxide, bosutinib, crizotinib, dasatinib, eribulin, fingolimod, lapatinib, nilotinib, pazopanib, sunitinib, vandetanib, vemurafenib 4. ANTIDEPRESSANTS—TCAs, venlafaxine 5. ANTIEMETICS—ondansetron 6. ANTIFUNGALS—fluconazole, posaconazole, voriconazole 7. ANTIHISTAMINES—terfenadine, hydroxyzine, mizolastine 8. ANTIHYPERTENSIVES—ketanserin	Risk of ventricular arrhythmias, particularly torsades de pointes	Additive effect; these drugs prolong the QT interval	Avoid coadministration

(*Continued*)

Primary Drug	Secondary Drug	Effect	Mechanism	Precautions
CNS STIMULANTS				
	9. ANTIMALARIALS—artemether with lumefantrine, chloroquine, halofantrine, hydroxychloroquine, mefloquine, quinine 10. ANTIPROTOZOALS—pentamidine isothionate 11. ANTIPSYCHOTICS—atypicals, phenothiazines, pimozide 12. ANTIVIRALS—boceprevir, rilpivirine, telaprevir 13. BETA-BLOCKERS—sotalol 14. BRONCHODILATORS—parenteral bronchodilators 15. RANOLAZINE			
ATOMOXETINE	ANALGESICS—methadone, tramadol	Risk of arrhythmias with methadone and possible risk of fits with tramadol	Atomoxetine is a selective noradrenaline re-uptake inhibitor. QT interval prolongation and serious arrhythmia (e.g., torsades de pointes) have occurred with methadone treatment	Avoid coadministration of atomoxetine with methadone or tramadol
ATOMOXETINE	**ANTIDEPRESSANTS**			
ATOMOXETINE	MAOIs	Risk of severe hypertensive reactions	Additive inhibition of norepinephrine reuptake	Avoid coadministration. MAOIs should not be started for at least 2 weeks after stopping atomoxetine; conversely, atomoxetine should not be started for at least 2 weeks after stopping MAOI
ATOMOXETINE	SSRIs	↑ Plasma concentrations and risk of adverse effects of atomoxetine (abdominal pain, vomiting, nausea, fatigue, irritability)	Atomoxetine is a selective norepinephrine reuptake inhibitor. ↑ plasma concentrations are due to inhibition of CYP2D6—it is inhibited by fluoxetine and paroxetine (potent), fluvoxamine and sertraline (less potent), and escitalopram and citalopram (weak)	Avoid coadministration. The interaction is usually severe with fluoxetine and paroxetine

(*Continued*)

Primary Drug	Secondary Drug	Effect	Mechanism	Precautions
CNS STIMULANTS				
ATOMOXETINE	BRONCHODILATORS—SALBUTAMOL	↑ Risk of arrhythmias with parenteral salbutamol	Additive effect	Avoid coadministration of atomoxetine with parenteral salbutamol
ATOMOXETINE	DRUG DEPENDENCE THERAPIES—BUPROPION	1. ↑ Plasma concentrations of atomoxetine with risk of toxic effects 2. ↑ Risk of seizures. This risk is marked in elderly people, in patients with a history of seizures, with addiction to opiates/cocaine/stimulants, and in diabetics treated with oral hypoglycemics or insulin	1. Bupropion and its metabolite hydroxybupropion inhibit CYP2D6 2. Bupropion is associated with a dose-related risk of seizures. These drugs, which lower seizure threshold, are individually epileptogenic. Additive effects when combined	1. Initiate therapy of these drugs, particularly those with a narrow therapeutic index at the lowest effective dose 2. Extreme caution. The dose of bupropion should not exceed 450 mg/day (or 150 mg/day in patients with severe hepatic cirrhosis)
ATOMOXETINE	DIURETICS—LOOP AND THIAZIDES	↑ Risk of arrhythmias with hypokalemia	These diuretics may cause hypokalemia	Monitor potassium levels closely
DEXAMFETAMINE ➢ ***Cardiovascular Drugs, Sympathomimetics***				
GUANFACINE				
GUANFACINE	CRIZOTINIB	Risk of excessive bradycardia	Additive effects	Caution with concurrent use
METHYLPHENIDATE ➢ ***Cardiovascular Drugs, Sympathomimetics***				
MODAFINIL				
MODAFINIL	**POTENT INDUCERS OF CYP3A4**			
MODAFINIL	ANTIEPILEPTICS—CARBAMAZEPINE, PHENOBARBITONE, RIFAMPICIN	↓ Plasma concentrations of modafinil with possibility of ↓ therapeutic effect	Induction of CYP3A4, which has a partial role in the metabolism of modafinil	Be aware

(*Continued*)

Primary Drug	Secondary Drug	Effect	Mechanism	Precautions
CNS STIMULANTS				
MODAFINIL	**OTHER INDUCERS OF CYP3A4**			
MODAFINIL	ANTIBIOTICS—RIFABUTIN ANTICANCER AND IMMUNOMODULATING DRUGS—CORTICOSTEROIDS ANTIDEPRESSANTS—ST. JOHN'S WORT ANTIEPILEPTICS—PHENYTOIN ANTIDIABETIC DRUGS—PIOGLITAZONE ANTIVIRALS—EFAVIRENZ, NEVIRAPINE	May ↓ modafinil levels	Induction of CYP3A4, which has a partial role in the metabolism of modafinil	Be aware
MODAFINIL	**POTENT INHIBITORS OF CYP3A4**			
MODAFINIL	ANTIBIOTICS—CLARITHROMYCIN, TELITHROMYCIN ANTIFUNGALS—ITRACONAZOLE, KETOCONAZOLE ANTIVIRALS—INDINAVIR, NELFINAVIR, RITONAVIR, SAQUINAVIR	↑ Plasma concentrations of modafinil, with risk of adverse effects	Due to inhibition of CYP3A4, which has a partial role in the metabolism of modafinil	Be aware. Warn patients to report dose-related adverse effects, e.g., headache, anxiety

(*Continued*)

Primary Drug	Secondary Drug	Effect	Mechanism	Precautions
CNS STIMULANTS				
MODAFINIL	**CYP2C19 SUBSTRATES**			
MODAFINIL	ANALGESICS—INDOMETACIN ANTIBIOTICS—CHLORAMPHENICOL ANTICANCER AND IMMUNOMODULATING DRUGS—CYCLOPHOSPHAMIDE ANTICOAGULANTS—WARFARIN ANTIDEPRESSANTS—MOCLOBEMIDE ANTIEPILEPTICS—PHENOBARBITONE, PRIMIDONE ANTIMALARIALS—PROGUANIL ANTIPLATELET AGENTS—CLOPIDOGREL ANTIVIRALS—NELFINAVIR ANXIOLYTICS AND HYPNOTICS—DIAZEPAM BETA-BLOCKERS—PROPANOLOL MUSCLE RELAXANTS—CARISOPRODOL PROTON PUMP INHIBITORS	May cause moderate ↑ plasma concentrations of these substrates	Modafinil is a reversible inhibitor of CYP2C19 when used in therapeutic doses	Be aware
MODAFINIL	**CYP2C9 SUBSTRATES**			
MODAFINIL	ANALGESICS—NSAIDs ANTICANCER AND IMMUNOMODULATING DRUGS—TAMOXIFEN ANTICOAGULANTS—WARFARIN	May cause ↑ plasma concentrations of these substrates if CYP2C9 is the predominant metabolic pathway and the alternative pathways are either genetically deficient or affected	Modafinil is a moderate inhibitor of CYP2C9	Be aware

(Continued)

Primary Drug	Secondary Drug	Effect	Mechanism	Precautions
CNS STIMULANTS				
	ANTIDEPRESSANTS—AMITRIPTYLINE ANTIDIABETIC DRUGS—NATEGLINIDE, ROSIGLITAZONE, SULFONYLUREAS			
MODAFINIL	**CYP1A2 SUBSTRATES**			
MODAFINIL	ANALGESICS—NAPROXEN, PARACETAMOL ANESTHETICS, LOCAL—ROPIVACAINE ANTIARRHYTHMICS—MEXILETINE ANTIDEPRESSANTS—AMITRIPTYLINE, CLOMIPRAMINE, FLUVOXAMINE, IMIPRAMINE ANTIEMETICS—ONDANSETRON ANTIMIGRAINE DRUGS—ZOLMITRIPTAN ANTIPSYCHOTICS—CLOZAPINE, HALOPERIDOL, OLANZAPINE BETA-BLOCKERS—PROPANOLOL BRONCHODILATORS—THEOPHYLLINE CALCIUM CHANNEL BLOCKERS—VERAPAMIL MUSCLE RELAXANTS—TIZANIDINE ESTROGENS RILUZOLE	May cause ↓ plasma concentrations of these substrates if CYP1A2 is the predominant metabolic pathway and alternative metabolic pathways are either genetically deficient or affected	Modafinil is moderate inducer of CYP1A2 in a concentration-dependent manner	Be aware. Patients who are using estrogen-containing contraceptives should be warned to use alternative forms of contraception during and for at least 1 month after cessation of modafinil

(*Continued*)

Primary Drug	Secondary Drug	Effect	Mechanism	Precautions
CNS STIMULANTS				
MODAFINIL	**ANTICANCER AND IMMUNOMODULATING DRUGS**			
MODAFINIL	BOSUTINIB	Reduced bosutinib levels	CYP3A induction	Manufacturer advises avoid concurrent use. Dose increase is unlikely to sufficiently compensate
MODAFINIL	CICLOSPORIN	↓ Ciclosporin levels up to 50%, with risk of lack of therapeutic effect	↑ Metabolism of ciclosporin. Modafinil is a moderate inducer of CYP3A4	Monitor ciclosporin levels
MODAFINIL	ANTIDEPRESSANTS—CLOMIPRAMINE, DESIPRAMINE ≻ CYP1A2 substrates, CYP2C9 substrates, above	↑ Of plasma concentrations of TCAs in a subset of the population (7%–10% of Caucasians) who are deficient in CYP2D6	CYP2C19 provides an ancillary pathway for the metabolism of clomipramine and desipramine. Modafinil inhibited CYP2C19 reversibly at pharmacologically relevant concentrations	↓ Dose of TCAs is often necessary
MODAFINIL	ANXIOLYTICS AND HYPNOTICS—TRIAZOLAM	May ↓ triazolam levels	Uncertain	Be aware
MODAFINIL	DRUG DEPENDENCE THERAPIES—BUPROPION	↑ Risk of seizures. This risk is marked in elderly people, in patients with a history of seizures, with addiction to opiates/cocaine/stimulants, and in diabetics treated with oral hypoglycemics or insulin	Bupropion is associated with a dose-related risk of seizures. These drugs, which lower seizure threshold, are individually epileptogenic. Additive effects when combined	Extreme caution. The dose of bupropion should not exceed 450 mg/day (or 150 mg/day in patients with severe hepatic cirrhosis)
MODAFINIL	LIPID-LOWERING DRUGS—STATINS	↓ Levels of atorvastatin and simvastatin	Induction of CYP 3A4-mediated metabolism of these statins	Monitor lipid profile closely and consider increasing the dose of statin
MODAFINIL	SYMPATHOMIMETICS—DEXAMFETAMINE, METHYLPHENIDATE	May ↓ modafinil levels	Due to delayed absorption	Be aware

Primary Drug	Secondary Drug	Effect	Mechanism	Precautions
DRUG DEPENDENCE THERAPIES				
BUPRENORPHINE ➢ *Analgesics, Opioids*				
BUPROPION				
BUPROPION	ALCOHOL	Rare reports of adverse neuropsychiatric events and ↓ alcohol tolerance	Uncertain	Warn patients to avoid or minimize alcohol intake during bupropion treatment
BUPROPION	ANTIDEPRESSANTS—PHENELZINE	↑ Acute toxicity of bupropion	Uncertain	Be aware
BUPROPION	ANTI-PARKINSON'S DRUGS—AMANTADINE, LEVODOPA	↑ CNS side effects	Additive effects	Initiate therapy with bupropion at the lowest dose and ↑ gradually
BUPROPION	**INHIBITORS OF CYP2B6**			
BUPROPION	ANTICANCER DRUGS—THIOTEPA ANTIDEPRESSANTS—FLUOXETINE, FLUVOXAMINE, PAROXETINE, SERTRALINE ANTIVIRALS—EFAVIRENZ, PROTEASE INHIBITORS	↑ Plasma concentrations of bupropion and risk of adverse effects	Inhibition of CYP2B6	Warn patients about adverse effects (dry mouth, taste disturbances, agitation, GI upset, insomnia), and use alternatives when possible. Avoid coadministration of bupropion with protease inhibitors. Coadminister efavirenz and bupropion with caution. A retrospective study showed that two patients received a combination without reported adverse effects. Potential ↑ risk of seizures
BUPROPION	**INDUCERS OF CYP2B6**			
BUPROPION	RIFAMPICIN	↓ Plasma concentrations of bupropion and lack of therapeutic effect	Induction of CYP2B6	↑ Dose of bupropion cautiously

(Continued)

DRUGS ACTING ON THE CENTRAL NERVOUS SYSTEM DRUG DEPENDENCE THERAPIES

Primary Drug	Secondary Drug	Effect	Mechanism	Precautions
DRUG DEPENDENCE THERAPIES				
BUPROPION	**DRUGS METABOLIZED BY CYP2D6**			
BUPROPION	ANALGESICS—CELECOXIB, OPIOIDS ANTIARRHYTHMICS—AMIODARONE, FLECAINIDE, PROPAFENONE ANTICANCER DRUGS—DOXORUBICIN, GEFITINIB ANTIDEPRESSANTS—DULOXETINE, MOCLOBEMIDE, SSRIs—ESCITALOPRAM, FLUOXETINE, FLUVOXAMINE, PAROXETINE, SERTRALINE, TCAs—AMITRIPTYLINE, CLOMIPRAMINE, DESIPRAMINE, DOXEPIN, IMIPRAMINE ANTIEMETICS—METOCLOPRAMIDE ANTIHISTAMINES—CHLORPHENAMINE, CLEMASTINE, HYDROXYZINE ANTIPSYCHOTICS—CHLORPROMAZINE, PERPHENAZINE, RISPERIDONE, THIORIDAZINE BETA-BLOCKERS—METOPROLOL, PROPRANOLOL, TIMOLOL CINACALCET CNS STIMULANTS—AMPHETAMINES, ATOMOXETINE ELIGLUSTAT H2 RECEPTOR BLOCKERS—CIMETIDINE, RANITIDINE	↑ Plasma concentrations of these substrates with risk of toxic effects	Bupropion and its metabolite hydroxybupropion inhibit CYP2D6	Initiate therapy of these drugs, particularly those with a narrow therapeutic index, at the lowest effective dose. Interaction is likely to be important with substrates for which CYP2D6 is considered the only metabolic pathway (e.g., hydrocodone, oxycodone, desipramine, paroxetine, chlorpheniramine, mesoridazine, alprenolol, amphetamines, atomoxetine)

(*Continued*)

Primary Drug	Secondary Drug	Effect	Mechanism	Precautions
DRUG DEPENDENCE THERAPIES				
BUPROPION	**DRUGS THAT LOWER THRESHOLD FOR SEIZURES**			
BUPROPION	ANTIBIOTICS—FLUOROQUINOLONES ANTICANCER AND IMMUNOMODULATING DRUGS—CORTICOSTEROIDS, INTERFERONS ANTIDEPRESSANTS—TCAs ANTIMALARIALS—CHLOROQUINE, MEFLOQUINE ANTIPSYCHOTICS BRONCHODILATORS—THEOPHYLLINE CNS STIMULANTS PARASYMPATHOMIMETICS	↑ Risk of seizures. This risk is marked in elderly people, in patients with a history of seizures, with addiction to opiates/cocaine/stimulants, and in diabetics treated with oral hypoglycemics or insulin	Bupropion is associated with a dose-related risk of seizures. These drugs, which lower seizure threshold, are individually epileptogenic. Additive effects occur when combined	Extreme caution. The dose of bupropion should not exceed 450 mg/day (or 150 mg/day in patients with severe hepatic cirrhosis)
BUPROPION	**DRUGS WHOSE METABOLISM WOULD ALTER AFTER CESSATION OF SMOKING**			
BUPROPION	ANTIARRHYTHMICS—FLECAINIDE, MEXILETINE ANTICOAGULANTS—WARFARIN ANTIDEPRESSANTS—FLUVOXAMINE ANTIPSYCHOTICS—CHLORPROMAZINE, CLOZAPINE, HALOPERIDOL, OLANZAPINE BETA-BLOCKERS—PROPANOLOL BRONCHODILATORS—THEOPHYLLINE	↑ Plasma concentrations of these drugs, with risk of toxic/adverse effects	Smoking induces mainly CYP1A2 and CYP2E1. Thus, deinduction takes place following cessation of smoking	Be aware, particularly with drugs with a narrow therapeutic index. Monitor clinically and biochemically (e.g., INR, plasma theophylline levels)
BUPROPION	ANTICANCER AND IMMUNOMODULATING DRUGS—CRIZOTINIB	Possible increased levels of CYP2B6 substrates	Crizotinib inhibits CYP2B6	Clinical significance uncertain; be aware of possible interaction

(*Continued*)

Primary Drug	Secondary Drug	Effect	Mechanism	Precautions
DRUG DEPENDENCE THERAPIES				
BUPROPION	ANXIOLYTICS AND HYPNOTICS—ZOLPIDEM	Cases of agitation ± hallucinations	Uncertain	Avoid coadministration
BUPROPION	DRUG DEPENDENCE THERAPIES—DISULFIRAM	Risk of psychosis	Additive effects; these drugs interfere with dopamine metabolism	Caution with coadministration. Warn patients and carers to watch for early features
CLONIDINE ➢ ***Cardiovascular Drugs, Antihypertensives and Heart Failure Drugs***				
DISULFIRAM				
DISULFIRAM	ALCOHOL	Disulfiram reaction	See above	Do not coadminister. Disulfiram must not be given within 12 h of ingestion of alcohol
DISULFIRAM	ANTIBIOTICS—METRONIDAZOLE	Report of psychosis	Additive effect; both drugs may cause neurological/psychiatric side effects (disulfiram by inhibiting the metabolism of dopamine, metronodazole by an unknown mechanism)	Caution with coadministration. Warn patients and carers to watch for early features
DISULFIRAM	ANTICANCER AND IMMUNOMODULATING DRUGS—THALIDOMIDE	Possible increased risk of peripheral neuropathy	Additive	Manufacturer advises caution
DISULFIRAM	ANTICOAGULANTS—WARFARIN	↑ Anticoagulant effect	Uncertain at present	Monitor INR at least weekly until stable
DISULFIRAM	ANTIEPILEPTICS—PHENYTOIN	↑ Phenytoin levels	Inhibited metabolism	Monitor phenytoin levels closely
DISULFIRAM	ANTIVIRALS—PROTEASE INHIBITORS	↑ Risk of disulfiram reaction with ritonavir (with or without lopinavir)	Ritonavir and lopinavir/ritonavir oral solutions contain 43% alcohol	Warn patients. Consider using capsule preparations as an alternative
DISULFIRAM	ANXIOLYTICS AND HYPNOTICS	↑ BZD levels	Inhibited metabolism	Warn patients of risk of excessive sedation
DISULFIRAM	BRONCHODILATORS—THEOPHYLLINE	↑ Theophylline levels	Disulfiram ↓ theophylline clearance by inhibiting hydroxylation and demethylation	Monitor theophylline levels before, during, and after coadministration
DISULFIRAM	DRUG DEPENDENCE THERAPIES—BUPROPION	Risk of psychosis	Additive effects; these drugs interfere with dopamine metabolism	Caution with coadministration. Warn patients and carers to watch for early features

(Continued)

DRUGS ACTING ON THE CENTRAL NERVOUS SYSTEM PARASYMPATHOMIMETICS

Primary Drug	Secondary Drug	Effect	Mechanism	Precautions
DRUG DEPENDENCE THERAPIES				
DISULFIRAM	MUSCLE RELAXANTS—CHLORZOXAZONE	↑ Chlorzoxazone levels	Inhibition of CYP2E1-mediated metabolism of chlorzoxazone	Warn patients to report side effects of chlorzoxazone (drowsiness, headache)
DISULFIRAM	PROTON PUMP INHIBITORS—OMEPRAZOLE	Possible ↑ adverse effects of disulfiram	Accumulation of metabolites	Monitor closely for ↑ side effects, although patients have received combinations without reported problems
DISULFIRAM	SYMPATHOMIMETICS—DEXAMFETAMINE, METHYLPHENIDATE	Risk of psychosis	Additive effects; these drugs interfere with dopamine metabolism	Caution with coadministration. Warn patients and carers to watch for early features
LOFEXIDINE				
LOFEXIDINE	ALCOHOL, BZDs, BARBITURATES	↑ Sedation	Additive effect	Warn patients of risk of excessive sedation
METHADONE ➢ ***Analgesics, Opioids***				
DRUGS USED TO TREAT NEUROMUSCULAR DISEASES AND MOVEMENT DISORDERS				
HALOPERIDOL ➢ ***Antipsychotics, above***				

Primary Drug	Secondary Drug	Effect	Mechanism	Precautions
PARASYMPATHOMIMETICS				
PARASYMPATHOMIMETICS	**ANTIARRHYTHMICS**			
PARASYMPATHOMIMETICS	PROPAFENONE	↓ Efficacy of neostigmine and pyridostigmine	Uncertain; propafenone has a degree of antinicotinic action that may oppose the action of parasympathomimetic therapy for myasthenia gravis	Watch for poor response to these parasympathomimetics and ↑ dose accordingly
DONEPEZIL, GALANTAMINE	QUINIDINE	Theoretical risk of ↑ donepezil and galantamine levels	Inhibition of CYP2D6-mediated metabolism	Warn patient to watch for development of side effects of donepezil and galantamine

(*Continued*)

Primary Drug	Secondary Drug	Effect	Mechanism	Precautions
PARASYMPATHOMIMETICS				
PARASYMPATHOMIMETICS	**ANTIBIOTICS**			
GALANTAMINE	ERYTHROMYCIN	↑ Galantamine levels	Inhibition of CYP3A4-mediated metabolism of galantamine	Be aware; watch for ↑ side effects from galantamine
NEOSTIGMINE, PYRIDOSTIGMINE	AMINOGLYCOSIDES, CLINDAMYCIN, COLISTIN	↓ Efficacy of neostigmine and pyridostigmine	Uncertain	Watch for poor response to these parasympathomimetics and ↑ dose accordingly
PARASYMPATHOMIMETICS	ANTICANCER AND IMMUNOMODULATING DRUGS			
PARASYMPATHOMIMETICS—PILOCARPINE	CRIZOTINIB	Risk of excessive bradycardia	Additive	Caution with concurrent use
PARASYMPATHOMIMETICS—PHYSOSTIGMINE	IRINOTECAN	Reduced levels of SN-38 (irinotecan metabolite) in vitro	Unknown	Clinical significance uncertain
PARASYMPATHOMIMETICS	**ANTIDEPRESSANTS**			
PARASYMPATHOMIMETICS	LITHIUM	↓ Efficacy of neostigmine and pyridostigmine	Uncertain	Watch for poor response to these parasympathomimetics and ↑ dose accordingly
GALANTAMINE	SSRIs	↑ Galantamine levels	Inhibition of CYP2D6-mediated metabolism of galantamine: Fluoxetine, paroxetine—potent Fluvoxamine, sertraline—less potent Escitalopram, citalopram—weak	Monitor PR and BP closely, watching for bradycardia and hypotension. Be aware that there is a theoretical risk with other SSRIs
GALANTAMINE	ANTIFUNGALS—KETOCONAZOLE	↑ Galantamine levels	Inhibition of 3A4-mediated metabolism of galantamine	Monitor PR and BP closely, watching for bradycardia and hypotension
PARASYMPATHOMIMETICS	ANTIMALARIALS—CHLOROQUINE, QUININE	↓ Efficacy of parasympathomimetics	These antimalarials occasionally cause muscle weakness, which may exacerbate the symptoms of myasthenia gravis	Watch for poor response to these parasympathomimetics and ↑ dose accordingly

(*Continued*)

Primary Drug	Secondary Drug	Effect	Mechanism	Precautions
PARASYMPATHOMIMETICS				
PARASYMPATHO-MIMETICS	ANTIMUSCARINICS	↓ Efficacy of parasympathomimetics	Parasympathomimetics and antimuscarinics have opposing effects	Avoid coadministration where possible
GALANTAMINE	ANTIVIRALS—RITONAVIR	Possibly ↑ plasma levels and side effects of galantamine, e.g., nausea and vomiting	Possibly inhibition of metabolism via CYP3A4	Monitor more closely
PARASYMPATHO-MIMETICS	**BETA-BLOCKERS**			
NEOSTIGMINE, PYRIDOSTIGMINE	BETA-BLOCKERS	1. Cases of bradycardia and ↓ BP when neostigmine or physostigmine is given to reverse anesthesia. This is a potential risk with all parasympathomimetics 2. ↓ Effectiveness of neostigmine and pyridostigmine in myasthenia gravis	1. Neostigmine and pyridostigmine causes an accumulation of ACh, which may cause additive bradycardia and ↓ BP 2. Beta-blockers are thought to have a depressant effect on the neuromuscular junction and thereby ↑ weakness	1. Monitor PR and BP closely when giving anticholinesterases to reverse anesthesia to patients on beta-blockers 2. Monitor the response to neostigmine and pyridostigmine when starting beta-blockers
PILOCARPINE	BETA-BLOCKERS	↑ Risk of arrhythmias	Additive bradycardia	Monitor PR and ECG closely
PARASYMPATHO-MIMETICS	CARDIAC GLYCOSIDES—DIGOXIN	Risk of bradycardia	Additive AV block	Avoid coadministration
DONEPEZIL, GALANTAMINE, RIVASTIGMINE	CALCIUM CHANNEL BLOCKERS	Risk of bradycardia	Additive effect	Monitor PR and BP closely until stable
PARASYMPATHO-MIMETICS	DRUG DEPENDENCE THERAPIES—BUPROPION	↑ Risk of seizures. This risk is marked in elderly people, in patients with a history of seizures, with addiction to opiates/cocaine/stimulants, and in diabetics treated with oral hypoglycemics or insulin	Bupropion is associated with a dose-related risk of seizures. These drugs, which lower seizure threshold, are individually epileptogenic. Additive effects occur when combined	Extreme caution. The dose of bupropion should not exceed 450 mg/day (or 150 mg/day in patients with severe hepatic cirrhosis)

(*Continued*)

DRUGS ACTING ON THE CENTRAL NERVOUS SYSTEM PARASYMPATHOMIMETICS

Primary Drug	Secondary Drug	Effect	Mechanism	Precautions
PARASYMPATHOMIMETICS				
PARASYMPATHO-MIMETICS	**MUSCLE RELAXANTS**			
DONEPEZIL	SUXAMETHONIUM	Possible ↑ efficacy of suxamethonium	Suxamethonium is metabolized by cholinesterase; parasympathomimetics inhibit cholinesterase and so prolong the action of suxamethonium	Avoid coadministration. Ensure that the effects of suxamethonium have worn off before administering a parasympathomimetic to reverse nondepolarizing muscle relaxants. A careful risk–benefit analysis should be made before considering the use of suxamethonium for emergency anesthesia in patients taking parasympathomimetics. The short half-life of edrophonium means that it can be used to diagnose suspected dual block with suxamethonium
PARASYMPATHO-MIMETICS	NONDEPOLARIZING	↓ Efficacy of nondepolarizing muscle relaxants	The anticholinesterases oppose the action of nondepolarising muscle relaxants	Used therapeutically
PIRACETAM				
PIRACETAM	ANTICOAGULANTS—ORAL	Case report of bleeding associated with ↑ INR in a patient taking warfarin 1 month after starting piracetam	Uncertain. Piracetam inhibits platelet aggregation but it is uncertain whether it has any effect on other aspects of the clotting cascade	Warn patient to report easy bruising, etc. Monitor INR closely
RILUZOLE				
RILUZOLE	MODAFINIL	May cause ↓ riluzole levels if CYP1A2 is the predominant metabolic pathway and alternative metabolic pathways are either genetically deficient or affected	Modafinil is a moderate inducer of CYP1A2 in a concentration-dependent manner	Be aware

(*Continued*)

Primary Drug	Secondary Drug	Effect	Mechanism	Precautions
PARASYMPATHOMIMETICS				
TETRABENAZINE				
TETRABENAZINE	ANTIDEPRESSANTS—MAOIs	Risk of confusion and agitation	Uncertain; although tetrabenazine depletes norepinephrine, if it is started on a patient who is already taking MAOIs, it may stimulate the release of accumulated neurotransmitter. This may not occur if a patient starts MAOI while taking tetrabenazine	Tetrabenazine may cause depression, so it should be used with caution in patients with depression. If necessary, consider using an alternative antidepressant or start an MAOI after tetrabenazine has been stabilized
TETRABENAZINE	ANTIEMETICS—METOCLOPRAMIDE	Risk of extrapyramidal symptoms	Additive effect	Avoid coadministration
TETRABENAZINE	ANTI-PARKINSON'S DRUGS—AMANTADINE	↓ Anti-Parkinson's efficacy of amantadine	Tetrabenazine may cause extrapyramidal symptoms	Use with caution; avoid in patients <20 years
TETRABENAZINE	ANTIPSYCHOTICS	Case report of extrapyramidal symptoms when tetrabenazine was given with chlorpromazine	Uncertain	Warn patients to report any extrapyramidal symptoms

PART 3

Anticancer and Immunomodulating Drugs

Patrick Yong

Primary Drug	Secondary Drug	Effect	Mechanism	Precautions
CYTOTOXICS				
ALL				
ALL	ANTIPSYCHOTICS—CLOZAPINE	↑ Risk of bone marrow toxicity	Additive effect	Avoid coadministration
ALL	CARDIAC GLYCOSIDES—DIGOXIN	Cytotoxics may ↓ levels of digoxin (by up to 50%) when digoxin is given in tablet form	Cytotoxic-induced damage to the mucosa of the intestine may ↓ absorption; this does not seem to be a problem with liquid or liquid-containing capsule formulations	Watch for poor response to digoxin; check levels if there are signs of ↓ effect and consider swapping to liquid digoxin or liquid-containing capsules
ALL	VACCINES—LIVE	Reduced efficacy of vaccines. Risk of contracting disease from live vaccines	↓ Immunity	Avoid live vaccines for at least 6 months after completing chemotherapy
ACLARUBICIN	MITOMYCIN	Increased risk of myelosuppression	Additive	Caution with concurrent use
AFATINIB				
AFATINIB	ANTIARRHYTHMICS—AMIODARONE, QUINIDINE	Possible increase in afatinib levels	P-glycoprotein inhibition	Manufacturer recommends staggered dosing 6–12 h apart or dose reduction
AFATINIB	**ANTIBIOTICS**			
AFATINIB	MACROLIDES—ERYTHROMYCIN	Possible increase in afatinib levels	P-glycoprotein inhibition	Manufacturer recommends staggered dosing 6–12 h apart or dose reduction
AFATINIB	RIFAMPICIN	Reduction in afatinib levels	P-glycoprotein induction	US manufacturer recommends dose increase
AFATINIB	ANTICANCER AND OTHER IMMUNOMODULATING DRUGS—CICLOSPORIN, TACROLIMUS, VALSPODAR	Possible increase in afatinib levels	P-glycoprotein inhibition	Manufacturer recommends staggered dosing 6–12 h apart or dose reduction
AFATINIB	ANTIDEPRESSANTS—ST. JOHN'S WORT	Reduction in afatinib levels	P-glycoprotein induction	US manufacturer recommends dose increase

(Continued)

Primary Drug	Secondary Drug	Effect	Mechanism	Precautions
CYTOTOXICS				
AFATINIB	ANTIEPILEPTICS—CARBAMAZEPINE, PHENOBARBITAL, PHENYTOIN	Reduction in afatinib levels	P-glycoprotein induction	US manufacturer recommends dose increase
AFATINIB	ANTIFUNGALS—ITRACONAZOLE, KETOCONAZOLE	Possible increase in afatinib levels	P-glycoprotein inhibition	Manufacturer recommends staggered dosing 6–12 h apart or dose reduction
AFATINIB	**ANTIVIRALS**			
AFATINIB	BOCEPREVIR	Predicted increased levels of afatinib	CYP3A4 inhibition	Manufacturer advises to avoid concurrent use
AFATINIB	NELFINAVIR, RITONAVIR, SAQUINAVIR, TELAPREVIR	Possible increase in afatinib levels	P-glycoprotein inhibition	Manufacturer recommends staggered dosing 6–12 h apart or dose reduction
AFATINIB	TIPRANAVIR	Reduction in afatinib levels	P-glycoprotein induction	US manufacturer recommends dose increase
AFATINIB	CALCIUM CHANNEL BLOCKERS—VERAPAMIL	Possible increase in afatinib levels	P-glycoprotein inhibition	Manufacturer recommends staggered dosing 6–12 h apart or dose reduction
AFATINIB	RANOLAZINE	Possible increase in afatinib levels	P-glycoprotein inhibition	Manufacturer recommends staggered dosing 6–12 h apart or dose reduction
ARSELNIC TRIOXIDE				
ARSENIC TRIOXIDE	**DRUGS THAT PROLONG THE QT INTERVAL**			
ARSENIC TRIOXIDE	1. ANTIARRHYTHMICS—ajmaline, amiodarone, azimilide, cibenzoline, disopyramide, dofetilide, dronedarone, ibutilide, procainamide, propafenone, quinidine 2. ANTIBIOTICS—macrolides (especially azithromycin, clarithromycin, parenteral erythromycin, telithromycin), quinolones (especially moxifloxacin), quinupristin/dalfopristin	Risk of ventricular arrhythmias, particularly torsades de pointes	Additive effect; these drugs prolong the QT interval Also, amitriptyline, clomipramine, and desipramine levels may be ↑ by propafenone Amitriptyline and clomipramine may ↑ propafenone levels Propafenone and these TCAs inhibit CYP2D6-mediated metabolism of each other	Avoid coadministration

(Continued)

Primary Drug	Secondary Drug	Effect	Mechanism	Precautions
CYTOTOXICS				
	3. ANTICANCER AND IMMUNOMODULATING DRUGS—bosutinib, crizotinib, dasatinib, eribulin, fingolimod, lapatinib, nilotinib, pazopanib, sunitinib, vandetanib, vemurafenib 4. ANTIDEPRESSANTS—TCAs, venlafaxine 5. ANTIEMETICS—ondansetron 6. ANTIFUNGALS—fluconazole, posaconazole, voriconazole 7. ANTIHISTAMINES—hydroxyzine, mizolastine 8. ANTIHYPERTENSIVES—ketanserin 9. ANTIMALARIALS—artemether with lumefantrine, chloroquine, halofantrine, hydroxychloroquine, mefloquine, quinine 10. ANTIPROTOZOALS—pentamidine isethionate 11. ANTIPSYCHOTICS—atypicals, phenothiazines, pimozide 12. ANTIVIRALS—boceprevir, rilpivirine, telaprevir 13. BETA-BLOCKERS—sotalol 14. BRONCHODILATORS—parenteral bronchodilators 15. CNS STIMULANTS—atomoxetine 16. RANOLAZINE			
ARSENIC TRIOXIDE	GENERAL ANESTHETICS—HALOTHANE	Risk of arrhythmias especially TdP	Arsenic trioxide may cause QT prolongation on its own but risk increased with halothane	Use an alternative inhalational anesthetic
ASPARAGINASE				
ASPARAGINASE	IMATINIB	Possible increased risk of hepatotoxicity	Unknown	Manufacturer advises caution with concurrent use

(*Continued*)

Primary Drug	Secondary Drug	Effect	Mechanism	Precautions
CYTOTOXICS				
AXITINIB				
AXITINIB	**ANTIBIOTICS**			
AXITINIB	MACROLIDES—CLARITHROMYCIN, ERYTHROMYCIN, TELITHROMYCIN	Increased levels of axitinib	CYP3A4/5 inhibition	Manufacturer advises to avoid concurrent use with strong CYP3A4/5 inhibitors if possible. If concurrent use is necessary, dose adjustment is recommended
AXITINIB	RIFAMPICIN, RIFABUTIN, RIFAPENTINE	Reduced axitinib levels	CYP3A4/5 induction	Manufacturer advises to avoid concurrent use if possible. If concurrent use is necessary, dose adjustment is recommended
AXITINIB	ANTICANCER AND OTHER IMMUNOMODULATING DRUGS—DEXAMETHASONE	Reduced axitinib levels	CYP3A4/5 induction	Manufacturer advises to avoid concurrent use if possible. If concurrent use is necessary, dose adjustment is recommended
AXITINIB	**ANTIDEPRESSANTS**			
AXITINIB	ST. JOHN'S WORT	Reduced axitinib levels	CYP3A4/5 induction	Manufacturer advises to avoid concurrent use if possible. If concurrent use is necessary, dose adjustment is recommended
AXITINIB	SSRIs—NEFAZODONE	Increased levels of axitinib	CYP3A4/5 inhibition	Manufacturer advises to avoid concurrent use with strong CYP3A4/5 inhibitors if possible. If concurrent use is necessary, dose adjustment is recommended
AXITINIB	ANTIEPILEPTICS—CARBAMAZEPINE, PHENOBARBITAL, PHENYTOIN	Reduced axitinib levels	CYP3A4/5 induction	Manufacturer advises to avoid concurrent if possible. If concurrent use is necessary, dose adjustment is recommended

(Continued)

Primary Drug	Secondary Drug	Effect	Mechanism	Precautions
CYTOTOXICS				
AXITINIB	ANTIFUNGALS—ITRACONAZOLE, KETOCONAZOLE	Increased levels of axitinib	CYP3A4/5 inhibition	Manufacturer advises to avoid concurrent use with strong CYP3A4/5 inhibitors if possible. If concurrent use is necessary, dose adjustment is recommended
AXITINIB	**ANTIVIRALS**			
AXITINIB	BOCEPREVIR	Predicted increased levels of axitinib	CYP3A4 inhibition	Manufacturer advises to avoid concurrent use
AXITINIB	ATAZANAVIR, INDINAVIR, NELFINAVIR, RITONAVIR, SAQUINAVIR	Increased levels of axitinib	CYP3A4/5 inhibition	Manufacturer advises to avoid concurrent use with strong CYP3A4/5 inhibitors if possible. If concurrent use is necessary, dose adjustment is recommended
AXITINIB	BRONCHODILATORS—THEOPHYLLINE	Possible increased levels of theophylline	Axitinib inhibits CYP1A2	Caution with concurrent use
AXITINIB	GRAPEFRUIT JUICE	Increased levels of axitinib	CYP3A4/5 inhibition	Manufacturer advises to avoid concurrent use with strong CYP3A4/5 inhibitors if possible. If concurrent use is necessary, dose adjustment is recommended
BENDAMUSTINE				
BENDAMUSTINE	ANTIBIOTICS—CIPROFLOXACIN	Theoretical risk of increased bendamustine levels	CYP1A2 inhibition	Monitor closely
BENDAMUSTINE	**ANTICANCER AND OTHER IMMUNOMODULATING DRUGS**			
BENDAMUSTINE	CICLOSPORIN	Risk of excessive immunosuppression and lymphoproliferation	Additive	Monitor closely

(*Continued*)

Primary Drug	Secondary Drug	Effect	Mechanism	Precautions
CYTOTOXICS				
BENDAMUSTINE	TACROLIMUS	Risk of excessive immunosuppression and lymphoproliferation	Additive	Monitor closely
BENDAMUSTINE	ANTIDEPRESSANTS—FLUVOXAMINE	Theoretical risk of increased bendamustine levels	CYP1A2 inhibition	Monitor closely
BENDAMUSTINE	ANTIVIRALS—ACICLOVIR	Theoretical risk of increased bendamustine levels	CYP1A2 inhibition	Monitor closely
BENDAMUSTINE	H2 RECEPTOR BLOCKERS—CIMETIDINE	Theoretical risk of increased bendamustine levels	CYP1A2 inhibition	Monitor closely
BEXAROTENE				
BEXAROTENE	ANTICANCER AND IMMUNOMODULATING DRUGS—CARBOPLATIN WITH PACLITAXEL	Carboplatin with paclitaxel may ↑ bexarotene levels	Unknown	Clinical significance unknown. Monitor more closely
BEXAROTENE	GRAPEFRUIT JUICE	Possibly ↑ efficacy and ↑ adverse effects	Possibly via inhibition of intestinal CYP3A4	Clinical significance unknown. Monitor more closely
BEXAROTENE	**LIPID-LOWERING DRUGS**			
BEXAROTENE	GEMFIBROZIL	Gemfibrozil may ↑ bexarotene levels	Uncertain at present	Avoid coadministration
BEXAROTENE	STATINS	Levels of atorvastatin reduced by bexarotene. Simvastatin and lovastatin may be affected	Possibly due to induction of CYP3A4	Atorvastatin dose increase may be necessary
BLEOMYCIN				
BLEOMYCIN	**ANTICANCER AND IMMUNOMODULATING DRUGS**			
BLEOMYCIN	BRENTUXIMAB VEDOTIN	Increased risk of pulmonary toxicity	Unknown	Avoid concomitant use

(*Continued*)

Primary Drug	Secondary Drug	Effect	Mechanism	Precautions
CYTOTOXICS				
BLEOMYCIN	CISPLATIN	↑ Bleomycin levels, with risk of pulmonary toxicity	Elimination of bleomycin is delayed by cisplatin due to ↓ glomerular filtration. This is most likely with accumulated doses of cisplatin in excess of 300 mg/m^2	Monitor renal function and adjust dose of bleomycin as per creatinine clearance. Monitor clinically, radiologically along with lung function tests for pulmonary toxicity
BLEOMYCIN	COLONY-STIMULATING FACTORS	Increased risk of pulmonary toxicity	Unknown	Monitor pulmonary function more closely
BLEOMYCIN	OXYGEN	Risk of potentially fatal pumonary toxicity with exposure to conventional oxygen concentrations in anesthesia	Unknown	Oxygen concentrations to be limited to <30%
BORTEZOMIB				
BORTEZOMIB	ANTIBIOTICS—RIFAMPICIN	Levels of bortezomib reduced	Induction of CYP3A4 and CYP2C19	Avoid concomitant use
BORTEZOMIB	**ANTICANCER AND IMMUNOMODULATING DRUGS**			
BORTEZOMIB	CICLOSPORIN	Possible increased risk of severe neuropathy in patients on long-term ciclosporin	Possible additive effect	Monitor closely. Dose of bortezomib may need to be modified
BORTEZOMIB	MELPHALAN	Slight increased bortezomib levels when used with melphalan and prednisolone	Uncertain	Be aware. Probably of no clinical significance
BORTEZOMIB	THALIDOMIDE	Possible increased risk of peripheral neuropathy	Additive	Manufacturer advises caution
BORTEZOMIB	ANTIDEPRESSANTS—ST. JOHN'S WORT	Levels of bortezomib reduced	Possibly due to induction of CYP3A4	Avoid concomitant use

(Continued)

ANTICANCER AND IMMUNOMODULATING DRUGS CYTOTOXICS Bortezomib

Primary Drug	Secondary Drug	Effect	Mechanism	Precautions
CYTOTOXICS				
BORTEZOMIB	ANTIDIABETIC DRUGS—CHLORPROPAMIDE	Likely to ↑ hypoglycemic effect of chlorpropamide	Unknown	Watch for and warn patients about symptoms of hypoglycemia. ➢ ***For signs and symptoms of hypoglycemia, see Clinical Features of Some Adverse Drug Interactions, Hypoglycemia***
BORTEZOMIB	ANTIEPILEPTICS—CARBAMAZEPINE, PHENOBARBITAL, PHENYTOIN	Levels of bortezomib possibly reduced by carbamazepine, phenobarbital, and phenytoin	Possibly due to induction of CYP3A4	Avoid concomitant use
BORTEZOMIB	ANTIHYPERTENSIVES AND HEART FAILURE DRUGS	↑ Hypotensive effect	Additive hypotensive effect	Monitor BP at least weekly until stable, particularly on initiation of therapy
BORTEZOMIB	BETA-BLOCKERS	↑ Hypotensive effect	Additive hypotensive effect	Monitor BP at least weekly until stable, particularly on initiation of therapy
BORTEZOMIB	CALCIUM CHANNEL BLOCKERS	↑ Hypotensive effect	Additive hypotensive effect	Monitor BP at least weekly until stable, particularly on initiation of therapy
BORTEZOMIB	DIURETICS—LOOP, THIAZIDES	↑ Hypotensive effect	Additive hypotensive effect	Monitor BP at least weekly until stable, particularly on initiation of therapy
BORTEZOMIB	NITRATES	↑ Hypotensive effect	Additive hypotensive effect	Monitor BP at least weekly until stable, particularly on initiation of therapy
BORTEZOMIB	POTASSIUM CHANNEL ACTIVATORS	↑ Hypotensive effect	Additive hypotensive effect	Monitor BP at least weekly until stable, particularly on initiation of therapy

(*Continued*)

Primary Drug	Secondary Drug	Effect	Mechanism	Precautions
CYTOTOXICS				
BOSUTINIB				
BOSUTINIB	**DRUGS THAT PROLONG THE QT INTERVAL**			
BOSUTINIB	1. ANTIARRHYTHMICS—ajmaline, amiodarone, azimilide, cibenzoline, disopyramide, dofetilide, dronedarone, ibutilide, procainamide, propafenone, quinidine 2. ANTIBIOTICS—macrolides (especially azithromycin, clarithromycin, parenteral erythromycin, telithromycin), quinolones (especially moxifloxacin), quinupristin/dalfopristin 3. ANTICANCER AND IMMUNOMODULATING DRUGS—arsenic trioxide, crizotinib, dasatinib, eribulin, fingolimod, lapatinib, nilotinib, pazopanib, sunitinib, vandetanib, vemurafenib 4. ANTIDEPRESSANTS—TCAs, venlafaxine 5. ANTIEMETICS—ondansetron 6. ANTIFUNGALS—fluconazole, posaconazole, voriconazole 7. ANTIHISTAMINES—terfenadine, hydroxyzine, mizolastine 8. ANTIHYPERTENSIVES—ketanserin 9. ANTIMALARIALS—artemether with lumefantrine, chloroquine, halofantrine, hydroxychloroquine, mefloquine, quinine 10. ANTIPROTOZOALS—pentamidine isethionate 11. ANTIPSYCHOTICS—atypicals, phenothiazines, pimozide 12. ANTIVIRALS—boceprevir, rilpivirine, telaprevir	Risk of ventricular arrhythmias, particularly torsades de pointes	Additive effect; these drugs prolong the QT interval Also, amitriptyline, clomipramine, and desipramine levels may be ↑ by propafenone Amitriptyline and clomipramine may ↑ propafenone levels Propafenone and these TCAs inhibit CYP2D6-mediated metabolism of each other	Avoid coadministration

(*Continued*)

Primary Drug	Secondary Drug	Effect	Mechanism	Precautions
CYTOTOXICS				
	13. BETA-BLOCKERS—sotalol 14. BRONCHODILATORS—parenteral bronchodilators 15. CNS STIMULANTS—atomoxetine 16. RANOLAZINE			
BOSUTINIB	ANTIARRHYTHMICS—DRONEDARONE	Increased bosutinib levels	CYP3A inhibition	Manufacturer advises to avoid concurrent use. If not possible, interruption of therapy or dose reduction should be considered
BOSUTINIB	**ANTIBIOTICS**			
BOSUTINIB	CIPROFLOXACIN	Increased bosutinib levels	CYP3A inhibition	Manufacturer advises to avoid concurrent use. If not possible, interruption of therapy or dose reduction should be considered
BOSUTINIB	MACROLIDES—ERYTHROMYCIN, CLARITHROMYCIN, TELITHROMYCIN, TROLEANDOMYCIN	Increased bosutinib levels	CYP3A inhibition	Manufacturer advises to avoid concurrent use. If not possible, interruption of therapy or dose reduction should be considered
BOSUTINIB	PENICILLINS—NAFCILLIN	Reduced bosutinib levels	CYP3A induction	Manufacturer advises to avoid concurrent use. Dose increase unlikely to sufficiently compensate
BOSUTINIB	RIFAMPICIN, RIFABUTIN	Reduced bosutininb levels	CYP3A induction	Manufacturer advises to avoid concurrent use. Dose increase unlikely to sufficiently compensate
BOSUTINIB	**ANTIDEPRESSANTS**			
BOSUTINIB	ST. JOHN'S WORT	Reduced bosutinib levels	CYP3A induction	Manufacturer advises to avoid concurrent use. Dose increase unlikely to sufficiently compensate

(*Continued*)

Primary Drug	Secondary Drug	Effect	Mechanism	Precautions
CYTOTOXICS				
BOSUTINIB	SSRIs—NEFAZODONE	Increased bosutinib levels	CYP3A inhibition	Manufacturer advises to avoid concurrent use. If not possible, interruption of therapy or dose reduction should be considered
BOSUTINIB	ANTIEMETIC—APREPITANT	Increased bosutinib levels	CYP3A inhibition	Manufacturer advises to avoid concurrent use. If not possible, interruption of therapy or dose reduction should be considered
BOSUTINIB	ANTIEPILEPTICS—CARBAMAZEPINE, PHENOBARBITAL, PHENYTOIN	Reduced bosutinib levels	CYP3A induction	Manufacturer advises to avoid concurrent use. Dose increase unlikely to sufficiently compensate
BOSUTINIB	ANTIHYPERTENSIVES AND HEART FAILURE DRUGS—BOSENTAN	Reduced bosutinib levels	CYP3A induction	Manufacturer advises to avoid concurrent use. Dose increase unlikely to sufficiently compensate
BOSUTINIB	ANTIFUNGALS—FLUCONAZOLE, ITRACONAZOLE, KETOCONAZOLE, VORICONAZOLE, POSACONAZOLE	Increased bosutinib levels	CYP3A inhibition	Manufacturer advises to avoid concurrent use. If not possible, interruption of therapy or dose reduction should be considered
BOSUTINIB	**ANTIVIRALS**			
BOSUTINIB	AMPRENAVIR, ATAZANAVIR, BOCEPREVIR, DARUNAVIR, FOSAMPRENAVIR, INDINAVIR, NELFINAVIR, RITONAVIR, SAQUINAVIR, TELAPREVIR	Increased bosutinib levels	CYP3A inhibition	Manufacturer advises to avoid concurrent use. If not possible, interruption of therapy or dose reduction should be considered
BOSUTINIB	EFAVIRENZ, ETRAVIRINE	Reduced bosutinib levels	CYP3A induction	Manufacturer advises to avoid concurrent use. Dose increase unlikely to sufficiently compensate

(*Continued*)

Primary Drug	Secondary Drug	Effect	Mechanism	Precautions
CYTOTOXICS				
BOSUTINIB	ANXIOLYTICS AND HYPNOTICS—TOFISOPAM	Increased bosutinib levels	CYP3A inhibition	Manufacturer advises to avoid concurrent use. If not possible, interruption of therapy or dose reduction should be considered
BOSUTINIB	CALCIUM CHANNEL BLOCKERS—DILTIAZEM, MIBEFRADIL, VERAPAMIL	Increased bosutinib levels	CYP3A inhibition	Manufacturer advises to avoid concurrent use. If not possible, interruption of therapy or dose reduction should be considered
BOSUTINIB	CONIVAPTAN	Increased bosutinib levels	CYP3A inhibition	Manufacturer advises to avoid concurrent use. If not possible, interruption of therapy or dose reduction should be considered
BOSUTINIB	GRAPEFRUIT JUICE	Increased bosutinib levels	CYP3A inhibition	Manufacturer advises to avoid concurrent use. If not possible, interruption of therapy or dose reduction should be considered
BOSUTINIB	CNS STIMULANTS—MODAFINIL	Reduced bosutinib levels	CYP3A induction	Manufacturer advises to avoid concurrent use. Dose increase unlikely to sufficiently compensate
BOSUTINIB	PROTON PUMP INHIBITORS	Reduced bosutinib levels	pH dependent solubility of bosutinib	Use short-acting antacids as alternative and administer separately to bosutinib
BUSULFAN				
BUSULFAN	**ANALGESICS**			
BUSULFAN	OPIOIDS—KETOBEMIDONE	Levels of busulfan may be increased	Unknown	Monitor carefully
BUSULFAN	PARACETAMOL	Busulfan levels may be ↑ by coadministration of paracetamol	Uncertain; paracetamol probably inhibits metabolism of busulfan	Manufacturers recommend that paracetamol should be avoided for 3 days before administering parenteral busulfan

(*Continued*)

Primary Drug	Secondary Drug	Effect	Mechanism	Precautions
CYTOTOXICS				
BUSULFAN	**ANTIBIOTICS**			
BUSULFAN	MACROLIDES—CLARITHROMYCIN, ERYTHROMYCIN, TELITHROMYCIN	↑ Plasma concentrations of busulfan and ↑ risk of toxicity of busulfan such as veno-occlusive disease and pulmonary fibrosis	Busulfan clearance may be ↓ by 25%, and the AUC of busulfan may ↑ by 1500 μmol/L	Monitor clinically for veno-occlusive disease and pulmonary toxicity in transplant patients. Monitor busulfan blood levels as AUC below 1500 μmol/L/min tends to prevent toxicity
BUSULFAN	METRONIDAZOLE	↑ Busulfan levels	Uncertain	Watch for early features of toxicity
BUSULFAN	**ANTICANCER AND IMMUNOMODULATING DRUGS**			
BUSULFAN	CYCLOPHOSPHAMIDE	↑ Incidence of veno-occlusive disease and mucositis when cyclophosphamide is given <24 h after the last dose of busulfan. Possibly also ↓ effect of cyclophosphamide	There is ↓ clearance and ↑ elimination half-life of cyclophosphamide, and ↑ concentrations of the active metabolite 4-hydroxycyclophosphamide	Administer cyclophosphamide at least 24 h after the last dose of busulfan
BUSULFAN	TIOGUANINE	↑ Risk of nodular regenerative hyperplasia of the liver, esophageal varices, and portal hypertension	Mechanism uncertain	Monitor liver function and for clinical and biochemical indices of liver toxicity (e.g., ascites, splenomegaly). Ask patients to report any symptoms suggestive of esophageal bleeding
BUSULFAN	BUSULFAN	↓ Levels of these drugs, with risk of therapeutic failure	Induction of hepatic metabolism	Monitor for ↓ clinical efficacy and ↑ their dose as required
BUSULFAN	ANTIFUNGALS—ITRACONAZOLE	↑ Busulfan levels, with risk of toxicity of busulfan, e.g., veno-occlusive disease and pulmonary fibrosis	Itraconazole is a potent inhibitor of CYP3A4. Busulfan clearance may be ↓ by 25%, and the AUC of busulfan may ↑ by 1500 μmol/L	Monitor clinically for veno-occlusive disease and pulmonary toxicity in transplant patients. Monitor busulfan blood levels as AUC below 1500 μmol/L/min tends to prevent toxicity

(*Continued*)

Primary Drug	Secondary Drug	Effect	Mechanism	Precautions
CYTOTOXICS				
BUSULFAN	CALCIUM CHANNEL BLOCKERS	↑ Busulfan levels, with risk of toxicity of busulfan, e.g., veno-occlusive disease and pulmonary fibrosis, when coadministered with diltiazem, nifedipine, or verapamil	Due to inhibition of CYP3A4-mediated metabolism of busulfan by these calcium channel blockers. Busulfan clearance may be ↓ by 25%, and the AUC of busulfan may ↑ by 1500 μmol/L	Monitor clinically for veno-occlusive disease and pulmonary toxicity in transplant patients. Monitor busulfan blood levels as AUC below 1500 μmol/L/min tends to prevent toxicity
BUSULFAN	H2 RECEPTOR BLOCKERS—CIMETIDINE	↑ Adverse effects of alkylating agent, e.g., myelosuppression	Additive toxicity	Monitor more closely; monitor FBC regularly
CABAZITAXEL				
CABAZITAXEL	**ANTIBIOTICS**			
CABAZITAXEL	CLARITHROMYCIN, TELITHROMYCIN	Increased cabazitaxel levels	CYP3A4 inhibition	Avoid coadministration
CABAZITAXEL	RIFABUTIN, RIFAMPICIN, RIFAPENTINE	Reduced cabazitaxel levels	CYP3A4 induction	Avoid coadministration
CABAZITAXEL	ANTICANCER AND OTHER IMMUNOMODULATING DRUGS—DABRAFENIB	Possible reduced levels of CYP3A4/CYP2Cs/CYP2B6 substrates. Level of reduction may vary	Dabrafenib induces CYP3A4/CYP2Cs/CYP2B6	Monitor closely or avoid concurrent use
CABAZITAXEL	**ANTIDEPRESSANTS**			
CABAZITAXEL	ST. JOHN'S WORT	Reduced cabazitaxel levels	CYP3A4 induction	Avoid coadministration
CABAZITAXEL	NEFAZODONE	Increased cabazitaxel levels	CYP3A4 inhibition	Avoid coadministration
CABAZITAXEL	ANTIEPILEPTICS—CARBAMAZEPINE, PHENYTOIN, PHENOBARBITAL	Reduced cabazitaxel levels	CYP3A4 induction	Avoid coadministration
CABAZITAXEL	ANTIFUNGALS—ITRACONAZOLE, KETOCONAZOLE, VORICONAZOLE,	Increased cabazitaxel levels	CYP3A4 inhibition	Avoid coadministration

(Continued)

Primary Drug	Secondary Drug	Effect	Mechanism	Precautions
CYTOTOXICS				
CABAZITAXEL	ANTIVIRALS—ATAZANAVIR, INDINAVIR, NELFINAVIR, RITONAVIR, SAQUINAVIR	Increased cabazitaxel levels	CYP3A4 inhibition	Avoid coadministration
CAPECITABINE				
Capecitabine is metabolized to fluorouracil ➢ ***Fluorouracil/capecitabine, below***				
CARBOPLATIN ➢ ***Platinum Compounds, below***				
CARMUSTINE				
CARMUSTINE	ANTICANCER AND IMMUNOMODULATING DRUGS—ETOPOSIDE (HIGH DOSE)	↑ Risk of liver toxicity, which usually occurs after 1–2 months after initiating treatment without an improvement in tumor response	Possible additive hepatotoxic effects	Avoid coadministration
CARMUSTINE	ANTIEPILEPTICS—PHENOBARBITAL	↓ Plasma concentrations of carmustine and ↓ antitumor effect in animal experiments	Attributed to induction of liver metabolizing enzymes of carmustine by phenobarbitone, particularly with long-term therapy	Avoid concurrent use. As this study did not show any interaction with phenytoin, phenytoin may be a suitable alternative antiepileptic
CARMUSTINE	H2 RECEPTOR BLOCKERS—CIMETIDINE	↑ Adverse effects of alkylating agent, e.g., myelosuppression	Additive toxicity	Monitor more closely; monitor FBC regularly
CHLORAMBUCIL				
CHLORAMBUCIL	**ANTICANCER AND OTHER IMMUNOMODULATING DRUGS**			
CHLORAMBUCIL	AZATHIOPRINE	↑ Risk of myelosuppression and immunosuppression. Deaths have occurred following profound myelosuppression and severe sepsis	Additive myelotoxic effects. Azathioprine is metabolized to 6-mercaptopurine in vivo, which results in additive myelosuppression, immunosuppression, and hepatotoxicity	Avoid coadministration

(Continued)

Primary Drug	Secondary Drug	Effect	Mechanism	Precautions
CYTOTOXICS				
CHLORAMBUCIL	CICLOSPORIN	Single report—reduced levels of ciclosporin	Unknown	Significance unclear
CHLORAMBUCIL	CORTICOSTEROIDS—PREDNISONE	Single report of seizures	Possibly additive effect	Combination widely used, assess seizure risk with drugs that reduce seizure threshold
CHLORAMBUCIL	H2 RECEPTOR BLOCKERS—CIMETIDINE	↑ Adverse effects of alkylating agent, e.g., myelosuppression	Additive toxicity	Monitor more closely; monitor FBC regularly
CHLORMETHINE (MUSTINE)				
CHLORMETHINE	ANTICANCER AND IMMUNOMODULATING DRUGS—PROCARBAZINE	Possible risk of neurological toxicity with high-dose procarbazine	Chlormethine may enhance effects of procarbazine	Avoid administration of drugs on same day
CHLORMETHINE	MUSCLE RELAXANTS—SUXAMETHONIUM	↑ Efficacy of suxamethonium	Uncertain; these drugs are likely to decrease plasma levels of pseudocholinesterase, enhancing the neuromuscular blockade	Caution with concurrent use. Reduce dosage or avoid suxamethonium
CISPLATIN ➢ ***Platinum Compounds, below***				
CLADRIBINE				
CLADRIBINE	**ANTIVIRALS**			
CLADRIBINE	NRTIs	Possible therapeutic failure of cladribine	Competition for intracellular activation via phosphorylation by deoxycytidine kinase. Adefovir, didanosine, and tenofovir inhibit adenosine uptake	Manufacturer advises to avoid concurrent use

(*Continued*)

Primary Drug	Secondary Drug	Effect	Mechanism	Precautions
CYTOTOXICS				
CLOFARABINE				
CLOFARABINE	ANALGESICS—NSAIDS	Possible increase in clofarabine levels	Clofarabine excreted primarily by kidneys	Manufacturer advises to avoid concurrent use. Monitor closely if this is unavoidable
CLOFARABINE	ANTIBIOTICS—AMINOGLYCOSIDES, PENTAMIDINE	Possible increase in clofarabine levels	Clofarabine excreted primarily by kidneys	Manufacturer advises to avoid concurrent use. Monitor closely if this is unavoidable
CLOFARABINE	ANTICANCER AND OTHER IMMUNOMODULATING DRUGS—PLATINUM COMPOUNDS, TACROLIMUS	Possible increase in clofarabine levels	Clofarabine excreted primarily by kidneys	Manufacturer advises to avoid concurrent use. Monitor closely if this is unavoidable
CLOFARABINE	ANTIVIRALS—ACICLOVIR	Possible increase in clofarabine levels	Clofarabine excreted primarily by kidneys	Manufacturer advises to avoid concurrent use. Monitor closely if this is unavoidable
CRISANTASPASE (ASPARAGINASE)				
CRISANTASPASE	**ANTICANCER AND IMMUNOMODULATING DRUGS**			
CRISANTASPASE	CORTICOSTEROIDS—DEXAMETHASONE	Dexamethasone clearance reduced	Related to serum albumin concentration, which is reduced by crisantaspase treatment	Be aware. Significance unclear
CRISANTASPASE	IMATINIB	Increased hepatotoxicity	Unknown	Caution regarding concurrent use
CRISANTASPASE	METHOTREXATE	Administration prior to or concurrently may ↓ efficacy of methotrexate	Crisantaspase inhibits protein synthesis and prevents cell entry to S phase, which leads to ↓ efficacy of methotrexate	Administer crisantaspase shortly after methotrexate or 9–10 days before methotrexate
CRISANTASPASE	VINCRISTINE	↑ Risk of neurotoxicity if concurrently administered or if crisantaspase is administered prior to vincristine	Uncertain but has been attributed by some to effects of crisantaspase on the metabolism of vincristine	Administer vincristine prior to crisantaspase

(*Continued*)

Primary Drug	Secondary Drug	Effect	Mechanism	Precautions
CYTOTOXICS				
CRIZOTINIB				
CRIZOTINIB	**DRUGS THAT PROLONG THE QT INTERVAL**			
CRIZOTINIB	1. ANTIARRHYTHMICS—ajmaline, amiodarone, azimilide, cibenzoline, disopyramide, dofetilide, dronedarone, ibutilide, procainamide, propafenone, quinidine 2. ANTIBIOTICS—macrolides (especially azithromycin, clarithromycin, parenteral erythromycin, telithromycin), quinolones (especially moxifloxacin), quinupristin/dalfopristin 3. ANTICANCER AND IMMUNOMODULATING DRUGS—arsenic trioxide, bosutinib, dasatinib, eribulin, fingolimod, lapatinib, nilotinib, pazopanib, sunitinib, vandetanib, vemurafenib 4. ANTIDEPRESSANTS—TCAs, venlafaxine 5. ANTIEMETICS—ondansetron 6. ANTIFUNGALS—fluconazole, posaconazole, voriconazole 7. ANTIHISTAMINES—terfenadine, hydroxyzine, mizolastine 8. ANTIHYPERTENSIVES—ketanserin 9. ANTIMALARIALS—artemether with lumefantrine, chloroquine, halofantrine, hydroxychloroquine, mefloquine, quinine 10. ANTIPROTOZOALS—pentamidine isethionate 11. ANTIPSYCHOTICS—atypicals, phenothiazines, pimozide 12. ANTIVIRALS—boceprevir, rilpivirine, telaprevir 13. BETA-BLOCKERS—sotalol 14. BRONCHODILATORS—parenteral bronchodilators 15. CNS STIMULANTS—atomoxetine 16. RANOLAZINE	Risk of ventricular arrhythmias, particularly torsades de pointes	Additive effect; these drugs prolong the QT interval Also, amitriptyline, clomipramine, and desipramine levels may be ↑ by propafenone Amitriptyline and clomipramine may ↑ propafenone levels Propafenone and these TCAs inhibit CYP2D6-mediated metabolism of each other	Avoid coadministration

(*Continued*)

Primary Drug	Secondary Drug	Effect	Mechanism	Precautions
CYTOTOXICS				
CRIZOTINIB	ANALGESICS—MORPHINE, NALOXONE, PARACETAMOL	Possible increased levels of UGT substrates	UGT (particularly UGT1A1, UGT2B7) inhibition	Caution with concurrent use
CRIZOTINIB	ANTIARRHYTHMICS—PROCAINAMIDE	Possible increased levels of OCT1 and OCT2 substrates	OCT1 and OCT2 inhibition	Clinical significance uncertain; be aware of possible interaction
CRIZOTINIB	**ANTIBIOTICS**			
CRIZOTINIB	MACROLIDES—CLARITHROMYCIN, TELITHROMYCIN, TROLEANDOMYCIN	Possible increased crizotinib levels	CYP3A inhibition	Manufacturer advises to avoid concurrent use
CRIZOTINIB	RIFABUTIN, RIFAMPICIN	Possible reduced crizotinib levels	CYP3A4 induction	Manufacturer advises to avoid concurrent use
CRIZOTINIB	ANTICANCER AND OTHER IMMUNOMODULATING DRUGS—IRINOTECAN	Possible increased levels of UGT substrates	UGT (particularly UGT1A1, UGT2B7) inhibition	Caution with concurrent use
CRIZOTINIB	ANTICOAGULANTS—DABIGATRAN	Possible increased levels of P-glycoprotein substrates	Crizotinib inhibits P-glycoprotein	Monitor closely
CRIZOTINIB	ANTIDEPRESSANTS—ST. JOHN'S WORT	Possible reduced crizotinib levels	CYP3A4 induction	Manufacturer advises to avoid concurrent use
CRIZOTINIB	ANTIDIABETICS—METFORMIN	Possible increased levels of OCT1 and OCT2 substrates	OCT1 and OCT2 inhibition	Clinical significance uncertain; be aware of possible interaction
CRIZOTINIB	ANTIEPILEPTICS—CARBAMAZEPINE, PHENOBARBITAL, PHENYTOIN	Possible reduced crizotinib levels	CYP3A4 induction	Manufacturer advises to avoid concurrent use
CRIZOTINIB	ANTIFUNGALS—ITRACONAZOLE, KETOCONAZOLE, VORICONAZOLE	Possible increased crizotinib levels	CYP3A inhibition	Manufacturer advises to avoid concurrent use
CRIZOTINIB	ANTIGOUTS—COLCHICINE	Possible increased levels of P-glycoprotein substrates	Crizotinib inhibits P-glycoprotein	Monitor closely
CRIZOTINIB	ANTIHYPERTENSIVES AND HEART FAILURE DRUGS—CLONIDINE	Risk of excessive bradycardia	Additive	Caution with concurrent use
CRIZOTINIB	ANTIMALARIALS—MEFLOQUINE	Risk of excessive bradycardia	Additive	Caution with concurrent use

(*Continued*)

Primary Drug	Secondary Drug	Effect	Mechanism	Precautions
CYTOTOXICS				
CRIZOTINIB	**ANTIVIRALS**			
CRIZOTINIB	EFAVIRENZ	Possible increased levels of CYP2B6 substrates	Crizotinib inhibits CYP2B6	Clinical significance uncertain; be aware of possible interaction
CRIZOTINIB	PROTEASE INHIBITORS—ATAZANAVIR, INDINAVIR, SAQUINAVIR	Possible increased crizotinib levels	CYP3A inhibition	Manufacturer advises to avoid concurrent use
CRIZOTINIB	RALTEGRAVIR	Possible increased levels of UGT substrates	UGT (particularly UGT1A1, UGT2B7) inhibition	Caution with concurrent use
CRIZOTINIB	ANXIOLYTICS AND HYPNOTICS—MIDAZOLAM	Midazolam levels increased	CYP3A4 inhibition	Closer monitoring and possible dose reduction of midazolam with concurrent use
CRIZOTINIB	BETA-BLOCKERS	Risk of excessive bradycardia	Additive	Caution with concurrent use
CRIZOTINIB	CALCIUM CHANNEL BLOCKERS—VERAPAMIL AND DILTIAZEM	Risk of excessive bradycardia	Additive	Caution with concurrent use
CRIZOTINIB	CARDIAC GLYCOSIDES—DIGOXIN	1. Possible increased levels of P-glycoprotein substrates 2. Risk of excessive bradycardia	1. Crizotinib inhibits P-glycoprotein 2. Additive	Monitor closely
CRIZOTINIB	CNS STIMULANTS—GUANFACINE	Risk of excessive bradycardia	Additive	Caution with concurrent use
CRIZOTINIB	DRUG DEPENDENCE THERAPIES—BUPROPION	Possible increased levels of CYP2B6 substrates	Crizotinib inhibits CYP2B6	Clinical significance uncertain; be aware of possible interaction
CRIZOTINIB	GRAPEFRUIT JUICE	Possible increased crizotinib levels	CYP3A inhibition	Manufacturer advises to avoid concurrent use
CRIZOTINIB	LIPID-LOWERING DRUGS—PRAVASTATIN	Possible increased levels of P-glycoprotein substrates	Crizotinib inhibits P-glycoprotein	Monitor closely
CRIZOTINIB	ORAL CONTRACEPTIVES	Possible reduced contraceptive effect	Induction of PXR and CAR-regulated enzymes	Use barrier contraceptive
CRIZOTINIB	PARASYMPATHOMIMETICS—PILOCARPINE	Risk of excessive bradycardia	Additive	Caution with concurrent use

(*Continued*)

Primary Drug	Secondary Drug	Effect	Mechanism	Precautions
CYTOTOXICS				
CYCLOPHOSPHAMIDE				
CYCLOPHOSPHAMIDE	ANTIARRHYTHMICS—AMIODARONE	Increased risk of pulmonary toxicity	Possible additive effect	Be aware of potential for increased pulmonary toxicity
CYCLOPHOSPHAMIDE	**ANTIBIOTICS**			
CYCLOPHOSPHAMIDE	CHLORAMPHENICOL	May reduce production of active metabolites of cyclophosphamide	Inhibition of cytochrome P450, which partially activates cyclophosphamide	Significance unclear, be aware of possible reduced response of cyclophosphamide
CYCLOPHOSPHAMIDE	METRONIDAZOLE	Single report of encephalopathy	Possibly due to inhibition of aldehyde dehydrogenase, resulting in toxic cyclophosphamide metabolites	Significance unclear
CYCLOPHOSPHAMIDE	**ANTICANCER AND IMMUNOMODULATING DRUGS**			
CYCLOPHOSPHAMIDE	AZATHIOPRINE	↑ Risk of myelosuppression and immunosuppression. Deaths have occurred following profound myelosuppression and severe sepsis	Additive myelotoxic effects. Azathioprine is metabolized to 6-mercaptopurine in vivo, which results in additive myelosuppression, immunosuppression, and hepatotoxicity	Avoid coadministration
CYCLOPHOSPHAMIDE	BUSULFAN	↑ Incidence of veno-occlusive disease and mucositis when cyclophosphamide is given <24 h after the last dose of busulfan. Possibly also ↓ effect of cyclophosphamide	There is ↓ clearance and ↑ elimination half-life of cyclophosphamide, and ↑ concentrations of the active metabolite 4-hydroxycyclophosphamide	Administer cyclophosphamide at least 24 h after the last dose of busulfan
CYCLOPHOSPHAMIDE	CICLOSPORIN	Cyclophosphamide reduces ciclosporin levels	Unknown	Significance unclear
CYCLOPHOSPHAMIDE	ETANERCEPT	Higher incidence of solid malignancy in patients with Wegener's granulomatosis	Unknown	Manufacturer advises to avoid concurrent use

(*Continued*)

Primary Drug	Secondary Drug	Effect	Mechanism	Precautions
CYTOTOXICS				
CYCLOPHOSPHAMIDE	NATALIZUMAB	Increased risk of opportunistic infection	Additive	Manufacturer advises to avoid concurrent use
CYCLOPHOSPHAMIDE	PACLITAXEL	↑ Risk of neutropenia, thrombocytopenia, and mucositis when paclitaxel is infused over 24 or 72 h prior to cyclophosphamide	Mechanism is uncertain	Administer cyclophosphamide first and then follow with paclitaxel
CYCLOPHOSPHAMIDE	PENTOSTATIN	↑ Risk of potentially fatal cardiac toxicity	Attributed to interference of adenosine metabolism by cyclophosphamide	Avoid coadministration
CYCLOPHOSPHAMIDE	THIOTEPA	Inhibition of cyclophosphamide metabolism if thiotepa is given first, potential reduction in efficacy and toxicity	Inhibition of CYP2B6	Order of administration may be of critical importance
CYCLOPHOSPHAMIDE	TRASTUZUMAB	↑ Risk of cardiac toxicity	Possibly additive cardiac toxic effect	Closely monitor cardiac function—clinically and electrocardiographically
CYCLOPHOSPHAMIDE	ANTICOAGULANTS—ORAL	Episodes of ↑ anticoagulant effect	Not understood but likely to be multifactorial	Monitor INR at least weekly until stable during administration of chemotherapy
CYCLOPHOSPHAMIDE	ANTIDIABETIC DRUGS—GLIPIZIDE	Blood sugar levels may be ↑ or ↓	Uncertain	Need to monitor blood glucose in patients with concomitant treatment at the beginning of treatment and after 1–2 weeks
CYCLOPHOSPHAMIDE	ANTIFUNGALS—FLUCONAZOLE, ITRACONAZOLE	Cyclophosphamide side effects possibly increased	Inhibition of CYP3A4 (and CYP2C9 byfluconazole)	Caution with concurrent use
CYCLOPHOSPHAMIDE	ANTIGOUT DRUGS—ALLOPURINOL	↑ Risk of bone marrow suppression	Uncertain but allopurinol seems to ↑ cyclophosphamide levels	Monitor FBC closely

(Continued)

Primary Drug	Secondary Drug	Effect	Mechanism	Precautions
CYTOTOXICS				
CYCLOPHOSPHAMIDE	CNS STIMULANTS—MODAFINIL	May cause moderate ↑ in plasma concentrations of cyclophosphamide	Modafinil is a reversible inhibitor of CYP2C19 when used in therapeutic doses	Be aware
CYCLOPHOSPHAMIDE	G-CSF	Increased risk of pulmonary toxicity	Unknown	Monitor pulmonary function more closely
CYCLOPHOSPHAMIDE	H2 RECEPTOR BLOCKERS—CIMETIDINE	↑ Adverse effects of alkylating agent, e.g., myelosuppression	1. Additive toxicity 2. Possible minor inhibition of cyclophosphamide metabolism via CYP2C9	Avoid coadministration of cimetidine with cyclophosphamide
CYCLOPHOSPHAMIDE	MUSCLE RELAXANTS—SUXAMETHONIUM	↑ Efficacy of suxamethonium	Uncertain; these drugs are likely to decrease plasma levels of pseudocholinesterase, enhancing the neuromuscular blockade	Caution with concurrent use. Reduce dosage or avoid suxamethonium
CYTARABINE				
CYTARABINE	**ANTICANCER AND IMMUNOMODULATING DRUGS**			
CYTARABINE	AZATHIOPRINE	↑ Risk of myelosuppression and immunosuppression. Deaths have occurred following profound myelosuppression and severe sepsis	Additive myelotoxic effects. Azathioprine is metabolized to 6-mercaptopurine in vivo, which results in additive myelosuppression, immunosuppression, and hepatotoxicity	Avoid coadministration
CYTARABINE	FLUDARABINE	↑ Efficacy of cytarabine	Uncertain	Watch for early features of toxicity of cytarabine
CYTARABINE	ANTIFUNGALS—FLUCYTOSINE	↓ Flucytosine levels	Uncertain	Watch for poor response to flucytosine
CYTARABINE	ANTIPLATELETS—DIPYRIDAMOLE	Single report of increased cytarabine toxicity	Dipyridamole inhibits the nucleoside transporter that transports cytarabine extracellularly, resulting in increased intracellular concentration in hepatocytes	Significance unclear, consider interaction if unexpected toxicity
CYTARABINE	ANTIPROTAZOALS—PYRIMETHAMINE	Increased risk of bone marrow aplasia	Additive	Caution with concurrent use

(Continued)

Primary Drug	Secondary Drug	Effect	Mechanism	Precautions
CYTOTOXICS				
DABRAFENIB				
DABRAFENIB	ANALGESICS—FENTANYL, METHADONE	Possible reduced levels of CYP3A4/CYP2Cs/CYP2B6 substrates. Level of reduction may vary	Dabrafenib induces CYP3A4/CYP2Cs/CYP2B6	Monitor closely or avoid concurrent use
DABRAFENIB	**ANTIBIOTICS**			
DABRAFENIB	DOXYCYCLINE	Possible reduced levels of CYP3A4/CYP2Cs/CYP2B6 substrates. Level of reduction may vary	Dabrafenib induces CYP3A4/CYP2Cs/CYP2B6	Monitor closely or avoid concurrent use
DABRAFENIB	MACROLIDES—CLARITHROMYCIN, TELITHROMYCIN	Predicted increased dabrafenib levels	CYP2C8/CYP3A4 inhibition	Avoid concurrent use if possible. Caution if concurrent use is necessary
DABRAFENIB	RIFAMPICIN	Predicted reduced dabrafenib levels	CYP2C8/CYP3A4 induction	Avoid concurrent use
DABRAFENIB	**ANTICANCER AND OTHER IMMUNOMODULATING DRUGS**			
DABRAFENIB	CABAZITAXEL	Possible reduced levels of CYP3A4/CYP2Cs/CYP2B6 substrates. Level of reduction may vary	Dabrafenib induces CYP3A4/CYP2Cs/CYP2B6	Monitor closely or avoid concurrent use
DABRAFENIB	CICLOSPORIN, SIROLIMUS, TACROLIMUS	Possible reduced levels of CYP3A4/CYP2Cs/CYP2B6 substrates. Level of reduction may vary	Dabrafenib induces CYP3A4/CYP2Cs/CYP2B6	Monitor closely or avoid concurrent use
DABRAFENIB	CORTICOSTEROIDS—DEXAMETHASONE, METHYLPREDNISOLONE	Possible reduced levels of CYP3A4/CYP2Cs/CYP2B6 substrates. Level of reduction may vary	Dabrafenib induces CYP3A4/CYP2Cs/CYP2B6	Monitor closely or avoid concurrent use

(Continued)

Primary Drug	Secondary Drug	Effect	Mechanism	Precautions
CYTOTOXICS				
DABRAFENIB	ANTICOAGULANTS—ACENOCOUMAROL, WARFARIN	Possible reduced levels of CYP3A4/CYP2Cs/CYP2B6 substrates. Level of reduction may vary	Dabrafenib induces CYP3A4/CYP2Cs/CYP2B6	Monitor closely or avoid concurrent use
DABRAFENIB	**ANTIDEPRESSANTS**			
DABRAFENIB	SSRIs—NEFAZODONE	Predicted increased dabrafenib levels	CYP2C8/CYP3A4 inhibition	Avoid concurrent use if possible. Caution if concurrent use necessary
DABRAFENIB	ST. JOHN'S WORT	Predicted reduced dabrafenib levels	CYP2C8/CYP3A4 induction	Avoid concurrent use
DABRAFENIB	**ANTIEPILEPTICS**			
DABRAFENIB	CARBAMAZEPINE, PHENOBARBITAL, PHENYTOIN	Predicted reduced dabrafenib levels	CYP2C8/CYP3A4 induction	Avoid concurrent use
DABRAFENIB	VALPROIC ACID	Possible reduced levels of CYP3A4/CYP2Cs/CYP2B6 substrates. Level of reduction may vary	Dabrafenib induces CYP3A4/CYP2Cs/CYP2B6	Monitor closely or avoid concurrent use
DABRAFENIB	ANTIFUNGALS—ITRACONAZOLE, KETOCONAZOLE, VORICONAZOLE, POSACONAZOLE	Predicted increased dabrafenib levels	CYP2C8/CYP3A4 inhibition	Avoid concurrent use if possible. Caution if concurrent use necessary
DABRAFENIB	ANTIPSYCHOTICS—HALOPERIDOL	Possible reduced levels of CYP3A4/CYP2Cs/CYP2B6 substrates. Level of reduction may vary	Dabrafenib induces CYP3A4/CYP2Cs/CYP2B6	Monitor closely or avoid concurrent use
DABRAFENIB	**ANTIVIRALS**			
DABRAFENIB	DELAVIRDINE, EFAVIRENZ	Possible reduced levels of CYP3A4/CYP2Cs/CYP2B6 substrates. Level of reduction may vary	Dabrafenib induces CYP3A4/CYP2Cs/CYP2B6	Monitor closely or avoid concurrent use

(*Continued*)

Primary Drug	Secondary Drug	Effect	Mechanism	Precautions
CYTOTOXICS				
DABRAFENIB	PROTEASE INHIBITORS—ATAZANAVIR, INDINAVIR, RITONAVIR, SQUINAVIR, TIPRANAVIR	Predicted increased dabrafenib levels	CYP2C8/CYP3A4 inhibition	Avoid concurrent use if possible. Caution if concurrent use necessary
DABRAFENIB	ANXIOLYTICS AND HYPNOTICS—DIAZEPAM, MIDAZOLAM, ZOLPIDEM	Possible reduced levels of CYP3A4/CYP2Cs/CYP2B6 substrates. Level of reduction may vary	Dabrafenib induces CYP3A4/CYP2Cs/CYP2B6	Monitor closely or avoid concurrent use
DABRAFENIB	CALCIUM CHANNEL BLOCKERS—DILTIAZEM, FELODIPINE, NICARDIPINE, NIFEDIPINE, VERAPAMIL	Possible reduced levels of CYP3A4/CYP2Cs/CYP2B6 substrates. Level of reduction may vary	Dabrafenib induces CYP3A4/CYP2Cs/CYP2B6	Monitor closely or avoid concurrent use
DABRAFENIB	CARDIAC GLYCOSIDES—DIGOXIN	Possible reduced levels of CYP3A4/CYP2Cs/CYP2B6 substrates. Level of reduction may vary	Dabrafenib induces CYP3A4/CYP2Cs/CYP2B6	Monitor closely or avoid concurrent use
DABRAFENIB	H2-RECEPTOR BLOCKERS	Theoretical risk of reduced dabrafenib levels	Dabrafenib solubility reduced at higher pH	Avoid concurrent use if possible
DABRAFENIB	**LIPID-LOWERING DRUGS**			
DABRAFENIB	GEMFIBROZIL	Predicted increased dabrafenib levels	CYP2C8/CYP3A4 inhibition	Avoid concurrent use if possible. Caution if concurrent use necessary
DABRAFENIB	ATORVASTATIN, SIMVASTATIN	Possible reduced levels of CYP3A4/CYP2Cs/CYP2B6 substrates. Level of reduction may vary	Dabrafenib induces CYP3A4/CYP2Cs/CYP2B6	Monitor closely or avoid concurrent use
DABRAFENIB	PROTON PUMP INHIBITORS	Theoretical risk of reduced dabrafenib levels	Dabrafenib's solubility is reduced at higher pH	Avoid concurrent use if possible
DABRAFENIB	ORAL CONTRACEPTIVES	Possible reduced efficacy of hormonal contraceptives	Dabrafenib induces CYP3A4/CYP2Cs/CYP2B6	Manufacturer recommends alternative contraceptive methods

(*Continued*)

Primary Drug	Secondary Drug	Effect	Mechanism	Precautions
CYTOTOXICS				
DACARBAZINE				
DACARBAZINE	ANTICANCER AND IMMUNOMODULATING DRUGS—IL-2	↓ Efficacy of dacarbazine	↓ AUC of dacarbazine due to ↓ volume of distribution	The clinical significance is uncertain as both drugs are used in the treatment of melanoma. It may be necessary to monitor clinically and by other appropriate measures the clinical response
DACARBAZINE	ANTI-PARKINSON'S DRUGS—LEVODOPA	Single report showed reduced effects of levodopa	Unknown	Be alert to need to increase levodopa dose
DACTINOMYCIN (ACTINOMYCIN D)				
DACTINOMYCIN	ANTICANCER AND IMMUNOMODULATING DRUGS—AZATHIOPRINE	↑ Risk of myelosuppression and immunosuppression. Deaths have occurred following profound myelosuppression and severe sepsis	Additive myelotoxic effects. Azathioprine is metabolized to 6-mercaptopurine in vivo, which results in additive myelosuppression, immunosuppression, and hepatotoxicity	Avoid coadministration
DASATINIB				
DASATINIB	**DRUGS THAT PROLONG THE QT INTERVAL**			
DASATINIB	1. ANTIARRHYTHMICS—ajmaline, amiodarone, azimilide, cibenzoline, disopyramide, dofetilide, dronedarone, ibutilide, procainamide, propafenone, quinidine 2. ANTIBIOTICS—macrolides (especially azithromycin, clarithromycin, parenteral erythromycin, telithromycin), quinolones (especially moxifloxacin), quinupristin/dalfopristin 3. ANTICANCER AND IMMUNOMODULATING DRUGS—arsenic trioxide, bosutinib, crizotinib, eribulin, fingolimod, lapatinib, nilotinib, pazopanib, sunitinib, vandetanib, vemurafenib	Risk of ventricular arrhythmias, particularly torsades de pointes	Additive effect; these drugs prolong the QT interval	Avoid coadministration

(Continued)

Primary Drug	Secondary Drug	Effect	Mechanism	Precautions
CYTOTOXICS				
	4. ANTIDEPRESSANTS—TCAs, venlafaxine 5. Antiemetics—ondansetron 6. ANTIFUNGALS—fluconazole, posaconazole, voriconazole 7. ANTIHISTAMINES—terfenadine, hydroxyzine, mizolastine 8. ANTIHYPERTENSIVES—ketanserin 9. ANTIMALARIALS—artemether with lumefantrine, chloroquine, halofantrine, hydroxychloroquine, mefloquine, quinine 10. ANTIPROTOZOALS—pentamidine isethionate 11. ANTIPSYCHOTICS—atypicals, phenothiazines, pimozide 12. ANTIVIRALS—boceprevir, rilpivirine, telaprevir 13. BETA-BLOCKERS—sotalol 14. BRONCHODILATORS—parenteral bronchodilators 15. CNS STIMULANTS—atomoxetine 16. RANOLAZINE			
DASATINIB	ANALGESICS—NSAIDs	Increased risk of bleeding	Additive	Caution with concurrent use
DASATINIB	ANTIARRHYTHMICS—QUINIDINE	Increased levels of quinidine	CYP3A4 inhibition	Caution with CYP3A4 substrates with narrow therapeutic window
DASATINIB	**ANTIBIOTICS**			
	MACROLIDES—CLARITHROMYCIN, ERYTHROMYCIN, TELITHROMYCIN	Predicted increased levels of dasatinib	CYP3A4 inhibition	Avoid concurrent use
DASATINIB	RIFAMPICIN	↓ Dasatinib levels	Rifampicin ↑ metabolism of dasatinib	Avoid coadministration
DASATINIB	ANTICANCER AND OTHER IMMUNOMODULATING DRUGS—DAUNORUBICIN, DOXORUBICIN, EPIRUBICIN, IDARUBICIN, VALRUBICIN	Increased risk of cardiac side effects	Dasatinib reported to cause QT prolongation	Avoid concurrent use

(Continued)

Primary Drug	Secondary Drug	Effect	Mechanism	Precautions
CYTOTOXICS				
DASATINIB	ANTICOAGULANTS—COUMARINS	Possible increased bleeding risk; particularly with dasatinib and also erlotinib, imatinib, nilotinib, pazopanib, sorafenib, sunitinib	Additive effect	Monitor closely with concurrent use
DASATINIB	ANTIDEPRESSANTS—ST. JOHN'S WORT	Possible increased levels of dasatinib inhibitors; evidence for imatinib only but dasatinib metabolized in a similar way	CYP3A4 induction	Avoid concurrent use
DASATINIB	ANTIFUNGALS—ITRACONAZOLE, KETOCONAZOLE, POSACONAZOLE, VORICONAZOLE	Increased levels of dasatinib	CYP3A4 inhibition	Avoid concurrent use Dose reduction if necessary
DASATINIB	ANTIHISTAMINES—ASTEMIZOLE, TERFENADINE	Increased levels of these antihistamines	CYP3A4 inhibition	Caution with CYP3A4 substrates with narrow therapeutic window
DASATINIB	ANTIMIGRAINE DRUGS—ERGOTAMINE, DIHYDROERGOTAMINE	Increased levels of these ergot alkaloids	CYP3A4 inhibition	Caution with CYP3A4 substrates with narrow therapeutic window
DASATINIB	ANTIPLATELET DRUGS	Increased risk of bleeding	Additive	Caution with concurrent use
DASATINIB	ANTIPSYCHOTICS—PIMOZIDE	Increased levels of pimozide	CYP3A4 inhibition	Caution with CYP3A4 substrates with narrow therapeutic window
DASATINIB	ANTIVIRALS—PROTEASE INHIBITORS	Predicted increased levels of dasatinib	CYP3A4 inhibition	Manufacturer advises to avoid concurrent use
DASATINIB	CALCIUM CHANNEL BLOCKERS—BEPRIDIL	Increased levels of bepridil	CYP3A4 inhibition	Caution with CYP3A4 substrates with narrow therapeutic window
DASATINIB	GRAPEFRUIT JUICE	Possible increased dasatinib levels	CYP3A4 inhibition	Avoid concurrent use
DASATINIB	H2 RECEPTOR BLOCKERS—FAMOTIDINE	Possible ↓ dasatinib levels	Famotidine ↑ metabolism of dasatinib	Consider using alternative acid-suppression therapy

(Continued)

ANTICANCER AND IMMUNOMODULATING DRUGS CYTOTOXICS

Primary Drug	Secondary Drug	Effect	Mechanism	Precautions
CYTOTOXICS				
DASATINIB	LIPID-LOWERING DRUGS—SIMVASTATIN	Possible ↓ simvastatin levels	↑ metabolism of simvastatin	Monitor lipid profile closely and adjust simvastatin dose accordingly when starting and stopping coadministration
DASATINIB	PROTON PUMP INHIBITORS	↓ Plasma concentration	↓ absorption as ↑ gastric pH	Avoid coadministration. Use an antacid if required but separate doses by at least 2 h before or after dasatinib administration
DAUNORUBICIN				
DAUNORUBICIN	**ANTICANCER AND IMMUNOMODULATING DRUGS**			
DAUNORUBICIN	AZATHIOPRINE	↑ Risk of myelosuppression and immunosuppression. Deaths have occurred following profound myelosuppression and severe sepsis	Additive myelotoxic effects. Azathioprine is metabolized to 6-mercaptopurine in vivo, which results in additive myelosuppression, immunosuppression, and hepatotoxicity	Avoid coadministration
DAUNORUBICIN	BEVACIZUMAB	Possible increased risk of cardiac failure	Additive	Be aware of interaction
DAUNORUBICIN	CICLOSPORIN	Increased daunorubicin levels	Uncertain	Monitor closely. Consider dose reduction
DAUNORUBICIN	DASATINIB	Increased risk of cardiac side effects	Dasatinib reported to cause QT prolongation	Avoid concurrent use
DAUNORUBICIN	LAPATINIB	Increased risk of cardiac side effects	Lapatinib reported to cause QT prolongation	Avoid concurrent use
DAUNORUBICIN	TRASTUZUMAB	↑ Risk of cardiac toxicity	Possibly additive cardiac toxic effect	Closely monitor cardiac function—clinically and electrocardiographically
DAUNORUBICIN	ANTIMALARIALS—PYRIMETHAMINE	Cases of fatal bone marrow aplasia reported with combined use of daunorubicin, cytarabine, and pyrimethamine	Additive	Monitor closely

(*Continued*)

Primary Drug	Secondary Drug	Effect	Mechanism	Precautions
CYTOTOXICS				
DOCETAXEL				
DOCETAXEL	**ANTIBIOTICS**			
DOCETAXEL	MACROLIDES—CLARITHROMYCIN, ERYTHROMYCIN, TELITHROMYCIN	↑ Docetaxel levels	Inhibition of CYP3A4-mediated metabolism of docetaxel	Avoid coadministration
DOCETAXEL	RIFAMPICIN	Predicted reduced docetaxel levels	CYP3A4 induction	Monitor closely Dose increase may be required
DOCETAXEL	**ANTICANCER AND IMMUNOMODULATING DRUGS**			
DOCETAXEL	AZATHIOPRINE	↑ Risk of myelosuppression, immunosuppression. Deaths have occurred following profound myelosuppression and severe sepsis	Additive myelotoxic effects. Azathioprine is metabolized to 6-mercaptopurine in vivo, which results in additive myelosuppression, immunosuppression, and hepatotoxicity	Avoid coadministration
DOCETAXEL	BEVACIZUMAB	Possible increased risk of cardiac failure	Additive	Be aware of interaction
DOCETAXEL	CICLOSPORIN	↑ Plasma concentrations of these drugs, with risk of toxic effects	Competitive inhibition of CYP3A4-mediated metabolism and Pgp transport of these drugs	Watch for toxic effects of these drugs
DOCETAXEL	CISPLATIN	↑ Docetaxel levels with ↑ risk of profound myelosuppression. Concurrent use also leads to ↑ risk of neurotoxicity	↓ Clearance of docetaxel when docetaxel is administered after cisplatin	Administer docetaxel first and follow it with cisplatin
DOCETAXEL	DOXORUBICIN	↑ Plasma concentrations of docetaxel (↑ AUC by 50%–70%) with ↑ efficacy and also ↑ risk of toxicity, particularly when docetaxel is administered after doxorubicin, compared with administration of docetaxel alone	Uncertain; possibly due to interference by hepatic microsomal enzymes	Monitor closely for ↑ incidence of bone marrow suppression, neurotoxicity, myalgia, and fatigue

(*Continued*)

ANTICANCER AND IMMUNOMODULATING DRUGS CYTOTOXICS

Primary Drug	Secondary Drug	Effect	Mechanism	Precautions
CYTOTOXICS				
DOCETAXEL	IFOSFAMIDE	Lower ifosfamide levels when given after docetaxel compared to before docetaxel	Unknown	Effects of interaction are schedule dependent
DOCETAXEL	SORAFENIB	Docetaxel levels increased	Possibly due to inhibition of P-glycoprotein, which transports docetaxel	Caution with concurrent use
DOCETAXEL	THALIDOMIDE	Possible increased risk of peripheral neuropathy	Additive	Manufacturer advises caution
DOCETAXEL	TOPOTECAN	↑ Risk of neutropenia when topotecan is administered on days 1–4 and docetaxel on day ↓	Attributed to ↓ clearance of docetaxel (by 50%) due to inhibition of hepatic metabolism of docetaxel by CYP3A4 by topotecan	Administer docetaxel on day 1 and topotecan on days 1–4
DOCETAXEL	VINFLUNINE	Reduced vinflunine levels in vitro	Unknown	Be aware. Clinical significance unknown
DOCETAXEL	VINORELBINE	Administration of docetaxel after vinorelbine ↑ plasma concentrations of vinorelbine, along with ↑ risk of neutropenia compared with giving docetaxel first	Docetaxel likely causes ↓ clearance of vinorelbine	Administer docetaxel first and follow it with vinorelbine
DOCETAXEL	ANTIDEPRESSANTS—ST. JOHN'S WORT	Predicted reduced docetaxel levels	CYP3A4 induction	Monitor closely Dose increase may be required
DOCETAXEL	ANTIEPILEPTICS—CARBAMAZEPINE, PHENOBARBITAL, PHENYTOIN	Predicted reduced docetaxel levels	CYP3A4 induction	Monitor closely Dose increase may be required
DOCETAXEL	ANTIFUNGALS—ITRACONAZOLE, FLUCONAZOLE, KETOCONAZOLE, POSACONAZOLE, VORICONAZOLE	Increased docetaxel levels	CYP3A4 inhibition	Avoid concurrent use If necessary, monitor closely and consider dose reduction
DOCETAXEL	ANTIHYPERTENSIVES AND HEART FAILURE DRUGS—BOSENTAN	Predicted reduced docetaxel levels	CYP3A4 induction	Monitor closely Dose increase may be required

(*Continued*)

Primary Drug	Secondary Drug	Effect	Mechanism	Precautions
CYTOTOXICS				
DOCETAXEL	ANTIVIRALS—PROTEASE INHIBITORS	↑ Risk of adverse effects of docetaxel	Inhibition of CYP3A4-mediated metabolism	Use with caution. Additional monitoring required. Monitor FBC weekly
DOCETAXEL	GRAPEFRUIT JUICE	↑ Docetaxel levels	Inhibition of CYP3A4-mediated metabolism of docetaxel	Warn patients to avoid grapefruit juice
DOXORUBICIN				
DOXORUBICIN	ANESTHETICS—GENERAL—INHALATIONAL	Risk of arrhythmias	Previous treatment with anthracyclines may enhance the myocardial depressive effect	Prevent hypotensive episodes and carbon dioxide retention (hypercapnia)
DOXORUBICIN	ANTIBIOTICS—CLARITHROMYCIN, ERYTHROMYCIN, TELITHROMYCIN	↑ Risk of myelosuppression due to ↑ plasma concentrations	Due to ↓ metabolism of doxorubicin by CYP3A4 isoenzymes owing to an inhibition of those enzymes	Monitor for ↑ myelosuppression, peripheral neuropathy, myalgias, and fatigue
DOXORUBICIN	**ANTICANCER AND IMMUNOMODULATING DRUGS**			
DOXORUBICIN	AZATHIOPRINE	↑ Risk of myelosuppression and immunosuppression. Deaths have occurred following profound myelosuppression and severe sepsis	Additive myelotoxic effects. Azathioprine is metabolized to 6-mercaptopurine in vivo, which results in additive myelosuppression, immunosuppression, and hepatotoxicity	Avoid coadministration
DOXORUBICIN	BEVACIZUMAB	Possible increased risk of cardiac failure	Additive	Be aware of interaction
DOXORUBICIN	CICLOSPORIN	High doses of ciclosporin ↑ AUC of doxorubicin by 48% and of a metabolite by 443%. Risk of severe myelosuppression and neurotoxicity	Ciclosporin inhibits Pgp and selectively inhibits cytochrome P450 isoenzymes, which results in ↓ clearance of doxorubicin	Advise patients to report symptoms such as sore throat, fever, bleeding and bruising (i.e., of myelosuppression) and confusion, headache, coma, and seizures (i.e., of neurotoxicity). ↓ dosage of doxorubicin is often necessary
DOXORUBICIN	DASATINIB	Increased risk of cardiac side effects	Dasatinib reported to cause QT prolongation	Avoid concurrent use

(Continued)

Primary Drug	Secondary Drug	Effect	Mechanism	Precautions
CYTOTOXICS				
DOXORUBICIN	DOCETAXEL	↑ Plasma concentrations of docetaxel (↑ AUC by 50%–70%) with ↑ efficacy and also ↑ risk of toxicity, particularly when docetaxel is administered after doxorubicin, compared with administration of docetaxel alone	Uncertain, possibly due to interference by hepatic microsomal enzymes	Monitor closely for ↑ incidence of bone marrow suppression, neurotoxicity, myalgia, and fatigue
DOXORUBICIN	IMATINIB	↑ Risk of myelosuppression due to ↑ plasma concentrations	Due to ↓ metabolism of doxorubicin by CYP3A4 isoenzymes owing to an inhibition of these enzymes	Monitor for ↑ myelosuppression, peripheral neuropathy, myalgias, and fatigue
DOXORUBICIN	LAPATINIB	Increased risk of cardiac side effects	Lapatinib reported to cause QT prolongation	Avoid concurrent use
DOXORUBICIN	MERCAPTOPURINE	↑ Risk of hepatotoxicity due to mercaptopurine	Uncertain, possibly due to previous treatment with mercaptopurine	Avoid coadministration—except in clinical trials
DOXORUBICIN	MITOMYCIN	Increased cardiotoxicity	Uncertain Possibly due to free radical generation	Monitor closely
DOXORUBICIN	PACLITAXEL	↑ Risk of neutropenia, stomatitis and cardiomyopathy due to ↑ plasma concentrations of doxorubicin	↑ Risk of neutropenia, stomatitis, and cardiomyopathy due to ↑ plasma concentrations of doxorubicin when paclitaxel is given before doxorubicin	Doxorubicin should be administered prior to paclitaxel. The cumulative dose of doxorubicin should be limited to 360 mg/m^2 when concurrently administered with paclitaxel
DOXORUBICIN	SORAFENIB	Slight increase in doxorubicin levels	Unknown	Be aware. Clinical relevance unknown
DOXORUBICIN	THALIDOMIDE	↑ Risk (up to sixfold) of deep venous thrombosis in patients with multiple myeloma compared with those treated without doxorubicin	Uncertain. Attributed to doxorubicin contributing to the thrombogenic activity	Avoid coadministration—except in clinical trials

(*Continued*)

Primary Drug	Secondary Drug	Effect	Mechanism	Precautions
CYTOTOXICS				
DOXORUBICIN	TRASTUZUMAB	When used in combination, the risk of cardiotoxicity due to trastuzumab is ↑ over fourfold	Due to additive cardiotoxic effects	Avoid coadministration—except in clinical trials
DOXORUBICIN	VINFLUNINE	Increased risk of neutropenia Increased vinflunine levels with liposomal doxorubicin	Additive Uncertain	Caution with concurrent use
DOXORUBICIN	ANTICOAGULANTS—ORAL	Episodes of ↑ anticoagulant effect	Not understood but likely to be multifactorial	Monitor INR at least weekly until stable during administration of chemotherapy
DOXORUBICIN	ANTIEPILEPTICS—BARBITURATES	↓ Doxorubicin levels	Induction of hepatic metabolism	Monitor for ↓ efficacy of doxorubicin
DOXORUBICIN	ANTIFUNGALS—ITRACONAZOLE, FLUCONAZOLE, KETOCONAZOLE, POSACONAZOLE, VORICONAZOLE	↑ Risk of myelosuppression due to ↑ plasma concentrations of doxorubicin	Due to ↓ metabolism of doxorubicin by CYP3A4 isoenzymes owing to an inhibition of those enzymes	Monitor for ↑ myelosuppression, peripheral neuropathy, myalgias, and fatigue
DOXORUBICIN	ANTIOBESITY—LORCASERIN	↑ Blood concentrations of captopril	Inhibition of CYP2D6-mediated metabolism	Monitor PR and BP closely until stable
DOXORUBICIN	**ANTIVIRALS**			
DOXORUBICIN	GANCICLOVIR VALGANCICLOVIR	Possibly increased ganciclovir toxicity	Additive effect on inhibition of rapidly dividing cell populations, e.g., bone marrow, tests, skin, GI mucosa	Monitor closely if concurrent use necessary
DOXORUBICIN	STAVUDINE, ZIDOVUDINE	1. Possibly reduced efficacy of stavudine 2. ↑ Adverse effects when doxorubicin is coadministered with zidovudine	1. Inhibition of activation via phosphorylation 2. Additive toxicity	Use with caution, monitor closely for treatment response, and monitor FBC and renal function closely. Adjust doses as necessary

(*Continued*)

Primary Drug	Secondary Drug	Effect	Mechanism	Precautions
CYTOTOXICS				
DOXORUBICIN	CALCIUM CHANNEL BLOCKERS	↑ Serum concentrations and efficacy of doxorubicin when coadministered with verapamil, nicardipine, and possibly diltiazem and nifedipine; however, no cases of doxorubicin toxicity have been reported	Uncertain; however, verapamil is known to inhibit intestinal Pgp, which may ↑ bioavailability of doxorubicin	Watch for symptoms/signs of toxicity (tachycardia, heart failure, and hand-foot syndrome)
DOXORUBICIN	DRUG DEPENDENCE THERAPIES—BUPROPION	↑ Plasma concentrations doxorubicin, with risk of toxic effects	Bupropion and its metabolite hydroxybupropion inhibit CYP2D6	Initiate therapy with doxorubicin at the lowest effective dose
DOXORUBICIN	GRAPEFRUIT JUICE	↑ Risk of myelosuppression due to ↑ plasma concentrations	Due to ↓ metabolism of doxorubicin by CYP3A4 isoenzymes owing to an inhibition of those enzymes	Monitor for ↑ myelosuppression, peripheral neuropathy, myalgias, and fatigue
EPIRUBICIN				
EPIRUBICIN	ANESTHETICS—GENERAL—ISOFLURANE	QT interval prolongation	Additive	Be aware of interaction
EPIRUBICIN	**ANTICANCER AND OTHER IMMUNOMODULATING DRUGS**			
EPIRUBICIN	BEVACIZUMAB	Possible increased risk of cardiac failure	Additive	Be aware of interaction
EPIRUBICIN	CICLOSPORIN	Increased epirubicin levels	Uncertain	Monitor closely. Consider dose reduction
EPIRUBICIN	DASATINIB	Increased risk of cardiac side effects	Dasatinib reported to cause QT prolongation	Avoid concurrent use
EPIRUBICIN	LAPATINIB	Increased risk of cardiac side effects	Lapatinib reported to cause QT prolongation	Avoid concurrent use
EPIRUBICIN	PACLITAXEL	↑ Plasma concentrations of epirubicin (↑ AUC by 37% and ↓ clearance by 25%), particularly following sequential administration of paclitaxel followed by epirubicin	Attributed to altered distribution of epirubicin in the plasma and inhibition of Pgp by Cremophor, the vehicle of paclitaxel formulation, resulting in ↓ clearance	Epirubicin should always be given prior to paclitaxel

(*Continued*)

Primary Drug	Secondary Drug	Effect	Mechanism	Precautions
CYTOTOXICS				
EPIRUBICIN	CALCIUM CHANNEL BLOCKERS	Cases of ↑ bone marrow suppression when verapamil added to epirubicin	Uncertain at present	Monitor FBC closely
EPIRUBICIN	H2 RECEPTOR BLOCKERS—CIMETIDINE	↑ Epirubicin levels, with risk of toxicity	Attributed to inhibition of hepatic metabolism of epirubicin by cimetidine	Avoid concurrent treatment and consider using an alternative H2 receptor blocker, e.g., ranitidine, famotidine
ERIBULIN				
ERIBULIN	**DRUGS THAT PROLONG THE QT INTERVAL**			
ERIBULIN	1. ANTIARRHYTHMICS—ajmaline, amiodarone, azimilide, cibenzoline, disopyramide, dofetilide, dronedarone, ibutilide, procainamide, propafenone, quinidine 2. ANTIBIOTICS—macrolides (especially azithromycin, clarithromycin, parenteral erythromycin, telithromycin), quinolones (especially moxifloxacin), quinupristin/dalfopristin 3. ANTICANCER AND IMMUNOMODULATING DRUGS—arsenic trioxide, bosutinib, crizotinib, dasatinib, fingolimod, lapatinib, nilotinib, pazopanib, sunitinib, vandetanib, vemurafenib 4. ANTIDEPRESSANTS—TCAs, venlafaxine 5. ANTIEMETICS—ondansetron 6. ANTIFUNGALS—fluconazole, posaconazole, voriconazole 7. ANTIHISTAMINES—terfenadine, hydroxyzine, mizolastine 8. ANTIHYPERTENSIVES—ketanserin	Risk of ventricular arrhythmias, particularly torsades de pointes	Additive effect; these drugs prolong the QT interval Also, amitriptyline, clomipramine, and desipramine levels may be ↑ by propafenone Amitriptyline and clomipramine may ↑ propafenone levels Propafenone and these TCAs inhibit CYP2D6-mediated metabolism of each other	Avoid coadministration

(Continued)

ANTICANCER AND IMMUNOMODULATING DRUGS CYTOTOXICS

Primary Drug	Secondary Drug	Effect	Mechanism	Precautions
CYTOTOXICS				
	9. ANTIMALARIALS—artemether with lumefantrine, chloroquine, halofantrine, hydroxychloroquine, mefloquine, quinine 10. ANTIPROTOZOALS—pentamidine isethionate 11. ANTIPSYCHOTICS—atypicals, phenothiazines, pimozide 12. ANTIVIRALS—boceprevir, rilpivirine, telaprevir 13. BETA-BLOCKERS—sotalol 14. BRONCHODILATORS—parenteral bronchodilators 15. CNS STIMULANTS—atomoxetine 16. RANOLAZINE			
ERIBULIN	ANTIBIOTICS—RIFAMPICIN	Possible reduced eribulin levels	CYP3A4 induction	Manufacturer recommends to avoid concurrent use
ERIBULIN	ANTIDEPRESSANTS—ST. JOHN'S WORT	Possible reduced eribulin levels	CYP3A4 induction	Manufacturer recommends to avoid concurrent use
ERIBULIN	ANTIEPILEPTICS—CARBAMAZEPINE, PHENYTOIN	Possible reduced eribulin levels	CYP3A4 induction	Manufacturer recommends to avoid concurrent use
ERLOTINIB				
ERLOTINIB	**ANALGESICS—NSAIDs**			
ERLOTINIB	NSAIDs	Risk of gastrointestinal bleeding	Additive effect	Avoid coadministration
ERLOTINIB	NSAIDs—CELECOXIB	↑ Celecoxib levels	Inhibition of CYP2D6-mediated metabolism	Use lowest effective dose of celecoxib when necessary
ERLOTINIB	**ANTIBIOTICS**			
ERLOTINIB	CIPROFLOXACIN	Increased levels of erlotinib	CYP1A2 inhibition	Caution with concurrent use. Consider dose reduction if toxicity occurs
ERLOTINIB	MACROLIDES	Predicted increased levels of erlotinib	CYP3A4 inhibition	Caution with concurrent use
ERLOTINIB	RIFAMPICIN	↓ Erlotinib levels	Rifampicin ↑ metabolism of erlotinib	Avoid coadministration

(*Continued*)

Primary Drug	Secondary Drug	Effect	Mechanism	Precautions
CYTOTOXICS				
ERLOTINIB	ANTICANCER AND OTHER IMMUNOMODULATING DRUGS			
ERLOTINIB	CICLOSPORIN	Altered distribution or elimination of erlotinib	P-glycoprotein inhibition	Caution with concurrent use
ERLOTINIB	IRINOTECAN	Increased concentration of irinotecan and SN-38 (its active metabolite), increased irinotecan toxicity	Inhibition of metabolism of SN-38	Caution with concurrent use, consider reduction in irinotecan dose, monitor for signs of toxicity
ERLOTINIB	SORAFENIB	Erlotinib levels possibly reduced	Unknown	Clinical significance uncertain
ERLOTINIB	VINFLUNINE	Increased bone marrow suppression	Unknown	Avoid concurrent use
ERLOTINIB	ANTICOAGULANTS—ORAL	Episodes of ↑ anticoagulant effect	Not understood but likely to be multifactorial	Monitor INR at least weekly until stable during administration of chemotherapy
ERLOTINIB	ANTIDEPRESSANTS—FLUVOXAMINE	Increased levels of erlotinib	CYP1A2 inhibition	Caution with concurrent use. Consider dose reduction if toxicity occurs
ERLOTINIB	ANTIEMETICS—APREPITANT	Single case of increased erlotinib levels	Possibly CYP3A4 inhibition	Be aware of possible interaction
ERLOTINIB	ANTIEPILEPTICS—CARBAMAZEPINE, OXCARBAZEPINE, PHENOBARBITAL, AND PRIMIDONE	Reduced levels of erlotinib	CYP3A4 induction	Avoid concurrent use. If not possible, consider dose increase of erlotinib
ERLOTINIB	PHENYTOIN	↓ Levels of these drugs, with risk of therapeutic failure	Induction of hepatic metabolism	↑ Dose of erlotinib (manufacturer advises starting at 300 mg)
ERLOTINIB	ANTIFUNGALS—FLUCONAZOLE, ITRACONAZOLE, KETOCONAZOLE, VORICONAZOLE	↑ Erlotinib levels	↓ Metabolism of erlotinib	Avoid coadministration

(*Continued*)

Primary Drug	Secondary Drug	Effect	Mechanism	Precautions
CYTOTOXICS				
ERLOTINIB	**ANTIVIRALS**			
ERLOTINIB	DIDANOSINE, STAVUDINE	↑ Risk of hematological toxicity	Additive toxicity	Avoid coadministration
ERLOTINIB	ANTIVIRALS—PROTEASE INHIBITORS	Predicted to inhibit metabolism of erlotinib, but no evidence	CYP3A4 inhibition	Manufacturer advises to exercise caution with concurrent use of HIV protease inhibitors; manufacturer of bocepravir advises against coadministration
ERLOTINIB	CALCIUM CHANNEL BLOCKERS—VERAPAMIL	Altered distribution or elimination of erlotinib	P-glycoprotein inhibition	Caution with concurrent use
ERLOTINIB	GRAPEFRUIT JUICE	Possible slight increased erlotinib levels	CYP3A4 inhibition	Caution with concurrent use
ERLOTINIB	H2-RECEPTOR BLOCKERS	Reduced erlotinib levels	Solubility reduced at higher pH	Avoid concurrent use of H2 antagonists
ERLOTINIB	LIPID-LOWERING DRUGS—SIMVASTATIN	Single case of rhabdomyolysis	Unknown	Significance unknown
ERLOTINIB	PROTON PUMP INHIBITORS	Reduced erlotinib levels	Solubility reduced at higher pH	Avoid concurrent use of PPIs
ESTRAMUSTINE				
ESTRAMUSTINE	ANTIHYPERTENSIVES AND HEART FAILURE DRUGS—ACE INHIBITORS	Possible increased risk of angioedema	Additive	Manufacturer recommends stopping treatment with estramustine if angioedema occurs
ESTRAMUSTINE	BISPHOSPONATES—CLODRONATE	Increased estramustine levels	Uncertain	Monitor closely with concurrent use
ESTRAMUSTINE	CALCIUM AND DAIRY PRODUCTS	↓ Plasma concentrations of estramustine and risk of poor therapeutic response	Due to ↓ absorption of estramustine owing to the formation of a calcium–phosphate complex	Administer estramustine 1 h before or 2 h after dairy products or calcium supplements
ESTRAMUSTINE	H2 RECEPTOR BLOCKERS—CIMETIDINE	↑ Adverse effects of alkylating agent, e.g., myelosuppression	Additive toxicity	Monitor more closely; monitor FBC regularly

(*Continued*)

Primary Drug	Secondary Drug	Effect	Mechanism	Precautions
CYTOTOXICS				
ETOPOSIDE				
ETOPOSIDE	**ANTICANCER AND IMMUNOMODULATING DRUGS**			
ETOPOSIDE	AZATHIOPRINE	↑ Risk of myelosuppression and immunosuppression. Deaths have occurred following profound myelosuppression and severe sepsis	Additive myelotoxic effects. Azathioprine is metabolized to 6-mercaptopurine in vivo, which results in additive myelosuppression, immunosuppression, and hepatotoxicity	Avoid coadministration
ETOPOSIDE	CARBOPLATIN	Slight increase in etoposide levels	Uncertain	Be aware. Probably not clinically significant
ETOPOSIDE (HIGH DOSE)	CARMUSTINE	↑ Risk of liver toxicity, which usually occurs after 1–2 months after initiating treatment without an improvement in tumor response	Possible additive hepatotoxic effects	Avoid coadministration
ETOPOSIDE	CICLOSPORIN	↑ Plasma concentrations of these drugs, with risk of toxic effects	Competitive inhibition of CYP3A4-mediated metabolism and Pgp transport of these drugs	Watch for toxic effects of these drugs
ETOPOSIDE	CISPLATIN	Slight increase in etoposide levels	Uncertain	Be aware. Probably not clinically significant
ETOPOSIDE	CORTICOSTEROIDS—PREDNISONE	Reduced etoposide levels	CYP3A4induction	Monitor closely
ETOPOSIDE	IMATINIB	Increased levels of etoposide	CYP3A4 inhibition	Animal data. Manufacturer advises to exercise caution with concurrent use
ETOPOSIDE	ANTICOAGULANTS—ORAL	Episodes of ↑ anticoagulant effect	Not understood but likely to be multifactorial	Monitor INR at least weekly until stable during administration of chemotherapy

(Continued)

Primary Drug	Secondary Drug	Effect	Mechanism	Precautions
CYTOTOXICS				
ETOPOSIDE	ANTIEPILEPTICS—CARBAMAZEPINE, PHENOBARBITAL	Significantly ↓ plasma concentrations of etoposide (clearance may be >170%) and considerable risk of loss of therapeutic efficacy	Due to potent induction of the hepatic microsomal enzymes that metabolize etoposide	Do not coadminister. Consider use of alternative antiepileptics that do not induce hepatic microsomal enzymes, e.g., valproic acid
PHENYTOIN	ETOPOSIDE	↓ Levels of etoposide, with risk of therapeutic failure	Induction of hepatic metabolism	Avoid coadministration of phenytoin with etoposide
ETOPOSIDE	ANTIFUNGALS—KETOCONAZOLE	Increased levels of etoposide	CYP3A4 inhibition	Clinical significance uncertain
ETOPOSIDE	ANTIMALARIALS—ATOVAQUONE	Possible increase in metabolite, etoposide catechol	Possible effect on CYP3A4 or P-glycoprotein	Caution with concurrent use
ETOPOSIDE	ANTIVIRALS—DIDANOSINE, STAVUDINE, ZIDOVUDINE	↑ Risk of hematological toxicity	Additive toxicity	Review for alternative treatment options, consider substitution of an alternative NRTI or antiretroviral
ETOPOSIDE	CALCIUM CHANNEL BLOCKERS	↑ Serum concentrations and risk of toxicity when verapamil is given to patients on etoposide	Verapamil inhibits CYP3A4-mediated metabolism of etoposide	Watch for symptoms/signs of toxicity (nausea, vomiting, bone marrow suppression) in patients taking calcium channel blockers
ETOPOSIDE	GRAPEFRUIT JUICE	Possibly ↓ efficacy	↓ Bioavailability; unclear	Interindividual variability is considerable. Monitor more closely
EVEROLIMUS				
EVEROLIMUS	ANTIARRHYTHMICS—DRONEDARONE	Predicted increased everolimus levels	CYP3A4 inhibition P-glycoprotein inhibition	Monitor closely with concurrent use
EVEROLIMUS	**ANTIBIOTICS**			
EVEROLIMUS	MACROLIDES ERYTHROMYCIN, CLARITHROMYCIN, TELITHROMYCIN, AZITHROMYCIN	Increased everolimus levels	CYP3A4 inhibition	Manufacturer advises to avoid concurrent use with clarithromycin and telithromycin Consider dose reduction and careful monitoring with others

(*Continued*)

Primary Drug	Secondary Drug	Effect	Mechanism	Precautions
CYTOTOXICS				
EVEROLIMUS	RIFAMPICIN, RIFABUTIN, RIFAPENTINE	Reduced everolimus levels	CYP3A4 and P-glycoprotein induction	Avoid concurrent use if possible If concurrent use is necessary, increase everolimus dose and monitor carefully
EVEROLIMUS	**ANTICANCER AND OTHER IMMUNOMODULATING DRUGS**			
EVEROLIMUS	CICLOSPORIN	Increased everolimus levels Possible increased risk of ciclosporin-induced renal toxicity	Not fully known	Monitor everolimus levels and adjust dose as necessary Monitor renal function and consider reduction in ciclosporin dose
EVEROLIMUS	CORTICOSTEROIDS—DEXAMETHASONE, PREDNISONE, PREDNISOLONE	Reduced everolimus levels	CYP3A4 induction	Avoid concurrent use Consider increasing dose of everolimus if concurrent use is necessary
EVEROLIMUS	IMATINIB	Possible increased everolimus levels	Unknown	Monitor everolimus levels and adjust dose as necessary
EVEROLIMUS	SUNITINIB	Clinically important toxicity in phase I trial	Unknown	Combination use likely to be limited
EVEROLIMUS	TACROLIMUS	Possible increased dose of tacrolimus required	Unknown	Monitor tacrolimus levels
EVEROLIMUS	VEMURAFENIB	Possible increased levels of P-glycoprotein substrates	Vemurafenib inhibits P-glycoprotein	Clinical significance is unknown
EVEROLIMUS	ANTIDEPRESSANTS—ST. JOHN'S WORT	Reduced everolimus levels	CYP3A4 induction	Avoid concurrent use Consider increasing dose of everolimus if concurrent use is necessary
EVEROLIMUS	ANTIEMETICS—APREPITANT, METOCLOPRAMIDE	Possible increased everolimus levels	CYP3A4 inhibition	Caution with concurrent use
EVEROLIMUS	ANTIEPILEPTICS—CARBAMAZEPINE, PHENYTOIN, PHENOBARBITAL	Reduced everolimus levels	CYP3A4 induction	Avoid concurrent use Consider increasing dose of everolimus if concurrent use is necessary

(*Continued*)

Primary Drug	Secondary Drug	Effect	Mechanism	Precautions
CYTOTOXICS				
EVEROLIMUS	ANTIFUNGALS—KETOCONAZOLE, ITRACONAZOLE, VORICONAZOLE, POSACONAZOLE, FLUCONAZOLE	Increased everolimus levels	CYP3A4 inhibition P-glycoprotein inhibition	Avoid concurrent use If concurrent use is necessary, consider dose reduction of everolimus
EVEROLIMUS	ANTIHYPERTENSIVES AND HEART FAILURE DRUGS—ACE INHIBITORS, ANGIOTENSIN II RECEPTOR ANTAGONISTS—LOSARTAN	Reports of angioedema	Uncertain—possibly additive effect (both can cause angioedema)	Warn patient to report facial swelling immediately
EVEROLIMUS	ANTI-PARKINSON'S DRUGS—BROMOCRIPTINE	Possible increased everolimus levels	CYP3A4 inhibition	Caution with concurrent use
EVEROLIMUS	**ANTIVIRALS**			
EVEROLIMUS	PROTEASE INHIBITORS	Predicted increase in everolimus levels	CYP3A4 inhibition	Avoid concurrent use
EVEROLIMUS	EFAVIRENZ, ETRAVIRINE, NEVIRAPINE	Reduced everolimus levels	CYP3A4 induction	Avoid concurrent use Consider increasing dose of everolimus if concurrent use is necessary
EVEROLIMUS	CALCIUM CHANNEL BLOCKERS VERAPAMIL DILTIAZEM	Increased levels of everolimus and verapamil Predicted increased levels of everolimus with diltiazem	CYP3A4 and P-glycoprotein inhibition (verapamil) CYP3A4 inhibition (diltiazem)	Monitor closely with concurrent use Consider dose reduction of everolimus
EVEROLIMUS	DANAZOL	Possible increased everolimus levels	CYP3A4 inhibition	Caution with concurrent use
EVEROLIMUS	GRAPEFRUIT JUICE	Possible increased everolimus levels	CYP3A4 inhibition	Caution with concurrent use
EVEROLIMUS	H2-RECEPTOR BLOCKERS—CIMETIDINE	↑ Adverse effects, e.g., thrombocytopenia, hepatotoxicity	Inhibition of metabolism via CYP3A4 and competition with tacrolimus for renal tubular secretion	Consider alternative acid suppression, e.g., alginate suspension, famotidine, nizatidine, or rabeprazole. Not thought to be clinically significant. Ensure close monitoring of immunosuppressant levels and renal function

(*Continued*)

Primary Drug	Secondary Drug	Effect	Mechanism	Precautions
CYTOTOXICS				
EXEMESTANE				
EXEMESTANE	PHENYTOIN	↓ Levels of exemestane, with risk of therapeutic failure	Induction of hepatic metabolism	↑ Dose of exemestane to 50 mg/day
FLUDARABINE				
FLUDARABINE	**ANTICANCER AND IMMUNOMODULATING DRUGS**			
FLUDARABINE	CYTARABINE	↑ Efficacy of cytarabine	Uncertain	Watch for early features of toxicity of cytarabine
FLUDARABINE	PENTOSTATIN	Risk of severe and potentially fatal pulmonary toxicity	Uncertain	Avoid coadministration
FLUDARABINE	ANTIPLATELET AGENTS—DIPYRIDAMOLE	Possible ↓ efficacy of fludarabine	Uncertain	Consider using an alternative antiplatelet drug
FLUOROURACIL/CAPECITABINE/TEGAFUR				
FLUOROURACIL	**ANTIBIOTICS**			
FLUOROURACIL	METRONIDAZOLE	↑ Risk of toxic effects of fluorouracil (>27%), e.g., bone marrow suppression, oral ulceration, nausea, and vomiting due to ↑ plasma concentrations of fluorouracil	Metronidazole ↓ clearance of fluorouracil	Avoid coadministration
FLUOROURACIL	ORAL NEOMYCIN	Delayed absorption of flourouracil	Neomycin results in malabsorption syndrome	Clinical significance uncertain
FLUOROURACIL	**ANTICANCER AND IMMUNOMODULATING DRUGS**			
FLUOROURACIL	AZATHIOPRINE	↑ Risk of myelosuppression and immunosuppression. Deaths have occurred following profound myelosuppression and severe sepsis	Additive myelotoxic effects. Azathioprine is metabolized to 6-mercaptopurine in vivo, which results in additive myelosuppression, immunosuppression, and hepatotoxicity	Avoid coadministration

(*Continued*)

Primary Drug	Secondary Drug	Effect	Mechanism	Precautions
CYTOTOXICS				
FLUOROURACIL	FOLINATE—CALCIUM FOLINATE, CALCIUM LEVOFOLINATE	Likely ↑ toxicity of leucovorin despite ↑ cytotoxic effects	↑ Cytotoxicity is attributed to maximized binding in the thymidylate synthase–fluorouracil complex (fluorouracil is thought to exert its cytotoxic effect by inhibiting thymidylate synthase, which in turn inhibits DNA synthesis)	Commonly used together for cytotoxic effects, but advise patients to report symptoms of hypersensitivity reactions (itching, wheezing) and fever
FLUOROURACIL	GEMCITABINE	Increased fluorouracil levels	Uncertain	Combination use being investigated for therapeutic potential
FLUOROURACIL	HYDROXYCARBAMIDE (HYDROXYUREA)	↑ Incidence of neurotoxicity (>20%)	Attributed to failure of conversion of fluorouracil to the active metabolite and an accumulation of neurotoxins	Avoid coadministration
CAPECITABINE	INTERFERON ALFA	Reduced maximum tolerated dose of capecitabine	Interferon alfa modulates fluorouracil activity	Reduce maximum capecitabine dose
TEGAFUR	IRINOTECAN	Reduced levels of SN-38 (metabolite of irinotecan)	Possible induction of enzyme responsible for biliary excretion of SN-38	Be aware. Clinical significance uncertain Findings require confirmation
FLUOROURACIL	METHOTREXATE	↓ Cytotoxic effect of methotrexate when fluorouracil is administered prior to methotrexate	Fluorouracil prevents the conversion of ↓ folates to dihydrofolate	Always administer methotrexate prior to fluorouracil
FLUOROURACIL	MITOMYCIN	Intravascular hemolysis and renal failure rarely	Uncertain	Stop drugs at first sign of hemolysis, proteinuria, or rising urea levels
FLUOROURACIL	PANITUMUMAB	High incidence of severe diarrhea with irinotecan, fluorouracil, and folinic acid regimens	Unknown	Manufacturer advises against this combination

(*Continued*)

Primary Drug	Secondary Drug	Effect	Mechanism	Precautions
CYTOTOXICS				
FLUOROURACIL (TOPICAL AND ORAL)	PORFIMER	↑ Risk of photosensitivity reactions	Attributed to additive effects	Avoid exposure of skin and eyes to direct sunlight for 30 days after porfimer therapy
CAPECITABINE	SORAFENIB	Levels of capecitabine increased	Unknown	Caution with concurrent use
FLUOROURACIL	SORAFENIB	Levels of fluorouracil increased	Unknown	Caution with concurrent use
FLUOROURACIL	TAMOXIFEN	Increased risk of thrombosis when used in chemotherapy regimens	Additive	Consider prophylactic anticoagulation
FLUOROURACIL	TEMOPORFIN	↑ Risk of photosensitivity with topical fluorouracil	Uncertain; possibly additive effect (topical fluorouracil can cause local irritation, while temoporfin is a photosensitizer)	Patients on temoporfin are advised to avoid direct sunlight for at least 15 days
FLUOROURACIL	THALIDOMIDE	↑ Risk of thromboembolism	Mechanism is uncertain; the endothelial damaging effect of fluorouracil may possibly initiate thalidomide-mediated thrombosis	Avoid coadministration
FLUOROURACIL (CONTINUOUS INFUSION BUT NOT BOLUS DOSES)	ANTICOAGULANTS—ORAL	Episodes of ↑ anticoagulant effect	Not understood but likely to be multifactorial	Monitor INR at least weekly until stable during administration of chemotherapy
FLUOROURACIL	ANTIDEPRESSANTS—TCAs	Possible ↑ fluorouracil levels	Inhibition of CYP2C9-mediated metabolism. The clinical significance of this depends upon whether alternative pathways of metabolism are also inhibited by coadministered drugs	Warn patients to report ↑ side effects and monitor blood count carefully
FLUOROURACIL, CAPECITABINE, TEGAFUR	ANTIEPILEPTICS—PHENYTOIN	Increased risk of phenytoin toxicitiy	Inhibition of CYP2C19	Avoid concurrent use If not possible, monitor phenytoin concentrations and adjust as necessary

(Continued)

Primary Drug	Secondary Drug	Effect	Mechanism	Precautions
CYTOTOXICS				
TEGAFUR	ANTIFUNGALS—CLOTRIMAZOLE, KETOCONAZOLE, MICONAZOLE	Possible increased levels of tegafur	Tegafur metabolized by CYP2A6	Clinical relevance remains to be determined Caution with concurrent use
CAPECITABINE	ANTIGOUT DRUGS—ALLOPURINOL	Possible ↓ efficacy of capecitabine	Capecitabine is a prodrug for fluorouracil; it is uncertain at which point allopurinol acts on the metabolic pathway	Manufacturers recommend avoiding coadministration
FLUOROURACIL	ANTIHYPERTENSIVE AND HEART FAILURE DRUGS—LOSARTAN	Inhibition of losartan by its active metabolite, E-3174	CYP2C9 inhibition	Clinical significance unclear
FLUOROURACIL	ANTIPROTOZOALS—LEVAMISOLE	↑ Risk of hepatotoxicity and neurotoxicity despite ↑ cytotoxic effects	Antiphosphatase activity of levamisole may ↑ fluorouracil cytotoxicity	This combination has been used successfully in the treatment of colon cancer. Monitor FBC and LFTs regularly. Advise patients to report symptoms such as diarrhea, numbness and tingling, and peeling of the skin of the hands and feet (hand-foot syndrome)
CAPECITABINE, TEGAFUR	**ANTIVIRALS**			
CAPECITABINE	BRIVUDINE	Serious and fatal toxcity	Conversion of brivudine to BVU, which inhibits dihydropyrimidine dehydrogenase, which is involved in fluorouracil metabolism	Avoid concurrent use
TEGAFUR	SORIVUDINE	Serious and fatal toxcity	Conversion of sorivudine to BVU, which inhibits dihydropyrimidine dehydrogenase, which is involved in fluorouracil metabolism	Avoid concurrent use
FLUOROURACIL	COLONY-STIMULATING FACTORS—FILGRASTIM	Possible ↑ risk of neutropenia	Uncertain	Monitor FBC regularly

(*Continued*)

Primary Drug	Secondary Drug	Effect	Mechanism	Precautions
CYTOTOXICS				
FLUOROURACIL	FOLIC ACID	Risk of fluorouracil toxicity	Folic acid exacerbates the inhibitory effect of fluorouracil on DNA	Avoid coadministration
FLUOROURACIL	H2 RECEPTOR BLOCKERS—CIMETIDINE	↑ Fluorouracil levels and altered efficacy of fluorouracil	Inhibition of metabolism and altered action	Monitor more closely. May be of clinical benefit. No additional toxicity was noted in one study
TEGAFUR	METHOXSALEN	Possible increased levels of tegafur	Tegafur metabolized by CYP2A6	Clinical relevance remains to be determined Caution with concurrent use
FOLINIC ACID AND FOLIC ACID				
FOLINATE—CALCIUM FOLINATE, CALCIUM LEVOFOLINATE	FLUOROURACIL	Likely ↑ toxicity of leucovorin despite↑ cytotoxic effects	↑ Cytotoxicity is attributed to maximized binding in the thymidylate synthase–fluorouracil complex (fluorouracil is thought to exert its cytotoxic effect by inhibiting thymidylate synthase, which in turn inhibits DNA synthesis)	Commonly used together for cytotoxic effects, but advise patients to report symptoms of hypersensitivity reactions (itching, wheezing) and fever
FOLINATE	PANITUMUMAB	High incidence of severe diarrhea with irinotecan, fluorouracil, and folinic acid regimens	Unknown	Manufacturer advises against this combination
FOLINATE	RALTITREXED	Folinates theoretically interfere with action of raltitrexed	Folinate antagonizes the anti-DNA effect of raltitrexed	Manufacturer advises to avoid concurrent use
FOLIC ACID	SULFASALAZINE	Possible reduced folic acid absorption	Sulfasalazine interferes with folic acid absorption	Monitor with regular FBC
GEFITINIB				
GEFITINIB	ANTIARRHYTHMICS—QUINIDINE	Increased levels of gefitinib	CYP2D6 inhibition	Monitor closely

(Continued)

ANTICANCER AND IMMUNOMODULATING DRUGS CYTOTOXICS

Primary Drug	Secondary Drug	Effect	Mechanism	Precautions
CYTOTOXICS				
GEFITINIB	**ANTIBIOTICS**			
GEFITINIB	MACROLIDES	Predicted increased levels of gefitinib	CYP3A4 inhibition	Caution with concurrent use
GEFITINIB	RIFAMPICIN	Reduced gefitinib levels	CYP3A4 induction	Avoid coadministration
GEFITINIB	**ANTICANCER AND OTHER IMMUNOMODULATING DRUGS**			
GEFITINIB	CARBOPLATIN	Increased gefitinib levels	Unknown	Unknown, increased toxicity not seen despite increased levels
GEFITINIB	GEMCITABINE	Levels of gemcitabine increased by high dose gefitinib	Unknown	Be aware. Clinical significance uncertain
GEFITINIB	IRINOTECAN	Increased concentration of irinotecan and SN-38 (its active metabolite) Increased irinotecan toxicity	Inhibition of metabolism of SN-38	Caution with concurrent use, consider reduction in irinotecan dose, monitor for signs of toxicity
GEFITINIB	PACLITAXEL	Gefitinib levels slightly increased	Unkonwn	Clinical significance uncertain
GEFITINIB	SORAFENIB	Gefitinib levels reduced	Unknown	Clinical significance uncertain
GEFITINIB	VINORELBINE	Increased risk of neutropenia	Unknown	Avoid concurrent use
GEFITINIB	ANTIDEPRESSANTS—FLUOXETINE, PAROXETINE	Increased levels of gefitinib	CYP2D6 inhibition	Monitor closely
GEFITINIB	PHENYTOIN	Gefitinib levels reduced	CYP3A4 induction	Avoid concurrent use. Consider dose increase if necessary
GEFITINIB	ANTIFUNGALS—KETOCONAZOLE, ITRACONAZOLE, POSACONAZOLE, VORICONAZOLE	Increased levels of gefitinib	CYP3A4 inhibition	Monitor closely with concurrent use Consider dose reduction if toxicity occurs
GEFITINIB	**ANTIVIRALS**			
GEFITINIB	DIDANOSINE, STAVUDINE	↑ Risk of hematological toxicity	Additive toxicity	Avoid coadministration

(Continued)

Primary Drug	Secondary Drug	Effect	Mechanism	Precautions
CYTOTOXICS				
GEFITINIB	PROTEASE INHIBITORS	Predicted to inhibit metabolism of gefitinib, but no evidence	CYP3A4 inhibition	Manufacturer advises caution with concurrent use of HIV protease inhibitors
GEFITINIB	CINACALCET	Increased levels of gefitinib	CYP2D6 inhibition	Monitor closely
GEFITINIB	DRUG DEPENDENCE THERAPIES—BUPROPION	Increased levels of gefitinib	CYP2D6 inhibition	Monitor closely
GEFITINIB	H2-RECEPTOR BLOCKERS	Reduced gefitinib levels	Solubility reduced at higher pH	Avoid concurrent use of H2 antagonists, and simultaneous use of antacids
GEFITINIB	PROTON PUMP INHIBITORS	Reduced gefitinib levels	Solubility reduced at higher pH	Avoid concurrent use of PPIs and simultaneous use of antacids
GEMCITABINE				
GEMCITABINE	**ANTICANCER AND IMMUNOMODULATING DRUGS**			
GEMCITABINE	FLUOROURACIL	Fluorouracil levels increased	Unknown	Combination use being investigated for therapeutic potential
GEMCITABINE	GEFITINIB	Levels of gemcitabine increased by high dose gefitinib	Unknown	Be aware. Clinical significance uncertain
GEMCITABINE	PACLITAXEL	Possibly ↓ antitumor effect in breast cancer	Based on experiments on breast cell lines	Avoid coadministration except in clinical trials
GEMCITABINE	SEMAXANIB	Combination of semaxanib, cisplatin, and gemcitabine resulted in increased thromboembolic events	Unknown	Caution with further studies using cytotoxics and angiogenesis inhibitors
GEMCITABINE	VANDETANIB	Increased levels and toxicity of cisplatin, mainly thromboembolic effects, when given together with gemcitabine and vandetanib	Unknown	Not suitable combination for chemotherapy

(Continued)

Primary Drug	Secondary Drug	Effect	Mechanism	Precautions
CYTOTOXICS				
GEMCITABINE	VINORELBINE	Gemcitabine and vinorelbine levels both reduced. Amount of reduction may depend on sequence of administration	Unknown	Further study required to establish the amount of effect
GEMCITABINE	ANTICOAGULANTS—ORAL	Episodes of ↑ anticoagulant effect	Not understood but likely to be multifactorial	Monitor INR at least weekly until stable during administration of chemotherapy
GEMCITABINE	ANTIVIRALS—DIDANOSINE, STAVUDINE, ZIDOVUDINE	↑ Risk of hematological and renal toxicity	Additive toxicity	Avoid coadministration with didanosine and stavudine. Monitor renal function closely
HYDROXYCARBAMIDE (HYDROXYUREA)				
HYDROXYCARBAMIDE	**ANTICANCER AND IMMUNOMODULATING DRUGS—FLUOROURACIL**			
HYDROXYCARBAMIDE	FLUOROURACIL	↑ Incidence of neurotoxicity (>20%)	Attributed to failure of conversion of fluorouracil to the active metabolite and an accumulation of neurotoxins	Avoid coadministration
HYDROXYCARBAMIDE	INTERFERON ALFA	Possible increased risk of vasculitis	Possibly additive	Caution with concurrent use
HYDROXYCARBAMIDE	**ANTIVIRALS—DIDANOSINE, ZIDOVUDINE**			
HYDROXYCARBAMIDE	DIDANOSINE, ZIDOVUDINE	↑ Adverse effects with didanosine and possibly zidovudine	Additive effects, enhanced antiretroviral activity via ↓ intracellular deoxynucleotides	Avoid coadministration
HYDROXYCARBAMIDE	GANCICLOVIR, VALGANCICLOVIR	Possible increased ganciclovir toxicity	Additive effect on inhibition of rapidly dividing cell populations, e.g., bone marrow, tests, skin, GI mucosa	Monitor closely if concurrent use is necessary
IDARUBICIN				
IDARUBICIN	**ANTICANCER AND IMMUNOMODULATING DRUGS**			
IDARUBICIN	ANESTHETICS, GENERAL—INHALATIONAL	Risk of arrhythmias	Previous treatment with anthracyclines may enhance the myocardial depressive effect	Prevent hypotensive episodes and carbon dioxide retention (hypercapnia)

(Continued)

Primary Drug	Secondary Drug	Effect	Mechanism	Precautions
CYTOTOXICS				
IDARUBICIN	BEVACIZUMAB	Possible increased risk of cardiac failure	Additive	Be aware of interaction
IDARUBICIN	CICLOSPORIN	Increased idarubicin levels	Uncertain	Monitor closely. Consider dose reduction
IDARUBICIN	DASATINIB	Increased risk of cardiac side effects	Dasatinib reported to cause QT prolongation	Avoid concurrent use
IDARUBICIN	LAPATINIB	Increased risk of cardiac side effects	Lapatinib reported to cause QT prolongation	Avoid concurrent use
IDARUBICIN	TRASTUZUMAB	↑ Risk of cardiotoxicity	Additive cardiotoxic effects	Avoid coadministration except in clinical trials
IFOSFAMIDE				
IFOSFAMIDE	**ANTIBIOTICS**			
IFOSFAMIDE	MACROLIDES—CLARITHROMYCIN, ERYTHROMYCIN, TELITHROMYCIN	↓ Plasma concentrations of 4-hydroxyifosfamide, the active metabolite of ifosfamide, and risk of inadequate therapeutic response	Due to inhibition of the isoenzymatic conversion to active metabolites	Monitor the efficacy of ifosfamide clinically and ↑ dose accordingly
IFOSFAMIDE	RIFAMPICIN	↑ Rate of biotransformation to 4-hydroxyifosfamide, the active metabolite, but there is no change in AUC of 4-hydroxyifosfamide	Due to ↑ rate of metabolism and of clearance owing to induction of CYP3A4 and CYP2D6	Be aware—clinical significance may be minimal or none
IFOSFAMIDE	**ANTICANCER AND IMMUNOMODULATING DRUGS**			
IFOSFAMIDE	CISPLATIN	↑ Risk of neurotoxicity, hematotoxicity and tubular nephrotoxicity of ifosfamide due to ↑ plasma concentrations of ifosfamide	Cisplatin tends to cause renal damage, which results in impaired clearance of ifosfamide	Do renal function tests before initiating therapy and during concurrent therapy, and adjust dosage based on creatinine clearance values. Advise patients to drink plenty of water—vigorous hydration—and consider mesna therapy for renal protection

(*Continued*)

Primary Drug	Secondary Drug	Effect	Mechanism	Precautions
CYTOTOXICS				
IFOSFAMIDE	CORTICOSTEROIDS—DEXAMETHASONE	↑ Rate of biotransformation to 4-hydroxyifosfamide, the active metabolite, but there is no change in AUC of 4-hydroxyifosfamide	Due to ↑ rate of metabolism and of clearance owing to induction of CYP3A4 and CYP2D6	Be aware—clinical significance may be minimal or none
IFOSFAMIDE	DOCETAXEL	Lower ifosfamide levels when given after docetaxel compared to before docetaxel	Unknown	Effects of interaction are schedule dependent
IFOSFAMIDE	IMATINIB	Increased levels of ifosfamide	CYP3A4 ihibition	Animal data. Manufacturer advises to exercise caution with concurrent use
IFOSFAMIDE	IRINOTECAN	Reduced levels of SN-38 (irinotecan metabolite) if ifosfamide given daily after irinotecan	Unknown	Avoid this administration's schedule
IFOSFAMIDE	SUNITINIB	Possible decreased sunitinib levels, possible increased risk of neutropenia	Unknown	Reduced maximum dose of ifofamide tolerated in single study due to neutropenia. Further investigation needed
IFOSFAMIDE	TOPOTECAN	Increased toxicity when used concurrently	Unknown	Doses limited for this combination
IFOSFAMIDE	ANTICOAGULANTS—ORAL	Episodes of ↑ anticoagulant effect	Not understood but likely to be multifactorial	Monitor INR at least weekly until stable during administration of chemotherapy
IFOSFAMIDE	ANTIDEPRESSANTS—ST. JOHN'S WORT	↑ Rate of biotransformation to 4-hydroxyifosfamide, the active metabolite, but there is no change in AUC of 4-hydroxyifosfamide	Due to ↑ rate of metabolism and of clearance owing to induction of CYP3A4 and CYP2D6	Be aware—clinical significance may be minimal or none

(Continued)

Primary Drug	Secondary Drug	Effect	Mechanism	Precautions
CYTOTOXICS				
IFOSFAMIDE	ANTIEPILEPTICS—CARBAMAZEPINE, PHENOBARBITAL	↑ Rate of biotransformation to 4-hydroxyifosfamide, the active metabolite, but there is no change in AUC of 4-hydroxyifosfamide	Due to ↑ rate of metabolism and of clearance owing to induction of CYP3A4 and CYP2D6	Be aware—clinical significance may be minimal or none
IFOSFAMIDE	PHENYTOIN	↓ Levels of ifosfamide, with risk of therapeutic failure	Induction of hepatic metabolism	Monitor for ↓ clinical efficacy and ↑ their dose as required
IFOSFAMIDE	**ANTIFUNGALS**			
IFOSFAMIDE	CONVENTIONAL AMPHOTERICIN B	May increase nephrotoxicity	Additive	Avoid concurrent use Consider use of liposomal amphotericin B with caution
IFOSFAMIDE	FLUCONAZOLE, ITRACONAZOLE, KETOCONAZOLE, VORICONAZOLE	↓ Plasma concentrations of 4-hydroxyifosfamide, the active metabolite of ifosfamide, and risk of inadequate therapeutic response	Due to inhibition of the isoenzymatic conversion to active metabolites	Monitor the efficacy of ifosfamide clinically and ↑ dose accordingly
IFOSFAMIDE	ANTIVIRALS—EFAVIRENZ, RITONAVIR	↓ Plasma concentrations of 4-hydroxyifosfamide, the active metabolite of ifosfamide, and risk of inadequate therapeutic response	Due to inhibition of the isoenzymatic conversion to active metabolites	Monitor the efficacy of ifosfamide clinically and ↑ dose accordingly

(Continued)

Primary Drug	Secondary Drug	Effect	Mechanism	Precautions
CYTOTOXICS				
IFOSFAMIDE	CALCIUM CHANNEL BLOCKERS	↓ Plasma concentrations of 4-hydroxyifosfamide, the active metabolite of ifosfamide, and risk of inadequate therapeutic response when coadministered with diltiazem, nifedipine, and verapamil	Due to inhibition of the isoenzymatic conversion to active metabolites by diltiazem	Monitor the efficacy of ifosfamide clinically and ↑ dose accordingly
IFOSFAMIDE	GRAPEFRUIT JUICE	↓ Plasma concentrations of 4-hydroxyifosfamide, the active metabolite of ifosfamide, and risk of inadequate therapeutic response	Due to inhibition of the isoenzymatic conversion to active metabolites	Monitor the efficacy of ifosfamide clinically and ↑ dose accordingly
IFOSFAMIDE	H2 RECEPTOR BLOCKERS—CIMETIDINE	↓ Plasma concentrations of 4-hydroxyifosfamide, the active metabolite of ifosfamide, and risk of inadequate therapeutic response	Due to inhibition of the isoenzymatic conversion to active metabolites	Monitor the efficacy of ifosfamide clinically and ↑ dose accordingly
IMATINIB				
IMATINIB	**ANALGESICS**			
IMATINIB	NSAIDs—CELECOXIB, DICLOFENAC, PIROXICAM	↑ Plasma concentrations, with risk of toxic effects of these drugs	Imatinib is a potent inhibitor of CYP2C9 isoenzymes, which metabolize these drugs	Watch for the early toxic effects of these drugs. If necessary, consider using alternative drugs while the patient is being given imatinib

(Continued)

Primary Drug	Secondary Drug	Effect	Mechanism	Precautions
CYTOTOXICS				
IMATINIB	OPIOIDS	Imatinib and nilotinib may cause ↑ plasma concentrations of codeine, dextromethorphan, hydroxycodone, methadone, morphine, oxycodone, pethidine fentanyl, alfentanil, and tramadol, with a risk of toxic effects	Inhibition of CYP2D6- and 3A4-mediated metabolism of these opioids by imatinib; nilotinib is an inhibitor of CYP3A4 and Pgp	Monitor for clinical efficacy and toxicity. Warn patients to report ↑ drowsiness, malaise, and anorexia Tramadol causes less respiratory depression than other opiates, but need to monitor BP and blood counts and advise patients to report wheezing, loss of appetite, and fainting attacks. Need to consider reducing dose Methadone may cause QT prolongation; the CSM has recommended that patients with heart and liver disease on methadone should be carefully monitored for heart conduction abnormalities such as QT prolongation on ECG, which may lead to sudden death. Also need to monitor patients on more than 100 mg methadone daily, and thus, ↑ plasma concentrations necessitates close monitoring of cardiac and respiratory functions
IMATINIB	PARACETAMOL	Possible increased risk of liver failure, but no pharmacokinetic interaction in studies	Inhibition of paracetamol glucuronidation, possible additive effect	Caution with concurrent use
IMATINIB	ANTIARRHYTHMICS—FLECAINIDE, MEXILETINE, PROPAFENONE	Imatinib may cause ↑ plasma concentrations of these drugs, with a risk of toxic effects	Inhibition of CYP2D6-mediated metabolism of these drugs	Watch for early features of toxicity of these drugs

(Continued)

Primary Drug	Secondary Drug	Effect	Mechanism	Precautions
CYTOTOXICS				
IMATINIB	**ANTIBIOTICS**			
IMATINIB	MACROLIDES—CLARITHROMYCIN, ERYTHROMYCIN	↑ Imatinib levels with ↑ risk of toxicity (e.g., abdominal pain, constipation, dyspnea) and of neurotoxicity (e.g., taste disturbances, dizziness, headache, paresthesia, peripheral neuropathy)	Due to inhibition of CYP3A4-mediated metabolism of imatinib	Monitor for clinical efficacy and for the signs of toxicity listed, along with convulsions, confusion, and signs of edema (including pulmonary edema). Monitor electrolytes and liver function, and for cardiotoxicity
IMATINIB	RIFAMPICIN	↓ Imatinib levels	Due to induction of CYP3A4-mediated metabolism of imatinib	Monitor for clinical efficacy and adjust dose as required. Avoid coadministration of imatinib and rifampicin
IMATINIB	**ANTICANCER AND IMMUNOMODULATING DRUGS**			
IMATINIB	ASPARAGINASE	Possible increased risk of hepatotoxicity	Unknown	Manufacturer advises caution with concurrent use
IMATINIB	CICLOSPORIN	↑ Plasma concentrations of ciclosporin, with risk of nephrotoxicity, myelosuppression, neurotoxicity, and excessive immunosuppression, with risk of infection and post-transplant lymphoproliferative disease	Inhibition of metabolism of ciclosporin	Monitor plasma ciclosporin levels to prevent toxicity
IMATINIB	CORTICOSTEROIDS	↑ Adrenal suppressive effects of corticosteroids, which may ↑ risk of infections and produce an inadequate response to stress scenarios	Due to inhibition of metabolism of corticosteroids	Monitor cortisol levels and warn patients to report symptoms such as fever and sore throat

(Continued)

Primary Drug	Secondary Drug	Effect	Mechanism	Precautions
CYTOTOXICS				
IMATINIB	CORTICOSTEROIDS—DEXAMETHASONE	↓ Imatinib levels	Due to induction of CYP3A4-mediated metabolism of imatinib	Monitor for clinical efficacy and adjust dose as required. Avoid coadministration of imatinib and rifampicin
IMATINIB	CRISANTASPASE	Increased hepatotoxicity	Unknown	Caution with concurrent use
IMATINIB	DOXORUBICIN	↑ Risk of myelosuppression due to ↑ plasma concentrations	Due to ↓ metabolism of doxorubicin by CYP3A4 isoenzymes owing to an inhibition of those enzymes	Monitor for ↑ myelosuppression, peripheral neuropathy, myalgias, and fatigue
IMATINIB	ETOPOSIDE	Increased levels of etoposide	CYP3A4 inhibition	Animal data. Manufacturer advises caution with concurrent use
IMATINIB	EVEROLIMUS	Possible increased everolimus levels	Unknown	Monitor everolimus levels and adjust dose as necessary
IMATINIB	IFOSFAMIDE	Increased levels of ifosfamide	CYP3A4 ihibition	Animal data. Manufacturer advises caution with concurrent use
IMATINIB	IRINOTECAN	↑ Plasma concentrations of SN-38 (the active metabolite of irinotecan) and ↑ toxicity of irinotecan, e.g., diarrhea, acute cholinergic syndrome, interstitial pulmonary disease	Inhibition of CYP3A4-mediated metabolism of SN-38	Peripheral blood counts should be checked before each course of treatment. Monitor lung function. The recommendation is to ↓ dose of irinotecan by 25%
IMATINIB	PONATINIB	Predicted increased in imatinib levels	P-glycoprotein inhibition	Be aware
IMATINIB	TACROLIMUS	Increased tracrolimus levels	CYP3A4 inhibition	Monitor tacrolimus levels
IMATINIB	VINCA ALKALOIDS	↑ Adverse effects of vinblastine and vincristine	Inhibition of CYP3A4-mediated metabolism. Also inhibition of Pgp efflux of vinblastine	Monitor FBCs and watch for early features of toxicity (pain, numbness, tingling in the fingers and toes, jaw pain, abdominal pain, constipation, ileus). Consider selecting an alternative drug

(*Continued*)

ANTICANCER AND IMMUNOMODULATING DRUGS CYTOTOXICS

Primary Drug	Secondary Drug	Effect	Mechanism	Precautions
CYTOTOXICS				
IMATINIB	ANTICOAGULANTS—ORAL	Episodes of ↑ anticoagulant effect	Not understood but likely to be multifactorial	Manufacturer recommends converting to LMWH from warfarin. However, if warfarin is considered essential, monitor INR at least weekly until stable during administration of chemotherapy
IMATINIB	**ANTIDEPRESSANTS**			
IMATINIB	ST. JOHN'S WORT	↓ Imatinib levels	Due to induction of CYP3A4-mediated metabolism of imatinib	Avoid concurrent use
IMATINIB	FLUOXETINE, PAROXETINE, TRAZODONE, VENLAFAXINE	Imatinib may cause ↑ plasma concentrations of these drugs, with a risk of toxic effects	Inhibition of CYP2D6-mediated metabolism of these drugs	Watch for early features of toxicity of these drugs
IMATINIB	SERTRALINE	↑ Plasma concentrations, with risk of toxic effects of sertraline	Imatinib is a potent inhibitor of CYP2C9 isoenzymes, which metabolize these drugs	Watch for the early toxic effects of these drugs. If necessary, consider using alternative drugs while the patient is being given imatinib
IMATINIB	TCAs	1. Imatinib may cause ↑ plasma concentrations of these drugs, with a risk of toxic effects 2. Possible ↑ imatinib levels	1. Inhibition of CYP2D6-mediated metabolism of these drugs 2. Inhibition of CYP2C9-mediated metabolism. The clinical significance of this depends upon whether alternative pathways of metabolism are also inhibited by coadministered drugs	1. Watch for early features of toxicity of these drugs 2. Warn patients to report ↑ side effects and monitor blood count carefully
IMANTINIB	**ANTIDIABETIC DRUGS**			
IMATINIB	GLIMEPIRIDE, GLIPIZIDE, TOLBUTAMIDE	↑ Plasma concentrations, with risk of toxic effects of these drugs	Imatinib is a potent inhibitor of CYP2C9 isoenzymes, which metabolize these drugs	Watch for the early toxic effects of these drugs. If necessary, consider using alternative drugs while the patient is being given imatinib

(Continued)

Primary Drug	Secondary Drug	Effect	Mechanism	Precautions
CYTOTOXICS				
IMATINIB	REPAGLINIDE	Likely to ↑ plasma concentrations of repaglinide and ↑ risk of hypoglycemic episodes	Due to inhibition of CYP3A4 isoenzymes, which metabolize repaglinide	Watch for and warn patients about hypoglycemia. ➢ ***For signs and symptoms of hypoglycemia, see Clinical Features of Some Adverse Drug Interactions, Hypoglycemia***
IMATINIB	**ANTIEPILEPTICS**			
IMATINIB	CARBAMAZEPINE, PHENOBARBITAL	↓ Imatinib levels	Due to induction of CYP3A4-mediated metabolism of imatinib	Monitor for clinical efficacy and adjust dose as required
IMATINIB	FOSPHENYTOIN, PHENYTOIN	1. ↓ Imatinib levels 2. ↑ Plasma concentrations, with risk of toxic effects of these drugs	1. Due to induction of CYP3A4-mediated metabolism of imatinib 2. Imatinib is a potent inhibitor of CYP2C9 isoenzymes, which metabolize these drugs	1. Monitor for clinical efficacy and adjust dose as required 2. Watch for the early toxic effects of these drugs. If necessary, consider using alternative drugs while the patient is being given imatinib
IMATINIB	TOPIRAMATE	↑ Plasma concentrations, with risk of toxic effects of topiramate	Imatinib is a potent inhibitor of CYP2C9	Watch for the early toxic effects of topiramate. If necessary, consider using alternative drugs while the patient is being given imatinib
IMATINIB	ANTIFUNGALS—FLUCONAZOLE, ITRACONAZOLE, KETOCONAZOLE VORICONAZOLE	↑ Imatinib levels with ↑ risk of toxicity (e.g., abdominal pain, constipation, dyspnea) and of neurotoxicity (e.g., taste disturbances, dizziness, headache, paresthesia, peripheral neuropathy)	Due to inhibition of CYP3A4-mediated metabolism of imatinib	Monitor for clinical efficacy and for the signs of toxicity listed, along with convulsions, confusion, and signs of edema (including pulmonary edema). Monitor electrolytes and liver function, and for cardiotoxicity
IMATINIB	ANTIHYPERTENSIVES AND HEART FAILURE DRUGS—IRBESARTAN, LOSARTAN, VALSARTAN	↑ Plasma concentrations, with risk of toxic effects of these drugs	Imatinib is a potent inhibitor of CYP2C9 isoenzymes, which metabolize these drugs	Watch for the early toxic effects of these drugs. If necessary, consider using alternative drugs while the patient is being given imatinib

(Continued)

ANTICANCER AND IMMUNOMODULATING DRUGS CYTOTOXICS

Primary Drug	Secondary Drug	Effect	Mechanism	Precautions
CYTOTOXICS				
IMATINIB	ANTIMIGRAINE DRUGS—ALMOTRIPTAN, ELETRIPTAN	↑ Plasma concentrations of almotriptan and risk of toxic effects of almotriptan, e.g., flushing, sensations of tingling, heat, heaviness, pressure, or tightness of any part of body including the throat and chest, dizziness	Almotriptan is metabolized mainly by CYP3A4 isoenzymes. Most CYP isoenzymes are inhibited by imatinib mesylate to varying degrees, and since there is an alternative pathway of metabolism by MAO-A, the toxicity responses will vary between individuals	The CSM has advised, particularly for sumatriptan, that if chest tightness or pressure is intense, triptan should be discontinued immediately and the patient investigated for ischemic heart disease by measuring cardiac enzymes and doing an ECG. Avoid concomitant use in patients with coronary artery disease and in those with severe or uncontrolled hypertension
IMATINIB	ANTIPSYCHOTICS—CLOZAPINE, HALOPERIDOL, PERPHENAZINE, RISPERIDONE, THIORIDAZINE	Imatinib may cause ↑ plasma concentrations of these drugs, with a risk of toxic effects	Inhibition of CYP2D6-mediated metabolism of these drugs	Watch for early features of toxicity of these drugs
IMATINIB	**ANTIVIRALS**			
IMATINIB	PROTEASE INHIBITORS—ATAZANAVIR, BOCEPREVIR, INDINAVIR, NELFINAVIR, RITONAVIR AND SAQUINAVIR	Predicted to increase imatinib levels	CYP3A4 inhibition	Manufacturer advises to avoid concurrent use
IMATINIB	EFAVIRENZ, RITONAVIR	↑ Imatinib levels with ↑ risk of toxicity (e.g., abdominal pain, constipation, dyspnea) and of neurotoxicity (e.g., taste disturbances, dizziness, headache, paresthesia, peripheral neuropathy)	Due to inhibition of CYP3A4-mediated metabolism of imatinib	Monitor for clinical efficacy and for the signs of toxicity listed, along with convulsions, confusion, and signs of edema (including pulmonary edema). Monitor electrolytes and liver function, and for cardiotoxicity
IMATINIB	BETA-BLOCKERS—METOPROLOL, PROPRANOLOL, TIMOLOL	Imatinib may cause ↑ plasma concentrations of these drugs, with a risk of toxic effects	Inhibition of CYP2D6-mediated metabolism of these drugs	Watch for early features of toxicity of these drugs

(*Continued*)

Primary Drug	Secondary Drug	Effect	Mechanism	Precautions
CYTOTOXICS				
IMATINIB	CALCIUM CHANNEL BLOCKERS	↑ Plasma concentrations of imatinib when coadministered with diltiazem, nifedipine, and verapamil. ↑ risk of toxicity (e.g., abdominal pain, constipation, dyspnea) and of neurotoxicity (e.g., taste disturbances, dizziness, headache, paresthesia, peripheral neuropathy)	Due to inhibition of hepatic metabolism of imatinib by the CYP3A4 isoenzymes by diltiazem	Monitor for clinical efficacy and for the signs of toxicity listed, along with convulsions, confusion, and signs of edema (including pulmonary edema). Monitor electrolytes and liver function, and for cardiotoxicity
IMATINIB	GRAPEFRUIT JUICE	Possible increased imatinib levels	CYP3A4 inhibition	Avoid concurrent use
IMATINIB	LEVOTHYROXINE	Hypothyroidism in thyroidectomy patients taking levothyroxine	Unknown	Monitor TSH levels and increase levothyroxine if necessary
IMATINIB	**LIPID-LOWERING DRUGS**			
IMATINIB	LOMITAPIDE	Predicted increased levels of imatinib	P-glycoprotein inhibition	Monitor closely with concurrent use
IMATINIB	STATINS	Imatinib may ↑ atorvastatin and simvastatin levels	Imatinib inhibits CYP3A4-mediated metabolism of simvastatin	Monitor LFTs, U&Es, and CK closely
IMATINIB	NEUROMUSCULAR DISEASES AND MOVEMENT DISORDERS—DONEPEZIL	Imatinib may cause ↑ plasma concentrations of donepezil, with a risk of toxic effects	Inhibition of CYP2D6-mediated metabolism of donepezil	Watch for early features of toxicity of donepezil
IMATINIB	PROTON PUMP INHIBITORS—OMEPRAZOLE	↑ Plasma concentrations, with risk of toxic effects of these drugs	Imatinib is a potent inhibitor of CYP2C9 isoenzymes, which metabolize these drugs	Watch for the early toxic effects of these drugs. If necessary, consider using alternative drugs while the patient is being given imatinib
IMATINIB	SYMPATHOMIMETICS—METHAMPHETAMINE	Imatinib may cause ↑ plasma concentrations of methamphetamine, with a risk of toxic effects	Inhibition of CYP2D6-mediated metabolism of methamphetamine	Watch for early features of toxicity of methamphetamine

(Continued)

ANTICANCER AND IMMUNOMODULATING DRUGS CYTOTOXICS Irinotecan

Primary Drug	Secondary Drug	Effect	Mechanism	Precautions
CYTOTOXICS				
IRINOTECAN				
IRINOTECAN	**ANTIBIOTICS**			
IRINOTECAN	MACROLIDES—CLARITHROMYCIN, ERYTHROMYCIN	↑ Plasma concentrations of SN-38 (↑ AUC by 100%) and ↑ toxicity of irinotecan, e.g., diarrhea, acute cholinergic syndrome, interstitial pulmonary disease	Due to inhibition of the metabolism of irinotecan by CYP3A4 isoenzymes by ketoconazole	Peripheral blood counts should be checked before each course of treatment. Monitor lung function. Recommendation is to ↓ dose of irinotecan by 25%
IRINOTECAN	RIFAMPICIN	↓ Plasma concentrations of irinotecan and risk of ↓ therapeutic efficacy. The effects may last for 3 weeks after discontinuation of CYP-inducer therapy	Due to induction of CYP3A4-mediated metabolism of irinotecan	Avoid concomitant use whenever possible; if not, ↑ dose of irinotecan by 50%
IRINOTECAN	**ANTICANCER AND IMMUNOMODULATING DRUGS**			
IRINOTECAN	CICLOSPORIN	Increased irinotecan levels, but reduced gastrointestinal toxicity	Possibly due to inhibition of irinotecan transporters	Combination used to improve irinotecan toxicity, but be aware of interaction when irinotecan is given to patient already taking ciclosporin
IRINOTECAN	CORTICOSTEROIDS—DEXAMETHASONE	↓ Plasma concentrations of irinotecan and risk of ↓ therapeutic efficacy. The effects may last for 3 weeks after discontinuation of CYP-inducer therapy	Due to induction of CYP3A4-mediated metabolism of irinotecan	Avoid concomitant use whenever possible; if not, ↑ dose of irinotecan by 50%
IRINOTECAN	CRIZOTINIB	Possible increased levels of UGT substrates	UGT (particularly UGT1A1, UGT2B7) inhibtion	Caution with concurrent use

(Continued)

Primary Drug	Secondary Drug	Effect	Mechanism	Precautions
CYTOTOXICS				
IRINOTECAN	ERLOTINIB	Increased concentration of irinotecan and SN-38 (its active metabolite), increased irinotecan toxicity	Inhibition of metabolism of SN-38	Caution with concurrent use, consider reduction in irinotecan dose, monitor for signs of toxicity
IRINOTECAN	GEFITINIB	Increased concentration of irinotecan and SN-38 (its active metabolite), increased irinotecan toxicity	Inhibition of metabolism of SN-38	Caution with concurrent use, consider reduction in irinotecan dose, monitor for signs of toxicity
IRINOTECAN	IFOSFAMIDE	Reduced levels of SN-38 (irinotecan metabolite) if ifosfamide given daily after irinotecan	Unknown	Avoid this administration schedule
IRINOTECAN	IMATINIB	↑ Plasma concentrations of SN-38 (↑ AUC by 100%) and ↑ toxicity of irinotecan, e.g., diarrhea, acute cholinergic syndrome, interstitial pulmonary disease	Due to inhibition of the metabolism of irinotecan by CYP3A4 isoenzymes by ketoconazole	Peripheral blood counts should be checked before each course of treatment. Monitor lung function. Recommendation is to ↓ dose of irinotecan by 25%
IRINOTECAN	PACLITAXEL	Possible increased irinotecan levels	Unknown	Clinical significance uncertain. Be aware of possible interaction
IRINOTECAN	PANITUMUMAB	High incidence of severe diarrhea with irinotecan, fluorouracil, and folinic acid regimens	Unknown	Manufacturer advises against this combination
IRINOTECAN	REGORAFENIB	Possible increased levels of UGT1A1 and UGT1A9 subtrates	UGT1A1 and UGT1A9 inhibition	Clinical significance not determined

(Continued)

Primary Drug	Secondary Drug	Effect	Mechanism	Precautions
CYTOTOXICS				
IRINOTECAN	SORAFENIB	Increased concentration of irinotecan and SN-38 (its active metabolite), increased irinotecan toxicity	Inhibition of metabolism of SN-38	Caution with concurrent use, consider reduction in irinotecan dose, monitor for signs of toxicity
IRINOTECAN	SUNITINIB	Increased concentration of irinotecan and SN-38 (its active metabolite), increased irinotecan toxicity	Inhibition of metabolism of SN-38	Caution with concurrent use, consider reduction in irinotecan dose, monitor for signs of toxicity
IRINOTECAN	TEGAFUR	Reduced levels of SN-38 (metabolite of irinotecan)	Possible induction of enzyme responsible for biliary excretion of SN-38	Be aware. Clinical significance uncertain Findings require confirmation
IRINOTECAN	VINORELBINE	Reduced levels of SN-38 (irinotecan metabolite) in vitro	Unknown	Be aware. Clinical significance uncertain
IRINOTECAN	ANTICOAGULANTS—WARFARIN	Episodes of increased anticoagulant effect	Not understood but likely to be multifactorial	Monitor INR at least weekly until stable during administration of chemotherapy
IRINOTECAN	ANTIDEPRESSANTS—ST. JOHN'S WORT	↓ Plasma concentrations of irinotecan and risk of ↓ therapeutic efficacy. The effects may last for 3 weeks after discontinuation of CYP-inducer therapy	Due to induction of CYP3A4-mediated metabolism of irinotecan	Avoid concomitant use whenever possible; if not, ↑ dose of irinotecan by 50%
IRINOTECAN	ANTIEPILEPTICS—CARBAMAZEPINE, PHENOBARBITAL	↓ Plasma concentrations of irinotecan and risk of ↓ therapeutic efficacy. The effects may last for 3 weeks after discontinuation of CYP-inducer therapy	Due to induction of CYP3A4-mediated metabolism of irinotecan	Avoid concomitant use whenever possible; if not, ↑ dose of irinotecan by 50%

(Continued)

Primary Drug	Secondary Drug	Effect	Mechanism	Precautions
CYTOTOXICS				
IRINOTECAN	PHENYTOIN	↓ Levels of irinotecan, with risk of therapeutic failure	Induction of hepatic metabolism	1. Avoid coadministration of phenytoin with irinotecan (if you not able to avoid, ↑ dose of irinotecan by 50%)
IRINOTECAN	ANTIFUNGALS—FLUCONAZOLE, ITRACONAZOLE, KETOCONAZOLE, VORICONAZOLE	↑ Plasma concentrations of SN-38 (↑ AUC by 100%) and ↑ toxicity of irinotecan, e.g., diarrhea, acute cholinergic syndrome, interstitial pulmonary disease	Due to inhibition of the metabolism of irinotecan by CYP3A4 isoenzymes	Peripheral blood counts should be checked before each course of treatment. Monitor lung function. Recommendation is to ↓ dose of irinotecan by 25%
IRINOTECAN	ANTIVIRALS—PROTEASE INHIBITORS—ATAZANAVIR/ RITONAVIR, LOPINAVIR/RITONAVIR, RITONAVIR	↑ Plasma concentrations of SN-38 (↑ AUC by 100%) and ↑ toxicity of irinotecan, e.g., diarrhea, acute cholinergic syndrome, interstitial pulmonary disease	Due to inhibition of the metabolism of irinotecan by CYP3A4 isoenzymes	Peripheral blood counts should be checked before each course of treatment. Monitor lung function. Recommendation is to ↓ dose of irinotecan by 25%
IRINOTECAN	CALCIUM CHANNEL BLOCKERS	Risk of ↑ serum concentrations of irinotecan with nifedipine. No cases of toxicity reported	Inhibition of hepatic microsomal enzymes, but exact mechanism is unknown	Watch for symptoms/signs of toxicity (especially diarrhea, an early manifestation of acute cholinergic syndrome)
IRINOTECAN	GRAPEFRUIT JUICE	↑ Plasma concentrations of SN-38 (↑ AUC by 100%) and ↑ toxicity of irinotecan, e.g., diarrhea, acute cholinergic syndrome, interstitial pulmonary disease	Due to inhibition of the metabolism of irinotecan by CYP3A4 isoenzymes	Peripheral blood counts should be checked before each course of treatment. Monitor lung function. Recommendation is to ↓ dose of irinotecan by 25%

(Continued)

Primary Drug	Secondary Drug	Effect	Mechanism	Precautions
CYTOTOXICS				
IRINOTECAN	H2 RECEPTOR BLOCKERS—CIMETIDINE	↑ Plasma concentrations of SN-38 (↑ AUC by 100%) and ↑ toxicity of irinotecan, e.g., diarrhea, acute cholinergic syndrome, interstitial pulmonary disease	Due to inhibition of the metabolism of irinotecan by CYP3A4 isoenzymes	Peripheral blood counts should be checked before each course of treatment. Monitor lung function. Recommendation is to ↓ dose of irinotecan by 25%
IRINOTECAN	MUSCLE RELAXANTS—SUXAMETHONIUM	Neuromuscular blocking effects may be prolonged	Irinotecan has anticholinesterase activity	Caution with concurrent use
IRINOTECAN	PARASYMPATHOMIMETICS—PHYSOSTIGMINE	Reduced levels of SN-38 (irinotecan metabolite) in vitro	Unknown	Clinical significance uncertain
LAPATINIB				
LAPATINIB	**DRUGS THAT PROLONG THE QT INTERVAL**			
LAPATINIB	1. ANTIARRHYTHMICS—ajmaline, amiodarone, azimilide, cibenzoline, disopyramide, dofetilide, dronedarone, ibutilide, procainamide, propafenone, quinidine 2. ANTIBIOTICS—macrolides (especially azithromycin, clarithromycin, parenteral erythromycin, telithromycin), quinolones (especially moxifloxacin), quinupristin/dalfopristin 3. ANTICANCER AND IMMUNOMODULATING DRUGS—arsenic trioxide, bosutinib, crizotinib, dasatinib, eribulin, fingolimod, nilotinib, pazopanib, sunitinib, vandetanib, vemurafenib 4. ANTIDEPRESSANTS—TCAs, venlafaxine	Risk of ventricular arrhythmias, particularly torsades de pointes	Additive effect; these drugs prolong the QT interval	Avoid coadministration

(Continued)

Primary Drug	Secondary Drug	Effect	Mechanism	Precautions
CYTOTOXICS				
	5. ANTIEMETICS—ondansetron 6. ANTIFUNGALS—fluconazole, posaconazole, voriconazole 7. ANTIHISTAMINES—terfenadine, hydroxyzine, mizolastine 8. ANTIHYPERTENSIVES—ketanserin 9. ANTIMALARIALS—artemether with lumefantrine, chloroquine, halofantrine, hydroxychloroquine, mefloquine, quinine 10. ANTIPROTOZOALS—pentamidine isethionate 11. ANTIPSYCHOTICS—atypicals, phenothiazines, pimozide 12. ANTIVIRALS—boceprevir, rilpivirine, telaprevir 13. BETA-BLOCKERS—sotalol 14. BRONCHODILATORS—parenteral bronchodilators 15. CNS STIMULANTS—atomoxetine 16. RANOLAZINE			
LAPATINIB	ANTACIDS	Reduced lapatinib levels	Solubility reduced at higher pH	Avoid concurrent use
LAPATINIB	**ANTIBIOTICS**			
LAPATINIB	MACROLIDES	Predicted increased levels of lapatinib	CYP3A4 inhibition	Avoid concurrent use
LAPATINIB	RIFAMPICIN	Predicted reduced lapatinib levels	CYP3A4 induction	Avoid coadministration
LAPATINIB	**ANTICANCER AND OTHER IMMUNOMODULATING DRUGS**			
LAPATINIB	CICLOSPORIN	Increased lapatinib levels	P-glycoprotein inhibition	Caution with concurrent use
LAPATINIB	DAUNORUBICIN, DOXORUBICIN, EPIRUBICIN, IDARUBICIN, VALRUBICIN	Increased risk of cardiac side effects	Lapatinib reported to cause QT prolongation	Avoid concurrent use

(*Continued*)

ANTICANCER AND IMMUNOMODULATING DRUGS CYTOTOXICS

ANTICANCER AND IMMUNOMODULATING DRUGS CYTOTOXICS Lapatinib

Primary Drug	Secondary Drug	Effect	Mechanism	Precautions
CYTOTOXICS				
LAPATINIB	PAZOPANIB	Increased pazopanib levels	Inhibition of P-glycoprotein or BCRP by lapatininb	Significance uncertain Clinical studies with pazopanib, pemetrexed, and lapatinib were stopped early because of increased toxicity
LAPATINIB	PONATINIB	Predicted increased in lapatinib levels	P-glycoprotein inhibition	Be aware
LAPATINIB	TOPOTECAN	Slightly reduced topotecan levels Lower tolerated dose of topotecan	Possible inhibition of drug transporter proteins by lapatinib	Caution with concurrent use
LAPATINIB	VALSPODAR	Increased lapatinib levels	P-glycoprotein inhibition	Caution with concurrent use
LAPATINIB	VINORELBINE	Reduced vinorelbine clearance	Possible CYP3A4 inhibition	Consider reduction in dosage of both drugs
LAPATINIB	ANTIDEPRESANTS—ST. JOHN'S WORT	Reduced lapatinib levels	P-glycoprotein induction	Caution with concurrent use
LAPATINIB	ANTIDIABETICS—REPAGLINIDE	Possible increased levels of CYP2C8 substrates	CYP2C8 inhibition	Avoid or caution with concurrent use
LAPATINIB	ANTIEPILEPTICS—CARBAMAZEPINE	Reduced lapatinib levels	CYP3A4 induction	Avoid concurrent use Consider dose increase if necessary
LAPATINIB	ANTIFUNGALS—KETOCONAZOLE, ITRACONAZOLE, POSACONAZOLE, VORICONAZOLE	Increased levels of lapatinib	CYP3A4 inhibition	Avoid concurrent use Consider dose reduction if concurrent use is necessary
LAPATINIB	**ANTIVIRALS**			
LAPATINIB	PROTEASE INHIBITORS	Predicted increased levels of lapatininb	CYP3A4 inhibition	Manufacturer advises to avoid concurrent use of HIV protease inhibitors, specifically ritonavir, atazanavir, indinavir, nelfinavir, and saquinavir

(Continued)

Primary Drug	Secondary Drug	Effect	Mechanism	Precautions
CYTOTOXICS				
LAPATINIB	BOCEPREVIR	Predicted increased levels of boceprevir	CYP3A4 inhibition	Manufacturer advises to avoid concurrent use
LAPATINIB	TIPRANAVIR	Reduced lapatinib levels	P-glycoprotein induction	Caution with concurrent use
LAPATINIB	ANXIOLYTICS AND HYPNOTICS—MIDAZOLAM	Midazolam levels slightly increased	CYP3A4 inhibition	Caution with concurrent use
LAPATINIB	**CALCIUM CHANNEL BLOCKERS**			
LAPATINIB	DIHYDROPYRIDINES	Possible increased levels of dihydropyridine calcium channel blockers	CYP3A4 inhibition	Interactions related to case reports. General relevance uncertain. Monitor concurrent use
LAPATINIB	VERAPAMIL	Increased lapatinib levels	P-glycoprotein inhibition	Caution with concurrent use
LAPATINIB	CARDIAC GLYCOSIDES—DIGOXIN	Increased levels of digoxin	P-glycoprotein inhibition	Monitor closely, measure digoxin levels, and consider dose reduction with digoxin
LAPATINIB	CONIVAPTAN	Increased lapatinib levels	P-glycoprotein inhibition	Caution with concurrent use
LAPATINIB	GRAPEFRUIT JUICE	Possible increased lapatinib levels	CYP3A4 inhibition	Avoid concurrent use
LAPATINIB	H2-RECEPTOR BLOCKERS	Reduced lapatinib levels	Solubility reduced at higher pH	Avoid concurrent use
LAPATINIB	LIPID-LOWERING DRUGS—LOMITAPIDE	Predicted increased levels of lapatinib	P-glycoprotein inhibition	Monitor closely with concurrent use
LAPATINIB	PROTON PUMP INHIBITORS	Reduced lapatinib levels	Solubility reduced at higher pH	Avoid concurrent use
LOMUSTINE				
LOMUSTINE	ANTIEPILEPTICS—PHENOBARBITAL	↓ Plasma concentrations of lomustine and risk of inadequate therapeutic response	Phenobarbital induces the metabolism of lomustine by the CYP450 isoenzymes	Avoid concurrent use. If necessary, ↑ dose of lomustine and monitor therapeutic effects
LOMUSTINE	BRONCHODILATORS—THEOPHYLLINE	Single case report of thrombocytopenia and bleeding	Inhibition of platelet phosphodiesterase activity by theophylline	Be aware. Clinical significance uncertain
LOMUSTINE	H2 RECEPTOR BLOCKERS—CIMETIDINE	↑ Adverse effects of alkylating agent, e.g., myelosuppression	Additive toxicity	Monitor more closely; monitor FBC regularly

(*Continued*)

Primary Drug	Secondary Drug	Effect	Mechanism	Precautions
CYTOTOXICS				
MELPHALAN				
MELPHALAN	ANTIBIOTICS—NALIDIXIC ACID	Risk of melphalan toxicity	Uncertain	Avoid coadministration
MELPHALAN	**ANTICANCER AND IMMUNOMODULATING DRUGS**			
MELPHALAN	BORTEZOMIB	Slight increased bortezomib levels when used with melphalan and prednisolone	Uncertain	Be aware. Probably of no clinical significance
MELPHALAN	CICLOSPORIN	Risk of renal toxicity	Additive effect	Monitor U&Es closely
MELPHALAN	INTERFERON ALFA	Reduced melphalan levels, but increased toxicity possibly due to interferon-induced fever	Uncertain	Be aware. Clinical importance uncertain
MELPHALAN	H2 RECEPTOR BLOCKERS—CIMETIDINE	↓ Plasma concentrations and bioavailability of melphalan by 30% and risk of poor therapeutic response to melphalan	Cimetidine causes a change in gastric pH, which ↓ absorption of melphalan	Avoid concurrent use
MERCAPTOPURINE				
MERCAPTOPURINE	ANTIBIOTICS—CO-TRIMOXAZOLE	↑ Risk of bone marrow toxicity	Additive effect	Avoid coadministration
MERCAPTOPURINE	**ANTICANCER AND IMMUNOMODULATING DRUGS**			
MERCAPTOPURINE	ADALIMUMAB	Cases of hepatosplenic T-cell lymphoma reported in adolescents and young adults	Unknown	Causal relationship unclear
MERCAPTOPURINE	AMINOSALICYLATES	↑ Risk of bone marrow suppression	Additive effect	Monitor FBC closely
MERCAPTOPURINE	AZATHIOPRINE	↑ Risk of myelosuppression and immunosuppression. Deaths have occurred following profound myelosuppression and severe sepsis	Additive myelotoxic effects. Azathioprine is metabolized to 6-mercaptopurine in vivo, which results in additive myelosuppression, immunosuppression, and hepatotoxicity	Avoid coadministration

(*Continued*)

Primary Drug	Secondary Drug	Effect	Mechanism	Precautions
CYTOTOXICS				
MERCAPTOPURINE	DOXORUBICIN	↑ Risk of hepatotoxicity due to mercaptopurine	Uncertain, possibly due to previous treatment with mercaptopurine	Avoid coadministration—except in clinical trials
MERCAPTOPURINE	INFLIXIMAB	Cases of hepatosplenic T-cell lymphoma reported in adolescents and young adults	Unknown	Causal relationship unclear
MERCAPTOPURINE	METHOTREXATE—ORAL	↑ Plasma concentrations of mercaptopurine (↑ AUC by 30%) and ↑ risk of myelotoxicity	Methotrexate ↑ oral bioavailability of mercaptopurine	↓ Dose of oral 6-mercaptopurine when used with doses of methotrexate >20 mg/m^2 or higher doses of methotrexate given intravenously
MERCAPTOPURINE	NATALIZUMAB	Potential increased risk of progressive multifocal leukoencephalopathy, although no increased risk of infection in available data	Additive	Manufacturer advises to avoid concurrent use
MERCAPTOPURINE	ANTICOAGULANTS—WARFARIN	Possible ↓ anticoagulant effect	Induction of metabolism of warfarin	Monitor INR closely
MERCAPTOPURINE	**ANTIGOUT DRUGS**			
MERCAPTOPURINE	ANTIGOUT DRUGS—ALLOPURINOL	↑ Mercaptopurine levels with risk of toxicity (e.g., myelosuppression, pancreatitis)	Azathioprine is metabolized to mercaptopurine. Allopurinol inhibits hepatic metabolism of mercaptopurine	↓ Doses of azathioprine and mercaptopurine to one-quarter of usual dose and monitor FBC, LFTs, and amylase carefully
MERCAPTOPURINE	FEBUXOSTAT	May increase azathioprine levels	Inhibition of xanthine oxidase	Avoid concurrent use If necessary, consider dose reduction and monitor closely
MESNA				
MESNA	CISPLATIN	Inactivation of cisplatin	Pharmaceutical interaction	Do not mix mesna with cisplatin infusions

(*Continued*)

Primary Drug	Secondary Drug	Effect	Mechanism	Precautions
CYTOTOXICS				
METHOTREXATE				
METHOTREXATE	ANESTHETICS—NITROUS OXIDE	↑ Antifolate effect of methotrexate	↑ Toxicity of methotrexate	Nitrous oxide is usually used for relatively brief durations when patients are anesthetized, and hence, this risk during anesthesia is minimal. However, nitrous oxide may be used as analgesia for longer durations, and this should be avoided
METHOTREXATE	ANALGESICS—NSAIDs	↑ Methotrexate levels, with reports of toxicity, with ibuprofen, indomethacin and possibly diclofenac, flurbiprofen, ketoprofen, and naproxen	Uncertain; postulated that an NSAID-induced ↓ in renal perfusion may have an effect	Consider using an alternative NSAID
METHOTREXATE	**ANTIBIOTICS**			
METHOTREXATE	CIPROFLOXACIN	↑ Plasma concentrations of methotrexate, with risk of toxic effects of methotrexate, e.g., liver cirrhosis, blood dyscrasias that may be fatal, pulmonary toxicity, and stomatitis. Hematopoietic suppression can occur abruptly. Other adverse effects include anorexia, dyspepsia, gastrointestinal ulceration and bleeding, and pulmonary edema	Ciprofloxacin ↓ renal elimination of methotrexate. Ciprofloxacin is known to cause renal failure and interstitial nephritis	Although the toxic effects of methotrexate are more frequent with high doses of methotrexate, it is necessary to do an FBC and liver and renal function tests before starting treatment even with low doses, and to repeat these tests weekly until therapy is stabilized and thereafter every 2–3 months. Patients should be advised to report symptoms such as sore throat and fever immediately, and also any gastrointestinal discomfort. A profound drop in white cell count or platelet count warrants immediate stoppage of methotrexate therapy and initiation of supportive therapy. Consider a nonreacting antibiotic

(*Continued*)

Primary Drug	Secondary Drug	Effect	Mechanism	Precautions
CYTOTOXICS				
METHOTREXATE	DOXYCYCLINE	↑ Plasma concentrations of methotrexate, with risk of toxic effects of methotrexate, e.g., liver cirrhosis, blood dyscrasias, which may be fatal, pulmonary toxicity, stomatitis. Hematopoietic suppression can occur abruptly. Other adverse effects include anorexia, dyspepsia, gastrointestinal ulceration and bleeding, and pulmonary edema	Tetracyclines destroy the bacterial flora necessary for the breakdown of methotrexate. This results in ↑ free methotrexate concentrations. Tetracyclines are also considered to inhibit the elimination of methotrexate and allow a buildup of methotrexate in the bladder. The effects of the interaction are often delayed	Although the toxic effects of methotrexate are more frequent with high doses of methotrexate, it is necessary to do an FBC, liver and renal function tests before starting treatment even with low doses, repeating these tests weekly until therapy is stabilized, and thereafter every 2–3 months. Patients should be advised to report symptoms such as sore throat and fever immediately, and also any gastrointestinal discomfort. A profound drop in white cell count or platelet count warrants immediate stoppage of methotrexate therapy and initiation of supportive therapy
METHOTREXATE—ORAL	NEOMYCIN, KANAMYCIN PAROMOMYCIN	↓ Plasma concentrations following oral methotrexate	Oral aminoglycosides ↓ absorption of oral methotrexate by 30%–50%	Separate doses of each drug by at least 2–4 h
METHOTREXATE	PENICILLINS	↑ Plasma concentrations of methotrexate and risk of toxic effects of methotrexate, e.g., myelosuppression, liver cirrhosis, pulmonary toxicity	Penicillins ↓ renal elimination of methotrexate by renal tubular secretion, which is the main route of elimination of methotrexate. Penicillins compete with methotrexate for renal elimination. Displacement from protein-binding sites may occur and is only a minor contribution to the interaction	Avoid concurrent use. If concurrent use is necessary, monitor clinically and biochemically for blood dyscrasia, liver toxicity, and pulmonary toxicity. Do FBCs and LFTs prior to concurrent treatment

(*Continued*)

Primary Drug	Secondary Drug	Effect	Mechanism	Precautions
CYTOTOXICS				
METHOTREXATE	SULFAMETHOXAZOLE/ TRIMETHOPRIM	↑ Plasma concentrations of methotrexate and risk of toxic effects of methotrexate, e.g., myelosuppression, liver cirrhosis, pulmonary toxicity	Sulfamethoxazole displaces methotrexate from plasma protein–binding sites and also ↓ renal elimination of methotrexate. Trimethoprim inhibits dihydrofolate reductase, which leads to additive toxic effects of methotrexate	Avoid concurrent use. If concurrent use is necessary, monitor clinically and biochemically for blood dyscrasias and liver, renal, and pulmonary toxicities
METHOTREXATE	SULFONAMIDES	↑ Plasma concentrations of methotrexate, with risk of toxic effects of methotrexate, e.g., liver cirrhosis, blood dyscrasias which may be fatal, pulmonary toxicity, stomatitis. Hematopoietic suppression can occur abruptly. Other adverse effects include anorexia, dyspepsia, gastrointestinal ulceration and bleeding, and pulmonary edema	The mechanism differs from that underlying the sulfamethoxazole/ trimethoprim interaction. Sulfonamides such as co-trimoxazole and sulfadiazine are known to cause renal dysfunction—interstitial nephritis and renal failure, which may ↓ excretion of methotrexate. Sulfonamides are also known to compete with methotrexate for renal elimination. Displacement from protein-binding sites of methotrexate is a minor contribution to the interaction	Although the toxic effects of methotrexate are more frequent with high doses of methotrexate, it is necessary to do an FBC, liver and renal function tests before starting treatment even with low doses, repeating these tests at 2–3 months. Patients should be advised to report symptoms such as sore throat and fever immediately, and also any gastrointestinal discomfort. A profound drop in white cell count or platelet count warrants immediate stoppage of methotrexate therapy and initiation of supportive therapy

(*Continued*)

Primary Drug	Secondary Drug	Effect	Mechanism	Precautions
CYTOTOXICS				
METHOTREXATE	TETRACYCLINE	↑ Plasma concentrations of methotrexate, with risk of toxic effects of methotrexate, e.g., liver cirrhosis, blood dyscrasias, which may be fatal, pulmonary toxicity, stomatitis. Hematopoietic suppression can occur abruptly. Other adverse effects include anorexia, dyspepsia, gastrointestinal ulceration and bleeding, and pulmonary edema	Tetracyclines destroy the bacterial flora necessary for the breakdown of methotrexate. This results in ↑ free methotrexate concentrations. Tetracyclines are also considered to inhibit the elimination of methotrexate and allow a buildup of methotrexate in the bladder. The effect of the interaction is often delayed	Although the toxic effects of methotrexate are more frequent with high doses of methotrexate, it is necessary to do an FBC, liver and renal function tests before starting treatment even with low doses, repeating these tests at 2–3 months. Patients should be advised to report symptoms such as sore throat and fever immediately, and also any gastrointestinal discomfort. A profound drop in white cell count or platelet count warrants immediate stoppage of methotrexate therapy and initiation of supportive therapy
METHOTREXATE	**ANTICANCER AND IMMUNOMODULATING DRUGS**			
METHOTREXATE	ADALIMUMAB	Increases clearance of adalimumab, reduces antibody formation, and increases elevation of liver enzymes	Unknown	Increase monitoring of liver function tests
METHOTREXATE	AMINOSALICYLATES—SULFASALAZINE	↑ Risk of hepatotoxicity with sulfasalazine and of folate deficiency anemia	Additive hepatotoxic effects. Sulfasalazine also competes with methotrexate for renal elimination	Monitor closely for symptoms of liver failure. Check LFTs at the beginning of treatment then weekly until stable, and repeat if there is clinical suspicion of liver disease
METHOTREXATE	AZATHIOPRINE	↑ Risk of hepatotoxicity	Additive hepatotoxic effects	Monitor closely for symptoms of liver failure, e.g., flu-like symptoms, abdominal pain, dark urine, pruritus, jaundice, ascites, and weight gain. Do LFTs at the beginning of treatment and weekly until stable, and repeat if there is clinical suspicion of liver disease

(*Continued*)

Primary Drug	Secondary Drug	Effect	Mechanism	Precautions
CYTOTOXICS				
METHOTREXATE	CICLOSPORIN	↑ Risk of renal toxicity and renal failure	Additive renal toxicity	Monitor renal function prior to and during therapy, and ensure an intake of at least 2L of fluid daily. Monitor serum potassium and magnesium and correct any deficiencies
METHOTREXATE	CISPLATIN	↑ Methotrexate levels, with ↑ risk of pulmonary toxicity	Cisplatin is the most common anticancer drug associated with renal proximal and distal tubular damage. Cisplatin could significantly ↓ renal elimination of methotrexate	It would be best to start with lower doses of methotrexate. It is necessary to assess renal function prior to and during concurrent treatment until stability is achieved. Monitor clinically and with pulmonary function tests
METHOTREXATE	CORTICOSTEROIDS	↑ Risk of bone marrow toxicity	Additive effect	Monitor FBC regularly
METHOTREXATE	CRISANTASPASE	Administration prior to or concurrently may ↓ efficacy of methotrexate	Crisantaspase inhibits protein synthesis and prevents cell entry to S phase, which leads to ↓ efficacy of methotrexate	Administer crisantaspase shortly after methotrexate or 9–10 days before methotrexate
METHOTREXATE	FLUOROURACIL	↓ Cytotoxic effect of methotrexate when fluorouracil is administered prior to methotrexate	Fluorouracil prevents the conversion of reduced folates to dihydrofolate	Always administer methotrexate prior to fluorouracil
METHOTREXATE	LEFLUNOMIDE	Possible increased leflunomide toxicity	Possibly additive	Avoid concurrent use If necessary, increase monitoring
METHOTREXATE—ORAL	MERCAPTOPURINE	↑ Plasma concentrations of mercaptopurine (↑ AUC by 30%) and ↑ risk of myelotoxicity	Methotrexate ↑ oral bioavailability of mercaptopurine	↓ Dose of oral 6-mercaptopurine when used with doses of methotrexate >20 mg/m^2 or higher doses of methotrexate given intravenously

(Continued)

Primary Drug	Secondary Drug	Effect	Mechanism	Precautions
CYTOTOXICS				
METHOTREXATE	NATALIZUMAB	Potential increased risk of progressive multifocal leukoencephalopathy, although no increased risk of infection in available data	Additive	Manufacturer advises to avoid concurrent use
METHOTREXATE	PONATINIB	Predicted increased in levels of these BCRP substrates	BCRP inhibition	Be aware
METHOTREXATE	PROCARBAZINE	↑ Risk of renal impairment if methotrexate infusion is given within 48 h of procarbazine administration. Also ↑ risk of methotrexate toxicity, particularly to the kidneys	Procarbazine has a transient effect on the kidneys, and this will delay the renal elimination of methotrexate	Do not start methotrexate infusion less than 72 h after the last dose of procarbazine. Hydrate patients aggressively (plenty of oral fluids or intravenous fluids), alkalinize the urine to pH > 7 and closely monitor renal function, e.g. blood urea and creatinine, before and after methotrexate infusion until methotrexate blood levels are <0.05 μmol/L
METHOTREXATE	REGORAFENIB	Possible increased levels of BCRP substrates	BCRP inhibition	Clinical significance not determined
METHOTREXATE	RETINOIDS—ACITRETIN, ETRETINATE	↑ Risk of hepatotoxicity	Additive hepatotoxic effects	Avoid coadministration
METHOTREXATE	TAMOXIFEN	Increased risk of thrombosis when used in chemotherapy regimens	Additive	Consider prophylactic anticoagulation
METHOTREXATE	VEMURAFENIB	Possible increased levels of BCRP substrates	Vemurafenib inhibits BCRP	Clinical significance unknown
METHOTREXATE	ANTICOAGULANTS—ORAL	Episodes of ↑ anticoagulant effect	Not understood but likely to be multifactorial	Monitor INR at least weekly until stable during administration of chemotherapy

(*Continued*)

ANTICANCER AND IMMUNOMODULATING DRUGS CYTOTOXICS Methotrexate

Primary Drug	Secondary Drug	Effect	Mechanism	Precautions
CYTOTOXICS				
METHOTREXATE	**ANTIEPILEPTICS**			
METHOTREXATE	PHENOBARBITAL CARBAMAZEPINE	Increased clearance of methotrexate (as 24 h infusion), reduced efficacy in combination therapy for B-cell leukemia	Unknown	Clinical significance uncertain—further study needed
METHOTREXATE	PHENYTOIN	1. Increased clearance of methotrexate (as 24 h infusion) reduced efficacy in combination therapy for B-cell leukemia 2. ↑ Plasma concentrations of phenytoin may occur and ↑ risk of toxic effects of phenytoin	High doses of methotrexate ↓ elimination of phenytoin	Monitor phenytoin levels and clinically watch for signs and symptoms of phenytoin toxicity, e.g., nausea, vomiting, insomnia, tremor, acne, hirsutism
METHOTREXATE	ANTIFUNGALS—AMPHOTERICIN B	Delayed clearance of methotrexate	Possibly due to amphotericin causing renal impairment	Monitor closely
METHOTREXATE	ANTIGOUT DRUGS—PROBENECID	↑ Methotrexate levels	Probenecid ↓ elimination of methotrexate renally by interfering with tubular secretion in the proximal tubule and also ↓ protein binding of methotrexate (a relatively minor effect). Probenecid competes with methotrexate for renal elimination	Avoid coadministration if possible; if not possible, ↓ dose of methotrexate and monitor FBC closely
METHOTREXATE	ANTIHYPERTENSIVES AND HEART FAILURE DRUGS—BOSENTAN	Reduced efficacy with oral methotrexate Case of hepatotoxicity with subcutaneous methotrexate	Reduced efficacy due to bosentan displacing methotrexate from its protein-binding sites, reducing conversion to active metabolites Heptatoxocity due to additive effects	Interaction not firmly established Caution with concurrent use

(Continued)

Primary Drug	Secondary Drug	Effect	Mechanism	Precautions
CYTOTOXICS				
METHOTREXATE	ANTIMALARIALS—PYRIMETHAMINE	↑ Antifolate effect of methotrexate	Pyrimethamine should not be used alone and is combined with sulfadoxine. Pyrimethamine and methotrexate synergistically induce folate deficiency	Although the toxic effects of methotrexate are more frequent with high doses of methotrexate, it is necessary to do an FBC, liver and renal function tests before starting treatment even with low doses, repeating these tests weekly until therapy is stabilized and thereafter every 2–3 months. Patients should be advised to report symptoms such as sore throat and fever immediately, and also any gastrointestinal discomfort. A profound drop in white cell count or platelet count warrants immediate stoppage of methotrexate therapy and initiation of supportive therapy
METHOTREXATE	ANTIPLATELET AGENTS—ASPIRIN	Risk of methotrexate toxicity when coadministered with high-dose aspirin. There is a risk of toxic effects of methotrexate, e.g., liver cirrhosis, blood dyscrasias, which may be fatal, pulmonary toxicity, stomatitis. Hematopoietic suppression can occur abruptly. Other adverse effects include anorexia, dyspepsia, gastrointestinal ulceration and bleeding, and pulmonary edema	Aspirin ↓ plasma protein binding of methotrexate (a relatively minor contribution to the interaction) and the renal excretion of high doses of methotrexate. Salicylates compete with methotrexate for renal elimination	Check FBC, U&Es, and LFTs before starting treatment, repeating weekly until stabilized, and then every 2–3 months. Patients should be advised to report symptoms such as sore throat, fever, or gastrointestinal discomfort immediately. Stop methotrexate and initiate supportive therapy if the white cell or platelet count drops. Do not administer aspirin within 10 days of high-dose methotrexate treatment

(*Continued*)

Primary Drug	Secondary Drug	Effect	Mechanism	Precautions
CYTOTOXICS				
METHOTREXATE	ANTIVIRALS—OSELTAMIVIR	Possible ↑ efficacy/toxicity	Competition for renal excretion	Monitor more closely for signs of immunosuppression. Predicted interaction
METHOTREXATE	BRONCHODILATORS—THEOPHYLLINE	Possible ↑ in theophylline levels	Possibly inhibition of CYP2D6-mediated metabolism of theophylline	Monitor clinically for toxic effects and advise patients to seek medical attention if they have symptoms suggestive of theophylline toxicity. Measure theophylline levels before, during, and after coadministration
METHOTREXATE	ELTROMBOPAG	Possible increased methotrexate levels	Inhibition of BCRP	Caution with concurrent use
METHOTREXATE	LIPID-LOWERING DRUGS—COLESTYRAMINE	Parenteral methotrexate levels may be ↓ by colestyramine	Colestyramine interrupts the enterohepatic circulation of methotrexate	Avoid coadministration
METHOTREXATE	PROTON PUMP INHIBITORS—OMEPRAZOLE	Likely ↑ plasma concentration of methotrexate and ↑ risk of toxic effects, e.g., blood dyscrasias, liver cirrhosis, pulmonary toxicity, and renal toxicity	Attributed to omeprazole decreasing the renal elimination of methotrexate	Monitor clinically and biochemically for blood dyscrasias and liver, renal, and pulmonary toxicities
METHOTREXATE	SAPROPTERIN	Predicted reduced sapropterin levels	Inhibition of dihydropteridine reductase, which reduces the regeneration of sapropterin by this enzyme	Caution with concurrent use
METHOTREXATE	URINARY ALKALINIZERS—SODIUM BICARBONATE ACETAZOLAMIDE	Increased urinary excretion of methotrexate	Methotrexate has increased solubility in alkaline fluids	Interaction normally used therapeutically to reduce toxicity
MITOMYCIN				
MITOMYCIN	**ANTICANCER AND IMMUNOMODULATING DRUGS**			
MITOMYCIN	ACLARUBICIN	Increased risk of myelosuppression	Additive	Caution with concurrent use

(Continued)

Primary Drug	Secondary Drug	Effect	Mechanism	Precautions
CYTOTOXICS				
MITOMYCIN	DOXORUBICIN	Increased cardiotoxicity	Uncertain Possibly due to free radical generation	Monitor closely
MITOMYCIN	FLUOROURACIL	Intravascular hemolysis and renal failure rarely	Uncertain	Stop drugs at first sign of hemolysis, proteinuria, or rising urea levels
MITOMYCIN	TAMOXIFEN	↑ Incidence of anemia and thrombocytopenia and risk of hemolytic-uremic syndrome	Mitomycin causes subclinical endothelial damage in addition to the thrombotic effect on platelets caused by tamoxifen, which leads to hemolytic-uremic syndrome	Monitor renal function at least twice weekly during concurrent therapy and watch clinically for bleeding episodes, e.g., nose bleeds, bleeding from the gums, skin bruising
MITOMYCIN	VINCA ALKALOIDS—VINBLASTINE, VINDESINE, VINORELBINE	↑ Risk of abrupt onset of pulmonary toxicity in 3%–6% of patients, when two courses of these drugs are administered concurrently	Mechanism is uncertain; possible additive pulmonary toxic effects	Monitor clinically and with lung function tests for pulmonary toxicity. Advise patients to report immediately symptoms such as shortness of breath and wheezing
MITOTANE				
MITOTANE	ANTIBIOTICS—RIFABUTIN, RIFAMPICIN	Possible reduction in levels of rifampicin	Induction of CYP450	Be aware; watch for poor response to these antibiotics
MITOTANE	ANTICOAGULANTS—WARFARIN	Possible ↓ anticoagulant effect	Induction of metabolism of warfarin	Monitor INR closely
MITOTANE	ANTIDEPRESSANTS—ST. JOHN'S WORT	Possible reduction in levels of St. John's wort	Induction of CYP450	Be aware; watch for poor response to St. John's wort
MITOTANE	ANTIEPILEPTICS	Possible reduction in levels of antiepileptics	Induction of CYP450	Be aware; watch for poor response to antiepileptics
MITOTANE	ANTIFUNGALS—GRISEOFULVIN	Possible reduction in levels of griseofulvin	Induction of CYP450	Be aware; watch for poor response to griseofulvin
MITOTANE	DIURETICS—SPIRONOLACTONE	Case report of reduced mitotane efficacy	Unknown	Avoid concurrent use

(*Continued*)

Primary Drug	Secondary Drug	Effect	Mechanism	Precautions
CYTOTOXICS				
MITOXANTRONE				
MITOXANTRONE	AZATHIOPRINE	↑ Risk of myelosuppression and immunosuppression. Deaths have occurred following profound myelosuppression and severe sepsis	Additive myelotoxic effects. Azathioprine is metabolized to 6-mercaptopurine in vivo, which results in additive myelosuppression, immunosuppression, and hepatotoxicity	Avoid coadministration
MITOXANTRONE	CICLOSPORIN—HIGH DOSES (leading to levels of ciclosporin from 3000 to 5000 ng/mL)	↑ Mitoxantrone levels; no ↑ toxicity has been reported	↓ Clearance (>40%) and ↑ terminal half-life (>50%) due to inhibition of Pgp in normal tissues	↓ Dose of mitoxantrone of ↓ 40% has been recommended in pediatric patients. Advisable to monitor mitoxantrone levels
MITOXANTRONE	FINGOLIMOD	Increased risk of opportunistic infections	Additive	Caution when switching to fingolimod due to long half-life of mitoxantrone
MITOXANTRONE	NATALIZUMAB	Potential increased risk of progressive multifocal leukoencephalopathy, although no increased risk of infection in available data	Additive	Manufacturer advises to avoid concurrent use
MITOXANTRONE	PONATINIB	Predicted increased in levels of these BCRP substrates	BCRP inhibition	Be aware
MITOXANTRONE	VEMURAFENIB	Possible increased levels of BCRP substrates	Vemurafenib inhibits BCRP	Clinical significance unknown
NELARABINE				
NELARABINE	PENTOSTATIN	Possible reduction in conversion of nelarabine to active metabolite and reduced efficacy	Inhibition of adenosine deaminase	Avoid concurrent use

(Continued)

Primary Drug	Secondary Drug	Effect	Mechanism	Precautions
CYTOTOXICS				
NILOTINIB				
NILOTINIB	**DRUGS THAT PROLONG THE QT INTERVAL**			
NILOTINIB	1. ANTIARRHYTHMICS—ajmaline, amiodarone, azimilide, cibenzoline, disopyramide, dofetilide, dronedarone, ibutilide, procainamide, propafenone, quinidine 2. ANTIBIOTICS—macrolides (especially azithromycin, clarithromycin, parenteral erythromycin, telithromycin), quinolones (especially moxifloxacin), quinupristin/dalfopristin 3. ANTICANCER AND IMMUNOMODULATING DRUGS—arsenic trioxide, bosutinib, crizotinib, dasatinib, eribulin, fingolimod, lapatinib, pazopanib, sunitinib, vandetanib, vemurafenib 4. ANTIDEPRESSANTS—TCAs, venlafaxine 5. ANTIEMETICS—ondansetron 6. ANTIFUNGALS—fluconazole, posaconazole, voriconazole 7. ANTIHISTAMINES—terfenadine, hydroxyzine, mizolastine 8. ANTIHYPERTENSIVES—ketanserin 9. ANTIMALARIALS—artemether with lumefantrine, chloroquine, halofantrine, hydroxychloroquine, mefloquine, quinine 10. ANTIPROTOZOALS—pentamidine isethionate 11. ANTIPSYCHOTICS—atypicals, phenothiazines, pimozide 12. ANTIVIRALS—boceprevir, rilpivirine, telaprevir 13. BETA-BLOCKERS—sotalol 14. BRONCHODILATORS—parenteral bronchodilators 15. CNS STIMULANTS—atomoxetine 16. RANOLAZINE	Risk of ventricular arrhythmias, particularly torsades de pointes	Additive effect; these drugs prolong the QT interval	Avoid coadministration

(*Continued*)

Primary Drug	Secondary Drug	Effect	Mechanism	Precautions
CYTOTOXICS				
NILOTINIB	ANALGESICS—OPIOIDS	Imatinib and nilotinib may cause ↑ plasma concentrations of codeine, dextromethorphan, hydroxycodone, methadone, morphine, oxycodone, pethidine fentanyl, alfentanil, and tramadol, with a risk of toxic effects	Inhibition of CYP2D6- and 3A4-mediated metabolism of these opioids by imatinib; nilotinib is an inhibitor of CYP3A4 and Pgp	Monitor for clinical efficacy and toxicity. Warn patients to report ↑ drowsiness, malaise, and anorexia Tramadol causes less respiratory depression than other opiates, but we need to monitor BP and blood counts and advise patients to report wheezing, loss of appetite, and fainting attacks. Need to consider reducing dose Methadone may cause QT prolongation; the CSM has recommended that patients with heart and liver disease on methadone should be carefully monitored for heart conduction abnormalities such as QT prolongation on ECG, which may lead to sudden death. Also need to monitor patients on more than 100 mg methadone daily, and thus, ↑ plasma concentrations necessitates close monitoring of cardiac and respiratory functions
NILOTINIB	ANTACIDS	Reduced nilotinib levels	Solubility reduced at higher pH	If necessary, antacids and nilotinib can be given separately
NILOTINIB	**ANTIBIOTICS**			
NILOTINIB	MACROLIDES	Predicted increased levels of nilotinib	CYP3A4 inhibition	Avoid concurrent use
NILOTINIB	RIFAMPICIN	Reduced nilotinib levels	CYP3A4 induction	Avoid coadministration

(*Continued*)

Primary Drug	Secondary Drug	Effect	Mechanism	Precautions
CYTOTOXICS				
NILOTINIB	**ANTICANCER AND OTHER IMMUNOMODULATING DRUGS**			
NILOTINIB	CICLOSPORIN	Increased nilotinib levels	P-glycoprotein inhibition	Caution with concurrent use
NILOTINIB	PONATINIB	Predicted increased in nilotinib levels	P-glycoprotein inhibition	Be aware
NILOTINIB	VALSPODAR	Increased nilotinib levels	P-glycoprotein inhibition	Caution with concurrent use
NILOTINIB	ANTICOAGULANTS—COUMARINS	Possible increased bleeding risk	Additive effect	Monitor closely with concurrent use
NILOTINIB	ANTIDEPRESSANTS—ST. JOHN'S WORT	Possible decreased levels of nilotinib; evidence for imatinib only but nilotinib metabolized in a similar way	CYP3A4 induction	Avoid concurrent use
NILOTINIB	ANTIFUNGALS—KETOCONAZOLE, ITRACONAZOLE, POSACONAZOLE, VORICONAZOLE	Increased levels of nilotinib	CYP3A4 inhibition	Avoid concurrent use Dose reduction if necessary
NILOTINIB	**ANTIVIRALS**			
NILOTINIB	PROTEASE INHIBITORS	Predicted increased nilotinib levels	CYP3A4 inhibition	Manufacturer advises to avoid concurrent use of HIV protease inhibitors, specifically ritonavir, atazanavir, indinavir, nelfinavir, and saquinavir
NILOTINIB	BOCEPREVIR	Predicted increased levels of nilotinib	CYP3A4 inhibition	Manufacturer advises to avoid concurrent use
NILOTINIB	TIPRANAVIR	Reduced nilotinib levels	P-glycoprotein induction	Caution with concurrent use
NILOTINIB	ANXIOLYTICS AND HYPNOTICS—MIDAZOLAM	Midazolam levels slightly increased	CYP3A4 inhibition	Caution with concurrent use
NILOTINIB	CALCIUM CHANNEL BLOCKERS—VERAPAMIL	Increased nilotinib levels	P-glycoprotein inhibition	Caution with concurrent use

(*Continued*)

Primary Drug	Secondary Drug	Effect	Mechanism	Precautions
CYTOTOXICS				
NILOTINIB	CARDIAC GLYCOSIDES—DIGOXIN	Increased levels of digoxin	P-glycoprotein inhibition	Monitor closely, measure digoxin levels and consider dose reduction with digoxin
NILOTINIB	CONIVAPTAN	Increased nilotinib levels	P-glycoprotein inhibition	Caution with concurrent use
NILOTINIB	GRAPEFRUIT JUICE	Increased nilotinib levels	CYP3A4 inhibition	Avoid concurrent use
NILOTINIB	H2-RECEPTOR BLOCKERS	Possible ↓ absorption of nilotinib	Nilotibin has reduced solubility at higher pH	If combined give nilotinib 2 h before or 10 h after H2 blocker
NILOTINIB	LIPID-LOWERING DRUGS—LOMITAPIDE	Predicted increased levels of nilotinib	P-glycoprotein inhibition	Monitor closely with concurrent use
NILOTINIB	PROTON PUMP INHIBITORS	Reduced nilotinib levels	Solubility reduced at higher pH	Caution with concurrent use of PPIs
OXALIPLATIN ➢ *Platinum Compounds, below*				
PACLITAXEL				
PACLITAXEL	ANTIARRHYTHMICS—QUINIDINE	Reduced paclitaxel levels	Unclear	Clinical relevance uncertain
PACLITAXEL	**ANTIBIOTICS**			
PACLITAXEL	MACROLIDES—CLARITHROMYCIN, ERYTHROMYCIN, TELITHROMYCIN	Predicted increased paclitaxel levels	CYP3A4 inhibition	Avoid concurrent use If necessary, monitor closely and consider dose reduction
PACLITAXEL	RIFAMPICIN	↓ Plasma concentration of paclitaxel and ↓ efficacy of paclitaxel	Due to induction of hepatic metabolism of paclitaxel by the CYP isoenzymes	Monitor for clinical efficacy and need to ↑ dose if inadequate response is due to interaction
PACLITAXEL	**ANTICANCER AND IMMUNOMODULATING DRUGS**			
PACLITAXEL WITH CARBOPLATIN	BEXAROTENE	Carboplatin with paclitaxel may ↑ bexarotene levels	Unknown	Clinical significance unknown. Monitor more closely
PACLITAXEL	CISPLATIN	↑ Risk of profound neutropenia	Prior administration of cisplatin tends to impair renal function and ↓ clearance of paclitaxel by approximately 25%	Advise administration of paclitaxel prior to cisplatin

(Continued)

Primary Drug	Secondary Drug	Effect	Mechanism	Precautions
CYTOTOXICS				
PACLITAXEL	CICLOSPORIN	↑ Plasma concentrations of these drugs, with risk of toxic effects	Competitive inhibition of CYP3A4-mediated metabolism and Pgp transport of these drugs	Watch for toxic effects of these drugs
PACLITAXEL	CORTICOSTEROIDS—DEXAMETHASONE	↓ Plasma concentrations of paclitaxel and ↓ efficacy of paclitaxel	Due to induction of hepatic metabolism of paclitaxel by the CYP isoenzymes	Monitor for clinical efficacy; need to ↑ dose if inadequate response is due to interaction
PACLITAXEL	CYCLOPHOSPHAMIDE	↑ Risk of neutropenia, thrombocytopenia, and mucositis when paclitaxel is infused over 24 or 72 h prior to cyclophosphamide	Mechanism is uncertain	Administer cyclophosphamide first and then follow with paclitaxel
PACLITAXEL	DOXORUBICIN	↑ Risk of neutropenia, stomatitis, and cardiomyopathy due to ↑ plasma concentrations of doxorubicin when paclitaxel is given before doxorubicin	This is possibly due to competitive inhibition of biliary excretion of doxorubicin by paclitaxel	Doxorubicin should be administered prior to paclitaxel. The cumulative dose of doxorubicin should be limited to 360 mg/m^2 when concurrently administered with paclitaxel
PACLITAXEL	EPIRUBICIN	↑ Plasma concentrations of epirubicin (↑ AUC by 37% and ↓ clearance by 25%), particularly following sequential administration of paclitaxel followed by epirubicin	Attributed to altered distribution of epirubicin in plasma and inhibition of Pgp by Cremophor, the vehicle of paclitaxel formulation, resulting in ↓ clearance	Epirubicin should always be given prior to paclitaxel
PACLITAXEL	GEFITINIB	Gefitinib levels slightly increased	Unknown	Clinical significance uncertain
PACLITAXEL	GEMCITABINE	Possibly ↓ antitumor effect in breast cancer	Based on experiments on breast cell lines	Avoid coadministration except in clinical trials
PACLITAXEL	IRINOTECAN	Possibly increased irinotecan levels	Unknown	Clinical significance uncertain. Be aware of possible interaction

(Continued)

Primary Drug	Secondary Drug	Effect	Mechanism	Precautions
CYTOTOXICS				
PACLITAXEL	PAZOPANIB	Paclitaxel levels slightly increased	Possible CYP3A4 and CYP2C8 inhibition	Caution with concurrent use
PACLITAXEL	PIXANTRONE	Theoretical risk of increased drug levels	Pixantrone inhibits CYP2C8	Manufacturer advises caution
PACLITAXEL	SORAFENIB	Paclitaxel and sorafenib levels slightly increased	Unknown	Unknown
PACLITAXEL	THALIDOMIDE	Possibly increased risk of peripheral neuropathy	Additive	Manufacturer advises caution
PACLITAXEL	TRASTUZUMAB	↑ Risk of cardiotoxicity	Possibly additive cardiac toxic effect	Closely monitor clinically and use ECGs for cardiotoxicity
PACLITAXEL	VINBLASTINE, VINCRISTINE	↓ Therapeutic efficacy of paclitaxel	Antagonistic effects	Avoid coadministration
PACLITAXEL	VINFLUNINE	Reduced vinflunine levels in vitro	Unknown	Clinical significance unknown
PACLITAXEL	VORINOSTAT	Slight increase in vorinostat levels	Uncertain	Further study needed
PACLITAXEL	ANTICOAGULANTS—WARFARIN	Episodes of increased anticoagulant effect	Not understood but likely to be multifactorial	Monitor INR at least weekly until stable during administration of chemotherapy
PACLITAXEL	ANTIDEPRESSANTS—ST. JOHN'S WORT	↓ Plasma concentration of paclitaxel and ↓ efficacy of paclitaxel	Due to induction of hepatic metabolism of paclitaxel by the CYP isoenzymes	Monitor for clinical efficacy and need to ↑ dose if inadequate response is due to interaction
PACLITAXEL	ANTIEPILEPTICS—CARBAMAZEPINE, PHENOBARBITAL	↓ Plasma concentration of paclitaxel and ↓ efficacy of paclitaxel	Due to induction of hepatic metabolism of paclitaxel by the CYP isoenzymes	Monitor for clinical efficacy and need to ↑ dose if inadequate response is due to interaction
PACLITAXEL	PHENYTOIN	↓ Levels of paclitaxel, with risk of therapeutic failure	Induction of hepatic metabolism	Monitor for ↓ clinical efficacy and ↑ dose as required
PACLITAXEL	ANTIFUNGALS—AZOLES	Predicted increased paclitaxel levels; however, there is no interaction with keloconazole	CYP3A4 inhibition	Avoid concurrent use If necessary, monitor closely and consider dose reduction

(*Continued*)

Primary Drug	Secondary Drug	Effect	Mechanism	Precautions
CYTOTOXICS				
PACLITAXEL	**ANTIVIRALS**			
PACLITAXEL	NNRTIS—EFAVIRENZ NEVIRAPINE	Predicted reduced paclitaxel levels	CYP3A4 induction	Monitor closely. Consider dose increase
PACLITAXEL	PROTEASE INHIBITORS	↑ Risk of adverse effects of docetaxel and paclitaxel	Inhibition of CYP3A4-mediated metabolism. Also inhibition of Pgp efflux of vinblastine	Use with caution. Additional monitoring required. Monitor FBC weekly
PACLITAXEL	CALCIUM CHANNEL BLOCKERS—R-VERAPAMIL (HIGH DOSE)	Increased paclitaxel levels increased hemtological toxicity	Inhibition of P-glycoprotein	Clinical relevance uncertain as R-verapamil usually used for investigational purposes only
PACLITAXEL	DEFERASIROX	Possible interaction with paclitaxel	Effects on CYP2C8	Caution with concurrent use
PACLITAXEL	LIPID-LOWERING DRUGS—GEMFIBROZIL	Possible raised paclitaxel levels	CYP2C8 inhibtion	Caution with concurrent use
PAZOPANIB				
PAZOPANIB	**DRUGS THAT PROLONG THE QT INTERVAL**			
PAZOPANIB	1. ANTIARRHYTHMICS—ajmaline, amiodarone, azimilide, cibenzoline, disopyramide, dofetilide, dronedarone, ibutilide, procainamide, propafenone, quinidine 2. ANTIBIOTICS—macrolides (especially azithromycin, clarithromycin, parenteral erythromycin, telithromycin), quinolones (especially moxifloxacin), quinupristin/dalfopristin 3. ANTICANCER AND IMMUNOMODULATING DRUGS—arsenic trioxide, bosutinib, crizotinib, dasatinib, eribulin, fingolimod, lapatinib, nilotinib, sunitinib, vandetanib, vemurafenib 4. ANTIDEPRESSANTS—TCAs, venlafaxine	Risk of ventricular arrhythmias, particularly torsades de pointes	Additive effect; these drugs prolong the QT interval	Avoid coadministration

(*Continued*)

Primary Drug	Secondary Drug	Effect	Mechanism	Precautions
CYTOTOXICS				
	5. ANTIEMETICS—ondansetron 6. ANTIFUNGALS—fluconazole, posaconazole, voriconazole 7. ANTIHISTAMINES—terfenadine, hydroxyzine, mizolastine 8. ANTIHYPERTENSIVES—ketanserin 9. Antimalarials—artemether with lumefantrine, chloroquine, halofantrine, hydroxychloroquine, mefloquine, quinine 10. ANTIPROTOZOALS—pentamidine isethionate 11. ANTIPSYCHOTICS—atypicals, phenothiazines, pimozide 12. Antivirals—boceprevir, rilpivirine, telaprevir 13. BETA-BLOCKERS—sotalol 14. BRONCHODILATORS—parenteral bronchodilators 15. CNS STIMULANTS—atomoxetine 16. RANOLAZINE			
PAZOPANIB	ANALGESICS—DEXTROMETHORPHAN	Increased levels of dextromethorphan	CYP2D6 inhibition	Be aware. Unknown significance
PAZOPANIB	**ANTIBIOTICS**			
PAZOPANIB	MACROLIDES	Predicted increased levels of pazopanib	CYP3A4 inhibition	Avoid concurrent use
PAZOPANIB	RIFAMPICIN	Predicted reduced pazopanib levels	CYP3A4 induction	Avoid coadministration
PAZOPANIB	**ANTICANCER AND OTHER IMMUNOMODULATING DRUGS**			
PAZOPANIB	LAPATINIB	Increased pazopanib levels	Inhibition of P-glycoprotein or BCRP by lapatininb	Significance uncertain Clinical studies with pazopanib, pemetrexed, and lapatinib were stopped early because of increased toxicity
PAZOPANIB	PACLITAXEL	Paclitaxel levels slightly increased	Possible CYP3A4 and CYP2C8 inhibition	Caution with concurrent use

(Continued)

Primary Drug	Secondary Drug	Effect	Mechanism	Precautions
CYTOTOXICS				
PAZOPANIB	ANTICOAGULANTS—COUMARINS	Possible increased bleeding risk	Additive effect	Monitor closely with concurrent use, Manufacturer of imatinib recommends LMWH to warfarin
PAZOPANIB	ANTIFUNGALS—KETOCONAZOLE, ITRACONAZOLE, POSACONAZOLE, VORICONAZOLE	Increased levels of pazopanib	CYP3A4 inhibition	Avoid concurrent use Consider dose reduction if concurrent use is necessary
PAZOPANIB	**ANTIVIRALS**			
PAZOPANIB	HIV PROTEASE INHIBITORS	Predicted to inhibit metabolism of pazopanib	CYP3A4 inhibition	Manufacturer advises to avoid concurrent use of HIV protease inhibitors, specifically ritonavir, atazanavir, indinavir, nelfinavir, and saquinavir
PAZOPANIB	BOCEPREVIR	Predicted increased levels of pazopanib	CYP3A4 inhibition	Manufacturer advises to avoid concurrent use
PAZOPANIB	ANXIOLYTICS AND HYPNOTICS—MIDAZOLAM	Midazolam levels slightly increased	CYP3A4 inhibition	Caution with concurrent use
PAZOPANIB	GRAPEFRUIT JUICE	Possible increased pazopanib levels	CYP3A4 inhibition	Avoid concurrent use
PAZOPANIB	H2 RECEPTOR BLOCKERS	Possible ↓ plasma concentrations	Possible ↓ absorption	If combined give pazopanib 2 h before or 10 h after H2 blocker
PAZOPANIB	LIPID-LOWERING DRUGS—SIMVASTATIN	Increased ALT levels	Possibly due to inhibition of organic anion transporting polypeptide (OATP) 1B1	Monitor ALT and stop simvastatin if ALT increases
PAZOPANIB	PROTON PUMP INHIBITORS	↓ Plasma concentration	↓ Absorption as ↑ gastric pH	Avoid coadministration if possible; otherwise, take pazopanib without food in the evening at the same time as the PPI

(*Continued*)

Primary Drug	Secondary Drug	Effect	Mechanism	Precautions
CYTOTOXICS				
PEMETREXED				
PEMETREXED	ANALGESICS—NSAIDs	Predicted reduced renal excretion of pemetrexed	Inhibition of prostaglandins by NSAIDs result in reduced renal perfusion	Manufacturer recommends caution with high doses of NSAIDs in patients with normal renal function. NSAIDs with short half-lives should be avoided 2 days before to 2 days after in patients with mild to moderate renal impairment. NSAIDs with longer half-lives should be avoided 5 days before to 2 days after pemetrexed. Manufacturer advises close monitoring if concurrent use is necessary
PEMETREXED	ANTIBIOTICS—AMINOGLYCOSIDES	Increased pemetrexed toxicity	Reduced renal clearance	Caution with concurrent use
PEMETREXED	ANTICANCER AND OTHER IMMUNOMODULATING DRUGS—CICLOSPORIN, PLATINUM COMPOUNDS	Increased pemetrexed toxicity	Reduced renal clearance	Caution with concurrent use
PEMETREXED	ANTIGOUT DRUGS—PROBENECID	↑ Pemetrexed levels	Probable ↓ renal excretion of pemetrexed	Avoid coadministration where possible. If both need to be given, monitor FBC and renal function closely and watch for gastrointestinal disturbance and features of myopathy
PEMETREXED	ANTIPLATELETS—ASPIRIN	Increased pemetrexed toxicity	Reduced renal clearance	Caution with concurrent use
PEMETREXED	ANTIMALARIALS—PYRIMETHAMINE	Effects of pemetrexed increased	Additive	Avoid concurrent use. If not possible, then folate supplementation preferably with folinic acid should be considered
PEMETREXED	DIURETICS—LOOP	Increased pemetrexed toxicity	Reduced renal clearance	Caution with concurrent use

(*Continued*)

Primary Drug	Secondary Drug	Effect	Mechanism	Precautions
CYTOTOXICS				
PENTOSTATIN				
PENTOSTATIN	**ANTICANCER AND IMMUNOMODULATING DRUGS**			
PENTOSTATIN	CYCLOPHOSPHAMIDE	↑ Risk of potentially fatal cardiac toxicity	Attributed to interference of adenosine metabolism by cyclophosphamide	Avoid coadministration
PENTOSTATIN	FLUDARABINE	Risk of severe and potentially fatal pulmonary toxicity	Uncertain	Avoid coadministration
PENTOSTATIN	NELARABINE	Possible reduction in conversion of nelarabine to active metabolite and reduced efficacy	Inhibition of adenosine deaminase	Avoid concurrent use
PIXANTRONE				
PIXANTRONE	ANTIBIOTICS—RIFAMPICIN	Theoretical risk of reduced pixantrone levels	Pixantrone excretion increased	Manufacturer advises caution
PIXANTRONE	**ANTICANCER AND OTHER IMMUNOMODULATING DRUGS**			
PIXANTRONE	CICLOSPORIN	Theoretical risk of increased pixantrone levels	Pixantrone is substrate for P-glycoprotein	Manufacturer advises to monitor
PIXANTRONE	CORTICOSTEROIDS	Theoretical risk of reduced pixantrone levels	Pixantrone excretion increased	Manufacturer advises to exercise caution
PIXANTRONE	PACLITAXEL	Theoretical risk of increased drug levels	Pixantrone inhibits CYP2C8	Manufacturer advises to exercise caution
PIXANTRONE	TACROLIMUS	Theoretical risk of increased pixantrone levels	Pixantrone is substrate for P-glycoprotein	Manufacturer advises to monitor closely
PIXANTRONE	ANTICOAGULANTS—WARFARIN	Theoretical risk of increased warfarin efficacy	Pixantrone inhibits CYP1A2	Manufacturer advises to monitor INR closely
PIXANTRONE	ANTIDEPRESSANTS—AMITRIPTYLINE	Theoretical risk of increased drug levels	Pixantrone inhibits CYP1A2	Manufacturer advises to monitor closely

(*Continued*)

Primary Drug	Secondary Drug	Effect	Mechanism	Precautions
CYTOTOXICS				
PIXANTRONE	ANTIDIABETICS—REPAGLINIDE, ROSIGLITAZONE	Theoretical risk of increased drug levels	Pixantrone inhibits CYP2C8	Manufacturer advises to exercise caution
PIXANTRONE	ANTIEMETICS—ONDANSETRON	Theoretical risk of increased drug levels	Pixantrone inhibits CYP1A2	Manufacturer advises to monitor closely
PIXANTRONE	ANTIEPILEPTICS—CARBAMAZEPINE	Theoretical risk of reduced pixantrone levels	Pixantrone excretion increased	Manufacturer advises to exercise caution
PIXANTRONE	ANTIPSYCHOTICS—HALOPERIDOL, CLOZAPINE	Theoretical risk of increased drug levels	Pixantrone inhibits CYP1A2	Manufacturer advises to monitor closely
PIXANTRONE	ANTIVIRALS—RITNOAVIR, SAQUINAVIR, NELFINAVIR	Theoretical risk of increased pixantrone levels	Inhibition of Pgp	Manufacturer advises to monitor closely
PIXANTRONE	BETA-BLOCKERS—PROPRANOLOL	Theoretical risk of increased drug levels	Pixantrone inhibits CYP1A2	Manufacturer advises to monitor closely
PIXANTRONE	BRONCHODILATORS—THEOPHYLLINE	Theoretical risk of increased theophylline levels	Pixantrone inhibits CYP1A2	Manufacturer advises to monitor closely
PLATINUM COMPOUNDS—CARBOPLATIN, CISPLATIN, OXALIPLATIN				
PLATINUM COMPOUNDS	**ANALGESICS**			
CISPLATIN	NSAIDs CELECOXIB, MELOXICAM PIROXICAM	Both celecoxib and cisplatin can lead to nephrotioxicity. Piroxicam increases blood concentrations of cisplatin	Additive nephrotoxic effects	Monitor renal function (creatinine, GFR) prior to and twice a week during therapy. Monitor toxic effects of cisplatin with piroxicam
PLATINUM COMPOUNDS	**ANTIBIOTICS**			
PLATINUM COMPOUNDS	AMINOGLYCOSIDES, CAPREOMYCIN, COLISTIN, STREPTOMYCIN, VANCOMYCIN	↑ Risk of renal toxicity and renal failure and of ototoxicity. The ototoxicity tends to occur when cisplatin is administered early during the course of aminoglycoside therapy	Additive renal toxicity	Monitor renal function prior to and during therapy, and ensure an intake of at least 2L of fluid daily. Monitor serum potassium and magnesium and correct any deficiencies. Most side effects of aminoglycosides are dose related, and it is necessary to ↑ interval between doses and ↓ dose of aminoglycoside if there is impaired renal function

(Continued)

Primary Drug	Secondary Drug	Effect	Mechanism	Precautions
CYTOTOXICS				
PLATINUM COMPOUNDS	**ANTICANCER AND IMMUNOMODULATING DRUGS**			
PLATINUM COMPOUNDS	AZATHIOPRINE	↑ Risk of myelosuppression and immunosuppression. Deaths have occurred following profound myelosuppression and severe sepsis	Additive myelotoxic effects. Azathioprine is metabolized to 6-mercaptopurine in vivo, which results in additive myelosuppression, immunosuppression, and hepatotoxicity	Avoid coadministration
CARBOPLATIN WITH PACLITAXEL	BEXAROTENE	Carboplatin with paclitaxel may ↑ bexarotene levels	Unknown	Clinical significance unknown. Monitor more closely
PLATINUM COMPOUNDS—CISPLATIN	BLEOMYCIN	↑ Bleomycin levels, with risk of pulmonary toxicity	Elimination of bleomycin is delayed by cisplatin due to ↓ glomerular filtration. This is most likely with accumulated doses of cisplatin in excess of 300 mg m^2	Monitor renal function and adjust the dose of bleomycin by creatinine clearance. Monitor clinically, radiologically, and with lung function tests to test for pulmonary toxicity
PLATINUM COMPOUNDS	CICLOSPORIN	↑ Risk of renal toxicity and renal failure	Additive renal toxicity	Monitor renal function prior to and during therapy, and ensure an intake of at least 2L of fluid daily. Monitor serum potassium and magnesium and correct any deficiencies
PLATINUM COMPOUNDS	CLOFARABINE	Possible increase in clofarabine levels	Clofarabine excreted primarily by kidneys	Manufacturer advises to avoid concurrent. Monitor closely if this is unavoidable
PLATINUM COMPOUNDS—CISPLATIN CARBOPLATIN	ETOPOSIDE	Slight increase in etoposide levels	Uncertain	Be aware. Probably not clinically significant
PLATINUM COMPOUNDS—CISPLATIN	DOCETAXEL	↑ Docetaxel levels, with ↑ risk of profound myelosuppression. Concurrent use also ↑ risk of neurotoxicity	↓ Clearance of docetaxel when docetaxel is administered after cisplatin	Administer docetaxel first and follow with cisplatin

(*Continued*)

ANTICANCER AND IMMUNOMODULATING DRUGS CYTOTOXICS

Primary Drug	Secondary Drug	Effect	Mechanism	Precautions
CYTOTOXICS				
PLATINUM COMPOUNDS—CARBOPLATIN	GEFITINIB	Increased gefitinib levels	Unknown	Unknown, increased toxicity not seen despite increased levels
PLATINUM COMPOUNDS—CISPLATIN	IFOSFAMIDE	↑ Risk of neurotoxicity, hematotoxicity, and tubular nephrotoxicity by ifosfamide due to ↑ plasma concentrations of ifosfamide	Cisplatin tends to cause renal damage, which results in impaired clearance of ifosfamide	Do renal function tests before initiating therapy and during concurrent therapy, and adjust the dosage based on creatinine clearance values. Advise patients to drink plenty of water—vigorous hydration—and consider mesna therapy for renal protection
PLATINUM COMPOUNDS—CISPLATIN	MESNA	Inactivation of cisplatin	Pharmaceutical interaction	Do not mix mesna with cisplatin infusions
PLATINUM COMPOUNDS—CISPLATIN	METHOTREXATE	↑ Methotrexate levels with ↑ risk of pulmonary toxicity	Cisplatin is the most common anticancer drug associated with renal proximal and distal tubular damage. Cisplatin could significantly ↓ renal elimination of methotrexate	It would be best to start with lower doses of methotrexate. It is necessary to assess renal function prior to and during concurrent treatment until stability is achieved. Monitor clinically and with pulmonary function tests
PLATINUM COMPOUNDS—CISPLATIN	PACLITAXEL	↑ Risk of profound neutropenia	Prior administration of cisplatin tends to impair renal function and ↓ clearance of paclitaxel by approximately 25%	Advise administration of paclitaxel prior to cisplatin
PLATINUM COMPOUNDS	PEMETREXED	Increased pemetrexed toxicity	Reduced renal clearance	Caution with concurrent use
PLATINUM COMPOUNDS	RITUXIMAB	↑ Risk of severe renal failure	Uncertain; possibly due to effects of tumor lysis syndrome (which is a result of a massive breakdown of cancer cells sensitive to chemotherapy). Features include hyperkalemia, hyperuricemia, hyperphosphatemia, and hypocalcemia	Monitor renal function closely. Hydrate with at least 2L of fluid before, during, and after therapy. Monitor potassium and magnesium levels in particular and correct deficits. Do an ECG as arrhythmias may accompany tumor lysis syndrome

(*Continued*)

Primary Drug	Secondary Drug	Effect	Mechanism	Precautions
CYTOTOXICS				
PLATINUM COMPOUNDS—CISPLATIN	SEMAXANIB	Combination of semaxanib, cisplatin, and gemcitabine resulted in increased thromboembolic events	Unknown	Caution with further studies using cytotoxics and angiogenesis inhibitors
PLATINUM COMPOUNDS—CARBOPLATIN	SORAFENIB	Increased levels of sorafenib in one study	Unknown	Significance unknown
PLATINUM COMPOUNDS	TACROLIMUS	↑ Risk of renal toxicity and renal failure	Additive renal toxicity	Monitor renal function prior to and during therapy, and ensure an intake of at least 2L of fluid daily. Monitor serum potassium and magnesium and correct any deficiencies
PLATINUM COMPOUNDS—CISPLATIN	THALIDOMIDE	Possible increased risk of peripheral neuropathy	Additive	Manufacturer advises to exercise caution
PLATINUM COMPOUNDS—CISPLATIN	TOPOTECAN	↑ Risk of bone marrow suppression, especially when topotecan is administered in doses >0.75 mg/m^2 on days 1–5 and cisplatin in doses >50 mg/m^2 on day 1 before topotecan	Attributed to cisplatin inducing subclinical renal toxicity, possibly causing ↓ clearance of topotecan	Administer cisplatin on day 5 after topotecan if dose of topotecan is >0.75 mg/m^2 and cisplatin dose is >50 mg/m^2 with the use of granulocyte colony–stimulating factors
PLATINUM COMPOUNDS—CISPLATIN	VANDETANIB	Increased levels and toxicity of cisplatin, mainly thromboembolic effects, when given together with gemcitabine	Unknown	Not suitable combination for chemotherapy
PLATINUM COMPOUNDS	VINORELBINE	↑ Incidence of grade III and grade IV granulocytopenia	Additive myelosuppressive effects	Monitor blood counts at least weekly and advise patients to report symptoms such as sore throat and fever
PLATINUM COMPOUNDS—CARBOPLATIN	ANTICOAGULANTS—ORAL	Episodes of ↑ anticoagulant effect	Not understood but likely to be multifactorial	Monitor INR at least weekly until stable during administration of chemotherapy

(*Continued*)

Primary Drug	Secondary Drug	Effect	Mechanism	Precautions
CYTOTOXICS				
PLATINUM COMPOUNDS—CISPLATIN	ANTIDEPRESSANTS—LITHIUM	Possible alteration in lithium levels	Unclear, possibly due to increased clearance due to cisplatin or hydration, or dilution	Monitor lithium levels closely
PLATINUM COMPOUNDS	ANTIDIABETIC DRUGS—METFORMIN	↑ Risk of lactic acidosis	↓ Renal excretion of metformin	Watch for lactic acidosis. The onset of lactic acidosis is often accompanied by symptoms, e.g., malaise, myalgia, respiratory distress, and ↑ nonspecific abdominal distress. There may be hypothermia and resistant bradyarrhythmias
PLATINUM COMPOUNDS	ANTIEPILEPTICS—CARBAMAZEPINE, PHENYTOIN, VALPROIC ACID	↓ Plasma concentrations of antiepileptic, which ↑ risk of seizures	Due to impaired absorption of antiepileptic	Monitor closely for seizure activity and warn patients and carers. Need to adjust dosage using parameters such as blood levels to ensure therapeutic levels
PLATINUM COMPOUNDS	ANTIFUNGALS—AMPHOTERICIN	↑ Risk of renal toxicity and renal failure	Additive renal toxicity	Monitor renal function prior to and during therapy, and ensure an intake of at least 2L of fluid daily. Monitor serum potassium and magnesium and correct any deficiencies
PLATINUM COMPOUNDS	DIURETICS—LOOP	Theoretical risk of auditory toxic effects with cisplatin	Loop diuretics cause tinnitus and deafness as side effects. Additive toxic effects on auditory system likely	Monitor hearing activity (auditory function) regularly, particularly if patients report symptoms such as tinnitus or impaired hearing
PONATINIB				
PONATINIB	**ANTIBIOTICS**			
PONATINIB	MACROLIDES—CLARITHROMYCIN, TELITHROMYCIN, TROLEANDOMYCIN	Possible increased ponatinib levels	CYP3A4 inhibition	Caution with concurrent use. Consider dose reduction
PONATINIB	RIFABUTIN, RIFAMPICIN	Possible reduced ponatinib levels	CYP3A4 induction	Avoid concurrent use if possible

(*Continued*)

Primary Drug	Secondary Drug	Effect	Mechanism	Precautions
CYTOTOXICS				
PONATINIB	**ANTICANCER AND OTHER IMMUNOMODULATING DRUGS**			
PONATINIB	IMATINIB, LAPATINIB, NILOTINIB	Predicted increase in levels of these P-glycoprotein substrates	P-glycoprotein inhibition	Be aware
PONATINIB	METHOTREXATE, MITOXANTRONE, SULFASALAZINE, AND TOPOTECAN	Predicted increase in levels of these BCRP substrates	BCRP inhibition	Be aware
PONATINIB	**ANTIDEPRESSANTS**			
PONATINIB	ST. JOHN'S WORT	Possible reduced ponatinib levels	CYP3A4 induction	Avoid concurrent use if possible
PONATINIB	NEFAZODONE	Possible increased ponatinib levels	CYP3A4 inhibition	Caution with concurrent use. Consider dose reduction
PONATINIB	ANTIDIABETICS—SAXAGLIPTIN, SITAGLIPTIN	Predicted increase in levels of these P-glycoprotein substrates	P-glycoprotein inhibition	Be aware
PONATINIB	ANTIEPILEPTICS—CARBAMAZEPINE, PHENOBARBITAL, PHENYTOIN	Possible reduction in ponatinib levels	CYP3A4 induction	Avoid concurrent use if possible
PONATINIB	**ANTIFUNGALS**			
PONATINIB	ITRACONAZOLE, KETOCONAZOLE, VORICONAZOLE	Possible increased ponatinib levels	CYP3A4 inhibition	Caution with concurrent use. Consider dose reduction
PONATINIB	POSACONAZOLE	Predicted increase in levels of posaconazole	P-glycoprotein inhibition	Be aware
PONATINIB	ANTIHYPERTENSIVES AND HEART FAILURE DRUGS—AMBRISENTAN	Predicted increase in levels of ambrisentan	P-glycoprotein inhibition	Be aware
PONATINIB	**ANTIVIRALS**			
PONATINIB	INDINAVIR, NELFINAVIR, RITONAVIR, SAQUINAVIR	Possible increased ponatinib levels	CYP3A4 inhibition	Caution with concurrent use. Consider dose reduction
PONATINIB	MARAVIROC	Predicted increase in levels of P-glycoprotein substrates	P-glycoprotein inhibition	Be aware

(Continued)

Primary Drug	Secondary Drug	Effect	Mechanism	Precautions
CYTOTOXICS				
PONATINIB	GRAPEFRUIT JUICE	Possible increased ponatinib levels	CYP3A4 inhibition	Caution with concurrent use. Consider dose reduction
PONATINIB	LIPID-LOWERING DRUGS—ROSUVASTATIN	Predicted increase in levels of rosuvastatin	BCRP inhibition	Be aware
PONATINIB	RANOLAZINE	Predicted increase in levels of ranolazine	P-glycoprotein inhibition	Be aware
PONATINIB	TOLVAPTAN	Predicted increase in levels of tolvaptan	P-glycoprotein inhibition	Be aware
PORFIMER				
PORFIMER	1. ACE INHIBITORS—enalapril 2. ANALGESICS—celecoxib, ibuprofen, ketoprofen, naproxen 3. ANTIARRHYTHMICS—amiodarone 4. ANTIBIOTICS—ciprofloxacin, dapsone, sulfonamides, tetracyclines 5. ANTICANCER AND IMMUNOMODULATING DRUGS—fluorouracil (topical and oral) 6. ANTIDIABETIC DRUGS—glipizide 7. ANTIMALARIALS—hydroxychloroquine, quinine 8. ANTIPSYCHOTICS—chlorpromazine, fluphenazine 9. CALCIUM CHANNEL BLOCKERS—diltiazem 10. DIURETICS—bumetanide, furosemide, hydrochlorothiazide 11. PARA-AMINOBENZOIC ACID (TOPICAL) 12. RETINOIDS—acitretin, isotretinoin 13. SALICYLATES (topical)	↑ Risk of photosensitivity reactions	Attributed to additive effects	Avoid exposure of skin and eyes to direct sunlight for 30 days after porfimer therapy
PROCARBAZINE				
PROCARBAZINE	ALCOHOL	May cause a disulfiram-like reaction, additive depression of the CNS, and postural hypotension	Some alcoholic beverages (beer, wine, ale) contain tyramine, which may induce hypertensive reactions	Avoid coadministration

(Continued)

Primary Drug	Secondary Drug	Effect	Mechanism	Precautions
CYTOTOXICS				
PROCARBAZINE	**ANESTHETICS—LOCAL**			
PROCARBAZINE	COCAINE	Risk of severe hypertensive episodes	The metabolism of sympathomimetics is impaired due to inhibition of MAO	Cocaine should not be administered during or within 14 days following administration of an MAOI
PROCARBAZINE	LOCAL ANESTHETICS WITH EPINEPHRINE	Risk of severe hypertension	Due to inhibition of MAO, which metabolizes epinephrine	No sympathomimetic should be administered to patients receiving drugs that inhibit one of the metabolizing enzymes, e.g., MAO
PROCARBAZINE	SPINAL ANESTHETICS	Risk of hypotensive episodes	Uncertain	Recommendation is to discontinue procarbazine for at least 10 days before elective spinal anesthesia
PROCARBAZINE	ANALGESICS—OPIOIDS	Unpredictable reactions may occur associated with hypotension and respiratory depression when procarbazine is coadministered with alfentanil, fentanyl, sufentanil, or morphine	Opioids cause hypotension due to arterial and venous vasodilatation, negative inotropic effects, and a vagally induced bradycardia. Procarbazine can cause postural hypotension. Also attributed to accumulation of serotonin due to inhibition of MAO	Recommended that a small test dose (one-quarter of the usual dose) be administered initially to assess response
PROCARBAZINE	**ANTICANCER AND IMMUNOMODULATING DRUGS**			
PROCARBAZINE	CHLORMETHINE (MUSTINE)	Possible risk of neurological toxicity with high-dose procarbazine	Chlormethine may enhance effects of procarbazine	Avoid administration of drugs on same day

(*Continued*)

Primary Drug	Secondary Drug	Effect	Mechanism	Precautions
CYTOTOXICS				
PROCARBAZINE	METHOTREXATE	↑ Risk of renal impairment if methotrexate infusion is given within 48 h of procarbazine administration. Also ↑ risk of methotrexate toxicity, particularly to the kidneys	Procarbazine has a transient effect on the kidneys, and this will delay the renal elimination of methotrexate	Do not start methotrexate infusion less than 72 h after the last dose of procarbazine. Hydrate patients aggressively (plenty of oral fluids or intravenous fluids), alkalinize the urine to pH > 7, and closely monitor renal function, e.g., blood urea and creatinine, before and after methotrexate infusion until methotrexate blood levels are <0.05 μmol/L
PROCARBAZINE	ANTICOAGULANTS—ORAL	Episodes of ↑ anticoagulant effect	Not understood but likely to be multifactorial	Monitor INR at least weekly until stable during administration of chemotherapy
PROCARBAZINE	**ANTIDEPRESSANTS**			
PROCARBAZINE	MAOIs	Concurrent therapy ↑ risk of hypertensive crisis and severe seizures	Additive effect on inhibiting MAO	Concurrent treatment should not be started on an outpatient basis. 14 days should elapse before starting these medications after procarbazine treatment
PROCARBAZINE	SSRIs	↑ Risk of serotonin syndrome and CNS toxicity	Additive toxicity. Procarbazine has MAOI activity	Monitor BP closely and also CNS side effects. Because of the long half-life of fluoxetine and its active metabolites, at least 5 weeks should elapse between discontinuation of fluoxetine and initiation of therapy with procarbazine
PROCARBAZINE	TCAs	Interaction similar to tricyclics with conventional MAOIs	Procarbazine is weak MAO inhibitor	Avoid concurrent use

(*Continued*)

Primary Drug	Secondary Drug	Effect	Mechanism	Precautions
CYTOTOXICS				
PROCARBAZINE	TRYPTOPHAN	Risk of hyperreflexia, shivering, hyperventilation, hyperthermia, mania or hypomania, disorientation/confusion	Tryptophan is a precursor of a number of neurotransmitters, including serotonin. Procarbazine has MAOI activity, which inhibits the breakdown of neurotransmitters	Tryptophan should be started under a specialist's supervision. Recommended to start with low doses and titrate upward with close monitoring of mental status and BP
PROCARBAZINE	ANTIDIABETIC DRUGS—INSULIN, SULFONYLUREAS	↑ Risk of hypoglycemic episodes	Procarbazine has mild MAOI properties. MAOIs have an intrinsic hypoglycemic effect and are considered to enhance the effect of hypoglycemic drugs	Watch for and warn patients about symptoms of hypoglycemia. ➢ ***For signs and symptoms of hypoglycemia, see Clinical Features of Some Adverse Drug Interactions, Hypoglycemia***
PROCARBAZINE	ANTIEPILEPTICS—CARBAMAZEPINE, PHENOBARBITAL, PHENYTOIN, VALPROIC ACID	↑ Risk of hypersensitivity reactions in patients with brain tumors	Strong correlation between the therapeutic antiepileptic level and the hypersensitivity reactions	Consider using nonenzyme-inducing agents
PROCARBAZINE	ANTIHISTAMINES—ALIMEMAZINE (TRIMEPRAZINE), CHLORPHENAMINE, PROMETHAZINE	1. The antimuscarinic effects (dry mouth, urinary retention, blurred vision, gastrointestinal disturbances) are ↑, as are the sedating effects of these older antihistamines 2. Excessive sedation may occur	1. MAOIs cause anticholinergic effects (including antimuscarinic effects), hence additive effects of both antimuscarinic activity and CNS depression 2. Additive effects on CNS, although on occasions chlorphenamine may cause CNS stimulation	Concurrent use is not recommended. If used together, patients should be warned to report any gastrointestinal problems as paralytic ileus has been reported. Also, caution is required when performing activities that requires alertness (e.g., driving, using sharp objects). Do not use OTC medications such as nasal decongestants or asthma and allergy remedies without consulting the pharmacist/doctor as these preparations may contain antihistamines
PROCARBAZINE	ANTIHYPERTENSIVES AND HEART FAILURE DRUGS	Hypotension	Additive	Monitor closely
PROCARBAZINE	ANTI-PARKINSON'S DRUGS—BROMOCRIPTINE	May cause ↑ serum prolactin levels and interfere with the effects of bromocriptine	Uncertain	Watch for ↓ effect of bromocriptine

(Continued)

Primary Drug	Secondary Drug	Effect	Mechanism	Precautions
CYTOTOXICS				
PROCARBAZINE	**ANTIPSYCHOTICS**			
PROCARBAZINE	CLOZAPINE	↑ Risk of bone marrow toxicity	Additive effect	Avoid coadministration
PROCARBAZINE	FLUPENTIXOL, PIMOZIDE, ZUCLOPENTHIXOL	Prolongation or greater intensity of sedative, hypotensive, and anticholinergic effects	Additive effect	Avoid coadministration
PROCARBAZINE	ANXIOLYTICS AND HYPNOTICS—BUSPIRONE	Risk of elevation of BP	Additive effect; buspirone acts at serotonin receptors; procarbazine inhibits breakdown of sympathomimetics	Avoid concurrent use
PROCARBAZINE	FOODS—TYRAMINE-CONTAINING—aged cheeses, aged pickles, smoked meats (e.g., salami), yeast extracts, beer (dark more than light and tap more than bottled), red wine more than white wine, avocado, sauerkraut, marmite, banana peel, soy bean products, broad bean pods, foods containing MSG	Risk of severe tyramine reactions—hypertension, occipital headaches, vomiting, palpitations, nausea, apprehension, chills, sweating. This reaction develops 20–60 min after ingestion of these foods	Tyramine has both direct and indirect sympathomimetic effects, and tyramine effects of foods may be potentiated by MAOIs 10–20-fold	Prompt treatment with phentolamine (0.5 mg intravenously) or nifedipine is effective, and death is rare (0.01%–0.02%). There is a recommendation that a 25 mg tablet of chlorpromazine be given to patients on MAOIs if a tyramine reaction occurs
PROCARBAZINE	SYMPATHOMIMETICS	Coadministration of ephedrine, metaraminol, methylphenidate, phenylephrine, or pseudoephedrine (including nasal and ophthalmic solutions) with procarbazine may cause prolongation and ↑ intensity of cardiac stimulant effects and effects on BP, which may cause headache, arrhythmias, and hypertensive or hyperpyretic crises	The metabolism of sympathomimetics is impaired due to inhibition of MAO	It is recommended that sympathomimetics not be administered during and within 14 days of stopping procarbazine. Do not use any OTC nasal decongestants (sprays or oral preparations) or asthma relief agents without consulting the pharmacist/doctor

(*Continued*)

Primary Drug	Secondary Drug	Effect	Mechanism	Precautions
CYTOTOXICS				
RALTITREXED				
RALTITREXED	FOLINIC ACID FOLIC ACID	Folinates theoretically interfere with action of raltitrexed	Folinate antagonizes the anti-DNA effect of raltitrexed	Manufacturer advises to avoid concurrent use
REGORAFENIB				
REGORAFENIB	ANALGESICS—MEFENAMIC ACID, DIFLUNISAL, AND NIFLUMIC ACID	Predicted increased regorafenib levels	UGT1A9 inhibition	Manufacturer advises to avoid concurrent use
REGORAFENIB	**ANTIBIOTICS**			
REGORAFENIB	CLARITHROMYCIN, TELITHROMYCIN	Predicted increased regorafenib levels	CYP3A4 inhibition	Manufacturer advises to avoid concurrent use
REGORAFENIB	RIFAMPICIN	Predicted reduced regorafenib levels	CYP3A4 induction	Manufacturer advises to avoid concurrent use
REGORAFENIB	**ANTICANCER AND OTHER IMMUNOMODULATING DRUGS**			
REGORAFENIB	IRINOTECAN	Possible increased levels of UGT1A1 and UGT1A9 substrates	UGT1A1 and UGT1A9 inhibition	Clinical significance not determined
REGORAFENIB	METHOTREXATE	Possible increased levels of BCRP substrates	BCRP inhibition	Clinical significance not determined
REGORAFENIB	ANTIDEPRESSANTS—ST. JOHN'S WORT	Predicted reduced regorafenib levels	CYP3A4 induction	Manufacturer advises to avoid concurrent use
REGORAFENIB	ANTIEPILEPTICS—PHENYTOIN, CARBAMAZEPINE, PHENOBARBITAL	Predicted reduced regorafenib levels	CYP3A4 induction	Manufacturer advises to avoid concurrent use
REGORAFENIB	ANTIFUNGALS—ITRACONAZOLE, KETOCONAZOLE, POSACONAZOLE, VORICONAZOLE	Predicted increased regorafenib levels	CYP3A4 inhibition	Manufacturer advises to avoid concurrent use
REGORAFENIB	CARDIAC GLYCOSIDES—DIGOXIN	Possible increased levels of digoxin	P-glycoprotein inhibition	Monitor PR and BP closely
REGORAFENIB	GRAPEFRUIT JUICE	Predicted increased regorafenib levels	CYP3A4 inhibition	Manufacturer advises to avoid concurrent use
REGORAFENIB	LIPID-LOWERING DRUGS—CHOLESTYRAMINE AND CHOLESTAGEL	Possible reduced regorafenib levels	Formation of insoluble complexes with regorafenib, reducing (re)absorption	Clinical significance unknown, but be aware of possible reduced efficacy of regorafenib. Consider separating doses

(*Continued*)

ANTICANCER AND IMMUNOMODULATING DRUGS CYTOTOXICS

Primary Drug	Secondary Drug	Effect	Mechanism	Precautions
CYTOTOXICS				
RUXOLITINIB				
RUXOLITINIB	**ANTIBIOTICS**			
RUXOLITINIB	CIPROFLOXACIN, CLARITHROMYCIN, ERYTHROMYCIN, TELITHROMYCIN	Increased levels of ruxolitinib	CYP3A4 inhibition	Manufacturer advises dose reduction Monitor closely
RUXOLITINIB	RIFABUTIN, RIFAMPICIN	Reduced levels of ruloxitinib	CYP3A4 induction	Monitor closely Titrate dose based on safety and efficacy
RUXOLITINIB	ANTICANCER AND OTHER IMMUNOMODULATING DRUGS—CICLOSPORIN	Predicted increase in P-glycoprotein or BCRP substrate levels	P-glycoprotein/BCRP inhibition	Monitor closely Separate administration of drugs
RUXOLITINIB	ANTICOAGULANTS—DABIGATRAN	Predicted increase in P-glycoprotein or BCRP substrate levels	P-glycoprotein/BCRP inhibition	Monitor closely Separate administration of drugs
RUXOLITINIB	**ANTIDEPRESSANTS**			
RUXOLITINIB	ST. JOHN'S WORT	Reduced levels of ruloxitinib	CYP3A4 induction	Monitor closely Titrate dose based on safety and efficacy
RUXOLITINIB	NEFAZODONE	Increased levels of ruxolitinib	CYP3A4 inhibition	Manufacturer advises dose reduction Monitor closely
RUXOLITINIB	ANTIEPILEPTICS—CARBAMAZEPINE, PHENOBARBITAL, PHENYTOIN	Reduced levels of ruloxitinib	CYP3A4 induction	Monitor closely Titrate dose based on safety and efficacy
RUXOLITINIB	ANTIFUNGALS—ITRACONAZOLE, KETOCONAZOLE, POSACONAZOLE, VORICONAZOLE	Increased levels of ruxolitinib	CYP3A4 inhibition	Manufacturer advises dose reduction Monitor closely
RUXOLITINIB	ANTIVIRALS—AMPRENAVIR, ATAZANAVIR, BOCEPREVIR, INDINAVIR, LOPINAVIR, RITONAVIR, NELFINAVIR, SAQUINAVIR, TELAPREVIR	Increased levels of ruxolitinib	CYP3A4 inhibition	Reduce dose of ruxolitinib by approximately 50%, give twice daily and monitor FBC twice weekly

(*Continued*)

Primary Drug	Secondary Drug	Effect	Mechanism	Precautions
CYTOTOXICS				
RUXOLITINIB	CALCIUM CHANNEL BLOCKERS—DILTIAZEM, MIBEFRADIL	Increased levels of ruxolitinib	CYP3A4 inhibition	Manufacturer advises dose reduction Monitor closely
RUXOLITINIB	CARDIAC GLYCOSIDES—DIGOXIN	Predicted increase in P-glycoprotein or BCRP substrate levels	P-glycoprotein/BCRP inhibition	Monitor closely Separate administration of drugs
RUXOLITINIB	H2-RECEPTOR BLOCKING DRUGS—CIMETIDINE	Increased levels of ruxolitinib	CYP3A4 inhibition	Monitor closely
RUXOLITINIB	**LIPID-LOWERING DRUGS**			
RUXOLITINIB	AVASIMIBE	Reduced levels of ruloxitinib	CYP3A4 induction	Monitor closely Titrate dose based on safety and efficacy
RUXOLITINIB	ROSUVASTATIN	Predicted increase in P-glycoprotein or BCRP substrate levels	P-glycoprotein/BCRP inhibition	Monitor closely Separate administration of drugs
SEMAXANIB				
SEMAXANIB	ANTICANCER AND IMMUNOMODULATING DRUGS—GEMCITABINE	Combination of semaxanib, cisplatin, and gemcitabine resulted in increased thromboembolic events	Unknown	Caution with further studies using cytotoxics and angiogenesis inhibitors
SEMAXANIB	PLATINUM COMPOUNDS—CISPLATIN	Combination of semaxanib, cisplatin, and gemcitabine resulted in increased thromboembolic events	Unknown	Caution with further studies using cytotoxics and angiogenesis inhibitors
SORAFENIB				
SORAFENIB	ANALGESICS—CELECOXIB, DICLOFENAC, PIROXICAM	Increased blood levels of these NSAIDs	Sorafenib inhibits CYP2C9	Monitor for toxic effects
SORAFENIB	ANTICOAGULANTS—ORAL	Episodes of ↑ anticoagulant effect	Not understood but likely to be multifactorial	Monitor INR at least weekly until stable during administration of chemotherapy

(Continued)

Primary Drug	Secondary Drug	Effect	Mechanism	Precautions
CYTOTOXICS				
SOREFENIB	**ANTIBIOTICS**			
SORAFENIB	NEOMYCIN	Sorafenib levels reduced	Reduced enterohepatic recycling of sorafenib, due to elimination of bacteria with glucuronidase activity	Monitor concurrent use for reduced effectiveness
SORAFENIB	RIFAMPICIN	Slight reduced sorafenib levels	CYP3A4 induction	Avoid coadministration
SORAFENIB	**ANTICANCER AND OTHER IMMUNOMODULATING DRUGS**			
SORAFENIB	BEVACIZUMAB	Lower maximum tolerated doses of bevacizumab and sorafenib, unexpected toxicity (hypertension, proteinuria, thrombocytopenia)	Unknown	Dose reduction required
SORAFENIB	CAPECITABINE	Levels of capecitabine increased	Unknown	Caution with concurrent use
SORAFENIB	CARBOPLATIN	Increased levels of sorafenib in one study	Unknown	Significance unknown
SORAFENIB	DOCETAXEL	Docetaxel levels increased	Possibly due to inhibition of P-glycoprotein, which transports docetaxel	Caution with concurrent use
SORAFENIB	DOXORUBICIN	Slight increase in doxorubicin levels	Unknown	Be aware. Clinical relevance unknown
SORAFENIB	ERLOTINIB	Erlotinib levels possibly reduced	Unknown	Clinical significance uncertain
SORAFENIB	FLUOROURACIL	Levels of fluorouracil increased	Unknown	Caution with concurrent use
SORAFENIB	GEFITINIB	Gefitinib levels reduced	Unknown	Clinical significance uncertain
SORAFENIB	IRINOTECAN	Increased concentration of irinotecan and SN-38 (its active metabolite) increased irinotecan toxicity	Inhibition of metabolism of SN-38	Caution with concurrent use, consider reduction in irinotecan dose, monitor for signs of toxicity

(*Continued*)

Primary Drug	Secondary Drug	Effect	Mechanism	Precautions
CYTOTOXICS				
SORAFENIB	PACLITAXEL	Paclitaxel and sorafenib levels slightly increased	Unknown	Unknown
SORAFENIB	TEMSIROLIMUS	Clinically important toxicity in phase I trial	Unknown	Not suitable regimen
SORAFENIB	ANTIEPILEPTICS—CARBAMAZEPINE, OXCARBAZEPINE, PHENYTOIN, PHENOBARBITAL, PRIMIDONE	Sorafenib levels reduced	CYP3A4 induction	Avoid concurrent use
SORAFENIB	ANTIVIRALS—BOCEPREVIR	Predicted increased levels of sorafenib	CYP3A4 inhibition	Manufacturer advises to avoid concurrent use
SUNITINIB				
SUNITINIB	**DRUGS THAT PROLONG THE QT INTERVAL**			
SUNITINIB	1. ANTIARRHYTHMICS—ajmaline, amiodarone, azimilide, cibenzoline, disopyramide, dofetilide, dronedarone, ibutilide, procainamide, propafenone, quinidine 2. ANTIBIOTICS—macrolides (especially azithromycin, clarithromycin, parenteral erythromycin, telithromycin), quinolones (especially moxifloxacin), quinupristin/dalfopristin 3. ANTICANCER AND IMMUNOMODULATING DRUGS—arsenic trioxide, bosutinib, crizotinib, dasatinib, eribulin, fingolimod, lapatinib, nilotinib, pazopanib, vandetanib, vemurafenib 4. ANTIDEPRESSANTS—TCAs, venlafaxine 5. ANTIEMETICS—ondansetron 6. ANTIFUNGALS—fluconazole, posaconazole, voriconazole 7. ANTIHISTAMINES—terfenadine, hydroxyzine, mizolastine	Risk of ventricular arrhythmias, particularly torsades de pointes	Additive effect; these drugs prolong the QT interval	Avoid coadministration

(Continued)

Primary Drug	Secondary Drug	Effect	Mechanism	Precautions
CYTOTOXICS				
	8. ANTIHYPERTENSIVES—ketanserin 9. ANTIMALARIALS—artemether with lumefantrine, chloroquine, halofantrine, hydroxychloroquine, mefloquine, quinine 10. ANTIPROTOZOALS—pentamidine isethionate 11. ANTIPSYCHOTICS—atypicals, phenothiazines, pimozide 12. ANTIVIRALS—boceprevir, rilpivirine, telaprevir 13. BETA-BLOCKERS—sotalol 14. BRONCHODILATORS—parenteral bronchodilators 15. CNS STIMULANTS—atomoxetine 16. RANOLAZINE			
SUNITINIB	ANALGESICS—PARACETAMOL	Single report of fatal liver failure	Unknown	Unknown
SUNITINIB	**ANTIBIOTICS**			
SUNITINIB	MACROLIDES	Predicted increased levels of sunitinib	CYP3A4 inhibition	Avoid concurrent use
SUNITINIB	RIFAMPICIN	↓ Sunitinib levels	Rifampicin ↑ metabolism of sunitinib	Avoid coadministration
SUNITINIB	**ANTICANCER AND OTHER IMMUNOMODULATING DRUGS**			
SUNITINIB	BEVACIZUMAB	Possible increased risk of microangiopathic hemolytic anemia	Unknown	Monitor concurrent use
SUNITINIB	EVEROLIMUS	Clinically important toxicity in phase I trial	Unknown	Combination use likely to be limited
SUNITINIB	IFOSFAMIDE	Possible decreased sunitinib levels, possible increased risk of neutropenia	Unknown	Reduced maximum dose of ifosfamide tolerated in single study due to neutropenia. Further investigation needed

(*Continued*)

Primary Drug	Secondary Drug	Effect	Mechanism	Precautions
CYTOTOXICS				
SUNITINIB	IRINOTECAN	Increased concentration of irinotecan and SN-38 (its active metabolite) increased irinotecan toxicity	Inhibition of metabolism of SN-38	Caution with concurrent use, consider reduction in irinotecan dose, monitor for signs of toxicity
SUNITINIB	TEMSIROLIMUS	Clinically important toxicity in phase I trial	Unknown	Not suitable regimen
SUNITINIB	ANTICOAGULANTS—COUMARINS	Possible increased bleeding risk	Additive effect	Monitor closely with concurrent use
SUNITINIB	ANTIFUNGALS—KETOCONAZOLE, ITRACONAZOLE, POSACONAZOLE, VORICONAZOLE	Increased levels of sunitinib Increased risk of QT prolongation	CYP3A4 inhibition	Avoid concurrent use Dose reduction if not possible
SUNITINIB	PROTEASE INHIBITORS	Predicted to inhibit metabolism of sunitinib, but no evidence	CYP3A4 inhibition	Manufacturer advises to avoid concurrent use of HIV protease inhibitors, specifically ritonavir, atazanavir, indinavir, nelfinavir, and saquinavir
SUNITINIB	BOCEPREVIR	Predicted increased levels of boceprevir	CYP3A4 inhibition	Manufacturer advises to avoid concurrent use
SUNITINIB	GRAPEFRUIT JUICE	Possible increased sunitinib levels	CYP3A4 inhibition	Avoid concurrent use
SUNITINIB	LEVOTHYROXINE	Single case of hypothyroidism in patients taking levothyroxine	Unknown	Monitor TSH levels and increase levothyroxine if necessary
TEGAFUR				
Tegafur is metabolized to fluorouracil ➢ ***Fluorouracil, above***				
TEMOPORFIN				
TEMOPORFIN	ANTICANCER AND OTHER IMMUNOMODULATING DRUGS—FLUOROURACIL	↑ Risk of photosensitivity with topical fluorouracil	Uncertain; possibly additive effect (topical fluorouracil can cause local irritation, while temoporfin is a photosensitizer)	Patients on temoporfin are advised to avoid direct sunlight for at least 15 days

(*Continued*)

Primary Drug	Secondary Drug	Effect	Mechanism	Precautions
CYTOTOXICS				
TEMOZOLOMIDE				
TEMOZOLOMIDE	VALPROATE	Increased temozolomide levels	Unknown	Oral clearance reduced by 5%—significance unclear. Be aware
TEMSIROLIMUS				
TEMSIROLIMUS	ANTIARRHYTHMICS—DRONEDARONE	Predicted increased temsirolimus levels	CYP3A4 inhibition P-glycoprotein inhibition	Monitor closely with concurrent use
TEMSIROLIMUS	ANTIBIOTICS—RIFAMPICIN	Reduced temsirolimus levels	CYP3A4 induction	Avoid concurrent use. If not possible, consider temsirolimus dose increase
TEMSIROLIMUS	ANTICANCER AND OTHER IMMUNOMODULATING DRUGS—SORAFENIB, SUNITINIB	Clinically important toxicity in phase I trial	Unknown	Not suitable regimen
TEMSIROLIMUS	ANTIEMETICS—METOCLOPRAMIDE	Possible increased temsirolimus levels	CYP3A4 inhibition	Caution with concurrent use
TEMSIROLIMUS	ANTIEPILEPTICS—CARBAMAZEPINE, PHENOBARBITOL, PHENYTOIN	Reduced temsirolimus levels	CYP3A4 induction	Avoid concurrent use. If not possible, consider temsirolimus dose increase
TEMSIROLIMUS	ANTIFUNGALS—ITRACONAZOLE, KETOCONAZOLE, POSACONAZOLE, VORICONAZOLE	Increased temsirolimus levels	CYP3A4 inhibition	Avoid concurrent use. If not possible, consider temsirolimus dose reduction. Washout period should be considered before increasing temsirolimus dose after CYP3A4 inhibitor is stopped
TEMSIROLIMUS	ANTIHYPERTENSIVES AND HEART FAILURE DRUGS—ACE INHIBITORS	Possible increased risk of angioedema	Additive	Monitor closely
TEMSIROLIMUS	ANTI-PARKINSON'S DRUGS—BROMOCRIPTINE	Possible increased temsirolimus levels	CYP3A4 inhibition	Caution with concurrent use
TEMSIROLIMUS	ANTIVIRALS—ETRAVIRINE	Possible increased temsirolimus levels	CYP3A4 inhibition	Caution with concurrent use
TEMSIROLIMUS	DANAZOL	Possible increased temsirolimus levels	CYP3A4 inhibition	Caution with concurrent use

(Continued)

Primary Drug	Secondary Drug	Effect	Mechanism	Precautions
CYTOTOXICS				
TEMSIROLIMUS	H2-RECEPTOR BLOCKERS—CIMETIDINE	↑ Adverse effects, e.g., thrombocytopenia, hepatotoxicity	Inhibition of metabolism via CYP3A4 and competition with tacrolimus for renal tubular secretion	Consider alternative acid suppression, e.g., alginate suspension, famotidine, nizatidine, or rabeprazole. Not thought to be clinically significant. Ensure close monitoring of immunosuppressant levels and renal function
THIOTEPA				
THIOTEPA	ANTICANCER AND OTHER IMMUNOMODULATING DRUGS—CYCLOPHOSPHAMIDE	Inhibition of cyclophosphamide metabolism if thiotepa given first, potential reduction in efficacy and toxicity	Inhibition of CYP2B6	Order of administration may be of critical importance
THIOTEPA	DRUG DEPENDENCE THERAPIES—BUPROPION	↑ Plasma concentrations of bupropion and risk of adverse effects	Inhibition of CYP2B6	Warn patients about adverse effects and use alternatives when possible
THIOTEPA	H2 RECEPTOR BLOCKERS—CIMETIDINE	↑ Adverse effects of alkylating agent, e.g., myelosuppression	Additive toxicity	Monitor more closely; monitor FBC regularly
THIOTEPA	MUSCLE RELAXANTS—DEPOLARIZING	↑ Efficacy of suxamethonium	Uncertain; these drugs are likely to decrease plasma levels of pseudocholinesterase, enhancing the neuromuscular blockade	Caution with concurrent use. Reduce dosage or avoid suxamethonium
TIOGUANINE (THIOGUANINE)				
TIOGUANINE	ANTICANCER AND IMMUNOMODULATING DRUGS—BUSULFAN	↑ Risk of hepatic nodular regenerative hyperplasia of the liver, esophageal varices, and portal hypertension	Mechanism is uncertain	Monitor liver function and clinical indices of liver toxicity, e.g., ascites, splenomegaly. Ask patients to report any symptoms suggestive of esophageal bleeding

(*Continued*)

Primary Drug	Secondary Drug	Effect	Mechanism	Precautions
CYTOTOXICS				
TOFACITINIB				
TOFACITINIB	**ANTICANCER AND IMMUNOMODULATING DRUGS**			
TOFACITINIB	AZATHIOPRINE	Increased risk of immunosuppression	Additive	Monitor closely
TOFACITINIB	CICLOSPORIN	Tofacitinib levels increased	Unknown	Caution with concurrent use
TOFACITINIB	TACROLIMUS	Slight increase in tofacitinib levels	Unknown	Caution with concurrent use
TOPOTECAN				
TOPOTECAN	**ANTICANCER AND IMMUNOMODULATING DRUGS**			
TOPOTECAN	CICLOSPORIN	Increased topotecan levels	P-glycoprotein and BCRP inhibition	Avoid concurrent use Monitor closely if necessary
TOPOTECAN	CISPLATIN	↑ Risk of bone marrow suppression, especially when topotecan is administered in doses >0.75 mg/m² on days 1–5 and cisplatin in doses >50 mg/m² on day 1 before topotecan	Attributed to cisplatin-induced subclinical renal toxicity, possibly causing ↓ clearance of topotecan	Administer cisplatin on day 5 after topotecan if dose of topotecan is >0.75 mg/m² and cisplatin dose is >50 mg/m² with the use of granulocyte colony–stimulating factor
TOPOTECAN	DOCETAXEL	↑ Risk of neutropenia when topotecan is administered on days 1–4 and docetaxel on day 4	Attributed to ↓ clearance of docetaxel (by 50%) due to inhibition of hepatic metabolism of docetaxel by CYP3A4 by topotecan	Administer docetaxel on day 1 and topotecan on day 1–4
TOPOTECAN	IFOSFAMIDE	Increased toxicity when used concurrently	Unknown	Doses limited with this combination
TOPOTECAN	LAPATINIB	Slight reduced topotecan levels Lower tolerated dose of topotecan	Possible inhibition of drug transporter proteins by lapatinib	Caution with concurrent use

(*Continued*)

Primary Drug	Secondary Drug	Effect	Mechanism	Precautions
CYTOTOXICS				
TOPETECAN	PONATINIB	Predicted increased in levels of these BCRP substrates	BCRP inhibition	Be aware
TOPOTECAN	ANTIEPILEPTICS—PHENYTOIN	↓ Levels of topetecan, with risk of therapeutic failure	Induction of hepatic metabolism	Monitor for ↓ clinical efficacy and ↑ their dose as required
TOPOTECAN	ELTROMBOPAG	Possible increased topotecan levels	Inhibition of BCRP	Caution with concurrent use
TRABECTEDIN				
TRABECTEDIN	ALCOHOL	Increased risk of hepatotoxicity	Additive	Avoid alcohol consumption
TRABECTEDIN	**ANTIBIOTICS**			
TRABECTEDIN	CLARITHROMYCIN, TELITHROMYCIN	Increased trabectedin levels	CYP3A4 inhibition	Avoid concurrent use with potent CP3A4 inhibitors if possible, monitor closely and consider dose reduction
TRABECTEDIN	RIFABUTIN, RIFAMPICIN, RIFAPENTINE	Reduced trabectedin levels	CYP3A4 induction	Monitor closely
TRABECTEDIN	CICLOSPORIN	Increased trabectedin levels	Inhibition of P-glycoprotein	Caution with concurrent use
TRABECTEDIN	**ANTIDEPRESSANTS**			
TRABECTEDIN	ST. JOHN'S WORT	Reduced trabectedin levels	CYP3A4 induction	Monitor closely
TRABECTEDIN	NEFAZODONE	Increased trabectedin levels	CYP3A4 inhibition	Avoid concurrent use with potent CP3A4 inhibitors if possible, monitor closely and consider dose reduction
TRABECTEDIN	**ANTIEPILEPTICS**			
TRABECTEDIN	ANTIEPILEPTICS—CARBAMAZEPINE, PHENYTOIN, PHENOBARBITAL	1. Reduced trabectedin levels 2. Reduced absorption of phenytoin	1. CYP3A4 induction 2. Trabectedin may damage gut mucosa, affecting absorption of phenytoin	1. Monitor closely 2. Monitor phenytoin levels

(*Continued*)

Primary Drug	Secondary Drug	Effect	Mechanism	Precautions
CYTOTOXICS				
TRABECTEDIN	ANTIFUNGALS—ITRACONAZOLE, KETOCONAZOLE, VORICONAZOLE	Increased trabectedin levels	CYP3A4 inhibition	Avoid concurrent use with potent CP3A4 inhibitors if possible, monitor closely and consider dose reduction
TRABECTEDIN	ANTIVIRALS—ATAZANAVIR, INDINAVIR, NELFINAVIR, RITONAVIR, SAQUINAVIR	Increased trabectedin levels	CYP3A4 inhibition	Avoid concurrent use with potent CP3A4 inhibitors if possible, monitor closely and consider dose reduction
TRABECTEDIN	CALCIUM CHANNEL BLOCKERS—VERAPAMIL	↑ Plasma concentrations of trabectin when coadministered with verapamil	Due to inhibition of Pgp	Warn patient to report features of toxicity (GI upset, headaches, edema). Monitor FBC, U&Es, and LFTs closely
TRABECTEDIN	LIPID-LOWERING DRUGS—STATINS	Possible increased risk of rhabdomyolysis	Additive	Caution with concurrent use
TRASTUZUMAB				
TRASTUZUMAB	**ANTICANCER AND IMMUNOMODULATING DRUGS**			
TRASTUZUMAB	CICLOSPORIN, SIROLIMUS	↑ Neutropenic effect of immunosuppressants	Additive effects	Warn patients to report symptoms such as sore throat and fever. ➢ ***For signs and symptoms of neutropenia, see Clinical Features of Some Adverse Drug Interactions, Immunosuppression and blood dyscrasias***
TRASTUZUMAB	CYCLOPHOSPHAMIDE, DAUNORUBICIN, IDARUBICIN, PACLITAXEL	↑ Risk of cardiac toxicity	Possibly additive cardiac toxic effect	Monitor cardiac function closely—clinically and electrocardiographically. Avoid coadministration of trastuzumab with idarubicin except in clinical trials
TRASTUZUMAB	DOXORUBICIN	When used in combination, the risk of cardiotoxicity due to trastuzumab is ↑ over fourfold	Due to additive cardiotoxic effects	Avoid coadministration except in clinical trials

(*Continued*)

Primary Drug	Secondary Drug	Effect	Mechanism	Precautions
CYTOTOXICS				
TREOSULFAN				
TREOSULFAN	H2 RECEPTOR BLOCKERS—CIMETIDINE	↑ Adverse effects of alkylating agent, e.g., myelosuppression	Additive toxicity	Monitor more closely; monitor FBC regularly
TRETAMINE				
TRETAMINE	MUSCLE RELAXANTS—SUXAMETHONIUM	↑ Efficacy of suxamethonium	Uncertain; these drugs are likely to decrease plasma levels of pseudocholinesterase, enhancing the neuromuscular blockade	Caution with concurrent use. Reduce dosage or avoid suxamethonium
TRETINOIN ➢ ***Other Immunomodulating Drugs, Retinoids below***				
VALRUBICIN				
VALRUBICIN	BEVACIZUMAB	Possible increased risk of cardiac failure	Additive	Be aware of interaction
VALRUBICIN	DASATINIB	Increased risk of cardiac side effects	Dasatinib reported to cause QT prolongation	Avoid concurrent use
VALRUBICIN	LAPATINIB	Increased risk of cardiac side effects	Lapatinib reported to cause QT prolongation	Avoid concurrent use
VANDETANIB				
VANDETANIB	**DRUGS THAT PROLONG THE QT INTERVAL**			
VANDETANIB	1. ANTIARRHYTHMICS—ajmaline, amiodarone, azimilide, cibenzoline, disopyramide, dofetilide, dronedarone, ibutilide, procainamide, propafenone, quinidine 2. ANTIBIOTICS—macrolides (especially azithromycin, clarithromycin, parenteral erythromycin, telithromycin), quinolones (especially moxifloxacin), quinupristin/dalfopristin	Risk of ventricular arrhythmias, particularly torsades de pointes	Additive effect; these drugs prolong the QT interval	Avoid coadministration

(*Continued*)

Primary Drug	Secondary Drug	Effect	Mechanism	Precautions
CYTOTOXICS				
	3. ANTICANCER AND IMMUNOMODULATING DRUGS—arsenic trioxide, bosutinib, crizotinib, dasatinib, eribulin, fingolimod, lapatinib, nilotinib, pazopanib, sunitinib, vemurafenib 4. ANTIDEPRESSANTS—TCAs, venlafaxine 5. ANTIEMETICS—ondansetron 6. ANTIFUNGALS—fluconazole, posaconazole, voriconazole 7. ANTIHISTAMINES—terfenadine, hydroxyzine, mizolastine 8. ANTIHYPERTENSIVES—ketanserin 9. ANTIMALARIALS—artemether with lumefantrine, chloroquine, halofantrine, hydroxychloroquine, mefloquine, quinine 10. ANTIPROTOZOALS—pentamidine isethionate 11. ANTIPSYCHOTICS—atypicals, phenothiazines, pimozide 12. ANTIVIRALS—boceprevir, rilpivirine, telaprevir 13. BETA-BLOCKERS—sotalol 14. BRONCHODILATORS—parenteral bronchodilators 15. CNS STIMULANTS—atomoxetine 16. RANOLAZINE			
VANDETANIB	ANTIBIOTICS—RIFAMPICIN	Slightly reduced vandetanib levels	CYP3A4 induction	Avoid coadministration
VANDETANIB	**ANTICANCER AND OTHER IMMUNOMODULATING DRUGS**			
VANDETANIB	CISPLATIN	Increased levels and toxicity of cisplatin, mainly thromboembolic effects, when given together with gemcitabine	Unknown	Not a suitable combination for chemotherapy

(Continued)

Primary Drug	Secondary Drug	Effect	Mechanism	Precautions
CYTOTOXICS				
VANDETANIB	GEMCITABINE	Increased levels and toxicity of cisplatin, mainly thromboembolic effects, when given together with gemcitabine and vandetanib	Unknown	Not a suitable combination for chemotherapy
VANDETANIB	VINORELBINE	Increased levels of toxicity (thromboembolic effects) when vandetanib, vinorelbine, and cisplation combined	Unknown	Not a suitable combination for chemotherapy
VANDETANIB	ANTIFUNGALS—KETOCONAZOLE	Possible increased levels of vandetanib	CYP3A4 inhibition	Caution with concurrent use
VANDETANIB	ANTIVIRALS—PROTEASE INHIBITORS	Predicted to increase vandetanib levels	CYP3A4 inhibition	Manufacturer advises caution with concurrent use of HIV protease inhibitors, specifically ritonavir
VANDETANIB	PROTON PUMP INHIBITORS	Possible ↓ plasma concentration	↓ Absorption	Manufacturer advises to avoid coadministration
VEMURAFENIB				
VEMURAFENIB	**DRUGS THAT PROLONG THE QT INTERVAL**			
VEMURAFENIB	1. ANTIARRHYTHMICS—ajmaline, amiodarone, azimilide, cibenzoline, disopyramide, dofetilide, dronedarone, ibutilide, procainamide, propafenone, quinidine 2. ANTIBIOTICS—macrolides (especially azithromycin, clarithromycin, parenteral erythromycin, telithromycin), quinolones (especially moxifloxacin), quinupristin/dalfopristin	Risk of ventricular arrhythmias, particularly torsades de pointes	Additive effect; these drugs prolong the QT interval	Avoid coadministration

(*Continued*)

ANTICANCER AND IMMUNOMODULATING DRUGS CYTOTOXICS

ANTICANCER AND IMMUNOMODULATING DRUGS CYTOTOXICS Vemurafenib

Primary Drug	Secondary Drug	Effect	Mechanism	Precautions
CYTOTOXICS				
	3. ANTICANCER AND IMMUNOMODULATING DRUGS—arsenic trioxide, bosutinib, crizotinib, dasatinib, eribulin, fingolimod, lapatinib, nilotinib, pazopanib, sunitinib, vandetanib 4. ANTIDEPRESSANTS—TCAs, venlafaxine 5. ANTIEMETICS—ondansetron 6. ANTIFUNGALS—fluconazole, posaconazole, voriconazole 7. ANTIHISTAMINES—terfenadine, hydroxyzine, mizolastine 8. ANTIHYPERTENSIVES—ketanserin 9. ANTIMALARIALS—artemether with lumefantrine, chloroquine, halofantrine, hydroxychloroquine, mefloquine, quinine 10. ANTIPROTOZOALS—pentamidine isethionate 11. ANTIPSYCHOTICS—atypicals, phenothiazines, pimozide 12. ANTIVIRALS—boceprevir, rilpivirine, telaprevir 13. BETA-BLOCKERS—sotalol 14. Bronchodilators—parenteral bronchodilators 15. CNS STIMULANTS—atomoxetine 16. RANOLAZINE			
VEMURAFENIB	**ANTIBIOTICS**			
VEMURAFENIB	MACROLIDES—TELITHROMYCIN	Possible increased levels of vemurafenib	CYP3A4 inhibition	Manufacturers caution against concurrent use
VEMURAFENIB	RIFAMPICIN, RIFABUTIN	Possible reduced levels of vemurafenib	CYP3A4 induction	Manufacturer recommends avoid concurrent use

(*Continued*)

Primary Drug	Secondary Drug	Effect	Mechanism	Precautions
CYTOTOXICS				
VEMURAFENIB	**ANTICANCER AND IMMUNOMODULATING DRUGS**			
VEMURAFENIB	EVEROLIMUS	Possible increased levels of P-glycoprotein substrates	Vemurafenib inhibits P-glycoprotein	Clinical significance unknown
VEMURAFENIB	IPILIMUMAB	Increased risk of raised liver function tests	Unknown	Avoid concurrent use
VEMURAFENIB	METHOTREXATE, MITOXANTRONE	Possible increased levels of BCRP substrates	Vemurafenib inhibits BCRP	Clinical significance unknown
VEMURAFENIB	ANTICOAGULANTS—WARFARIN	Possible increased warfarin levels	CYP2C9 inhibition	Monitor INR closely
VEMURAFENIB	**ANTIDEPRESSANTS**			
VEMURAFENIB	NEFAZODONE	Possible increased levels of vemurafenib	CYP3A4 inhibition	Manufacturers caution against concurrent use
VEMURAFENIB	ST. JOHN'S WORT	Possible reduced levels of vemurafenib	CYP3A4 induction	Manufacturer recommends to avoid concurrent use
VEMURAFENIB	ANTIEPILEPTICS—CARBAMAZEPINE, PHENYTOIN	Possible reduced levels of vemurafenib	CYP3A4 induction	Manufacturer recommends to avoid concurrent use
VEMURAFENIB	ANTIFUNGALS—KETOCONAZOLE, ITRACONAZOLE, VORICONAZOLE, POSACONAZOLE	Possible increased levels of vemurafenib	CYP3A4 inhibition	Manufacturers caution against concurrent use
VEMURAFENIB	ANTIGOUTS—COLCHICINE	Possible increased levels of P-glycoprotein substrates	Vemurafenib inhibits P-glycoprotein	Be aware. Clinical significance unknown
VEMURAFENIB	ANTIHISTAMINES—FEXOFENADINE	Possible increased levels of P-glycoprotein substrates	Vemurafenib inhibits P-glycoprotein	Be aware. Clinical significance unknown
VEMURAFENIB	ANTIHYPERTENSIVES AND HEART FAILURE DRUGS—ALISKIREN	Possible increased levels of P-glycoprotein substrates	Vemurafenib inhibits P-glycoprotein	Be aware. Clinical significance unknown
VEMURAFENIB	ANTIVIRALS—ATAZANAVIR, RITONAVIR, SAQUINAVIR	Possible increased levels of vemurafenib	CYP3A4 inhibition	Manufacturers caution against concurrent use
VEMURAFENIB	CARDIAC GLYCOSIDES—DIGOXIN	Possible increased levels of P-glycoprotein substrates	Vemurafenib inhibits P-glycoprotein	Clinical significance unknown

(Continued)

ANTICANCER AND IMMUNOMODULATING DRUGS CYTOTOXICS Vinca alkaloids

Primary Drug	Secondary Drug	Effect	Mechanism	Precautions
CYTOTOXICS				
VEMURAFENIB	LIPID-LOWERING DRUGS—ROSUVASTATIN	Possible increased levels of BCRP substrates	Vemurafenib inhibits BCRP	Clinical significance unknown
VEMURAFENIB	ESTROGENS—ORAL CONTRACEPTION	Possible reduced efficacy of contraception	CYP3A4 induction	Alternative contraception may be required
VINCA ALKALOIDS				
VINCA ALKALOIDS	**ANTIBIOTICS**			
VINCA ALKALOIDS	ISONIAZID	Increased vincristine neurotoxicity	Uncertain	Monitor closely with concurrent use
VINCA ALKALOIDS	MACROLIDES—CLARITHROMYCIN, ERYTHROMYCIN	↑ Adverse effects of vinblastine and vincristine	Inhibition of CYP3A4-mediated metabolism. Also inhibition of Pgp efflux of vinblastine	Monitor FBC. Watch for early features of toxicity (pain, numbness, tingling in the fingers and toes, jaw pain, abdominal pain, constipation, ileus). Consider selecting an alternative drug
VINCA ALKALOIDS	PENICILLINS—PIPERACILLIN AND TAZOBACTAM	Single case of autonomic neuropathy and cholestasis	Uncertain	Clinical significance uncertain Be aware of possible interaction
VINBLASTINE, VINCRISTINE	RIFAMPICIN	↓ Plasma concentrations of vinblastine and vincristine, with risk of inadequate therapeutic response. Reports of ↓ AUC by 40% and elimination half-life by 35%, and ↑ clearance by 63%, in patients with brain tumors taking vincristine, which could lead to dangerously inadequate therapeutic responses	Due to induction of CYP3A4-mediated metabolism	Monitor for clinical efficacy, and ↑ dose of vinblastine and vincristine as clinically indicated; in the latter case, monitor clinically and radiologically for clinical efficacy in patients with brain tumors and ↑ dose to obtain desired response
VINFLUNINE, VINORELBINE	RIFAMPICIN	Possible reduced levels of vinflunine and vinorelbine Animal data only	Uncertain, CYP3A4 induction may play a role	Caution with concurrent use

(*Continued*)

Primary Drug	Secondary Drug	Effect	Mechanism	Precautions
CYTOTOXICS				
VINCA ALKALOIDS	**ANTICANCER AND OTHER IMMUNOMODULATING DRUGS**			
VINCA ALKALOIDS	AZATHIOPRINE	↑ Risk of myelosuppression and immunosuppression. Deaths have occurred following profound myelosuppression and severe sepsis	Additive myelotoxic effects. Azathioprine is metabolized to 6-mercaptopurine in vivo, which results in additive myelosuppression, immunosuppression, and hepatotoxicity	Avoid coadministration
VINCRISTINE	CICLOSPORIN	High doses of ciclosporin (7.5–10 mg/kg/day intravenously) tend to ↑ plasma concentrations of vincristine and ↑ risk of neurotoxicity and musculoskeletal pain	Due to a combination, to varying degrees, of inhibition of CYP3A4 metabolism and Pgp inhibition. Vinblastine and vincristine are known substrates of Pgp	Monitor for neurotoxicity and myelosuppression. The dose-limiting effect of all is myelosuppression. Monitor blood counts and clinically watch for and ask patients to report infections
VINORELBINE	CISPLATIN	↑ Incidence of grade III and grade IV granulocytopenia	Additive myelosuppressive effects	Monitor blood counts at least weekly and advise patients to report symptoms such as sore throat and fever
VINBLASTINE, VINCRISTINE	CORTICOSTEROIDS—DEXAMETHASONE	↓ Plasma concentrations of vinblastine and vincristine, with risk of inadequate therapeutic response. Reports of ↓ AUC by 40% and elimination half-life by 35%, and ↑ clearance by 63%, in patients with brain tumors taking vincristine, which could lead to dangerously inadequate therapeutic responses	Due to induction of CYP3A4-mediated metabolism	Monitor for clinical efficacy, and ↑ dose of vinblastine and vincristine as clinically indicated; in the latter case, monitor clinically and radiologically for clinical efficacy in patients with brain tumors and ↑ dose to obtain desired response

(Continued)

Primary Drug	Secondary Drug	Effect	Mechanism	Precautions
CYTOTOXICS				
VINCRISTINE	CRISANTASPASE	↑ Risk of neurotoxicity if concurrently administered or if crisantaspase is administered prior to vincristine	Uncertain but attributed by some to effects of asparaginase on the metabolism of vincristine	Administer vincristine prior to asparaginase
VINFLUNINE	DOCETAXEL	Reduced vinflunine levels in vitro	Unknown	Be aware. Clinical significance unknown
VINORELBINE	DOCETAXEL	Administration of docetaxel after vinorelbine ↑ plasma concentrations of vinorelbine, along with ↑ risk of neutropenia compared with giving docetaxel first	Docetaxel likely causes ↓ clearance of vinorelbine	Administer docetaxel first and follow with vinorelbine
VINFLUNINE	DOXORUBICIN	Increased risk of neutropenia Increased vinflunine levels with liposomal doxorubicin	Additive Uncertain	Caution with concurrent use
VINFLUNINE	ERLOTINIB	Increased bone marrow suppression	Unknown	Avoid concurrent use
VINORELBINE	GEFITINIB	Increased risk of neutropenia	Unknown	Avoid concurrent use
VINORELBINE	GEMCITABINE	Gemcitabine and vinorelbine levels both reduced. Amount of reduction may depend on sequence of administration	Unknown	Further study required to establish the amount of effect
VINCA ALKALOIDS	IMATINIB	↑ Adverse effects of vinblastine and vincristine	Inhibition of CYP3A4-mediated metabolism. Also inhibition of Pgp efflux of vinblastine	Monitor FBC. Watch for early features of toxicity (pain, numbness, tingling in the fingers and toes, jaw pain, abdominal pain, constipation, ileus). Consider selecting an alternative drug

(*Continued*)

Primary Drug	Secondary Drug	Effect	Mechanism	Precautions
CYTOTOXICS				
VINORELBINE	IRINOTECAN	Reduced levels of SN-38 (irinotecan metabolite) in vitro	Unknown	Be aware. Clinical significance uncertain
VINORELBINE	LAPATINIB	Reduced vinorelbine clearance	Possible CYP3A4 inhibition	Consider reduction in dosage of both drugs
VINBLASTINE, VINDESINE, VINORELBINE	MITOMYCIN	↑ Risk of abrupt onset of pulmonary toxicity in 3%–6% of patients, when two courses of these drugs are administered concurrently	Mechanism is uncertain; possible additive pulmonary toxic effects	Monitor clinically and with lung function tests for pulmonary toxicity. Advise patients to report immediately symptoms such as shortness of breath and wheezing
VINBLASTINE, VINCRISTINE	PACLITAXEL	↓ Therapeutic efficacy of paclitaxel	Antagonistic effects	Avoid coadministration
VINFLUNINE	PACLITAXEL	Reduced vinflunine levels in vitro	Unknown	Clinical significance unknown
VINCRISTINE	THALIDOMIDE	Possible increased risk of peripheral neuropathy	Additive	Manufacturer advises caution
VINORELBINE	VANDETANIB	Increased levels of toxicity (thromboembolic effects) when vandetanib, vinorelbine, and cisplation are combined	Unknown	Not suitable combination for chemotherapy
VINCA ALKALOIDS	**ANTIDEPRESSANTS**			
VINBLASTINE, VINCRISTINE, VINFLUNINE	ST. JOHN'S WORT	↓ Plasma concentrations of vinblastine and vincristine, with risk of inadequate therapeutic response. Reports of ↓ AUC by 40% and elimination half-life by 35%, and ↑ clearance by 63%, in patients with brain tumors taking vincristine, which could lead to dangerously inadequate therapeutic responses	Due to induction of CYP3A4-mediated metabolism	Monitor for clinical efficacy, and ↑ dose of vinblastine and vincristine as clinically indicated; in the latter case, monitor clinically and radiologically for clinical efficacy in patients with brain tumors and ↑ dose to obtain desired response

(Continued)

Primary Drug	Secondary Drug	Effect	Mechanism	Precautions
CYTOTOXICS				
VINBLASTINE	TCAs	Possible ↑ plasma concentrations of vinblastine	Inhibition of CYP2D6-mediated metabolism of vinblastine. The clinical significance of this depends upon whether vinblastine's alternative pathways of metabolism are also inhibited by coadministered drugs	Warn patients to report ↑ side effects of vinblastine, and monitor blood count carefully
VINCA ALKALOIDS—VINBLASTINE, VINCRISTINE	ANTIEPILEPTICS—CARBAMAZEPINE, PHENOBARBITAL	↓ Plasma concentrations of vinblastine and vincristine, with risk of inadequate therapeutic response. Reports of ↓ AUC by 40% and elimination half-life by 35%, and ↑ clearance by 63%, in patients with brain tumors taking vincristine, which could lead to dangerously inadequate therapeutic responses	Due to induction of CYP3A4-mediated metabolism	Monitor for clinical efficacy, and ↑ dose of vinblastine and vincristine as clinically indicated; in the latter case, monitor clinically and radiologically for clinical efficacy in patients with brain tumors and ↑ dose to obtain desired response
VINCA ALKALOIDS	PHENYTOIN	↓ Levels of vinca alkaloids, with risk of therapeutic failure	Induction of hepatic metabolism	Monitor for ↓ clinical efficacy and ↑ dose as required
VINCA ALKALOIDS	ANTIFUNGALS—FLUCONAZOLE, ITRACONAZOLE, KETOCONAZOLE, VORICONAZOLE (POSSIBLY POSACONAZOLE)	↑ Adverse effects of vinblastine and vincristine	Inhibition of CYP3A4-mediated metabolism. Also inhibition of Pgp efflux of vinblastine	Monitor FBC. Watch for early features of toxicity (pain, numbness, tingling in the fingers and toes, jaw pain, abdominal pain, constipation, ileus). Consider selecting an alternative drug
VINCA ALKALOIDS	**ANTIVIRALS**			
VINCA ALKALOIDS—VINBLASTINE, VINCRISTINE	GANCICLOVIR, VALGANCICLOVIR	Possible increased ganciclovir toxicity	Additive effect on inhibition of rapidly dividing cell populations, e.g., bone marrow, tests, skin, GI mucosa	Monitor closely if concurrent use necessary

(*Continued*)

Primary Drug	Secondary Drug	Effect	Mechanism	Precautions
CYTOTOXICS				
VINCA ALKALOIDS	NNRTIs—EFAVIRENZ	↑ Adverse effects of vinblastine and vincristine	Inhibition of CYP3A4-mediated metabolism. Also inhibition of Pgp efflux of vinblastine	Monitor FBC. Watch for early features of toxicity (pain, numbness, tingling in the fingers and toes, jaw pain, abdominal pain, constipation, ileus). Consider selecting an alternative drug
VINCA ALKALOIDS	NRTIs—DIDANOSINE, STAVUDINE, ZIDOVUDINE	1. ↑ Risk of peripheral neuropathy particularly with didanosine and stavudine 2. ↑ Adverse effects when vincristine and possibly vinblastine are coadministered with zidovudine	Additive toxicity	Review for alternative treatment options, consider substitution of an alternative NRTI or antiretroviral. Use with caution. Monitor FBC and renal function closely. ↓ doses as necessary
VINBLASTINE VINCRISTINE	PROTEASE INHIBITORS	↑ Adverse effects of vinblastine and vincristine	Inhibition of CYP3A4-mediated metabolism. Also inhibition of Pgp efflux of vinblastine	Monitor FBC. Watch for early features of toxicity (pain, numbness, tingling in the fingers and toes, jaw pain, abdominal pain, constipation, ileus). Consider selecting an alternative drug
VINFLUNINE	RITONAVIR	Possible ↑ plasma concentrations of vinflunine	Uncertain	Avoid coadministration
VINCA ALKALOIDS	CALCIUM CHANNEL BLOCKERS	1. ↑ Risk of bone marrow depression, neurotoxicity, and ileus due to ↑ plasma concentrations of vinblastine when coadministered with diltiazem, nifedipine, or verapamil	1. Inhibition of CYP3A4-mediated metabolism of vinblastine and ↓ efflux of vinblastine due to inhibition of renal Pgp 2. ↓ Clearance, but exact mechanism is not known	1. Avoid concurrent use of CYP3A4 inhibitors and Pgp efflux inhibitors with vinblastine. Select an alternative drug of the same group with ↓ effects on enzyme inhibition and Pgp inhibition 2. Watch for symptoms/signs of toxicity

(Continued)

Primary Drug	Secondary Drug	Effect	Mechanism	Precautions
CYTOTOXICS				
		2. Verapamil ↑ vincristine levels; no cases of toxicity have been reported 3. ↑ Plasma concentrations of vinorelbine and ↑ risk of bone marrow and neurotoxicity when coadministered with diltiazem, nifedipine, or verapamil	3. Due to inhibition of CYP3A4-mediated metabolism of vinorelbine by these calcium channel blockers	3. Monitor for clinical efficacy and monitor FBCs and for neurotoxicity (pain, numbness, tingling in the fingers and toes, jaw pain, abdominal pain, constipation, ileus)
VINCRISTINE	COLONY-STIMULATING FACTORS—FILGRASTIM, SARGRAMOSTIM	A high incidence of severe atypical neuropathy (excruciating foot pain associated with marked motor weakness)	Synergistic neurotoxicity, which was related to the cumulative dose of vincristine and the number of doses given in cycle 1	A modification in administration of two doses given on days 1 and 8, instead of three doses given on days 1, 8, and 15, in the cycle has been suggested to minimize neurotoxicity
VINCA ALKALOIDS	GRAPEFRUIT JUICE	↑ Adverse effects of vinblastine and vincristine	Inhibition of CYP3A4-mediated metabolism. Also inhibition of Pgp efflux of vinblastine	Monitor FBC. Watch for early features of toxicity (pain, numbness, tingling in the fingers and toes, jaw pain, abdominal pain, constipation, ileus). Consider selecting an alternative drug
VINCA ALKALOIDS	H2 RECEPTOR BLOCKERS—CIMETIDINE	↑ Adverse effects of vinblastine and vincristine	Inhibition of CYP3A4-mediated metabolism. Also inhibition of Pgp efflux of vinblastine	Monitor FBC. Watch for early features of toxicity (pain, numbness, tingling in the fingers and toes, jaw pain, abdominal pain, constipation, ileus). Consider selecting an alternative drug
VORINOSTAT				
VORINOSTAT	PACLITAXEL	Slight increase in vorinostat levels	Uncertain	Further study needed

Primary Drug	Secondary Drug	Effect	Mechanism	Precautions
HORMONES AND HORMONE ANTAGONISTS				
AMINOGLUTETHIMIDE				
AMINOGLUTETHIMIDE	DEXAMETHASONE	Effects of dexamethasone reduced or abolished	Aminoglutethimide increases dexamethasone metabolism	Consider dose increase of dexamethsone Use hydrocortisone, which is not affected by aminoglutethimide
ANASTRAZOLE				
ANASTRAZOLE	ANTICOAGULANTS—WARFARIN	↑ Anticoagulant effect	Uncertain; possibly inhibition of hepatic enzymes. Anastrazole is a known inhibitor of CYP1A2, CYP2C9, and CYP3A4	Monitor INR at least weekly until stable at initiation and discontinuation of concurrent therapy
ANASTRAZOLE	ANTIDIABETIC DRUGS—REPAGLINIDE	Risk of hypoglycemia	Mechanism unknown	Watch for hypoglycemia Warn patients about hypoglycemia. ➢ ***For signs and symptoms of hypoglycemia, see Clinical Features of Some Adverse Drug Interactions, Hypoglycemia***
BICALUTAMIDE				
BICALUTAMIDE	ANTICANCER AND IMMUNOMODULATING DRUGS—CICLOSPORIN	Predicted increased ciclosporin levels	CYP3A4 inhibition	Monitor ciclosporin concentration closely
BICALUTAMIDE	ANTICOAGULANTS—WARFARIN	↑ Plasma concentrations of warfarin	Bicalutamide displaces warfarin from protein-binding sites	Monitor INR at least weekly until stable at initiation and discontinuation of concurrent therapy
FLUTAMIDE				
FLUTAMIDE	ANTICOAGULANTS—WARFARIN	↑ Anticoagulant effect	Uncertain; possibly inhibition of hepatic enzymes	Monitor INR at least weekly until stable at initiation and discontinuation of concurrent therapy

(*Continued*)

ANTICANCER AND IMMUNOMODULATING DRUGS HORMONES AND HORMONE ANTAGONISTS 525

Primary Drug	Secondary Drug	Effect	Mechanism	Precautions
HORMONES AND HORMONE ANTAGONISTS				
LANREOTIDE				
LANREOTIDE	ANTICANCER AND IMMUNOMODULATING DRUGS—CICLOSPORIN	↓ Plasma concentrations of ciclosporin and risk of transplant rejection	Lanreotide possibly induces CYP3A4-mediated metabolism of ciclosporin	Avoid coadministration if possible; if not, monitor ciclosporin levels closely
LANREOTIDE	ANTIDIABETIC DRUGS	Likely to alter hypoglycemic agent requirements	Octreotide and lanreotide suppress pancreatic insulin and counterregulatory hormones (glucagon, growth hormone), and delay or ↓ absorption of glucose from the intestine	Essential to monitor blood sugar at least twice a week after initiating concurrent treatment until blood sugar levels are stable. Advise self-monitoring, and warn patients about hypoglycemia. ➢ ***For signs and symptoms of hypoglycemia, see Clinical Features of Some Adverse Drug Interactions, Hypoglycemia***
LETROZOLE				
LETROZOLE	TAMOXIFEN	↓ Plasma concentrations of letrozole (by approximately 40%) and ↓ efficacy of letrozole	Attributed to induction of enzymes metabolizing letrozole by tamoxifen	Avoid concurrent use outside clinical trials
MEGESTROL				
MEGESTROL	ANTIARRHYTHMICS—DOFETILIDE	↑ Dofetilide levels with risk of ↑ QT prolongation	Megestrol reduces renal excretion of dofetilide	Avoid coadministration
PASIREOTIDE				
PASIREOTIDE	BETA-BLOCKERS	Risk of bradycardia	Additive effect	Monitor PR closely until stable
PASIREOTIDE	CALCIUM CHANNEL BLOCKERS—VERAPAMIL	1. Risk of bradycardia 2. Increased pasireotide levels	1. Additive effect 2. Inhibition of Pgp	1. Monitor PR closely until stable 2. Warn patient to report adverse effects of pasireotide

(*Continued*)

Primary Drug	Secondary Drug	Effect	Mechanism	Precautions
HORMONES AND HORMONE ANTAGONISTS				
SOMATOSTATIN ANALOGUES				
SOMATOSTATIN ANALOGUES—LANREOTIDE, OCTREOTIDE, PASIREOTIDE	ANTICANCER AND IMMUNOMODULATING DRUGS—CICLOSPORIN	↓ Plasma concentrations of ciclosporin and risk of transplant rejection	Octreotide is a strong inducer of CYP3A4-mediated metabolism of ciclosporin	Avoid coadministration if possible; if not, monitor ciclosporin levels closely
SOMATOSTATIN ANALOGUES	**ANTIDIABETIC DRUGS**			
SOMATOSTATIN ANALOGUES—OCTREOTIDE	ANTIDIABETIC DRUGS	Likely to alter hypoglycemic agent requirements	Octreotide and lanreotide suppress pancreatic insulin and counterregulatory hormones (glucagon, growth hormone), and delay or ↓ absorption of glucose from the intestine	Essential to monitor blood sugar at least twice a week after initiating concurrent treatment until blood sugar levels are stable. Advice self-monitoring. Warn patients regarding hypoglycemia. ➢ ***For signs and symptoms of hypoglycemia, see Clinical Features of Some Adverse Drug Interactions, Hypoglycemia***
OCTREOTIDE, LANTREOTIDE	THIAZOLIDINEDIONES	Requirements of antidiabetic agents possibly reduced	Decreased insulin secretion	Consider lowering dose of thiazolidinedione
SOMATOSTATIN ANALOGUES—OCTREOTIDE	ANTI-PARKINSON'S DRUGS—BROMOCRIPTINE	↑ Bromocriptine levels	Uncertain	Be aware
TAMOXIFEN				
TAMOXIFEN	ANTIARRHYTHMIAS—QUINIDINE	Theoretcial risk of reduced efficacy of tamoxifen with increased recurrence of breast cancer	↓ CYP2D6-mediated metabolism of tamoxifen to its active metabolite	Avoid coadministration
TAMOXIFEN	ANTIBIOTICS—RIFAMPICIN	↓ Plasma concentrations of tamoxifen and risk of inadequate therapeutic response	Due to induction of metabolism of tamoxifen by the CYP3A isoenzymes by rifampicin	Avoid concurrent use if possible. Otherwise, monitor for clinical efficacy of tamoxifen by ↑ dose of tamoxifen

(Continued)

ANTICANCER AND IMMUNOMODULATING DRUGS HORMONES AND HORMONE ANTAGONISTS 527

Primary Drug	Secondary Drug	Effect	Mechanism	Precautions
HORMONES AND HORMONE ANTAGONISTS				
TAMOXIFEN	ANTICANCER AND IMMUNOMODULATING DRUGS			
TAMOXIFEN	AZATHIOPRINE	↑ Risk of myelosuppression and immunosuppression. Deaths have occurred following profound myelosuppression and severe sepsis	Additive myelotoxic effects. Azathioprine is metabolized to 6-mercaptopurine in vivo, which results in additive myelosuppression, immunosuppression, and hepatotoxicity	Avoid coadministration
TAMOXIFEN	CICLOSPORIN	↑ Plasma concentrations of ciclosporin, with risk of toxic effects	Competitive inhibition of CYP3A4-mediated metabolism and Pgp transport of these drugs	Watch for toxic effects of ciclosporin
TAMOXIFEN	CORTICOSTEROIDS	↓ Plasma concentrations of tamoxifen and risk of inadequate therapeutic response	Due to induction of metabolism of tamoxifen by the CYP3A isoenzymes by dexamethasone	Avoid concurrent use if possible. Otherwise, monitor for clinical efficacy of tamoxifen by ↑ dose of tamoxifen
TAMOXIFEN	FLUOROURACIL	Increased risk of thrombosis when used in chemotherapy regimens	Additive	Consider prophylactic anticoagulation
TAMOXIFEN	LETROZOLE	↓ Plasma concentrations of letrozole (by approximately 40%) and ↓ efficacy of letrozole	Attributed to induction of enzymes metabolizing letrozole by tamoxifen	Avoid concurrent use outside clinical trials
TAMOXIFEN	METHOTREXATE	Increased risk of thrombosis when used in chemotherapy regimens	Additive	Consider prophylactic anticoagulation
TAMOXIFEN	MITOMYCIN	↑ Incidence of anemia and thrombocytopenia and risk of hemolytic–uremic syndrome	Mitomycin causes subclinical endothelial damage in addition to the thrombotic effect on platelets caused by tamoxifen, which leads to the hemolytic-uremic syndrome	Monitor renal function at least twice weekly during concurrent therapy and clinically watch for bleeding episodes, e.g., nose bleeds, bleeding from gums, skin bruising

(*Continued*)

Primary Drug	Secondary Drug	Effect	Mechanism	Precautions
HORMONES AND HORMONE ANTAGONISTS				
TAMOXIFEN	ANTICOAGULANTS—WARFARIN	↑ Anticoagulant effect	Uncertain; possibly inhibition of hepatic enzymes. Tamoxifen inhibits CYP3A4	Monitor INR at least weekly until stable at initiation and discontinuation of concurrent therapy
TAMOXIFEN	ANTIDEPRESSANTS—ST. JOHN'S WORT	↓ Plasma concentrations of tamoxifen and risk of inadequate therapeutic response	Due to induction of metabolism of tamoxifen by the CYP3A isoenzymes by St. John's wort	Avoid concurrent use
TAMOXIFEN	ANTIEPILEPTICS—CARBAMAZEPINE, PHENOBARBITAL	↓ Plasma concentrations of tamoxifen and risk of inadequate therapeutic response	Due to induction of metabolism of tamoxifen by the CYP3A isoenzymes by phenytoin	Avoid concurrent use if possible. Otherwise, monitor for clinical efficacy of tamoxifen by ↑ dose of tamoxifen
TAMOXIFEN	PHENYTOIN	↓ Levels of these drugs, with risk of therapeutic failure	Induction of hepatic metabolism	Avoid coadministration of phenytoin with tamoxifen
TAMOXIFEN	ANTIVIRALS—RITONAVIR	Possible ↓ plasma levels of active metabolite, so reducing therapeutic efficacy	Inhibition of metabolism via CYP2D6	Avoid coadministration
TAMOXIFEN	CNS STIMULANTS—MODAFINIL	May cause↑ plasma concentrations of these substrates if CYP2C9 is the predominant metabolic pathway and the alternative pathways are either genetically deficient or affected	Modafinil is a moderate inhibitor of CYP2C9	Be aware
TAMOXIFEN	H2-RECEPTOR BLOCKERS—CIMETIDINE	↓ Plasma concentrations of active metabolite endoxifen	Inhibition of metabolism via CYP2D6 and CYP3A4 by cimetidine	Poorer outcomes for treatment of breast cancer not proven but increasing evidence to avoid combination. Use alternatives, e.g., famotidine or nizatidine
TAMOXIFEN	TIBOLONE	↓ Efficacy of tamoxifen with risk of recurrence of breast cancer	Tibolone has estrogenic effects, which oppose the effects of tamoxifen	Avoid coadministration

(*Continued*)

Primary Drug	Secondary Drug	Effect	Mechanism	Precautions
HORMONES AND HORMONE ANTAGONISTS				
TOREMIFENE				
TOREMIFENE	ANTIBIOTICS—MACROLIDES	↑ Plasma concentrations of toremifene with clarithromycin and erythromycin	Due to inhibition of metabolism of toremifene by the CYP3A4 isoenzymes by clarithromycin	Clinical relevance is uncertain. Necessary to monitor for clinical toxicities
TOREMIFENE	ANTICOAGULANTS—WARFARIN	↑ Anticoagulant effect	Uncertain; possibly inhibition of hepatic enzymes	Monitor INR at least weekly until stable at initiation and discontinuation of concurrent therapy
TOREMIFENE	ANTIEPILEPTICS—BARBITURATES, CARBAMAZEPINE	↓ Plasma concentrations of toremifene	Due to induction of metabolism of toremifene	Watch for poor response to toremifene
TOREMIFENE	PHENYTOIN	↓ Levels of toremifene, with risk of therapeutic failure	Induction of hepatic metabolism	Monitor for ↓ clinical efficacy and ↑ their dose as required
TOREMIFENE	ANTIFUNGALS—AZOLES	↑ Plasma concentrations of toremifene	Due to inhibition of metabolism of toremifene by the CYP3A4 isoenzymes by ketoconazole	Clinical relevance is uncertain. Necessary to monitor for clinical toxicities
TOREMIFENE	**ANTIVIRALS**			
TOREMIFENE	NNRTIs—EFAVIRENZ	↑ Plasma concentrations of toremifene	Due to inhibition of metabolism of toremifene by the CYP3A4 isoenzymes by efavirenz	Clinical relevance is uncertain. Necessary to monitor for clinical toxicities
TOREMIFENE	PROTEASE INHIBITORS—RITONAVIR	↑ Plasma concentrations of toremifene	Due to inhibition of metabolism of toremifene by the CYP3A4 isoenzymes by ritonavir	Clinical relevance is uncertain. Necessary to monitor for clinical toxicities
TOREMIFENE	CALCIUM CHANNEL BLOCKERS	↑ Plasma concentrations of toremifene when coadministered with diltiazem, nifedipine, or verapamil	Due to inhibition of CYP3A4-mediated metabolism of toremifene	Clinical relevance is uncertain. Necessary to monitor for clinical toxicities

(*Continued*)

Primary Drug	Secondary Drug	Effect	Mechanism	Precautions
HORMONES AND HORMONE ANTAGONISTS				
TOREMIFENE	DIURETICS—THIAZIDES	Risk of hypercalcemia	Additive effect	Monitor calcium levels closely. Warn patients about the symptoms of hypercalcemia
TOREMIFENE	GRAPEFRUIT JUICE	↑ Plasma concentrations of toremifene	Inhibition of CYP3A4-mediated metabolism of toremifene	Clinical relevance is uncertain. Necessary to monitor for clinical toxicities
TOREMIFENE	H2 RECEPTOR BLOCKERS—CIMETIDINE	↑ Plasma concentrations of toremifene	Due to inhibition of metabolism of toremifene by the CYP3A4 isoenzymes by cimetidine	Clinical relevance is uncertain. Necessary to monitor for clinical toxicities

Primary Drug	Secondary Drug	Effect	Mechanism	Precautions
OTHER IMMUNOMODULATING DRUGS				
ALL	VACCINES—LIVE	Risk of contracting disease from the vaccine	↓ Immunity	Avoid live vaccines for at least 3 months after completing immunomodulating therapy
ABATACEPT				
ABATACEPT	ANAKINRA	Insufficient information about safety	Unknown	Manufacturer recommends to avoid concurrent use
ABATACEPT	ADALIMUMAB CERTOLIZUMAB PEGOL ETANERCEPT GOLIMUMAB INFLIXIMAB	Increased risk of serious infection	Additive	Avoid concurrent use
ACITRETIN ➢ *Other Immunomodulating Drugs, Retinoids below*				
ADALIMUMAB				
ADALIMUMAB	**ANTICANCER AND OTHER IMMUNOMODULATING DRUGS**			
ADALIMUMAB	ANAKINRA	↑ Risk of bone marrow suppression	Additive effect	Avoid coadministration
ADALIMUMAB	ABATACEPT	Increased risk of serious infection	Additive	Avoid concurrent use

(Continued)

Primary Drug	Secondary Drug	Effect	Mechanism	Precautions
OTHER IMMUNOMODULATING DRUGS				
ADALIMUMAB	AZATHIOPRINE	Cases of hepatosplenic T-cell lymphoma reported in adolescents and young adults	Unknown	Causal relationship unclear
ADALIMUMAB	CICLOSPORIN	Possible reduced levels of ciclosporin	Reversal of cytochrome P450 suppression by adalimumab. Ciclosporin has a narrow therapeutic index	Monitor closely, dose adjustment may be needed
ADALIMUMAB	MERCAPTOPURINE	Cases of hepatosplenic T-cell lymphoma reported in adolescents and young adults	Unknown	Causal relationship unclear
ADALIMUMAB	METHOTREXATE	Increases clearance of adalimumab, reduces antibody formation, and increases elevation of liver enzymes	Unknown	Increase monitoring of liver function tests
ADALIMUMAB	ANTICOAGULANTS—WARFARIN	Possible reduced levels of warfarin	Reversal of cytochrome P450 suppression by adalimumab. Warfarin has a narrow therapeutic index	Monitor closely, dose adjustment may be needed
ADALIMUMAB	ANTIEPILEPTICS—PHENYTOIN	Possible reduced levels of phenytoin	Reversal of cytochrome P450 suppression by adalimumab. Phenytoin has a narrow therapeutic index	Monitor closely, dose adjustment may be needed
ADALIMUMAB	BRONCHODILATORS—THEOPHYLLINE	Possible reduced levels of theophylline	Reversal of cytochrome P450 suppression by adalimumab. Theophylline has a narrow therapeutic index	Monitor closely, dose adjustment may be needed
ALDESLEUKIN ➢ *Other Immunomodulating Drugs, Interleukin-2, below*				
AMINOSALICYLATES				
AMINOSALICYLATES—SULFASALAZINE	ANTIBIOTICS—AMPICILLIN RIFAMPICIN	Reduced colonic release of sulfasalazine	Antibacterials reduce anaerobic bacteria in gut, which are responsible for conversion of sulfasalazine to active metabolite	Clinical significance uncertain

(Continued)

Primary Drug	Secondary Drug	Effect	Mechanism	Precautions
OTHER IMMUNOMODULATING DRUGS				
AMINOSALICYLATES	**ANTICANCER AND IMMUNOMODULATING DRUGS**			
AMINOSALICYLATES	AZATHIOPRINE	↑ Blood levels of azathioprine and ↑ risk of side effects	Due to inhibition of metabolism of purines by these aminosalicylates	Monitor FBC closely
AMINOSALICYLATES	MERCAPTOPURINE	↑ Risk of bone marrow suppression	Additive effect	Monitor FBC closely
AMINOSALICYLATES	METHOTREXATE	↑ Risk of hepatotoxicity with sulfasalazine	Additive hepatotoxic effects. Sulfasalazine competes with methotrexate for renal elimination	Monitor closely for symptoms of liver failure. Check LFTs at beginning of treatment and then weekly until stable, and repeat if there is clinical suspicion of liver disease
AMINOSALICYLATES—SULFASALAZINE	PONATINIB	Predicted increased in levels of these BCRP substrates	BCRP inhibition	Be aware
SALICYLATES—TOPICAL	PORFIMER	↑ Risk of photosensitivity reactions when porfimer is coadministered with hydrochlorothiazide	Attributed to additive effects	Avoid exposure of skin and eyes to direct sunlight for 30 days after porfimer therapy
AMINOSALICYLATES	ANTIGOUT DRUGS—PROBENECID	Aminosalicylate levels ↑ by probenecid	Probenecid competes with aminosalicylate for active renal excretion	Watch for early features of toxicity of aminosalicylate. Consider ↓ dose of aminosalicylate
AMINOSALICYLATES—BALSALAZIDE, SULFASALAZINE	CARDIAC GLYCOSIDES—DIGOXIN	Sulfasalazine may ↓ digoxin levels. The manufacturers of balsalazide also warn against the possibility of this interaction despite a lack of case reports	Uncertain at present	Watch for poor response to digoxin; check levels if there are signs of ↓ effect
AMINOSALICYLATES—SULFASALAZINE	FOLIC ACID	Possible reduced folic acid absorption	Sulfasalazine interferes with folic acid absorption	Monitor with regular FBC

(Continued)

Primary Drug	Secondary Drug	Effect	Mechanism	Precautions
OTHER IMMUNOMODULATING DRUGS				
ANAKINRA				
ANAKINRA	**ANTICANCER AND OTHER IMMUNOMODULATING DRUGS**			
ANAKINRA	ABATACEPT	Insufficent information about safety	Unknown	Manufacturer recommends avoiding concurrent use
ANAKINRA	ADALIMUMAB, ETANERCEPT, INFLIXIMAB	↑ Risk of bone marrow suppression	Additive effect	Avoid coadministration
ANAKINRA	CERTOLIZUMAB PEGOL	Increased risk of serious infection	Additive	Avoid concurrent use
ANAKINRA	CICLOSPORIN	Possible reduced levels of ciclosporin	Reversal of cytochrome P450 suppression by anakinra. Ciclosporin has a narrow therapeutic index	Monitor closely, dose adjustment may be needed
ANAKINRA	GOLIMUMAB	Increased risk of serious infection	Additive	Avoid concurrent use
ANAKINRA	ANTICOAGULANTS—WARFARIN	Possible reduced levels of warfarin	Reversal of cytochrome P450 suppression by anakinra. Warfarin has a narrow therapeutic index	Monitor closely, dose adjustment may be needed
ANAKINRA	ANTIEPILEPTICS—PHENYTOIN	Possible reduced levels of phenytoin	Reversal of cytochrome P450 suppression by anakinra. Phenytoin has a narrow therapeutic index	Monitor closely, dose adjustment may be needed
ANAKINRA	BRONCHODILATORS—THEOPHYLLINE	Possible reduced levels of theophylline	Reversal of cytochrome P450 suppression by anakinra. Theophylline has a narrow therapeutic index	Monitor closely, dose adjustment may be needed
AZATHIOPRINE/MERCAPTOPURINE				
AZATHIOPRINE	ANTIBIOTICS—CO-TRIMOXAZOLE	↑ Risk of leukopenia	Additive effects, as co-trimoxazole inhibits white cell production	Caution. ➢***For signs and symptoms of leukopenia, see Clinical Features of Some Adverse Drug Interactions, Immunosuppression and blood dyscrasias***

(Continued)

Primary Drug	Secondary Drug	Effect	Mechanism	Precautions
OTHER IMMUNOMODULATING DRUGS				
AZATHIOPRINE	**ANTICANCER AND IMMUNOMODULATING DRUGS**			
AZATHIOPRINE	**CYTOTOXICS**			
AZATHIOPRINE	ADALIMUMAB	Cases of hepatosplenic T-cell lymphoma reported in adolescents and young adults	Unknown	Causal relationship unclear
AZATHIOPRINE	AMINOSALICYLATES	↑ Blood levels of azathioprine and ↑ risk of side effects	Due to inhibition of metabolism of purines by these aminosalicylates	Monitor FBC closely
AZATHIOPRINE	CHLORAMBUCIL, CISPLATIN, CYCLOPHOSPHAMIDE, CYTARABINE, DACTINOMYCIN (ACTINOMYCIN D), DAUNORUBICIN, DOCETAXEL, DOXORUBICIN, ETOPOSIDE, FLUOROURACIL, MELPHALAN, MERCAPTOPURINE, MITOXANTRONE, VINCA ALKALOIDS	↑ Risk of myelosuppression and immunosuppression. Deaths have occurred following profound myelosuppression and severe sepsis	Additive myelotoxic effects. Azathioprine is metabolized to 6-mercaptopurine in vivo, which results in additive myelosuppression, immunosuppression, and hepatotoxicity	Avoid coadministration
AZATHIOPRINE	INFLIXIMAB	Increase in azathioprine metabolites Hepatosplenic T-cell lymphoma reported in adolescents and young adults	Unknown	Increase in metabolites associated with good tolerance and favorable response to inflixmab Causal relationship unclear

(*Continued*)

Primary Drug	Secondary Drug	Effect	Mechanism	Precautions
OTHER IMMUNOMODULATING DRUGS				
AZATHIOPRINE	LEFLUNOMIDE	↑ Risk of serious infections (sepsis) and of opportunistic infections (*Pneumocystis jiroveci* pneumonia, tuberculosis, aspergillosis)	Additive immunosuppression	Monitor platelets, white bloods cell, hemoglobin, and hematocrit at baseline and regularly—weekly, during concomitant therapy. With evidence of bone marrow suppression, discontinue leflunomide and administer colestyramine or charcoal to ↑ elimination of leflunomide. ➢ ***For signs and symptoms of immunosuppression, see Clinical Features of Some Adverse Drug Interactions, Immunosuppression and Blood Dyscrasias***
AZATHIOPRINE	METHOTREXATE	↑ Risk of hepatotoxicity	Additive hepatotoxic effects	Monitor closely for symptoms of liver failure, e.g., flu-like symptoms, abdominal pain, dark urine, pruritus, jaundice, ascites, and weight gain. Do LFTs at the beginning of treatment and weekly until stable, and repeat if there is clinical suspicion of liver disease
AZATHIOPRINE	MYCOPHENOLATE	Increased risk of bone marrow suppression	Additive, both are purine inhibitors	Avoid concurrent use
AZATHIOPRINE	NATALIZUMAB	↑ Risk of myelosuppression and immunosuppression. Deaths have occurred following profound myelosuppression and severe sepsis	Additive myelotoxic effects. Azathioprine is metabolized to 6-mercaptopurine in vivo, which results in additive myelosuppression, immunosuppression, and hepatotoxicity	Avoid coadministration

(*Continued*)

Primary Drug	Secondary Drug	Effect	Mechanism	Precautions
OTHER IMMUNOMODULATING DRUGS				
AZATHIOPRINE	TAMOXIFEN	↑ Risk of myelosuppression and immunosuppression. Deaths have occurred following profound myelosuppression and severe sepsis	Additive myelotoxic effects. Azathioprine is metabolized to 6-mercaptopurine in vivo, which results in additive myelosuppression, immunosuppression, and hepatotoxicity	Avoid coadministration
AZATHIOPRINE	TOFACITINIB	Increased risk of immunosuppression	Additive	Monitor closely
AZATHIOPRINE	ANTICOAGULANTS—WARFARIN	Possible ↓ anticoagulant effect	Induction of metabolism of warfarin	Monitor INR closely
AZATHIOPRINE	**ANTIGOUT DRUGS**			
AZATHIOPRINE	ALLOPURINOL	↑ Mercaptopurine levels, with risk of toxicity (e.g., myelosuppression, pancreatitis)	Azathioprine is metabolized to mercaptopurine. Allopurinol inhibits hepatic metabolism of mercaptopurine	↓ Doses of azathioprine and mercaptopurine to one-quarter of usual dose and monitor FBC, LFTs, and amylase carefully
AZATHIOPRINE	FEBUXOSTAT	May increase azathioprine levels	Inhibition of xanthine oxidase	Avoid concurrent use If necessary, consider dose reduction and monitor closely
AZATHIOPRINE	ANTIHYPERTENSIVES AND HEART FAILURE DRUGS—ACE INHIBITORS	Risk of anemia with captopril and enalapril, and leukopenia with captopril	Exact mechanism is uncertain. Azathioprine-induced impairment of hematopoiesis and ACE inhibitor induced ↓ in erythropoietin may cause additive effects. Enalapril has been used to treat postrenal transplant erythrocytosis	Monitor blood counts regularly
AZATHIOPRINE	ANTIVIRALS—LAMIVUDINE	1. ↑ Adverse effects with lamivudine 2. Single case of pancreatitis	1. Unclear 2. Unclear	1. Monitor closely 2. Clinical significance uncertain

(*Continued*)

Primary Drug	Secondary Drug	Effect	Mechanism	Precautions
OTHER IMMUNOMODULATING DRUGS				
AZATHIOPRINE	VACCINES	↓ Effectiveness of vaccines. ↑ risk of adverse/toxic effects of live vaccines (e.g., measles, mumps, rubella, oral polio, BCG, yellow fever, varicella, TY21a typhoid), and vaccinal infections may develop	Disseminated infection due to enhanced replication of vaccine virus in the presence of diminished immunocompetence	Do not vaccinate when patients are on immunosuppressants. Vaccination should be deferred for at least 3 months after discontinuing immunosuppressants/myelosuppressants. If an individual has been recently vaccinated, do not initiate therapy for at least 2 weeks after vaccination
AZATHIOPRINE	ELTROMBOPAG	May result in higher than desired platelet counts in patients with ITP	Additive	Monitor closely
AZATHIOPRINE	ROMIPLOSTIM	May result in higher than desired platelet counts in patients with ITP	Additive	Monitor closely
BALSALAZIDE ➢ *Other Immunomodulating Drugs, Aminosalicylates, above*				
BASILIXIMAB				
BASILIXIMAB	**ANTICANCER AND IMMUNOMODULATING DRUGS**			
BASILIXIMAB	CICLOSPORIN	Ciclosporin levels and adverse effects may be altered	Unknown	Monitor closely
BASILIXIMAB	TACROLIMUS	Possible increased tacrolimus levels	Unknown	Tacrolimus dose may need adjusting more than normal
BEVACIZUMAB				
BEVACIZUMAB	ANTICOAGULANTS	Theoretical risk of increased bleeding, limited evidence suggests this might not be the case	Additive, bevacizumab associated with increased risk of hemorrhage	Monitor concurrent use

(Continued)

Primary Drug	Secondary Drug	Effect	Mechanism	Precautions
OTHER IMMUNOMODULATING DRUGS				
BEVACIZUMAB	**ANTICANCER AND IMMUNOMODULATING DRUGS**			
BEVACIZUMAB	DAUNORUBICIN, DOXORUBICIN, EPIRUBICIN, IDARUBICIN, VALRUBICIN	Possible increased risk of cardiac failure	Additive	Be aware of interaction
BEVACIZUMAB	PANITUMUMAB	Reduced panitumumab efficacy with increased toxicity, when given with chemotherapy regimes containing bevacizumab	Unknown	Manufacturer advises against this combination
BEVACIZUMAB	SORAFENIB	Lower maximum tolerated doses of bevacizumab and sorafenib, unexpected toxicity (hypertension, proteinuria, thrombocytopenia)	Unknown	Dose reduction required
BEVACIZUMAB	SUNITINIB	Possible increased risk of microangiopathic hemolytic anemia	Unknown	Monitor concurrent use
BRENTUXIMAB VEDOTIN				
BRENTUXIMAB VEDOTIN	ANTICANCER AND IMMUNOMODULATING DRUGS—BLEOMYCIN	Increased risk of pulmonary toxicity	Unknown	Avoid concomitant use
BRENTUXIMAB VEDOTIN	ANTIBIOTICS—RIFAMPICIN	Possible reduction in efficacy of brentuximab	CYP3A4 induction	Monitor concurrent use
BRENTUXIMAB VEDOTIN	ANTIFUNGALS—KETOCONAZOLE	Increased levels of monomethyl auristatin E (MMAE) from brentuximab vedotin, increased risk of neutropenia	CYP3A4 inhibition	Monitor FBC
CERTOLIZUMAB PEGOL				
CERTOLIZUMAB PEGOL	ABATACEPT	Increased risk of serious infection	Additive	Avoid concurrent use
CERTOLIZUMAB PEGOL	ANAKINRA	Increased risk of serious infection	Additive	Avoid concurrent use

(Continued)

Primary Drug	Secondary Drug	Effect	Mechanism	Precautions
OTHER IMMUNOMODULATING DRUGS				
CICLOSPORIN				
CICLOSPORIN	ANALGESICS—NSAIDs	1. ↑ Risk of renal failure with NSAIDs 2. Diclofenac levels ↑ by ciclosporin 3. Rofecoxib ↓ plasma concentrations of ciclosporin, with risk of transplant rejection	1. Additive effect; both can cause renal insufficiency; ciclosporin may cause direct renal toxicity-acute tubular necrosis 2. Uncertain; possibly due to ↑ bioavailability 3. Rofecoxib is a mild inducer of CYP3A4 and not a substrate of CYP3A4	1. Monitor renal function closely 2. Halve the dose of diclofenac 3. Be aware. May not be clinically significant
CICLOSPORIN	**ANTIARRHYTHMICS**			
CICLOSPORIN	AMIODARONE	Ciclosporin levels may be ↑ by amiodarone; but there is a risk of nephrotoxicity	Uncertain; ciclosporin is metabolized by CYP3A4, which is markedly inhibited by amiodarone. Amiodarone also interferes with the renal elimination of ciclosporin and inhibits intestinal Pgp, which may ↑ bioavailability of ciclosporin	Monitor renal function closely; consider ↓ dose of ciclosporin when coadministering amiodarone
CICLOSPORIN	PROPAFENONE	Possible ↑ ciclosporin levels	Uncertain	Watch for signs of ciclosporin toxicity
CICLOSPORIN	**ANTIBIOTICS**			
CICLOSPORIN	AMINOGLYCOSIDES, COLISTIN	↑ Risk of nephrotoxicity	Additive nephrotoxic effects	Monitor renal function
CICLOSPORIN	CLINDAMYCIN	Two cases of reduced ciclosporin levels	Uncertain	Monitor closely
CICLOSPORIN	CO-TRIMOXAZOLE	Exacerbates hyperkalemia induced by ciclosporin	Additive effect	Monitor serum potassium levels during coadministration. ➢ ***For signs and symptoms of hyperkalemia, see Clinical Features of Some Adverse Drug Interactions, Hyperkalemia***
CICLOSPORIN	DAPTOMYCIN	Risk of myopathy	Additive effect	Avoid coadministration

(*Continued*)

Primary Drug	Secondary Drug	Effect	Mechanism	Precautions
OTHER IMMUNOMODULATING DRUGS				
CICLOSPORIN	FIDAXOMICIN	Increased fidaxomicin levels	P-glycoprotein inhibition	US manufacturer advises that no dose adjustment is necessary UK manufacturer advises to avoid concurrent use
CICLOSPORIN	MACROLIDES—CLARITHROMYCIN, ERYTHROMYCIN, TELITHROMYCIN	↑ Plasma concentrations of ciclosporin, with risk of nephrotoxicity, myelosuppression, neurotoxicity, excessive immunosuppression, with risk of infection and posttransplant lymphoproliferative disease	Inhibition of CYP3A4-mediated metabolism of ciclosporin; these inhibitors vary in potency. Clarithromycin and telithromycin are classified as potent inhibitors	Avoid coadministration with clarithromycin and telithromycin. Consider alternative antibiotics but need to monitor plasma ciclosporin levels to prevent toxicity
CICLOSPORIN	METRONIDAZOLE	Possible increased ciclosporin levels	Uncertain	General significance uncertain Be aware of interaction
CICLOSPORIN	**QUINOLONES**			
CICLOSPORIN	CIPROFLOXACIN	Ciprofloxacin may ↓ immunosuppressive effect (pharmacodynamic interaction)	Ciprofloxacin ↓ inhibitory effect of ciclosporin on IL-2 production, resulting in ↓ immunosuppressive effect	Avoid coadministration
CICLOSPORIN	NORFLOXACIN	↑ Plasma concentrations of ciclosporin, with risk of nephrotoxicity, myelosuppression, neurotoxicity, excessive immunosuppression, with risk of infection and posttransplant lymphoproliferative disease	Inhibition of CYP3A4-mediated metabolism of ciclosporin; these inhibitors vary in potency	Monitor plasma ciclosporin levels to prevent toxicity. Monitor renal function

(*Continued*)

ANTICANCER AND IMMUNOMODULATING DRUGS OTHER IMMUNOMODULATING DRUGS

Primary Drug	Secondary Drug	Effect	Mechanism	Precautions
OTHER IMMUNOMODULATING DRUGS				
CICLOSPORIN	QUINUPRISTIN/DALFOPRISTIN	↑ Plasma concentrations of immunosuppressants. ↑ risk of infections and toxic effects of ciclosporin	Due to inhibition of CYP3A4-mediated metabolism of ciclosporin	Monitor renal function prior to concurrent therapy, and blood count and ciclosporin levels during therapy. Warn patients to report symptoms (fever, sore throat) immediately
CICLOSPORIN	RIFAMYCINS	↓ Plasma concentrations of ciclosporin, with risk of transplant rejection	Due to induction of CYP3A4-mediated metabolism of ciclosporin by these drugs. The potency of induction varies	Monitor for signs of rejection of transplants. Monitor ciclosporin levels to ensure adequate therapeutic concentrations and ↑ dose when necessary
CICLOSPORIN	TETRACYCLINES—DOXYCYCLINE	↑ Levels of ciclosporin leading to risk of nephrotoxicity, hepatotoxicity, and possible neurotoxicity such as hallucinations, convulsions, and coma	The mechanism is not known, but doxycycline is thought to ↑ ciclosporin levels	Concomitant use in transplant patients should be well monitored, with frequent ciclosporin levels. In nontransplant patients, renal function should be monitored closely and patients warned about potential side effects such as back pain, flushing, and gastrointestinal upset. The dose of ciclosporin should be ↓ appropriately
CICLOSPORIN	VANCOMYCIN	Risk of renal toxicity	Additive effect	Monitor renal function closely
CICLOSPORIN	**ANTICANCER AND OTHER IMMUNOMODULATING DRUGS**			
CICLOSPORIN	ADALIMUMAB	Possible reduced levels of ciclosporin	Reversal of cytochrome P450 suppression by adalimumab. Ciclosporin has a narrow therapeutic index	Monitor closely, dose adjustment may be needed
CICLOSPORIN	AFATINIB	Possible increase in afatinib levels	P-glycoprotein inhibition	Manufacturer recommends staggered dosing 6–12 h apart or dose reduction
CICLOSPORIN	ANAKINRA	Possible reduced levels of ciclosporin	Reversal of cytochrome P450 suppression by adalimumab. Ciclosporin has a narrow therapeutic index	Monitor closely, dose adjustment may be needed

(*Continued*)

Primary Drug	Secondary Drug	Effect	Mechanism	Precautions
OTHER IMMUNOMODULATING DRUGS				
CICLOSPORIN	BASILIXIMAB	Ciclosporin levels and adverse effects may be altered	Unknown	Monitor closely
CICLOSPORIN	BENDAMUSTINE	Risk of excessive immunosuppression and lymphoproliferation	Additive	Monitor closely
CICLOSPORIN	BICALUTAMIDE	Predicted increased ciclosporin levels	CYP3A4 inhibition	Monitor ciclosporin concentration closely
CICLOSPORIN	BORTEZOMIB	Possible increased risk of severe neuropathy in patients on long-term ciclosporin	Possible additive effect	Monitor closely. Dose of bortezomib may need to be modified
CICLOSPORIN	CHLORAMBUCIL	Single report—reduced levels of ciclosporin	Unknown	Significance unclear
CICLOSPORIN	CISPLATIN	↑ Risk of renal toxicity and renal failure	Additive renal toxicity	Monitor renal function prior to and during therapy, and ensure an intake of at least 2L of fluid daily. Monitor serum potassium and magnesium and correct any deficiencies
CICLOSPORIN	CORTICOSTEROIDS	↓ Plasma concentrations of ciclosporin, with risk of transplant rejection	Due to induction of metabolism of ciclosporin by these drugs. The potency of induction varies	Monitor for signs of rejection of transplants. Monitor ciclosporin levels to ensure adequate therapeutic concentrations and ↑ dose when necessary
CICLOSPORIN	CYCLOPHOSPHAMIDE	Cyclophosphamide reduces ciclosporin levels	Unknown	Significance unclear
CICLOSPORIN	DABRAFENIB	Possible reduced levels of CYP3A4/CYP2Cs/CYP2B6 substrates. Level of reduction may vary	Dabrafenib induces CYP3A4/CYP2Cs/CYP2B6	Monitor closely or avoid concurrent use
CICLOSPORIN	DAUNORUBICIN	Increased daunorubicin levels	Uncertain	Monitor closely Consider dose reduction

(Continued)

Primary Drug	Secondary Drug	Effect	Mechanism	Precautions
OTHER IMMUNOMODULATING DRUGS				
CICLOSPORIN	DOCETAXEL	↑ Plasma concentrations of these drugs, with risk of toxic effects	Competitive inhibition of CYP3A4-mediated metabolism and Pgp transport of these drugs	Watch for toxic effects of these drugs
CICLOSPORIN	DOXORUBICIN	High doses of ciclosporin ↑ AUC of doxorubicin by 48% and of a metabolite by 443%. Risk of severe myelosuppression and neurotoxicity	Ciclosporin inhibits Pgp and cytochrome P450, which results in ↓ clearance of doxorubicin	Advise patients to report symptoms such as sore throat, fever, bleeding, and bruising. ➢ ***For signs and symptoms of immunosuppression, see Clinical Features of Some Adverse Drug Interactions, Immunosuppression and blood dyscrasias***
CICLOSPORIN	EPIRUBICIN	Increased epirubicin levels	Uncertain	Monitor closely Consider dose reduction
CICLOSPORIN	ERLOTINIB	Altered distribution or elimination of erlotinib	P-glycoprotein inhibition	Caution with concurrent use
CICLOSPORIN	ETOPOSIDE	↑ Plasma concentrations of these drugs, with risk of toxic effects	Competitive inhibition of CYP3A4-mediated metabolism and Pgp transport of these drugs	Watch for toxic effects of these drugs
CICLOSPORIN	EVEROLIMUS	Increased everolimus levels Possible increased risk of ciclosporin induced renal toxicity	Not fully known	Monitor everolimus levels and adjust dose as necessary Monitor renal function and consider reduction in ciclosporin dose
CICLOSPORIN	GOLIMUMAB	Possible reduced levels of ciclosporin	Induction of metabolism	Monitor closely, dose adjustment may be needed
CICLOSPORIN	IDARUBICIN	Increased idarubicin levels	Uncertain	Monitor closely Consider dose reduction

(Continued)

Primary Drug	Secondary Drug	Effect	Mechanism	Precautions
OTHER IMMUNOMODULATING DRUGS				
CICLOSPORIN	IMATINIB	↑ Plasma concentrations of ciclosporin, with risk of nephrotoxicity, myelosuppression, neurotoxicity, excessive immunosuppression, with risk of infection and posttransplant lymphoproliferative disease	Inhibition of metabolism of ciclosporin	Monitor plasma ciclosporin levels to prevent toxicity
CICLOSPORIN	INFLIXIMAB	Possible reduced levels of ciclosporin	Reversal of cytochrome P450 suppression by adalimumab. Ciclosporin has a narrow therapeutic index	Monitor closely, dose adjustment may be needed
CICLOSPORIN	IRINOTECAN	Increased irinotecan levels, but reduced gastrointestinal toxicity	Possibly due to inhibition of irinotecan transporters	Combination used to improve irinotecan toxicity, but be aware of interaction when irinotecan given to patient already taking ciclosporin
CICLOSPORIN	LAPATINIB	Increased lapatinib levels	P-glycoprotein inhibition	Caution with concurrent use
CICLOSPORIN	LEFLUNOMIDE	↑ Risk of serious infections (sepsis) and of opportunistic infections (*Pneumocystis jiroveci* pneumonia, tuberculosis, aspergillosis)	Additive immunosuppression	Monitor platelets, white blood cells, hemoglobin, and hematocrit at baseline and regularly—weekly—during concomitant therapy. With evidence of bone marrow suppression, discontinue leflunomide and administer colestyramine and charcoal to ↑ elimination of leflunomide. ➢ ***For signs and symptoms of immunosuppression, see Clinical Features of Some Adverse Drug Interactions, Immunosuppression and blood dyscrasias***

(*Continued*)

ANTICANCER AND IMMUNOMODULATING DRUGS OTHER IMMUNOMODULATING DRUGS

Primary Drug	Secondary Drug	Effect	Mechanism	Precautions
OTHER IMMUNOMODULATING DRUGS				
CICLOSPORIN	LENALIDOMIDE	Lenalidomide levels increased, risk of toxicity	Inhibition of P-glycoprotein	Monitor closely and adjust dose as necessary
CICLOSPORIN	MELPHALAN	Risk of renal toxicity	Additive effect	Monitor U&Es closely
CICLOSPORIN	METHOTREXATE	↑ Risk of renal toxicity and renal failure	Additive renal toxicity	Monitor renal function prior to and during therapy, and ensure an intake of at least 2L of fluid daily. Monitor serum potassium and magnesium levels and correct any deficiencies
CICLOSPORIN	MIFAMURTIDE	Potentially interferes with mifamurtide	Theoretical effect on macrophage and mononuclear phagocytic function	Manufacturer advises to avoid concurrent use
CICLOSPORIN	MITOXANTRONE	High-dose ciclosporin (leading to levels of ciclosporin from 3000 to 5000 ng/mL) ↑ plasma concentrations of mitoxantrone	Due to inhibition by ciclosporin of Pgp leading to ↓ clearance (by >40%) and ↑ terminal half-life (>50%)	↓ Dose of mitoxantrone of 40% has been recommended in pediatric patients. Advisable to monitor mitoxantrone levels
CICLOSPORIN	MYCOPHENOLATE	↓ Plasma concentrations of mycophenolate and of the active metabolite mycophenolic acid	Ciclosporin is thought to interrupt the enterohepatic circulation of mycophenolate by inhibiting MRP-2 in the biliary tract, which prevents the excretion of its glucuronide	Watch for poor response to mycophenolate if ciclosporin is added; conversely, watch for early features of toxicity if ciclosporin is stopped
CICLOSPORIN	NATALIZUMAB	↑ Risk of adverse effects of natalizumab and ↑ risk of concurrent infections	Additive effect	Monitor FBC closely. Warn patient to report early features suggestive of infection
CICLOSPORIN	NILOTINIB	Increased nilotinib levels	P-glycoprotein inhibition	Caution with concurrent use
CICLOSPORIN	PACLITAXEL	↑ Plasma concentrations of these drugs, with risk of toxic effects	Competitive inhibition of CYP3A4-mediated metabolism and Pgp transport of these drugs	Watch for toxic effects of these drugs

(Continued)

Primary Drug	Secondary Drug	Effect	Mechanism	Precautions
OTHER IMMUNOMODULATING DRUGS				
CICLOSPORIN	PEMETREXED	Increased pemetrexed toxicity	Reduced renal clearance	Caution with concurrent use
CICLOSPORIN	PIXANTRONE	Theoretical risk of increased pixantrone levels	Pixantrone is substrate for P-glycoprotein	Manufacturer advises monitor
CICLOSPORIN	RUXOLITINIB	Predicted increase in P-glycoprotein or BCRP substrate levels	P-glycoprotein/BCRP inhibition	Monitor closely Separate administration of drugs
CICLOSPORIN	SIROLIMUS	↑ Bioavailability of sirolimus (30%–40% when drug administrations are separated by 4 h and 100% when administered together)	Due to inhibition of Pgp by ciclosporin and competition for metabolism by CYP3A4	Be aware of toxic effects of sirolimus and monitor blood levels
CICLOSPORIN	SOMATOSTATIN ANALOGUES—LANREOTIDE, OCTREOTIDE, PASIREOTIDE	↓ Plasma concentrations of ciclosporin and risk of transplant rejection	Probable induction of CYP3A4-mediated metabolism of ciclosporin	Avoid coadministration if possible; if not, monitor ciclosporin levels closely
CICLOSPORIN	TACROLIMUS	↑ Plasma concentrations of ciclosporin	Tacrolimus is probably a more powerful inhibitor of CYP3A4 than ciclosporin	Avoid coadministration
CICLOSPORIN	TAMOXIFEN	↑ Plasma concentrations of ciclosporin, with risk of toxic effects	Competitive inhibition of CYP3A4-mediated metabolism and Pgp transport of these drugs	Watch for toxic effects of ciclosporin
CICLOSPORIN	TOCILIZUMAB	Reduced levels of ciclosporin	Tocilizumab reverses cytochrome P450 isoenzyme suppression by IL-6	Monitor closely and consider dose adjustment
CICLOSPORIN	TOFACITINIB	Tofacitinib levels increased	Unknown	Caution with concurrent use
CICLOSPORIN	TOPOTECAN	Increased topotecan levels	P-glycoprotein and BCRP inhibition	Avoid concurrent use Monitor closely if necessary
CICLOSPORIN	TRABECTEDIN	Increased trabectedin levels	Inhibition of P-glycoprotein	Caution with concurrent use

(Continued)

Primary Drug	Secondary Drug	Effect	Mechanism	Precautions
OTHER IMMUNOMODULATING DRUGS				
CICLOSPORIN	TRASTUZUMAB	↑ Neutropenic effect of immunosuppressants	Additive effects	Warn patients to report symptoms such as sore throat and fever. ➢ ***For signs and symptoms of neutropenia, see Clinical Features of Some Adverse Drug Interactions, Immunosuppression and blood dyscrasias***
CICLOSPORIN	VINCA ALKALOIDS	High doses of ciclosporin (7.5–10 mg/kg/day intravenously) ↑ plasma concentrations of vincristine. The predominant toxic effect of vincristine is peripheral neuropathy, and the toxic effect of the rest is myelosuppression	Due to a combination, to varying degrees, of inhibition of CYP3A4 metabolism and Pgp inhibition. Vinblastine and vincristine are known substrates of Pgp	Monitor for neurotoxicity and myelosuppression. The dose-limiting effect of all vinca alkaloids is myelosuppression. Monitor blood counts and clinically watch for and ask patients to report infections
CICLOSPORIN	**ANTICOAGULANTS**			
CICLOSPORIN	ANTICOAGULANTS—ORAL	1. ↓ Ciclosporin levels when coadministered with warfarin or acenocoumarol 2. ↓ Anticoagulant effect with warfarin and variable effect with acenocoumarol	Competitive metabolism by CYP3A4	1. Watch for ↓ efficacy of ciclosporin 2. Monitor INR at least weekly until stable
CICLOSPORIN	DABIGATRAN	↑ Dabigatran levels	Inhibition of Pgp	Manufacturers advises against coadministration
CICLOSPORIN	**ANTIDEPRESSANTS**			
CICLOSPORIN	ST. JOHN'S WORT	↓ Plasma concentrations of ciclosporin, with risk of transplant rejection	Due to induction of metabolism of ciclosporin by these drugs. The potency of induction varies. St. John's wort may produce its effects due to an effect on Pgp	Avoid coadministration

(*Continued*)

Primary Drug	Secondary Drug	Effect	Mechanism	Precautions
OTHER IMMUNOMODULATING DRUGS				
CICLOSPORIN	SSRIs	↑ Plasma concentrations of ciclosporin with risk of nephrotoxicity, myelosuppression, and neurotoxicity	Inhibition of CYP3A4-mediated metabolism of ciclosporin; these inhibitors vary in potency Potent—fluoxetine, nefazodone Moderate—fluvoxamine Weak—paroxetine, sertraline	Monitor plasma ciclosporin levels to prevent toxicity. Use SSRI with weak or no CYP3A4 inhibition
CICLOSPORIN	**ANTIDIABETIC DRUGS**			
CICLOSPORIN	REPAGLINIDE	↑ Plasma concentrations of repaglinide	Hepatic metabolism inhibited	Watch for hypoglycemia. ➢ ***For signs and symptoms of hypoglycemia, see Clinical Features of Some Adverse Drug Interactions, Hypoglycemia***
CICLOSPORIN	SULFONYLUREAS—GLIPIZIDE	May ↑ plasma concentrations of ciclosporin	Glipizide inhibits CYP3A4-mediated metabolism of ciclosporin	Monitor plasma ciclosporin levels to prevent toxicity
CICLOSPORIN	ANTIEMETICS—METOCLOPRAMIDE	Slight increase in ciclosporin levels	Increased ciclosporin absorption due to metoclopramide increasing gastric emptying	Clinical significance uncertain
CICLOSPORIN	**ANTIEPILEPTICS**			
CICLOSPORIN	BARBITURATES, CARBAMAZEPINE	↓ Plasma concentrations of ciclosporin, with risk of transplant rejection	Due to induction of metabolism of ciclosporin by these drugs. The potency of induction varies	Monitor for signs of rejection of transplants. Monitor ciclosporin levels to ensure adequate therapeutic concentrations and ↑ dose when necessary
CICLOSPORIN	PHENYTOIN	↓ Levels of ciclosporin, with risk of therapeutic failure	Induction of hepatic metabolism	Monitor for ↓ clinical efficacy and ↑ dose as required. Monitor ciclosporin levels
CICLOSPORIN	**ANTIFUNGALS**			
CICLOSPORIN	AMPHOTERICIN	↑ Risk of nephrotoxicity	Additive nephrotoxic effects	Monitor renal function

(Continued)

Primary Drug	Secondary Drug	Effect	Mechanism	Precautions
OTHER IMMUNOMODULATING DRUGS				
CICLOSPORIN	AZOLES—ITRACONAZOLE, KETOCONAZOLE, VORICONAZOLE	↑ Plasma concentrations of ciclosporin, with risk of nephrotoxicity, myelosuppression, neurotoxicity, excessive immunosuppression, with risk of infection and posttransplant lymphoproliferative disease	Inhibition of CYP3A4-mediated metabolism of ciclosporin; these inhibitors vary in potency. Ketoconazole and itraconazole are classified as potent inhibitors. Effect not clinically relevant with fluconazole	Avoid coadministration with itraconazole or ketoconazole. Consider alternative azole but need to monitor plasma ciclosporin levels to prevent toxicity
CICLOSPORIN	CASPOFUNGIN	1. ↓ Plasma concentrations of ciclosporin, with risk of transplant rejection 2. Enhanced toxic effects of caspofungin and ↑ alanine transaminase levels	1. Due to induction of metabolism of ciclosporin by these drugs. The potency of induction varies 2. Uncertain	1. Monitor for signs of rejection of transplants. Monitor ciclosporin levels to ensure adequate therapeutic concentrations and ↑ dose when necessary 2. Monitor LFTs
CICLOSPORIN	GRISEOFULVIN	↓ Plasma concentrations of ciclosporin (may be as much as 40%) and risk of rejection in patients who have received transplants	Induction of ciclosporin metabolism	Monitor ciclosporin levels closely
CICLOSPORIN	**ANTIGOUT DRUGS**			
CICLOSPORIN	ALLOPURINOL	Ciclosporin levels may be ↑	Uncertain	Monitor renal function closely
CICLOSPORIN	COLCHICINE	↑ Colchicine plasma concentrations and ↑ toxic effects (hepatotoxicity, nephrotoxicity, myopathy). ↑ penetration of ciclosporin through blood–brain barrier and ↑ risk of neurotoxicity	Competitive inhibition of Pgp with ↑ penetrations of ciclosporin to tissues. Ciclosporin inhibits transport of colchicine	Avoid concurrent use, especially in hepatic or renal impairment Watch for signs of colchicine toxicity if concomitant use is necessary

(Continued)

Primary Drug	Secondary Drug	Effect	Mechanism	Precautions
OTHER IMMUNOMODULATING DRUGS				
CICLOSPORIN	SULFINPYRAZONE	Cases of ↓ ciclosporin levels with transplant rejection	Uncertain	Monitor ciclosporin levels
CICLOSPORIN	**ANTIHYPERTENSIVE AND HEART FAILURE DRUGS**			
CICLOSPORIN	ACE INHIBITORS, ANGIOTENSIN—II RECEPTOR ANTAGONISTS	↑ Risk of hyperkalemia and renal failure	Ciclosporin causes a dose-dependent ↑ in serum creatinine, urea, and potassium, especially in renal dysfunction	Monitor renal function and serum potassium weekly until stable and then at least every 3–6 months
CICLOSPORIN	ALISKIREN	Likely to ↑ plasma concentrations of aliskiren	Uncertain	Avoid coadministration
CICLOSPORIN	ALPHA BLOCKERS	1. Slight reduced GFR with prazosin in renal transplants 2. Predicted increase in silodosin levels	1. Uncertain 2. P-glycoprotein inhibtion	1. Prazosin not ideal antihypertensive 2. Avoid concurrent use
CICLOSPORIN	CENTRALLY-ACTING ANTIHYPERTENSIVES—CLONIDINE	Single case of increased ciclosporin levels	Uncertain	Be aware of interaction
CICLOSPORIN	VASODILATOR ANTIHYPERTENSIVES	1. Coadministration of bosentan and ciclosporin leads to ↑ bosentan and ↓ ciclosporin levels 2. Ciclosporin moderately ↑ ambrisentan levels 3. Risk of hypertrichosis when minoxidil given with ciclosporin	1. Additive effect; both drugs inhibit the bile sodium export pump, which is associated with hepatotoxicity 2. Uncertain 3. Additive effect	1. Avoid coadministration of bosentan and ciclosporin 2. Limit ambrisentan to 5 mg/day and monitor BP closely until stable 3. Warn patients of the potential interaction
CICLOSPORIN	ANTIMALARIALS—(HYDROXY) CHLOROQUINE	↑ Plasma concentrations of ciclosporin	Likely inhibition of ciclosporin	Monitor renal function weekly
CICLOSPORIN	ANTIMUSCARINICS—DARIFENACIN	↑ Levels of darifenacin	Ciclosporin inhibits Pgp and CYP3A4, which results in ↓ clearance of darifenacin	Avoid coadministration

(*Continued*)

Primary Drug	Secondary Drug	Effect	Mechanism	Precautions
OTHER IMMUNOMODULATING DRUGS				
CICLOSPORIN	ANTIPLATELETS DRUGS—TICAGRELOR	Risk of ↑ ticagrelor levels	Inhibition of Pgp	Manufacturer recommends avoid coadministration
CICLOSPORIN	**ANTIOBESITY DRUGS**			
CICLOSPORIN	ORLISTAT	↓ Plasma concentrations of ciclosporin and risk of transplant rejection	↓ Absorption of ciclosporin	Avoid coadministration
CICLOSPORIN	RIMONABANT	Slight increase in ciclosporin levels	Uncertain	Monitor ciclosporin levels closely
CICLOSPORIN	**ANTIVIRALS**			
CICLOSPORIN	ACICLOVIR	↑ Risk of nephrotoxicity and ↑ risk of neurotoxicity with ciclosporin	Additive effect	Monitor renal function prior to concomitant therapy and monitor ciclosporin levels
CICLOSPORIN	ADEFOVIR DIPIVOXIL	Possible ↑ efficacy and side effects	Competition for renal excretion	Monitor renal function weekly
CICLOSPORIN	BIFENDATE	Reduced ciclosporin levels	Possible CYP3A4 induction	Monitor concurrent use
CICLOSPORIN	FOSCARNET, GANCICLOVIR	↑ Risk of nephrotoxicity	Additive nephrotoxic effects	Monitor renal function
CICLOSPORIN	MARAVIROC	Possible ↑ plasma levels of maraviroc	Inhibition of metabolism via CYP3A	Monitor more closely
CICLOSPORIN	NNRTIs—EFAVIRENZ, ETRAVIRINE, NEVIRAPINE	↓ Efficacy of ciclosporin	Possibly ↑ CYP3A4-mediated metabolism of ciclosporin	Use combination with caution, monitor closely for clincial response and check immunosuppreasant levels for at least 2 weeks when treatment with NNRTIs is started or stopped
CICLOSPORIN	PROTEASE INHIBITORS, COBICISTAT	↑ Ciclosporin levels with protease inhibitors	Inhibition of CYP3A4-mediated metabolism of ciclosporin	Monitor clinical effects closely and check levels
CICLOSPORIN	TENOFOVIR	Possibly ↑ adverse effects	Additive renal toxicity	Monitor renal function

(*Continued*)

Primary Drug	Secondary Drug	Effect	Mechanism	Precautions
OTHER IMMUNOMODULATING DRUGS				
CICLOSPORIN	**ANXIOLYTICS AND HYPNOTICS**			
CICLOSPORIN	BZDs—ALPRAZOLAM, MIDAZOLAM, DIAZEPAM	Likely ↑ plasma concentrations and risk of ↑ sedation	These BZDs are metabolized primarily by CYP3A4, which is moderately inhibited by ciclosporin	Warn patients about ↑ sedation. Consider using alternative drugs, e.g., flurazepam, quazepam. Warn about activities requiring attention. ➢ ***For signs and symptoms of CNS depression, see Clinical Features of Some Adverse Drug Interactions, Central nervous system depression***
CICLOSPORIN	**BETA-BLOCKERS**			
CICLOSPORIN	ACEBUTOLOL, ATENOLOL, BETAXOLOL, BISOPROLOL, METOPROLOL, PROPRANOLOL	↑ Risk of hyperkalemia	Beta-blockers cause an efflux of potassium from cells, which has been observed during ciclosporin therapy	Monitor serum potassium levels during coadministration. ➢ ***For signs and symptoms of hyperkalemia, see Clinical Features of Some Adverse Drug Interactions, Hyperkalemia***
CICLOSPORIN	CARVEDILOL	Possible ↑ in plasma concentrations of ciclosporin	Carvedilol is metabolized primarily by CYP2D6 and CYP2D9, with a minor contribution from CYP3A4	Usually ↓ dose of ciclosporin (20%) is required
CICLOSPORIN	CALCIUM CHANNEL BLOCKERS	1. Plasma concentrations of ciclosporin are ↑ when coadministered with diltiazem, nicardipine, verapamil, and possibly amlodipine and nisoldipine. However, calcium channel blockers seem to protect renal function 2. Ciclosporin ↑ nifedipine levels	1. Uncertain; presumed to be due to impaired hepatic metabolism. Also diltiazem and verapamil inhibit intestinal Pgp, which may ↑ bioavailability of ciclosporin. Uncertain mechanism of renal protection 2. Uncertain effect of ciclosporin on nifedipine	1. Monitor ciclosporin levels and ↓ dose accordingly (possibly by up to 25%–50% with nicardipine) 2. Monitor BP closely and warn patients to watch for signs of nifedipine toxicity

(Continued)

Primary Drug	Secondary Drug	Effect	Mechanism	Precautions
OTHER IMMUNOMODULATING DRUGS				
CICLOSPORIN	CARDIAC GLYCOSIDES—DIGOXIN	↑ Plasma digoxin levels, with risk of toxicity. Digoxin may ↑ ciclosporin bioavailability (15%–20%)	Attributed to inhibition of intestinal and renal Pgp, which ↑ bioavailability and renal elimination. Digoxin ↑ bioavailability of ciclosporin due to substrate competition for Pgp	Watch for digoxin toxicity. Monitor plasma digoxin and ciclosporin levels
CICLOSPORIN	**CNS STIMULANTS**			
CICLOSPORIN	MODAFINIL	↓ Ciclosporin levels up to 50%, with risk of lack of therapeutic effect	↑ Metabolism of ciclosporin. Modafinil is a moderate inducer of CYP3A4	Monitor ciclosporin levels
CICLOSPORIN	DANAZOL	↑ Plasma concentrations of ciclosporin, with risk of toxic effects	Inhibition of ciclosporin metabolism	Watch for toxic effects of ciclosporin
CICLOSPORIN	**DIURETICS**			
CICLOSPORIN	CARBONIC ANHYDRASE INHIBITORS—ACETAZOLAMIDE	Reports of rapid ↑ in ciclosporin levels	Uncertain	Monitor ciclosporin dose closely—consider reducing dose of ciclosporin and titrating to blood levels
CICLOSPORIN	LOOP DIURETICS, THIAZIDES	Risk of nephrotoxicity	Additive effect	Monitor renal function weekly
CICLOSPORIN	POTASSIUM-SPARING DIURETICS	↑ Risk of hyperkalemia	Additive effect	Avoid coadministration
CICLOSPORIN	GRAPEFRUIT JUICE	↑ Plasma concentrations of ciclosporin, with risk of nephrotoxicity, myelosuppression, neurotoxicity, excessive immunosuppression, and posttransplant lymphoproliferative disease	Inhibition of CYP3A4-mediated metabolism of ciclosporin; these inhibitors vary in potency. Grapefruit juice is classified as a potent inhibitor	Avoid grapefruit juice while taking ciclosporin
CICLOSPORIN	HERBAL REMEDIES—BERBERINE	Increased ciclosporin levels	Possibly due to CYP3A inhibition	Monitor closely

(*Continued*)

Primary Drug	Secondary Drug	Effect	Mechanism	Precautions
OTHER IMMUNOMODULATING DRUGS				
CICLOSPORIN	H2 RECEPTOR BLOCKERS—CIMETIDINE	↑ Plasma concentrations of ciclosporin, with risk of nephrotoxicity, myelosuppression, neurotoxicity, excessive immunosuppression, with risk of infection and posttransplant lymphoproliferative disease	Inhibition of CYP3A4-mediated metabolism of ciclosporin; these inhibitors vary in potency. Cimetidine is classified as a potent inhibitor	Avoid coadministration with cimetidine. Consider an alternative H2-blocker, but need to monitor plasma ciclosporin levels to prevent toxicity
CICLOSPORIN	IVACAFTOR	Possible increased ciclosporin levels	P-glycoprotein inhibition	Caution with concurrent use
CICLOSPORIN	**LIPID-LOWERING DRUGS**			
CICLOSPORIN	EZETIMIBE	↑ Levels of both drugs when ezetimibe is coadministered with ciclosporin	Uncertain	Watch for signs of ciclosporin toxicity
CICLOSPORIN	FIBRATES	↑ Risk with renal failure	Uncertain at present	Monitor renal function closely
CICLOSPORIN	PROBUCOL	Slight increase in ciclosporin levels	Unknown	Monitor concurrent use
CICLOSPORIN	STATINS—ATORVASTATIN, LOVASTATIN, ROSUVASTATIN, SIMVASTATIN	↑ Plasma concentrations of these statins, with risk of myopathy and rhabdomyolysis	Ciclosporin is a moderate inhibitor of CYP3A4, which metabolizes these statins	↓ Statins to lowest possible dose (do not give simvastatin in doses >10 mg). Monitor LFTs and CK closely; warn patients to report any features of rhabdomyolysis. This interaction does not occur with pravastatin
CICLOSPORIN	METHOXSALEN	Slight increase in ciclosporin levels	Methoxsalen possibly increases ciclosporin absorption	General significance uncertain Be aware of interaction
CICLOSPORIN	NANDROLONE	Cases of hepatotoxicity	Uncertain	Monitor LFTs closely

(*Continued*)

Primary Drug	Secondary Drug	Effect	Mechanism	Precautions
OTHER IMMUNOMODULATING DRUGS				
CICLOSPORIN	ESTROGENS	Possibly ↑ plasma concentrations of ciclosporin	Estradiol and immunosuppressants are substrates of CYP3A4 and Pgp. Estradiol is an inhibitor of Pgp	Monitor blood ciclosporin concentrations. Monitor renal function prior to concurrent therapy. Be aware that infections in immunocompromised patients carry a serious threat to life
CICLOSPORIN	PHOSPHODIESTERASE TYPE 5 INHIBITORS—SILDENAFIL	↑ Plasma concentrations of ciclosporin, with risk of adverse effects	Competitive inhibition of CYP3A4-mediated metabolism of ciclosporin	Be aware. Sildenafil is taken intermittently and is unlikely to be of clinical significance unless concomitant therapy is given on a long-term basis
CICLOSPORIN	POTASSIUM	↑ Risk of hyperkalemia	Additive effect	Monitor electrolytes closely. ➢ ***For signs and symptoms of hyperkalemia, see Clinical Features of Some Adverse Drug Interactions, Hyperkalemia***
CICLOSPORIN	PROGESTOGENS	↑ Plasma concentrations of ciclosporin	Inhibition of metabolism of ciclosporin	Monitor blood ciclosporin concentrations. Monitor renal function prior to concurrent therapy. Be aware that infections in immunocompromised patients carry a serious threat to life
CICLOSPORIN	PROTON PUMP INHIBITORS—OMEPRAZOLE	Conflicting information. Possible altered efficacy of ciclosporin	Unclear	Monitor closely. Studies have reported combination use with no significant changes in ciclosporin levels
CICLOSPORIN	RANOLAZINE	↑ Levels of both ciclosporin and ranolazine when coadministered	Mutual inhibition of Pgp	1. Watch for ciclosporin toxicity; ↓ dose as necessary and monitor levels if available 2. Monitor ECG carefully—titrate dose accordingly
CICLOSPORIN	SOMATROPIN	Predicted reduced ciclosporin levels	CYP3A4 induction	Monitor closely

(*Continued*)

Primary Drug	Secondary Drug	Effect	Mechanism	Precautions
OTHER IMMUNOMODULATING DRUGS				
CICLOSPORIN	SYMPATHOMIMETICS	Methylphenidate may ↑ ciclosporin levels	Uncertain at present	Watch for ciclosporin toxicity; ↓ levels as necessary and monitor levels if available
CICLOSPORIN	URSODEOXYCHOLIC ACID	↑ Ciclosporin levels	↑ Absorption	Watch for early features of ciclosporin toxicity; monitor FBC closely
CICLOSPORIN	VACCINES	Immunosuppressants diminish effectiveness of vaccines. There is ↑ risk of adverse/toxic effects of live vaccines, and vaccinal infections may develop	Disseminated infection due to enhanced replication of vaccine virus in the presence of diminished immunocompetence	Do not vaccinate when patients are on immunosuppressants. Vaccination should be deferred for at least 3 months after discontinuing immunosuppressants/myelosuppressants. If an individual has been recently vaccinated, do not initiate therapy for at least 2 weeks after vaccination
CORTICOSTEROIDS				
CORTICOSTEROIDS	ANALGESICS—NSAIDs	1. ↑ Risk of gastrointestinal ulceration and bleeding 2. Parecoxib levels may be ↓ by dexamethasone	1. Additive effect 2. Dexamethasone induces CYP3A4-mediated metabolism of parecoxib	1. Watch for early signs of gastrointestinal upset; remember that corticosteroids may mask these features 2. Watch for poor response to parecoxib
CORTICOSTEROIDS	ANTACIDS (LARGE DOSES)	Prednisone, prdnisolone, and deamethasone absorption reduced	Possibly due to adsorption on to surface of antacid	Consider separating administration
CORTICOSTEROIDS	**ANTIARRHYTHMICS**			
CORTICOSTEROIDS	AMIODARONE	Risk of arrhythmias	Cardiac toxicity directly related to hypokalemia	Monitor potassium levels every 4–6 weeks until stable, then at least annually
CORTICOSTEROIDS	DISOPYRAMIDE	Risk of hypokalemia	Additive effect	Monitor potassium levels closely
CORTICOSTEROIDS	FLECAINIDE	Risk of arrhythmias	Cardiac toxicity directly related to hypokalemia	Monitor potassium levels closely; watch for hypokalemia

(Continued)

ANTICANCER AND IMMUNOMODULATING DRUGS OTHER IMMUNOMODULATING DRUGS Corticosteroids

Primary Drug	Secondary Drug	Effect	Mechanism	Precautions
OTHER IMMUNOMODULATING DRUGS				
CORTICOSTEROIDS	**ANTIBIOTICS**			
CORTICOSTEROIDS	MACROLIDES—CLARITHROMYCIN, ERYTHROMYCIN, TELITHROMYCIN	↑ Adrenal suppressive effects of corticosteroids, which may ↑ risk of infections and produce an inadequate response to stress scenarios	Due to inhibition of metabolism of corticosteroids	Monitor cortisol levels and warn patients to report symptoms such as fever and sore throat
CORTICOSTEROIDS	RIFAMPICIN	↓ Plasma concentrations of corticosteroids and risk of poor or inadequate therapeutic response, which would be undesirable if used for, e.g., cerebral edema	Due to induction of hepatic metabolism by the CYP3A4 isoenzymes	Closely monitor therapeutic response—clinically, by ophthalmoscopy and radiologically—and ↑ dose of corticosteroids for desired therapeutic effect
CORTICOSTEROIDS	**ANTICANCER AND IMMUNOMODULATING DRUGS**			
DEXAMETHASONE	AMINOGLUTETHIMIDE	Effects of dexamethasone reduced or abolished	Aminoglutethimide increases dexamethasone metabolism	Consider dose increase of dexamethsone Use hydrocortisone, which is not affected by aminoglutethimide
DEXAMETHASONE	AXITINIB	Reduced axitinib levels	CYP3A4/5 induction	Manufacturer advises to avoid concurrent use if possible. If concurrent use is necessary, dose adjustment is recommended
CORTICOSTEROIDS—PREDNISONE	CHLORAMBUCIL	Single report of seizures	Possibly additive effect	Combination widely used, assess seizure risk with drugs that reduce seizure threshold
CORTICOSTEROIDS	CICLOSPORIN	↓ Plasma concentrations of ciclosporin, with risk of transplant rejection	Due to induction of metabolism of ciclosporin by these drugs. The potency of induction varies	Monitor for signs of rejection of transplants. Monitor ciclosporin levels to ensure adequate therapeutic concentrations, and ↑ dose when necessary

(Continued)

Primary Drug	Secondary Drug	Effect	Mechanism	Precautions
OTHER IMMUNOMODULATING DRUGS				
DEXAMETHASONE	CRISANTASPASE	Dexamethasone clearance reduced	Related to serum albumin concentration, which is reduced by crisantaspase treatment	Be aware. Significance unclear
DEXAMETHASONE, METHYLPREDNISOLONE	DABRAFENIB	Possible reduced levels of CYP3A4/CYP2Cs/CYP2B6 substrates. Level of reduction may vary	Dabrafenib induces CYP3A4/CYP2Cs/CYP2B6	Monitor closely or avoid concurrent use
PREDNISONE	ETOPOSIDE	Reduced etoposide levels	CYP3A4 induction	Monitor closely
DEXAMETHASONE, PREDNISONE, PREDNISOLONE	EVEROLIMUS	Reduced everolimus levels	CYP3A4 induction	Avoid concurrent use Consider increasing dose of everolimus if concurrent use necessary
DEXAMETHASONE	IFOSFAMIDE	↑ Rate of biotransformation to 4-hydroxyifosfamide, the active metabolite, but no change in AUC of 4-hydroxyifosfamide	Due to ↑ rate of metabolism and clearance due to induction of CYP3A4 and CYP2D6	Be aware—the clinical significance may be minimal or none
CORTICOSTEROIDS	IL-2	↓ Antitumor effect of IL-2	Corticosteroids inhibit the release of IL-2-induced tumor necrosis factor, thus opposing the pharmacological effect of IL-2	Avoid concurrent use if possible
CORTICOSTEROIDS	IMATINIB	↑ Adrenal suppressive effects of corticosteroids, which may ↑ risk of infections and then produce an inadequate response to stress scenarios	Due to inhibition of metabolism of corticosteroids	Monitor cortisol levels and warn patients to report symptoms such as fever and sore throat
DEXAMETHASONE	IRINOTECAN	↓ Plasma concentrations of irinotecan and risk of ↓ therapeutic efficacy. The effects may last for 3 weeks after discontinuation of CYP-inducer therapy	Due to induction of CYP3A4-mediated metabolism of irinotecan	Avoid concomitant use whenever possible; if not, ↑ dose of irinotecan by 50%

(Continued)

Primary Drug	Secondary Drug	Effect	Mechanism	Precautions
OTHER IMMUNOMODULATING DRUGS				
CORTICOSTEROIDS	METHOTREXATE	↑ Risk of bone marrow toxicity	Additive effect	Monitor FBC regularly
CORTICOSTEROIDS	MIFAMURTIDE	Potentially interferes with mifamurtide	Inhibits immune system	Manufacturer advises to avoid concurrent use
CORTICOSTEROIDS	MYCOPHENOLATE	↓ Plasma concentrations of mycophenolate and risk of transplant rejection	Corticosteroids induce UGT enzymes and multidrug resistance-associated protein 2, involved in disposition of mycophenolate	Intervention to prevent rejection is mandatory. ↑ mycophenolate dosage to maintain therapeutic blood levels. It is important is to monitor levels following steroid withdrawal to prevent adverse outcomes
DEXAMETHASONE	PACLITAXEL	↓ Plasma concentration of paclitaxel and ↓ efficacy of paclitaxel	Due to induction of hepatic metabolism of paclitaxel by the CYP isoenzymes	Monitor for clinical efficacy and need to ↑ dose if inadequate response is due to interaction
CORTICOSTEROIDS	PIXANTRONE	Theoretical risk of reduced pixantrone levels	Pixantrone excretion increased	Manufacturer advises caution
CORTICOSTEROIDS	TAMOXIFEN	↓ Plasma concentrations of tamoxifen and risk of inadequate therapeutic response	Due to induction of metabolism of tamoxifen by the CYP3A isoenzymes by dexamethasone	Avoid concurrent use if possible. Otherwise, monitor for clinical efficacy of tamoxifen by ↑ dose of tamoxifen
DEXAMETHASONE	VINCA ALKALOIDS	↓ Of plasma concentrations of vinblastine and vincristine, with risk of inadequate therapeutic response. Reports of ↓ AUC by 40% and elimination half-life by 35%, and ↑ clearance by 63%, in patients with brain tumors taking vincristine, which could lead to dangerously inadequate therapeutic responses	Due to induction of CYP3A4-mediated metabolism	Monitor for clinical efficacy, and ↑ dose of vinblastine and vincristine as clinically indicated; in the latter case, monitor clinically and radiologically for clinical efficacy in patients with brain tumors, and ↑ dose to obtain desired response

(*Continued*)

Primary Drug	Secondary Drug	Effect	Mechanism	Precautions
OTHER IMMUNOMODULATING DRUGS				
CORTICOSTEROIDS	**ANTICOAGULANTS**			
CORTICOSTEROIDS	ANTICOAGULANTS—ORAL	↑ Anticoagulant effect	Uncertain at present	Monitor INR at least weekly until stable
DEXAMETHASONE	APIXABAN	1. ↓ Apixaban levels 2. ↓ Dexamethasone levels	1. Induction of CYP3A4-mediated metabolism and Pgp-mediated transport of apixaban 2. Apixaban induces hepatic/intestinal CYP3A4 metabolism	Avoid coadministration
CORTICOSTEROIDS	ANTIDEPRESSANTS—ST. JOHN'S WORT	↓ Plasma concentrations of corticosteroids and risk of poor or inadequate therapeutic response, which would be undesirable if used for, e.g., cerebral edema	Due to induction of the hepatic metabolism by the CYP3A4 isoenzymes	Closely monitor therapeutic response—clinically, by ophthalmoscopy and radiologically—and ↑ dose of corticosteroids for desired therapeutic effect
CORTICOSTEROIDS	**ANTIDIABETIC DRUGS**			
CORTICOSTEROIDS	ANTIDIABETIC DRUGS	Often ↑ hypoglycemic agent requirements, particularly of those with high glucocorticoid activity	Corticosteroids, particularly the glucocorticoids (betamethasone, dexamethasone, deflazacort, prednisolone > cortisone, hydrocortisone), have intrinsic hyperglycemic activity in both diabetic and nondiabetic subjects	Monitor blood sugar during concomitant treatment, weekly if possible, or advise self-monitoring, until blood sugar levels are stable. Larger doses of insulin are often needed
CORTICOSTEROIDS	THIAZOLIDINEDIONES	Antihyperglycemic effect of antidiabetic agent antagonized	Increased gluconeogenesis from the liver	Monitor blood glucose closely
CORTICOSTEROIDS	ANTIEMETICS—APREPITANT	↑ Dexamethasone and methylprednisolone levels	Inhibition of CYP3A4-mediated metabolism of these corticosteroids	Be aware

(*Continued*)

Primary Drug	Secondary Drug	Effect	Mechanism	Precautions
OTHER IMMUNOMODULATING DRUGS				
CORTICOSTEROIDS	ANTIEPILEPTICS—CARBAMAZEPINE, PHENOBARBITAL	↓ Plasma concentrations of corticosteroids and risk of poor or inadequate therapeutic response, which would be undesirable if used for, e.g., cerebral edema	Due to induction of the hepatic metabolism by the CYP3A4 isoenzymes	Closely monitor therapeutic response—clinically, by ophthalmoscopy and radiologically—and ↑ dose of corticosteroids for desired therapeutic effect
CORTICOSTEROIDS	PHENYTOIN	↓ Levels of steroids, with risk of therapeutic failure	Induction of hepatic metabolism	Monitor for ↓ clinical efficacy and ↑ their dose as required
CORTICOSTEROIDS	**ANTIFUNGALS**			
CORTICOSTEROIDS	AMPHOTERICIN	Risk of hypokalemia	Additive effect	Avoid coadministration
DEXAMETHASONE	CASPOFUNGIN	↓ Caspofungin levels, with risk of therapeutic failure	Induction of caspofungin metabolism	↑ dose of caspofungin to 70 mg daily
CORTICOSTEROIDS	AZOLES—FLUCONAZOLE, ITRACONAZOLE, KETOCONAZOLE, POSACONAZOLE, VORICONAZOLE	↑ Adrenal suppressive effects of corticosteroids, which may ↑ risk of infections and produce inadequate response to stress scenarios	Due to inhibition of metabolism of corticosteroids	Monitor cortisol levels and warn patients to report symptoms such as fever and sore throat
CORTICOSTEROIDS	**ANTIHYPERTENSIVES AND HEART FAILURE DRUGS**			
CORTICOSTEROIDS	ANTIHYPERTENSIVES AND HEART FAILURE DRUGS	↓ Hypotensive effect	Corticosteroids cause sodium and water retention leading to ↑ BP	Monitor BP at least weekly until stable
CORTICOSTEROIDS	VASODILATOR ANTIHYPERTENSIVES	Risk of hyperglycemia when diazoxide is coadministered with corticosteroids	Additive effect; both drugs have a hyperglycemic effect	Monitor blood glucose closely, particularly with diabetics

(*Continued*)

Primary Drug	Secondary Drug	Effect	Mechanism	Precautions
OTHER IMMUNOMODULATING DRUGS				
CORTICOSTEROIDS—DEXAMETHASONE	ANTIMIGRAINE DRUGS—ALMOTRIPTAN, ELETRIPTAN	Possible ↓ plasma concentrations of almotriptan and risk of inadequate therapeutic efficacy	One of the major metabolizing enzymes of almotriptan; CYP3A4 isoenzymes are induced by rifampicin. As there are alternative metabolic pathways, the effect may not be significant and could vary from individual to individual	Be aware of possibility of ↓ response to triptan and consider ↑ dose if considered due to interaction
CORTICOSTEROIDS	**ANTIPLATELET AGENTS**			
CORTICOSTEROIDS	ANTIPLATELET AGENTS—ASPIRIN	Corticosteroids ↓ aspirin levels, and therefore, there is a risk of salicylate toxicity when withdrawing corticosteroids. Risk of gastric ulceration when aspirin is coadministered with corticosteroids	Uncertain	Watch for features of salicylate toxicity when withdrawing corticosteroids. Use aspirin in the lowest dose. Remember that corticosteroids may mask the features of peptic ulceration
CORTICOSTEROIDS	**ANTIVIRALS**			
DEXAMETHASONE	COBICISTAT	Possible ↓ plasma levels of cobicistat, risk of treatment failure and resistance	Induction of metabolism via CYP3A	Use with caution
FLUTICASONE	COBICISTAT	Possible ↑ plasma concentration from inhaled fluticasone, risk of increased steroid exposure and systemic effects	Inhibition of metabolism via CYP3A4	Use with caution if patient is on high-dose fluticasone. Monitor closely for signs of corticosteroid toxicity, adrenal suppression and immunosupression, review alternatives or ↓ dose as necessary. Short term, low dose or as required use will have less risk of adverse effects. Consider using inhaled beclometasone as an alternative as it is not metabolized via CYP3A4 or mometasone as it shows very low systemic bioavailablity

(Continued)

Primary Drug	Secondary Drug	Effect	Mechanism	Precautions
OTHER IMMUNOMODULATING DRUGS				
CORTICOSTEROIDS	NNRTIs—EFAVIRENZ	↑ Adrenal suppressive effects of corticosteroids, which may ↑ risk of infections and then produce an inadequate response to stress scenarios	Due to inhibition of metabolism of corticosteroids	Monitor cortisol levels and warn patients to report symptoms such as fever and sore throat
CORTICOSTEROIDS	PROTEASE INHIBITORS—RITONAVIR	↑ Plasma levels of betamethasone, dexamethasone, hydrocortisone, prednisolone, and both inhaled and intranasal budesonide and fluticasone with ritonavir (with or without lopinavir)	Inhibition of CYP3A4-mediated metabolism	Monitor closely for signs of corticosteroid toxicity and immunosupression, and ↓ dose as necessary. Consider using inhaled beclometasone
CORTICOSTEROIDS	BETA-BLOCKERS	↓ Efficacy of beta-blockers	Mineralocorticoids cause ↑ BP as a result of sodium and water retention	Watch for poor response to beta-blockers
CORTICOSTEROIDS	BRONCHODILATORS—BETA AGONISTS (HIGH-DOSE), THEOPHYLLINE	Risk of hypokalemia	Additive effect. The CSM notes that this effect occurs with beta-2 agonists, theophyllines, and corticosteroids, all of which may be given during severe asthma; hypoxia exacerbates this effect	Monitor blood potassium levels prior to concomitant administration and during therapy (monitor 1–2-hourly during parenteral administration). Administer potassium supplements to prevent hypokalemia, which may also be worsened by hypoxia during severe attacks of asthma
CORTICOSTEROIDS	CALCITRIOL	Possible antagonism of activity by corticosteroids	Antagonism of increased calcium absorption by calcitriol	Be aware of interaction
CORTICOSTEROIDS	CALCIUM	↓ Calcium levels	↓ Intestinal absorption and ↑ excretion	Separate doses as much as possible

(*Continued*)

Primary Drug	Secondary Drug	Effect	Mechanism	Precautions
OTHER IMMUNOMODULATING DRUGS				
CORTICOSTEROIDS	CALCIUM CHANNEL BLOCKERS	1. Antihypertensive effect of calcium channel blockers are antagonized by corticosteroids 2. ↑ adrenal suppressive effects of corticosteroids, methylprednisolone, and prednisolone when coadministered with diltiazem, nifedipine, and verapamil. This may ↑ risk of infections and produce an inadequate response to stress scenarios	1. Mineralocorticoids cause sodium and water retention, which antagonizes the hypotensive effects of calcium channel blockers 2. Due to inhibition of metabolism of these corticosteroids	1. Monitor BP at least weekly until stable 2. Monitor cortisol levels and warn patients to report symptoms such as fever and sore throat
CORTICOSTEROIDS	CARBIMAZOLE	Reduced prednisolone levels	Uncertain	Higher doses of prednisolone may be needed
CORTICOSTEROIDS	CARDIAC GLYCOSIDES—DIGOXIN	Risk of digoxin toxicity due to hypokalemia	Corticosteroids may cause hypokalemia	Monitor potassium levels closely. Monitor digoxin levels; watch for digoxin toxicity
CORTICOSTEROIDS	CNS STIMULANTS—MODAFINIL	May ↓ modafinil levels	Induction of CYP3A4, which has a partial role in the metabolism of modafinil	Be aware
CORTICOSTEROIDS	**DIURETICS**			
CORTICOSTEROIDS	POTASSIUM-SPARING—EPLERENONE	Reduced antihypertensive effect	Corticosteroids cause fluid and sodium retention	Be aware of interaction
CORTICOSTEROIDS	DIURETICS—LOOP AND THIAZIDES	Risk of hypokalemia	Additive effect	Monitor serum potassium weekly until stable
CORTICOSTEROIDS	DRUG DEPENDENCE THERAPIES—BUPROPION	↑ Risk of seizures. This risk is marked in elderly people, in patients with a history of seizures, with addiction to opiates/cocaine/stimulants, and in diabetics treated with oral hypoglycemics or insulin	Bupropion is associated with a dose-related risk of seizures. These drugs, which lower seizure threshold, are individually epileptogenic. Additive effects occur when combined	Extreme caution. The dose of bupropion should not exceed 450 mg/day (or 150 mg/day in patients with severe hepatic cirrhosis)

(Continued)

Primary Drug	Secondary Drug	Effect	Mechanism	Precautions
OTHER IMMUNOMODULATING DRUGS				
CORTICOSTEROIDS	GRAPEFRUIT JUICE	↑ Adrenal suppressive effects of corticosteroids, which may ↑ risk of infections and produce an inadequate response to stress scenarios	Due to inhibition of metabolism of corticosteroids	Monitor cortisol levels and warn patients to report symptoms such as fever and sore throat
CORTICOSTEROIDS	H2 RECEPTOR BLOCKERS—CIMETIDINE	↑ Adrenal suppressive effects of corticosteroids, which may ↑ risk of infections and produce an inadequate response to stress scenarios	Due to inhibition of metabolism of corticosteroids	Monitor cortisol levels and warn patients to report symptoms such as fever and sore throat
CORTICOSTEROIDS—HYDROCORTISONE	LIPID-LOWERING DRUGS—COLESTYRAMINE, COLESTIPOL	↓ Absorption of oral hydrocortisone and possibly budesonide and dexamethasone with colestyramine and colestipol. Prednisolone is not affected	↓ Absorption	Give steroid 1 h before or 4–6 h after colestyramine or colestipol
CORTICOSTEROIDS	LIQUORICE	Delayed clearance of prednisolone and hydrocortisone Risk of hypokalemia in large quantities	Inhibition of 11 β-hydroxysteroid dehydrogenase Additive	Monitor concurrent use
CORTICOSTEROIDS	MIFEPRISTONE	Reduced effects of corticosteroids	Antiglucocorticoid activity of mifepristone	Avoid concurrent use Monitor closely if necessary
CORTICOSTEROIDS	NEUROMUSCULAR BLOCKERS	Reduced effect of neuromusuclar blockers Risk of myopathy with prolonged use of corticosteroids	Uncertain	Dosage of neuromuscular blocker may need to be increased Be aware of interaction, particularly in patients in intensive care
CORTICOSTEROIDS	NICORANDIL	Possible increased risk of gastric perforation	Uncertain	Monitor closely

(Continued)

Primary Drug	Secondary Drug	Effect	Mechanism	Precautions
OTHER IMMUNOMODULATING DRUGS				
CORTICOSTEROIDS	NITRATES	Antihypertensive effect of nitrates are antagonized by corticosteroids	Mineralocorticoids cause sodium and water retention	Monitor BP at least weekly until stable
CORTICOSTEROIDS	ESTROGENS	Possibly ↑ corticosteroid levels	Uncertain	Warn patients to report symptoms such as fever and sore throat
CORTICOSTEROIDS	SODIUM PHENYLBUTYRATE	Possibly ↓ efficacy of sodium phenylbutyrate	These drugs are associated with ↑ ammonia levels	Avoid coadministration
CORTICOSTEROIDS	SOMATROPIN	Possible ↓ efficacy of somatropin	Uncertain	Watch for poor response to somatropin
CORTICOSTEROIDS	SYMPATHOMIMETICS—EPHEDRINE	Ephedrine may ↓ dexamethasone levels	Uncertain at present	Watch for poor response to dexamethasone. Uncertain at present if other corticosteroids are similarly affected
CORTICOSTEROIDS	TOBACCO	Reduced steroid efficacy in asthma	Uncertain	Smoking cessation
ETANERCEPT				
ETANERCEPT	**ANTICANCER AND OTHER IMMUNOMODULATING DRUGS**			
ETANERCEPT	ABATACEPT	Increased risk of serious infection	Additive	Avoid concurrent use
ETANERCEPT	ANAKINRA	↑ Risk of bone marrow suppression	Additive effect	Avoid coadministration
ETANERCEPT	CYCLOPHOSPHAMIDE	Higher incidence of solid malignancy in patients with Wegener's granulomatosis	Unknown	Manufacturer advises to avoid concurrent use
FAMPRIDINE				
FAMPRIDINE	CIMETIDINE	↑ Plasma concentrations	Inhibition of active renal tubular secretion via organic ion transporters	Avoid coadministration

(Continued)

ANTICANCER AND IMMUNOMODULATING DRUGS OTHER IMMUNOMODULATING DRUGS Fingolimod

Primary Drug	Secondary Drug	Effect	Mechanism	Precautions
OTHER IMMUNOMODULATING DRUGS				
FINGOLIMOD				
FINGOLIMOD	**DRUGS THAT PROLONG THE QT INTERVAL**			
FINGOLIMOD	1. ANTIARRHYTHMICS—ajmaline, amiodarone, azimilide, cibenzoline, disopyramide, dofetilide, dronedarone, ibutilide, procainamide, propafenone, quinidine 2. ANTIBIOTICS—macrolides (especially azithromycin, clarithromycin, parenteral erythromycin, telithromycin), quinolones (especially moxifloxacin), quinupristin/dalfopristin 3. ANTICANCER AND IMMUNOMODULATING DRUGS—arsenic trioxide, bosutinib, crizotinib, dasatinib, eribulin, lapatinib, nilotinib, pazopanib, sunitinib, vandetanib, vemurafenib 4. ANTIDEPRESSANTS—TCAs, venlafaxine 5. ANTIEMETICS—ondansetron 6. ANTIFUNGALS—fluconazole, posaconazole, voriconazole 7. ANTIHISTAMINES—terfenadine, hydroxyzine, mizolastine 8. ANTIHYPERTENSIVES—ketanserin 9. ANTIMALARIALS—artemether with lumefantrine, chloroquine, halofantrine, hydroxychloroquine, mefloquine, quinine 10. ANTIPROTOZOALS—pentamidine isethionate 11. ANTIPSYCHOTICS—atypicals, phenothiazines, pimozide 12. ANTIVIRALS—boceprevir, rilpivirine, telaprevir 13. BETA-BLOCKERS—sotalol 14. BRONCHODILATORS—parenteral bronchodilators 15. CNS STIMULANTS—atomoxetine 16. RANOLAZINE	Risk of ventricular arrhythmias, particularly torsades de pointes	Additive effect; these drugs prolong the QT interval	Avoid coadministration

(*Continued*)

Primary Drug	Secondary Drug	Effect	Mechanism	Precautions
OTHER IMMUNOMODULATING DRUGS				
FINGOLIMOD	**ANTIBIOTICS**			
FINGOLIMOD	MACROLIDES—CLARITHROMYCIN, ERYTHROMYCIN, TELITHROMYCIN	Fingolimod levels increased	Inhibition of CYP3A4	Monitor for adverse effects
FINGOLIMOD	RIFAMPICIN	Fingolimod levels reduced	Induction of CYP3A4	Uncertain
FINGOLIMOD	**ANTICANCER AND OTHER IMMUNOMODULATING DRUGS**			
FINGOLIMOD	MITOXANTRONE	Increased risk of opportunistic infections	Additive	Caution when switching to fingolimod due to long half-life of mitoxantrone
FINGOLIMOD	NATALIZUMAB	Increased risk of opportunistic infections	Additive	Caution when switching to fingolimod due to long half-life of mitoxantrone
FINGOLIMOD	ANTIDEPRESSANTS—ST. JOHN'S WORT	Fingolimod levels reduced	Induction of CYP3A4	Manufacturer advises to avoid concurrent use
FINGOLIMOD	ANTIEPILEPTICS—CARBAMAZEPINE, PHENOBARBITAL, PHENYTOIN	Fingolimod levels reduced	Induction of CYP3A4	Uncertain
FINGOLIMOD	ANTIFUNGALS—ITRACONAZOLE, KETOCONAZOLE, POSICONAZOLE, VORACONAZOLE	Fingolimod levels increased	Inhibition of CYP3A4	Monitor for adverse effects
FINGOLIMOD	BETA-BLOCKERS	Possible increased risk of bradycardia	Additive	Monitor for bradycardia, ECG prior to starting fingolimod
FINGOLIMOD	CALCIUM CHANNEL BLOCKERS—DILTIAZEM, VERAPAMIL	Possible increased risk of bradycardia	Additive	Monitor for bradycardia, ECG prior to starting fingolimod
GLATIRAMER ACETATE				
GLATIRAMER ACETATE	NATALIZUMAB	Increased risk of infections	Additive	Avoid concurrent use
GOLD (SODIUM AUROTHIOMALATE)				
GOLD	ANALGESICS—NSAIDs	Gold may cause interstitial nephritis. Risk of renal failure	Additive renal toxicity	Monitor renal function prior to and during gold therapy
GOLD	ANTICANCER AND OTHER IMMUNOMODULATING DRUGS—PENICILLAMINE	Possible increased risk of side effects	Uncertain	Avoid concurrent use

(*Continued*)

ANTICANCER AND IMMUNOMODULATING DRUGS OTHER IMMUNOMODULATING DRUGS

ANTICANCER AND IMMUNOMODULATING DRUGS OTHER IMMUNOMODULATING DRUGS Histamine

Primary Drug	Secondary Drug	Effect	Mechanism	Precautions
OTHER IMMUNOMODULATING DRUGS				
GOLD	ANTIHYPERTENSIVES AND HEART FAILURE DRUGS—ACE INHIBITORS	Cases of ↓ BP. May be delayed by several months	Additive vasodilating effects	Monitor BP at least weekly until stable. Warn patients to report symptoms of hypotension (light-headedness, dizziness on standing, etc.). If a reaction occurs, consider changing to an alternative gold formulation or stopping ACE inhibitor
GOLD	ANTIPLATELET DRUGS—ASPIRIN (ANALGESIC DOSES)	Increased risk of aspirin-induced hepatotoxicity compared to fenoprofen	Uncertain	Safer with fenoprofen
GOLIMUMAB				
GOLIMUMAB	**ANTICANCER AND OTHER IMMUNOMODULATING DRUGS**			
GOLIMUMAB	ABATACEPT	Increased risk of serious infection	Additive	Avoid concurrent use
GOLIMUMAB	ANAKINRA	Increased risk of serious infection	Additive	Avoid concurrent use
GOLIMUMAB	CICLOSPORIN	Possible reduced levels of ciclosporin	Induction of metabolism	Monitor closely, dose adjustment may be needed
GOLIMUMAB	ANTICOAGULANTS—WARFARIN	Possible reduced levels of warfarin	Induction of metabolism	Monitor closely, dose adjustment may be needed
GOLIMUMAB	ANTIEPILEPTICS—PHENYTOIN	Possible reduced levels of phenytoin	Induction of metabolism	Monitor closely, dose adjustment may be needed
GOLIMUMAB	BRONCHODILATORS—THEOPHYLLINE	Possible reduced levels of theophylline	Induction of metabolism	Monitor closely, dose adjustment may be needed
HISTAMINE				
HISTAMINE	ANALGESICS—OPIOIDS	Can releases endogenous histamine, potential additive effects	Additive effect	Consider potential additive effect
HISTAMINE	**ANTIDEPRESSANTS**			
HISTAMINE	MAOIs	Alter histamine metabolism	Altered histamine metabolism	Avoid concurrent use

(Continued)

Primary Drug	Secondary Drug	Effect	Mechanism	Precautions
OTHER IMMUNOMODULATING DRUGS				
HISTAMINE	TRICYCLIC ANTIDEPRESSANTS	Effects of histamine antagonized	Histamine blockade	Avoid concurrent use
HISTAMINE	ANTIHISTAMINES	Effects of histamine antagonized	Histamine blockade	Avoid concurrent use
HISTAMINE	ANTIHYPERTENSIVES AND HEART FAILURE DRUGS—CLONIDINE	Possible increased toxicity of histamine	Additive effect on lowering blood pressure	Avoid concurrent use
HISTAMINE	ANTIMALARIALS—ATOVAQUONE	Alter histamine metabolism	Altered histamine metabolism	Avoid concurrent use
HISTAMINE	ANTIPSYCHOTICS	Effects of histamine antagonized	Histamine blockade	Avoid concurrent use
HISTAMINE	H2-RECEPTOR RECEPTOR BLOCKERS	Effects of histamine antagonized	Histamine blockade	Avoid concurrent use
HISTAMINE	X-RAY CONTRAST MEDIA	Can releases endogenous histamine, potential additive effects	Additive effect	Consider potential additive effect
HYDROXYCHLOROQUINE ➢ ***Drugs to Treat Infections, Antimalarials***				
INFLIXIMAB				
INFLIXIMAB	**ANTICANCER AND OTHER IMMUNOMODULATING DRUGS**			
INFLIXIMAB	ABATACEPT	Increased risk of serious infection	Additive	Avoid concurrent use
INFLIXIMAB	ANAKINRA	↑ Risk of bone marrow suppression	Additive effect	Avoid coadministration
INFLIXIMAB	AZATHIOPRINE	Increase in azathioprine metabolites Hepatosplenic T-cell lymphoma reported in adolescents and young adults	Unknown	Increase in metabolites associated with good tolerance and favorable response to inflixmab Causal relationship unclear
INFLIXIMAB	CICLOSPORIN	Possible reduced levels of ciclosporin	Reversal of cytochrome P450 suppression by infliximab. Ciclosporin has a narrow therapeutic index	Monitor closely, dose adjustment may be needed

(Continued)

Primary Drug	Secondary Drug	Effect	Mechanism	Precautions
OTHER IMMUNOMODULATING DRUGS				
INFLIXIMAB	MERCAPTOPURINE	Cases of hepatosplenic T-cell lymphoma reported in adolescents and young adults	Unknown	Causal relationship unclear
INFLIXIMAB	ANTICOAGULANTS—WARFARIN	Possible reduced levels of warfarin	Reversal of cytochrome P450 suppression by infliximab. Warfarin has a narrow therapeutic index	Monitor closely, dose adjustment may be needed
INFLIXIMAB	ANTIEPILEPTICS—PHENYTOIN	Possible reduced levels of phenytoin	Reversal of cytochrome P450 suppression by infliximab. Phenytoin has a narrow therapeutic index	Monitor closely, dose adjustment may be needed
INFLIXIMAB	BRONCHODILATORS—THEOPHYLLINE	Possible reduced levels of theophylline	Reversal of cytochrome P450 suppression by infliximab. Theophylline has a narrow therapeutic index	Monitor closely, dose adjustment may be needed
INTERFERONS—(PEG)INTERFERON ALFA, INTERFERON BETA, INTERFERON GAMMA				
INTERFERON	**ANTICANCER AND OTHER IMMUNOMODULATING DRUGS**			
INTERFERON ALFA	CAPECITABINE	Maximum tolerated dose of capecitabine reduced	Affects fluorouracil metabolism	Reduce maximum capecitabine dose
INTERFERON ALFA	HYDROXYCARBAMIDE	Possible increased risk of vasculitis	Possibly additive	Caution with concurrent use
INTERFERON ALFA	MELPHALAN	Reduced melphalan levels, but increased toxcity possibly due to interferon-induced fever	Uncertain	Be aware. Clinical importance uncertain
INTERFERON BETA	NATALIZUMAB	2 cases of progressive multifocal encephalopathy	Uncertain	Avoid concurrent use
PEGINTERFERON ALFA	THALIDOMIDE	Severe bone marrow suppression in one case	Additive	Caution with concurrent use
INTERFERON ALFA	ANTICOAGULANTS—ORAL	↑ Anticoagulant effect	Uncertain at present	Monitor INR at least weekly until stable

(*Continued*)

Primary Drug	Secondary Drug	Effect	Mechanism	Precautions
OTHER IMMUNOMODULATING DRUGS				
INTERFERON ALFA	ACE INHIBITORS	Risk of severe granulocytopenia	Possibly due to synergistic hematological toxicity	Monitor blood counts frequently; warn patients to report promptly any symptoms of infection
INTERFERON	**ANTIVIRALS**			
INTERFERON	TELBIVUDINE	Peripheral neuropathy	Unclear	Use with caution
INTERFERONS ALFA AND BETA	ZIDOVUDINE	Increased zidovudine levels HIV positive patients with hepatitis C may be at increased risk of lactic acidosis and hepatic decompensation	Inhibition of zidovudine glucuronidation by liver	Monitor closely
INTERFERON—INTERFERONS ALFA AND BETA	BRONCHODILATORS—THEOPHYLLINE	↑ Theophylline levels	Inhibition of theophylline metabolism	Monitor theophylline levels before, during, and after coadministration
INTERFERON GAMMA	CARDIAC GLYCOSIDES—DIGOXIN	↑ Plasma concentrations of digoxin may occur with interferon gamma	Interferon gamma ↓ Pgp-mediated renal and biliary excretion of digoxin	Monitor digoxin levels; watch for digoxin toxicity
INTERFERON	DRUG DEPENDENCE THERAPIES—BUPROPION	↑ Risk of seizures. This risk is marked in elderly people, in patients with history of seizures, with addiction to opiates/cocaine/stimulants, and in diabetics treated with oral hypoglycemics or insulin	Bupropion is associated with dose-related risk of seizures. These drugs, which lower seizure threshold, are individually epileptogenic. Additive effects occur when combined	Extreme caution. The dose of bupropion should not exceed 450 mg/day (or 150 mg/day in patients with severe hepatic cirrhosis)
INTERFERON ALFA	LIPID-LOWERING DRUGS—GEMFIBROZIL	Case reports of raised liver enzymes	Unknown	Monitor closely

(*Continued*)

Primary Drug	Secondary Drug	Effect	Mechanism	Precautions
OTHER IMMUNOMODULATING DRUGS				
INTERFERON GAMMA	VACCINES	Immunosuppressants diminish the effectiveness of vaccines. There is ↑ risk of adverse/toxic effects of live vaccines, and vaccinal infections may develop	Disseminated infection due to enhanced replication of vaccine virus in the presence of diminished immunocompetence	Do not vaccinate when patients are on immunosuppressants. Vaccination should be deferred for at least 3 months after discontinuing suppressants/ myelosuppressants. If an individual has been recently vaccinated, do not initiate therapy for at least 2 weeks after vaccination
INTERLEUKIN-2 (ALDESLEUKIN)				
IL-2	**ANTICANCER AND IMMUNOMODULATING DRUGS**			
IL-2	CYTOTOXICS—DACARBAZINE	↓ Efficacy of dacarbazine	↓ AUC of dacarbazine due to ↓ volume of distribution	The clinical significance is uncertain as both drugs are used in the treatment of melanoma. It may be necessary to monitor clinically and by other appropriate measures of clinical response
IL-2	IMMUNOMODULATING DRUGS—CORTICOSTEROIDS	↓ Efficacy of interleukin-2	Corticosteroids inhibit release of aldesleukin-induced tumor necrosis factor, thus opposing the action of aldesleukin	Avoid concurrent use if possible
IL-2	ANTIHYPERTENSIVE AND HEART FAILURE DRUGS	↑ Hypotensive effect	Additive hypotensive effect; may be used therapeutically. Aldesleukin causes ↓ vascular resistance and ↑ capillary permeability	Monitor BP at least weekly until stable. Warn patients to report symptoms of hypotension (light-headedness, dizziness on standing, etc.)
IL-2	**ANTIVIRALS**			
IL-2	NUCLEOSIDE REVERSE TRANSCRIPTASE INHIBITORS—TENOFOVIR	↑ Adverse effects with tenofovir	Uncertain	Avoid if possible; otherwise, monitor renal function weekly

(*Continued*)

Primary Drug	Secondary Drug	Effect	Mechanism	Precautions
OTHER IMMUNOMODULATING DRUGS				
IL-2	PROTEASE INHIBITORS	↑ Protease inhibitor levels, with risk of toxicity	Aldesleukin induces formation of IL-6, which inhibits the metabolism of protease inhibitors by the CYP3A4 isoenzymes	Warn patients to report symptoms such as nausea, vomiting, flatulence, dizziness, and rashes. Monitor blood sugar at initiation of and on discontinuing treatment
IL-2	BETA-BLOCKERS, CALCIUM CHANNEL BLOCKERS, DIURETICS, NITRATES, POTASSIUM CHANNEL ACTIVATORS	↑ Hypotensive effect	Additive hypotensive effect; may be used therapeutically. Aldesleukin causes ↓ vascular resistance and ↑ capillary permeability	Monitor BP at least weekly until stable. Warn patients to report symptoms of hypotension (light-headedness, dizziness on standing, etc.)
IPILIMUMAB				
IPILIMUMAB	ANTICOAGULANTS	Increased risk of bleeding	Additive	Monitor closely
IPILIMUMAB	ANTICANCER AND OTHER IMMUNOMODULATING DRUGS—VEMURAFENIB	Increased risk of raised liver function tests	Unknown	Avoid concurrent use
IPILIMUMAB	VEMURAFENIB	Increased risk of raised liver function tests	Unknown	Avoid concurrent use
LEFLUNOMIDE				
LEFLUNOMIDE	**ANTICANCER AND IMMUNOMODULATING DRUGS**			
LEFLUNOMIDE	AZATHIOPRINE	↑ Risk of serious infections (sepsis) and of opportunistic infections (*Pneumocystis jiroveci* pneumonia, tuberculosis, aspergillosis)	Additive immunosuppression	Monitor platelets, white blood cells, hemoglobin, and hematocrit at baseline and regularly—weekly—during concomitant therapy. With evidence of bone marrow suppression, discontinue leflunomide and administer colestyramine and charcoal to ↑ elimination of leflunomide. ➢ ***For signs and symptoms of immunosuppression, see Clinical Features of Some Adverse Drug Interactions, Immunosuppression and blood dyscrasias***

(*Continued*)

Primary Drug	Secondary Drug	Effect	Mechanism	Precautions
OTHER IMMUNOMODULATING DRUGS				
LEFLUNOMIDE	CICLOSPORIN	↑ Risk of serious infections (sepsis) and of opportunistic infections (*Pneumocystis jiroveci* pneumonia, tuberculosis, aspergillosis)	Additive immunosuppression	Monitor platelets, white blood cells, hemoglobin, and hematocrit at baseline and regularly—weekly—during concomitant therapy. With evidence of bone marrow suppression, discontinue leflunomide and administer colestyramine and charcoal to ↑ elimination of leflunomide. ➢ ***For signs and symptoms of immunosuppression, see Clinical Features of Some Adverse Drug Interactions, Immunosuppression and blood dyscrasias***
LEFLUNOMIDE	METHOTREXATE	Possible increased leflunomide toxicity	Possibly additive	Avoid concurrent use If necessary, increase monitoring
LEFLUNOMIDE	MYCOPHENOLATE	↑ Risk of serious infections (sepsis) and of opportunistic infections (*Pneumocystis jiroveci* pneumonia, tuberculosis, aspergillosis)	Additive immunosuppression	Monitor platelets, white blood cells, hemoglobin, and hematocrit at baseline and regularly—weekly—during concomitant therapy. With evidence of bone marrow suppression, discontinue leflunomide and administer colestyramine and charcoal to ↑ elimination of leflunomide. ➢ ***For signs and symptoms of immunosuppression, see Clinical Features of Some Adverse Drug Interactions, Immunosuppression and blood dyscrasias***
LEFLUNOMIDE	ANTICOAGULANTS—ORAL	↑ Anticoagulant effect	Uncertain at present	Monitor INR at least weekly until stable

(*Continued*)

Primary Drug	Secondary Drug	Effect	Mechanism	Precautions
OTHER IMMUNOMODULATING DRUGS				
LEFLUNOMIDE	ANTIDEPRESSANTS—TCAs	Possible ↑ leflunomide levels	Inhibition of CYP2C9-mediated metabolism. The clinical significance of this depends upon whether alternative pathways of metabolism are also inhibited by coadministered drugs	Warn patients to report ↑ side effects and monitor blood count carefully
LEFLUNOMIDE	ANTIDIABETIC DRUGS—TOLBUTAMIDE	Possible ↑ effect of tolbutamide	Uncertain	Monitor blood sugar closely. Watch for and warn patients about symptoms of hypoglycemia. ➢ ***For signs and symptoms of hypoglycemia, see Clinical Features of Some Adverse Drug Interactions, Hypoglycemia***
LEFLUNOMIDE	ANTIEPILEPTICS—PHENYTOIN	Possible increase in phenytoin toxicity	CYP2C9 inhibition by leflunomide metabolite	Monitor closely
LEFLUNOMIDE	LIPID-LOWERING DRUGS—CHOLESTYRAMINE	↓ Levels of leflunomide	↓ Absorption	Avoid coadministration
NANDROLONE	LEFLUNOMIDE	Cases of hepatotoxicity	Uncertain	Monitor LFTs closely
LENALIDOMIDE				
LENALIDOMIDE	ANTIBIOTICS—CLARITHROMYCIN	Lenalidomide levels increased, risk of toxicity	Inhibition of P-glycoprotein	Monitor closely and adjust dose as necessary
LENALIDOMIDE	ANTICANCER AND IMMUNOMODULATING DRUGS—CICLOSPORIN	Lenalidomide levels increased, risk of toxicity	Inhibition of P-glycoprotein	Monitor closely and adjust dose as necessary
LENALIDOMIDE	ANTIFUNGALS—ITRACONAZOLE, KETOCONAZOLE	Lenalidomide levels increased, risk of toxicity	Inhibition of P-glycoprotein	Monitor closely and adjust dose as necessary
LENALIDOMIDE	CALCIUM CHANNEL BLOCKERS—VERAPAMIL	Lenalidomide levels increased, risk of toxicity	Inhibition of P-glycoprotein	Monitor closely and adjust dose as necessary
LENALIDOMIDE	EPOETINS	Increased risk of thromboembolic events	Additive	Caution with concurrent use
LENALIDOMIDE	LIPID-LOWERING DRUGS—STATINS	Increased risk of rhabdomyolysis	Additive	Monitor closely

(*Continued*)

Primary Drug	Secondary Drug	Effect	Mechanism	Precautions
OTHER IMMUNOMODULATING DRUGS				
LENALIDOMIDE	**ESTROGENS**			
LENALIDOMIDE	COMBINED ORAL CONTRACEPTIVE	Theoretical increased risk of thrombolic events	Additive	Contraception must be used as lenalidomide is a teratogen, but UK manufacturer advises to avoid combined hormonal contraceptive
LENALIDOMIDE	HRT	Possible increased risk of thromboembolic events	Additive	Caution with concurrent use
MESALAZINE ➢ *Other Immunomodulating Drugs, Aminosalicylates, above*				
MIFAMURTIDE				
MIFAMURTIDE	ANALGESICS—NSAIDs	Inhibits mechanism of mifamurtide in vitro	Uncertain	Manufacturer advises to avoid concurrent use with high doses of NSAIDs
MIFAMURTIDE	**ANTICANCER AND OTHER IMMUNOMODULATING DRUGS**			
MIFAMURTIDE	CICLOSPORIN	Potentially interferes with mifamurtide	Theoretical effect on macrophage and mononuclear phagocytic function	Manufacturer advises to avoid concurrent use
MIFAMURTIDE	CORTICOSTEROIDS	Potentially interferes with mifamurtide	Inhibits immune system	Manufacturer advises to avoid concurrent use
MIFAMURTIDE	TACROLIMUS	Potentially interferes with mifamurtide	Theoretical effect on macrophage and mononuclear phagocytic function	Manufacturer advises to avoid concurrent use
MYCOPHENOLATE				
MYCOPHENOLATE	ANALGESICS—NSAIDs	↑ Risk of nephrotoxicity	Additive effect	Monitor renal function closely
MYCOPHENOLATE	ANTACIDS	↓ Plasma concentrations of mycophenolate (may be 30%)	↓ Absorption	Do not coadminister simultaneously—separate by at least 4s hours

(*Continued*)

Primary Drug	Secondary Drug	Effect	Mechanism	Precautions
OTHER IMMUNOMODULATING DRUGS				
MYCOPHENOLATE	**ANTIBIOTICS**			
MYCOPHENOLATE	CO-TRIMOXAZOLE	Exacerbates neutropenia caused by mycophenolate	Additive effect	➢ ***For signs and symptoms of neutropenia, see Clinical Features of Some Adverse Drug Interactions, Immunosuppression and blood dyscrasias***
MYCOPHENOLATE	METRONIDAZOLE, NORFLOXACIN, RIFAMPICIN	Significant ↓ plasma mycophenolate concentrations (>60% with rifampicin)	Inhibition of metabolism of mycophenolate	Avoid coadministration
MYCOPHENOLATE	ANTIVIRALS—ACICLOVIR, GANCICLOVIR	↑ Plasma concentrations of both drugs. Toxic effects of both drugs likely	Attributed to competition for renal tubular excretion	Monitor blood counts. ➢***For signs and symptoms of immunosuppression, see Clinical Features of Some Adverse Drug Interactions, Immunosuppression and blood dyscrasias***
MYCOPHENOLATE	**ANTICANCER AND IMMUNOMODULATING DRUGS**			
MYCOPHENOLATE	AZATHIOPRINE	Increased risk of bone marrow suppression	Additive, both are purine inhibitors	Avoid concurrent use
MYCOPHENOLATE	CICLOSPORIN	↓ Plasma concentrations of mycophenolate and of its active metabolite mycophenolic acid	Ciclosporin is thought to interrupt the enterohepatic circulation of mycophenolate by inhibiting MRP-2 in the biliary tract, which prevents the excretion of its glucuronide	Watch for poor response to mycophenolate if ciclosporin is added; conversely, watch for early features of toxicity if ciclosporin is stopped
MYCOPHENOLATE	CORTICOSTEROIDS	↓ Plasma concentrations of mycophenolate and risk of transplant rejection	Corticosteroids induce UGT enzymes and multidrug resistance associated protein 2, involved in disposition of mycophenolate	Intervention to prevent rejection is mandatory. ↑ tacrolimus dosage to maintain therapeutic blood levels (see below). It is important to monitor levels following steroid withdrawal to prevent adverse outcomes

(Continued)

Primary Drug	Secondary Drug	Effect	Mechanism	Precautions
OTHER IMMUNOMODULATING DRUGS				
MYCOPHENOLATE	LEFLUNOMIDE	↑ Risk of serious infections (sepsis) and of opportunistic infections (*Pneumocystis jiroveci* pneumonia, tuberculosis, aspergillosis)	Additive immunosuppression	Monitor platelets, white blood cells, hemoglobin, and hematocrit at baseline and regularly—weekly—during concomitant therapy. With evidence of bone marrow suppression, discontinue leflunomide and administer cholestyramine and charcoal to ↑ elimination of leflunomide. ➢ ***For signs and symptoms of immunosuppression, see Clinical Features of Some Adverse Drug Interactions, Immunosuppression and blood dyscrasias***
MYCOPHENOLATE	NATALIZUMAB	↑ Risk of infections including progressive multifocal leuko-encephalopathy, a potentially fatal virus infection of the brain	Due to additive immunosuppressant effects. Natalizumab inhibits migration of leukocytes into the CNS	Avoid coadministration
MYCOPHENOLATE	SIROLIMUS	Higher mycophenolic acid levels compared to when taken with ciclosporin	Ciclosporin inhibits mycophenolate metabolism	Monitor closely if switching from ciclosporin to sirolimus, and adjust dose if toxicity occurs
MYCOPHENOLATE	ANTIGOUT DRUGS—PROBENICID	Possible increased mycophenolate levels	Probenicid inhibits renal excretion of mycophenolate metabolite	Be aware. Clinical significance uncertain
MYCOPHENOLATE	ANTIHYPERTENSIVES AND HEART FAILURE DRUGS—TELMISARTAN	Reduced mycophenolic acid levels	Unknown	Consider monitoring mycophenolate levels
MYCOPHENOLATE	ANTIVIRALS—ACICLOVIR, GANCICLOVIR	Possible ↑ efficacy	Competition for renal excretion	Monitor renal function, particularly if on >4 g valaciclovir. ↓ dose of aciclovir if there is a background of renal failure

(*Continued*)

Primary Drug	Secondary Drug	Effect	Mechanism	Precautions
OTHER IMMUNOMODULATING DRUGS				
MYCOPHENOLATE	IRON—ORAL	↓ Plasma concentrations of mycophenolate and risk of transplant rejection	↓ Absorption	Avoid coadministration
MYCOPHENOLATE	LIPID-LOWERING DRUGS—COLESTYRAMINE	↓ Plasma concentrations of mycophenolate by approximately 40%. Risk of therapeutic failure	Due to interruption of enterohepatic circulation due to binding of recirculating mycophenolate with cholestyramine in intestine	Avoid coadministration
MYCOPHENOLATE	ESTROGENS	Possible altered efficacy of contraceptive	Unclear	Clinical significance uncertain. It would seem wise to advise patients to use an alternative form of contraception during and for 1 month after stopping coadministration of these drugs
MYCOPHENOLATE	PROTON PUMP INHIBITORS	↓ Plasma concentration of mycophenolic acid (active metabolite)	Unclear	Be aware and monitor for ↓ efficacy though no difference in rejection rates noted in studies
MYCOPHENOLATE	SEVELAMER	↓ Plasma concentrations of mycophenolate	Attributed to binding of mycophenolate to calcium-free phosphate binders	Separate administration by at least 2 h
MYCOPHENOLATE	VACCINES	Immunosuppressants diminish effectiveness of vaccines. ↑ risk of adverse/toxic effects of live vaccines, and vaccinal infections may develop	Disseminated infection due to enhanced replication of vaccine virus in the presence of diminished immunocompetence	Do not vaccinate when patients are on immunosuppressants. Vaccination should be deferred for at least 3 months after discontinuing immunosuppressants/myelosuppressants. If an individual has recently been vaccinated, do not initiate therapy for at least 2 weeks after vaccination

(Continued)

Primary Drug	Secondary Drug	Effect	Mechanism	Precautions
OTHER IMMUNOMODULATING DRUGS				
NATALIZUMAB				
NATALIZUMAB	ANTICANCER AND OTHER IMMUNOMODULATING DRUGS			
NATALIZUMAB	CYTOTOXICS	Increased risk of infections, particularly progressive multifocal leukoencephalopathy	Additive	Avoid concurrent use wherever possible
NATALIZUMAB	AZATHIOPRINE	↑ Risk of myelosuppression, immunosuppression. Deaths have occurred following profound myelosuppression and severe sepsis	Additive myelotoxic effects. Azathioprine is metabolized to 6-mercaptopurine in vivo, which results in additive myelosuppression, immunosuppression, and hepatotoxicity	Avoid coadministration
NATALIZUMAB	CICLOSPORIN	↑ Risk of adverse effects of natalizumab and ↑ risk of concurrent infections	Additive effect	Monitor FBC closely. Warn patients to report early features suggestive of infection
NATALIZUMAB	CYCLOPHOSPHAMIDE	Increased risk of opportunistic infection	Additive	Manufacturer advises to avoid concurrent use
NATALIZUMAB	FINGOLIMOD	Increased risk of opportunistic infections	Additive	Caution when switching to fingolimod due to long half-life of natalizumab
NATALIZUMAB	GLATIRAMER ACETATE	Increased risk of infections	Additive	Avoid concurrent use
NATALIZUMAB	INTERFERON BETA	2 cases of progressive multifocal leukoencephalopathy	Uncertain if causal link exists	UK manufacturer contraindicates concurrent use
NATALIZUMAB	MERCAPTOPURINE	Potential increased risk of progressive multifocal leukoencephalopathy, although no increased risk of infection in available data	Additive	Manufacturer advises to avoid concurrent use

(*Continued*)

Primary Drug	Secondary Drug	Effect	Mechanism	Precautions
OTHER IMMUNOMODULATING DRUGS				
NATALIZUMAB	METHOTREXATE MITOXANTRONE	Potential increased risk of progressive multifocal leukoencephalopathy, although no increased risk of infection in available data	Additive	Manufacturer advises to avoid concurrent use
NATALIZUMAB	MYCOPHENOLATE	↑ Risk of infections, including progressive multifocal leuko-encephalopathy, a potentially fatal virus infection of the brain	Due to additive immunosuppressant effects. Natalizumab inhibits migration of leukocytes in to the CNS	Avoid coadministration
OLSALAZINE ➢ ***Other Immunomodulating Drugs, Aminosalicylates, above***				
PANITUMUMAB				
PANITUMUMAB	**ANTICANCER AND OTHER IMMUNOMODULATING DRUGS**			
PANITUMUMAB	BEVACIZUMAB	Reduced panitumumab efficacy with increased toxicity, when given with chemotherapy regimens containing bevacizumab	Unknown	Manufacturer advises against this combination
PANITUMUMAB	IRINOTECAN, FLUOROURACIL AND FOLINIC ACID REGIMENS	High incidence of severe diarrhea	Unknown	Manufacturer advises against this combination
PENICILLAMINE				
PENICILLAMINE	ANALGESICS—NSAIDs	↑ Risk of nephrotoxicity	Additive effect	Monitor renal function closely
PENICILLAMINE	ANTACIDS	↓ Penicillamine levels	↓ Absorption of penicillamine	Avoid coadministration
PENICILLAMINE	ANTICANCER AND OTHER IMMUNOMODULATING DRUGS—GOLD	Possible increased risk of side effects	Uncertain	Avoid concurrent use
PENICILLAMINE	ANTIMALARIALS—CHLOROQUINE	Increased penicllamine levels	Uncertain	Be alert for increased toxicity

(*Continued*)

Primary Drug	Secondary Drug	Effect	Mechanism	Precautions
OTHER IMMUNOMODULATING DRUGS				
PENICILLAMINE	ANTI-PARKINSON'S DRUGS—LEVODOPA	Possible increased levodopa levels	Uncertain	Parkinsonian symptoms may improve Monitor closely for increased levodopa side effects
PENICILLAMINE	ANTIPSYCHOTICS—CLOZAPINE	Risk of bone marrow suppression	Additive effect	Avoid coadministration
PENICILLAMINE	CARDIAC GLYCOSIDES—DIGOXIN	Plasma concentrations of digoxin may be ↓ by penicillamine	Uncertain at present	Watch for poor response to digoxin
PENICILLAMINE	IRON—ORAL	↓ Penicillamine levels	↓ Absorption of penicillamine	Avoid coadministration
PENICILLAMINE	ZINC	↓ Penicillamine and zinc levels	Mutual ↓ absorption	Avoid coadministration
RETINOIDS				
RETINOIDS	ANTIBIOTICS—TETRACYCLINE	Risk of benign intracranial hypertension with tetracycline	Unknown	Avoid coadministration
RETINOIDS	**ANTICANCER AND IMMUNOMODULATING DRUGS**			
RETINOIDS—ACITRETIN, ETRETINATE	METHOTREXATE	↑ Risk of hepatotoxicity	Additive hepatotoxic effects	Avoid coadministration
RETINOIDS	PORFIMER	↑ Risk of photosensitivity reactions when porfimer is coadministered with hydrochlorothiazide	Attributed to additive effects	Avoid exposure of skin and eyes to direct sunlight for 30 days after porfimer therapy
ORAL RETINOIDS	ANTIDIABETICS—GLP-1 ANALOGUES	Potential increased risk of pancreatitis	Retinoids can result in hypertriglyceridemia, which together with a GLP-1 analogue may cause pancreatitis	Avoid concomitant use unless triglyceride levels are unaffected by retinoid
ALITRETINOIN	ANTIVIRALS—INDINAVIR	Possibly ↑ plasma levels	Possibly inhibition of metabolism via CYP3A4	Be aware

(*Continued*)

Primary Drug	Secondary Drug	Effect	Mechanism	Precautions
OTHER IMMUNOMODULATING DRUGS				
RETINOIDS—TRETINOIN	CALCIUM CHANNEL BLOCKERS	↓ Plasma tretinoin levels and risk of ↓ antitumor activity when coadministered with diltiazem, nifedipine, or verapamil	Due to induction of CYP3A4-mediated metabolism of tretinoin	Avoid coadministration if possible
RETINOIDS—TRETINOIN	TRANEXAMIC ACID, OTHER INTRAVENOUS ANTIFIBRINOLYTICS	Increased risk of fatal thrombotic complications in acute promyelocytic leukemia	Additive	Caution with concurrent use
RETINOIDS	VITAMIN A	Risk of vitamin A toxicity	Additive effect; tretinoin is a form of vitamin A	Avoid coadministration
RITUXIMAB				
RITUXIMAB	CISPLATIN	↑ Risk of severe renal failure	Uncertain, possibly due to effects of tumor lysis syndrome (which is a result of massive breakdown of cancer cells sensitive to chemotherapy). Features include hyperkalemia, hyperuricemia, hyperphosphatemia, and hypocalcemia	Monitor renal function closely. Hydrate with at least 2L of fluid before, during, and after therapy. Monitor potassium and magnesium levels in particular and correct deficits. Do an ECG as arrhythmias may accompany tumor lysis syndrome
SIROLIMUS				
SIROLIMUS	ANALGESICS—NSAIDs	↑ Risk of nephrotoxicity	Additive effect	Monitor renal function closely
SIROLIMUS	**ANTIARRHYTHMICS**			
SIROLIMUS	AMIODARONE	Increased sirolimus levels	CYP3A4 inhibition	Monitor closely
SIROLIMUS	DRONEDARONE	↑ Plasma levels of sirolimus	Inhibition of CYP3A4-mediated metabolism of sirolimus	Monitor blood sirolimus levels closely

(*Continued*)

Primary Drug	Secondary Drug	Effect	Mechanism	Precautions
OTHER IMMUNOMODULATING DRUGS				
SIROLIMUS	**ANTIBIOTICS**			
SIROLIMUS	CO-TRIMOXAZOLE	Exacerbates neutropenia caused by sirolimus	Additive effect	Monitor blood count closely. ➢***For signs and symptoms of neutropenia, see Clinical Features of Some Adverse Drug Interactions, Immunosuppression and blood dyscrasias***
SIROLIMUS	MACROLIDES—CLARITHROMYCIN, ERYTHROMYCIN, TELITHROMYCIN	↑ Sirolimus levels	Inhibition of metabolism of sirolimus	Avoid coadministration
SIROLIMUS	RIFAMPICIN	↓ Sirolimus levels	Induction of CYP3A4-mediated metabolism of sirolimus	Avoid coadministration
SIROLIMUS	**ANTICANCER AND OTHER IMMUNOMODULATING DRUGS**			
SIROLIMUS	CICLOSPORIN	↑ Bioavailability of sirolimus (30%–40% when drug administrations are separated by 4 h and 100% when administered together)	Due to inhibition of Pgp by ciclosporin and competition for metabolism by CYP3A4	Be aware of toxic effects of sirolimus and monitor blood levels
SIROLIMUS	DABRAFENIB	Possible reduced levels of CYP3A4/CYP2Cs/CYP2B6 substrates. Level of reduction may vary	Dabrafenib induces CYP3A4/CYP2Cs/CYP2B6	Monitor closely or avoid concurrent use
SIROLIMUS	MYCOPHENOLATE	Higher mycophenolic acid levels compared to when taken with ciclosporin	Ciclosporin inhibits mycophenolate metabolism	Monitor closely if switching from ciclosporin to sirolimus, and adjust dose if toxicity occurs

(*Continued*)

Primary Drug	Secondary Drug	Effect	Mechanism	Precautions
OTHER IMMUNOMODULATING DRUGS				
SIROLIMUS	TRASTUZUMAB	↑ Neutropenic effect of immunosuppressants	Additive effect	Warn patients to report symptoms such as sore throat and fever. ➢ ***For signs and symptoms of neutropenia, see Clinical Features of Some Adverse Drug Interactions, Immunosuppression and blood dyscrasias***
SIROLIMUS	ANTIEMETICS—METOCLOPRAMIDE	Possible increased sirolimus levels	CYP3A4 inhibition	Caution with concurrent use
SIROLIMUS	ANTIEPILEPTICS—PHENYTOIN	Possible reduced sirolimus levels	CYP3A4 and P-glycoprotein induction	Monitor closely with concurrent use
SIROLIMUS	**ANTIFUNGALS**			
SIROLIMUS	AZOLES	↑ Sirolimus levels	Inhibition of metabolism of sirolimus	Avoid coadministration
SIROLIMUS	MICAFUNGIN	Possible increased sirolimus levels	Uncertain	Monitor closely
SIROLIMUS	ANTIHYPERTENSIVES AND HEART FAILURE DRUGS—ACE INHIBITORS	Reports of angioedema	Uncertain—possibly additive effect (both can cause angioedema)	Warn patient to report facial swelling immediately
SIROLIMUS	ANTI-PARKINSON'S DRUGS—BROMOCRIPTINE	Possible increased sirolimus levels	CYP3A4 inhibition	Caution with concurrent use
SIROLIMUS	**ANTIVIRALS**			
SIROLIMUS	EFAVIRENZ, ETRAVIRINE, NEVIRAPINE	Possible increased sirolimus levels	CYP3A4 inhibition	Caution with concurrent use
SIROLIMUS	ANTIVIRALS—PROTEASE INHIBITORS, COBICISTAT	↑ Levels with protease inhibitors	Inhibition of CYP3A4-mediated metabolism of sirolimus	Monitor clinical effects closely; check levels
SIROLIMUS	CALCIUM CHANNEL BLOCKERS	Plasma concentrations of sirolimus are ↑ when given with diltiazem. Plasma concentrations of both drugs are ↑ when verapamil and sirolimus are coadministered	Diltiazem and verapamil inhibit intestinal CYP3A, which is the main site of sirolimus metabolism	Watch for side effects of sirolimus when it is coadministered with diltiazem or verapamil; monitor renal and hepatic function. Monitor PR and BP closely when sirolimus is given with verapamil

(Continued)

Primary Drug	Secondary Drug	Effect	Mechanism	Precautions
OTHER IMMUNOMODULATING DRUGS				
SIROLIMUS	DANAZOL	Possible increased sirolimus levels	CYP3A4 inhibition	Caution with concurrent use
SIROLIMUS	GRAPEFRUIT JUICE	Possibly ↑ efficacy and ↑ adverse effects	Possibly ↑ bioavailability via inhibition of intestinal CYP3A4 and effects of Pgp	Avoid coadministration
SIROLIMUS	H2 RECEPTOR BLOCKERS	↑ Adverse effects of sirolimus, e.g., thrombocytopenia, hepatotoxicity	Sirolimus is metabolized primarily by CYP3A4 isoenzymes, which are inhibited by cimetidine. Cimetidine is also an inhibitor of CYP2D6, CYP2C19, and CYP1A2	Consider alternative acid suppression, e.g., alginate suspension or rabeprazole. Not thought to be clinically significant, although ensure close monitoring of immunosuppressant levels and renal function
SIROLIMUS	STATINS	Reports of rhabdomyolysis when sirolimus is coadministered with simvastatin or fluvastatin	Uncertain	Warn patients to report immediately muscle pain
SULFASALAZINE ➢ ***Other Immunomodulating Drugs, Aminosalicylates, above***				
TACROLIMUS				
TACROLIMUS	ANALGESICS—NSAIDs	↑ Risk of nephrotoxicity	Additive effect	Monitor renal function closely
TACROLIMUS	**ANTIARRHYTHMICS**			
TACROLIMUS	AMIODARONE	Increased tacrolimus levels	CYP3A4 inhibition	Monitor closely
TACROLIMUS	DRONEDARONE	Possibly ↑ plasma levels of tacrolimus	Inhibition of CYP3A4-mediated metabolism of tacrolimus	Monitor blood tacrolimus levels closely
TACROLIMUS	**ANTIBIOTICS**			
TACROLIMUS	AMINOGLYCOSIDES	Risk of renal toxicity	Additive effect	Monitor renal function closely
TACROLIMUS	CHLORAMPHENICOL	Toxic blood levels of tacrolimus, usually on the second day of starting chloramphenicol	Attributed to impaired clearance of tacrolimus by chloramphenicol	Dose ↓ of nearly 80% of tacrolimus may be required to prevent toxicity. Watch for adverse effects. Monitor tacrolimus plasma concentrations

(Continued)

Primary Drug	Secondary Drug	Effect	Mechanism	Precautions
OTHER IMMUNOMODULATING DRUGS				
TACROLIMUS	CO-TRIMOXAZOLE	Exacerbates hyperkalemia induced by tacrolimus	Additive hyperkalemic effects	Monitor electrolytes closely. ➢ ***For signs and symptoms of hyperkalemia, see Clinical Features of Some Adverse Drug Interactions, Hyperkalemia***
TACROLIMUS	MACROLIDES	↑ Plasma concentrations of tacrolimus, with risk of toxic effect	Clarithromycin, erythromycin, and telithromycin inhibit the CYP3A4-mediated metabolism of tacrolimus. Azithromycin, mildly if at all, inhibits CYP3A4; marked ↑ in tacrolimus levels is attributed to inhibition of Pgp	Be aware, and monitor tacrolimus plasma concentrations
TACROLIMUS	METRONIDAZOLE	Possible increased tacrolimus levels	Unknown	Be aware of interaction
TACROLIMUS	QUINUPRISTIN WITH DALFOPRISTIN	Slight increase in tacrolimus levels Possible increased risk of myalgia and arthralgia	CYP3A4 inhibition	Be aware of interaction
TACROLIMUS	RIFAMPICIN	↓ Tacrolimus levels	Induction of CYP3A4-mediated metabolism of tacrolimus	Avoid coadministration
TACROLIMUS	TIGECYCLINE	Increased tacrolimus levels in single case	Possibly CYP3A4 inhibition	Monitor closely
TACROLIMUS	VANCOMYCIN	Risk of renal toxicity	Additive effect	Monitor renal function closely
TACROLIMUS	**ANTICANCER AND OTHER IMMUNOMODULATING DRUGS**			
TACROLIMUS	AFATINIB	Possible increase in afatinib levels	P-glycoprotein inhibition	Manufacturer recommends staggered dosing 6–12 h apart or dose reduction
TACROLIMUS	BASILIXIMAB	Possible increased tacrolimus levels	Unknown	Tacrolimus dose may need adjusting more than normal
TACROLIMUS	BENDAMUSTINE	Risk of excessive immunosuppression and lymphoproliferation	Additive	Monitor closely

(*Continued*)

Primary Drug	Secondary Drug	Effect	Mechanism	Precautions
OTHER IMMUNOMODULATING DRUGS				
TACROLIMUS	CICLOSPORIN	↑ Plasma concentrations of ciclosporin	Tacrolimus is probably a more powerful inhibitor of CYP3A4 than ciclosporin	Avoid coadministration
TACROLIMUS	CISPLATIN	↑ Risk of renal toxicity and renal failure	Additive renal toxicity	Monitor renal function prior to and during therapy, and ensure an intake of at least 2L of fluid daily. Monitor serum potassium and magnesium levels and correct any deficiencies
TACROLIMUS	CLOFARABINE	Possible increase in clofarabine levels	Clofarabine excreted primarily by kidneys	Manufacturer advises to avoid concurrent use. Monitor closely if this is unavoidable
TACROLIMUS	DABRAFENIB	Possible reduced levels of CYP3A4/CYP2Cs/CYP2B6 substrates. Level of reduction may vary	Dabrafenib induces CYP3A4/CYP2Cs/CYP2B6	Monitor closely or avoid concurrent use
TACROLIMUS	EVEROLIMUS	Possible increased dose of tacrolimus required	Unknown	Monitor tacrolimus levels
TACROLIMUS	MIFAMURTIDE	Potentially interferes with mifamurtide	Theoretical effect on macrophage and mononuclear phagocytic function	Manufacturer advises to avoid concurrent use
TACROLIMUS	IMATINIB	Increased tracrolimus levels	CYP3A4 inhibition	Monitor tacrolimus levels
TACROLIMUS	PIXANTRONE	Theoretical risk of increased pixantrone levels	Pixantrone is substrate for P-glycoprotein	Manufacturer advises to monitor closely
TACROLIMUS	TOFACITINIB	Slight increase in tofacitinib levels	Unknown	Caution with concurrent use
TACROLIMUS	ANTICOAGULANTS—DABIGATRAN	↑ Dabigatran levels	Inhibition of Pgp	Manufacturers advises against coadministration
TACROLIMUS	**ANTIDEPRESSANTS**			
TACROLIMUS	ST. JOHN'S WORT	↓ Tacrolimus levels	Induction of CYP3A4-mediated metabolism of tacrolimus	Avoid coadministration

(Continued)

Primary Drug	Secondary Drug	Effect	Mechanism	Precautions
OTHER IMMUNOMODULATING DRUGS				
TACROLIMUS	SSRIs	↑ Plasma concentrations of tacrolimus with risk of nephrotoxicity, myelosuppression, and neurotoxicity	• Inhibition of CYP3A4-mediated metabolism of tacrolimus; these inhibitors vary in potency • Potent—fluoxetine, nefazodone • Moderate—fluvoxamine • Weak—paroxetine, sertraline	Monitor closely to prevent toxicity. Use SSRI with weak or no CYP3A4 inhibition
TACROLIMUS	ANTIDIABETIC DRUGS—METFORMIN	↑ Level of metformin	↓ Renal excretion of metformin	Watch for and warn patients about hypoglycemia. ➢ ***For signs and symptoms of hypoglycemia, see Clinical Features of Some Adverse Drug Interactions, Hypoglycemia***
TACROLIMUS	ANTIEPILEPTICS—PHENOBARBITAL	↓ Tacrolimus levels	Induction of CYP3A4-mediated metabolism of tacrolimus	Avoid coadministration
TACROLIMUS	PHENYTOIN	↓ Levels of tacrolimus, with risk of therapeutic failure	Induction of hepatic metabolism	Avoid coadministration of phenytoin with tacrolimus
TACROLIMUS	**ANTIFUNGALS**			
TACROLIMUS	AMPHOTERICIN	Risk of renal toxicity	Additive effect	Monitor renal function closely
TACROLIMUS	AZOLES	↑ Levels with azoles	Inhibition of CYP3A4-mediated metabolism of tacrolimus	Monitor clinical effects closely, check levels
TACROLIMUS	CASPOFUNGIN	↓ Tacrolimus levels	Induction of CYP3A4-mediated metabolism of tacrolimus	Avoid coadministration
TACROLIMUS	ANTIHYPERTENSIVES AND HEART FAILURE DRUGS—ANGIOTENSIN II RECEPTOR ANTAGONISTS	↑ Risk of hyperkalemia	Uncertain	Monitor serum potassium weekly until stable and then every ↑ months
TACROLIMUS	**ANTIVIRALS**			
TACROLIMUS	ADEFOVIR DIPIVOXIL	Possible ↑ efficacy and side effects	Competition for renal excretion	Monitor renal function weekly

(*Continued*)

Primary Drug	Secondary Drug	Effect	Mechanism	Precautions
OTHER IMMUNOMODULATING DRUGS				
TACROLIMUS	GANCICLOVIR/VALGANCICLOVIR	Possible ↑ nephrotoxicity/ neurotoxicity	Additive side effects	Monitor more closely; check tacrolimus levels
TACROLIMUS	MARAVIROC	↑ Plasma levels of maraviroc	Inhibition of metabolism via CYP3A	Monitor tacrolimus levels closely, reduced dose likely to be required
TACROLIMUS	NNRTIs—EFAVIRENZ, ETRAVIRINE, NEVIRAPINE	May affect tacrolimus levels	Possibly CYP3A4 induction	Monitor closely
TACROLIMUS	NRTIs—TENOFOVIR	Possbly ↑ adverse effects	Additive renal toxicity	Monitor renal function
TACROLIMUS	PROTEASE INHIBITORS, COBICISTAT	↑ Levels with protease inhibitors	Inhibition of CYP3A4-mediated metabolism of tacrolimus	Monitor clinical effects closely; check levels
TACROLIMUS	CALCIUM CHANNEL BLOCKERS	Plasma concentrations of tacrolimus are ↑ when given with diltiazem, felodipine, and nifedipine; however, they appear to protect renal function	Uncertain, but presumed to be due to inhibition of CYP3A4-mediated tacrolimus metabolism	Watch for side effects of tacrolimus; monitor ECG, blood count, and renal and hepatic functions
TACROLIMUS	CARDIAC GLYCOSIDES—DIGOXIN	Digoxin toxicity (pharmacodynamic)	Possibly due to tacrolimus-induced hyperkalemia and hypomagnesemia	Watch for digoxin toxicity. Monitor potassium and magnesium levels
TACROLIMUS	DANAZOL	Cases of ↑ tacrolimus levels	Uncertain	Watch for early features of tacrolimus toxicity
TACROLIMUS	DIURETICS—POTASSIUM-SPARING DIURETICS AND ALDOSTERONE ANTAGONISTS	Risk of hyperkalemia	Additive effect	Monitor potassium levels closely
TACROLIMUS	ECHINACEA	May ↓ immunosuppressant effect	Considered to improve immunity and is usually taken in the long term	Be aware
TACROLIMUS	GRAPEFRUIT JUICE	↑ Efficacy and ↑ adverse effects of tacrolimus	Unclear but probably due to inhibition of metabolism	Avoid concomitant use. Measure levels if toxicity is suspected, ↓ dose as necessary, and monitor levels closely

(Continued)

Primary Drug	Secondary Drug	Effect	Mechanism	Precautions
OTHER IMMUNOMODULATING DRUGS				
TACROLIMUS	H2 RECEPTOR BLOCKERS	↑ Adverse effects of tacrolimus, e.g., thrombocytopenia, hepatotoxicity	Tacrolimus is metabolized primarily by CYP3A4 isoenzymes, which are inhibited by cimetidine. Cimetidine is also an inhibitor of CYP2D6, CYP2C19, and CYP1A2. Sirolimus has multiple pathways of metabolism that would be inhibited by cimetidine	Consider alternative acid suppression, e.g., alginate suspension or rabeprazole. Not thought to be clinically significant, although ensure close monitoring of immunosuppressant levels and renal function
TACROLIMUS	IVACAFTOR	Possible increased ciclosporin and tacrolimus levels	P-glycoprotein inhibition	Caution with concurrent use
TACROLIMUS	**LIPID-LOWERING DRUGS**			
TACROLIMUS	EZETIMIBE	Possible slight increase in ezetimibe levels	P-glycoprotein inhibition	Unlikely to be of clinical significance
TACROLIMUS	STATINS	Single case report of rhabdomyolysis when simvastatin was added to tacrolimus	Uncertain at present	Monitor LFTs and CK closely; warn patients to report any features of rhabdomyolysis
TACROLIMUS	ESTROGENS	May ↑ plasma tacrolimus concentrations	Due to inhibition of CYP3A4	Be aware. Monitor plasma tacrolimus concentrations and watch for adverse effects
TACROLIMUS	PHOSPHODIESTERASE TYPE-5 INHIBITORS—SILDENAFIL	Increased sildenafil levels, reduction in blood pressure	Uncertain	Start on lower dose of sildenafil if needed
TACROLIMUS	POTASSIUM	Risk of hyperkalemia	Additive effect	Monitor potassium levels closely
TACROLIMUS	PROTON PUMP INHIBITORS	Possible ↑ efficacy and adverse effects of immunosuppression	Altered metabolism from CYP2C19 to CYP3A4 in patients with low CYP2C19 levels	Monitor tacrolimus levels and renal function more closely, dose adjustment may be needed
TACROLIMUS	RANOLAZINE	↑ Tacrolimus levels	Possibly CYP3A4 and P-glycoprotein inhibition	Monitor tacrolimus levels closely
TACROLIMUS	SEVELAMER	Possible reduced tacrolimus absorption	Sevelamer binds tacrolimus in gut	Avoid giving drugs at same time and monitor closely

(Continued)

ANTICANCER AND IMMUNOMODULATING DRUGS OTHER IMMUNOMODULATING DRUGS

Primary Drug	Secondary Drug	Effect	Mechanism	Precautions
OTHER IMMUNOMODULATING DRUGS				
THALIDOMIDE				
THALIDOMIDE	ANALGESICS—OPIOIDS	Increased sedation	Additive	Caution with concurrent use
THALIDOMIDE	ANTIARRYHYTHMICS—AMIODARONE	Possible increased risk of peripheral neuropathy	Additive	Manufacturer advises caution
THALIDOMIDE	ANTIBIOTICS—METRONIDAZOLE	Possible increased risk of peripheral neuropathy	Additive	Manufacturer advises caution
THALIDOMIDE	**ANTICANCER AND IMMUNOMODULATING DRUGS**			
THALIDOMIDE	BORTEZOMIB	Possible increased risk of peripheral neuropathy	Additive	Manufacturer advises caution
THALIDOMIDE	CISPLATIN	Possible increased risk of peripheral neuropathy	Additive	Manufacturer advises caution
THALIDOMIDE	DOCETAXEL	Possible increased risk of peripheral neuropathy	Additive	Manufacturer advises caution
THALIDOMIDE	DOXORUBICIN	↑ Risk (up to sixfold) of deep venous thrombosis in patients with multiple myeloma compared with those treated without doxorubicin	Uncertain. Attributed to doxorubicin contributing to the thrombogenic activity	Avoid coadministration except in clinical trials
THALIDOMIDE	FLUOROURACIL	↑ Risk of thromboembolism	Mechanism is uncertain; possibly the endothelium-damaging effect of fluorouracil may initiate thalidomide-mediated thrombosis	Avoid coadministration
THALIDOMIDE	PEGINTERFERON ALFA	Case report of bone marrow depression	Additive	Caution with concurrent use

(Continued)

Primary Drug	Secondary Drug	Effect	Mechanism	Precautions
OTHER IMMUNOMODULATING DRUGS				
THALIDOMIDE	PACLITAXEL	Possible increased risk of peripheral neuropathy	Additive	Manufacturer advises caution
THALIDOMIDE	VINCRISTINE	Possible increased risk of peripheral neuropathy	Additive	Manufacturer advises caution
THALIDOMIDE	ANTIDEPRESSANTS	Increased sedation	Additive	Caution with concurrent use
THALIDOMIDE	ANTIEPILEPTICS—PHENYTOIN	Possible increased risk of peripheral neuropathy	Additive	Manufacturer advises caution
THALIDOMIDE	ANTIHYPERTENSIVES AND HEART FAILURE DRUGS—ALPHA-BLOCKERS	Excessive bradycardia	Additive effect	Monitor BP and PR closely
THALIDOMIDE	ANTIPSYCHOTICS	Increased sedation	Additive	Caution with concurrent use
THALIDOMIDE	ANXIOLYTICS AND HYPNOTICS	Increased sedation	Additive	Caution with concurrent use
THALIDOMIDE	BETA-BLOCKERS	Excessive bradycardia	Additive effect	Monitor BP and PR closely
THALIDOMIDE	CALCIUM CHANNEL BLOCKERS	Risk of bradycardia	Additive effect	Monitor BP and PR closely
THALIDOMIDE	CARDIAC GLYCOSIDES—DIGOXIN	Excessive bradycardia	Additive effect	Monitor BP and PR closely
THALIDOMIDE	EPOETINS	Possible increased thromboembolic risk	Additive	Monitor closely Consider thromboprophylaxis
THALIDOMIDE	DRUG DEPENDENCE THERAPIES—DISULFIRAM	Possible increased risk of peripheral neuropathy	Additive	Manufacturer advises caution
THALIDOMIDE	**ESTROGENS**			
THALIDOMIDE	COMBINED ORAL CONTRACEPTIVE	Theoretical increased risk of thrombolic events	Additive	Contraception must be used as thalidomide is a teratogen, but UK manufacturer advises to avoid combined hormonal contraceptive
THALIDOMIDE	HRT	Possible increased risk of thromboembolic events	Additive	Caution with concurrent use

(Continued)

Primary Drug	Secondary Drug	Effect	Mechanism	Precautions
OTHER IMMUNOMODULATING DRUGS				
TOCILIZUMAB				
TOCILIZUMAB	ANALGESICS—DEXTROMETHORPHAN	Reduced levels	Tocilizumab reverses cytochrome P450 isoenzyme suppression by IL-6	Monitor closely and consider dose adjustment
TOCILIZUMAB	ANTICANCER AND OTHER IMMUNOMODULATING DRUGS—CICLOSPORIN	Reduced levels	Tocilizumab reverses cytochrome P450 isoenzyme suppression by IL-6	Monitor closely and consider dose adjustment
TOCILIZUMAB	ANTICOAGULANTS—WARFARIN	Reduced levels	Tocilizumab reverses cytochrome P450 isoenzyme suppression by IL-6	Monitor closely and consider dose adjustment
TOCILIZUMAB	ANTIEPILEPTICS—PHENYTOIN	Reduced levels	Tocilizumab reverses cytochrome P450 isoenzyme suppression by IL-6	Monitor closely and consider dose adjustment
TOCILIZUMAB	BRONCHODILATORS—THEOPHYLLINE	Reduced levels	Tocilizumab reverses cytochrome P450 isoenzyme suppression by IL-6	Monitor closely and consider dose adjustment
TOCILIZUMAB	CALCIUM CHANNEL BLOCKERS	Reduced levels	Tocilizumab reverses cytochrome P450 isoenzyme suppression by IL-6	Monitor closely and consider dose adjustment
TOCILIZUMAB	LIPID-LOWERING DRUGS—STATINS	Reduced levels of simvastatin. Other statins may be affected	Tocilizumab reverses cytochrome P450 isoenzyme suppression by IL-6	Monitor closely. Consider increasing statin dose
TOCILIZUMAB	ESTROGENS—ORAL CONTRACEPTIVES	Reduced levels	Tocilizumab reverses cytochrome P450 isoenzyme suppression by IL-6	Monitor closely and consider dose adjustment
TOCILIZUMAB	PROTON PUMP INHIBITORS—OMEPRAZOLE	Reduced levels	Tocilizumab reverses cytochrome P450 isoenzyme suppression by IL-6	Monitor closely and consider dose adjustment
VALSPODAR	**ANTICANCER AND IMMONOMODULATING DRUGS**			
VALSPODAR	AFATINIB	Possible increase in afatinib levels	P-glycoprotein inhibition	Manufacturer recommends staggered dosing 6–12 h apart or dose reduction
VALSPODAR	LAPATINIB	Increased lapatinib levels	P-glycoprotein inhibition	Caution with concurrent use
VALSPODAR	NILOTINIB	Increased nilotinib levels	P-glycoprotein inhibition	Caution with concurrent use

PART 4

Anticoagulants

Rebecca Chanda

1. APIXABAN
2. COUMARINS
3. DABIGATRAN
4. FONDAPARINUX
5. HEPARINS
6. RIVAROXABAN
7. THROMBOLYTICS

Primary Drug	Secondary Drug	Effect	Mechanism	Precautions
APIXABAN				
APIXABAN	ANALGESICS—NSAIDs	1. Risk of gastrointestinal bleeding with all NSAIDs 2. Possible ↑ anticoagulant effect with diclofenac, ketorolac, naproxen	1. NSAIDs irritate the gastric mucosa and can cause bleeding, which is exacerbated by anticoagulants 2. Uncertain	1. Avoid coadministration
APIXABAN	ANTIARRHYTHMICS—QUINIDINE	↑ Quinidine levels	Inhibition of CYP3A4-mediated metabolism	Avoid coadministration
APIXABAN	**ANTIBIOTICS**			
APIXABAN	RIFABUTIN, RIFAMPRICIN	1. ↓ Apixaban levels 2. ↓ Rifabutin and rifampicin levels	1. Induction of CYP3A4-mediated metabolism and Pgp-mediated transport of apixaban 2. Apixaban induces hepatic/intestinal CYP3A4 metabolism	Avoid coadministration
APIXABAN	**ANTICANCER AND OTHER IMMUNOMODULATING DRUGS**			
APIXABAN	BEVACIZUMAB	Theoretical risk of ↑ bleeding; limited evidence suggests this might not be the case	Additive, bevacizumab associated with ↑ risk of hemorrhage	Monitor concurrent use
APIXABAN	DEXAMETHASONE	1. ↓ Apixaban levels 2. ↓ Dexamethasone levels	1. Induction of CYP3A4-mediated metabolism and Pgp-mediated transport of apixaban. 2. Apixaban induces hepatic/intestinal CYP3A4 metabolism	Avoid coadministration
APIXABAN	IPILIMUMAB	Increased risk of bleeding	Additive	Monitor closely
APIXABAN	ANTICOAGULANTS	↑ Risk of hemorrhage	Additive effect	Avoid coadministration

(Continued)

Primary Drug	Secondary Drug	Effect	Mechanism	Precautions
APIXABAN				
APIXABAN	**ANTIDEPRESSANTS**			
APIXABAN	ST. JOHN'S WORT	↓ Apixaban levels	Induction of CYP3A4-mediated metabolism and Pgp-mediated transport of apixaban	Avoid coadministration
APIXABAN	SSRIs, SNRIs	↑ Effect of dabigatran	Uncertain	Warn patients to report early evidence of bleeding
APIXABAN	ANTIEPILEPTICS—CARBAMAZEPINE, PHENOBARBITAL, PHENYTOIN	↓ Apixaban levels	Induction of CYP3A4-mediated metabolism and Pgp-mediated transport of apixaban	Avoid coadministration
APIXABAN	**ANTIFUNGALS**			
APIXABAN	ITRACONAZOLE, POSACONAZOLE, POSSIBLY VORICONAZOLE	↑ Apixaban levels	Inhibition of CYP3A4-mediated metabolism and Pgp-mediated transport of apixaban	Avoid coadministration
APIXABAN	KETOCONAZOLE	↑ Apixaban levels	Inhibition of CYP3A4-mediated metabolism and Pgp-mediated transport of apixaban	Dosage of apixaban should be reduced to 2.5 mg twice daily with such concomitant therapy. Concomitant use of apixaban and ketoconazole should be avoided in patients who have two or more of the following characteristics: Age ≥ 80 Body weight ≥ 60 kg Serum creatinine ≥ 1.5 mg/dL
APIXABAN	ANTIGOUTS—SULFINPYRAZONE	↑ Risk of bleeding	Uncertain	Manufacturers of apixaban do not recommend concomitant use
APIXABAN	ANTIPLATELETS	Risk of bleeding when prasugrel is coadministered with anticoagulants	Additive effect on different parts of the clotting mechanism	Closely monitor effects; watch for signs of excess bleeding
APIXABAN	**ANTIVIRALS**			
APIXABAN	COBICISTAT	Possible ↑ plasma levels of apixaban and ↑ clinical effect	Inhibition of metabolism via CYP3A4	Use with caution, advise patients to report unusual bruising/bleeding, monitor anti-factor Xa levels if overanticoagulation is suspected

(*Continued*)

Primary Drug	Secondary Drug	Effect	Mechanism	Precautions
APIXABAN				
APIXABAN	PROTEASE INHIBITORS—ATAZANAVIR, BOCEPREVIR, DARUNAVIR, FOSAMPRENAVIR, INDINAVIR, LOPINAVIR, RITONAVIR, SAQUINAVIR, TELAPREVIR, TIPRANAVIR	↑ Apixaban levels	Inhibition of CYP3A4-mediated metabolism and Pgp-mediated transport of apixaban	No specific information on apixaban

Primary Drug	Secondary Drug	Effect	Mechanism	Precautions
COUMARINS				
COUMARINS	ALCOHOL	Fluctuations in anticoagulant effect in heavy drinkers or patients with liver disease who drink alcohol	Alcohol may reduce the half-life of oral anticoagulants by inducing hepatic enzymes. They may also alter hepatic synthesis of clotting factors	Caution should be taken when prescribing oral anticoagulants to alcoholics, particularly those who binge drink or have liver damage
COUMARINS	**ANALGESICS**			
COUMARINS	NSAIDs	1. Risk of gastrointestinal bleeding with all NSAIDs 2. Possible ↑ anticoagulant effect with celecoxib, etoricoxib, flurbiprofen, piroxicam, sulindac, and valdecoxib	1. NSAIDs irritate the gastric mucosa and can cause bleeding, which is exacerbated by anticoagulants 2. Uncertain but possibly a combination of impaired hepatic metabolism and displacement of anticoagulants from their plasma proteins	1. Extreme caution when coadministering; monitor patients closely 2. Monitor INR before and during therapy until stable. Ask patients to report increased bruising, bleeding from gums while brushing teeth, etc.
COUMARINS	OPIOIDS	Cases of ↑ anticoagulant effect with tramadol	Likely to be seen mainly in CYP2D6-depleted individuals. Thereby tramadol metabolism is shunted to CYP3A4 resulting in competitive inhibition of warfarin	Monitor INR at least weekly until stable

(Continued)

Primary Drug	Secondary Drug	Effect	Mechanism	Precautions
COUMARINS				
COUMARINS	PARACETAMOL	Possible ↑ anticoagulant effect when paracetamol is taken regularly (but not occasionally)	Uncertain; possibly due to competitive inhibition of CYP-mediated metabolism of warfarin	Monitor INR closely for the first 1–2 weeks of starting or stopping regular paracetamol
COUMARINS	**ANTIARRHYTHMICS**			
COUMARINS	AMIODARONE	Cases of bleeding within ↓ weeks of starting amiodarone in patients previously stabilized on warfarin. The effect was seen to last up to 16 weeks after stopping amiodarone	Amiodarone inhibits CYP2C9- and CYP3A4-mediated metabolism of warfarin	Reduce the dose of anticoagulant by 30%–50% and monitor INR closely for at least the first month of starting amiodarone and for ↓ months after stopping amiodarone. If the INR suddenly ↑ after being initially stabilized, check TSH
COUMARINS	DRONEDARONE	Case reports of ↑ INR when dronedarone given with warfarin	Likely inhibition of metabolism of warfarin	Monitor INR closely until stable in patients on warfarin when starting and stopping dronedarone
COUMARINS	PROPAFENONE	Warfarin levels may be ↑ by propafenone	Propafenone seems to inhibit warfarin metabolism	Monitor INR at least weekly until stable
COUMARINS	**ANTIBIOTICS**			
COUMARINS	AMINOGLYCOSIDES—NEOMYCIN	Elevated prothrombin times and ↑ risk of bleeding	The mechanism is not fully understood, but it is thought that neomycin may reduce the number of vitamin K–producing bacteria in the gastrointestinal tract and/or that absorption of vitamin K may be ↓ by neomycin	The INR should be monitored in all patients starting or stopping neomycin therapy. Patients more at risk are those with an inadequate diet
COUMARINS	CEPHALOSPORINS	Certain cephalosporins (cefaclor, cefixime, ceftriaxone) may ↑ efficacy of oral anticoagulants	These cephalosporins have vitamin K-antagonistic activity, which adds to the action of oral anticoagulants	Monitor INR closely; any significant ↑ INR may require vitamin K therapy. If possible, use an alternative cephalosporin
COUMARINS	METRONIDAZOLE, SULFONAMIDES, TRIMETHOPRIM	↑ Anticoagulant effect	Inhibition of CYP2C9-mediated metabolism of oral anticoagulants	Monitor INR every 2–3 days

(Continued)

Primary Drug	Secondary Drug	Effect	Mechanism	Precautions
COUMARINS				
COUMARINS	CHLORAMPHENICOL, MACROLIDES, PENICILLINS, QUINOLONES	Occasional episodes of ↑ anticoagulant effect	Uncertain at present	Monitor INR every 2–3 days
COUMARINS	RIFAMPICIN	↓ Anticoagulant effect	Rifampicin induces CYP2C9-mediated metabolism of warfarin	Monitor INR closely for at least 1 week after starting rifampicin and up to 5 weeks after stopping it. During coadministration, the warfarin dose may need to be markedly ↑
COUMARINS	TETRACYCLINES	Additive effects of warfarin and oxytetracycline leading to prolongation of the prothrombin time or INR and bleeding	Tetracyclines have been associated with ↓ prothrombin activity, causing hypoprothrombinemia and bleeding. Tetracyclines may also decrease the intestinal flora of the gut, depleting the body of vitamin K2; this may only be significant if the patient's diet is low in vitamin K1	Monitor INR closely and adjust the dose of warfarin accordingly. Patients should be alert for signs of overanticoagulation, bleeding from the gums when brushing their teeth, nose bleeds, unusual bruising, and weakness
COUMARINS	**ANTICANCER AND IMMUNOMODULATING DRUGS**			
COUMARINS	**CYTOTOXICS**			
COUMARINS	ADALIMUMAB	Possible ↓ levels of warfarin	Reversal of cytochrome P450 suppression by adalimumab. Warfarin has a narrow therapeutic index	Monitor closely, dose adjustment may be needed
COUMARINS	ANAKINRA	Possible ↓ levels of warfarin	Reversal of cytochrome P450 suppression by adalimumab. Warfarin has a narrow therapeutic index	Monitor closely, dose adjustment may be needed

(Continued)

Primary Drug	Secondary Drug	Effect	Mechanism	Precautions
COUMARINS				
COUMARINS	AZATHIOPRINE, MERCAPTOPURINE, MITOTANE	Possible ↓ anticoagulant effect	Induction of metabolism of warfarin	Monitor INR closely
COUMARINS	BEVACIZUMAB	Theoretical risk of increased bleeding; limited evidence suggests this might not be the case	Additive, bevacizumab associated with an increased risk of hemorrhage	Monitor concurrent use
COUMARINS	CAPECITABINE, CARBOPLATIN, CYCLOPHOSPHAMIDE, DASATINIB, DOXORUBICIN, ERLOTINIB, ETOPOSIDE, FLUOROURACIL (continuous infusion but not bolus doses), GEMCITABINE, IFOSFAMIDE, METHOTREXATE, PROCARBAZINE, SORAFENIB, TEGAFUR WITH URACIL	Episodes of ↑ anticoagulant effect	Not understood but likely to be multifactorial, including CYP interactions (e.g., capecitabine/imatinib inhibits CYP2C9, ifosfamide inhibits CYP3A4), ↓ protein binding of warfarin (e.g., etoposide, flutamide), and ↓ absorption of anticoagulant or vitamin K	Monitor INR at least weekly until stable during administration of chemotherapy
COUMARINS—ACENOCOUMAROL, WARFARIN	DABRAFENIB	Possible ↓ levels of CYP3A4/CYP2Cs/CYP2B6 substrates. Level of reduction may vary	Dabrafenib induces CYP3A4/CYP2Cs/CYP2B6	Monitor closely or avoid concurrent use
COUMARINS	IMINITIB	Episodes of ↑ anticoagulant effect	Not understood but likely to be multifactorial, including CYP interactions (e.g., capecitabine/imatinib inhibits CYP2C9, ifosfamide inhibits CYP3A4), ↓ protein binding of warfarin (e.g., etoposide, flutamide), and ↓ absorption of anticoagulant or vitamin K	Manufacturer recommends converting to LMWH from warfarin. However, if warfarin is considered essential, monitor INR at least weekly until stable during the administration of chemotherapy

(Continued)

Primary Drug	Secondary Drug	Effect	Mechanism	Precautions
COUMARINS				
COUMARINS	INFLIXIMAB	Possible ↓ levels of warfarin	Reversal of cytochrome P450 suppression by adalimumab. Warfarin has a narrow therapeutic index	Monitor closely, dose adjustment may be needed
COUMARINS	IRINOTECAN	Episodes of ↑ anticoagulant effect	Not understood but likely to be multifactorial	Monitor INR at least weekly until stable during administration of chemotherapy
COUMARINS	NILOTINIB	Possible ↑ bleeding risk	Additive effect	Monitor closely with concurrent use
COUMARINS	PACLITAXEL	Episodes of ↑ anticoagulant effect	Not understood but likely to be multifactorial	Monitor INR at least weekly until stable during administration of chemotherapy
COUMARINS	PAZOPANIB	Possible ↑ bleeding risk	Additive effect	Monitor closely with concurrent use Manufacturer of imatinib recommends LMWH to warfarin
COUMARINS	PIXANTRONE	Theoretical risk of ↑ warfarin efficacy	Pixantrone inhibits CYP1A2	Manufacturer advises to monitor INR closely
COUMARINS	SUNITINIB	Possible ↑ bleeding risk	Additive effect	Monitor closely with concurrent use
COUMARINS	TOCILIZUMAB	↓ Levels	Tocilizumab reverses cytochrome P450 isoenzyme suppression by IL-6	Monitor closely and consider dose adjustment
COUMARINS	VEMURAFENIB	Possible ↑ warfarin levels	CYP2C9 inhibition	Monitor INR closely
COUMARINS	**HORMONES AND HORMONE ANTAGONISTS**			
COUMARINS	BICALUTAMIDE	↑ Plasma concentrations of warfarin	Bicalutamide displaces warfarin from protein-binding sites	Monitor INR at least weekly until stable at initiation and discontinuation of concurrent therapy
COUMARINS	FLUTAMIDE, TAMOXIFEN, POSSIBLY ANASTROZOLE AND TOREMIFENE	↑ Anticoagulant effect	Uncertain; possibly inhibition of hepatic enzymes. Anastrozole is a known inhibitor of CYP1A2, CYP2C9, and CYP3A4. Tamoxifen inhibits CYP3A4	Monitor INR at least weekly until stable at initiation and discontinuation of concurrent therapy

(*Continued*)

Primary Drug	Secondary Drug	Effect	Mechanism	Precautions
COUMARINS				
COUMARINS	**IMMUNOMODULATING DRUGS**			
COUMARINS	ACITRETIN, CORTICOSTEROIDS, INTERFERON ALFA, LEFLUNOMIDE	↑ Anticoagulant effect	Uncertain at present	Monitor INR at least weekly until stable
COUMARINS	CICLOSPORIN	1. ↓ Ciclosporin levels when coadministered with warfarin or acenocoumarol 2. ↓ Anticoagulant effect with warfarin and variable effect with acenocoumarol	Competitive metabolism by CYP3A4	1. Watch for ↓ efficacy of ciclosporin. 2. Monitor INR at least weekly until stable
COUMARINS	GOLIMUMAB	Possible ↓ levels of warfarin	Induction of metabolism	Monitor closely, dose adjustment may be needed
COUMARINS	IPILIMUMAB	↑ Risk of bleeding	Additive	Monitor closely
COUMARINS	ANTIDEMENTIA DRUGS-MEMANTINE	Possible ↑ anticoagulant effect	Uncertain at present	Monitor INR at least weekly until stable
COUMARINS	**ANTIDEPRESSANTS**			
COUMARINS	MIRTAZAPINE	↑ Anticoagulant effect of warfarin	Inhibition of metabolism of warfarin	Monitor INR at least weekly until stable
COUMARINS	ST. JOHN'S WORT	↓ Warfarin levels	Induction of metabolism	Avoid coadministration
COUMARINS	SSRIs	Possible ↑ in anticoagulant effect with fluoxetine, fluvoxamine, paroxetine, and sertraline	Uncertain at present	Monitor INR at least weekly until stable
COUMARINS	TCAs	Cases of both ↑ and ↓ effect of warfarin	Uncertain at present	Monitor INR at least weekly until stable
COUMARINS	**ANTIDIABETIC DRUGS**			
COUMARINS	GLP-1 ANALOGUES—EXENATIDE	Exenatide possibly enhances the anticoagulant effect of warfarin	Unknown mechanism	Monitor INR closely on concomitant prescribing

(*Continued*)

Primary Drug	Secondary Drug	Effect	Mechanism	Precautions
COUMARINS				
COUMARINS	SULFONYLUREAS	Cases reported of hypoglycemia when coumarins are started in patients on tolbutamide. Conversely, there are several case reports of bleeding when patients taking tolbutamide are started on oral anticoagulants	Oral anticoagulants inhibit hepatic metabolism of tolbutamide and ↑ its half-life threefold. Tolbutamide possibly alters the plasma protein binding of anticoagulants	Use alternative sulfonylurea or another class of hypoglycemic
COUMARINS	**ANTIEPILEPTICS**			
COUMARINS	BARBITURATES	↓ Anticoagulant effect. This reaches a maximum after 3 weeks and can last up to 6 weeks after stopping the barbiturates	Barbiturates induce CYP2B6- and CYP2C9-mediated metabolism of warfarin	Monitor INR carefully. Dose of anticoagulant may need to be ↑ by up to 60%
COUMARINS	CARBAMAZEPINE	Carbamazepine ↓ effect of warfarin	Uncertain; carbamazepine probably ↑ hepatic metabolism of warfarin	Monitor INR at least weekly until stable
COUMARINS	PHENYTOIN	Initial ↑ in warfarin levels, then ↓ level with risk of therapeutic failure	Potential induction and inhibition of CYP2C9 by phenytoin—possibly leading to a biphasic interaction	Requires monitoring of INR at least three times a week until stable
COUMARINS	**ANTIFUNGALS**			
COUMARINS	AZOLES—FLUCONAZOLE, ITRACONAZOLE, KETOCONAZOLE, MICONAZOLE, VORICONAZOLE	↑ Anticoagulant effect with azole antifungals. There have been cases of bleeding when topical miconazole (oral gel or pessaries) has been used by patients on warfarin. Posaconazole may be a safer alternative	Itraconazole potently inhibits CYP3A4, which metabolizes both R-warfarin (also metabolized by CYP1A2) and the more active S-warfarin (also metabolized by CYP2C9)	Necessary to monitor the effects of warfarin closely (weekly INR) and to warn patients to report any symptoms of bleeding ➢ ***For signs and symptoms of hypoglycemia, see Clinical Features of Some Adverse Drug Interactions, Bleeding disorders***

(Continued)

Primary Drug	Secondary Drug	Effect	Mechanism	Precautions
COUMARINS				
COUMARINS	GRISEOFULVIN	Possible ↓ anticoagulant effect coumarins and phenindione	Uncertain at present	Necessary to monitor the effects of warfarin closely (weekly INR) and to warn patients to report any symptoms of bleeding ➢ ***For signs and symptoms of hypoglycemia, see Clinical Features of Some Adverse Drug Interactions, Bleeding disorders***
COUMARINS	**ANTIGOUT DRUGS**			
COUMARINS	ALLOPURINOL	Uncommon instances of ↑ anticoagulant effect in patients on warfarin who have started allopurinol	Allopurinol possibly ↓ hepatic metabolism of warfarin but is considerable individual variation	Monitor INR at least weekly until stable
COUMARINS	BENZBROMARONE	↑ Warfarin levels	Inhibition of CYP2D6-mediated metabolism of warfarin	Monitor INR closely until stabilized—consider ↓ warfarin dose (one study suggested ↓ dose by 1/3)
COUMARINS	SULFINPYRAZONE	↑ Anticoagulant effect of warfarin	Uncertain; possibly displacement of anticoagulant from plasma proteins, possibly inhibition of CYP2C9-mediated metabolism of warfarin	Monitor INR until stable
COUMARINS	ANTIHYPERTENSIVES AND HEART FAILURE DRUGS—VASODILATOR ANTIHYPERTENSIVES	Bosentan may ↓ warfarin levels Iloprost and sitaxentan may ↑ warfarin levels	1. Uncertain; postulated that bosentan induces CYP3A4 and CYP2C9 2. Uncertain	Monitor INR closely
COUMARINS	ANTIOBESITY DRUGS—ORLISTAT	↓ Anticoagulant effect	Probably ↓ absorption of coumarins	Monitor INR closely until stable
COUMARINS	ANTI-PARKINSON'S DRUGS—ENTACAPONE	↑ Anticoagulant effect	Uncertain at present	Monitor INR at least weekly until stable
COUMARINS	**ANTIPLATELET AGENTS**			
COUMARINS	ASPIRIN	Risk of bleeding when high-dose aspirin is coadministered with anticoagulants; less risk with low-dose aspirin	Antiplatelet effects of aspirin add to the anticoagulant effects. Aspirin also irritates the gastric mucosa	Avoid coadministration of anticoagulants and high-dose aspirin. Patients on warfarin should be warned that many OTCs and some herbal remedies contain aspirin

(Continued)

Primary Drug	Secondary Drug	Effect	Mechanism	Precautions
COUMARINS				
COUMARINS	CLOPIDOGREL	Risk of bleeding when clopidogrel coadministered with anticoagulants	Additive effect on different parts of the clotting mechanism	Closely monitor effects; watch for signs of excess bleeding
COUMARINS	DIPYRIDAMOLE	Cases of mild bleeding when dipyridamole is added to warfarin	Antiplatelet effects of dipyridamole add to the anticoagulant effects	Warn patients to report early signs of bleeding
COUMARINS	PRASUGREL	Risk of bleeding when prasugrel is coadministered with anticoagulants	Additive effect on different parts of the clotting mechanism	Closely monitor effects; watch for signs of excess bleeding
COUMARINS	ANTIPROTOZOALS—LEVAMISOLE	Possible ↑ anticoagulant effect	Uncertain	Monitor INR closely
COUMARINS	**ANTIVIRALS**			
COUMARINS	NNRTIs	↓ Efficacy of warfarin with nevirapine	Altered metabolism. S-warfarin is metabolized by CYP2D6, R-warfarin by CYP3A4	Monitor INR every 3–7 days when starting or altering treatment and adjust dose by 10% as necessary. May need an approximately twofold increase in dose
COUMARINS	PROTEASE INHIBITORS	1. Anticoagulant effect may be altered (cases of both ↑ and ↓) when ritonavir and possibly saquinavir are given with warfarin 2. Reduced anticoagulant effect with tipranavir/ritonavir after 10 days 3. Possibly ↓ anticoagulant effect when ritonavir and nelfinavir are given with acenocoumarol	1 and 2. Complex interaction. Ritonavir initially inhibits CYP3A4 and CYP2C9 and then induces these and CYP1A2 3. Probably competition for metabolism via CYP2C9 (nelfinavir) or CYP2C9 induction (ritonavir)	Monitor INR closely, adjust anticoagulant doses as needed. Consider alternative anticoagulation
COUMARINS	APREPITANT	Possible ↓ in INR when aprepitant is added to warfarin	Aprepitant ↑ CYP2C9-mediated metabolism of warfarin	Monitor INR carefully for 2 weeks after completing each course of aprepitant
COUMARINS	CNS STIMULANTS—MODAFINIL	May cause moderate ↑ plasma concentrations of warfarin	Modafinil is a reversible inhibitor of CYP2C9 and CYP2C19 when used in therapeutic doses	Be aware

(Continued)

ANTICOAGULANTS COUMARINS

Primary Drug	Secondary Drug	Effect	Mechanism	Precautions
COUMARINS				
COUMARINS	CRANBERRY JUICE	Cases of markedly ↑ anticoagulant effect (including fatal hemorrhage) with regular cranberry juice ingestion	Uncertain; possibly due to inhibition of CYP-mediated metabolism of warfarin	Patients taking warfarin should avoid cranberry juice
COUMARINS	DANAZOL	Possible ↓ anticoagulant effect	Uncertain	Monitor INR at least weekly until stable
COUMARINS	DISULFIRAM	↑ Anticoagulant effect	Uncertain at present	Monitor INR at least weekly until stable
COUMARINS	GESTRINONE	Possible ↓ anticoagulant effect	Uncertain	Monitor INR at least weekly until stable
COUMARINS	GLUCAGON	↑ Anticoagulant effect	Uncertain at present	Monitor INR after administration of glucagon
COUMARINS	GLUCOSAMINE	↑ Anticoagulant effect	Uncertain at present	Avoid coadministration
COUMARINS	GRAPEFRUIT JUICE	↑ Efficacy and ↑ adverse effects of warfarin, e.g., ↑ INR, hemorrhage	Unclear. Possibly via inhibition of intestinal CYP3A4	Monitor INR more closely. Avoid concomitant use if unstable INR
COUMARINS	H2 RECEPTOR BLOCKERS	↑ Anticoagulant effect with cimetidine and possibly famotidine	Inhibition of metabolism via CYP1A2, CYP2C9, and CYP2C19	Use alternative acid suppression, e.g., other H2 antagonist or protein pump inhibitor (not esomeprazole, lansoprazole or omeprazole) or monitor INR more closely; ↓ dose may be required. Take acid suppression regularly and not PRN if it affects INR control
COUMARINS	IVACAFTOR	Theoretical risk of ↑ warfarin levels	Ivacator inhibits CYP2C9 which metabolizes warfarin	Monitor INR closely until stable
COUMARINS	LEUKOTRIENE ANTAGONISTS	Zafirlukast ↑ anticoagulant effect	Zafirlukast inhibits CYP2C9-mediated metabolism of warfarin	Monitor INR at least weekly until stable
COUMARINS	**LIPID-LOWERING DRUGS**			
COUMARINS	ANION EXCHANGE RESINS	↓ Anticoagulant effect with colestyramine	↓ Absorption of warfarin	Give warfarin 1 h before or 4–6 h after colestyramine
COUMARINS	FIBRATES	↑ Efficacy of warfarin and phenindione	Uncertain; postulated that fibrates displace anticoagulants from their binding sites	Monitor INR closely

(*Continued*)

Primary Drug	Secondary Drug	Effect	Mechanism	Precautions
COUMARINS				
COUMARINS	STATINS	Possible ↑ anticoagulant effect with fluvastatin and simvastatin	Uncertain; possibly due to inhibition of CYP2C9-mediated metabolism of warfarin	Monitor INR at least weekly until stable
COUMARINS	NANDROLONE	Episodes of bleeding when patients on oral anticoagulants are started on anabolic steroids	Not understood	Reduce the dose of anticoagulant by 50% and monitor INR closely until stabilized
COUMARINS	ESTROGENS	↑ Anticoagulant effect	Uncertain at present	Estrogens are usually not recommended in those with a history of thromboembolism; if they are used, monitor INR closely
COUMARINS	PERIPHERAL VASODILATORS	Cases of major hemorrhage when pentoxifylline is given with acenocoumarol	Uncertain; possibly additive effect (pentoxifylline has an antiplatelet action)	Monitor INR closely
COUMARINS	PIRACETAM	Case of bleeding associated with ↑ INR in a patient taking warfarin 1 month after starting piracetam	Uncertain; piracetam inhibits platelet aggregation but uncertain whether it has any effect on other aspects of the clotting cascade	Warn patients to report easy bruising, etc. Monitor INR closely
COUMARINS	PROGESTOGENS	↓ Anticoagulant effect	Uncertain at present	Monitor INR closely
COUMARINS	PROTON PUMP INHIBITORS	Possibly ↑ anticoagulant effect particularly when esomeprazole, lansoprazole, or omeprazole is added to warfarin	Omeprazole and lansoprazole induce CYP1A2, which plays a role in the activation of coumarins. Inhibition of anticoagulant metabolism via CYP2C9 and CYP2C19 likely to be involved	Monitor INR more closely. ↓ dose may be required. If values are 10% or 20%–30% over range, omit the dose for 1 or 2 days respectively, and consider ↓ maintenance dose by 10%. Regular dosing of a proton pump inhibitor is preferable if it affects INR significantly. Not reported with pantoprazole or rabeprazole
COUMARINS	RALOXIFENE	Possible ↓ anticoagulant effect, which may take several weeks to develop	Uncertain at present	Monitor INR closely for several weeks
COUMARINS	SUCRALFATE	Possible ↓ anticoagulant effect	↓ Absorption of warfarin	Monitor INR at least weekly until stable

(*Continued*)

ANTICOAGULANTS DABIGATRAN

Primary Drug	Secondary Drug	Effect	Mechanism	Precautions
COUMARINS				
COUMARINS	SYMPATHOMIMETICS—INDIRECT	Methylphenidate may increase the efficacy of warfarin	Uncertain at present	Monitor INR at least weekly until stable
COUMARINS	TESTOSTERONE	Possible ↑ anticoagulant effect	Uncertain	Monitor INR at least weekly until stable
COUMARINS	THYROID HORMONES	Possible ↑ anticoagulant effect	Uncertain	Monitor INR at least weekly until stable
COUMARINS	VITAMIN E	Case of ↑ anticoagulant effect	Uncertain	Monitor INR closely for 1–2 weeks after starting and stopping vitamin E

Primary Drug	Secondary Drug	Effect	Mechanism	Precautions
DABIGATRAN				
DABIGATRAN	ANAGRELIDE	Theoretical ↑ risk of bleeding	Additive effect; both drugs have the potential to cause bleeding	Warn patients to report early evidence of bleeding
DABIGATRAN	ANALGESICS—NSAIDs	↑ Risk of bleeding	Uncertain	Avoid coadministration
DABIGATRAN	**ANTIARRHYTHMICS**			
DABIGATRAN	AMIODARONE	↑ Dabigatran levels	Inhibition of Pgp	Reduce dose of dabigatran to 150 mg/day (75 mg in renal failure)
DABIGATRAN	DRONEDARONE	↑ Dabigatran levels	Possible inhibition of Pgp Coadministration increases dabigatran exposure by 70%–140%; when dronedarone administered 2 h after dabigatran, exposure ↑ only 30%–60%	Reduce dose of dabigatran to 150 mg/day (75 mg in renal failure)
DABIGATRAN	QUINIDINE	↑ Dabigatran levels	Inhibition of Pgp	Reduce dose of dabigatran to 150 mg/day (75 mg in renal failure)
DABIGATRAN	**ANTIBIOTICS**			
DABIGATRAN	CLARITHROMYCIN	Theoretical risk of ↑ dabigatran levels	Possible inhibition of Pgp	Warn patients to report early evidence of bleeding. Manufacturers state that ↑ dabigatran levels are not clinically significant

(*Continued*)

Primary Drug	Secondary Drug	Effect	Mechanism	Precautions
DABIGATRAN				
DABIGATRAN	RIFAMPICIN	↓ Dabigatran levels	Induction of Pgp	Manufacturers advise against coadministration
DABIGATRAN	**ANTICANCER AND IMMUNOMODULATING DRUGS**			
DABIGATRAN	BEVACIZUMAB	Theoretical risk of increased bleeding; limited evidence suggests this might not be the case	Additive, bevacizumab associated with increased risk of hemorrhage	Monitor concurrent use
DABIGATRAN	CICLOSPORIN, CRIZOTINIB, TACROLIMUS	↑ Dabigatran levels	Induction of Pgp	Manufacturers advise against coadministration
DABIGATRAN	IPILIMUMAB	↑ Risk of bleeding	Additive	Monitor closely
DABIGATRAN	RUXOLITINIB	Predicted increase in Pgp or BCRP substrate levels	P-glycoprotein/BCRP inhibition	Monitor closely Separate administration of drugs
DABIGATRAN	ANTICOAGULANTS	↑ Risk of bleeding	Additive effect	Avoid coadministration
DABIGATRAN	**ANTIDEPRESSANTS**			
DABIGATRAN	ST. JOHN'S WORT	↓ Dabigatran levels	Induction of Pgp	Manufacturers recommend avoiding coadministration
DABIGATRAN	SSRIs, SNRIs	↑ Effect of dabigatran	Uncertain	Warn patients to report early evidence of bleeding
DABIGATRAN	ANTIEPILEPTICS—CARBAMAZEPINE, PHENYTOIN	↓ Dabigatran levels	Induction of Pgp	Manufacturers advise against coadministration
DABIGATRAN	**ANTIFUNGALS**			
DABIGATRAN	ITRACONAZOLE, POSACONAZOLE	↑ Dabigatran levels	Inhibition of Pgp	Manufacturers advise against coadministration
DABIGATRAN	KETOCONAZOLE	↑ Dabigatran levels	Inhibition of Pgp	UK manufacturer advises against coadministration; U.S. manufacturer recommends reducing dose to 75 mg bd
DABIGATRAN	ANTIGOUT DRUGS—SULFINPYRAZONE	Possible ↑ risk of bleeding	Uncertain	Manufacturers of dabigatran advise caution with concomitant use
DABIGATRAN	ANTIPLATELETS	↑ Risk of bleeding	Additive effect	Avoid coadministration
DABIGATRAN	ANTIVIRALS—PROTEASE INHIBITORS, RILPIVIRINE	↑ Dabigatran levels	Inhibition of Pgp	Avoid coadministration

(Continued)

ANTICOAGULANTS DABIGATRAN

Primary Drug	Secondary Drug	Effect	Mechanism	Precautions
DABIGATRAN				
DABIGATRAN	CALCIUM CHANNEL BLOCKERS—VERAPAMIL	↑ Dabigatran levels	Inhibition of Pgp	Reduce dose: 1. VTE prophylaxis—150 mg od (taken at the same time as verapamil)—reduce further to 75 mg od in presence of renal impairment 2. Stroke prophylaxis—110 mg bd
DABIGATRAN	ELIGLUSTAT	↑ Dabigatran levels	Inhibition of Pgp	Reduce dose of dabigatran; warn patients to report bleeding
DABIGATRAN	H2-RECEPTOR BLOCKERS	↓ Dabigatran levels	Dabigatran capsules require an acidic environment for dissolution; increasing gastric pH reduces this process	Avoid coadministration
DABIGATRAN	PROTON PUMP INHIBITORS	↓ Dabigatran levels	Dabigatran capsules require an acidic environment for dissolution; increasing gastric pH reduces this process	Avoid coadministration
DABIGATRAN	ULIPRISTAL	↑ Dabigatran levels	Inhibition of Pgp	Avoid coadministration

Primary Drug	Secondary Drug	Effect	Mechanism	Precautions
FONDAPARINUX				
FONDAPARINUX	ANTICOAGULANTS—PARENTERAL	↑ Risk of bleeding when heparins are given with fondaparinux	Combined anticoagulant effect	Manufacturers recommend avoiding coadministration

Primary Drug	Secondary Drug	Effect	Mechanism	Precautions
HEPARINS				
HEPARINS	ALISKIREN	Risk of hyperkalemia with heparin	Additive effect	Monitor serum potassium closely

(*Continued*)

Primary Drug	Secondary Drug	Effect	Mechanism	Precautions
HEPARINS				
HEPARINS	ANALESICS—NSAIDS	1. Risk of prolonged bleeding when ketorolac is coadministered with dalteparin (but not enoxaparin), and intravenous diclofenac is given with heparins 2. ↑ Risk of hyperkalemia when ketorolac is given with heparin	1. Uncertain 2. Heparin inhibits aldosterone secretion, causing hyperkalemia	1. Avoid coadministration 2. Monitor potassium levels closely
HEPARINS	ANTICOAGULANTS—PARENTERAL	↑ Risk of bleeding when heparins are given with fondaparinux	Combined anticoagulant effect	Manufacturers recommend avoiding coadministration
HEPARINS	**ANTIHYPERTENSIVES AND HEART FAILURE DRUGS**			
HEPARINS	ACE INHIBITORS, ANGIOTENSIN II RECEPTOR ANTAGONISTS	↑ Risk of hyperkalemia	Heparin inhibits aldosterone secretion, causing hyperkalemia	Monitor potassium levels closely
HEPARINS	VASODILATOR ANTIHYPERTENSIVES	Possible ↑ risk of bleeding with iloprost	Anticoagulant effects of heparins ↑ by a mechanism that is uncertain at present	Monitor APTT closely
HEPARINS	ANTIOBESITY DRUGS—SIBUTRAMINE	Possible ↑ risk of bleeding	Uncertain	Monitor APTT closely
HEPARINS	ANTIPLATELET AGENTS	↑ Risk of bleeding when heparins are coadministered with glycoprotein IIb/IIIa inhibitors, dipyridamole, clopidogrel, or high-dose aspirin	Additive effect on different parts of the clotting mechanism. Aspirin also irritates the gastric mucosa	Closely monitor effects; watch for signs of excess bleeding. Avoid coadministration of heparins with high-dose aspirin
HEPARINS	DROTRECOGIN ALFA (recombinant activated protein C)	↑ Risk of bleeding	Drotrecogin alfa ↓ prothrombin production and has fibrinolytic/antithrombotic effects	Avoid coadministration of drotrecogin alfa with high-dose heparin (>15 IU/kg/h). Carefully consider the risk–benefit ratio when giving lower doses of heparin
HEPARINS	NITRATES	Possible ↓ efficacy of heparin with GTN infusion	Uncertain	Monitor APTT closely

(*Continued*)

ANTICOAGULANTS HEPARINS

ANTICOAGULANTS RIVAROXABAN

Primary Drug	Secondary Drug	Effect	Mechanism	Precautions
HEPARINS				
HEPARINS	THROMBOLYTICS	Heparin requirements are ↑ when administered after streptokinase	Uncertain at present	Monitor APTT closely when starting heparin after streptokinase
HIRUDINS				
HIRUDINS	THROMBOLYTICS	↑ Risk of bleeding complications when alteplase or streptokinase is coadministered with lepirudin	Additive effect on clotting cascade	Watch for bleeding complications. Risk–benefit analysis is needed before coadministering; this will involve availability of alternative therapies such as primary angioplasty

Primary Drug	Secondary Drug	Effect	Mechanism	Precautions
RIVAROXABAN				
RIVAROXABAN	ANTIARRHYTHMICS—DRONEDARONE	No information on specific effect with rivaroxaban	No specific information relating to mechanism	Manufacturer of rivaroxaban advises avoid concomitant use with dronedarone
RIVAROXABAN	ANTIBIOTICS—RIFAMPICIN	↓ Rivaroxaban plasma concentrations	Induction of P-glycoprotein and CYP3A4-mediated metabolism of rivaroxaban	Concomitant use of rifampin and rivaroxaban should be avoided
RIVAROXABAN	**ANTICANCER AND IMMUNOMODULATING DRUGS**			
RIVAROXABAN	BEVACIZUMAB	Theoretical risk of increased bleeding; limited evidence suggests this might not be the case	Additive, bevacizumab associated with increased risk of hemorrhage	Monitor concurrent use
RIVAROXABAN	IPILIMUMAB	↑ Risk of bleeding	Additive	Monitor closely
RIVAROXABAN	ANTICOAGULANTS	↑ Risk of bleeding	Additive effect	Avoid coadministration
RIVAROXABAN	ANTIDEPRESSANTS—ST. JOHN'S WORT	↓ Rivaroxaban exposure	Induction of CYP3A4-mediated metabolism and Pgp-mediated efflux transport	Avoid coadministration
RIVAROXABAN	ANTIEPILEPTICS—CARBAMAZEPINE, PHENOBARBITAL, PHENYTOIN	↓ Rivaroxaban exposure	Induction of CYP3A4-mediated metabolism and Pgp-mediated efflux transport	Avoid coadministration

(*Continued*)

Primary Drug	Secondary Drug	Effect	Mechanism	Precautions
RIVAROXABAN				
RIVAROXABAN	ANTIFUNGALS—ITRACONAZOLE, KETOCONAZOLE, POSACONAZOLE, VORICONAZOLE	↑ Rivaroxaban exposure	Inhibition of CYP3A4-mediated metabolism and Pgp-mediated efflux transport	Avoid coadministration
RIVAROXABAN	ANTIPLATELETS—PRASUGREL	Risk of bleeding when prasugrel is coadministered with anticoagulants	Additive effect on different parts of the clotting mechanism	Closely monitor effects; watch for signs of excess bleeding
RIVAROXABAN	ANTIVIRALS—COBICISTAT, PROTEASE INHIBITORS	↑ Plasma levels of rivaroxaban, ↑ risk of overanticoagulation and bleeding	Inhibition of metabolism via CYP3A and Pgp	Avoid coadministration

Primary Drug	Secondary Drug	Effect	Mechanism	Precautions
THROMBOLYTICS				
THROMBOLYTICS	**ANTICOAGULANTS—PARENTERAL**			
THROMBOLYTICS	HEPARINS	Heparin requirements are ↑ when administered after streptokinase	Uncertain at present	Monitor APTT closely when starting heparin after streptokinase
THROMBOLYTICS	HIRUDINS	↑ Risk of bleeding complications when alteplase or streptokinase coadministered with lepirudin	Additive effect on clotting cascade	Watch for bleeding complications. Risk–benefit analysis is needed before coadministering; this will involve the availability of alternative therapies such as primary angioplasty
THROMBOLYTICS	**ANTIPLATELET AGENTS**			
THROMBOLYTICS	ASPIRIN	↑ Risk of intracerebral bleeding when streptokinase is coadministered with high-dose (300 mg) aspirin	Additive effect	Avoid coingestion when streptokinase is given for cerebral infarction; use low-dose aspirin when coadministered for myocardial infarction

(Continued)

Primary Drug	Secondary Drug	Effect	Mechanism	Precautions
THROMBOLYTICS				
THROMBOLYTICS	GLYCOPROTEIN Iib/IIia INHIBITORS	1. ↑ Risk of major hemorrhage when coadministered with alteplase 2. Possible ↑ risk of bleeding complications when streptokinase is coadministered with eptifibatide	1. Uncertain; other thrombolytics do not seem to interact 2. Additive effect	1. Avoid coadministration 2. Watch for bleeding complications. Risk–benefit analysis is needed before coadministering; this will involve the availability of alternative therapies such as primary angioplasty
THROMBOLYTICS	THROMBOLYTICS	Repeated doses of streptokinase are ineffective, and there is ↑ risk of allergic reactions	Antistreptococcal antibodies are formed within a few days of administering a dose; these neutralize subsequent doses	Do not give more than one dose of streptokinase

ANTICOAGULANTS THROMBOLYTICS

PART 5

Antidiabetic Drugs

Yohan P. Samarasinghe, Ming Ming Teh, and Janaka Karalliedde

1. ACARBOSE
2. BIGUANIDES—METFORMIN
3. DIPEPTIDYL PEPTIDASE-4 (DDP-4) INHIBITORS (GLIPTINS)
4. GLUCAGON-LIKE PEPTIDE-1 (GLP-1) ANALOGUES
5. INSULIN
6. MEGLITINIDE DERIVATIVES—NATEGLINIDE, REPAGLINIDE
7. SODIUM-GLUCOSE CO-TRANSPORTER 2 (SGLT-2) INHIBITORS (GLIFLOZINS)
8. SULFONYLUREAS
9. THIAZOLIDINEDIONES (GLITAZONES)—PIOGLITAZONE, ROSIGLITAZONE

Primary Drug	Secondary Drug	Effect	Mechanism	Precautions
ACARBOSE				
ACARBOSE	ALCOHOL	Tends to mask signs of hypoglycemia and ↑ risk of hypoglycemic episodes	Inhibits glucose production and release from many sources, including the liver	Watch for and warn patients about symptoms of hypoglycemia. ➢ ***For signs and symptoms of hypoglycemia, see Clinical Features of Some Adverse Drug Interactions, Hypoglycemia***
ACARBOSE	**ANTIBIOTICS**			
ACARBOSE	AMINOGLYCOSIDES—NEOMYCIN	↑ Postprandial hypoglycemia and ↑ Gastrointestinal effects as a result of concurrent use of acarbose and neomycin	Neomycin is known to cause a drop in blood glucose levels after meals; when used concomitantly with acarbose, this ↓ may be ↑. Neomycin also exacerbates the adverse gastrointestinal effects caused by acarbose	Blood glucose levels should be closely monitored; if gastrointestinal signs are severe, the dose of acarbose should be ↓
ACARBOSE	QUINOLONES—CIPROFLOXACIN, NORFLOXACIN, OFLOXACIN	↑ Risk of hypoglycemic episodes	Mechanism uncertain. Ciprofloxacin is a potent inhibitor of CYP1A2. Norfloxacin is a weak inhibitor of CYP1A2, but these drugs may inhibit other CYP isoenzymes to varying degrees	Watch for and warn patients about symptoms of hypoglycemia. ➢ ***For signs and symptoms of hypoglycemia, see Clinical Features of Some Adverse Drug Interactions, Hypoglycemia***
ACARBOSE	**ANTIDEPRESSANTS**			
ACARBOSE	SSRIs	Fluctuations in blood sugar are very likely, with both hypoglycemic and hyperglycemic events being reported in diabetics receiving hypoglycemic treatment	Brain serotonin and corticotropin-releasing hormone systems participate in the control of blood sugar levels. ↑ (usually acute) in brain serotonergic activity induces a hyperglycemic response	Both hyper- and hypoglycemic responses have been reported with SSRIs; there is a need to monitor blood glucose closely prior to, during, and after discontinuing SSRI treatment. ➢ ***For signs and symptoms of hypoglycemia and hpyerglycemia, see Clinical Features of Some Adverse Drug Interactions, Hypoglycemia, Hpyerglycemia***

(*Continued*)

Primary Drug	Secondary Drug	Effect	Mechanism	Precautions
ACARBOSE				
ACARBOSE	TCAs	Likely to impair control of diabetes	TCAs may ↑ serum glucose levels by up to 150%, ↑ appetite (particularly carbohydrate craving), and ↓ metabolic rate	Be aware and monitor blood sugar weekly until stable. They are generally considered safe unless diabetes is poorly controlled or is associated with significant cardiac or renal disease. Amitriptyline, imipramine, and citalopram are also used to treat painful diabetic neuropathy
ACARBOSE	ANTIDIABETIC DRUGS	↑ Risk of hypoglycemic episodes	Due to additive effects by similar or differing mechanisms to lower blood sugar	Combinations are often used and useful. Warn patients about hypoglycemia. ➢ ***For signs and symptoms of hypoglycemia, see Clinical Features of Some Adverse Drug Interactions, Hypoglycemia***
ACARBOSE	ANTIEPILEPTICS—VALPROATE	Case of ↓ valproate levels	Uncertain	Monitor valproate levels
ACARBOSE	ANTIHYPERTENSIVES AND HEART FAILURE DRUGS—ADRENERGIC NEURONE BLOCKERS	↑ Hypoglycemic effect	Catecholamines are diabetogenic; guanethidine blocks the release of catecholamines from nerve endings	Monitor blood glucose closely
ACARBOSE	ANTIOBESITY DRUGS—ORLISTAT, RIMONABANT, SIBUTRAMINE	Tendency for blood glucose levels to fluctuate	These agents change dietary intake of carbohydrates and other foods, and the risk of fluctuations in blood glucose is greater if there is a concurrent dietary regimen. A side effect of orlistat is hypoglycemia	These agents are used often in patients with type II diabetes who are on hypoglycemic therapy. Need to monitor blood sugar twice weekly until stable. Advise self-monitoring. Watch for and warn patients about symptoms of hypoglycemia. Avoid coadministration of acarbose and orlistat. ➢ ***For signs and symptoms of hypoglycemia, see Clinical Features of Some Adverse Drug Interactions, Hypoglycemia***

(Continued)

Primary Drug	Secondary Drug	Effect	Mechanism	Precautions
ACARBOSE				
ACARBOSE	ANTIPLATELET AGENTS—ASPIRIN	Risk of hypoglycemia when high-dose aspirin (3.5–7.5 g/day) is given with antidiabetic drugs	Additive effect; aspirin has a hypoglycemic effect	Avoid high-dose aspirin
ACARBOSE	ANTIPROTOZOALS—PENTAMIDINE	May alter acarbose requirements due to altered glycemic control	Attributed to pancreatic beta cell toxicity	Need to monitor blood sugar until stable and the following withdrawal of pentamidine
ACARBOSE	CARDIAC GLYCOSIDES	Acarbose may ↓ plasma levels of digoxin	Uncertain; possibly ↓ absorption of digoxin	Monitor digoxin levels; watch for ↓ levels
ACARBOSE	H2 RECEPTOR BLOCKERS—RANITIDINE	↓ Blood levels of ranitidine	Possibly due to ↓ absorption of ranitidine	Be aware
ACARBOSE	LIPID-LOWERING DRUGS—ANION EXCHANGE RESINS	↑ Hypoglycemic effect of acarbose	Uncertain	Monitor blood glucose during coadministration and after discontinuation of concurrent therapy
ACARBOSE	MUSCLE RELAXANTS—BACLOFEN	↓ Hypoglycemic effect	Due to these drugs causing hyperglycemia, the mechanism is uncertain at present	↑ Doses of antidiabetic drugs are often required for adequate glycemic control
ACARBOSE	NANDROLONE	↑ Effect of antidiabetic drugs	Uncertain	Monitor blood sugar closely. Banned by sporting authorities
ACARBOSE	NIACIN	↓ Hypoglycemic effect	Uncertain at present. The effects of niacin (< or = 2.5 g/d), alone or in combination with statins, on fasting glucose (an increase of 4%–5%) and hemoglobin A1c levels (an increase of < or = 0.3%) are modest, transient or reversible	Typically amenable to adjustments in oral hypoglycemic regimens without discontinuing niacin. Benefits outweigh risks. ↑ Doses of antidiabetics are often necessary

(*Continued*)

ANTIDIABETIC DRUGS ACARBOSE

Primary Drug	Secondary Drug	Effect	Mechanism	Precautions
ACARBOSE				
ACARBOSE	NICOTINE	↓ Hypoglycemic effect	Uncertain at present. Exposure of human blood samples to nicotine raised the level of hemoglobin A1c. The higher the nicotine dose, the more the A1c level rose. Cigarettes, by working through a drug interaction cause the body to release its own stores of sugar usually in a matter of seconds	↑ Doses of antidiabetic drugs are often required for adequate glycemic control
ACARBOSE	ESTROGENS	Altered glycemic control	Uncertain at present. Significantly high or low levels of estrogen could both be involved in the development of insulin resistance. Higher than normal estrogen appears to be linked with increased insulin resistance, yet other studies have shown that low estrogen levels, are linked with greater insulin resistance	Monitor blood glucose closely
ACARBOSE	PANCREATIN	Theoretical risk of ↓ efficacy of acarbose	↓ Absorption	Watch for poor response to acarbose; monitor capillary blood glucose closely
ACARBOSE	PROGESTOGENS	Altered glycemic control	Uncertain at present. One study revealed that low progesterone levels, cause over-production of insulin, leading to hypoglycemia and an outpouring of adrenaline to bring sugar levels up	Monitor blood glucose closely
ACARBOSE	SOMATROPIN	↓ Hypoglycemic effect	Due to these drugs causing hyperglycemia, the mechanism is uncertain at present	↑ Doses of antidiabetic drugs are often required for adequate glycemic control
ACARBOSE	THYROID HORMONES	↓ Hypoglycemic effect	Due to these drugs causing hyperglycemia, the mechanism is uncertain at present	↑ Doses of antidiabetic drugs are often required for adequate glycemic control

Primary Drug	Secondary Drug	Effect	Mechanism	Precautions
BIGUANIDES—METFORMIN				
METFORMIN	ALCOHOL	Enhanced effect of metformin and ↑ risk of lactic acidosis. May mask signs and symptoms of hypoglycemia	Alcohol is known to influence the effect of metformin on lactate metabolism. Inhibits glucose production and release from many sources, including the liver and release	Watch for and warn patients about symptoms of hypoglycemia. The onset of lactic acidosis is often subtle with symptoms of malaise, myalgia, respiratory distress, and ↑ nonspecific abdominal distress. There may be hypothermia and resistant bradyarrhythmias. ➢ ***For signs and symptoms of hypoglycemia, see Clinical Features of Some Adverse Drug Interactions, Hypoglycemia***
METFORMIN	**ANALGESICS**			
METFORMIN	NSAIDs	Possibility of ↑ plasma levels of metformin if there is renal impairment due to NSAIDs. High metformin levels cause lactic acidosis	NSAIDs can cause renal dysfunction and lead to accumulation of metformin, which is mainly excreted unchanged via kidneys	Do not use metformin if serum creatinine is >1.5 mg/dL in males and >1.4 mg/dL in females, or creatinine clearance is <30 mL/min. Use with caution in patients who have a creatinine clearance of 30–60 mL/min. Warn patients about hypoglycemia. ➢ ***For signs and symptoms of hypoglycemia, see Clinical Features of Some Adverse Drug Interactions, Hypoglycemia***
METFORMIN	MORPHINE	↑ Level of metformin and risk of lactic acidosis. The onset of lactic acidosis is often subtle with symptoms of malaise, myalgia, respiratory distress, and ↑ nonspecific abdominal distress. There may be hypothermia and resistant bradyarrhythmias	Metformin is not metabolized in humans and is not protein bound. Competition for renal tubular excretion is the basis for ↑ activity or retention of metformin	A theoretical possibility. Need to consider ↓ of metformin dose or avoidance of coadministration. Warn patients about hypoglycemia. ➢ ***For signs and symptoms of hypoglycemia, see Clinical Features of Some Adverse Drug Interactions, Hypoglycemia***

(*Continued*)

ANTIDIABETIC DRUGS BIGUANIDES—METFORMIN

ANTIDIABETIC DRUGS BIGUANIDES—METFORMIN

Primary Drug	Secondary Drug	Effect	Mechanism	Precautions
BIGUANIDES—METFORMIN				
METFORMIN	ANTIARRHYTHMICS—DISOPYRAMIDE	↑ Risk of hypoglycemic episodes	Disopyramide and its metabolite mono-isopropyl disopyramide ↑ secretion of insulin (considered to be due to inhibition of potassium-ATP channels). Suggestion that disopyramide causes an impairment of the counterregulatory (homeostatic) mechanisms that follow hypoglycemia	The risk of this interaction is high. Recommended that if disopyramide is absolutely necessary, doses in the lower range (1–4 ng/mL) be used. Watch for and warn patients about symptoms of hypoglycemia. ➢ ***For signs and symptoms of hypoglycemia, see Clinical Features of Some Adverse Drug Interactions, Hypoglycemia***
METFORMIN	**ANTIBIOTICS**			
METFORMIN	AMINOGLYCOSIDES	Risk of hypoglycemia due to ↑ plasma concentrations of metformin	Mechanism uncertain. Metformin does not undergo hepatic metabolism. Renal tubular secretion is the major route of metformin elimination. Aminoglycosides are also principally excreted via the kidney, and nephrotoxicity is an important side effect	Watch and monitor for hypoglycemia, and warn patients about it. ➢ ***For signs and symptoms of hypoglycemia, see Clinical Features of Some Adverse Drug Interactions, Hypoglycemia***
METFORMIN	ISONIAZID	↓ Efficacy of antidiabetic drugs	Isoniazid causes hyperglycemia, the mechanism is uncertain at present	Monitor capillary blood glucose closely; ↑ doses of antidiabetic drugs may be needed
METFORMIN	QUINOLONES	↑ Risk of hypoglycemic episodes	Mechanism uncertain	Watch for and warn patients about symptoms of hypoglycemia. ➢ ***For signs and symptoms of hypoglycemia, see Clinical Features of Some Adverse Drug Interactions, Hypoglycemia***

(*Continued*)

Primary Drug	Secondary Drug	Effect	Mechanism	Precautions
BIGUANIDES—METFORMIN				
METFORMIN	**ANTICANCER AND IMMUNOMODULATING DRUGS**			
METFORMIN	CYTOTOXICS—PLATINUM COMPOUNDS	↑ Risk of lactic acidosis	Renal excretion of metformin is ↓	Watch for lactic acidosis. The onset of lactic acidosis is often subtle with symptoms of malaise, myalgia, respiratory distress, and ↑ nonspecific abdominal distress. There may be hypothermia and resistant bradyarrhythmias
METFORMIN	HORMONES AND HORMONE ANTAGONISTS—LANREOTIDE, OCTREOTIDE	Likely to alter metformin requirements	Octreotide and lanreotide suppress pancreatic insulin and counterregulatory hormones (glucagon, growth hormone) and delay or ↓ absorption of glucose from the intestine	Essential to monitor blood sugar at least twice a week after initiating concurrent treatment until blood sugar levels are stable. Advise self-monitoring. Warn patients about hypoglycemia. ➢ ***For signs and symptoms of hypoglycemia, see Clinical Features of Some Adverse Drug Interactions, Hypoglycemia***
METFORMIN	**IMMUNOMODULATING DRUGS**			
METFORMIN	CORTICOSTEROIDS	Often ↑ requirements of hypoglycemic agent, particularly with high glucocorticoid activity steroids	Corticosteroids, particularly the glucocorticoids (betamethasone, dexamethasone, deflazacort, prednisolone > cortisone, hydrocortisone), have intrinsic hyperglycemic activity in both diabetic and nondiabetic subjects	Monitor blood sugar during concomitant treatment, weekly if possible, or advise self-monitoring, until blood sugar levels are stable. Larger doses of glimepiride are often needed
METFORMIN	CRIZOTINIB	Possibly increased crizotinib levels	Attributed to decreased elimination due to interference with transporters	Clinical significance uncertain; be aware of possible interaction
METFORMIN	TACROLIMUS	↑ Level of metformin	↓ Renal excretion of metformin	Watch for and warn patients about hypoglycemia. ➢ ***For signs and symptoms of hypoglycemia, see Clinical Features of Some Adverse Drug Interactions, Hypoglycemia***

(Continued)

ANTIDIABETIC DRUGS BIGUANIDES—METFORMIN

Primary Drug	Secondary Drug	Effect	Mechanism	Precautions
BIGUANIDES—METFORMIN				
METFORMIN	**ANTIDEPRESSANTS**			
METFORMIN	SSRIs	Fluctuations in blood sugar are very likely, with both hypoglycemic and hyperglycemic events being reported in diabetics receiving hypoglycemic treatment	Brain serotonin- and corticotropin-releasing hormone systems participate in the control of blood sugar levels. ↑ (usually acute) in brain serotonergic activity induces a hyperglycemic response	Both hyper- and hypoglycemic responses have been reported with SSRIs, and there is a need to monitor blood glucose closely prior to, during, and after discontinuing SSRI treatment. ➢ ***For signs and symptoms of hypoglycemia, see Clinical Features of Some Adverse Drug Interactions, Hypoglycemia***
METFORMIN	TCAs	Likely to impair control of diabetes	TCAs may ↑ serum glucose levels by up to 150%, ↑ appetite (particularly carbohydrate craving) and ↓ metabolic rate	Be aware and monitor blood sugar weekly until stable. They are generally considered safe unless diabetes is poorly controlled or is associated with significant cardiac or renal disease. Amitriptyline, imipramine, and citalopram are also used to treat painful diabetic neuropathy
METFORMIN	**ANTIEPILEPTICS**			
METFORMIN	HYDANTOINS	↓ Hypoglycemic efficacy	Hydantoins are considered to ↓ release of insulin	Monitor capillary blood glucose closely; higher doses of antidiabetic drugs will be needed
METFORMIN	TOPIRAMATE	↑ Level of metformin	Unknown mechanism	Watch for and warn patients about hypoglycemia. ➢ ***For signs and symptoms of hypoglycemia, see Clinical Features of Some Adverse Drug Interactions, Hypoglycemia***
METFORMIN	ANTIGOUT DRUGS—PROBENECID	↑ Level of metformin and risk of lactic acidosis. The onset of lactic acidosis is often subtle with symptoms of malaise, myalgia, respiratory distress, and ↑ nonspecific abdominal distress. There may be hypothermia and resistant bradyarrhythmias	↓ Renal excretion of metformin	Watch for hypoglycemia and lactic acidosis. Warn patients about hypoglycemia. ➢ ***For signs and symptoms of hypoglycemia, see Clinical Features of Some Adverse Drug Interactions, Hypoglycemia***

(*Continued*)

Primary Drug	Secondary Drug	Effect	Mechanism	Precautions
BIGUANIDES—METFORMIN				
METFORMIN	ANTIHISTAMINES—KETOTIFEN	↓ Platelet count	Unknown	Avoid coadministration (manufacturers' recommendation)
METFORMIN	**ANTIHYPERTENSIVES AND HEART FAILURE DRUGS**			
METFORMIN	ACE INHIBITORS	↑ Risk of hypoglycemic episodes	Mechanism uncertain. ACE inhibitors possibly ↑ insulin sensitivity and glucose utilization. Altered renal function may also be a factor. ACE inhibitors may ↑ bradykinin levels, which ↓ production of glucose by the liver. Hypoglycemia is reported as a (rare) side effect of ACE inhibitors. It is suggested that the occurrence of hypoglycemia is greater with captopril than enalapril. Captopril and enalapril are used in the treatment of diabetic nephropathy	Concurrent treatment need not be avoided and is often beneficial in type II diabetes. Watch for and warn patients about symptoms of hypoglycemia. Be aware that the risk of hypoglycemia is greater in the elderly and in those with poor glycemic control. ➢ ***For signs and symptoms of hypoglycemia, see Clinical Features of Some Adverse Drug Interactions, Hypoglycemia***
METFORMIN	ADRENERGIC NEURON BLOCKERS	↑ Hypoglycemic effect	Catecholamines are diabetogenic; guanethidine blocks the release of catecholamines from nerve endings	Monitor blood glucose closely
METFORMIN	VASODILATOR ANTIHYPERTENSIVES—DIAZOXIDE	May ↑ metformin requirements	Diazoxide causes hyperglycemia by inhibiting insulin release and probably by a catecholamine-induced extrahepatic effect. Used in the treatment of hypoglycemia due to insulinomas	Larger doses of metformin are often required; need to monitor blood sugar until adequate control of blood sugar is achieved
METFORMIN	ANTIPLATELET AGENTS—ASPIRIN	Risk of hypoglycemia when high-dose aspirin (3.5–7.5 g/day) is given with antidiabetic drugs	Additive effect; aspirin has a hypoglycemic effect	Avoid high-dose aspirin

(Continued)

ANTIDIABETIC DRUGS BIGUANIDES—METFORMIN

Primary Drug	Secondary Drug	Effect	Mechanism	Precautions
BIGUANIDES—METFORMIN				
METFORMIN	**ANTIPSYCHOTICS**			
METFORMIN	CLOZAPINE	May cause ↑ blood sugar and loss of control of blood sugar	Clozapine can cause resistance to the action of insulin	Watch and monitor for diabetes mellitus in patients on long-term clozapine treatment
METFORMIN	PHENOTHIAZINES	May ↑ blood sugar-lowering effect and risk of hypoglycemic episodes. Likely to occur with doses exceeding 100 mg/day	Phenothiazines such as chlorpromazine inhibit the release of epinephrine and ↑ risk of hypoglycemia. May inhibit the release of insulin	Chlorpromazine is nearly always used in the long term. Watch for and warn patients about symptoms of hypoglycemia. ➢ ***For signs and symptoms of hypoglycemia, see Clinical Features of Some Adverse Drug Interactions, Hypoglycemia***
ANTIVIRALS				
METFORMIN	CIDOFOVIR	↑ Risk of lactic acidosis	↓ Renal excretion of metformin	Watch for lactic acidosis. The onset of lactic acidosis is often subtle with symptoms of malaise, myalgia, respiratory distress, and ↑ nonspecific abdominal distress. There may be hypothermia and resistant bradyarrhythmias
METFORMIN	DOLUTEGRAVIR	Possible increased plasma concentration of metformin	Inhibition of metformin transport via OCT-2	Monitor for increased side effects of metformin
METFORMIN	RILPIVIRINE	Potential for plasma concentration of metformin to increase	Unknown mechanism	Monitor blood glucose levels
METFORMIN	BETA-BLOCKERS	Beta-blockers may mask the symptoms and signs of hypoglycemia, such as tachycardia and tremor; there have even been cases of bradycardia and ↑ BP during hypoglycemic episodes in patients on beta-blockers	Beta-blockers prevent or inhibit the normal physiological response to hypoglycemia by interfering with catecholamine-induced mobilization—glycogenolysis and mobilization of glucose—thereby prolonging the time taken by the body to achieve normal (euglycemic) blood sugar levels	Warn patients about the masking of signs of hypoglycemia. Cardioselective beta-blockers are preferred, and all beta-blockers should be avoided in those having frequent hypoglycemic attacks; otherwise monitor glycemic control, especially during initiation of therapy. ➢ ***For signs and symptoms of hypoglycemia, see Clinical Features of Some Adverse Drug Interactions, Hypoglycemia***

(*Continued*)

Primary Drug	Secondary Drug	Effect	Mechanism	Precautions
BIGUANIDES—METFORMIN				
METFORMIN	BRONCHODILATORS—BETA AGONISTS	↑ Risk of hyperglycemia. If administered during pregnancy, there is a risk of hypoglycemia in the fetus, independent of maternal blood glucose levels. ↑ risk of ketoacidosis when administered intravenously	By inducing glycogenolysis, beta-adrenergic agonists cause elevation of blood sugar in adults. In the fetus, these agents cause a depletion of fetal glycogen stores	Monitor blood sugar closely during concomitant administration until blood sugar levels are stable. Be cautious during use in pregnancy. Formoterol and salmeterol are long-acting beta-agonists
METFORMIN	DIURETICS—AMILORIDE	↑ Metformin levels and risk of lactic acidosis	Metformin is not metabolized in humans and is not protein bound. Competition for renal tubular excretion is the basis for ↑ activity or retention of metformin	A theoretical possibility. Need to consider ↓ dose of metformin or avoidance of coadministration
METFORMIN	H2 RECEPTOR BLOCKERS—CIMETIDINE, NIZATIDINE	↑ Level of metformin and risk of lactic acidosis. The onset of lactic acidosis is often subtle with symptoms of malaise, myalgia, respiratory distress, and ↑ nonspecific abdominal distress. There may be hypothermia and resistant bradyarrhythmias	1. Cimetidine competes for renal tubular excretion with metformin, which is not metabolized in humans and is not protein bound 2. Nizatidine inhibits MATE2K, altering metforim secretion and reabsorption	Requires ↓ metformin dose to be considered or to avoid coadministration
METFORMIN	MUSCLE RELAXANTS—BACLOFEN	↓ Hypoglycemic effect of metformin	Due to these drugs causing hyperglycemia, the mechanism is uncertain at present	↑ Doses of metformin are often required for adequate glycemic control
METFORMIN	NANDROLONE	↑ Effect of antidiabetic drugs	Uncertain	Monitor blood sugar closely. Banned by sporting authorities
METFORMIN	NIACIN	↓ Hypoglycemic effect of metformin	Uncertain at present. The effects of niacin (< or = 2.5 g/d), alone or in combination with statins, on fasting glucose (an increase of 4%–5%) and hemoglobin A1c levels (an increase of < or = 0.3%) are modest, transient or reversible	Typically amenable to adjustments in oral hypoglycemic regimens without discontinuing niacin. Benefits outweigh risks. ↑ Doses of antidiabetics are often necessary
METFORMIN	NICOTINIC ACID	↓ Hypoglycemic effect of metformin	Due to these drugs causing hyperglycemia, the mechanism is uncertain at present	↑ Doses of metformin are often required for adequate glycemic control

(Continued)

Primary Drug	Secondary Drug	Effect	Mechanism	Precautions
BIGUANIDES—METFORMIN				
METFORMIN	SOMATROPIN	↓ Hypoglycemic effect of metformin	Growth hormone is considered to have anti-insulin activity by suppressing the ability of insulin to stimulate uptake of glucose in peripheral tissues and enhance glucose synthesis in the liver. Paradoxically, administration of growth hormone stimulates insulin secretion, leading to hyperinsulinemia	↑ Doses of metformin are often required for adequate glycemic control
METFORMIN	SYMPATHOMIMETICS—EPINEPHRINE	May ↑ antidiabetic requirements	Epinephrine causes the release of glucose from the liver and is an important defense/homeostatic mechanism. Hyperglycemia due to an antagonistic effect	Larger doses of antidiabetic therapy may be needed during the period of epinephrine use, which is usually in the short term or in emergency situations
METFORMIN	TESTOSTERONE	↑ Hypoglycemic effect and ↑ risk of hypoglycemic episodes	Exact mechanism is uncertain. Low testosterone levels are associated with type II diabetes. Experimental work has suggested that testosterone may play a role in glucose efflux from cells	Warn patients about symptoms of hypoglycemia. ➢ ***For signs and symptoms of hypoglycemia, see Clinical Features of Some Adverse Drug Interactions, Hypoglycemia***
METFORMIN	THYROID HORMONES	↓ Hypoglycemic effect of metformin	Due to these drugs causing hyperglycemia, the mechanism is uncertain at present	↑ Doses of metformin are often required for adequate glycemic control

Primary Drug	Secondary Drug	Effect	Mechanism	Precautions
DIPEPTIDYL PEPTIDASE-4 (DDP-4) INHIBITORS (GLIPTINS)				
LINAGLIPTIN	ANTIBIOTICS—RIFAMPICIN	Effect of linagliptin possibly reduced	Both metabolized by the CYP450 3A4 system	Monitor blood glucose closely
SAXAGLIPTIN, SITAGLIPTIN	ANTICANCER AND IMMUNOMODULATING DRUGS—PONATINIB	Predicted increase in levels of these P-glycoprotein substrates	P-glycoprotein inhibition	Be aware

(*Continued*)

Primary Drug	Secondary Drug	Effect	Mechanism	Precautions
DIPEPTIDYL PEPTIDASE-4 (DDP-4) INHIBITORS (GLIPTINS)				
DDP-4 INHIBITORS	**ANTIDIABETIC DRUGS**			
DDP-4 INHIBITORS	ANTIDIABETIC DRUGS	↑ Risk of hypoglycemic episodes	Due to additive effects by similar or differing mechanisms to lower blood sugar	Combinations may be used therapeutically. Warn patients about hypoglycemia. ➢ ***For signs and symptoms of hypoglycemia, see Clinical Features of Some Adverse Drug Interactions, Hypoglycemia***
SAXAGLIPTAN	THIAZOLIDINEDIONES	Peripheral edema with saxagliptin	Unknown mechanism	Monitor for signs of edema and stop if necessary
SITAGLIPTIN	ANTIHYPERTENSIVE AND HEART FAILURE DRUGS—ENALAPRIL	Hypotensive effects altered with Sitagliptin	Mechanism unknown	Monitor blood pressure
SAXAGLIPTIN	CALCIUM CHANNEL BLOCKERS	Likely to ↑ plasma concentrations of saxagliptin and ↑ risk of hypoglycemic episodes with diltiazem and verapamil	Inhibition of CYP3A4-mediated metabolism of saxagliptin	Watch for and warn patients about hypoglycemia. ➢ ***For signs and symptoms of hypoglycemia, see Clinical Features of Some Adverse Drug Interactions, Hypoglycemia***
SITAGLIPTIN	CARDIAC GLYCOSIDES—DIGOXIN	Possibly ↑ levels of digoxin	Uncertain at present	Monitor digoxin levels; watch for ↑ levels
Gliflozins—see SGLT2 INHIBITORS that follows				
Glitazones—see THIAZOLIDINEDIONES that follows				

Primary Drug	Secondary Drug	Effect	Mechanism	Precautions
GLUCAGON-LIKE PEPTIDE-1 (GLP-1) ANALOGUES				
GLP-1 ANALOGUES	DRUGS THAT REQUIRE RAPID ONSET OF ACTION OR ACHIEVEMENT OF TARGET PEAK CONCENTRATIONS	GLP-1 agonists may delay absorption	As a result of gastric stasis	Give such drugs 1 h before or 4 h after GLP-1 injection
LIXISENATIDE	ANALGESICS—PARACETAMOL	Lixisenatide possibly reduces absorption of paracetamol when given 1–4 h before	Possibly caused by gastric stasis and decreased stomach motility	Consider injecting lixisenatide after paracetamol administration

(Continued)

ANTIDIABETIC DRUGS GLUCAGON-LIKE PEPTIDE-1 (GLP-1) ANALOGUES

Primary Drug	Secondary Drug	Effect	Mechanism	Precautions
GLUCAGON-LIKE PEPTIDE-1 (GLP-1) ANALOGUES				
GLP-1 ANALOGUES	ANTICANCER AND OTHER IMMUNOMODULATING DRUGS—ORAL RETINOIDS	Potential increased risk of pancreatitis	Retinoids can result in hypertriglyceridemia, which together with a GLP-1 agonist may cause pancreatitis	Avoid concomitant use unless triglyceride levels are unaffected by retinoid
GLP-1 ANALOGUES—EXENATIDE	ANTICOAGULANTS—WARFARIN	Exenatide possibly enhances the anticoagulant effect of warfarin	Unknown mechanism	Monitor INR closely on concomitant prescribing
GLP-1 ANALOGUES	LIPID-LOWERING DRUGS—LOVASTATIN	AUC and C_{max} reduced by 40% and 28%, respectively	Unknown mechanism	Monitor lipid levels

Primary Drug	Secondary Drug	Effect	Mechanism	Precautions
INSULIN				
INSULIN	ALCOHOL	Tends to mask signs of hypoglycemia and ↑ risk of hypoglycemic episodes	Inhibits glucose production and release from many sources, including the liver	Watch for and warn patients about symptoms of hypoglycemia ➢ ***For signs and symptoms of hypoglycemia, see Clinical Features of Some Adverse Drug Interactions, Hypoglycemia***
INSULIN	ANTIARRHYTHMICS—DISOPYRAMIDE	↑ Risk of hypoglycemic episodes—particularly in patients with impaired renal function. Hypoglycemic attacks may occur even when plasma levels of disopyramide are within the normal range (attacks occurring with plasma disopyramide levels of 1–4 ng/mL)	Disopyramide and its metabolite mono-isopropyl disopyramide ↑ secretion of insulin (considered to be due to inhibition of potassium-ATP channels). Suggestion that disopyramide causes an impairment of the counter regulatory (homeostatic) mechanisms that follow hypoglycemia	In patients receiving antidiabetic drugs, start with the lowest dose of disopyramide if there is no alternative. Measure creatinine clearance. If creatinine clearance is 40 mL/min or less, the dose of disopyramide should not exceed 100 mg and should be administered once daily if creatinine clearance is <15 mL/min. Watch for and warn patients about symptoms of hypoglycemia. ➢ ***For signs and symptoms of hypoglycemia, see Clinical Features of Some Adverse Drug Interactions, Hypoglycemia***

(Continued)

Primary Drug	Secondary Drug	Effect	Mechanism	Precautions
INSULIN				
INSULIN	**ANTIBIOTICS**			
INSULIN	ISONIAZID	↓ Efficacy of antidiabetic drugs	Isoniazid causes hyperglycemia, the mechanism is uncertain at present	Monitor capillary blood glucose closely; ↑ doses of antidiabetic drugs may be needed
INSULIN	**QUINOLONES**			
INSULIN	LEVOFLOXACIN	Altered insulin requirements	Both hyperglycemia and hypoglycemia	Altered glycemic control requires frequent monitoring
INSULIN	OFLOXACIN	↑ Risk of hypoglycemic episodes	Mechanism underlying hypoglycemia is not known	Watch for and warn patients about symptoms of hypoglycemia ➢ ***For signs and symptoms of hypoglycemia, see Clinical Features of Some Adverse Drug Interactions, Hypoglycemia***
INSULIN	**ANTICANCER AND IMMUNOMODULATING DRUGS**			
INSULIN	CYTOTOXICS—PROCARBAZINE	↑ Risk of hypoglycemic episodes	Procarbazine has mild MAO properties. MAOIs have an intrinsic hypoglycemic effect and are considered to enhance the effect of hypoglycemic drugs	Watch for and warn patients about symptoms of hypoglycemia ➢ ***For signs and symptoms of hypoglycemia, see Clinical Features of Some Adverse Drug Interactions, Hypoglycemia***
INSULIN	HORMONE ANTAGONISTS—OCTREOTIDE, LANREOTIDE	Likely to alter insulin requirements	Octreotide and lanreotide suppress pancreatic insulin and counter-regulatory hormones (glucagon, growth hormone) and delay or ↓ absorption of glucose from the intestine	Essential to monitor blood sugar at least twice a week after initiating concurrent treatment until blood sugar levels are stable. Advise self-monitoring. Warn patients regarding hypoglycemia. ➢ ***For signs and symptoms of hypoglycemia, see Clinical Features of Some Adverse Drug Interactions, Hypoglycemia***

(Continued)

ANTIDIABETIC DRUGS INSULIN

Primary Drug	Secondary Drug	Effect	Mechanism	Precautions
INSULIN				
INSULIN	IMMUNOMODULATING DRUGS—CORTICOSTEROIDS	Often ↑ insulin requirements, particularly with those with high glucocorticoid activity	Corticosteroids, particularly the glucocorticoids (betamethasone, dexamethasone, deflazacort, prednisolone > cortisone, hydrocortisone), have intrinsic hyperglycemic activity in both diabetic and nondiabetic subjects	Monitor blood sugar during concomitant treatment, weekly if possible, or advise self-monitoring, until blood sugar levels are stable. Larger doses of insulin are often needed
INSULIN	**ANTIDEPRESSANTS**			
INSULIN	MAOIs	↑ Risk of hypoglycemic episodes	MAOIs have an intrinsic hypoglycemic effect and are considered to enhance the effect of hypoglycemic drugs	Watch for and warn patients about symptoms of hypoglycemia. ➢ ***For signs and symptoms of hypoglycemia, see Clinical Features of Some Adverse Drug Interactions, Hypoglycemia***
INSULIN	SSRIs	Fluctuations in blood sugar are very likely, with both hypoglycemic and hyperglycemic events being reported in diabetics receiving hypoglycemic treatment	Brain serotonin- and corticotropin-releasing hormone systems participate in the control of blood sugar levels. An ↑ (usually acute) in brain serotonergic activity induces a hyperglycemic response	Both hyper- and hypoglycemic responses have been reported with SSRIs, and there is a need to monitor blood glucose closely prior to, during, and after discontinuing SSRI treatment. ➢ ***For signs and symptoms of hypoglycemia and hyperglycemia, see Clinical Features of Some Adverse Drug Interactions, Hypoglycemia, Hyperglycemia***
INSULIN	TCAs	Likely to impair control of diabetes	TCAs may ↑ serum glucose levels by up to 150%, and ↑ appetite (particularly carbohydrate craving) and ↓ metabolic rate	Be aware and monitor blood sugar weekly until stable. They are generally considered safe unless diabetes is poorly controlled or is associated with significant cardiac or renal disease. Amitriptyline, imipramine, and citalopram are also used to treat painful diabetic neuropathy

(*Continued*)

Primary Drug	Secondary Drug	Effect	Mechanism	Precautions
INSULIN				
INSULIN	**ANTIDIABETIC DRUGS**			
INSULIN	ANTIDIABETIC DRUGS	↑ Risk of hypoglycemic episodes	Due to additive effects by similar or differing mechanisms to lower blood sugar	Combinations may be used therapeutically. Warn patients about hypoglycemia. ➢ ***For signs and symptoms of hypoglycemia, see Clinical Features of Some Adverse Drug Interactions, Hypoglycemia***
INSULIN	THIAZOLIDEDIONES	1. Edema 2. Hypoglycemia	1. Exacerbated by salt retaining potential of insulin 2. Due to increased insulin sensitivity	1. Warn patients to report increasing peripheral edema and symptoms such as shortness of breath/reduced exercise tolerance 2. May be used therapeutically; monitor blood glucose closely
INSULIN	**ANTIHYPERTENSIVES AND HEART FAILURE DRUGS**			
INSULIN	ACE INHIBITORS	↑ Risk of hypoglycemic episodes	Mechanism uncertain. ACE inhibitors possibly ↑ insulin sensitivity and glucose utilization. Altered renal function may also be factor. ACE inhibitors may ↑ bradykinin levels, which ↓ production of glucose by the liver. Hypoglycemia is reported as a (rare) side effect of ACE inhibitors. Suggested that occurrence of hypoglycemia is greater with captopril than enalapril. Captopril and enalapril are used in the treatment of diabetic nephropathy	Concurrent treatment need not be avoided and is often beneficial in type II diabetes. Watch for and warn patients about symptoms of hypoglycemia. Be aware that the risk of hypoglycemia is greater in elderly people and in patients with poor glycemic control. ➢ ***For signs and symptoms of hypoglycemia, see Clinical Features of Some Adverse Drug Interactions, Hypoglycemia***
INSULIN	ADRENERGIC NEURONE BLOCKERS	↑ Hypoglycemic effect	Catecholamines are diabetogenic; guanethidine blocks the release of catecholamines from nerve endings	Monitor blood glucose closely

(*Continued*)

ANTIDIABETIC DRUGS INSULIN

Primary Drug	Secondary Drug	Effect	Mechanism	Precautions
INSULIN				
INSULIN	VASODILATOR ANTIHYPERTENSIVES—DIAZOXIDE	May ↑ insulin requirement	Diazoxide causes hyperglycemia by inhibiting insulin release and probably by a catecholamine-induced extrahepatic effect. Used in the treatment of hypoglycemia due to insulinomas	Larger doses of insulin are often required, and there is a need to monitor blood sugar until adequate control of blood sugar is achieved
INSULIN	ANTIOBESITY DRUGS—ORLISTAT, RIMONABANT, SIBUTRAMINE	Tendency for blood glucose levels to fluctuate	These agents change dietary intake of carbohydrates and other foods, and the risk of such fluctuations in blood glucose is greater if there is a concurrent dietary regimen. A side effect of orlistat is hypoglycemia	These agents are used often in patients with type II diabetes who are on hypoglycemic therapy. Need to monitor blood sugar twice weekly until stable. Advise self-monitoring and watch for and warn about symptoms of hypoglycemia. ➢ ***For signs and symptoms of hypoglycemia, see Clinical Features of Some Adverse Drug Interactions, Hypoglycemia***
INSULIN	ANTI-PARKINSON'S DRUGS—RASAGILINE, SELEGILINE	↑ Risk of hypoglycemic episodes	These drugs are MAO-B inhibitors. MAOIs have an intrinsic hypoglycemic effect and are considered to enhance the effect of hypoglycemic drugs	Watch for and warn patients about symptoms of hypoglycemia. ➢ ***For signs and symptoms of hypoglycemia, see Clinical Features of Some Adverse Drug Interactions, Hypoglycemia***
INSULIN	ANTIPLATELET AGENTS—ASPIRIN	Risk of hypoglycemia when high-dose aspirin (3.5–7.5 g/day) is given with antidiabetic drugs	Additive effect; aspirin has a hypoglycemic effect	Avoid high-dose aspirin
INSULIN	ANTIPROTOZOALS—PENTAMIDINE	Altered insulin requirement	Attributed to pancreatic beta cell toxicity	Altered glycemic control; need to monitor blood sugar until stable and following withdrawal of pentamidine
INSULIN	ANTIPSYCHOTICS—CLOZAPINE	May cause ↑ blood sugar and loss of control of blood sugar	Clozapine can cause resistance to the action of insulin	Watch for diabetes mellitus in patients on long-term clozapine treatment

(*Continued*)

Primary Drug	Secondary Drug	Effect	Mechanism	Precautions
INSULIN				
INSULIN	ANTIVIRALS—PROTEASE INHIBITORS	↓ Efficacy of insulin	Several mechanisms considered include insulin resistance, impaired insulin-stimulated glucose uptake by skeletal muscle cells, ↓ insulin binding to receptors, and inhibition of intrinsic transport activity of glucose transporters in the body	Necessary to establish baseline values for blood sugar before initiating therapy with a protease inhibitor. Atazanavir, darunavir, fosamprenavir, or tipranavir may be safer. ➢ ***For signs and symptoms of hyperglycemia, see Clinical Features of Some Adverse Drug Interactions, Hyperglycemia***
INSULIN	APROTININ	↑ Availability of insulin and risk of hypoglycemic episodes	Aprotinin ↑ availability of insulin injected subcutaneously. The mechanism is uncertain	Watch for and warn patients about symptoms of hypoglycemia. ➢ ***For signs and symptoms of hypoglycemia, see Clinical Features of Some Adverse Drug Interactions, Hypoglycemia***
INSULIN	**BETA-BLOCKERS**			
INSULIN	BETA-BLOCKERS	Beta-blockers may mask the symptoms and signs of hypoglycemia. They also ↓ insulin sensitivity; however, beta-blockers that also have vasodilating properties (carvedilol, celiprolol, labetalol, nebivolol) seem to ↑ sensitivity to insulin	Beta-blockers ↓ glucose tolerance and interfere with the metabolic and autonomic responses to hypoglycemia	Warn patients about the masking of signs of hypoglycemia. Vasodilating beta-blockers are preferred in patients with diabetes, and all beta-blockers should be avoided in those having frequent hypoglycemic attacks. Monitor capillary blood glucose closely, especially during initiation of therapy. ➢ ***For signs and symptoms of hypoglycemia, see Clinical Features of Some Adverse Drug Interactions, Hypoglycemia***
INSULIN	BETA-BLOCKERS—PINDOLOL, PROPRANOLOL, TIMOLOL EYE DROPS	Hypoglycemia has occurred in patients on insulin also taking oral propanolol and pindolol, propanolol, and timolol eye drops	These beta-blockers inhibit the rebound in blood glucose that occurs as a response to a fall in blood glucose levels	Cardioselective beta-blockers are preferred, and all beta-blockers should be avoided in those having frequent hypoglycemic attacks. Monitor capillary blood glucose closely, especially during initiation of therapy. ➢ ***For signs and symptoms of hypoglycemia, see Clinical Features of Some Adverse Drug Interactions, Hypoglycemia***

(Continued)

ANTIDIABETIC DRUGS INSULIN

ANTIDIABETIC DRUGS INSULIN

Primary Drug	Secondary Drug	Effect	Mechanism	Precautions
INSULIN				
INSULIN	BRONCHODILATORS—BETA-AGONISTS	↑ Risk of hyperglycemia. ↑ risk of hypoglycemia in the fetus when administered during pregnancy even with normal maternal blood sugar levels. ↑ risk of ketoacidosis when administered intravenously	By inducing glycogenolysis, beta-adrenergic agonists cause an elevation of blood sugar in adults. In the fetus, these agents cause a depletion of fetal glycogen stores	Monitor blood sugar closely during concomitant administration until blood sugar levels are stable. Be cautious during use in pregnancy. Formoterol and salmeterol are long-acting beta-agonists
INSULIN	CALCIUM CHANNEL BLOCKERS—DILTIAZEM, NIFEDIPINE	Single case reports of impaired glucose intolerance requiring ↑ insulin requirements with diltiazem and nifedipine	Uncertain at present	Evidence suggests that calcium channel blockers are safe in diabetics; monitor blood glucose levels when starting calcium channel blockers
INSULIN	MUSCLE RELAXANTS—BACLOFEN	↓ Hypoglycemic effect of insulin	Due to these drugs causing hyperglycemia, the mechanism is uncertain at present	↑ Doses of insulin are often required for adequate glycemic control
INSULIN	NANDROLONE	↑ Effect of antidiabetic drugs	Uncertain	Monitor blood sugar closely. Banned by sporting authorities
INSULIN	NIACIN	↓ Hypoglycemic effect of insulin	Uncertain at present. The effects of niacin (< or = 2.5 g/d), alone or in combination with statins, on fasting glucose (an increase of 4%–5%) and hemoglobin A1c levels (an increase of < or = 0.3%) are modest, transient or reversible	Typically amenable to adjustments in oral hypoglycemic regimens without discontinuing niacin. Benefits outweigh risks. ↑ Doses of antidiabetics are often necessary
INSULIN	NICOTINE	↓ Hypoglycemic effect of insulin	Uncertain at present. Exposure of human blood samples to nicotine raised the level of hemoglobin A1c. The higher the nicotine dose, the more the A1c level rose. Cigarettes, by working through a drug interaction cause the body to release its own stores of sugar usually in a matter of seconds	↑ Doses of insulin are often required for adequate glycemic control

(*Continued*)

Primary Drug	Secondary Drug	Effect	Mechanism	Precautions
INSULIN				
INSULIN	ESTROGENS	Altered glycemic control	Uncertain at present. Significantly high or low levels of estrogen could both be involved in the development of insulin resistance. Higher than normal estrogen appears to be linked with increased insulin resistance, yet other studies have shown that low estrogen levels, are linked with greater insulin resistance	Monitor blood glucose closely
INSULIN	PROGESTOGENS	Altered glycemic control	Uncertain at present. One study revealed that low progesterone levels, cause over-production of insulin, leading to hypoglycemia and an outpouring of adrenaline to bring sugar levels up	Monitor blood glucose closely
INSULIN	SOMATROPIN	↓ Hypoglycemic effect of insulin	Growth hormone is considered to have anti-insulin activity by suppressing the ability of insulin to stimulate uptake of glucose in peripheral tissues and enhance glucose synthesis in the liver. Paradoxically, administration of growth hormone stimulates insulin secretion, leading to hyperinsulinemia	↑ Doses of insulin are often required for adequate glycemic control
INSULIN	SYMPATHOMIMETICS—EPINEPHRINE	May ↑ insulin requirement	Epinephrine causes the release of glucose from the liver and is an important defense/homeostatic mechanism. Hyperglycemia due to an antagonistic effect	Larger doses of insulin may be needed during the period of epinephrine use, which is usually in the short term or in emergency situations

(Continued)

ANTIDIABETIC DRUGS INSULIN

Primary Drug	Secondary Drug	Effect	Mechanism	Precautions
INSULIN				
INSULIN	TESTOSTERONE	↑ Hypoglycemic effect and ↑ risk of hypoglycemic episodes	Exact mechanism is uncertain. Low testosterone levels are associated with type II diabetes. Experimental work has suggested that testosterone may play a role in glucose efflux from cells	Warn patients about symptoms of hypoglycemia. ➢ ***For signs and symptoms of hypoglycemia, see Clinical Features of Some Adverse Drug Interactions, Hypoglycemia***
INSULIN	THYROID HORMONES	↓ Hypoglycemic effect of insulin	Due to these drugs causing hyperglycemia, the mechanism is uncertain at present	↑ doses of insulin are often required for adequate glycemic control

Primary Drug	Secondary Drug	Effect	Mechanism	Precautions
MEGLITINIDE DERIVATIVES—NATEGLINIDE, REPAGLINIDE				
NATEGLINIDE, REPAGLINIDE	ALCOHOL	Tends to mask signs of hypoglycemia and ↑ risk of hypoglycemic episodes	Inhibits glucose production and release from many sources, including the liver and release	Watch for and warn patients about symptoms of hypoglycemia. ➢ ***For signs and symptoms of hypoglycemia, see Clinical Features of Some Adverse Drug Interactions, Hypoglycemia***
NATEGLINIDE, REPAGLINIDE	ANTIARRHYTHMICS—DISOPYRAMIDE	↑ Risk of hypoglycemic episodes—particularly in patients with impaired renal function. Hypoglycemic attacks may occur even when plasma levels of disopyramide are within the normal range (attacks occurring with plasma disopyramide levels of 1–4 ng/mL)	Disopyramide and its metabolite mono-isopropyl disopyramide ↑ secretion of insulin (considered to be due to inhibition of potassium-ATP channels). Suggestion that disopyramide causes an impairment of the counterregulatory (homeostatic) mechanisms that follow hypoglycemia	In patients receiving antidiabetic drugs, start with the lowest dose of disopyramide if there is no alternative. Measure creatinine clearance. If creatinine clearance is 40 mL/min or less, the dose of disopyramide should not exceed 100 mg and should be administered once daily if creatinine clearance is <15 mL/min. Watch for and warn patients about symptoms of hypoglycemia. ➢ ***For signs and symptoms of hypoglycemia, see Clinical Features of Some Adverse Drug Interactions, Hypoglycemia***

(Continued)

Primary Drug	Secondary Drug	Effect	Mechanism	Precautions
MEGLITINIDE DERIVATIVES—NATEGLINIDE, REPAGLINIDE				
NATEGLINIDE, REPAGLINIDE	**ANTIBIOTICS**			
NATEGLINIDE, REPAGLINIDE	ISONIAZID	↓ Efficacy of antidiabetic drugs	Isoniazid causes hyperglycemia, the mechanism is uncertain at present	Monitor capillary blood glucose closely; ↑ doses of antidiabetic drugs may be needed
REPAGLINIDE	MACROLIDES—ERYTHROMYCIN, CLARITHROMYCIN, TELITHROMYCIN	Likely to ↑ plasma concentrations of repaglinide and ↑ risk of hypoglycemic episodes. ↑ risk of gastrointestinal side effects with clarithromycin	Due to inhibition of CYP3A4 isoenzymes, which metabolize repaglinide. These drugs vary in potency as inhibitors (clarithromycin is a potent inhibitor), and ↑ plasma concentrations will vary. Clarithromycin ↑ plasma concentrations by 60%. However, the alternative pathway—CYP2C8—is unaffected by these inhibitors	Watch for and warn patients about hypoglycemia. ➢ ***For signs and symptoms of hypoglycemia, see Clinical Features of Some Adverse Drug Interactions, Hypoglycemia***
NATEGLINIDE, REPAGLINIDE	QUINOLONES—CIPROFLOXACIN, LEVOFLOXACIN, NORFLOXACIN, OFLOXACIN	↑ Risk of hypoglycemic episodes	Mechanism uncertain. Ciprofloxacin is a potent inhibitor of CYP1A2. Norfloxacin is a weak inhibitor of CYP1A2, but these drugs may inhibit other CYP isoenzymes to varying degrees	Watch for and warn patients about symptoms of hypoglycemia. ➢ ***For signs and symptoms of hypoglycemia, see Clinical Features of Some Adverse Drug Interactions, Hypoglycemia***
REPAGLINIDE	RIFAMPICIN	↓ Plasma concentrations of repaglinide likely. Rifampicin ↓ AUC of repaglinide by 25%	Due to inducing CYP3A4 isoenzymes, which metabolize repaglinide. However, the alternative pathway—CYP2C8—is unaffected by these inducers except by rifampicin	The interaction is likely to be most severe with rifampicin. Be aware and monitor for hyperglycemia. ➢ ***For signs and symptoms of hyperglycemia, see Clinical Features of Some Adverse Drug Interactions, Hyperglycemia***
MEGLITINIDE DERIVATIVES	SULFONAMIDES	Increased hypoglycemic effect	Displaced from protein binding	Monitor glucose levels closely
REPAGLINIDE	TRIMETHOPRIM	↑ Repaglinide levels (by approximately 40%); risk of hypoglycemia	Hepatic metabolism inhibited	Manufacturers do not recommend concurrent use

(*Continued*)

ANTIDIABETIC DRUGS MEGLITINIDE DERIVATIVES—NATEGLINIDE, REPAGLINIDE

Primary Drug	Secondary Drug	Effect	Mechanism	Precautions
MEGLITINIDE DERIVATIVES—NATEGLINIDE, REPAGLINIDE				
NATEGLINIDE, REPAGLINIDE	**ANTICANCER AND IMMUNOMODULATING DRUGS**			
REPAGLINIDE	ANASTROZOLE	Risk of hypoglycemia	Mechanism unknown	Watch for and warn patients about hypoglycemia. ➢ ***For signs and symptoms of hypoglycemia, see Clinical Features of Some Adverse Drug Interactions, Hypoglycemia***
REPAGLINIDE	CICLOSPORIN	↑ Repaglinide levels, with ↑ risk of hypoglycemia	Hepatic metabolism inhibited	Watch for and warn patients about hypoglycemia ➢ ***For signs and symptoms of hypoglycemia, see Clinical Features of Some Adverse Drug Interactions, Hypoglycemia***
REPAGLINIDE	IMATINIB	Likely to ↑ plasma concentrations of repaglinide and ↑ risk of hypoglycemic episodes	Due to inhibition of CYP3A4 isoenzymes, which metabolize repaglinide	Watch for and warn patients about hypoglycemia. ➢ ***For signs and symptoms of hypoglycemia, see Clinical Features of Some Adverse Drug Interactions, Hypoglycemia***
NATEGLINIDE, REPAGLINIDE	LANREOTIDE, OCTREOTIDE	Likely to alter antidiabetic requirements	Octreotide and lanreotide suppress pancreatic insulin and counter-regulatory hormones (glucagon, growth hormone) and delay or ↓ absorption of glucose from the intestine	Essential to monitor blood sugar at least twice a week after initiating concurrent treatment until blood sugar levels are stable. Advise self-monitoring. Warn patients about hypoglycemia. ➢ ***For signs and symptoms of hypoglycemia, see Clinical Features of Some Adverse Drug Interactions, Hypoglycemia***
REPAGLINIDE	LAPATINIB	Possible increased levels of CYP2C8 substrates	CYP2C8 inhibition	Avoid or caution with concurrent use
REPAGLINIDE	PIXANTRONE	Theoretical risk of increased drug levels	Pixantrone inhibits CYP2C8	Manufacturer advises caution

(Continued)

Primary Drug	Secondary Drug	Effect	Mechanism	Precautions
MEGLITINIDE DERIVATIVES—NATEGLINIDE, REPAGLINIDE				
NATEGLINIDE, REPAGLINIDE	**ANTIDEPRESSANTS**			
NATEGLINIDE, REPAGLINIDE	SSRIs	Fluctuations in blood sugar are very likely, with both hypoglycemic and hyperglycemic events being reported in diabetics receiving hypoglycemic treatment	Brain serotonin- and corticotropin-releasing hormone systems participate in the control of blood sugar levels. ↑ (usually acute) in brain serotonergic activity induces a hyperglycemic response	Both hyper- and hypoglycemic responses have been reported with SSRIs; there is a need to monitor blood glucose closely prior to, during, and after discontinuing SSRI treatment. ➢ ***For signs and symptoms of hypoglycemia and hpyerglycemia, see Clinical Features of Some Adverse Drug Interactions, Hypoglycemia, Hyperglycemia***
REPAGLINIDE	ST. JOHN'S WORT	↓ Plasma concentrations of repaglinide likely	Due to inducing CYP3A4 isoenzymes, which metabolize repaglinide. However, the alternative pathway—CYP2C8—is unaffected by these inducers	Be aware and monitor for hyperglycemia. ➢ ***For signs and symptoms of hyperglycemia, see Clinical Features of Some Adverse Drug Interactions, Hyperglycemia***
NATEGLINIDE, REPAGLINIDE	TCAs	Likely to impair control of diabetes	TCAs may ↑ serum glucose levels by up to 150%, ↑ appetite (particularly carbohydrate craving) and ↓ metabolic rate	Be aware and monitor blood sugar weekly until stable. They are generally considered safe unless diabetes is poorly controlled or is associated with significant cardiac or renal disease. Amitriptyline, imipramine, and citalopram are also used to treat painful diabetic neuropathy
NATEGLINIDE, REPAGLINIDE	ANTIDIABETIC DRUGS	↑ Risk of hypoglycemic episodes	Due to additive effects by similar or differing mechanisms to lower blood sugar	Combinations are often used and useful. Warn patients about hypoglycemia. ➢ ***For signs and symptoms of hypoglycemia, see Clinical Features of Some Adverse Drug Interactions, Hypoglycemia***

(*Continued*)

ANTIDIABETIC DRUGS MEGLITINIDE DERIVATIVES—NATEGLINIDE, REPAGLINIDE

Primary Drug	Secondary Drug	Effect	Mechanism	Precautions
MEGLITINIDE DERIVATIVES—NATEGLINIDE, REPAGLINIDE				
REPAGLINIDE	ANTIEPILEPTICS—CARBAMAZEPINE, PHENOBARBITONE, HYDANTOINS	↓ Plasma concentrations of repaglinide likely	Due to inducing CYP3A4 isoenzymes, which metabolize repaglinide. However, the alternative pathway—CYP2C8—is unaffected by these inducers	Be aware and monitor for hyperglycemia. ➢ ***For signs and symptoms of hyperglycemia, see Clinical Features of Some Adverse Drug Interactions, Hyperglycemia***
NATEGLINIDE, REPAGLINIDE	**ANTIFUNGALS**			
NATEGLINIDE, REPAGLINIDE	AZOLES—KETOCONAZOLE, FLUCONAZOLE, ITRACONAZOLE, VORICONAZOLE	Likely to ↑ plasma concentrations of repaglinide and ↑ risk of hypoglycemic episodes	Due to inhibition of CYP3A4-mediated metabolism. These drugs vary in potency as inhibitors (ketoconazole and itraconazole are potent inhibitors) and ↑ plasma concentrations will vary	Watch for and warn patients of hypoglycemia. ➢ ***For signs and symptoms of hypoglycemia, see Clinical Features of Some Adverse Drug Interactions, Hypoglycemia***
REPAGLINIDE	GRISEOFULVIN	↓ Repaglinide levels	Hepatic metabolism is induced	Watch for and warn patients of hypoglycemia. ➢ ***For signs and symptoms of hypoglycemia, see Clinical Features of Some Adverse Drug Interactions, Hypoglycemia***
NATEGLINIDE	ANTIGOUT DRUGS—SULFINPYRAZONE	↑ Blood levels of nateglinide	Sulfinpyrazone is a selective CYP2C9 inhibitor	Need to monitor blood sugar weekly in patients receiving both drugs. Watch for and warn patients of hypoglycemia. ➢ ***For signs and symptoms of hypoglycemia, see Clinical Features of Some Adverse Drug Interactions, Hypoglycemia***

(*Continued*)

Primary Drug	Secondary Drug	Effect	Mechanism	Precautions
MEGLITINIDE DERIVATIVES—NATEGLINIDE, REPAGLINIDE				
NATEGLINIDE, REPAGLINIDE	**ANTIHYPERTENSIVES AND HEART FAILURE DRUGS**			
NATEGLINIDE, REPAGLINIDE	ACE INHIBITORS	↑ Risk of hypoglycemic episodes	Mechanism uncertain. ACE inhibitors possibly ↑ insulin sensitivity and glucose utilization. Altered renal function may also be factor. ACE inhibitors may ↑ bradykinin levels, which ↓ production of glucose by the liver. Hypoglycemia is reported as a (rare) side effect of ACE inhibitors. Suggestion that the occurrence of hypoglycemia is greater with captopril than enalapril. Captopril and enalapril are used in the treatment of diabetic nephropathy	Concurrent treatment need not be avoided and is often beneficial in type II diabetes. Watch for and warn patients of hypoglycemia. Be aware that the risk of hypoglycemia is greater in elderly people and in patients with poor glycemic control. ➢ ***For signs and symptoms of hypoglycemia, see Clinical Features of Some Adverse Drug Interactions, Hypoglycemia***
NATEGLINIDE, REPAGLINIDE	ADRENERGIC NEURONE BLOCKERS	↑ Hypoglycemic effect	Catecholamines are diabetogenic; guanethidine blocks release of catecholamines from nerve endings	Monitor blood glucose closely
NATEGLINIDE, REPAGLINIDE	VASODILATOR ANTIHYPERTENSIVES—DIAZOXIDE	May ↑ antidiabetic requirements	Diazoxide causes hyperglycemia by inhibiting insulin release and probably by a catecholamine-induced extrahepatic effect. Used in the treatment of hypoglycemia due to insulinomas	Larger doses of antidiabetic drugs are often required; need to monitor blood sugar until adequate control of blood sugar is achieved

(Continued)

ANTIDIABETIC DRUGS MEGLITINIDE DERIVATIVES—NATEGLINIDE, REPAGLINIDE

ANTIDIABETIC DRUGS MEGLITINIDE DERIVATIVES—NATEGLINIDE, REPAGLINIDE

ANTIDIABETIC DRUGS MEGLITINIDE DERIVATIVES—NATEGLINIDE, REPAGLINIDE

Primary Drug	Secondary Drug	Effect	Mechanism	Precautions
MEGLITINIDE DERIVATIVES—NATEGLINIDE, REPAGLINIDE				
NATEGLINIDE, REPAGLINIDE	ANTIOBESITY DRUGS—ORLISTAT, RIMONABANT, SIBUTRAMINE	Tendency for blood glucose levels to fluctuate	These agents change dietary intake of carbohydrates and other foods, and the risk of fluctuations in blood glucose is greater if there is a concurrent dietary regimen. A side effect of orlistat is hypoglycemia	These agents are used often in patients with type II diabetes who are on hypoglycemic therapy. Need to monitor blood sugar twice weekly until stable. Advise self-monitoring. Watch for and warn patients about symptoms of hypoglycemia. ➢ ***For signs and symptoms of hypoglycemia, see Clinical Features of Some Adverse Drug Interactions, Hypoglycemia***
NATEGLINIDE, REPAGLINIDE	ANTIPLATELET AGENTS—ASPIRIN	Risk of hypoglycemia when high-dose aspirin (3.5–7.5 g/day) is given with antidiabetic drugs	Additive effect; aspirin has a hypoglycemic effect	Avoid high-dose aspirin
NATEGLINIDE, REPAGLINIDE	ANTIPROTOZOALS—PENTAMIDINE	May alter antidiabetic requirements due to altered glycemic control	Attributed to pancreatic beta cell toxicity	Need to monitor blood sugar until stable and following withdrawal of pentamidine
NATEGLINIDE, REPAGLINIDE	**ANTIPSYCHOTICS**			
REPAGLINIDE	PHENOTHIAZINES, CLOZAPINE, OLANZAPINE	↓ Hypoglycemic effect	Antagonistic effect	Higher doses of repaglinide needed
NATEGLINIDE, REPAGLINIDE	RISPERIDONE	↑ Risk of hypoglycemic episodes	Attributed to a synergistic effect	Watch for and warn patients about symptoms of hypoglycemia. ➢ ***For signs and symptoms of hypoglycemia, see Clinical Features of Some Adverse Drug Interactions, Hypoglycemia***
NATEGLINIDE, REPAGLINIDE	**ANTIVIRALS**			
REPAGLINIDE	NNRTIs—EFAVIRENZ	Likely to ↑ plasma concentrations of repaglinide and ↑ risk of hypoglycemic episodes	Due to inhibition of CYP3A4 isoenzymes, which metabolize repaglinide	Watch for and warn patients about hypoglycemia. ➢ ***For signs and symptoms of hypoglycemia, see Clinical Features of Some Adverse Drug Interactions, Hypoglycemia***

(Continued)

Primary Drug	Secondary Drug	Effect	Mechanism	Precautions
MEGLITINIDE DERIVATIVES—NATEGLINIDE, REPAGLINIDE				
NATEGLINIDE, REPAGLINIDE	PROTEASE INHIBITORS	↑ Levels of these antidiabetic drugs	Inhibition of CYP2C9- and CYP3A4-mediated metabolism of nateglinide and CYP3A4-mediated metabolism of repaglinide	Monitor blood sugar closely
NATEGLINIDE, REPAGLINIDE	BETA-BLOCKERS	Beta-blockers may mask the symptoms and signs of hypoglycemia. They also ↓ insulin sensitivity; however, beta-blockers that also have vasodilating properties (carvedilol, celiprolol, labetalol, nebivolol) seem to ↑ sensitivity to insulin	Beta-blockers ↓ glucose tolerance and interfere with metabolic and autonomic responses to hypoglycemia	Warn patients about the masking of signs of hypoglycemia. Vasodilating beta-blockers are preferred in patients with diabetes, and all beta-blockers should be avoided in those having frequent hypoglycemic attacks. Monitor capillary blood glucose closely, especially during initiation of therapy. ➢ ***For signs and symptoms of hypoglycemia, see Clinical Features of Some Adverse Drug Interactions, Hypoglycemia***
NATEGLINIDE	CNS STIMULANTS—MODAFINIL	May cause ↑ plasma concentrations of nateglinide if CYP2C9 is the predominant metabolic pathway and the alternative pathways are either genetically deficient or affected	Modafinil is a moderate inhibitor of CYP2C9	Be aware
REPAGLINIDE	DEFERASIROX	Increased risk of hypoglycemia	Plasma concentration of repaglinide increased	Monitor blood glucose levels closely if used concomitantly
REPAGLINIDE	DIURETICS—POTASSIUM-SPARING	↓ Hypoglycemic effect	Antagonistic effect	Higher doses of repaglinide are needed
REPAGLINIDE	GRAPEFRUIT JUICE	Possibly ↑ repaglinide levels	Due to inhibition of CYP3A4 isoenzymes, which metabolize repaglinide	Uncertain if clinically significant. May need to monitor blood glucose more closely
MEGLITINIDE DERIVATIVES	HERBAL REMEDIES—GINSENG	Increased hypoglycemic effect	Increasing insulin sensitivity and secretion	Monitor glucose levels
NATEGLINIDE, REPAGLINIDE	H2 RECEPTOR BLOCKERS—CIMETIDINE	Likely to ↑ plasma concentrations of these antidiabetic drugs and ↑ risk of hypoglycemic episodes	Due to inhibition of CYP3A4-mediated metabolism of nateglinide and repaglinide	Watch for and warn patients about hypoglycemia. ➢ ***For signs and symptoms of hypoglycemia, see Clinical Features of Some Adverse Drug Interactions, Hypoglycemia***

(Continued)

ANTIDIABETIC DRUGS MEGLITINIDE DERIVATIVES—NATEGLINIDE, REPAGLINIDE

ANTIDIABETIC DRUGS MEGLITINIDE DERIVATIVES—NATEGLINIDE, REPAGLINIDE

Primary Drug	Secondary Drug	Effect	Mechanism	Precautions
MEGLITINIDE DERIVATIVES—NATEGLINIDE, REPAGLINIDE				
NATEGLINIDE, REPAGLINIDE	**LIPID-LOWERING DRUGS**			
REPAGLINIDE	FIBRATES—GEMFIBROZIL	Marked ↑ in repaglinide levels, with risk of severe hypoglycemia	Gemfibrozil is a relatively selective inhibitor of CYP2C8. Also drug transportation may have a role	Avoid coadministration. Bezafibrate and fenofibrate are suitable alternatives if a fibric acid derivative is required
NATEGLINIDE, REPAGLINIDE	STATINS	↑ Incidence of adverse effects such as myalgia. There was ↑ maximum concentration of repaglinide by 25%, with high variability	Uncertain. Statins are also substrates for CYP3A4, and competition for metabolism by the enzyme system may be a factor	Clinical significance of the effect is uncertain, but it is necessary to be aware of it. Warn patients about adverse effects of statins and repaglinide
REPAGLINIDE	MONTELUKAST	↑ Repaglinide levels; risk of hypoglycemia	Hepatic metabolism inhibited	Watch for and warn patients about hypoglycemia. ➢ ***For signs and symptoms of hypoglycemia, see Clinical Features of Some Adverse Drug Interactions, Hypoglycemia***
NATEGLINIDE, REPAGLINIDE	MUSCLE RELAXANTS—BACLOFEN	↓ Hypoglycemic effect	Due to these drugs causing hyperglycemia, the mechanism is uncertain at present	↑ Doses of antidiabetic are often required for adequate glycemic control
NATEGLINIDE, REPAGLINIDE	NANDROLONE	↑ Effect of antidiabetic drugs	Uncertain	Monitor blood sugar closely. Banned by sporting authorities
NATEGLINIDE, REPAGLINIDE	NIACIN	↓ Hypoglycemic effect	Uncertain at present. The effects of niacin (< or = 2.5 g/d), alone or in combination with statins, on fasting glucose (an increase of 4%–5%) and hemoglobin A1c levels (an increase of < or = 0.3%) are modest, transient or reversible	Typically amenable to adjustments in oral hypoglycemic regimens without discontinuing niacin. Benefits outweigh risks. ↑ Doses of antidiabetics are often necessary

(Continued)

Primary Drug	Secondary Drug	Effect	Mechanism	Precautions
MEGLITINIDE DERIVATIVES—NATEGLINIDE, REPAGLINIDE				
NATEGLINIDE, REPAGLINIDE	NICOTINE	↓ Hypoglycemic effect	Uncertain at present. Exposure of human blood samples to nicotine raised the level of hemoglobin A1c. The higher the nicotine dose, the more the A1c level rose. Cigarettes, by working through a drug interaction cause the body to release its own stores of sugar usually in a matter of seconds	↑ Doses of antidiabetic are often required for adequate glycemic control
NATEGLINIDE, REPAGLINIDE	ESTROGENS	Altered glycemic control	Uncertain at present. Significantly high or low levels of estrogen could both be involved in the development of insulin resistance. Higher than normal estrogen appears to be linked with increased insulin resistance, yet other studies have shown that low estrogen levels, are linked with greater insulin resistance	Monitor blood glucose closely
NATEGLINIDE, REPAGLINIDE	PROGESTOGENS	Altered glycemic control	Uncertain at present. One study revealed that low progesterone levels, cause over-production of insulin, leading to hypoglycemia and an outpouring of adrenaline to bring sugar levels up	Monitor blood glucose closely
NATEGLINIDE, REPAGLINIDE	SOMATROPIN	↓ Hypoglycemic effect	Growth hormone is considered to have anti-insulin activity by suppressing the ability of insulin to stimulate uptake of glucose in peripheral tissues and enhance glucose synthesis in the liver. Paradoxically, administration of growth hormone stimulates insulin secretion, leading to hyperinsulinemia	↑ Doses of antidiabetic are often required for adequate glycemic control
NATEGLINIDE, REPAGLINIDE	THYROID HORMONES	↓ Hypoglycemic effect	Due to these drugs causing hyperglycemia, the mechanism is uncertain at present	↑ Doses of antidiabetic are often required for adequate glycemic control

ANTIDIABETIC DRUGS MEGLITINIDE DERIVATIVES—NATEGLINIDE, REPAGLINIDE

ANTIDIABETIC DRUGS SODIUM-GLUCOSE CO-TRANSPORTER 2 (SGLT-2) INHIBITORS

Primary Drug	Secondary Drug	Effect	Mechanism	Precautions
SODIUM-GLUCOSE CO-TRANSPORTER 2 (SGLT-2) INHIBITORS (GLIFLOZINS)				
SGLT2 INHIBITORS	ANALGESICS—NSAIDs—MEFENAMIC ACID	Possible increased effect of dapagliflozin	AUC increased by 51%	No significant change of dose required as interaction probably not clinically significant
SGLT2 INHIBITORS	ANTIBIOTICS—RIFAMPICIN	Possible decreased effect of dapagliflozin	AUC decreased by 22%	No significant change of dose required as interaction probably not clinically significant
SGLT2 INHIBITORS	**ANTIDIABETIC DRUGS**			
SGLT2 INHIBITORS	INSULINS	↑ Risk of hypoglycemic episodes	Increased glucose excretion in urine combined with exogenous insulin	Lower insulin doses when combining agents
SGLT2 INHIBITORS	METEGLINIDES	↑ Risk of hypoglycemic episodes	Increased glucose excretion in urine combined with increased insulin secretion by secretagogue	Lower doses when combining agents
SGLT2 INHIBITORS	SULFONYLUREAS	↑ Risk of hypoglycemic episodes	Increased glucose excretion in urine combined with increased insulin secretion by secretagogue	Lower doses when combining agents
SGLT2 INHIBITORS—DAPAGLIFLOZIN	THIAZOLIDEDIONES	Potential risk of urogenital malignancies	Both drugs in clinical trial program have identified a signal of increased bladder cancer	Avoid concomitant prescribing
SGLT2 INHIBITORS	ANTIHYPERTENSIVE AND HEART FAILURE DRUGS	Potential for hypotension	Osmotic (natriuresis) effects of drug enhance diuresis and hypotension	Monitor blood pressure closely; warn patients about the symptoms of orthostatic hypotension. Manufacturer does not recommend use in combination with loop diuretics
SGLT2 INHIBITORS	DIURETICS—LOOP	Potential for intravascular depletion and hypotension	Osmotic (natriuresis) effects of both classes of drug enhance diuresis	Manufacturer does not recommend use in combination with loop diuretics

Primary Drug	Secondary Drug	Effect	Mechanism	Precautions
SULFONYLUREAS				
SULFONYLUREAS	**SULFONYLUREAS ARE METABOLIZED MAINLY BY CYP2C9. POLYMORPHISMS, CYP2C9*3 (Ile359Leu) AND TO A LESSER EXTENT CYP2C9*2 (ARG144Cys), INFLUENCE THE PHARMACOKINETICS OF MANY SULFONYLUREAS**			
SULFONYLUREAS	ALCOHOL	Tends to mask signs of hypoglycemia and ↑ risk of hypoglycemic episodes	Inhibits glucose production and release from many sources, including the liver and release	Watch for and warn patients about symptoms of hypoglycemia. ➢ ***For signs and symptoms of hypoglycemia, see Clinical Features of Some Adverse Drug Interactions, Hypoglycemia***
SULFONYLUREAS	ANALGESICS—NSAIDs	Enhanced hypoglycemic effect of sulfonylureas with most NSAIDs, which are highly protein bound. There have been reports of hyperglycemia and hypoglycemia (e.g., with diclofenac)	Attributed to displacement of sulfonylureas from protein-binding sites, thus ↑ plasma concentration. Some NSAIDs may impair the renal elimination of sulfonylureas particularly chlorpropamide	Be aware. There are conflicting reports. Suggestions that sulindac and diclofenac with misoprostol may interact minimally
SULFONYLUREAS	ANTIARRHYTHMICS—DISOPYRAMIDE	↑ Risk of hypoglycemic episodes—particularly in patients with impaired renal function. Hypoglycemic attacks may occur even when plasma levels of disopyramide are within the normal range (attacks occurring with plasma disopyramide levels of 1–4 ng/mL)	Disopyramide and its metabolite mono-isopropyl disopyramide ↑ secretion of insulin (considered to be due to inhibition of potassium-ATP channels). Suggestion that disopyramide causes an impairment of the counter-regulatory (homeostatic) mechanisms that follow hypoglycemia	In patients receiving antidiabetic drugs, start with the lowest dose of disopyramide if there is no alternative. Measure creatinine clearance. If creatinine clearance is 40 mL/min or less, the dose of disopyramide should not exceed 100 mg and should be administered once daily if creatinine clearance is <15 mL/min. Watch for and warn patients about symptoms of hypoglycemia. ➢ ***For signs and symptoms of hypoglycemia, see Clinical Features of Some Adverse Drug Interactions, Hypoglycemia***
SULFONYLUREAS	**ANTIBIOTICS**			
SULFONYLUREAS	CHLORAMPHENICOL	Possibly ↓ hypoglycemic effect of sulfonylureas	Chloramphenicol is an inhibitor of cytochromes including 3A4 and 2C9	Be aware

(Continued)

Primary Drug	Secondary Drug	Effect	Mechanism	Precautions
SULFONYLUREAS				
SULFONYLUREAS	ISONIAZID	↓ Efficacy of antidiabetic drugs	Isoniazid is a cytochrome inhibitor and increased serum glimepiride concentration, resulting in hyperinsulinemia	Monitor capillary blood glucose closely; ↑ doses of antidiabetic drugs may be needed
SULFONYLUREAS	QUINOLONES	↑ Risk of hypoglycemic episodes	Recently reported was the eighth case of levofloxacin-induced hypoglycemia—an uncommon but potentially fatal side effect of this antibiotic. Report of one case was with 1 dose of ciprofloxacin in combination with glipizide	Watch for and warn patients about symptoms of hypoglycemia. ➢ ***For signs and symptoms of hypoglycemia, see Clinical Features of Some Adverse Drug Interactions, Hypoglycemia***
SULFONYLUREAS	RIFAMPICIN	↓ Hypoglycemic efficacy	CYP2C9 is induced by rifampicin. Clearance of drugs such as tolbutamide are doubled during therapy with rifampicin	Watch for and warn patients about symptoms of hyperglycemia. ➢ ***For signs and symptoms of hypoglycemia, see Clinical Features of Some Adverse Drug Interactions, Hypoglycemia***
SULFONYLUREAS	SULFONAMIDES, TRIMETHOPRIM	↑ Risk of hypoglycemia	18 cases of trimethoprim-sulfamethoxazole associated hypoglycemia are reported in the literature. Because of their structural similarities to sulfonylureas, sulfonamides are liable to facilitate hypoglycemia by increasing insulin release in susceptible individuals. Sulfonamides can potentiate the hypoglycemic effect of sulfonylurea agents when given in combination	Monitor blood glucose levels closely

(*Continued*)

Primary Drug	Secondary Drug	Effect	Mechanism	Precautions
SULFONYLUREAS				
SULFONYLUREAS	TUMOUR NECROSIS FACTOR ALPHA INHIBITORS-INFLIXIMAB, CERTLIZUMAB, ETANERCEPT, ADALIMUBAB, GOLIMUMAB	↑ Risk of hypoglycemia	Hypoglycemia is a possible side-effect tumor necrosis factor-alpha inhibitors. Attributed by some to increased sensitivity to insulin. Prolonged use of infliximab and etanercept can cause a therapeutic side effect of higher insulin sensitivity, suggesting a therapeutic potential of TNF-α inhibitors in diabetes. On the molecular level, through mouse models, TNF-α is known to downregulate GLUT-4 (GLUT-4 is a transporter which allows for uptake of glucose into adipose tissue)	Monitor blood sugars daily until stable. Changes in blood sugar usually occur after about a month but be aware from beginning of combined therapy
SULFONYLUREAS	**ANTICANCER AND IMMUNOMODULATING DRUGS**			
SULFONYLUREAS	**CYTOTOXICS**			
CHLORPROPAMIDE	BORTEZOMIB	Likely to ↑ hypoglycemic effect of chlorpropamide	Unknown. Both hypo and hyperglycemia may occur with bortezomib. May worsen diabetic peripheral neuropayhy	Watch for and warn patients about symptoms of hypoglycemia. Caution in patients with diabetic peripheral neuropathy. Decreased dose of bortexomib has to be considered. ➢ ***For signs and symptoms of hypoglycemia, see Clinical Features of Some Adverse Drug Interactions, Hypoglycemia***
GLIPIZIDE	CYCLOPHOSPHAMIDE	Blood sugar levels may be ↑ or ↓	Uncertain	Need to monitor blood glucose in patients with concomitant treatment at the beginning of treatment and after 1–2 weeks

(Continued)

ANTIDIABETIC DRUGS SULFONYLUREAS

Primary Drug	Secondary Drug	Effect	Mechanism	Precautions
SULFONYLUREAS				
SULFONAMIDES—GLIMEPIRIDE, GLIPIZIDE, TOLBUTAMIDE	IMATINIB	↑ Plasma concentrations, with risk of toxic effects of these drugs	Imatinib is a potent inhibitor of CYP2C9 isoenzymes, which metabolize these drugs	Watch for the early toxic effects of these drugs. If necessary, consider using alternative drugs while the patient is being given imatinib
GLIPIZIDE	PORFIMER	↑ Risk of photosensitivity reactions	Attributed to additive effects	Avoid exposure of skin and eyes to direct sunlight for 30 days after porfimer therapy
SULFONYLUREAS	PROCARBAZINE	↑ Risk of hypoglycemic episodes	MAOIs have an intrinsic hypoglycemic effect. MAOIs are considered to enhance the effect of hypoglycemic drugs	Watch for and warn patients about symptoms of hypoglycemia. ➢ ***For signs and symptoms of hypoglycemia, see Clinical Features of Some Adverse Drug Interactions, Hypoglycemia***
SULFONYLUREAS	**HORMONES AND HORMONE ANTAGONISTS**			
SULFONYLUREAS	LANREOTIDE, OCTREOTIDE	Likely to alter insulin requirements	Octreotide and lanreotide suppress pancreatic insulin and counter-regulatory hormones (glucagon, growth hormone) and delay or ↓ absorption of glucose from the intestine	Essential to monitor blood sugar at least twice a week after initiating concurrent treatment until blood sugar levels are stable. Advise self-monitoring
SULFONYLUREAS	**IMMUNOMODULATING DRUGS**			
GLIPIZIDE	CICLOSPORIN	May ↑ plasma concentrations of ciclosporin	Glipizide inhibits CYP3A4-mediated metabolism of ciclosporin	Monitor plasma ciclosporin levels to prevent toxicity
SULFONYLUREAS	CORTICOSTEROIDS	Often ↑ requirements of hypoglycemic agent, particularly with high glucocorticoid activity steroids	Corticosteroids, particularly the glucocorticoids (betamethasone, dexamethasone, deflazacort, prednisolone > cortisone, hydrocortisone), have intrinsic hyperglycemic activity in both diabetic and nondiabetic subjects	Monitor blood sugar during concomitant treatment, weekly if possible, or advise self-monitoring, until blood sugar levels are stable. Larger doses of glimepiride are often needed

(*Continued*)

Primary Drug	Secondary Drug	Effect	Mechanism	Precautions
SULFONYLUREAS				
TOLBUTAMIDE	LEFLUNOMIDE	Possible ↑ effect of tolbutamide	Uncertain	Monitor blood sugar closely. Watch for and warn patients about symptoms of hypoglycemia. ➢ ***For signs and symptoms of hypoglycemia, see Clinical Features of Some Adverse Drug Interactions, Hypoglycemia***
SULFONYLUREAS	ANTICOAGULANTS—ORAL	Cases reported of hypoglycemia when coumarins started in patients on tolbutamide. Conversely, there are several case reports of bleeding when tolbutamide was started in patients on oral anticoagulants	Oral anticoagulants inhibit hepatic metabolism of tolbutamide and ↑ its half-life threefold. Tolbutamide possibly alters the plasma protein binding of anticoagulants	Use an alternative sulfonylurea or another class of hypoglycemic
SULFONYLUREAS	**ANTIDEPRESSANTS**			
SULFONYLUREAS	MAOIs	↑ Risk of hypoglycemic episodes	MAOIs have an intrinsic hypoglycemic effect and are considered to enhance the effect of hypoglycemic drugs	Watch for and warn patients about symptoms of hypoglycemia. ➢ ***For signs and symptoms of hypoglycemia, see Clinical Features of Some Adverse Drug Interactions, Hypoglycemia***
SULFONYLUREAS	SSRIs	Fluctuations in blood sugar are very likely, with both hypoglycemic and hyperglycemic events being reported in diabetics receiving hypoglycemic treatment. ↑ plasma concentrations of sulfonylureas (e.g., tolbutamide) may occur	Brain serotonin- and corticotropin-releasing hormone systems participate in the control of blood sugar levels. ↑ (usually acute) in brain serotonergic activity induces a hyperglycemic response	Both hyper- and hypoglycemic responses have been reported with SSRIs; there is a need to monitor blood glucose closely prior to, during, and after discontinuing SSRI treatment. ➢ ***For signs and symptoms of hypoglycemia and hyperglycemia, see Clinical Features of Some Adverse Drug Interactions, Hypoglycemia, Hyperglycemia***

(Continued)

Primary Drug	Secondary Drug	Effect	Mechanism	Precautions
SULFONYLUREAS				
SULFONYLUREAS	ST. JOHN'S WORT	↓ Hypoglycemic efficacy	Plasma levels of sulfonylureas are ↓ by induction of CYP-mediated metabolism	Watch for and warn patients about symptoms of hyperglycemia. ➢ ***For signs and symptoms of hyperglycemia, see Clinical Features of Some Adverse Drug Interactions, Hyperglycemia***
SULFONYLUREAS	TCAs	Likely to impair control of diabetes	TCAs may ↑ serum glucose levels by up to 150%, ↑ appetite (particularly carbohydrate craving) and ↓ metabolic rate	Be aware and monitor blood sugar weekly until stable. They are generally considered safe unless diabetes is poorly controlled or is associated with significant cardiac or renal disease. Amitriptyline, imipramine, and citalopram are also used to treat painful diabetic neuropathy
SULFONYLUREAS	**OTHER ANTIDIABETIC DRUGS**			
SULFONYLUREAS	ANTIDIABETIC DRUGS	↑ Risk of hypoglycemic episodes	Due to additive effects by similar or differing mechanisms to lower blood sugar	Combinations may be used therapeutically. Warn patients about hypoglycemia. ➢ ***For signs and symptoms of hypoglycemia, see Clinical Features of Some Adverse Drug Interactions, Hypoglycemia***
SULFONYLUREAS	THIAZOLIDEDIONES	1. Edema 2. Hypoglycemia	1. Exacerbated by salt retaining potential of insulin 2. Due to increased insulin sensitivity	1. Warn patients to report increasing peripheral edema and symptoms such as shortness of breath/reduced exercise tolerance 2. May be used therapeutically; monitor blood glucose closely
TOLBUTAMIDE	ANTIEMETICS—APREPITANT	↓ Tolbutamide levels	Aprepitant ↑ CYP2C9-mediated metabolism of tolbutamide	Monitor blood glucose closely

(Continued)

Primary Drug	Secondary Drug	Effect	Mechanism	Precautions
SULFONYLUREAS				
SULFONYLUREAS	**ANTIEPILEPTICS**			
SULFONYLUREAS	BARBITURATES	↓ Hypoglycemic efficacy	Plasma levels of sulfonylureas are ↓ by induction of CYP-mediated metabolism	Watch for and warn patients about symptoms of hyperglycemia. ➢ ***For signs and symptoms of hyperglycemia, see Clinical Features of Some Adverse Drug Interactions, Hyperglycemia***
GLIPIZIDE	CARBAMAZEPINE	↓ Blood sugar-lowering effect of glipizide due to ↓ blood levels	↑ Metabolism of glipizide due to ↑ activity of the enzymes that metabolize glipizide by carbamazepine	A higher dose of glipizide may be needed for adequate control of high blood sugar
SULFONYLUREAS	HYDANTOINS	↓ Hypoglycemic efficacy	Hydantoins are considered to ↓ release of insulin	Monitor capillary blood glucose closely; higher doses of antidiabetic drugs are needed
SULFONYLUREAS	ANTIFUNGALS—ITRACONAZOLE, FLUCONAZOLE, MICONAZOLE, VORICONAZOLE	↑ Risk of hypoglycemic episodes	Inhibition of CYP2C9-mediated metabolism of sulfonylureas	Watch for and warn patients about symptoms of hypoglycemia. ➢ ***For signs and symptoms of hypoglycemia, see Clinical Features of Some Adverse Drug Interactions, Hypoglycemia***
SULFONYLUREAS	**ANTIGOUT DRUGS**			
CHLORPROPAMIDE	ALLOPURINOL	↑ Risk of prolonged hypoglycemic effect in the presence of renal impairment	Possible competition for renal excretion	Monitor blood glucose closely
SULFONYLUREAS	PROBENECID	↑ Risk of hypoglycemic episodes due to ↑ plasma levels of glimepiride	Attributed to ↓ renal excretion of sulfonylureas by probenecid. Probenecid is also an inhibitor of CYP2C9 isoenzymes	Watch for and warn patients about symptoms of hypoglycemia. ➢ ***For signs and symptoms of hypoglycemia, see Clinical Features of Some Adverse Drug Interactions, Hypoglycemia***
SULFONYLUREAS	SULFINPYRAZONE	↑ Hypoglycemic effect of sulfonylureas	Uncertain	Monitor blood glucose regularly

(Continued)

ANTIDIABETIC DRUGS SULFONYLUREAS

Primary Drug	Secondary Drug	Effect	Mechanism	Precautions
SULFONYLUREAS				
SULFONYLUREAS	**ANTIHYPERTENSIVES AND HEART FAILURE DRUGS**			
SULFONYLUREAS	ACE INHIBITORS	↑ Risk of hypoglycemic episodes	Mechanism uncertain. ACE inhibitors possibly ↑ insulin sensitivity and glucose utilization. Altered renal function may also be factor. ACE inhibitors may ↑ bradykinin levels, which ↓ production of glucose by the liver. Hypoglycemia is reported as a (rare) side effect of ACE inhibitors. Suggested that the occurrence of hypoglycemia is greater with captopril than enalapril. Captopril and enalapril are used in the treatment of diabetic nephropathy	Concurrent treatment need not be avoided and is often beneficial in type II diabetes. Watch for and warn patients about symptoms of hypoglycemia. Be aware that the risk of hypoglycemia is greater in elderly people and in patients with poor glycemic control. ➢ ***For signs and symptoms of hypoglycemia, see Clinical Features of Some Adverse Drug Interactions, Hypoglycemia***
SULFONYLUREAS	ADRENERGIC NEURONE BLOCKERS	↑ Hypoglycemic effect	Catecholamines are diabetogenic; guanethidine blocks the release of catecholamines from nerve endings	Monitor blood glucose closely
SULFONYLUREAS—TOLBUTAMIDE	ANGIOTENSIN II RECEPTOR ANTAGONISTS—IRBESARTAN	Possible ↑ hypotensive effect of irbesartan	Tolbutamide competitively inhibits CYP2C9-mediated metabolism of irbesartan	Monitor BP at least weekly until stable. Warn patients to report symptoms of hypotension (light-headedness, dizziness on standing, etc.)

(*Continued*)

659

Primary Drug	Secondary Drug	Effect	Mechanism	Precautions
SULFONYLUREAS				
SULFONYLUREAS	VASODILATOR ANTIHYPERTENSIVES—BOSENTAN	1. Risk of hepatotoxicity when bosentan is given with glibenclamide 2. ↑ Risk of hypoglycemic episodes when bosentan is given with tolbutamide	1. Additive effect: both drugs inhibit the bile sodium export pump 2. Bosentan may inhibit CYP2C9-mediated metabolism of tolbutamide	1. Avoid coadministration of bosentan and glibenclamide 2. Monitor blood glucose levels closely. Warn patients about the signs and symptoms of hypoglycemia. ➢ ***For signs and symptoms of hypoglycemia, see Clinical Features of Some Adverse Drug Interactions, Hypoglycemia***
SULFONYLUREAS	DIAZOXIDE	May ↑ Sulfonylurea requirements	Diazoxide causes hyperglycemia by inhibiting insulin release and probably by a catecholamine-induced extrahepatic effect. Sulfonylureas act by ↑ insulin release. Used in the treatment of hypoglycemia due to insulinomas	Larger doses of sulfonylureas are often required; need to monitor blood sugar until adequate control of blood sugar is achieved
SULFONYLUREAS	ANTIOBESITY DRUGS—ORLISTAT, RIMONABANT, SIBUTRAMINE	Tendency for blood glucose levels to fluctuate. There may be a tendency to enhance the hypoglycemic effect	These agents change dietary intake of carbohydrates and other foods, and the risk of fluctuations of blood glucose is greater if there is a concurrent dietary regimen. A side effect of orlistat is hypoglycemia	These agents are used often in type II diabetics on hypoglycemic therapy. Need to monitor blood sugar twice weekly until stable. Advise self-monitoring. Warn patients about hypoglycemia. ➢ ***For signs and symptoms of hypoglycemia, see Clinical Features of Some Adverse Drug Interactions, Hypoglycemia***
SULFONYLUREAS	ANTI-PARKINSON'S DRUGS—RASAGILINE, SELEGILINE	↑ Risk of hypoglycemic episodes	These drugs are MAO-B inhibitors. MAOIs have an intrinsic hypoglycemic effect and are considered to enhance the effect of hypoglycemic drugs	Watch for and warn patients about symptoms of hypoglycemia. ➢ ***For signs and symptoms of hypoglycemia, see Clinical Features of Some Adverse Drug Interactions, Hypoglycemia***

(Continued)

ANTIDIABETIC DRUGS SULFONYLUREAS

Primary Drug	Secondary Drug	Effect	Mechanism	Precautions
SULFONYLUREAS				
SULFONYLUREAS	ANTIPLATELET AGENTS—ASPIRIN	Risk of hypoglycemia when high-dose aspirin (3.5–7.5 g/day) is given with antidiabetic drugs	Additive effect; aspirin has a hypoglycemic effect	Avoid high-dose aspirin
SULFONYLUREAS	ANTIPROTOZOALS—PENTAMIDINE	May alter sulfonylurea requirements due to altered glycemic control	Attributed to pancreatic beta cell toxicity	Need to monitor blood sugar until stable and following withdrawal of pentamidine
SULFONYLUREAS	**ANTIPSYCHOTICS**			
SULFONYLUREAS	CLOZAPINE	May cause ↑ blood sugar and loss of control of blood sugar	Clozapine can cause resistance to the action of insulin	Watch/monitor for diabetes mellitus in subjects on long-term clozapine treatment
SULFONYLUREAS	PHENOTHIAZINES	May ↑ blood sugar-lowering effect and risk of hypoglycemic episodes. Likely to occur with doses exceeding 100 mg/day per day	Phenothiazines such as chlorpromazine inhibit the release of epinephrine and ↑ risk of hypoglycemia. May inhibit release of insulin, which is the mechanism by which sulfonylureas act	Chlorpromazine is nearly always used in the long term. Watch for and warn patients about symptoms of hypoglycemia. ➢ ***For signs and symptoms of hypoglycemia, see Clinical Features of Some Adverse Drug Interactions, Hypoglycemia***
SULFONYLUREAS	ANTIVIRALS—PROTEASE INHIBITORS	↑ Adverse effects of tolbutamide with ritonavir (e.g., myelosuppression, peripheral neuropathy, mucositis)	Uncertain	Monitor blood sugar closely
SULFONYLUREAS	APROTININ	↑ Availability of insulin and risk of hypoglycemic episodes	Aprotinin ↑ availability of insulin injected subcutaneously. The mechanism is uncertain. Sulfonylureas augment insulin release	Watch for and warn patients about symptoms of hypoglycemia. ➢ ***For signs and symptoms of hypoglycemia, see Clinical Features of Some Adverse Drug Interactions, Hypoglycemia***

(*Continued*)

Primary Drug	Secondary Drug	Effect	Mechanism	Precautions
SULFONYLUREAS				
SULFONYLUREAS	BETA-BLOCKERS	Beta-blockers may mask the symptoms and signs of hypoglycemia, such as tachycardia and tremor; there have even been cases of bradycardia and ↑ BP during hypoglycemic episodes in patients on beta-blockers	Beta-blockers prevent or inhibit the normal physiological response to hypoglycemia by interfering with catecholamine-induced mobilization—glycogenolysis and mobilization of glucose—thereby prolonging the time taken by the body to achieve normal (euglycemic) blood sugar levels	Warn patients about the masking of signs of hypoglycemia. Cardioselective beta-blockers are preferred, and all beta-blockers should be avoided in patients having frequent hypoglycemic attacks; otherwise, monitor glycemic control, especially during initiation of therapy. ➢ ***For signs and symptoms of hypoglycemia, see Clinical Features of Some Adverse Drug Interactions, Hypoglycemia***
SULFONYLUREAS	BRONCHODILATORS—BETA-AGONISTS	↑ Risk of hyperglycemia. If administered during pregnancy, there is a risk of hypoglycemia in the fetus, independent of maternal blood glucose levels. ↑ risk of ketoacidosis when administered intravenously	By inducing glycogenolysis, beta-adrenergic agonists cause elevation of blood sugar in adults. In the fetus, these agents cause a depletion of fetal glycogen stores	Monitor blood sugar closely during concomitant administration until blood sugar levels are stable. Be cautious during use in pregnancy. Formoterol and salmeterol are long-acting beta agonists
SULFONYLUREAS	CNS STIMULANTS—MODAFINIL	May cause ↑ plasma concentrations of sulfonylureas if CYP2C9 is the predominant metabolic pathway and the alternative pathways are either genetically deficient or affected	Modafinil is a moderate inhibitor of CYP2C9	Be aware
SULFONYLUREAS	**THIAZIDES**			
SULFONYLUREAS	THIAZIDES	↓ Hypoglycemic efficacy	Hyperglycemia due to antagonistic effect	Monitor blood glucose regularly until stable. A higher dose of oral antidiabetic is often needed
CHLORPROPAMIDE	THIAZIDES	Risk of hyponatremia when chlorpropamide is given to a patient taking both potassium-sparing diuretics/aldosterone antagonists and thiazides	Additive effect; chlorpropamide enhances ADH secretion	Monitor serum sodium regularly

(Continued)

ANTIDIABETIC DRUGS SULFONYLUREAS

Primary Drug	Secondary Drug	Effect	Mechanism	Precautions
SULFONYLUREAS				
SULFONYLUREAS	H2-RECEPTOR BLOCKERS—CIMETIDINE, RANITIDINE	Altered plasma concentrations of glimepride, risk of unstable blood sugar control and hypoglycemic episodes with glipizide and glimepride and of adverse effects with glibenclamide	Cimetidine and ranitidine ↓ renal elimination of glimepride and ↑ intestinal absorption of glimepride. Cimetidine also inhibits metabolism via CYP2C9	Avoid coadministration with cimetidine if possible. Consider alternative acid suppression, e.g., a proton pump inhibitor (not omeprazole), and monitor more closely
SULFONYLUREAS	**LIPID-LOWERING DRUGS**			
SULFONYLUREAS	ANION EXCHANGE RESINS	1. Glipizide absorption may be ↓ by colestyramine 2. Glibenclamide absorption may be ↓ by colesevelam	1. Colestyramine interrupts the enterohepatic circulation of glipizide 2. Likely colesevelam binds glibenclamide in the stomach and small bowel	1. Avoid coadministration 2. Take glibenclamide 4 h before colesevelam
TOLBUTAMIDE	FIBRATES	Fibrates may ↑ efficacy of sulfonylureas	Uncertain; postulated that fibrates displace sulfonylureas from plasma proteins and ↓ their hepatic metabolism. In addition, fenofibrate may inhibit CYP2C9-mediated metabolism of tolbutamide	Monitor blood glucose levels closely. Warn patients about hypoglycemia. ➢ ***For signs and symptoms of hypoglycemia, see Clinical Features of Some Adverse Drug Interactions, Hypoglycemia***
SULFONYLUREAS	MUSCLE RELAXANTS—BACLOFEN	↓ Hypoglycemic effect of sulfonylureas	Due to these drugs causing hyperglycemia, the mechanism is uncertain at present	↑ Doses of sulfonylureas are often required for adequate glycemic control
SULFONYLUREAS	NANDROLONE	↑ Effect of antidiabetic drugs	Uncertain	Monitor blood sugar closely. Banned by sporting authorities.
SULFONYLUREAS	NIACIN	↓ Hypoglycemic effect of sulfonylureas	Uncertain at present. The effects of niacin (< or = 2.5 g/d), alone or in combination with statins, on fasting glucose (an increase of 4%–5%) and hemoglobin A1c levels (an increase of < or = 0.3%) are modest, transient or reversible	Typically amenable to adjustments in oral hypoglycemic regimens without discontinuing niacin. Benefits outweigh risks. ↑ Doses of antidiabetics are often necessary

(*Continued*)

Primary Drug	Secondary Drug	Effect	Mechanism	Precautions
SULFONYLUREAS				
SULFONYLUREAS	NICOTINE	↓ Hypoglycemic effect of sulfonylureas	Uncertain at present. Exposure of human blood samples to nicotine raised the level of hemoglobin A1c. The higher the nicotine dose, the more the A1c level rose. Cigarettes, by working through a drug interaction cause the body to release its own stores of sugar usually in a matter of seconds	↑ Doses of sulfonylureas are often required for adequate glycemic control
SULFONYLUREAS	ESTROGENS	Altered glycemic control	Uncertain at present. Significantly high or low levels of estrogen could both be involved in the development of insulin resistance. Higher than normal estrogen appears to be linked with increased insulin resistance, yet other studies have shown that low estrogen levels, are linked with greater insulin resistance	Monitor blood glucose closely
SULFONYLUREAS	PROGESTOGENS	Altered glycemic control	Uncertain at present. One study revealed that low progesterone levels, cause over-production of insulin, leading to hypoglycemia and an outpouring of adrenaline to bring sugar levels up	Monitor blood glucose closely
SULFONYLUREAS	PROTON PUMP INHIBITORS	Possible ↑ efficacy and adverse effects of sulfonylurea, e.g., hypoglycemia	Possible ↑ absorption	Monitor capillary blood glucose more closely; ↓ dose may be required

(*Continued*)

ANTIDIABETIC DRUGS THIAZOLIDINEDIONES (GLITAZONES)—PIOGLITAZONE, ROSIGLITAZONE

Primary Drug	Secondary Drug	Effect	Mechanism	Precautions
SULFONYLUREAS				
SULFONYLUREAS	SOMATROPIN	↓ Hypoglycemic effect of sulfonylureas	Due to these drugs causing hyperglycemia, the mechanism is uncertain at present	↑ Doses of sulfonylureas are often required for adequate glycemic control
SULFONYLUREAS	SYMPATHOMIMETICS—EPINEPHRINE	May ↑ antidiabetic therapy requirement	Epinephrine causes the release of glucose from the liver and is an important defense/homeostatic mechanism. Hyperglycemia due to antagonistic effect	Larger doses of antidiabetic therapy may be needed during the period of epinephrine use, which is usually in the short term or in emergency situations
SULFONYLUREAS	TESTOSTERONE	↑ Hypoglycemic effect and ↑ of hypoglycemic episodes	Exact mechanism is uncertain. Low testosterone levels are associated with type II diabetes. Experimental work has suggested that testosterone may play a role in glucose efflux from cells	Warn patients about symptoms of hypoglycemia. ➢ ***For signs and symptoms of hypoglycemia, see Clinical Features of Some Adverse Drug Interactions, Hypoglycemia***
SULFONYLUREAS	THYROID HORMONES	↓ Hypoglycemic effect of sulfonylureas	Due to these drugs causing hyperglycemia, the mechanism is uncertain at present	↑ Doses of sulfonylureas are often required for adequate glycemic control

Primary Drug	Secondary Drug	Effect	Mechanism	Precautions
THIAZOLIDINEDIONES (GLITAZONES)—PIOGLITAZONE, ROSIGLITAZONE				
PIOGLITAZONE, ROSIGLITAZONE	ALCOHOL	Tends to mask signs of hypoglycemia and ↑ risk of hypoglycemic episodes	Inhibits glucose production and release from many sources, including the liver and release	Watch for and warn patients about hypoglycemia. ➢ ***For signs and symptoms of hypoglycemia, see Clinical Features of Some Adverse Drug Interactions, Hypoglycemia***

(*Continued*)

Primary Drug	Secondary Drug	Effect	Mechanism	Precautions
THIAZOLIDINEDIONES (GLITAZONES)—PIOGLITAZONE, ROSIGLITAZONE				
PIOGLITAZONE, ROSIGLITAZONE	ANTIARRHYTHMICS—DISOPYRAMIDE	↑ Risk of hypoglycemic episodes—particularly in patients with impaired renal function. Hypoglycemic attacks may occur even when plasma levels of disopyramide are within the normal range (attacks occurring with plasma disopyramide levels of 1–4 ng/mL)	Disopyramide and its metabolite mono-isopropyl disopyramide ↑ secretion of insulin (considered to be due to inhibition of potassium-ATP channels). Suggestion that disopyramide causes an impairment of the counter-regulatory (homeostatic) mechanisms that follow hypoglycemia	In patients receiving antidiabetic drugs, start with the lowest dose of disopyramide if there is no alternative. Measure creatinine clearance. If creatinine clearance is 40 mL/min or less, the dose of disopyramide should not exceed 100 mg and should be administered once daily if creatinine clearance is <15 mL/min. Watch for and warn patients about symptoms of hypoglycemia. ➢ ***For signs and symptoms of hypoglycemia, see Clinical Features of Some Adverse Drug Interactions, Hypoglycemia***
PIOGLITAZONE, ROSIGLITAZONE	**ANTIBIOTICS**			
PIOGLITAZONE, ROSIGLITAZONE	ISONIAZID	↓ Efficacy of antidiabetic drugs	Isoniazid causes hyperglycemia, the mechanism is uncertain at present	Monitor capillary blood glucose closely; ↑ doses of antidiabetic drugs may be needed
PIOGLITAZONE, ROSIGLITAZONE	QUINOLONES—CIPROFLOXACIN, NORFLOXACIN, OFLOXACIN	↑ Risk of hypoglycemic episodes	Mechanism uncertain. Ciprofloxacin is a potent inhibitor of CYP1A2. Norfloxacin is a weak inhibitor of CYP1A2, but these may inhibit other CYP isoenzymes to varying degrees	Watch for and warn patients about hypoglycemia. ➢ ***For signs and symptoms of hypoglycemia, see Clinical Features of Some Adverse Drug Interactions, Hypoglycemia***
PIOGLITAZONE, ROSIGLITAZONE	RIFAMPICIN	Significant ↓ in blood levels of rosiglitazone. Metabolism and clearance is ↑, the latter threefold	Rosiglitazone is metabolized primarily by CYP2C8, with a minor contribution from CYP2C9. Rifampicin is a potent inducer of CYP2C8 and CYP2C9 and ↑ the formation of *N*-desmethyl-rosiglitazone by about 40%	May need to use an alternative drug or ↑ dose of rosiglitazone

(*Continued*)

Primary Drug	Secondary Drug	Effect	Mechanism	Precautions
THIAZOLIDINEDIONES (GLITAZONES)—PIOGLITAZONE, ROSIGLITAZONE				
PIOGLITAZONE, ROSIGLITAZONE	TRIMETHOPRIM	↑ In blood levels of rosiglitazone by nearly 40%	Trimethoprim is a relatively selective inhibitor of CYP2C8	Watch for hypoglycemic events and ↓ dose of rosiglitazone after repeated blood sugar measurements. Warn patients about hypoglycemia. ➢ ***For signs and symptoms of hypoglycemia, see Clinical Features of Some Adverse Drug Interactions, Hypoglycemia***
THIAZOLIDINEDIONES	**ANTICANCER AND IMMUNOMODULATING DRUGS**			
THIAZOLIDINEDIONES	CORTICOSTEROIDS	Antihyperglycemic effect of antidiabetic agent antagonized	Increased gluconeogenesis from the liver	Monitor blood glucose closely
THIAZOLIDINEDIONES	OCTREOTIDE, LANTREOTIDE	Requirements of antidiabetic agents possibly reduced	Decreased insulin secretion	Consider lowering dose of thiazolidinedione
ROSIGLITAZONE	PIXANTRONE	Theoretical risk of increased drug levels	Pixantrone inhibits CYP2C8	Manufacturer advises caution
PIOGLITAZONE, ROSIGLITAZONE	**ANTIDEPRESSANTS**			
PIOGLITAZONE, ROSIGLITAZONE	SSRIs	Fluctuations in blood sugar are very likely, with both hypoglycemic and hyperglycemic events being reported in diabetics receiving hypoglycemic treatment	Brain serotonin- and corticotropin-releasing hormone systems participate in the control of blood sugar levels. ↑ (usually acute) in brain serotonergic activity induces a hyperglycemic response	Both hyper- and hypoglycemic responses have been reported with SSRIs, and there is a need to monitor blood glucose closely prior to, during, and after discontinuing SSRI treatment. ➢ ***For signs and symptoms of hypoglycemia and hpyerglycemia, see Clinical Features of Some Adverse Drug Interactions, Hypoglycemia, Hyperglycemia***

(*Continued*)

Primary Drug	Secondary Drug	Effect	Mechanism	Precautions
THIAZOLIDINEDIONES (GLITAZONES)—PIOGLITAZONE, ROSIGLITAZONE				
PIOGLITAZONE, ROSIGLITAZONE	TCAs	Likely to impair control of diabetes	TCAs may ↑ serum glucose levels by up to 150%, ↑ appetite (particularly carbohydrate craving) and ↓ metabolic rate	Be aware and monitor blood sugar weekly until stable. They are generally considered safe unless diabetes is poorly controlled or is associated with significant cardiac or renal disease. Amitriptyline, imipramine, and citalopram are also used to treat painful diabetic neuropathy
THIAZOLIDINEDIONES	**OTHER ANTIDIABETIC DRUGS**			
THIAZOLIDINEDIONES	DDP-4 INHIBITORS—SAXAGLIPTIN	Peripheral edema with saxagliptin	Unknown mechanism	Monitor for signs of edema and stop if necessary
THIAZOLIDEDIONES	INSULIN	1. Edema 2. Hypoglycemia	1. Exacerbated by salt retaining potential of insulin 2. Due to increased insulin sensitivity	1. Warn patients to report increasing peripheral edema and symptoms such as shortness of breath/reduced exercise tolerance 2. May be used therapeutically; monitor blood glucose closely
THIAZOLIDEDIONES	SGLT-2 INHIBITORS—DAPAGLIFLOZIN	Potential risk of urogenital malignancies	Both drugs in clinical trial program have identified a signal of increased bladder cancer	Avoid concomitant prescribing
THIAZOLIDEDIONES	SULFONYLUREAS	1. Edema 2. Hypoglycemia		1. Warn patients to report increasing peripheral edema and symptoms such as shortness of breath/reduced exercise tolerance 2. May be used therapeutically; monitor blood glucose closely

(*Continued*)

Primary Drug	Secondary Drug	Effect	Mechanism	Precautions
THIAZOLIDINEDIONES (GLITAZONES)—PIOGLITAZONE, ROSIGLITAZONE				
PIOGLITAZONE, ROSIGLITAZONE	**ANTIHYPERTENSIVES AND HEART FAILURE DRUGS**			
PIOGLITAZONE, ROSIGLITAZONE	ADRENERGIC NEURONE BLOCKERS	↑ Hypoglycemic effect	Catecholamines are diabetogenic; guanethidine blocks the release of catecholamines from nerve endings	Monitor blood glucose closely
PIOGLITAZONE, ROSIGLITAZONE	VASODILATOR ANTIHYPERTENSIVES—DIAZOXIDE	May ↑ antidiabetic requirements; hypoglycemic effect of antidiabetics antagonized by diazoxide	Diazoxide causes hyperglycemia by inhibiting insulin release and probably by a catecholamine-induced extrahepatic effect	Higher doses of antidiabetic agents are often required. Diazoxide should not be used to treat low blood sugar from poor nutrition/diet (functional hypoglycemia)
PIOGLITAZONE, ROSIGLITAZONE	ANTIPLATELET AGENTS—ASPIRIN	Risk of hypoglycemia when high-dose aspirin (3.5–7.5 g/day) is given with antidiabetic drugs	Additive effect; aspirin has a hypoglycemic effect	Avoid high-dose aspirin
PIOGLITAZONE	ANTIVIRALS—PROTEASE INHIBITORS	↑ Levels of these antidiabetic drugs	Inhibition of CYP3A4-mediated metabolism of pioglitazone	Monitor blood sugar closely
THIAZOLIDINEDIONES	ANXIOLYTICS AND HYPNOTICS—MIDAZOLAM	Reduction in AUC of midazolam (syrup)	Possibly related to metabolism using the same CYP3A4 pathway	Midazolam dose may need compensatory increase when coadministered
PIOGLITAZONE, ROSIGLITAZONE	BETA-BLOCKERS	Beta-blockers may mask the symptoms and signs of hypoglycemia. They also ↓ insulin sensitivity; however, beta-blockers that also have vasodilating properties (carvedilol, celiprolol, labetalol, nebivolol) seem to ↑ sensitivity to insulin	Beta-blockers ↓ glucose tolerance and interfere with the metabolic and autonomic responses to hypoglycemia	Warn patients about the masking of signs of hypoglycemia. Vasodilating beta-blockers are preferred in patients with diabetes, and all beta-blockers should be avoided in those having frequent hypoglycemic attacks. Monitor capillary blood glucose closely, especially during initiation of therapy. ➢ ***For signs and symptoms of hypoglycemia, see Clinical Features of Some Adverse Drug Interactions, Hypoglycemia***

(Continued)

Primary Drug	Secondary Drug	Effect	Mechanism	Precautions
THIAZOLIDINEDIONES (GLITAZONES)—PIOGLITAZONE, ROSIGLITAZONE				
THIAZOLIDINEDIONES	CALCIUM CHANNEL BLOCKERS—NIFEDIPINE	Decreased levels of Nifedipine in the blood	Possibly related to metabolism using the same CYP3A4 pathway	Nifedipine dose may need to be increased
PIOGLITAZONE, ROSIGLITAZONE	**CNS STIMULANTS**			
PIOGLITAZONE	MODAFINIL	May ↓ modafinil levels	Induction of CYP3A4, which has a partial role in the metabolism of modafinil	Be aware
ROSIGLITAZONE	MODAFINIL	May cause ↑ plasma concentrations of rosiglitazone if CYP2C9 is the predominant metabolic pathway and the alternative pathways are either genetically deficient or affected	Modafinil is a moderate inhibitor of CYP2C9	Be aware
ROSIGLITAZONE	LIPID-LOWERING DRUGS—GEMFIBROZIL	↑ In blood levels of rosiglitazone—often doubled	Gemfibrozil is a relatively selective inhibitor of CYP2C8	Watch for hypoglycemic events and ↓ dose of rosiglitazone after repeated blood sugar measurements. Warn patients about hypoglycemia. ➢ ***For signs and symptoms of hypoglycemia, see Clinical Features of Some Adverse Drug Interactions, Hypoglycemia***
THIAZOLIDINEDIONES	STATINS—ATORVASTATIN	Decreased levels of both pioglitazone and atorvastatin in the blood	Possibly related to metabolism using the same CYP3A4 pathway	Consider increasing doses of both agents
PIOGLITAZONE, ROSIGLITAZONE	MUSCLE RELAXANTS—BACLOFEN	↓ Hypoglycemic effect	Due to these drugs causing hyperglycemia, the mechanism is uncertain at present	↑ Doses of antidiabetic are often required for adequate glycemic control
PIOGLITAZONE, ROSIGLITAZONE	NANDROLONE	↑ Effect of antidiabetic drugs	Uncertain	Monitor blood sugar closely. Banned by sporting authorities.

(Continued)

ANTIDIABETIC DRUGS THIAZOLIDINEDIONES (GLITAZONES)—PIOGLITAZONE, ROSIGLITAZONE

Primary Drug	Secondary Drug	Effect	Mechanism	Precautions
THIAZOLIDINEDIONES (GLITAZONES)—PIOGLITAZONE, ROSIGLITAZONE				
PIOGLITAZONE, ROSIGLITAZONE	NIACIN	↓ Hypoglycemic effect	Uncertain at present. The effects of niacin (< or = 2.5 g/d), alone or in combination with statins, on fasting glucose (an increase of 4%–5%) and hemoglobin A1c levels (an increase of < or = 0.3%) are modest, transient or reversible	↑ Typically amenable to adjustments in oral hypoglycemic regimens without discontinuing niacin. Benefits outweigh risks. ↑ Doses of antidiabetics are often necessary
PIOGLITAZONE, ROSIGLITAZONE	NICOTINE	↓ Hypoglycemic effect	Uncertain at present. Exposure of human blood samples to nicotine raised the level of hemoglobin A1c. The higher the nicotine dose, the more the A1c level rose. Cigarettes, by working through a drug interaction cause the body to release its own stores of sugar usually in a matter of seconds	↑ Doses of antidiabetic are often required for adequate glycemic control
PIOGLITAZONE, ROSIGLITAZONE	ESTROGENS	Altered glycemic control	Uncertain at present. Significantly high or low levels of estrogen could both be involved in the development of insulin resistance. Higher than normal estrogen appears to be linked with increased insulin resistance, yet other studies have shown that low estrogen levels, are linked with greater insulin resistance	Monitor blood glucose closely

(*Continued*)

Primary Drug	Secondary Drug	Effect	Mechanism	Precautions
THIAZOLIDINEDIONES (GLITAZONES)—PIOGLITAZONE, ROSIGLITAZONE				
PIOGLITAZONE, ROSIGLITAZONE	PROGESTOGENS	Altered glycemic control	Uncertain at present. One study revealed that low progesterone levels,cause over-production of insulin, leading to hypoglycemia and an outpouring of adrenaline to bring sugar levels up	Monitor blood glucose closely
PIOGLITAZONE, ROSIGLITAZONE	SOMATROPIN	↓ Hypoglycemic effect	Growth hormone is considered to have anti-insulin activity by suppressing the ability of insulin to stimulate uptake of glucose in peripheral tissues and enhance glucose synthesis in the liver. Paradoxically, administration of growth hormone stimulates insulin secretion, leading to hyperinsulinemia	↑ Doses of antidiabetic are often required for adequate glycemic control
PIOGLITAZONE, ROSIGLITAZONE	THYROID HORMONES	↓ Hypoglycemic effect	Due to these drugs causing hyperglycemia, the mechanism is uncertain at present	↑ Doses of antidiabetic are often required for adequate glycemic control

PART 6

Other Endocrine Drugs

Ming Ming Teh, Yohan P. Samarasinghe, and Janaka Karalliedde

Primary Drug	Secondary Drug	Effect	Mechanism	Precautions
BISPHOSPHONATES				
ALENDRONATE, ETIDRONATE, IBANDRONATE, RISEDRONATE, ZOLEDRONIC ACID	ANALGESICS—NSAIDs	Risk of esophagitis/peptic ulceration. ↑ Risk of renal damage	Additive effect. A recent study showed that GI ulcers occurred in 17% of patients on NSAIDs without concurrent bisphosphonates, and in 31% of patients receiving bisphosphonates with NSAIDs. The i.v. bisphosphonates are not metabolized, do not interact with or affect the P450 enzyme system, and are excreted unchanged by the kidneys by glomerular filtration, without a significant component of tubular secretion	Avoid coadministration. Risk probably less for ibandronate. Monitoring serum creatinine prior to each treatment, temporarily withholding therapy in the setting of renal insufficiency, and adjusting doses in patients with pre-existing chronic kidney disease. Zoledronate is not recommended for use in patients with a creatinine clearance (CrCl) <30ml/min, and the dose should be adjusted for CrCl values between 30–60cc/min. Renal damage is minimized by administering IV bisphosphonates to well hydrated patients. These include swallowing the drug with a large glass of water and remaining in the upright position for at least 30 min after intake (60 min for ibandronate). One case of transient elevated liver enzymes has been reported with zoledronic acid and ibuprofen
BISPHOSPHONATES	ANTACIDS	↓ Bisphosphonate levels	↓ Absorption	Separate doses by at least 30 min
CLODRONATE	ANTIBIOTICS—AMINOGLYCOSIDES	Medications containing divalent/trivalent cations Ca, Mg, Al, Fe, Zn, e.g., antacids	Chelation occurs decreasing drug absorption	Monitor calcium levels closely
BISPHOSPHONATES	**ANTICANCER AND OTHER IMMUNOMODULATING DRUGS**			
CLODRONATE	ESTRAMUSTINE	Increased estramustine levels	Uncertain	Monitor closely with concurrent use

(Continued)

Primary Drug	Secondary Drug	Effect	Mechanism	Precautions
BISPHOSPHONATES				
BISPHOSPHONATES	AMINOGLYCOSIDES	Renal damage due to bisphosphonates could be exacerbated by aminoglycoside antibiotics. Impaired renal function ↓ bisphosphonate excretion and can lead to excessive serum (and bone) levels with resultant toxicity	Additive renal toxicity	Monitor renal function prior to and during coadministration and alter dosage as required
BISPHOSPHONATES	DEFERASIROX	May increase risk of gastrointestinal bleeds	Both drugs can cause GI bleeding	Avoid concomitant prescribing
BISPHOSPHONATES	PROTON PUMP INHIBITORS	An apparent increase in the risk of fracture has been reported in individuals receiving acid-proton pump inhibitors	Unclear	Not reported with histamine H_2-receptor antagonists
BISPHOSPHONATES	VITAMIN D	May cause hypercalcemia	Both drugs increase calcium levels	Monitor calcium and phosphorus levels

Primary Drug	Secondary Drug	Effect	Mechanism	Precautions
CARBIMAZOLE				
CARBIMAZOLE	CORTICOSTEROIDS	Reduced prednisolone levels	Uncertain	Higher doses of prednisolone may be needed

Primary Drug	Secondary Drug	Effect	Mechanism	Precautions
CONIVAPTAN				
CONIVAPTAN	**ANTICANCER AND OTHER IMMUNOMODULATING DRUGS**			
CONIVAPTAN	BOSUTINIB, SUNITINIB	Increased bosutinib levels; levels may ↑ by 50%	CYP3A inhibition	Manufacturer advises avoid concurrent use. If not possible, interruption of therapy or dose reduction should be considered
CONIVAPTAN	LAPATINIB	Increased lapatinib levels	P-glycoprotein inhibition and inhibition of CYP3A4	Caution with concurrent use
CONIVAPTAN	NILOTINIB	Increased nilotinib levels	P-glycoprotein inhibition and inhibition of CYP3A4	Caution with concurrent use

(*Continued*)

Primary Drug	Secondary Drug	Effect	Mechanism	Precautions
CONIVAPTAN				
CONIVAPATAN	IMANITIB, ITRACONAZOLE, KETCONAZOLE-See other strong inhibitors of CYP3A4 in CYP section	↑ Levels of conivapatan	Imanitib would inhibits metabolism of conivapatan by CYP3A4	Avoid coadministration with strong CYP3A4 inhibitors
CONIVAPATAN	CYP3A4 INDUCRS	↓ Levels of conivapatan	Due ↑ metabolism of conivapatan	Be aware
CONIVAPATAN	PIMOZIDE, ASTEMIZOLE	↑ Levels of pimozide and risk of dangerous arrhythmias	Decreased metabolism of pimozide	Avoid coadministration
CONIVAPATAN	LOMITAPIDE	↑ Levels of lomitapide	↑ Levels of lomitapide	Monitor for lomitapide toxicity (e.g.) liver injury, GI disturbances
CONIVAPTAN	ELIGLUSTAT	↑ Eliglustat levels	Inhibition of CYP3A4-mediated metabolism	Reduce dose to 85 mg od in extensive metabolizers. Avoid coadministration in intermediate and poor metabolizers; Eliglustat is contraindicated if strong or moderate inhibitors of CYP2D6 are coadministered with strong or moderate inhibitors of CYP3A4
CONIVAPTAN	NITISINONE	Possible ↑ nitisinone levels	Inhibition of limited CYP3A4-mediated metabolism	Monitor carefully

Primary Drug	Secondary Drug	Effect	Mechanism	Precautions
DANAZOL ➢ *Drugs Used in Obstetrics and Gynaecology*				

Primary Drug	Secondary Drug	Effect	Mechanism	Precautions
DESMOPRESSIN				
DESMOPRESSIN	**ANALGESICS**			
DESMOPRESSIN	NSAIDs	↑ Efficacy of desmopressin with indomethacin	Additive water retention effect	Monitor U&Es and BP closely
DESMOPRESSIN	OPIOIDS	May enhance the adverse/ toxic effect of desmopressin	May contribute to hyponatremia. Mechanism uncertain	Monitor serum sodium before and after concurrent treatment

(Continued)

Primary Drug	Secondary Drug	Effect	Mechanism	Precautions
DESMOPRESSIN				
DESMOPRESSIN	ANTIDIARRHEAL DRUGS—LOPERAMIDE	↑ Desmopressin levels when given orally	Delayed intestinal transit time t absorption of desmopressin	Watch for early features of desmopressin toxicity (e.g., abdominal pain, headaches)

Primary Drug	Secondary Drug	Effect	Mechanism	Precautions
DIAZOXIDE ➢ *Cardiovascular Drugs, Antihypertensives, and Heart Failure Drugs*				
DUTASTERIDE ➢ *Urological Drugs*				
FEMALE SEX HORMONES ➢ *Drugs Used in Obstetrics and Gynaecology*				
GESTRINONE ➢ *Drugs Used in Obstetrics and Gynaecology*				

Primary Drug	Secondary Drug	Effect	Mechanism	Precautions
GLUCAGON				
GLUCAGON	ANTICOAGULANTS—ORAL AND HEPARIN	↑ Anticoagulant effect	Uncertain at present	Monitor INR after administration of glucagon
GLUCAGON	BETA-BLOCKERS	↓ Hyperglycemic effect of glucagon	Uncertain; Beta blockers may mask signs of hypoglycemia	Monitor blood sugar closely
GLUCAGON	DICHLORPHENAMIDE	Additive hypokalemia	Uncertain	Monitor serum potassium closely
GLUCAGON	ANTIDEPRESSANTS- TCA's, SSRIs (FLUOXETINE)	Fluoxetine can sometimes enhance the effects of desmopressin. May increase the risk of developing water retention and hyponatremia	Uncertain	Seek medical attention if there is loss of appetite, nausea, vomiting, headache, lethargy, irritability, difficulty concentrating, memory impairment, confusion, muscle spasm, weakness, unsteadiness, decreased urination, and/or sudden weight gain. These may be symptoms of water intoxication and hyponatremia

Primary Drug	Secondary Drug	Effect	Mechanism	Precautions
NANDROLONE				
NANDROLONE	ANTICOAGULANTS—ORAL	Episodes of bleeding when patients on oral anticoagulants are started on anabolic steroids	Not understood	↓ Dose of anticoagulant by 50% and monitor INR closely until stabilized
NANDROLONE	ANTICANCER AND IMMUNOMODULATING DRUGS—CICLOSPORIN, LEFLUNOMIDE	Cases of hepatotoxicity	Uncertain	Monitor LFTs closely
NANDROLONE	ANTIDIABETIC DRUGS	↑ Effect of antidiabetic drugs	Uncertain	Monitor blood sugar closely

Primary Drug	Secondary Drug	Effect	Mechanism	Precautions
PEGVISOMANT (GROWTH HORMONE RECEPTOR ANTAGONIST)				
PEGVISOMANT	OPIOIDS	May diminish the therapeutic effect of pegvisomant	Narcotic medicines, e.g., opioids decrease effect—the mechanism for relative resistance is uncertain	Need higher doses of pegvisomant for therapeutic results during concomitant use
PEGVISOMANT	INSULIN AND/OR ORAL HYPOGLYCEMIC AGENTS	Glucose tolerance may increase in some patients treated with pegvisomant	GH opposes the effects of http://www.rxlist.com/script/main/art.asp?articlekey=3989 insulin on carbohydrate metabolism by ↓ insulin sensitivity	Patients on pegvisomant therapy with acromegaly and diabetes mellitus treated with http://www.rxlist.com/script/main/art.asp?articlekey=3989 insulin and/or oral http://www.rxlist.com/script/main/art.asp?articlekey=18046 hypoglycemic agents may require dose reductions of insulin and/or oral hypoglycemic agents
RALOXIFENE	CHOLESTYRAMINE, COLESTIPOL ANTICOAGULANTS e.g., warfarin	↓ Efficacy of raloxifene ↓ Efficacy of anticoagulants	↓ Absorption of raloxifene Raloxifene may increase the risk of blood clot in legs or lungs	Separate drug intake by at least 2 h Monitor efficacy of anticoagulant
RALOXIFENE	DIAZEPAM, DIAZOXIDE LIDOCAINE	↑ Risk of adverse effects of these drugs due to raloxifene	Raloxifene displaces these drugs from plasma proteins increasing their free fraction	Warn patients re adverse effects of coadministered drugs

OTHER ENDOCRINE DRUGS PEGVISOMANT (GROWTH HORMONE RECEPTOR ANTAGONIST)

Primary Drug	Secondary Drug	Effect	Mechanism	Precautions
SOMATROPIN (GROWTH HORMONE)				
SOMATROPIN	**ANTICANCER AND IMMUNOMODULATING DRUGS**			
SOMATROPIN	CICLOSPORIN	Predicted reduced ciclosporin levels	CYP3A4 induction	Monitor closely
SOMATROPIN	CORTICOSTEROIDS	Possible ↓ efficacy of somatropin	Uncertain	Watch for poor response to somatropin
SOMATROPIN	ANTIDIABETIC DRUGS	↓ Hypoglycemic effect of insulin	GH opposes the effects of insulin on carbohydrate metabolism by ↓ insulin sensitivity	↑ Doses of antidiabetic agents are often required for adequate glycemic control
SOMATROPIN	ESTROGENS	Possible ↓ efficacy of somatropin	Uncertain; Evidence that estrogen modulates GH action independent of secretion	↑ Dose of somatropin may be needed

Primary Drug	Secondary Drug	Effect	Mechanism	Precautions
STEROID REPLACEMENT THERAPY ➢ *Anticancer and Immunomodulating Drugs, Other Immunomodulating Drugs*				
STRONTIUM RANELATE				
STRONTIUM RANELATE	ANTIBIOTICS—QUINOLONES, TETRACYCLINES	↓ Levels of these antibiotics	↓ Absorption	Avoid coadministration
STRONTIUM RANELATE	ANTIPSYCHOTICS—CLOZAPINE	Increased risk of bone marrow toxicity	Uncertain	Monitor FBC closely
STRONTIUM RANELATE	RANELATECALCIUM SUPPLEMENTS, ANTACIDS (MEDICATIONS CONTAINING ALUMINUM, CALCIUM, OR MAGNESIUM)	↓ Effect of strontium ranelate	Possibly due to ↓ absorption	Take these products 2 hours after strontium ranelate

Primary Drug	Secondary Drug	Effect	Mechanism	Precautions
TESTOSTERONE				
TESTOSTERONE	ANTICOAGULANTS—ORAL	Possible ↑ anticoagulant effect	Uncertain	Monitor INR at least weekly until stable

(Continued)

Primary Drug	Secondary Drug	Effect	Mechanism	Precautions
TESTOSTERONE				
TESTOSTERONE	ANTIDIABETIC DRUGS	↑ Hypoglycemic effect and ↑ risk of hypoglycemic episodes	Exact mechanism is uncertain. Low testosterone levels are associated with type II diabetes. Experimental work has suggested that testosterone may play a role in glucose efflux from cells	Warn patients about symptoms of hypoglycemia; Reduced doses of hypoglycemic drugs are often required ➢ ***For signs and symptoms of hypoglycemia, see clinical features of some adverse drug interactions, hypoglycemia***
TESTOSTERONE	DUTASTERIDE, FINASTERIDE	↑ Testosterone levels when testosterone administered orally	↑ Bioavailability	May be used therapeutically
TESTOSTERONE	ADRENOCORTICOTROPIC HORMONE (ACTH) OR CORTICOSTEROIDS	May result in increased fluid retention	Additive effect of fluid retention	Requires careful monitoring particularly in patients with cardiac, renal or hepatic disease
TESTOSTERONE	SEVELAMER HYDROCHLORIDE, CHROMIUM PICOLINATE	↓ Absorption of thyroid hormone preparations	Each significantly ↓ thyroxine AUC	Hypothyroid patients taking sevelamer hydrochloride or chromium picolinate should be advised to separate the time of ingestion of these drugs from their thyroid hormone preparation by several hours. Ezetimibe had no effect

Primary Drug	Secondary Drug	Effect	Mechanism	Precautions
THYROID HORMONES AND IODINE				
POTASSIUM IODIDE	ANTIDEPRESSANTS—LITHIUM	Hypothyroidism	Uncertain	Be aware—monitor TFTs
THYROID HORMONES	ANESTHETICS—GENERAL—KETAMINE	Cases of tachycardia and hypertension when ketamine was given to patients on thyroxine; this required treatment with propranolol	Uncertain	Monitor PR and BP closely

(Continued)

OTHER ENDOCRINE DRUGS THYROID HORMONES AND IODINE

Primary Drug	Secondary Drug	Effect	Mechanism	Precautions
THYROID HORMONES AND IODINE				
THYROID HORMONES	ANTIARRHYTHMICS—AMIODARONE	Risk of either under- or overtreatment of thyroid function	Amiodarone contains iodine and has been reported to cause both hyper- and hypothyroidism; May be due to inhibition of T4 transport and T4 deiodination into T3	Monitor triiodothyronine, thyroxine, and TSH levels at least 6 months
THYROID HORMONES	BETA ADRENERGIC BLOCKERS—PROPRANOLOL, ALPRENOLOL, SOTALOL, ATENOLOL, METOPROLOL	Significant ↓ in serum T3 after propranolol, alprenolol, atenolol, and metoprolol. A significant increase in rT3 was found in the propranolol and alprenolol treated groups whereas a significant fall in rT3 was found in the atenolol and metoprolol treated groups	The changes observed in serum T3 and in rT3 could be explained by an inhibition of the 5′deiodinase enzyme by propranolol and alprenolol and an inhibition of both the 5′deiodinase and 5 deiodinase enzymes caused by atenolol and metoprolol	Monitor thyroid function tests before and after initiating therapy until stable. No change was found in the sotalol treated group
THYROID HORMONES	**ANTIBIOTICS**			
THYROID HORMONES	QUINOLONES—CIPROFLOXACIN	↓ Levels of levothyroxine and possible therapeutic failure	The mechanism has not been elucidated; the concurrent administration of ciprofloxacin with levothyroxine may interfere with the absorption of levothyroxine and result in lower than expected levels	The interaction may be minimized by separating dosing of the two agents; ciprofloxacin should be taken several hours before or after taking levothyroxine
THYROID HORMONES	RIFAMPICIN	↓ Levothyroxine levels	Induction of metabolism	Monitor TFTs regularly and consider ↑ dose of levothyroxine

(*Continued*)

Primary Drug	Secondary Drug	Effect	Mechanism	Precautions
THYROID HORMONES AND IODINE				
THYROID HORMONES	**ANTICANCER AND IMMUNOMODULATING DRUGS (IMATINIB)**			
THYROID HORMONES	ANTICANCER AND IMMUNOMODULATING DRUGS—IMANITIB, SUNITIB, VANDETANIB, MOTESANIB, SORAFENIB	Sunitinib-a first-generation tyrosine kinase inhibitors (TKIs) likely causes thyroid dysfunction more frequently than other TKI classes, leading to hypothyroidism, but also to thyrotoxicosis. Symptoms of hypothyroidism in all patients who had undergone thyroidectomy, whereas patients with the thyroid in situ remained clinically and biochemically euthyroid. Imatinib in L-T4 treated hypothyroid patients increases serum TSH in all patients (towards five times the upper normal limit), and FT4 values are reduced by about 60% but remain within the normal range. Motesanib in L-T4 treated hypothyroid patients is associated with TSH concentrations ten times higher than baseline on at least one occasion in 50% of patients. Sorafenib induces hypothyroidism in euthroid patients with intact thyroid glands in 18%. In another study, sorafenib ↓ serum FT4 and T3 by 11% and 18% respectively, whereas TSH levels ↑ (requiring a slight increase of L-T4 dose of 10%)	Considered to be brought about by sunitinib-induced thyrotoxicosis or the direct effects of sunitinib that lead to degeneration of thyroid follicular cells. Effects of imatinib are due to stimulation of T4 and T3 clearance by the induction of uridine diphosphate-glucuronosyltransferases	Hypothyroid subjects receiving imatinib have a high likelihood for increased levothyroxine replacement and should be closely monitored for elevations in thyrotropin indicating worsening hypothyroidism. Vandetanib increases thyroid hormone, calcium, and vitamin D analog requirements. Imatinib and motesanib do not affect serum TSH in euthyroid subjects with an intact thyroid gland. With imanitib-the required L-T4 dose has to be ↑ by 210%. The effect appears rapidly after initiation of therapy and is reversible, since TSH normalized after discontinuation of imatinib

(*Continued*)

OTHER ENDOCRINE DRUGS THYROID HORMONES AND IODINE

OTHER ENDOCRINE DRUGS THYROID HORMONES AND IODINE

Primary Drug	Secondary Drug	Effect	Mechanism	Precautions
THYROID HORMONES AND IODINE				
THYROID HORMONES	BEXAROTENE	Hypothyroidism may develop in patients with cutaneous T-cell lymphoma who are treated with high-dose bexarotene	Most likely because the retinoid X receptor-selective ligand suppresses thyrotropin secretion	Be aware and monitor requirement for thyroid hormone therapy
THYROID HORMONES	ANTICOAGULANTS—ORAL	Possible ↑ anticoagulant effect	Uncertain	Monitor INR at least weekly until stable
THYROID HORMONES	DENILEUKIN, DIFTITOX, ALEMTUZUMAB, INTERFERON-A, INTERLEUKIN-2, IPILIMUMAB, TREMELIMUMAB, THALIDOMIDE, LENALIDOMIDE	Primary hypothyroidism is the most common side effect, although thyrotoxicosis and effects on thyroid-stimulating hormone secretion and thyroid hormone metabolism have also been described. Alemtuzumab ↑ the risk of thyroid dysfunction in relapsing-remitting multiple sclerosis. Ten percent of alemtuzumab patients had more than one episode of thyroid dysfunction-Graves' hyperthyroidism occurred in 22%, hypothyroidism in 7%, and subacute thyroiditis in 4%. Of patients with overt Graves' hyperthyroidism, 23% spontaneously became euthyroid and an additional 15% spontaneously developed hypothyroidism. The annual incidence of a first episode of thyroid dysfunction increased each year through year 3 and then decreased each subsequent study year	Most agents cause thyroid dysfunction in 20%–50% of patients, although some have even higher rates	Physicians may overlook drug-induced thyroid dysfunction because of the complexity of the clinical picture in the cancer patient. Symptoms of hypothyroidism, such as fatigue, weakness, depression, memory loss, cold intolerance, and cardiovascular effects, may be incorrectly attributed to the primary disease or to the antineoplastic agent. Underdiagnosis of thyroid dysfunction can have important consequences for cancer patient management. Alternatively, such symptoms can lead to dose reductions of potentially life-saving therapies. Thyrotoxicosis can be mistaken for sepsis or a nonendocrinologic drug side effect. Recommend routine testing for thyroid abnormalities in patients receiving these antineoplastic agents
THYROID HORMONES	ANTIDEPRESSANTS—TCAs	Possible ↑ antidepressant effect; possibility of spurious hyperthyroidism	Uncertain; Thyroid hormones ↑ receptor sensitivity to catecholamines	May be beneficial but reported cases of nausea and dizziness; warn patients to report these symptoms

(*Continued*)

Primary Drug	Secondary Drug	Effect	Mechanism	Precautions
THYROID HORMONES AND IODINE				
THYROID HORMONES	ANTIDIABETIC DRUGS	↓ Hypoglycemic effect	Due to these a drugs causing hyperglycemia, the mechanism being uncertain at present	↑ Doses of antidiabetic drug are often required for adequate glycemic control
THYROID HORMONES	ANTIEPILEPTICS—BARBITURATES, CARBAMAZEPINE, PHENYTOIN, OXCARBAMAZEPINE	Antiepileptics cause an ↑ free hormone fractions and free T4 and T3. Three patients developed central hypothyroidism associated with oxcarbazepine treatment	Therapeutic levels of phenytoin and carbamazepine displace T4 and T3 from serum binding proteins. Several antiepileptic induce mixed function oxygenases responsible for hepatic drug oxidation, which accelerates thyroxine clearance via pathways that do not lead to T3 production. Oxcarbazepine is suggested to interfere with the hypothalamic-pituitary axis	In drug-treated patients, increased free T4 and T3 fractions offset the significant decrease in serum T4 and T3, resulting in normal free T4 and free T3 concentrations. Since currently available clinical tests will continue to show decreased free T4 concentrations in patients taking phenytoin or carbamazepine, clinicians should rely on serum TSH measurements to confirm the euthyroid status of these patients. Because of enzyme induction L-T4 dosage must be increased
THYROID HORMONES	ANTIOBESITY DRUGS—ORLISTAT	Possible risk of hypothyroidism	Uncertain	Monitor TFTs closely
THYROID HORMONES	ANTIVIRALS—PROTEASE INHIBITORS	Altered efficacy of levothyroxine by lopinavir/ritonavir or ritonavir and possibly indinavir and nelfinavir	Uncertain; possibly altered metabolism via induction of glucuronosyltransferases	Monitor thyroid function closely, adjust levothyroxine doses as needed
THYROID HORMONES	BRONCHODILATORS—THEOPHYLLINE	Altered theophylline levels (↑ or ↓) when thyroid status was altered therapeutically	Uncertain	Monitor theophylline levels closely during changes in treatment of abnormal thyroid function. Watch for early features of theophylline toxicity

(*Continued*)

OTHER ENDOCRINE DRUGS TRILOSTANE

Primary Drug	Secondary Drug	Effect	Mechanism	Precautions
THYROID HORMONES AND IODINE				
THYROID HORMONES	IRON, LIPID LOWERING DRUGS, ANION EXCHANGE RESINS, SODIUM POLYSTYRENE SULFONATE, SUCRALFATE, CALCIUM, H2 RECEPTOR BLOCKERS (CIMETIDINE), BILE-ACID SEQUESTRANTS: COLESTIPOL, CHOLESTYRAMINE, COLESEVELAM	↓ Effect of thyroid hormone preparations	Due to ↓ absorption	Monitor TFTs regularly. Consider ↑ doses of levothyroxine. Separate doses of drugs by at least two hours
THYROID HORMONES	NSAIDs	Single-dose aspirin or salsalate decreased, whereas meclofenamate increased, various total and free thyroid hormone measurements. One week of aspirin or salsalate decreased total T(4), free T(4) (salsalate only), total T(3), free T(3), and TSH	These data confirm that aspirin, salsalate, and meclofenamate affect total and free thyroid hormone measurements. TSH remained within the normal range during acute or 1-wk administration of all of the NSAIDs	Be aware

Primary Drug	Secondary Drug	Effect	Mechanism	Precautions
TOLVAPTAN				
TOLVAPTAN	PONATINIB	Predicted increased in levels of tolvaptan	P-glycoprotein inhibition	Be aware

Primary Drug	Secondary Drug	Effect	Mechanism	Precautions
TRILOSTANE				
TRILOSTANE	DIURETICS—POTASSIUM—SPARING	Risk of hyperkalemia	Additive effect	Monitor potassium levels regularly during coadministration

PART 7

Analgesics

Ruwan Parakramawansha

Primary Drug	Secondary Drug	Effect	Mechanism	Precautions
ACETAMINOPHEN ➢ *See Paracetamol*				
NEFOPAM				
NEFOPAM	**ADDITIVE ANTIMUSCARINIC EFFECTS**			
NEFOPAM	1. ANTIARRHYTHMICS—disopyramide, propafenone 2. ANTIDEPRESSANTS—TCAs 3. ANTIEMETICS—cyclizine 4. ANTIHISTAMINES—chlorphenamine, cyproheptadine, hydroxyzine 5. ANTIMUSCARINICS—atropine, benzatropine, cyclopentolate, dicycloverine, flavoxate, homatropine, hyoscine, orphenadrine, oxybutynin, procyclidine, propantheline, tolterodine, trihexyphenidyl, or tropicamide 6. ANTI-PARKINSON'S DRUGS—dopaminergics 7. ANTIPSYCHOTICS—phenothiazines, clozapine, pimozide 8. MUSCLE RELAXANTS—baclofen 9. NITRATES—isosorbide dinitrate	↑ Risk of antimuscarinic side effects. *NB ↓ efficacy of sublingual nitrate tablets*	Additive effect; both drugs cause antimuscarinic side-effects. *Antimuscarinic effects ↓ saliva production, which ↓ dissolution of the tablet*	Warn patients of this additive effect. *Consider using sublingual nitrate spray*
NEFOPAM	**ANTIDEPRESSANTS**			
NEFOPAM	TCAs	1. Risk of seizures with TCAs 2. ↑ Antimuscarinic effects (from Stockley's DIs)	Additive effect; both drugs lower the seizure threshold	Avoid coadministration
NEFOPAM	MAOIs	Hypertensive crises (from Stockley's DIs)	Additive effect; both drugs have sympathomimetic effects	Avoid coadministration

ANALGESICS NEFOPAM

Primary Drug	Secondary Drug	Effect	Mechanism	Precautions
NONSTEROIDAL ANTI-INFLAMMATORY DRUGS (NSAIDs)				
NSAIDs	**ANALGESICS**			
NSAIDs	ANTACIDS	1. Magnesium hydroxide ↑ absorption of ibuprofen, flurbiprofen, mefenamic acid, and tolfenamic acid 2. Aluminum-containing antacids ↓ absorption of these NSAIDs	Uncertain	These effects are ↓ by taking these drugs with food
NSAIDs	NSAIDs	↑ Risk of gastrointestinal bleeding	Additive effect. The more an NSAID blocks COX-1, there is a greater tendency to cause ulcers and promote bleeding. Celecoxib blocks COX-2 but has little effect on COX-1, and is further classified as a selective COX-2 inhibitor. Selective COX-2 inhibitors cause less bleeding and fewer ulcers than other NSAIDs	Combination of NSAID therapy cannot be justified as toxicity may be increased without any improvement in efficacy. Avoid coadministration
PARECOXIB, CELECOXIB	ANTIARRHYTHMICS—FLECAINIDE, PROPAFENONE	Possible ↑ flecainide or propafenone levels	Parecoxib and celecoxib inhibits CYP2D6	Monitor PR and BP closely. If possible, use only short courses of NSAID
NSAIDs	**ANTIBIOTICS**			
INDOMETHACIN	AMINOGLYCOSIDES	↑ Amikacin, gentamicin, and vancomycin levels in neonates	Uncertain; indomethacin possibly ↓ renal clearance of these aminoglycosides. Aminoglycosides cause direct renal toxicity: acute tubular necrosis	Halve the dose of antibiotic. This interaction is reported in premature infants. Therefore it is uncertain whether this applies to adults. Otherwise use an alternative NSAID
INDOMETHACIN	CEPHALOSPORINS	Indomethacin ↑ ceftazidime levels in neonates	Indomethacin ↓ clearance of ceftazidime	↓ Dose of ceftazidime

(*Continued*)

Primary Drug	Secondary Drug	Effect	Mechanism	Precautions
NONSTEROIDAL ANTI-INFLAMMATORY DRUGS (NSAIDs)				
NSAIDs	QUINOLONES	Reports of convulsions when NSAIDs are added to quinolones in epileptic patients	Unknown	Take care in coadministering antiepileptics and NSAIDs in epileptic patients
NSAIDs	RIFAMPICIN	Rifampicin ↓ diclofenac, celecoxib, etoricoxib, and parecoxib levels	Rifampicin ↑ CYP2C9-mediated metabolism of these NSAIDs	Monitor analgesic effects; consider using alternative NSAIDs
NSAIDs	**ANTICANCER AND IMMUNOMODULATING DRUGS**			
NSAIDs	CICLOSPORIN	1. ↑ Risk of renal failure with NSAIDs 2. Diclofenac levels ↑ by ciclosporin	1. Additive effect; both can cause renal insufficiency; ciclosporin may cause direct renal toxicity: acute tubular necrosis 2. Uncertain; possibly due to ↑ bioavailability	1. Monitor renal function closely 2. Halve the dose of diclofenac
NSAIDs, CELECOXIB, MELOXICAM, PIROXICAM	CISPLATIN	Both celecoxib and cisplatin can lead to nephrotoxicity. Piroxicam increases blood concentrations of cisplatin	Additive nephrotoxic effects	Monitor renal function (creatinine, GFR) prior to twice a week during therapy. Monitor toxic effects of cisplatin with piroxicam
NSAIDs	CLOFARABINE	Possible increase in clofarabine levels	Clofarabine excreted primarily by kidneys	Manufacturer advises to avoid concurrent use. Monitor closely if this is unavoidable
NSAIDs	CORTICOSTEROIDS	1. ↑ Risk of gastrointestinal ulceration and bleeding 2. Parecoxib levels may be ↓ by dexamethasone	1. Additive effect 2. Dexamethasone induces CYP3A4-mediated metabolism of parecoxib	1. Watch for early signs of gastrointestinal upset; remember that corticosteroids may mask these features. Consider using gastroprotection with a proton pump inhibitor 2. Watch for poor response to parecoxib
NSAIDs	DASATINIB	↑ Risk of bleeding	Additive effect; thrombocytopenia with dasatinib	Avoid coadministration

(*Continued*)

ANALGESICS NONSTEROIDAL ANTI-INFLAMMATORY DRUGS (NSAIDs)

ANALGESICS NONSTEROIDAL ANTI-INFLAMMATORY DRUGS (NSAIDs)

Primary Drug	Secondary Drug	Effect	Mechanism	Precautions
NONSTEROIDAL ANTI-INFLAMMATORY DRUGS (NSAIDs)				
NSAIDs	ERLOTINIB	↑ Risk of bleeding	Additive effect	Avoid coadministration
NSAIDs—CELECOXIB	ERLOTINIB	↑ Celecoxib levels	Inhibition of CYP2D6-mediated metabolism	Use lowest effective dose of celecoxib when necessary
NSAIDs	GOLD	Gold may cause interstitial nephritis. Risk of renal failure	Additive renal toxicity	Monitor renal function prior to and during gold therapy
NSAIDs	METHOTREXATE	↑ Methotrexate levels, with reports of toxicity, with ibuprofen, indomethacin, and possibly diclofenac, flurbiprofen, ketoprofen, meloxicam, and naproxen	Uncertain; postulated that an NSAID-induced ↓ in renal perfusion may have an effect	Consider using an alternative NSAID
NSAIDs	MIFAMURTIDE	Inhibits mechanism of mifamurtide in vitro	Uncertain	Manufacturer advises to avoid concurrent use with high doses of NSAIDs
NSAIDs	MYCOPHENOLATE, PENICILLAMINE, SIROLIMUS, TACROLIMUS	↑ Risk of nephrotoxicity	Additive effect	Monitor renal function closely
NSAIDs	PEMETREXED	Predicted reduced renal excretion of pemetrexed	Inhibition of prostaglandins by NSAIDs results in reduced renal perfusion	Manufacturer recommends to exercise caution with high doses of NSAIDs in patients with normal renal function. NSAIDs with short half-lives should be avoided 2 days before to 2 days after in patients with mild to moderate renal impairment. NSAIDs with longer half-lives should be avoided 5 days before to 2 days after pemetrexed. Manufacturer advises close monitoring if concurrent use is necessary

(*Continued*)

Primary Drug	Secondary Drug	Effect	Mechanism	Precautions
NONSTEROIDAL ANTI-INFLAMMATORY DRUGS (NSAIDs)				
NSAIDS—CELECOXIB, IBUPROFEN, KETOPROFEN, OR NAPROXEN	PORFIMER	↑ Risk of photosensitivity reactions when porfimer is coadministered with celecoxib, ibuprofen, ketoprofen, or naproxen	Attributed to additive effects	Avoid exposure of skin and eyes to direct sunlight for 30 days after porfimer therapy
MEFENAMIC ACID, DIFLUNISAL, AND NIFLUMIC ACID	REGORAFENIB	Predicted increased regorafenib levels	UGT1A9 inhibition	Manufacturer advises to avoid concurrent use
NSAIDs—CELECOXIB, DICLOFENAC, PIROXICAM	SORAFENIB	Increased blood levels of these NSAIDs	Sorafenib inhibits CYP2C9	Monitor for toxic effects
NSAIDs	**ANTICOAGULANTS**			
NSAIDs	**ANTICOAGULANTS—ORAL**			
NSAIDs	APIXABAN	1. Risk of gastrointestinal bleeding with all NSAIDs 2. Possible ↑ anticoagulant effect with diclofenac, ketorolac, naproxen	1. NSAIDs irritate the gastric mucosa and can cause bleeding, which is exacerbated by anticoagulants 2. Uncertain	1. Extreme caution when coadministering; monitor patients closely 2. Avoid coadministration
NSAIDs	DABIGATRAN, RIVAROXABAN	↑ Risk of bleeding	Uncertain	A careful benefit-risk assessment. Close observation for signs of bleeding and The considering co-administration of a PPI to prevent GI bleeding are recommended
NSAIDs	WARFARIN	1. Risk of gastrointestinal bleeding with all NSAIDs 2. Possible ↑ anticoagulant effect with celecoxib, etoricoxib, flurbiprofen, piroxicam, sulindac, veldecoxib, ibuprofen, and naproxen	1. NSAIDs irritate the gastric mucosa and can cause bleeding, which is exacerbated by anticoagulants 2. Uncertain but possibly a combination of impaired hepatic metabolism through competitive inhibition of CYP2C9 and displacement of anticoagulants from their plasma proteins	1. To avoid the combination whenever possible; extreme caution when co-administering with gastroprotection 2. Monitor INR before and during therapy until stable. Ask patients to report increased bruising, bleeding from gums while brushing teeth, etc.

(*Continued*)

ANALGESICS NONSTEROIDAL ANTI-INFLAMMATORY DRUGS (NSAIDs)

ANALGESICS NONSTEROIDAL ANTI-INFLAMMATORY DRUGS (NSAIDs)

Primary Drug	Secondary Drug	Effect	Mechanism	Precautions
NONSTEROIDAL ANTI-INFLAMMATORY DRUGS (NSAIDs)				
NSAIDs	ANTICOAGULANTS—PARENTERAL	1. Risk of prolonged bleeding when ketorolac is coadministered with dalteparin (but not enoxaparin), and intravenous diclofenac is given with heparins 2. ↑ Risk of hyperkalemia when ketorolac is given with heparin	1. Uncertain 2. Heparin inhibits aldosterone secretion, causing hyperkalemia	1. Avoid coadministration 2. Monitor potassium levels closely
NSAIDs	**ANTIDEPRESSANTS**			
NSAIDs	LITHIUM	NSAIDs may ↑ lithium levels; cases of toxicity have been reported	Uncertain; possibly NSAIDs ↓ renal clearance of lithium by reducing renal prostaglandin synthesis	Avoid coadministration when possible. If not possible, monitor lithium levels closely; note blood concentrations of lithium may need to be measured for 4–7 days after an NSAID is either added or stopped
NSAIDs	SSRIs, VENLAFAXINE	Slight ↑ risk of bleeding. SSRIs increase the risk of gastrointestinal adverse effects in first time users as compared with nonselective antidepressants	1. Additive pharmacodynamics interaction; SSRIs inhibit serotonin medicated platelet aggregation 2. Paroxetine, sertraline, and fluvoxamine inhibit CYP2C9 mediated metabolism of NSAIDs causing their accumulation	Warn patients to watch if possible to avoid the combination and use alternative analgesics; Use gastroprotection when used together; Warn patients to watch for early signs of bleeding
NSAIDs	**ANTIDIABETIC DRUGS**			
ANALGESICS—NSAIDs—MEFENAMIC ACID	DAPAGLIFLOZIN	Possible increased effect of dapagliflozin	AUC increased by 51%	No significant change of dose required as interaction probably not clinically significant

(*Continued*)

Primary Drug	Secondary Drug	Effect	Mechanism	Precautions
NONSTEROIDAL ANTI-INFLAMMATORY DRUGS (NSAIDs)				
NSAIDs	METFORMIN	Possibility of ↑ plasma levels of metformin if there is renal impairment due to NSAIDs. High metformin levels cause lactic acidosis	NSAIDs can cause renal dysfunction and lead to accumulation of metformin which is mainly excreted unchanged via kidneys	Do not use metformin if serum creatinine is >1.5 mg/dL in males and >1.4 mg/dL in females, or creatinine clearance is <30 mL/min. Use with caution in patients who have a creatinine clearance of 30–60 mL/min. Warn patients about hypoglycemia and lactic acidosis. ➢ ***For signs and symptoms of hypoglycemia, see Clinical Features of Some Adverse Drug Interactions, Hypoglycemia***
NSAIDs	SULFONYLUREAS	Enhanced hypoglycemic effect of sulfonylureas with most NSAIDs, which are highly protein bound. There have been reports of hyper- and hypoglycemia (e.g., with diclofenac)	Attributed to displacement of sulfonylureas from protein-binding sites, thus increasing the plasma concentration. Some NSAIDs may impair the renal elimination of sulfonylureas, particularly chlorpropamide	Be aware. Conflicting reports.
NSAIDs	ANTIEMETICS	1. Metoclopramide speeds up the onset of action of tolfenamic acid 2. Metoclopramide ↓ efficacy of ketoprofen	Metoclopramide promotes gastric emptying 1. Tolfenamic acid reaches its main site of absorption in the small intestine more rapidly 2. Ketoprofen has low solubility and has less time to dissolve in the stomach; therefore, less ketoprofen is absorbed	1. This interaction can be used beneficially to hasten the onset of analgesia 2. Take ketoprofen at least 2 h before metoclopramide

(*Continued*)

ANALGESICS NONSTEROIDAL ANTI-INFLAMMATORY DRUGS (NSAIDs)

ANALGESICS NONSTEROIDAL ANTI-INFLAMMATORY DRUGS (NSAIDs)

Primary Drug	Secondary Drug	Effect	Mechanism	Precautions
NONSTEROIDAL ANTI-INFLAMMATORY DRUGS (NSAIDs)				
NSAIDs	CARBAMAZEPINE	Parecoxib and celecoxib levels may be ↓ by carbamazepine	1. Carbamazepine and phenytoin induce CYP2C9-mediated metabolism of celecoxib and parecoxib 2. Uncertain; possibly competitive inhibition of CYP2C9-mediated	Watch for poor response
NSAIDs—CELECOXIB, PARECOXIB	PHENYTOIN	1. ↓ Levels of these drugs, with risk of therapeutic failure 2. Report of ↑ phenytoin levels parecoxib	1. Induction of hepatic metabolism 2. Inhibition of CYP2C9-mediated metabolism of phenytoin by parecoxib	1. Monitor for ↓ clinical efficacy and ↑ their dose as required 2. Monitor phenytoin levels when coadministered with parecoxib
NSAIDs	**ANTIFUNGALS**			
NSAIDs	AMPHOTERICIN	Amphotericin may cause direct renal toxicity (acute tubular necrosis)	Additive renal toxicity	Monitor renal function
NSAIDs	FLUCONAZOLE	Fluconazole ↑ celecoxib and possibly parecoxib levels	Fluconazole inhibits CYP2C9-mediated metabolism of celecoxib and parecoxib	Halve the dose of celecoxib and start parecoxib at the lowest dose
NSAIDs	ANTIGOUT DRUGS—PROBENECID	↑ Levels of acemetacin, diflunisal, indomethacin, ketoprofen, ketorolac, naproxen, tenoxicam, and tiaprofenic acid	Probenecid competitively inhibits renal clearance of these NSAIDs	Watch for signs of toxicity of these NSAIDs. Consider using an alternative NSAID. The manufacturers of ketorolac advise avoiding coadministration of ketorolac and probenecid

(*Continued*)

Primary Drug	Secondary Drug	Effect	Mechanism	Precautions
NONSTEROIDAL ANTI-INFLAMMATORY DRUGS (NSAIDs)				
NSAIDs	**ANTIHYPERTENSIVES AND HEART FAILURE DRUGS**			
NSAIDs	ANTIHYPERTENSIVES AND HEART FAILURE DRUGS	↓ Hypotensive effect, especially with indomethacin. The effect is variable among different ACE inhibitors and NSAIDs, but is most notable between captopril and indomethacin	NSAIDs cause sodium and water retention and raise BP by inhibiting vasodilating renal prostaglandins. ACE inhibitors metabolize tissue kinins (e.g., bradykinin), and this may be the basis for indomethacin attenuating the hypotensive effect of captopril	Monitor BP at least weekly until stable. Avoid coadministering indomethacin with captopril
NSAIDs	ACE INHIBITORS, ANGIOTENSIN II RECEPTOR ANTAGONISTS	1. ↓ Hypotensive effect 2. ↑ Risk of renal impairment 3. ↑ Risk of hyperkalemia	1. NSAIDs cause sodium and water retention and raise BP by inhibiting vasodilating renal prostaglandins 2. Additive effect 3. Additive effect	Benefits often outweigh risks for short-term NSAID use, but exercise particular caution in the elderly. For longer-term use, monitor BP, renal function, and serum potassium at least weekly until stable
NSAIDs	ADRENERGIC NEURONE BLOCKERS	↓ Hypotensive effect reported with phenylbutazone. Theoretical risk of similar effect with other NSAIDs	NSAIDs cause sodium and water retention and raise BP by inhibiting vasodilating renal prostaglandins	Benefits often outweigh risks for short-term NSAID use, but exercise particular caution in the elderly. For longer-term use, monitor BP, renal function, and serum potassium at least weekly until stable
NSAIDs	ALISKIREN	1. ↓ Hypotensive effect 2. ↑ Risk of renal impairment 3. ↑ Risk of hyperkalemia	1. NSAIDs cause sodium and water retention and raise BP by inhibiting vasodilating renal prostaglandins 2. Additive effect 3. Additive effect	Benefits often outweigh risks for short-term NSAID use, but exercise particular caution in the elderly. For longer-term use, monitor BP, renal function, and serum potassium at least weekly until stable

(*Continued*)

ANALGESICS NONSTEROIDAL ANTI-INFLAMMATORY DRUGS (NSAIDs)

ANALGESICS NONSTEROIDAL ANTI-INFLAMMATORY DRUGS (NSAIDs)

Primary Drug	Secondary Drug	Effect	Mechanism	Precautions
NONSTEROIDAL ANTI-INFLAMMATORY DRUGS (NSAIDs)				
NSAIDs	VASODILATOR ANTIHYPERTENSIVES	1. Etoricoxib may ↑ minoxidil levels 2. Indomethacin opposes the hypotensive effect of IV hydralazine	1. Etoricoxib inhibits sulfotransferase activity 2. Unknown mechanism	1. Monitor BP closely 2. Monitor BP closely
NSAIDs	ANTIOBESITY DRUGS—SIBUTRAMINE	↑ Risk of bleeding	Additive effect	Avoid coadministration
NSAIDs	**ANTIPLATELET AGENTS**			
NSAIDs	ASPIRIN	1. Risk of gastrointestinal bleeding when aspirin, even low dose, is coadministered with NSAIDs 2. Ibuprofen ↓ antiplatelet effect of aspirin 3. Reduced cardioprotective effect of aspirin when taken with NSAIDs, including COXIBs	1. Additive effect 2. Ibuprofen competitively inhibits binding of aspirin to platelets 3. Uncertain; possibly related to variable inhibition of cyclo-oxygenase 1 and 2 isoenzymes	1. Avoid coadministration; if essential to coprescribe, add a proton pump inhibitor 2. Avoid coadministration; if there is no alternative, low-dose aspirin (81 mg daily) should be taken 30 min before or 8 h after taking ibuprofen 3. Avoid coadministration
NSAIDs	CLOPIDOGREL	1. Risk of gastrointestinal bleeding when clopidogrel is coadministered with NSAIDs 2. Case report of intracerebral hemorrhage when clopidogrel is given with celecoxib	1. NSAIDs may cause gastric mucosal irritation/ulceration; clopidogrel inhibits platelet aggregation 2. Uncertain; possible that celecoxib inhibits CYP2D6-mediated metabolism of clopidogrel	1. Warn patients to report immediately about any gastrointestinal symptoms; use NSAIDs for as short a course as possible 2. Avoid coingestion of clopidogrel and celecoxib
NSAIDs	PRASUGREL, TICAGRELOR	↑ Risk of gastrointestinal bleeding	Pharmacodynamic additive effect on GI mucosal irritation and bleeding	Watch for features of gastrointestinal bleeding. Be careful about gastroprotection if combination cannot be avoided

(Continued)

Primary Drug	Secondary Drug	Effect	Mechanism	Precautions
NONSTEROIDAL ANTI-INFLAMMATORY DRUGS (NSAIDs)				
NSAIDs	ANTIPSYCHOTICS	1. Reports of ↑ sedation when indomethacin was added to haloperidol 2. Risk of agranulocytosis when azapropazone is given with clozapine	1. Unknown 2. Unknown	1. Avoid coadministration 2. Avoid coadministration
NSAIDs	**ANTIVIRALS**			
NSAIDs	NRTIs—ZIDOVUDINE	↑ Risk of hematological effects of zidovudine and ↑ risk of bleeding with NSAIDs	Unknown	Avoid coadministration if possible. If not, use NSAIDs for as short a duration as possible and monitor closely
NSAIDs	PROTEASE INHIBITORS—RITONAVIR, TENOFOVIR	1. Ritonavir ↑ piroxicam levels 2. ↑ Risk of renal impairment with tenofovir	1. Uncertain; ritonavir is known to inhibit CYP2C9, for which NSAIDs are substrates 2. Additive effect	Avoid coadministration; monitor renal function if coadministration unavoidable
NSAIDs	**BETA-BLOCKERS**			
NSAIDs	BETA-BLOCKERS	↓ Hypotensive efficacy of beta-blockers with indomethacin, piroxicam, and possibly ibuprofen and naproxen. Other NSAIDs do not seem to show this effect	Additive toxic effects on kidney, salt, and water retention by NSAIDs. NSAIDs can raise BP by inhibiting the renal synthesis of vasodilating prostaglandins. Uncertain why this effect is specific to these NSAIDs	Watch for ↓ response to beta-blockers with indomethacin, piroxicam, ibuprofen, and naproxen
NSAIDs—CELECOXIB, VALDECOXIB, CELECOXIB	METOPROLOL	Risk of ↑ hypotensive efficacy of metoprolol	Inhibition of CYP2D6-mediated metabolism of metoprolol	Monitor BP at least weekly until stable. Warn patients to report symptoms of hypotension (light headedness, dizziness on standing, etc.)
NSAIDs	BISPHOSPHONATES—ALENDRONATE	Risk of esophagitis/peptic ulceration	Additive effect	Avoid coadministration
NSAIDs	BRONCHODILATORS—BETA-2 AGONISTS	Etoricoxib may ↑ oral salbutamol levels	Etoricoxib inhibits sulfotransferase activity	Monitor PR and BP closely

(Continued)

ANALGESICS NONSTEROIDAL ANTI-INFLAMMATORY DRUGS (NSAIDs)

Primary Drug	Secondary Drug	Effect	Mechanism	Precautions
NONSTEROIDAL ANTI-INFLAMMATORY DRUGS (NSAIDs)				
NSAIDs	CALCIUM CHANNEL BLOCKERS	↓ Antihypertensive effect of calcium channel blockers	NSAIDs cause salt retention and vasoconstriction at possibly both renal and endothelial sites	Monitor BP at least weekly until stable
NSAIDs	CARDIAC GLYCOSIDES	Diclofenac, indomethacin, and possibly fenbufen, ibuprofen, and tiaprofenic ↑ plasma concentrations of digoxin and ↑ Risk of precipitating cardiac failure and renal dysfunction	Uncertain. Postulated that NSAID-induced renal impairment plays a role; however, since all NSAIDs have this effect, it is not understood why only certain NSAIDs actually influence digoxin levels	Monitor renal function closely; watch for digoxin toxicity and check levels if necessary
NSAIDs	**CNS STIMULANTS**			
INDOMETHACIN	MODAFINIL	May cause ↑ indomethacin levels if CYP2C9 is the predominant metabolic pathway and the alternative pathways are either genetically deficient or affected	Modafinil is a moderate inhibitor of CYP2C9	Be aware
NAPROXEN	MODAFINIL	May cause ↓ naproxen levels if CYP1A2 is the predominant metabolic pathway and alternative metabolic pathways are either genetically deficient or affected	Modafinil is moderate inducer of CYP1A2 in a concentration-dependent manner	Be aware
NSAIDs	DESMOPRESSIN	↑ Efficacy of desmopressin with indomethacin	Additive water retention effect	Monitor U&Es and BP closely
NSAIDs	**DIURETICS**			
NSAIDs	LOOP, THIAZIDES	1. Reduced efficacy of diuretics 2. ↑ Risk of nephrotoxicity	1. NSAIDs cause sodium and water retention 2. Additive effect	Monitor BP and U&Es closely
NSAIDs	POTASSIUM-SPARING AND ALDOSTERONE ANTAGONISTS	1. Risk of hyperkalemia with NSAIDs 2. Reports of acute renal failure when triamterene coadministered with indomethacin	1. Renal insufficiency caused by NSAIDs can exacerbate potassium retention by these diuretics 2. Uncertain	1. Monitor renal function and potassium closely 2. Avoid coadministration of triamterene and indomethacin

(*Continued*)

Primary Drug	Secondary Drug	Effect	Mechanism	Precautions
NONSTEROIDAL ANTI-INFLAMMATORY DRUGS (NSAIDs)				
NSAIDs—CELECOXIB	DRUG DEPENDENCE THERAPIES—BUPROPION	↑ Plasma concentrations of these substrates, with risk of toxic effects	Bupropion and its metabolite hydroxybupropion inhibit CYP2D6	Initiate therapy of these drugs at the lowest effective dose
NSAIDs	LIPID-LOWERING DRUGS	Cholestyramine ↓ absorption of some NSAIDs	Colestyramine binds NSAIDs in the intestine, reducing their absorption; it also binds those NSAIDs with a significant enterohepatic recirculation (meloxicam, piroxicam, sulindac, tenoxicam)	Give NSAID 1 h before or 4–6 h after colestyramine; however, meloxicam, piroxicam, sulindac, or tenoxicam should not be given with colestyramine
NSAIDs	MIFEPRISTONE	↓ Efficacy of mifepristone	NSAIDs have an antiprostaglandin effect	Avoid coadministration
NSAIDs	MUSCLE RELAXANTS—SKELETAL	↑ Baclofen levels with ibuprofen	↓ Renal excretion of baclofen	Avoid coadministration
NSAIDs	NITRATES	Hypotensive effects of hydralazine, minoxidil, and nitroprusside are antagonized by NSAIDs	NSAIDs cause salt and water retention in the kidney and can raise BP due to ↓ production of vasodilating renal prostaglandins	Monitor BP at least weekly until stable
NSAIDs	ESTROGENS	Etoricoxib may ↑ ethinylestradiol levels	Etoricoxib inhibits sulfotransferase activity	Consider using a formulation with a lower dose of ethinylestradiol
NSAIDs	PERIPHERAL VASODILATORS	Risk of bleeding when pentoxifylline is given with ketorolac post surgery	Possibly additive antiplatelet effect	Avoid coadministration
NSAIDs	PROGESTOGENS	↑ Risk of hyperkalemia	Drospirenone (component of the Yasmin brand of combined contraceptive pill) is a progestogen derived from spironolactone that can cause potassium retention	Monitor serum potassium weekly until stable, and then every 6 months
NSAIDs	PROSTAGLANDINS—DINOPROSTONE	Theoretical risk of ↓ efficacy of dinoprost; not confirmed in clinical studies	Antagonism of effect	UK manufacturers recommend stopping NSAIDs before administering dinoprostone. U.S. manufacturer does not give this advice

ANALGESICS NONSTEROIDAL ANTI-INFLAMMATORY DRUGS (NSAIDs)

Primary Drug	Secondary Drug	Effect	Mechanism	Precautions
OPIOIDS				
OPIOIDS	ALCOHOL	↑ Sedation	Additive CNS depression effect	Warn Patient
OPIOIDS	**ANTIARRHYTHMICS**			
FENTANYL	AMIODARONE	Profound bradycardia, sinus arrest, and hypotension have reported	Exact mechanism is uncertain	Coadministration of fentanyl and amiodarone should be avoided wherever possible. Fentanyl should not be used as an adjunct to sedation or analgesic in any patient who may reasonably be foreseen as requiring amiodarone. Fentanyl should never be administered following amiodarone administration
METHADONE, TRAMADOL	FLECAINIDE, PROCAINAMIDE, PROPAFENONE	Possible ↑ flecainide, procainamide, and propafenone levels	Methadone and tramadol inhibit CYP2D6	Monitor PR and BP closely
OPIOIDS	MEXILETINE	1. Absorption of oral mexiletine is ↓ by coadministration with morphine or diamorphine 2. Methadone may ↑ mexiletine levels	1. Uncertain but thought to be due to an opioid-induced delay in gastric emptying 2. Methadone inhibits CYP2D6-mediated metabolism of mexiletine	1. Watch for poor response to mexiletine; consider starting at a higher or using the intravenous route 2. Monitor PR, BP, and ECG closely; watch for mexiletine toxicity
CODEINE	QUINIDINE	↓ Analgesic effect of codeine	Inhibition of CYP2D6-mediated conversion of codeine to its active metabolite	Be aware that codeine may be less effective in patients taking codeine; there is a theoretical risk that dihydrocodeine and hydrocodone may be similarly affected
FENTANYL, PETHIDINE, TRAMADOL	QUINIDINE	↑ Fentanyl, pethidine, and tramadol levels	Quinidine inhibits CYP2D6	Theoretical drug interaction; watch for excessive narcotization

(*Continued*)

Primary Drug	Secondary Drug	Effect	Mechanism	Precautions
OPIOIDS				
OPIOIDS	**ANTIBIOTICS**			
OPIOIDS	CIPROFLOXACIN	1. Effects of methadone ↑ by ciprofloxacin 2. ↓ Levels of ciprofloxacin with opioids	1. Ciprofloxacin inhibits CYP1A2-, CYP2D6-, and CYP3A4-mediated metabolism of methadone 2. Uncertain	1. Watch for ↑ effects of methadone 2. Avoid opioid premedication when ciprofloxacin is used as surgical prophylaxis
OPIOIDS	MACROLIDES	Effects of alfentanil, fentanyl, and methadone ↑ by erythromycin, telithromycin, and clarithromycin	These macrolides inhibit CYP3A4-mediated metabolism of alfentanil, fentanyl, and methadone	Monitor for effects of opioid toxicity (especially when alfentanil given as an infusion)
OPIOIDS	RIFAMPICIN	↓ Effect of alfentanil, codeine, methadone, and morphine	Rifampicin ↑ hepatic metabolism of these opioids (alfentanil by CYP3A4, codeine by CYP2D6, morphine unknown) Rifampicin is also known to induce intestinal Pgp, which may ↓ bioavailability of oral morphine	Be aware that alfentanil, codeine, methadone, and morphine doses may need to be ↑.
OPIOIDS	**ANTICANCER AND IMMUNOMODULATING DRUGS**			
OPIOIDS—KETOBEMIDONE	BUSULFAN	Levels of busulfan may be increased	Unknown	Monitor carefully
MORPHINE, NALOXONE	CRIZOTINIB	Possible increased levels of UGT substrates	UGT (particularly UGT1A1, UGT2B7) inhibition	Caution with concurrent use
FENTANYL, METHADONE	DABRAFENIB	Possible reduced levels of CYP3A4/CYP2Cs/CYP2B6 substrates. Level of reduction may vary	Dabrafenib induces CYP3A4/CYP2Cs/CYP2B6	Monitor closely or avoid concurrent use
OPIOIDS	HISTAMINE	Can releases endogenous histamine; potential additive effects	Additive effect	Consider potential additive effect

(*Continued*)

ANALGESICS OPIOIDS

Primary Drug	Secondary Drug	Effect	Mechanism	Precautions
OPIOIDS				
OPIOIDS	IMATINIB, NILOTINIB	Imatinib and nilotinib may cause ↑ plasma concentrations of codeine, dextromethorphan, hydroxycodone, methadone, morphine, oxycodone, pethidine fentanyl, alfentanil, and tramadol, with a risk of toxic effects	Inhibition of CYP2D6- and 3A4-mediated metabolism of these opioids by imatinib; nilotinib is an inhibitor of CYP3A4 and Pgp	Monitor for clinical efficacy and toxicity. Warn patients to report ↑ drowsiness, malaise, and anorexia Tramadol causes less respiratory depression than other opiates, but need to monitor BP and blood counts and advise patients to report wheezing, loss of appetite, and fainting attacks. Need to consider reducing dose Methadone may cause QT prolongation; the CSM has recommended that patients with heart and liver disease on methadone should be carefully monitored for heart conduction abnormalities such as QT prolongation on ECG, which may lead to sudden death. Also need to monitor patients on more than 100 mg methadone daily, and thus ↑ plasma concentrations necessitate close monitoring of cardiac and respiratory functions
DEXTROMETHORPHAN	PAZOPANIB	Increased levels of dextromethorphan	CYP2D6 inhibition	Be aware. Unknown significance

(*Continued*)

Primary Drug	Secondary Drug	Effect	Mechanism	Precautions
OPIOIDS				
OPIOIDS	PROCARBAZINE	Unpredictable reactions may occur associated with hypotension and respiratory depression when procarbazine is coadministered with alfentanil, fentanyl, sufentanil, or morphine	Opioids cause hypotension due to arterial and venous vasodilatation, negative inotropic effects, and a vagally induced bradycardia. Procarbazine can cause postural hypotension. Also attributed to accumulation of serotonin due to inhibition of MAO	Recommended that a small test dose (one-quarter of the usual dose) be administered initially to assess response
OPIOIDS	THALIDOMIDE	Increased sedation	Additive	Caution with concurrent use
DEXTROMETHORPHAN	TOCILIZUMAB	Reduced levels	Tocilizumab reverses cytochrome P450 isoenzyme suppression by IL-6	Monitor closely and consider dose adjustment
OPIOIDS	ANTICOAGULANTS—ORAL	Cases of ↑ anticoagulant effect with tramadol	Likely to be seen mainly in CYP2D6 depleted individuals. Thereby, tramadol metabolism is shunted to CYP3A4, resulting in competitive inhibition of warfarin	Monitor INR at least weekly until stable
DEXTROMETHORPHAN	ANTIDEMENTIA DRUGS—MEMANTINE	↑ CNS side effects	Additive effects on NMDA receptors	Avoid coadministration
OPIOIDS	**ANTIDEPRESSANTS**			
OPIOIDS—DEXTROMETHORPHAN, PENTAZOCINE, TRAMADOL	LITHIUM	Possible risk of serotonin syndrome	Additive effect of increased serotonin levels in brain	Be aware of the possibility of serotonin syndrome. Also need to monitor lithium levels with appropriate dose adjustments during coadministration. ➢ ***For signs and symptoms of serotonin toxicity, see Clinical Features of Some Adverse Drug Interactions, Serotonin toxicity and serotonin syndrome***

(Continued)

ANALGESICS OPIOIDS

Primary Drug	Secondary Drug	Effect	Mechanism	Precautions
OPIOIDS				
OPIOIDS	MAOIs	Additive depression of CNS ranging from drowsiness to coma and respiratory depression. Opioids may enhance the serotonergic effect of MAO inhibitors. This could result in serotonin syndrome	Synergistic depressant effects on CNS function	Necessary to warn patients, particularly regards activities that require attention, e.g., driving or using machinery and equipment that could cause self-harm. Avoid use of fentanyl (and other anilidopiperidine opioids when possible) in patients who have used a monoamine oxidase inhibitor within the past 14 days due to reports of unpredictable but severe adverse effects
DEXTROMETHORPHAN, MORPHINE, PETHIDINE, PHENOPERIDINE, TRAMADOL	MAOIS	Two types of reactions are reported: 1. Risk of serotonin syndrome with dextromethorphan, pethidine, phenoperidine or tramadol, and MAOIs 2. Depressive—respiratory depression, hypotension, coma	Type I reactions are attributed to an inhibition of reuptake of serotonin; this is more common with pethidine, phenoperidine, dextromethorphan, and tramadol Type II reactions, attributed to MAOI inhibition of metabolism of opioids, are more common with morphine	Avoid coadministration; do not give dextromethorphan, pethidine or tramadol for at least 2 weeks after cessation of MAOI
OPIOIDS—TRAMADOL	REBOXETINE	Risk of ↑ reboxetine levels	Possibly inhibition of CYP3A4-mediated metabolism of reboxetine	Avoid coadministration
OPIOIDS	SSRIs	1. Possible ↓ analgesic effect of codeine, and tramadol 2. ↑ Serotonin effects, including possible cases of serotonin syndrome, when opioids (oxycodone, pethidine, pentazocine, tramadol) are coadministered with SSRIs (fluoxetine, sertraline) 3. SSRIs may ↑ codeine, fentanyl, methadone, oxycodone, pethidine, and tramadol levels	1. Some SSRIs like paroxetine inhibit CYP2D6, which is required to produce the active form of codeine and tramadol 2. Additive effect; these opioids inhibit reuptake of serotonin 3. SSRIs inhibit CYP2D6-mediated metabolism of these opioids	1. Consider using an alternative opioid 2. Look for signs of ↑ serotonin activity, particularly on initiating therapy 3. Watch for excessive narcotization

(*Continued*)

Primary Drug	Secondary Drug	Effect	Mechanism	Precautions
OPIOIDS				
OPIOIDS	SNRIs—DULOXETINE	↑ Serotonin effects, including possible cases of serotonin syndrome, when opioids (oxycodone, pethidine, pentazocine, tramadol) are given	Uncertain	Look for signs of ↑ serotonin activity, particularly on initiating therapy
OPIOIDS	TCAS	1. Risk of ↑ respiratory depression and sedation 2. ↑ Levels of morphine 3. Cases of seizures when tramadol is coadministered with TCAs 4. TCAs may ↑ codeine, fentanyl, pethidine, and tramadol levels 5. Serotonin syndrome	1. Additive effect 2. Uncertain; likely to ↑ bioavailability of morphine 3. Unknown 4. TCAs inhibit CYP2D6-mediated metabolism of these opioids 5. Inhibit reuptake of serotonin with tramadol	1. Warn patients of this effect Titrate doses carefully 2. Warn patients of this effect. Titrate doses carefully 3. Consider an alternative opioid 4. Watch for excessive narcotization 5. Consider an alternative opioid; monitor for signs of serotonin syndrome
TRAMADOL	TRYPTOPHAN	Risk of serotonin syndrome	Additive effect	Use with caution
MORPHINE	ANTIDIABETIC DRUGS—METFORMIN	↑ Level of metformin and risk of lactic acidosis. The onset of lactic acidosis is often subtle with symptoms of malaise, myalgia, respiratory distress, and increasing nonspecific abdominal distress. There may be hypothermia and resistant bradyarrhythmias	Metformin is not metabolized in humans and is not protein bound. Competition for renal tubular excretion is the basis for ↑ activity or retention of metformin	Theoretical possibility. Requires ↓ of metformin dose to be considered or to avoid coadministration. Warn patients re hypoglycemia ➢ ***For signs and symptoms of hypoglycemia, see Clinical Features of Some Adverse Drug Interactions, Hypoglycemia***

(Continued)

Primary Drug	Secondary Drug	Effect	Mechanism	Precautions
OPIOIDS				
OPIOIDS	ANTIEMETICS	1. Ondansetron seems to ↓ analgesic effect of tramadol 2. ↓ Efficacy of domperidone and metoclopramide on gut motility by opioids 3. Metoclopramide ↑ speed of onset and effect of oral morphine	1. Uncertain; tramadol exerts its analgesic properties via serotoninergic pathways in addition to stimulation of opioid receptors. Ondansetron is a serotonin receptor antagonist. 2. Antagonist effect. 3. Uncertain; possibly metoclopramide promotes absorption of morphine by increasing gastric emptying	1. Avoid coadministration. Although increasing the dose of tramadol restored the analgesic effect, it also caused a poor response to an antiemetic 2. Caution with coadministration 3. Be aware that the effects of oral morphine are ↑
OPIOIDS	**ANTIEPILEPTICS**			
OPIOIDS	BARBITURATES	1. Barbiturates ↑ sedative effects of opioids 2. ↓ Efficacy of fentanyl and methadone	1. Additive sedative effect 2. ↑ Hepatic metabolism of fentanyl and methadone, and possibly an effect at the opioid receptor	1. Monitor respiratory rate and conscious levels 2. Be aware that the dose of fentanyl and methadone may need to be ↑.
OPIOIDS	CARBAMAZEPINE	1. ↓ Efficacy of fentanyl and methadone 2. ↓ Tramadol levels	1. Additive sedative effect 2. Carbamazepine ↑ metabolism of tramadol	1. Monitor respiratory rate and conscious levels 2. Watch for poor effect of tramadol. Consider using an alternative opioid
OPIOIDS—MORPHINE	GABAPENTIN	1. CNS depression 2. ↑ Analgesic effect	1. Pharmacodynamic additive CNS depression 2. Uncertain; partly due to ↑ plasma concentration of gabapentin due to ↓ gut mobility with morphine	Monitor for signs of CNS depression; titrate doses of gabapentin and/or morphine
OPIOIDS	PHENYTOIN	1. ↓ Efficacy of fentanyl and methadone with carbamazepine, phenytoin 2. Risk of pethidine toxicity	1. ↑ Hepatic metabolism of fentanyl and methadone, and possibly an effect at the opioid receptor 2. Phenytoin induces metabolism of pethidine, which causes ↑ level of a neurotoxic metabolite	1. Be aware that the dose of fentanyl and methadone may need to be ↑ 2. Coadminister with caution; the effect may be ↓ by administering pethidine intravenously

(*Continued*)

Primary Drug	Secondary Drug	Effect	Mechanism	Precautions
OPIOIDS				
OPIOIDS	ANTIFUNGALS—AZOLES	1. Ketoconazole ↑ effect of buprenorphine 2. Fluconazole and itraconazole ↑ the effect of alfentanil 3. Fluconazole, itraconazole, and possibly voriconazole ↑ effect of methadone with a risk of ventricular arrhythmias	1. Ketoconazole ↓ the CYP3A4-mediated metabolism of buprenorphine 2. ↓ Clearance of alfentanil 3. Inhibition of CYP3A4-mediated metabolism	1. The dose of buprenorphine needs to be ↓ (by up to 50%) 2. ↓ Dose of alfentanil 3. Watch for ↑ effects of methadone
OPIOIDS	ANTIHISTAMINES	Promethazine ↑ analgesic and anesthetic effects of opioids. However, it has an additive sedative effect	Unknown	Monitor vital signs closely during coadministration
OPIOIDS	ANTIMALARIALS—QUININE	↑ Codeine, fentanyl, pethidine, and tramadol levels	Quinine inhibits CYP2D6	Watch for excessive narcotization
OPIOIDS	**ANTIOBESITY DRUGS**			
DEXTROMETHORPHAN, TRAMADOL	LOCASERIN	Risk of serotonin syndrome	Additive effect	Be aware of the possibility of serotonin syndrome. ➢ ***For signs and symptoms of serotonin toxicity, see Clinical Features of Some Adverse Drug Interactions, Serotonin toxicity and serotonin syndrome***
OPIOIDS—DEXTROMETHORPHAN, FENTANYL, PETHIDINE, PENTAZOCINE	SIBUTRAMINE	Risk of serotonin syndrome	Additive effect	Manufacturer advises against coadministration
PETHIDINE, TRAMADOL	ANTI-PARKINSON'S DRUGS—RASAGILINE, SELEGILINE	1. Risk of neurological toxicity when pethidine is coadministered with rasagiline 2. Risk of hyperpyrexia when pethidine and possibly tramadol is coadministered with selegiline	Unknown	1. Avoid coadministration; do not use pethidine for at least 2 weeks after stopping rasagiline 2. Avoid coadministration

(Continued)

ANALGESICS OPIOIDS

Primary Drug	Secondary Drug	Effect	Mechanism	Precautions
OPIOIDS				
OPIOIDS	ANTIPSYCHOTICS	Risk of ↑ respiratory depression, sedation, and ↓ BP. This effect seems to be particularly marked with clozapine	Additive effects	Warn patients of these effects. Monitor BP closely. Titrate doses carefully
TRAMADOL	ANTIPSYCHOTICS	↑ Risk of fits	Additive effects	Consider using an alternative analgesic
OPIOIDS	**ANTIVIRALS**			
METHADONE	NNRTIs	Methadone levels may be significantly ↓ by efavirenz and nevirapine	↑ CYP3A4- and 2B6-mediated metabolism of methadone	Monitor closely for opioid withdrawal; ↑ dose as necessary. Likely to need dose titration of methadone (mean 22% but up to 186% ↑)
METHADONE	NUCLEOSIDE REVERSE TRANSCRIPTASE INHIBITORS	↓ Efficacy of methadone when coadministered with abacavir	Uncertain; possibly enzyme induction	Monitor for opioid withdrawal and consider increasing dose
OPIOIDS	**PROTEASE INHIBITORS**			
ALFENTANIL, BUPRENORPHINE, FENTANYL, TRAMADOL	PROTEASE INHIBITORS	Possibly ↑ adverse effects when buprenorphine is coadministered with indinavir, ritonavir (with or without lopinavir), or saquinavir	Inhibition of CYP3A4 (CYP2D6 in the case of tramadol)	Halve the starting dose and titrate to effect. For single injection of fentanyl, monitor sedation and respiratory function closely. If continued use of fentanyl, ↓ dose may be required. Concomitant use of ritonavir and transdermal fentanyl is not recommended
CODEINE, DIHYDROCODEINE	PROTEASE INHIBITORS	↓ Efficacy of codeine and dihydrocodeine when given with ritonavir	Inhibition of CYP2D6-mediated metabolism of codeine to its active metabolites	Use an alternative opioid

(Continued)

ANALGESICS OPIOIDS

Primary Drug	Secondary Drug	Effect	Mechanism	Precautions
OPIOIDS				
METHADONE, PETHIDINE	PROTEASE INHIBITORS	↓ Efficacy of methadone, with risk of withdrawal, when coadministered with amprenavir, nelfinavir, ritonavir (with or without lopinavir), or saquinavir	Uncertain; possibly due to induction of CYP3A4 and CYP2D6	Monitor closely for opioid withdrawal, and ↑ dose of methadone as necessary. This advice includes coadministration of methadone with low-dose ritonavir. Short-term use of pethidine is unlikely to cause a problem
OPIOIDS	**ANXIOLYTICS AND HYPNOTICS**			
OPIOIDS	ANXIOLYTICS AND HYPNOTICS	1. ↑ Sedation with BZDs 2. Respiratory depressant effect of morphine antagonized by lorazepam	1. Additive effect; both drugs are sedatives 2. Uncertain	1. Closely monitor vital signs during coadministration 2. Although this effect may be considered to be beneficial, risk of additive effects should be borne in mind if the combination of an opioid and BZDs is used for sedation for painful procedures
OPIOIDS	ANXIOLYTICS AND HYPNOTICS—SODIUM OXYBATE	Risk of CNS depression—coma, respiratory depression	Additive effect	Avoid coadministration
OPIOIDS	BETA-BLOCKERS	1. Risk of ↑ plasma concentrations and effects of labetalol, metoprolol, and propranolol; ↑ systemic effects of timolol eye drops 2. ↑ Plasma concentrations of esmolol when morphine added 3. ↑ Plasma concentrations of metoprolol and propranolol when dextropropoxyphene added	1. Methadone inhibits CYP2D6, which metabolizes these beta-blockers 2. Unknown 3. ↓ Hepatic clearance of metoprolol and propanolol	1. Monitor BP at least weekly until stable 2. Monitor BP closely 3. Monitor BP at least weekly until stable. Warn patients to report symptoms of hypotension (light headedness, dizziness on standing, etc.)

(*Continued*)

Primary Drug	Secondary Drug	Effect	Mechanism	Precautions
OPIOIDS				
OPIOIDS	CALCIUM CHANNEL BLOCKERS	Diltiazem prolongs the action of alfentanil, fentanyl, and methadone	Diltiazem inhibits CYP3A4-mediated metabolism	Watch for the prolonged action of alfentanil and features of toxicity in patients taking calcium channel blockers; case reports of delayed extubation in patients recovering from anesthetics involving large doses of alfentanil in patients on diltiazem
OPIOIDS	CARDIAC GLYCOSIDES	↑ Concentrations of digoxin may occur with tramadol	Unknown	Watch for digoxin toxicity; check levels and ↓ dose of digoxin as necessary
OPIOIDS	CNS STIMULANTS—ATOMOXETINE	Risk of arrhythmias with methadone and possible risk of fits with tramadol	Uncertain	Avoid coadministration of atomoxetine with methadone or tramadol
OPIOIDS	DESMOPRESSIN	May enhance the adverse/toxic effect of desmopressin	May contribute to hyponatremia. Mechanism uncertain	Monitor serum sodium before and after concurrent treatment
OPIODS	DIURETICS	Opioids may enhance the orthostatic hypotensive effect of diuretics	Additive hypotensive effect	Warn about dizziness when standing up suddenly and warn also about other symptoms of orthostatic hypotension
OPIOIDS	DRUG DEPENDENCE THERAPIES—BUPROPION	↑ Plasma concentrations of these substrates, with risk of toxic effects	Bupropion and its metabolite hydroxybupropion inhibit CYP2D6	Initiate therapy of these drugs at the lowest effective dose
METHADONE	GRAPEFRUIT JUICE	↑ Plasma concentrations and ↑ risk of adverse effects. There is a rapid onset of interaction, but it is of minor clinical significance	Methadone is metabolized by intestinal CYP3A4, which is inhibited by grapefruit juice	Prudent to be aware and warn users and carers of rapid onset of drowsiness and difficulty in breathing
MORPHINE	GRAPEFRUIT JUICE	Grapefruit juice ↑ morphine antinociception. Gradually ↓ CSF and blood concentrations following repeated treatment with morphine	Grapefruit juice is considered to ↑ intestinal absorption of morphine due to inhibition of Pgp, which also probably contributes to ↓ CSF concentrations	This interaction is unlikely to be of clinical significance, but be aware. Warn patients and carers to report any difficulty in breathing and excessive drowsiness

(*Continued*)

Primary Drug	Secondary Drug	Effect	Mechanism	Precautions
OPIOIDS				
OPIOIDS	**H2 RECEPTOR BLOCKERS**			
ALFENTANIL, FENTANYL, PETHIDINE, TRAMADOL	CIMETIDINE	↑ Levels and risk of adverse effects, including respiratory depression	Inhibition of CYP3A4 mediated metabolism and reduced pethidine clearance	Watch for excessive narcotization; monitor pain, sedation scores, and respiratory rate closely
CODEINE	CIMETIDINE	Cimetidine may ↓ efficacy of codeine	Due to inhibition of enzymatic conversion to active metabolite via CYP2D6	Watch for poor response to codeine. Consider using an alternative opioid or acid suppression therapy; famotidine, nizatidine, and PPIs are not likely to interact significantly
OPIOIDS	**MUSCLE RELAXANTS—NONDEPOLARIZING**			
SUFENTANIL	MUSCLE RELAXANTS—NONDEPOLARIZING	Initial requirement of neuromuscular blockers may be decreased	Uncertain	Monitor neuromuscular block closely
SUFENTANIL	PANCURONIUM	The vagolytic effects of pancuronium may produce a dose-dependent elevation in heart rate during sufentanil-oxygen anesthesia	The use of moderate doses of pancuronium or of a less vagolytic neuromuscular blocking agent may be used to maintain a stable lower heart rate and blood pressure during sufentanil-oxygen anesthesia	Monitor heart rate and titrate doses
OPIOIDS	ESTROGENS	Effect of morphine may be ↓ by combined oral contraceptives	Hepatic metabolism of morphine is ↑	Be aware that morphine dose may need to be ↑. Consider using an alternative opioid such as pethidine
OPIOIDS	PEGVISOMANT (GROWTH HORMONE RECEPTOR ANTAGONIST)	May diminish the therapeutic effect of pegvisomant	Narcotic medicines, e.g., opioids, decrease effect—the mechanism for relative resistance is uncertain	Need higher doses of pegvisomant for therapeutic results during concomitant use
OPIOIDS	PROGESTOGENS	Gestodene ↑ effect of buprenorphine	Gestodene ↓ the CYP3A4-mediated metabolism of buprenorphine	The dose of buprenorphine needs to be ↓ (by up to 50%)

(Continued)

ANALGESICS OPIOIDS

Primary Drug	Secondary Drug	Effect	Mechanism	Precautions
OPIOIDS				
OPIOIDS	SYMPATHOMIMETICS—INDIRECT	Dexamfetamine and methylphenidate ↑ analgesic effects and ↓ sedation of opioids, when used for chronic pain	Uncertain; complex interaction between the sympathetic nervous system and opioid receptors	Opioid requirements may be ↓ when patients also take indirect sympathomimetics

Primary Drug	Secondary Drug	Effect	Mechanism	Precautions
PARACETAMOL (ACETAMINOPHEN)				
PARACETAMOL	ANTIARRHYTHMICS	Disopyramide and propafenone may slow the onset of action of intermittent-dose paracetamol	Anticholinergic effects delay gastric emptying and absorption	Warn patients that the action of paracetamol may be delayed. This will not be the case when paracetamol is taken regularly
PARACETAMOL	**ANTIBIOTICS**			
PARACETAMOL	ISONIAZID	Risk of paracetamol toxicity at regular, therapeutic doses when coadministered with isoniazid	Uncertain; it seems that formation of toxic metabolites is ↑ in fast acetylators when isoniazid levels ↓ (i.e., at the end of a dosing period)	There have been cases of hepatic pathology; regular paracetamol should be avoided in patients taking isoniazid
PARACETAMOL	RIFAMPICIN	Rifampicin ↓ paracetamol levels	Rifampicin ↑ glucuronidation of paracetamol	Warn patients that paracetamol may be less effective
PARACETAMOL	**ANTICANCER AND IMMUNOMODULATING DRUGS—BUSULFAN**			
PARACETAMOL	BUSULFAN	Busulfan levels may be ↑ by coadministration of paracetamol	Uncertain; paracetamol probably inhibits metabolism of busulfan	Manufacturers recommend that paracetamol should be avoided for 3 days before administering parenteral busulfan
PARACETAMOL	CRIZOTINIB	Possible increased levels of UGT substrates	UGT (particularly UGT1A1, UGT2B7) inhibition	Caution with concurrent use
PARACETAMOL	IMANITIB	Possible increased risk of liver failure, but no pharmacokinetic interaction in studies	Inhibition of paracetamol glucuronidation, possible additive effect	Caution with concurrent use

(Continued)

Primary Drug	Secondary Drug	Effect	Mechanism	Precautions
PARACETAMOL (ACETAMINOPHEN)				
PARACETAMOL	SUNITINIB	Single report of fatal liver failure	Unknown	Unknown
PARACETAMOL	ANTICOAGULANTS—ORAL	Possible ↑ anticoagulant effect when paracetamol is taken regularly (but not occasionally)	Uncertain; possibly due to competitive inhibition of CYP-mediated metabolism of warfarin	Monitor INR closely for the first 1–2 weeks of starting or stopping regular paracetamol
PARACETAMOL	ANTIDEPRESSANTS—TCAs	TCAs may slow the onset of action of intermittent-dose paracetamol	Anticholinergic effects delay gastric emptying and absorption	Warn patients that the action of paracetamol may be delayed. This will not be the case when paracetamol is taken regularly
PARACETAMOL	ANTIDIABETICS—LIXISENATIDE	Lixisenatide possibly reduces absorption of paracetamol when given 1–4 h before	Possibly caused by gastric stasis and decreased stomach motility	Consider injecting lixisenatide after paracetamol administration
PARACETAMOL	ANTIEMETICS	Cyclizine may slow the onset of action of intermittent-dose paracetamol	Anticholinergic effects delay gastric emptying and absorption	Warn patients that the action of paracetamol may be delayed. This will not be the case when paracetamol is taken regularly
PARACETAMOL	ANTIHISTAMINES	Chlorphenamine, cyproheptadine, and hydroxyzine may slow the onset of action of intermittent-dose paracetamol	Anticholinergic effects delay gastric emptying and absorption	Warn patients that the action of paracetamol may be delayed. This will not be the case when paracetamol is taken regularly
PARACETAMOL	ANTIMUSCARINICS	Atropine, benzatropine, orphenadrine, procyclidine, and trihexyphenidyl may slow the onset of action of intermittent-dose paracetamol	Anticholinergic effects delay gastric emptying and absorption	Warn patients that the action of paracetamol may be delayed. This will not be the case when paracetamol is taken regularly

(*Continued*)

ANALGESICS PARACETAMOL (ACETAMINOPHEN)

ANALGESICS PARACETAMOL (ACETAMINOPHEN)

Primary Drug	Secondary Drug	Effect	Mechanism	Precautions
PARACETAMOL (ACETAMINOPHEN)				
PARACETAMOL	ANTI-PARKINSON'S DRUGS—DOPAMINERGICS	Amantadine, bromocriptine, levodopa, pergolide, pramipexole, and selegiline may slow the onset of action of intermittent-dose paracetamol	Anticholinergic effects delay gastric emptying and absorption	Warn patients that the action of paracetamol may be delayed. This will not be the case when paracetamol is taken regularly
PARACETAMOL	ANTIVIRALS	Cases of hepatotoxicity have been reported when paracetamol was added to either didanosine or zidovudine	Uncertain; possible additive hepatotoxic effect	Monitor liver function regularly during coadministration
PARACETAMOL	CNS STIMULANTS—MODAFINIL	May cause ↓ paracetamol levels if CYP1A2 is the predominant metabolic pathway and alternative metabolic pathways are either genetically deficient or affected	Modafinil is moderate inducer of CYP1A2 in a concentration-dependent manner	Be aware
PARACETAMOL	LIPID-LOWERING DRUGS	Colestyramine ↓ paracetamol by 60% when they are given together	Colestyramine binds paracetamol in the intestine	Give colestyramine and paracetamol at least 1 h apart
PARACETAMOL	MUSCLE RELAXANTS—SKELETAL	Baclofen may slow the onset of action of intermittent-dose paracetamol	Anticholinergic effects delay gastric emptying and absorption	Warn patients that the action of paracetamol may be delayed. This will not be the case when paracetamol is taken regularly

PART 8

Musculoskeletal Drugs

Wing Lam Yeung

1. ANTIGOUT DRUGS
2. DRUGS AFFECTING BONE METABOLISM ➢ *Other Endocrine Drugs*
3. DRUGS TREATING INFLAMMATORY ARTHROPATHIES
   - CORTICOSTEROIDS ➢ *Anticancer and Immunomodulating Drugs, Other Immunomodulating Drugs*
   - DISEASE-MODIFYING DRUGS ➢ *Anticancer and Immunomodulating Drugs; Drugs to Treat Infections, Antimalarial Drugs*
   - NONSTEROIDAL ANTI-INFLAMMATORY DRUGS ➢ *Analgesics, Nonsteroidal Anti-inflammatory Drugs*
4. SKELETAL MUSCLE RELAXANTS

Primary Drug	Secondary Drug	Effect	Mechanism	Precautions
ANTIGOUT DRUGS				
ALLOPURINOL				
ALLOPURINOL	**ANTIBIOTICS**			
ALLOPURINOL	AMOXICILLIN, AMPICILLIN	↑ Risk of rash with amoxicillin and ampicillin (over 20% incidence in one study)	Uncertain	Reassure patients that the rash is unlikely to have clinical significance
ALLOPURINOL	PYRAZINAMIDE	↓ Efficacy of antigout drugs	Pyrazinamide can induce hyperuricemia	Pyrazinamide should not be used in patients with gout
ALLOPURINOL	**ANTICANCER AND IMMUNOMODULATING DRUGS**			
ALLOPURINOL	AZATHIOPRINE/ MERCAPTOPURINE	↑ Mercaptopurine levels, with risk of toxicity (e.g., myelosuppression, pancreatitis)	Azathioprine is metabolized to mercaptopurine. Allopurinol inhibits hepatic metabolism of mercaptopurine	↓ Doses of azathioprine and mercaptopurine to one-quarter of usual dose, and monitor FBC, LFTs, and amylase carefully
ALLOPURINOL	CAPECITABINE/ FLUOROURACIL	Possible ↓ efficacy of capecitabine	Capecitabine is a prodrug for fluorouracil; uncertain at which point allopurinol acts on the metabolic pathway	Manufacturers recommend avoiding coadministration
ALLOPURINOL	CICLOSPORIN	Ciclosporin levels may be ↑	Uncertain	Monitor renal function closely
ALLOPURINOL	CYCLOPHOSPHAMIDE	↑ Risk of bone marrow suppression	Uncertain but allopurinol seems to ↑ cyclophosphamide levels	Monitor FBC closely
ALLOPURINOL	ANTICOAGULANTS—ORAL	Uncommon instances of ↑ anticoagulant effect in patients on warfarin who started allopurinol	Allopurinol possibly ↓ hepatic metabolism of warfarin but with considerable individual variation	Monitor INR at least weekly until stable
ALLOPURINOL	**ANTIEPILEPTICS**			
ALLOPURINOL	CARBAMAZEPINE	High-dose allopurinol (600 mg/day) may ↑ carbamazepine levels over a period of several weeks. 300 mg/day allopurinol does not seem to have this effect	Uncertain	Monitor carbamazepine levels in patients taking long-term, high-dose allopurinol

(*Continued*)

Primary Drug	Secondary Drug	Effect	Mechanism	Precautions
ANTIGOUT DRUGS				
ALLOPURINOL	PHENYTOIN	Phenytoin levels may be ↑ in some patients	Uncertain	Monitor phenytoin levels
ALLOPURINOL	ANTIHYPERTENSIVES AND HEART FAILURE DRUGS—ACE INHIBITORS	Risk of serious hypersensitivity with captopril and enalapril. ↑ Risk of leukopenia	Uncertain. Both drugs can cause hypersensitivity reactions	Warn patient to look for clinical features of hypersensitivity and Stevens–Johnson syndrome
ALLOPURINOL	ANTIVIRALS—DIDANOSINE	↑ Levels of didanosine	Probably altered metabolism via xanthine oxidase	Coadministration not recommended, consider alternative regimens. Watch for early signs of toxicity, especially in patients with renal impairment. A dose reduction of didanosine may be required if combination essential
ALLOPURINOL	BRONCHODILATORS—THEOPHYLLINE	May ↑ theophylline levels	Probable inhibition of theophylline metabolism	Watch for early features of toxicity of theophylline (headache, nausea) Monitor theophylline levels when starting or increasing allopurinol
ALLOPURINOL	DIURETICS—THIAZIDES	Possible ↑ risk of severe allergic reactions when allopurinol is given with thiazides in the presence of renal impairment	Uncertain	Caution in coadministering allopurinol with thiazides in the presence of renal insufficiency
ALLOPURINOL	ANTIDIABETICS—CHLORPROPAMIDE	↑ Risk of prolonged hypoglycemic effect in the presence of renal impairment	Possible competition for renal excretion	Monitor blood glucose closely
BENZBROMARONE				
BENZBROMARONE	ANTIBIOTICS—PYRAZINAMIDE	↓ Efficacy of antigout drugs	Pyrazinamide can induce hyperuricemia	Pyrazinamide should not be used in patients with gout
BENZBROMARONE	ANTICOAGULANTS—WARFARIN	↑ Warfarin levels	Inhibition of CYP2D6-mediated metabolism of warfarin	Monitor INR closely until stabilized—consider ↓ warfarin dose (one study suggested ↓ dose by 1/3)
BENZBROMARONE	ANTIPLATELET AGENTS—ASPIRIN	High doses of aspirin antagonize the effects of benzbromarone	Uncertain	Watch for poor response to benzbromarone

(*Continued*)

Primary Drug	Secondary Drug	Effect	Mechanism	Precautions
ANTIGOUT DRUGS				
COLCHICINE				
COLCHICINE	ANTIARRHYTHMICS—QUINIDINE	Colchicine levels ↑ by quinidine	Quinidine is a moderate P-glycoprotein (Pgp) inhibitor	Avoid coadministration in the presence of renal failure. In the presence of normal renal function, UK manufacturer recommends reducing dose and/or increasing dosing interval. The U.S. manufacturer recommends more specific dosage adjustments: for treatment of gout stat dose of 0.6 mg not to be repeated for 3 days. For gout prophylaxis: 0.6 mg bd –> 0.3 mg od; 0.6 mg od –> 0.3 mg alternate days
COLCHICINE	**ANTIBIOTICS**			
COLCHICINE	MACROLIDES	Case reports of colchicine toxicity when macrolides were added	Uncertain; macrolides possibly inhibit hepatic metabolism of colchicine. Clarithromycin and erythromycin both inhibit intestinal Pgp, which may ↑ bioavailability of colchicine	Monitor FBC and renal function closely Consider ↓ colchicine dose or withhold colchicine Concomitant use is contraindicated in hepatic or renal impairment
COLCHICINE	PYRAZINAMIDE	↓ Efficacy of antigout drugs	Pyrazinamide can induce hyperuricemia	Pyrazinamide should not be used in patients with gout
COLCHICINE	**ANTICANCER AND IMMUNOMODULATING DRUGS**			
COLCHICINE	CICLOSPORIN	↑ Colchicine plasma concentrations and ↑ toxic effects (hepatotoxicity, nephrotoxicity, myopathy). ↑ Penetration of ciclosporin through blood–brain barrier and ↑ risk of neurotoxicity	Competitive inhibition of Pgp with ↑ penetrations of ciclosporin to tissues. Ciclosporin inhibits transport of colchicine	Avoid concurrent use, especially in hepatic or renal impairment Watch for signs of colchicine toxicity if concomitant use necessary
COLCHICINE	CRIZOTINIB	Possible increased levels of Pgp substrates	Crizotinib inhibits Pgp	Monitor closely

(Continued)

Primary Drug	Secondary Drug	Effect	Mechanism	Precautions
ANTIGOUT DRUGS				
COLCHICINE	VEMURAFENIB	Possible increased levels of Pgp substrates	Vemurafenib inhibits Pgp	Be aware. Clinical significance unknown
COLCHICINE	ANTIFUNGALS—ITRACONAZOLE	↑ Risk of colchicine toxicity	CYP3A4 inhibition	Watch for signs of colchicine toxicity Consider ↓ colchicine dose or withhold colchicine Concomitant use is contraindicated in hepatic or renal impairment
COLCHICINE	ANTIVIRALS—ATAZANAVIR, INDINAVIR, RITONAVIR, TELAPREVIR	↑ Risk of colchicine toxicity	CYP3A4 inhibition	Watch for signs of colchicine toxicity Consider ↓ colchicine dose or withhold colchicine Concomitant use is contraindicated in hepatic or renal impairment
COLCHICINE	CALCIUM—CHANNEL BLOCKERS—DILTIAZEM, VERAPAMIL	↑ Colchicine levels by diltiazem and verapamil—reports of toxicity	Combination of inhibition of CYP 3A4 and Pgp	Reduce dose of colchicine—monitor FBC regularly and warn patients to report features of colchicine toxicity (GI upset, muscle aches, sore throat)
COLCHICINE	CARDIAC GLYCOSIDES—DIGOXIN	↑ Risk of myopathy	Possible competition for Pgp	Ask patients to report signs of myopathy
COLCHICINE	ELIGLUSTAT	↑ Colchicine levels	Inhibition of Pgp	Reduce dose of colchicine; watch for adverse effects
COLCHICINE	LIPID-LOWERING DRUGS—STATINS	↑ Risk of myopathy	Uncertain. Both drugs can cause myopathy	Ask patients to report signs of myopathy
COLCHICINE	RANOLAZINE	↑ Colchicine levels	Combination of inhibition of CYP 3A4 and Pgp	Reduce dose of colchicine—monitor FBC regularly and warn patients to report features of colchicine toxicity (GI upset, muscle aches, sore throat)
FEBUXOSTAT				
FEBUXOSTAT	AZATHIOPRINE/ MERCAPTOPURINE	May increase azathioprine levels	Inhibition of xanthine oxidase	Avoid concurrent use If necessary, consider dose reduction and monitor closely

(Continued)

Primary Drug	Secondary Drug	Effect	Mechanism	Precautions
ANTIGOUT DRUGS				
PROBENECID				
PROBENECID	ACE INHIBITORS	↑ Plasma concentrations of captopril and enalapril; uncertain clinical significance	Renal excretion of captopril and enalapril ↓ by probenecid	Monitor BP closely
PROBENECID	ANALGESICS—NSAIDs	↑ Levels of acemetacin, diflunisal, indomethacin, ketoprofen, ketorolac, naproxen, tenoxicam, and tiaprofenic acid	Probenecid competitively inhibits renal clearance of these NSAIDs	Watch for signs of toxicity of these NSAIDs. Consider using an alternative NSAID. The manufacturers of ketorolac advise avoiding coadministration of ketorolac and probenecid
PROBENECID	**ANTIBIOTICS**			
PROBENECID	CEPHALOSPORINS	↑ Cephalosporin levels	↓ Renal clearance of cephalosporins	Watch for ↑ incidence of side effects of antibiotic
PROBENECID	DAPSONE	↑ Dapsone levels, with risk of bone marrow suppression	↓ Excretion of dapsone	Monitor FBC closely
PROBENECID	MEROPENEM	↑ Meropenem levels	↓ Renal excretion of meropenem	Manufacturers advise caution with coadministration
PROBENECID	NITROFURANTOIN	↓ Efficacy of nitrofurantoin in urinary tract infections and ↑ risk of side effects	↓ Urinary excretion of nitrofurantoin	Watch for poor response to nitrofurantoin
PROBENECID	PENICILLINS	↑ Penicillin levels	↓ Renal excretion of penicillins	Watch for ↑ incidence of side effects of antibiotic
PROBENECID	PYRAZINAMIDE	↓ Efficacy of antigout drugs	Pyrazinamide can induce hyperuricemia	Pyrazinamide should not be used in patients with gout
PROBENECID	QUINOLONES—CIPROFLOXACIN, LEVOFLOXACIN, NALIDIXIC ACID, NORFLOXACIN	↑ Ciprofloxacin, nalidixic acid, and norfloxacin levels	↓ Renal excretion of quinolones	Watch for ↑ incidence of side effects. Moxifloxacin does not seem to interact and could be used as alternative therapy
PROBENECID	**ANTICANCER AND IMMUNOMODULATING DRUGS**			
PROBENECID	AMINOSALICYLATES	Aminosalicylate levels are ↑ by probenecid	Probenecid competes with aminosalicylate for active renal excretion	Watch for early features of toxicity of aminosalicylate. Consider ↓ dose of aminosalicylate

(Continued)

MUSCULOSKELETAL DRUGS ANTIGOUT DRUGS Probenecid

Primary Drug	Secondary Drug	Effect	Mechanism	Precautions
ANTIGOUT DRUGS				
PROBENECID	METHOTREXATE	↑ Methotrexate levels	Probenecid ↓ elimination of methotrexate renally by interfering with tubular secretion in the proximal tubule and also ↓ protein binding of methotrexate (a relatively minor effect). Probenecid competes with methotrexate for renal elimination	Avoid coadministration if possible; if not possible, ↓ dose of methotrexate and monitor FBC closely
PROBENECID	MYCOPHENOLATE	Possible increased mycophenolate levels	Probenecid inhibits renal excretion of mycophenolate metabolite	Be aware. Clinical significance uncertain
PROBENECID	PEMETREXED	↑ Pemetrexed levels	Probable ↓ renal excretion of pemetrexed	Avoid coadministration where possible. If both need to be given, monitor FBC and renal function closely and watch for gastrointestinal disturbances and features of myopathy
PROBENECID	**ANTIDIABETIC DRUGS**			
PROBENECID	METFORMIN	↑ Level of metformin and risk of lactic acidosis. The onset of lactic acidosis is often subtle with symptoms of malaise, myalgia, respiratory distress, and ↑ nonspecific abdominal distress. There may be hypothermia and resistant bradyarrhythmias	↓ Renal excretion of metformin	Watch for hypoglycemia and lactic acidosis. Warn patients about hypoglycemia ➢ ***For signs and symptoms of hypoglycemia, see clinical features of some adverse drug interactions, hypoglycemia***
PROBENECID	SULFONYLUREAS	↑ Risk of hypoglycemic episodes due to ↑ plasma levels of glimepiride	Attributed to ↓ renal excretion of sulfonylureas by probenecid. Probenecid is also an inhibitor of CYP2C9 isoenzymes	Watch for and warn patients about symptoms of hypoglycemia ➢ ***For signs and symptoms of hypoglycemia, see clinical features of some adverse drug interactions, hypoglycemia***
PROBENECID	ANTIPLATELET AGENTS	High doses of aspirin antagonize the effects of probenecid	Uncertain	Watch for poor response to probenecid

(*Continued*)

Primary Drug	Secondary Drug	Effect	Mechanism	Precautions
ANTIGOUT DRUGS				
PROBENECID	**ANTIVIRALS**			
PROBENECID	ANTIVIRALS	↑ Levels of acyclovir, famciclovir, valacyclovir, ganciclovir, and valganciclovir	Competitive inhibition of renal excretion	Care with coadministering probenecid with high-dose antivirals Monitor for toxicity
PROBENECID	ZIDOVUDINE	↑ Levels of zidovudine with cases of toxicity	Competition for renal tubular secretion via OATs	Avoid coadministration if possible; if not possible, ↓ dose of zidovudine and monitor for hematological toxicity
PROBENECID	ANXIOLYTICS AND HYPNOTICS—NITRAZEPAM	Possibly ↑ nitrazepam levels	Possibly ↓ renal excretion of nitrazepam	Consider ↓ dose of nitrazepam Watch for excessive sedation
PROBENECID	H2-RECEPTOR BLOCKERS—CIMETIDINE, FAMOTIDINE	↑ Plasma concentrations of cimetidine or famotidine	↓ Renal tubular secretion	Avoid concomitant use
PROBENECID	SODIUM PHENYLBUTYRATE	Possibly ↑ sodium phenylbutyrate levels	Possibly ↓ excretion of the conjugation product of sodium phenylbutyrate	Watch for signs of sodium phenylbutyrate toxicity. Monitor FBC, U&Es, and ECG
SULFINPYRAZONE				
SULFINPYRAZONE	**ANTIBIOTICS DRUGS**			
SULFINPYRAZONE	NITROFURANTOIN	↓ Efficacy of nitrofurantoin in urinary tract infections and ↑ risk of side effects	↓ Urinary excretion of nitrofurantoin	Watch for poor response to nitrofurantoin
SULFINPYRAZONE	PENICILLINS	↑ Penicillin levels	↓ Renal excretion of penicillins	Watch for ↑ incidence of side effects
SULFINPYRAZONE	PYRAZINAMIDE	↓ Efficacy of antigout drugs	Pyrazinamide can induce hyperuricemia	Pyrazinamide should not be used in patients with gout
SULFINPYRAZONE	ANTICANCER AND IMMUNOMODULATING DRUGS—CICLOSPORIN	Cases of ↓ ciclosporin levels with transplant rejection	Uncertain	Monitor ciclosporin levels
SULFINPYRAZONE	**ANTICOAGULANTS**			
SULFINPYRAZONE	APIXABAN	↑ Risk of bleeding	Uncertain	Manufacturers of apixaban do not recommend concomitant use

(Continued)

Primary Drug	Secondary Drug	Effect	Mechanism	Precautions
ANTIGOUT DRUGS				
SULFINPYRAZONE	DABIGATRAN	Possible ↑ risk of bleeding	Uncertain	Manufacturers of dabigatran advise caution with concomitant use
SULFINPYRAZONE	WARFARIN	↑ Anticoagulant effect of warfarin	Uncertain; possibly displacement of anticoagulant from plasma proteins, possibly inhibition of CYP2C9-mediated metabolism of warfarin	Monitor INR closely until stable
SULFINPYRAZONE	**ANTIDIABETIC DRUGS**			
SULFINPYRAZONE	NATEGLINIDE	↑ Blood levels of nateglinide	Sulfinpyrazone is a selective CYP2C9 inhibitor	Need to monitor blood sugar weekly in patients receiving both drugs. Warn patients about hypoglycemia. ➢ ***For signs and symptoms of hypoglycemia, see clinical features of some adverse drug interactions, hypoglycemia***
SULFINPYRAZONE	SULFONYLUREAS	↑ Hypoglycemic effect of sulfonylureas	Uncertain	Monitor blood glucose regularly
SULFINPYRAZONE	ANTIEPILEPTICS	Phenytoin levels may be ↑ in some patients	Possible displacement of phenytoin from its plasma protein-binding sites; inhibition of phenytoin metabolism by the liver	Monitor phenytoin levels
SULFINPYRAZONE	ANTIPLATELET AGENTS	High-dose aspirin antagonizes the urate-lowering effect of sulfinpyrazone	Salicylates block the sulfinpyrazone-induced inhibition of renal tubular reabsorption of urate	Avoid long-term coadministration of high-dose aspirin with sulfinpyrazone. Low-dose aspirin does not seem to have this effect
SULFINPYRAZONE	BETA-BLOCKERS	Antihypertensive effects of oxprenolol ↓ by sulfinpyrazone	Unknown	Monitor PR and BP closely; consider starting an alternative beta-blocker
SULFINPYRAZONE	BRONCHODILATORS—THEOPHYLLINE	↓ Theophylline levels	Due to ↑ demethylation and hydroxylation, and thus ↑ clearance of theophylline	May need to ↑ dose of theophylline by 25%
SULFINPYRAZONE	CALCIUM CHANNEL BLOCKERS	Serum concentrations of verapamil are significantly ↓ when it is coadministered with sulfinpyrazone	Uncertain, but presumed to be due to ↑ hepatic metabolism	Monitor PR and BP closely; watch for poor response to verapamil

Primary Drug	Secondary Drug	Effect	Mechanism	Precautions
DRUGS AFFECTING BONE METABOLISM ➢ *Other Endocrine Drugs*				

Primary Drug	Secondary Drug	Effect	Mechanism	Precautions
DRUGS TREATING INFLAMMATORY ARTHROPATHIES				
CORTICOSTEROIDS ➢ *Anticancer and Immunomodulating Drugs, Other Immunomodulating Drugs*				
DISEASE-MODIFYING DRUGS ➢ *Anticancer and Immunomodulating Drugs; Drugs to Treat Infections, Antimalarial Drugs*				
NONSTEROIDAL ANTI-INFLAMMATORY DRUGS ➢ *Analgesics, Nonsteroidal Anti-inflammatory Drugs*				

Primary Drug	Secondary Drug	Effect	Mechanism	Precautions
SKELETAL MUSCLE RELAXANTS				
BACLOFEN				
BACLOFEN	**ADDITIVE ANTIMUSCARINIC EFFECTS**			
BACLOFEN	1. ANALGESICS—nefopam 2. ANTIARRHYTHMICS—disopyramide, propafenone 3. ANTIDEPRESSANTS—TCAs 4. ANTIEMETICS—cyclizine 5. ANTIHISTAMINES—Chlorpheniramine, cyproheptadine, hydroxyzine 6. ANTIMUSCARINICS—atropine, benztropine, cyclopentolate, dicycloverine, flavoxate, homatropine, hyoscine, orphenadrine, oxybutynin, procyclidine, propantheline, tolterodine, trihexyphenidyl, tropicamide 7. ANTI-PARKINSON'S DRUGS—dopaminergics 8. ANTIPSYCHOTICS—phenothiazines, clozapine, pimozide 9. NITRATES	↑ Risk of antimuscarinic side effects. **NB ↓ efficacy of sublingual nitrate tablets**	Additive effect; both drugs cause antimuscarinic side effects. **Antimuscarinic effects ↓ saliva production, which ↓ dissolution of the tablet**	Warn patients of this additive effect. **Consider using sublingual nitrate spray**

(*Continued*)

Primary Drug	Secondary Drug	Effect	Mechanism	Precautions
SKELETAL MUSCLE RELAXANTS				
BACLOFEN	**ADDITIVE HYPOTENSIVE EFFECTS**			
BACLOFEN	ALCOHOL	↑ Sedation	Additive effect	Warn patients; advise them to drink alcohol only in moderation and not to drive if they have drunk any alcohol and are taking these muscle relaxants
BACLOFEN	**ANALGESICS**			
BACLOFEN	NSAIDs	↑ Baclofen levels with ibuprofen	↓ Renal excretion of baclofen	Avoid coadministration
BACLOFEN	PARACETAMOL	Baclofen may slow the onset of action of intermittent-dose paracetamol	Anticholinergic effects delay gastric emptying and absorption	Warn patients that the action of paracetamol may be delayed. This will not be the case when paracetamol is taken regularly
BACLOFEN	ANESTHETICS—GENERAL	↑ Hypotensive effect	Additive hypotensive effect	Be aware; monitor BP closely
BACLOFEN	ANTICANCER AND IMMUNOMODULATING DRUGS—IL-2	↑ Hypotensive effect	Additive hypotensive effect	Monitor BP at least weekly until stable. Warn patients to report symptoms of hypotension (light-headedness, dizziness on standing, etc.)
BACLOFEN	**ANTIDEPRESSANTS**			
BACLOFEN	LITHIUM	Enhancement of hyperkinesias associated with lithium	Uncertain	Consider alternative skeletal muscle relaxant
BACLOFEN	MAOIs	↑ Hypotensive effect	Additive hypotensive effect	Monitor BP at least weekly until stable. Warn patients to report symptoms of hypotension (light-headedness, dizziness on standing, etc.)
BACLOFEN	ANTIDIABETIC DRUGS	↓ Hypoglycemic effect	Due to these drugs causing hyperglycemia, the mechanism being uncertain at present	↑ Doses of antidiabetic drugs are often required for adequate glycemic control

(*Continued*)

Primary Drug	Secondary Drug	Effect	Mechanism	Precautions
SKELETAL MUSCLE RELAXANTS				
BACLOFEN	ANTIHYPERTENSIVES AND HEART FAILURE DRUGS	↑ Hypotensive effect	Additive hypotensive effect	Monitor BP at least weekly until stable. Warn patients to report symptoms of hypotension (light-headedness, dizziness on standing, etc.)
BACLOFEN	ANTI-PARKINSON'S DRUGS—LEVODOPA	Reports of CNS agitation and ↓ efficacy of levodopa	Uncertain	Avoid coadministration
BACLOFEN	ANTIPSYCHOTICS	↑ Hypotensive effect	Additive hypotensive effect	Monitor BP at least weekly until stable. Warn patients to report symptoms of hypotension (light-headedness, dizziness on standing, etc.)
BACLOFEN	ANXIOLYTICS AND HYPNOTICS	1. ↑ Sedation 2. ↑ Hypotensive effect	1. Additive effect 2. Additive hypotensive effect	1. Warn patients; advise them to drink alcohol only in moderation and not to drive if they have drunk any alcohol and are taking these muscle relaxants 2. Monitor BP at least weekly until stable. Warn patients to report symptoms of hypotension (light-headedness, dizziness on standing, etc.)
BACLOFEN	BETA-BLOCKERS	↑ Hypotensive effect	Additive hypotensive effect	Monitor BP at least weekly until stable. Warn patients to report symptoms of hypotension (light-headedness, dizziness on standing, etc.)
BACLOFEN	CALCIUM CHANNEL BLOCKERS	↑ Hypotensive effect	Additive hypotensive effect	Monitor BP at least weekly until stable. Warn patients to report symptoms of hypotension (light-headedness, dizziness on standing, etc.)
BACLOFEN	DIURETICS—LOOP, THIAZIDES	↑ Hypotensive effect	Additive hypotensive effect	Monitor BP at least weekly until stable. Warn patients to report symptoms of hypotension (light-headedness, dizziness on standing, etc.)

(Continued)

Primary Drug	Secondary Drug	Effect	Mechanism	Precautions
SKELETAL MUSCLE RELAXANTS				
BACLOFEN	NITRATES	↑ Hypotensive effect	Additive hypotensive effect	Monitor BP at least weekly until stable. Warn patients to report symptoms of hypotension (light-headedness, dizziness on standing, etc.)
BACLOFEN	PERIPHERAL VASODILATORS—MOXISYLYTE (THYMOXAMINE)	↑ Hypotensive effect	Additive hypotensive effect	Monitor BP at least weekly until stable. Warn patients to report symptoms of hypotension (light-headedness, dizziness on standing, etc.)
BACLOFEN	POTASSIUM CHANNEL ACTIVATORS	↑ Hypotensive effect	Additive effect	Monitor BP closely
CARISOPRODOL				
CARISOPRODOL	CNS STIMULANTS—MODAFINIL	May cause moderate ↑ in carisoprodol levels	Modafinil is a reversible inhibitor of CYP2C19 when used in therapeutic doses	Be aware
CHLORZOXAZONE				
CHLORZOXAZONE	ANTIBIOTICS—ISONIAZID	↑ Chlorzoxazone levels	Inhibition of CYP2E1-mediated metabolism of chlorzoxazone	Warn patients to report side effects of chlorzoxazone (drowsiness, headache)
CHLORZOXAZONE	DRUG DEPENDENCE THERAPIES—DISULFIRAM	↑ Chlorzoxazone levels	Inhibition of CYP2E1-mediated metabolism of chlorzoxazone	Warn patients to report side effects of chlorzoxazone (drowsiness, headache).
CYCLOBENZAPRINE				
CYCLOBENZAPRINE	**ANTIDEPRESSANTS**			
CYCLOBENZAPRINE	MAOIs	↑ Risk of serotonin syndrome and of adrenergic syndrome ➢ ***For signs and symptoms of serotonin toxicity, see clinical features of some adverse drug interactions, serotonin toxicity, and serotonin syndrome***	Cyclobenzaprine is structurally similar to tricyclic antidepressants. TCAs are believed to act also by inhibiting the reuptake of serotonin and norepinephrine, increasing the risk of serotonin and adrenergic syndromes	Avoid coadministration

(Continued)

Primary Drug	Secondary Drug	Effect	Mechanism	Precautions
SKELETAL MUSCLE RELAXANTS				
CYCLOBENZAPRINE	SNRIs, SSRIs	↑ Risk of serotonin syndrome ➢ ***For signs and symptoms of serotonin toxicity, see clinical features of some adverse drug interactions, serotonin toxicity, and serotonin syndrome***	Additive effect. Cyclobenzaprine is structurally similar to tricyclic antidepressants. TCAs block uptake reuptake of serotonin	Caution with coadministration Specialist advice should be sought and alternatives considered
CYCLOBENZAPRINE	TCAs, including Trazodone	↑ Risk of serotonin syndrome and of adrenergic syndrome	Cyclobenzaprine is structurally similar to tricyclic antidepressants and may have an additive effect	Avoid coadministration
DANTROLENE				
DANTROLENE	ANTIEMETICS—METOCLOPRAMIDE	Possibly ↑ dantrolene levels	Uncertain	Be aware; monitor BP and LFTs closely
DANTROLENE	CALCIUM CHANNEL BLOCKERS	Risk of arrhythmias when diltiazem is given with intravenous dantrolene. Risk of ↓ BP, myocardial depression, and hyperkalemia when verapamil is given with intravenous dantrolene	Uncertain at present	Extreme caution must be exercised when administering parenteral dantrolene to patients on diltiazem or verapamil. Monitor BP and cardiac rhythm closely; watch for hyperkalemia
METHOCARBAMOL				
METHOCARBAMOL	ALCOHOL	↑ Sedation	Additive effect	Warn patients; advise them to drink alcohol only in moderation and not to drive if they have drunk any alcohol and are taking these muscle relaxants
METHOCARBAMOL	ANXIOLYTICS AND HYPNOTICS	↑ Sedation	Additive effect	Warn patients; advise them to drink alcohol only in moderation and not to drive if they have drunk any alcohol and are taking these muscle relaxants

(*Continued*)

Primary Drug	Secondary Drug	Effect	Mechanism	Precautions
SKELETAL MUSCLE RELAXANTS				
TIZANIDINE				
TIZANIDINE	ALCOHOL	↑ Sedation	Additive effect	Warn patients; advise them to drink alcohol only in moderation and not to drive if they have drunk any alcohol and are taking these muscle relaxants
TIZANIDINE	ANESTHETICS—GENERAL	↑ Hypotensive effect	Additive hypotensive effect	Be aware; monitor BP closely
TIZANIDINE	ANTIBIOTICS—CIPROFLOXACIN	↑ Tizanidine levels	Tizanidine is a substrate for CYP1A2; ciprofloxacin is a potent inhibitor of CYP1A2 and is thought to inhibit presystemic metabolism of tizanidine, resulting in ↑ absorption and ↑ levels	Avoid coadministration
TIZANIDINE	ANTICANCER AND IMMUNOMODULATING DRUGS—IL-2	↑ Hypotensive effect	Additive hypotensive effect	Monitor BP at least weekly until stable. Warn patients to report symptoms of hypotension (light-headedness, dizziness on standing, etc.)
TIZANIDINE	ANTIDEPRESSANTS—MAOIs	↑ Hypotensive effect	Additive hypotensive effect	Monitor BP at least weekly until stable. Warn patients to report symptoms of hypotension (light-headedness, dizziness on standing, etc.)
TIZANIDINE	**ANTIHYPERTENSIVES AND HEART FAILURE DRUGS**			
TIZANIDINE	ANTIHYPERTENSIVES AND HEART FAILURE DRUGS	↑ Hypotensive effect	Additive hypotensive effect	Monitor BP at least weekly until stable. Warn patients to report symptoms of hypotension (light-headedness, dizziness on standing, etc.)
TIZANIDINE	CLONIDINE	Theoretical risk of marked hypotension	Additive effect—tizanidine is structurally related to clonidine	Manufacturers recommend avoiding coadministration

(Continued)

Primary Drug	Secondary Drug	Effect	Mechanism	Precautions
SKELETAL MUSCLE RELAXANTS				
TIZANIDINE	ANTI-PSYCHOTICS	↑ Hypotensive effect	Additive hypotensive effect	Monitor BP at least weekly until stable. Warn patients to report symptoms of hypotension (light-headedness, dizziness on standing, etc.)
TIZANIDINE	ANXIOLYTICS AND HYPNOTICS	1. ↑ Sedation 2. ↑ Hypotensive effect	1. Additive effect 2. Additive hypotensive effect	1. Warn patients; advise them to drink alcohol only in moderation and not to drive if they have drunk any alcohol and are taking these muscle relaxants 2. Monitor BP at least weekly until stable. Warn patients to report symptoms of hypotension (light-headedness, dizziness on standing, etc.)
TIZANIDINE	BETA-BLOCKERS	↑ Hypotensive effect	Additive hypotensive effect. Tizanidine also has a negative chronotropic effect and may cause additive bradycardia with beta-blockers	Monitor BP at least weekly until stable. Warn patients to report symptoms of hypotension (light-headedness, dizziness on standing, etc.)
TIZANIDINE	CALCIUM CHANNEL BLOCKERS	↑ Hypotensive effect	Additive hypotensive effect. Tizanidine also has a negative chronotropic effect and may cause additive bradycardia with calcium channel blockers	Monitor BP at least weekly until stable. Warn patients to report symptoms of hypotension (light-headedness, dizziness on standing, etc.)
TIZANIDINE	CARDIAC GLYCOSIDES—DIGOXIN	Risk of bradycardia when tizanidine is given with digoxin	Tizanidine has a negative inotropic effect	Monitor PR closely
TIZANIDINE	CNS STIMULANTS—MODAFINIL	Possibly ↓ tizanidine levels	Modafinil is moderate inducer of CYP1A2 in a concentration-dependent manner	Be aware. Watch for poor response to tizanidine
TIZANIDINE	DIURETICS—LOOP, THIAZIDES	↑ Hypotensive effect	Additive hypotensive effect	Monitor BP at least weekly until stable. Warn patients to report symptoms of hypotension (light-headedness, dizziness on standing, etc.)

(Continued)

Primary Drug	Secondary Drug	Effect	Mechanism	Precautions
SKELETAL MUSCLE RELAXANTS				
TIZANIDINE	NITRATES	↑ Hypotensive effect	Additive hypotensive effect	Monitor BP at least weekly until stable. Warn patients to report symptoms of hypotension (light-headedness, dizziness on standing, etc.)
TIZANIDINE	PERIPHERAL VASODILATORS—MOXISYLYTE (THYMOXAMINE)	↑ Hypotensive effect	Additive hypotensive effect	Monitor BP at least weekly until stable. Warn patients to report symptoms of hypotension (light-headedness, dizziness on standing, etc.)
TIZANIDINE	POTASSIUM CHANNEL ACTIVATORS	↑ Hypotensive effect	Additive hypotensive effect	Monitor BP at least weekly until stable. Warn patients to report symptoms of hypotension (light-headedness, dizziness on standing, etc.)

PART 9

Anesthetic Drugs

Vasanthi Pinto and E. Queenie Veerasingham

1. ANESTHETICS—General
2. ANESTHETICS—Local
3. ANTICHOLINESTERASES ➢ *Drugs Acting on the Nervous System, Drugs used to Treat Neuromuscular Diseases and Movement Disorders*
4. ANTIMUSCARINICS ➢ *Drugs Acting on the Nervous System, Anti-Parkinson's Drugs*
5. BENZODIAZEPINES ➢ *Drugs Acting on the Nervous System, Anxiolytics and Hypnotics*
6. DANTROLENE ➢ *Musculoskeletal Drugs, Skeletal Muscle Relaxants*
7. MUSCLE RELAXANTS—Depolarizing
8. MUSCLE RELAXANTS—Nondepolarizings
9. OPIOIDS ➢ *Analgesics, Opioids*

Primary Drug	Secondary Drug	Effect	Mechanism	Precautions
ANESTHETICS—GENERAL				
INHALATIONAL ANESTHETICS	ANTIARRHYTHMICS—AMIODARONE	Amiodarone may ↑ myocardial depressant effects of inhalational anesthetics	Additive effect	Monitor PR, BP, and ECG closely
ANESTHETICS—GENERAL	**ANTIBIOTICS**			
INHALATIONAL ANESTHETICS, e.g., HALOTHANE, ISOFLURANE, SEVOFLURANE	AMINOGLYCOSIDES	↑ Potential for nephrotoxicity	Attributed to fluoride production having an additive nephrotoxic effect on aminoglycosides	Monitor renal function postoperatively
INTRAVENOUS—THIOPENTONE	SULFONAMIDES	↑ Effect of thiopentone but ↓ duration of action	Uncertain; possibly displacement from protein-binding sites	Be aware that ↓ dose may be needed
ANESTHETICS—GENERAL	**ANTICANCER AND IMMUNOMODULATING DRUGS**			
HALOTHANE	ARSENIC TRIOXIDE	Risk of arrhythmias especially TdP	Arsenic trioxide may cause QT prolongation on its own but risk ↑ with halothane	Use an alternative inhalational anesthetic
INHALATIONAL ANESTHETICS	DAUNORUBICIN, DOXORUBICIN, IDARUBICIN	Risk of arrhythmias	Previous treatment with anthracyclines may enhance the myocardial depressive effect	Prevent hypotensive episodes and carbon dioxide retention (hypercapnia)
INHALATIONAL—ISOFLURANE	EPIRUBICIN	QT interval prolongation	Additive	Be aware of interaction
NITROUS OXIDE	METHOTREXATE	↑ Antifolate effect of methotrexate	↑ Toxicity of methotrexate	Nitrous oxide is usually used for relatively brief durations when patients are anesthetized, and hence this risk during anesthesia is minimal. However, nitrous oxide may be used for analgesia for longer durations, and this should be avoided

(Continued)

Primary Drug	Secondary Drug	Effect	Mechanism	Precautions
ANESTHETICS—GENERAL				
ANESTHETICS—GENERAL	**ANTIDEPRESSANTS**			
ANESTHETICS—GENERAL	LITHIUM	1. Risk of hemodynamic instability and a range of arrhythmias 2. ↓ Anesthetic requirements 3. Risk of lithium toxicity	1. Due to impaired renal excretion and interference with sodium and potassium levels 2. Sedative effect of lithium ↓ anesthetic requirements 3. Sodium depletion ↓ renal excretion of lithium and can lead to lithium toxicity	Discontinue lithium 72 h before surgery. The only reason not to stop lithium is minor surgery under local anesthesia. Lithium can be stopped abruptly because no withdrawal symptoms occur To prevent significant renal absorption of lithium, administer sodium-based intravenous fluids during the perioperative period Lithium should be restarted, with monitoring of blood levels within 1 week. This is most important because the psychiatric risk of recurrence or relapse is hazardous
ANESTHETICS—GENERAL	MAOIs	Some cases of both ↑ and ↓ BP on induction of anesthesia. Mostly no significant changes	Uncertain; may cause hypotensive effects	Some recommend stopping MAOIs 2 weeks before surgery. Others suggest no need for this; monitor BP closely, especially during induction of anesthesia
ANESTHETICS—GENERAL (BALANCED ANESTHESIA) SUPPLEMENTED BY OPIOIDS, MUSCLE RELAXANTS, SYMPATHOMIMETICS	MAOIs	1. General anesthetics: • ↓ Dose requirements of thiopentone • Risk of hypertensive crises with ketamine 2. Muscle relaxants: • Phenelzine prolongs the action of suxamethonium • Risk of hypertensive crises with pancuronium	1. General anesthetics: • MAOIs may cause a reduction in hepatic metabolism of barbiturates • Ketamine causes sympathetic stimulation • Benzodiazepines, inhalational anesthetic agents, anticholinergic drugs, and nonsteroidal anti-inflammatory drugs can be used safely in patients taking MAOIs	The decision to stop MAOI therapy preoperatively for elective surgery should be made in advance on an individual basis after discussion between the anesthesiologist, psychiatric team, and patient. Although continuation of MAOIs carries risks, by careful anesthetic technique, these risks can be minimized and must be balanced against the risks of relapse and discontinuation syndrome

(*Continued*)

Primary Drug	Secondary Drug	Effect	Mechanism	Precautions
ANESTHETICS—GENERAL				
		3. Opioids: • Additive depression of CNS ranging from drowsiness to coma and respiratory depression • Risk of serotonin syndrome with dextromethorphan, pethidine, phenoperidine, or tramadol 4. Sympathomimetics: • Risk of adrenergic syndrome • Unlikely to occur with moclobemide and selegiline	2. Muscle relaxants: • Phenelzine decreases plasma cholinesterase concentration • Pancuronium releases stored noradrenaline 3. Opioids: • Synergistic depressant effects on CNS function; in addition, MAOIs inhibit metabolism of opioids especially morphine • Additive effect: dextromethorphan, pethidine, phenoperidine, or tramadol inhibits serotonin reuptake 4. Sympathomimetics: • Due to inhibition of MAOI, which breaks down sympathomimetics • Moclobemide is involved in the breakdown of serotonin, while selegiline is mainly involved in the breakdown of dopamine	If MAOIs are continued, consider the following: 1. General anesthetics: • Be aware—reduce dose of thiopentone, or use an alternative induction agent • Ketamine should be avoided as it causes sympathetic stimulation. Local anesthetics containing adrenaline should be used with caution 2. Muscle relaxants: • Be aware of the potential for prolonged relaxation with suxamethonium • Pancuronium should be avoided 3. Opioids: • Avoid coadministration of MAOIs with dextromethorphan, pethidine, phenoperidine or tramadol for at least 2 weeks after cessation of MAOI • Other opioids are safe 4. Indirect-acting sympathomimetics are absolutely contraindicated with any MAOIs. Titrate doses of direct-acting sympathomimetics

(Continued)

ANESTHETIC DRUGS ANESTHETICS—GENERAL

Primary Drug	Secondary Drug	Effect	Mechanism	Precautions
ANESTHETICS—GENERAL				
ANESTHETICS—GENERAL	TCAs	1. ↑ Availability of neurotransmitters in the CNS can result in ↑ anesthetic requirements 2. TCAs may result in ↑ response to intraoperatively administered anticholinergics and those that cross the blood–brain barrier, such as atropine 3. May cause postoperative confusion 4. Exaggerated BP responses following administration of indirect-acting vasopressors such as ephedrine 5. Chronic therapy depletes cardiac catecholamines, potentiating the cardiac depressant effects of anesthetic agents	Given chronically, TCAs 1. ↓ Stores of noradrenergic catecholamines 2. Cause changes on the ECG (changes in the T wave, widening of the QRS complex, and prolongation of QT interval; bundle branch block or other conduction abnormalities, or PVCs) 3. Predispose to ventricular arrhythmias 4. Refractory hypotension may occur in higher doses 5. Exaggerated responses to vasopressors due to ↑ availability of norepinephrine at the post-synaptic nervous system	The most important interaction between anesthetic agents and tricyclic antidepressant drugs is an exaggerated response to both indirect-acting vasopressors and sympathetic stimulation Pancuronium-, ketamine-, meperidine-, and epinephrine-containing solutions should be avoided Avoid use of vasopressors—necessary to maintain BP with accurate replacement of blood or fluids During anesthesia and surgery, it is important to avoid stimulating the sympathetic nervous system. If hypotension occurs and vasopressors are needed, direct-acting drugs such as phenylephrine are recommended. The dose should probably be decreased to minimize the likelihood of an exaggerated hypertensive response
ANESTHETICS—GENERAL	SSRIs, SNRIs	No interactions with general anesthetics Note when considering balanced anesthesia, there is a risk of serotonin syndrome when dextromethorphan, pethidine, phenoperidine or tramadol is used with patients taking SSRIs/SNRIs	Additive effect: these opioids inhibit serotonin uptake	SSRIs should be continued throughout the perioperative period to prevent discontinuation syndrome Avoid the use of dextromethorphan, pethidine, phenoperidine or tramadol

(*Continued*)

ANESTHETIC DRUGS ANESTHETICS—GENERAL

Primary Drug	Secondary Drug	Effect	Mechanism	Precautions
ANESTHETICS—GENERAL				
INTRAVENOUS—KETAMINE	ANTIDEMENTIA DRUGS—MEMANTINE	↑ CNS side effects	Additive effects on NMDA receptors	Avoid coadministration
INTRAVENOUS ANESTHETICS	ANTIHYPERTENSIVES AND HEART FAILURE DRUGS	Risk of severe hypotensive episodes during induction of anesthesia	Most general anesthetics are myocardial depressants and vasodilators. Additive hypotensive effect	Monitor BP closely, especially during induction of anesthesia
INHALATIONAL AGENTS	ANTI-PARKINSON'S DRUGS—LEVODOPA	Possible risk of arrhythmias	Uncertain	Monitor ECG and BP closely. Consider using intravenous agents for maintenance of anesthesia
INTRAVENOUS—THIOPENTONE	ANTIPLATELET AGENTS—ASPIRIN	↓ Requirements of thiopentone when aspirin (1 g) used during premedication	Uncertain at present	Be aware of possible ↓ dose requirements for thiopentone
ANESTHETICS—GENERAL	ANTIPSYCHOTICS	Risk of hypotension	Additive effect	Monitor BP closely, especially during induction of anesthesia
INTRAVENOUS ANESTHETICS (e.g., THIOPENTONE SODIUM, PROPOFOL)	BETA-BLOCKERS	Risk of severe hypotensive episodes during induction of anesthesia (including patients taking timolol eye drops)	Most intravenous anesthetic agents are myocardial depressants and vasodilators, and additive ↓ BP may occur	Monitor BP closely, especially during induction of anesthesia
ANESTHETICS—GENERAL	**BRONCHODILATORS**			
INHALATIONAL—HALOTHANE	TERBUTALINE, THEOPHYLLINE	Cases of arrhythmias when these bronchodilators are coadministered with halothane	Possibly due to sensitization of the myocardium to circulating catecholamines by the volatile anesthetics to varying degrees	Risk of cardiac events is higher with halothane. Desflurane is irritant to the upper respiratory tract, and ↑ secretions can occur and are best avoided in patients with bronchial asthma. Sevoflurane is nonirritant and unlikely to cause serious adverse effects

(*Continued*)

ANESTHETIC DRUGS ANESTHETICS—GENERAL

Primary Drug	Secondary Drug	Effect	Mechanism	Precautions
ANESTHETICS—GENERAL				
INTRAVENOUS—KETAMINE	THEOPHYLLINE	Risk of fits	Uncertain	A careful risk–benefit assessment should be made before using ketamine. However, there are significant benefits for the use of ketamine to anesthetize patients for emergency management of life-threatening asthma
INHALATIONAL ANESTHETICS	CALCIUM CHANNEL BLOCKERS	↑ Hypotensive effects of dihydropyridines and hypotensive/bradycardic effects of diltiazem and verapamil	Additive hypotensive and negative inotropic effects. General anesthetics tend to be myocardial depressants and vasodilators; they also ↓ sinus automaticity and AV conduction	Monitor BP and ECG closely
INHALATIONAL AND INTRAVENOUS ANESTHETICS	DIURETICS	↑ Hypotensive effect	Additive effect as the anesthetics cause varying degrees of myocardial depression and/or vasodilatation, while diuretics tend to ↓ circulatory volume	Monitor BP closely, especially during induction of anesthesia
HALOTHANE	ERGOT DERIVATIVES	↓ Efficacy of ergometrine on uterus	Halothane ↓ muscle tone of the pregnant uterus; generally, its use in obstetric anesthesia is not recommended as it ↑ risk of postpartum hemorrhage, for which ergot derivatives are commonly used	Use alternative form of anesthesia for surgery requiring use of ergotamine
ANESTHETICS—GENERAL	**MUSCLE RELAXANTS**			
ANESTHETICS—GENERAL	MUSCLE RELAXANTS—BACLOFEN, TIZANIDINE	↑ Hypotensive effect	Additive hypotensive effect. Tizanidine also has a negative chronotropic effect and may cause additive bradycardia with beta-blockers and calcium channel blockers	Monitor BP closely, especially during induction of anesthesia

(*Continued*)

Primary Drug	Secondary Drug	Effect	Mechanism	Precautions
ANESTHETICS—GENERAL				
ANESTHETICS—ISOFLURANE AND ENFLURANE	NONDEPOLARIZING—MIVACURIUM	The neuromuscular blocking action of mivacurium chloride is potentiated; the ED50 of mivacurium is reduced by as much as 25%. The clinically effective duration of action is prolonged and the average infusion requirement of mivacurium is ↓ by as much as 35%–40%	A greater potentiation of the neuromuscular blocking effects is expected with higher concentrations of enflurane or isoflurane. Halothane has little or no effect on the ED50, but may prolong the duration of action and ↓ the average infusion requirement by as much as 20%	Monitoring neuromuscular blockade carefully
ANESTHETICS—GENERAL	NITRATES	↑ Hypotensive effect	Additive effect (vasodilatation and/or depression of myocardial contractility)	Monitor BP closely, especially during induction of anesthesia
INHALATIONAL—HALOTHANE	OXYTOCICS	Report of arrhythmias and cardiovascular collapse when halothane was given to patients taking oxytocin	Uncertain; possibly additive effect. High-dose oxytocin may cause hypotension and arrhythmias	Monitor PR, BP, and ECG closely; give oxytocin in the lowest possible dose. Otherwise, consider using an alternative inhalational anesthetic
ANESTHETICS—GENERAL	PERIPHERAL VASODILATORS—MOXISYLYTE	↑ Hypotensive effect	Additive effect	Monitor BP closely, especially during induction of anesthesia
ANESTHETICS—GENERAL	POTASSIUM CHANNEL ACTIVATORS	↑ Hypotensive effect	Additive effect	Monitor BP closely
ANESTHETICS—GENERAL	**SYMPATHOMIMETICS**			
ANESTHETICS—GENERAL	DIRECT-ACTING SYMPATHOMIMETICS (e.g., EPINEPHRINE)	1. Risk of arrhythmias when inhalational anesthetics are coadministered with epinephrine or norepinephrine 2. Case report of marked ↑ BP when phenylephrine eye drops were given during general anesthesia	1. The arrhythmogenic threshold with injected epinephrine is lower with halothane than isoflurane or enflurane, which is attributed to sensitization to beta-adrenoceptor stimulation 2. Uncertain. Phenylephrine produces its effects by acting on alpha-adrenergic receptors; possible that these effects are enhanced	1. Use epinephrine in the smallest possible dose (when using 1:100,000 = 10 μg/mL infiltration to ↓ intraoperative bleeding, no more than 10 mL/10 min and less than 30 mL/h should be given). Prevent carbon dioxide retention during anesthesia as carbon dioxide increases sensitizing effect 2. Avoid use of phenylephrine eye drops during anesthesia

(*Continued*)

ANESTHETIC DRUGS ANESTHETICS—GENERAL

Primary Drug	Secondary Drug	Effect	Mechanism	Precautions
ANESTHETICS—GENERAL				
ANESTHETICS—GENERAL	INDIRECT-ACTING SYMPATHOMIMETICS (e.g., METHYLPHENIDATE)	1. Risk of arrhythmias when inhalational anesthetics are coadministered with methylphenidate 2. Case report of ↓ sedative effect of midazolam and ketamine by methylphenidate	1. Uncertain; attributed by some to sensitization of the myocardium to sympathomimetics by inhalational anesthetics 2. Uncertain at present; possibly due to CNS stimulation caused by methylphenidate (hence its use in narcolepsy)	Avoid giving methylphenidate on the day of elective surgery
INTRAVENOUS—KETAMINE	THYROID HORMONES	Case reports of tachycardia and hypertension when ketamine was given to patients on thyroxine; treatment with propanolol	Uncertain	Monitor PR and BP closely

Primary Drug	Secondary Drug	Effect	Mechanism	Precautions
ANESTHETICS—LOCAL				
PHARMACEUTICAL INTERACTIONS				
LIDOCAINE SOLUTIONS	AMPHOTERICIN, AMPICILLIN, PHENYTOIN, SULFADIAZINE	Precipitation of drugs, which may not be immediately apparent	A pharmaceutical interaction	Do not mix in the same infusion or syringe
PROCAINE SOLUTIONS	AMINOPHYLLINE, AMPHOTERICIN, BARBITURATES, MAGNESIUM SULFATE, PHENYTOIN, SODIUM BICARBONATE	Precipitation of drugs, which may not be immediately apparent	A pharmaceutical interaction	Do not mix in the same infusion or syringe
PROCAINE SOLUTIONS	CALCIUM-, MAGNESIUM-, AND SODIUM SALT–CONTAINING SOLUTIONS	A temperature-dependent incompatibility that causes a physicochemical reaction	A pharmaceutical interaction	Do not mix in the same infusion or syringe

(*Continued*)

Primary Drug	Secondary Drug	Effect	Mechanism	Precautions
ANESTHETICS—LOCAL				
OTHER INTERACTIONS				
ANESTHETICS—LOCAL	**ANTIARRHYTHMICS**			
ANESTHETICS—LOCAL	ADENOSINE	↑ Myocardial depression	Additive effect; local anesthetics and adenosine are myocardial depressants	Monitor PR, BP, and ECG closely
ANESTHETICS—LOCAL	AMIODARONE, DISOPYRAMIDE, FLECAINIDE, MEXILETINE, PROCAINAMIDE, PROPAFENONE	Risk of ↓ BP	Additive myocardial depression	Particular care should be taken to avoid inadvertent intravenous administration during bupivacaine infiltration; monitor PR, BP, and ECG during epidural administration of bupivacaine
LIDOCAINE	MEXILETINE	Mexiletine ↑ lidocaine levels (with cases of toxicity when lidocaine is given intravenously)	Mexiletine displaces lidocaine from its tissue binding sites; it also seems to ↓ its clearance, but the exact mechanism is uncertain at present	Watch for the early symptoms/signs of lidocaine toxicity (perioral paresthesia)
LIDOCAINE	PROCAINAMIDE	Case report of neurotoxicity when intravenous lidocaine administered with procainamide. No significant interaction expected when lidocaine is used for local anesthetic infiltration	Likely to be an additive effect; both may cause neurotoxicity in overdose	Care should be taken when administering lidocaine as an infusion for patients taking procainamide
ANESTHETICS—LOCAL	**ANTIBIOTICS**			
LIDOCAINE	QUINUPRISTIN/DALFOPRISTIN	Risk of arrhythmias	Additive effect when lidocaine given intravenously	Avoid coadministration of quinupristin/dalfopristin with intravenous lidocaine
PRILOCAINE	SULFONAMIDES	Risk of methemoglobinemia; a case report of methemoglobinemia with topical prilocaine in a patient taking sulfonamides	Additive effect	Avoid coadministration

(Continued)

Primary Drug	Secondary Drug	Effect	Mechanism	Precautions
ANESTHETICS—LOCAL				
ANESTHETICS—LOCAL	**ANTICANCER AND IMMUNOMODULATING DRUGS**			
LOCAL ANESTHETICS WITH EPINEPHRINE	PROCARBAZINE	Risk of severe hypertension	Due to inhibition of MAO, which metabolizes epinephrine	
SPINAL ANESTHETICS	PROCARBAZINE	Risk of hypotensive episodes	Uncertain	Recommendation is to discontinue procarbazine for at least 10 days before elective spinal anesthesia
ROPIVACAINE	ANTIDEPRESSANTS—FLUVOXAMINE	↑ Plasma concentrations and prolonged effects of ropivacaine, a local anesthetic related to bupivacaine but less potent and cardiotoxic than bupivacaine. Adverse effects include nausea, vomiting, tachycardia, headache, and rigors	Fluvoxamine inhibits metabolism of ropivacaine	Be aware of the possibility of prolonged effects and of toxicity. Take note of any numbness or tingling around the lips and mouth or slurring of speech after administration as they may be warning signs of more severe toxic effects such as seizures or loss of consciousness
ANESTHETICS—LOCAL	**ANTIHYPERTENSIVES AND HEART FAILURE DRUGS**			
ANESTHETICS—LOCAL	ACE INHIBITORS	Risk of profound ↓ BP with epidural bupivacaine in patients on captopril	Additive hypotensive effect; epidural bupivacaine causes vasodilatation in the lower limbs	Monitor BP closely. Ensure that the patient is preloaded with fluids
ANESTHETICS—LOCAL	ADRENERGIC NEURON BLOCKERS—GUANETHIDINE	↓ Clinical efficacy of guanethidine when used in the treatment of complex regional pain syndrome type I	The local anesthetic ↓ reuptake of guanethidine	Be aware. Consider use of a local anesthetic that minimally inhibits reuptake, e.g., lidocaine, when possible
ANESTHETICS—LOCAL, SYSTEMIC LIDOCAINE	ANTIVIRAL DRUGS (PROTEASE INHIBITORS), ATAZANAVIR/RITONAVIR, DARUNAVIR, FOSAMPRENAVIR/RITONAVIR, LOPINAVIR/RITONAVIR, SAQUINAVIR/RITONAVIR	Lidocaine levels may be ↑ with risk of ventricular arrhythmias	Uncertain but postulated to be due to ↓ metabolism via CYP3A	Avoid combination with saquinavir/ritonavir. For others, use with caution, watch closely for lidocaine toxicity, and monitor lidocaine levels. Consider ↓ initial lidocaine dose and titrate more slowly

(*Continued*)

Primary Drug	Secondary Drug	Effect	Mechanism	Precautions
ANESTHETICS—LOCAL				
ANESTHETICS—LOCAL	**BETA-BLOCKERS**			
↑ BP is likely when epinephrine-containing local anesthetics are used in patients on treatment with beta-adrenergic blockers **Remember that ↑ BP can occur when epinephrine-containing local anesthetics are used with patients on beta-blockers** **➢ *Sympathomimetics, as follows***				
BUPIVACAINE	BETA-BLOCKERS	Risk of bupivacaine toxicity	Beta-blockers, particularly propranolol, inhibit the hepatic microsomal metabolism of bupivacaine	Watch for bupivacaine toxicity—monitor ECG and BP
LIDOCAINE	BETA-BLOCKERS	1. Risk of bradycardia (occasionally severe), ↓ BP, and heart failure with intravenous lidocaine 2. Risk of lidocaine toxicity due to ↑ plasma concentrations of lidocaine, particularly with propranolol and nadolol 3. ↑ Plasma concentrations of propranolol and possibly some other beta-blockers	1. Additive negative inotropic and chronotropic effects 2. Uncertain, but possibly a combination of beta-blocker-induced ↓ hepatic blood flow (due to ↓ cardiac output) and inhibition of metabolism of lidocaine 3. Attributed to inhibition of metabolism by lidocaine	1. Monitor PR, BP, and ECG closely; watch for development of heart failure when intravenous lidocaine is administered to patients on beta-blockers 2. Watch for lidocaine toxicity 3. Be aware. Regional anesthetics should be used cautiously in patients with bradycardia. Beta-blockers could cause dangerous hypertension due to stimulation of alpha receptors if adrenaline is used with local anesthetic
ANESTHETICS—LOCAL	CALCIUM CHANNEL BLOCKERS	Case reports of severe ↓ BP when a bupivacaine epidural was administered to patients on calcium channel blockers	Additive hypotensive effect; both bupivacaine and calcium channel blockers are cardiodepressant. In addition, epidural anesthesia causes sympathetic block in the lower limbs, which leads to vasodilatation and ↓ BP	Monitor BP closely. Preload intravenous fluids prior to the epidural
ANESTHETICS—LOCAL, ROPIVACAINE	CNS STIMULANTS—MODAFINIL	May cause ↓ plasma concentrations of these substrates if CYP1A2 is the predominant metabolic pathway and alternative metabolic pathways are either genetically deficient or affected	Modafinil is moderate inducer of CYP1A2 in a concentration-dependent manner	Be aware

(Continued)

ANESTHETIC DRUGS ANTIMUSCARINICS

Primary Drug	Secondary Drug	Effect	Mechanism	Precautions
ANESTHETICS—LOCAL				
PROCAINE	ECOTHIOPATE	↑ Plasma concentrations and risk of unconsciousness and cardiovascular collapse with injections of prilocaine	Ecothiopate inhibits pseudocholinesterase, which metabolizes prilocaine	Do not coadminister. Use an alternative local anesthetic not subject to metabolism by pseudocholinesterases
LIDOCAINE	**H2-RECEPTOR BLOCKERS**			
LIDOCAINE	CIMETIDINE, RANITIDINE	↑ Efficacy and adverse effects of lidocaine and bupivacaine, e.g., light-headedness, paresthesia	Not fully established but likely to be reduced clearance and altered metabolism via CYP enzymes	Uncertain. Consider alternative acid suppression or monitor more closely, ↓ dose may be required. No toxicity reported to date with bupivacaine
ANESTHETICS—INTRAVENOUS, LIDOCAINE	CIMETIDINE	↑ Efficacy and adverse effects	Not fully established but likely to be reduced clearance and altered metabolism via CYP enzymes	Avoid coadministration, or if essential monitor closely for symptoms of toxicity, and check lidocaine levels
PROCAINE	LARONIDASE	Possibly ↓ efficacy of laronidase	Uncertain	Avoid coadministration
ANESTHETICS—LOCAL	**MUSCLE RELAXANTS**			
PROCAINE	DEPOLARIZING	Possibly ↑ plasma concentrations of both drugs, with risk of toxic effects	Due to competition for metabolism by pseudocholinesterase	Avoid coadministration
LIDOCAINE (INTRAVENOUS), COCAINE	DEPOLARIZING	↑ Efficacy of suxamethonium	Uncertain	Monitor neuromuscular blockade carefully

Primary Drug	Secondary Drug	Effect	Mechanism	Precautions
ANTICHOLINESTERASES ➢ *Drugs Acting on the Nervous System, Drugs Used to Treat Neuromuscular Diseases and Movement Disorders*				

Primary Drug	Secondary Drug	Effect	Mechanism	Precautions
ANTIMUSCARINICS ➢ *Drugs Acting on the Nervous System, Anti-Parkinson's Drugs*				

Primary Drug	Secondary Drug	Effect	Mechanism	Precautions
BENZODIAZEPINES ➢ *Drugs Acting on the Nervous System, Anxiolytics and Hypnotics*				

Primary Drug	Secondary Drug	Effect	Mechanism	Precautions
DANTROLENE ➢ *Musculoskeletal Drugs, Skeletal Muscle Relaxants*				

Primary Drug	Secondary Drug	Effect	Mechanism	Precautions
MUSCLE RELAXANTS—DEPOLARIZING				
SUXAMETHONIUM	**ANESTHETICS—LOCAL**			
SUXAMETHONIUM	LIDOCAINE (INTRAVENOUS), COCAINE	↑ Efficacy of suxamethonium	Uncertain	Monitor neuromuscular blockade carefully
SUXAMETHONIUM	PROCAINE	Possibly ↑ plasma concentrations of both drugs, with risk of toxic effects	Due to competition for metabolism by pseudocholinesterase	Avoid coadministration
SUXAMETHONIUM	ANTIARRHYTHMICS—PROCAINAMIDE, QUINIDINE	Possibility of ↑ neuromuscular blockade	Uncertain; procainamide may ↓ plasma cholinesterase levels	Be aware of the possibility of a prolonged effect of suxamethonium
SUXAMETHONIUM	**ANTIBIOTICS**			
SUXAMETHONIUM	AMINOGLYCOSIDES	↑ Neuromuscular block	Aminoglycosides ↓ release of ACh at neuromuscular junctions by altering the influx of calcium. It is also thought to alter the sensitivity of the postsynaptic receptors/membrane, with ↓ transmission. These effects are additive to those of nondepolarizing muscle relaxants/neuromuscular blockers, which essentially prevents ACh acting on postsynaptic nicotinic receptors	Monitor neuromuscular blockade closely. Aminoglycosides vary in their potency to block neuromuscular junctions, with neomycin having the highest potency, then streptomycin, gentamicin, and kanamycin

(Continued)

ANESTHETIC DRUGS MUSCLE RELAXANTS—DEPOLARIZING

Primary Drug	Secondary Drug	Effect	Mechanism	Precautions
MUSCLE RELAXANTS—DEPOLARIZING				
SUXAMETHONIUM	AZLOCILLIN, CLINDAMYCIN, COLISTIN, PIPERACILLIN	↑ Efficacy of muscle relaxants	Piperacillin has some neuromuscular blocking activity	Monitor neuromuscular blockade carefully
SUXAMETHONIUM	VANCOMYCIN	1. ↑ Efficacy of these muscle relaxants 2. Possible risk of hypersensitivity reactions	1. Vancomycin has some neuromuscular blocking activity 2. Animal studies suggest additive effect on histamine release	1. Monitor neuromuscular blockade carefully 2. Be aware
SUXAMETHONIUM	**ANTICANCER AND IMMUNOMODULATING DRUGS**			
SUXAMETHONIUM	CHLORMETHINE, CYCLOPHOSPHAMIDE, THIOTEPA, TRETAMINE	↑ Efficacy of suxamethonium	Uncertain; these drugs are likely to decrease plasma levels of pseudocholinesterase, enhancing the neuromuscular blockade	Caution with concurrent use. Reduce dosage or avoid suxamethonium
SUXAMETHONIUM	IRINOTECAN	Neuromuscular blocking effects may be prolonged	Irinotecan has anticholinesterase activity	Caution with concurrent use
SUXAMETHONIUM	ANTIEMETICS—METOCLOPRAMIDE	Possible ↑ efficacy of suxamethonium	Uncertain	Be aware and monitor effects of suxamethonium closely
SUXAMETHONIUM	BRONCHODILATORS—BAMBUTEROL	↑ Effect of suxamethonium	Bambuterol is an inhibitor of pseudocholinesterase, which hydrolyzes suxamethonium	Be cautious of prolonged periods of respiratory muscle paralysis, and monitor respiration closely until complete recovery
SUXAMETHONIUM	CALCIUM CHANNEL BLOCKERS	↑ Effect of suxamethonium with parenteral, but not oral, calcium channel blockers	Uncertain; postulated that ACh release at the synapse is calcium dependent. ↓ calcium concentrations at the nerve ending may ↓ ACh release, which in turn prolongs the nerve blockade	Monitor nerve blockade carefully particularly during short procedures
SUXAMETHONIUM	CARDIAC GLYCOSIDES—DIGOXIN	Risk of ventricular arrhythmias when suxamethonium is given to patients taking digoxin	Uncertain; postulated that the mechanism involves a rapid efflux of potassium from cells	Use caution, and monitor ECG closely if suxamethonium needs to be used in patients taking digoxin

(Continued)

Primary Drug	Secondary Drug	Effect	Mechanism	Precautions
MUSCLE RELAXANTS—DEPOLARIZING				
SUXAMETHONIUM	MAGNESIUM (PARENTERAL)	↑ Efficacy of these muscle relaxants, with risk of prolonged neuromuscular blockade	Additive effect; magnesium inhibits ACh release and ↓ postsynaptic receptor sensitivity	Monitor nerve blockade closely
SUXAMETHONIUM	PARASYMPATHOMIMETICS—DONEPEZIL	Possible ↑ efficacy of suxamethonium	Suxamethonium is metabolized by cholinesterase; parasympathomimetics inhibit cholinesterase and so prolong the action of suxamethonium	Avoid coadministration. Ensure that the effects of suxamethonium have worn off before administering a parasympathomimetic to reverse nondepolarizing muscle relaxants. A careful risk–benefit analysis should be made before considering the use of suxamethonium
SUXAMETHONIUM	PESTICIDES—ORGANOPHOSPHATE AND CARBAMATE	↑ and prolonged response to suxamethonium	↓ Pseudocholinesterase activity	Suxamethonium is best avoided in patients requiring anesthetics if they had been exposed to pesticides

Primary Drug	Secondary Drug	Effect	Mechanism	Precautions
MUSCLE RELAXANTS—NONDEPOLARIZINGS				
NONDEPOLARIZING—MIVACURIUM	ANESTHETICS—ISOFLURANE AND ENFLURANE	The neuromuscular blocking action of mivacurium chloride is potentiated; the ED50 of mivacurium is ↓ by as much as 25%. The clinically effective duration of action is prolonged, and the average infusion requirement of mivacurium is ↓ by as much as 35%–40%	A greater potentiation of the neuromuscular blocking effects is expected with higher concentrations of enflurane or isoflurane. Halothane has little or no effect on the ED50, but may prolong the duration of action and ↓ the average infusion requirement by as much as 20%	Monitoring neuromuscular blockade carefully

(Continued)

Primary Drug	Secondary Drug	Effect	Mechanism	Precautions
MUSCLE RELAXANTS—NONDEPOLARIZINGS				
NONDEPOLARIZING	**ANALGESICS—OPIOIDS**			
MUSCLE RELAXANTS—NONDEPOLARIZING	SUFENTANIL	Initial requirement of neuromuscular blockers may be ↓	Uncertain	Monitor neuromuscular block closely
PANCURONIUM	SUFENTANIL	The vagolytic effects of pancuronium may produce a dose-dependent elevation in heart rate during sufentanil–oxygen anesthesia	The use of moderate doses of pancuronium or of a less vagolytic neuromuscular blocking agent may be used to maintain a stable lower heart rate and BP during sufentanil–oxygen anesthesia	Monitor heart rate and titrate doses
MUSCLE RELAXANTS—DEPOLARIZING AND NONDEPOLARIZING	ANTIARRHYTHMICS—QUINIDINE	↑ Effect and duration of both depolarizing and nondepolarizing muscle relaxants	Uncertain	Be aware of possible prolonged neuromuscular blockade in patients taking quinidine
NONDEPOLARIZING	**ANTIBIOTICS**			
NONDEPOLARIZING	AMINOGLYCOSIDES	↑ Neuromuscular block	Aminoglycosides ↓ release of ACh at neuromuscular junctions by altering the influx of calcium. It is also thought to alter the sensitivity of the postsynaptic receptors/membrane, with ↓ transmission. These effects are additive to those of nondepolarizing muscle relaxants/neuromuscular blockers, which essentially prevents ACh acting on postsynaptic nicotinic receptors	Monitor neuromuscular blockade closely. Aminoglycosides vary in their potency to block neuromuscular junctions, with neomycin having the highest potency, then streptomycin, gentamicin, and kanamycin
NONDEPOLARIZING	AZLOCILLIN, CLINDAMYCIN, COLISTIN, PIPERACILLIN	↑ Efficacy of muscle relaxants	Piperacillin has some neuromuscular blocking activity	Monitor neuromuscular blockade carefully

(*Continued*)

Primary Drug	Secondary Drug	Effect	Mechanism	Precautions
MUSCLE RELAXANTS—NONDEPOLARIZINGS				
NONDEPOLARIZING	VANCOMYCIN	1. ↑ Efficacy of these muscle relaxants 2. Possible risk of hypersensitivity reactions	1. Vancomycin has some neuromuscular blocking activity 2. Animal studies suggest additive effect on histamine release	1. Monitor neuromuscular blockade carefully 2. Be aware
NEUROMUSCULAR BLOCKERS	ANTICANCER AND IMMUNOMODULATING DRUGS—CORTICOSTEROIDS	Reduced effect of neuromuscular blockers Risk of myopathy with prolonged use of corticosteroids	Uncertain	Dosage of neuromuscular blocker may need to be increased Be aware of interaction, particularly in patients in intensive care
NONDEPOLARIZING	**ANTIDEPRESSANTS**			
NONDEPOLARIZING	LITHIUM	Antagonism of effects of nondepolarizing muscle relaxants	Uncertain	Monitor intraoperative muscle relaxation closely; may need ↑ doses of muscle relaxants
NONDEPOLARIZING—PANCURONIUM	MAOIs	Risk of severe hypertension	Pancuronium releases stored noradrenaline	Pancuronium should be avoided
NONDEPOLARIZING	**ANTIEPILEPTICS**			
NONDEPOLARIZING—MIVACURIUM	BARBITURATES—THIOPENTONE	Inactivation of mivacurium in the presence of an alkaline environment—pH > 8.5. In the presence of an alkaline solution, there is a risk that mivacurium may be inactivated and a free acid precipitated	Mivacurium injection is acidic (pH 3.5–5.5) and should not be mixed in the same syringe with highly alkaline solutions (e.g., some barbiturate solutions) or administered simultaneously through the same needle during intravenous infusion	Avoid mixing with alkaline solutions
NONDEPOLARIZING	CARBAMAZEPINE, PHENYTOIN	Resistance to neuromuscular blocking action may occur in patients who are taking regular carbamazepine or phenytoin. This results in a shorter duration of neuromuscular blockade	Unknown	Infusion rates of nondepolarizing muscle relaxants may need to be increased

(*Continued*)

Primary Drug	Secondary Drug	Effect	Mechanism	Precautions
MUSCLE RELAXANTS—NONDEPOLARIZINGS				
NONDEPOLARIZING	BETA-BLOCKERS	1. Modest ↑ efficacy of muscle relaxants, particularly with propanolol 2. Risk of ↓ BP with atracurium and alcuronium	1 and 2. Uncertain	1. Watch for prolonged muscular paralysis after use of muscle relaxants 2. Monitor BP at least weekly until stable
NONDEPOLARIZING—PANCURONIUM	BRONCHODILATORS—THEOPHYLLINE	Antagonism of neuromuscular blockade	Uncertain	Larger doses of pancuronium may be needed to obtain the desired muscle relaxation during anesthesia; other nondepolarizing muscle relaxants do not seem to be affected
NONDEPOLARIZING	CALCIUM CHANNEL BLOCKERS—DILTIAZEM, VERAPAMIL	↑ Effect of nondepolarizing muscle relaxants with parenteral calcium channel blockers; the effect is less certain with oral therapy. In two cohort studies, vecuronium requirements were halved in patients on diltiazem. Nimodipine does not seem to share this effect	Uncertain; postulated that ACh release at the synapse is calcium dependent. ↓ calcium concentrations at the nerve ending may ↓ ACh release, which in turn prolongs the nerve blockade	Monitor nerve blockade carefully in patients on calcium channel blockers, particularly near to the end of surgery, when muscle relaxation may be prolonged and difficult to reverse
NONDEPOLARIZING	CARDIAC GLYCOSIDES—DIGOXIN	Case reports of S–T segment/T wave changes and sinus/atrial tachycardia when pancuronium was given to patients on digoxin	Uncertain	Avoid pancuronium in patients taking digoxin
NONDEPOLARIZING—MIVACURIUM	DIURETICS	↑ Neuromuscular block	Uncertain; multiple factors likely, including electrolyte disturbances and possible direct effect on muscle contractility	Monitor neuromuscular block and titrate doses of mivacurium
NONDEPOLARIZING—VECURONIUM	H2-RECEPTOR BLOCKERS—CIMETIDINE	↑ Efficacy of vecuronium	Unclear	Potential for slightly prolonged recovery time (minutes)

(Continued)

Primary Drug	Secondary Drug	Effect	Mechanism	Precautions
MUSCLE RELAXANTS—NONDEPOLARIZINGS				
NONDEPOLARIZING	MAGNESIUM (PARENTERAL)	↑ Efficacy of these muscle relaxants, with risk of prolonged neuromuscular blockade	Additive effect; magnesium inhibits ACh release and ↓ postsynaptic receptor sensitivity	Monitor nerve blockade closely
NONDEPOLARIZING	PARASYMPATHOMIMETICS	↓ Efficacy of nondepolarizing muscle relaxants	Anticholinesterases oppose the action of nondepolarizing muscle relaxants	Used therapeutically
NONDEPOLARIZING—VECURONIUM	PROTON PUMP INHIBITORS—LANSOPRAZOLE	Possible ↑ efficacy and adverse effects of vecuronium	Unclear	Altered duration of action. May need ↑ recovery time
NONDEPOLARIZING MIVACURIUM	SODIUM BICARBONATE	Inactivation of mivacurium in the presence of an alkaline environment—pH > 8.5. In the presence of an alkaline solution, there is a risk that mivacurium may be inactivated and a free acid precipitated	Mivacurium injection is acidic (pH 3.5–5.5) and should not be mixed in the same syringe with highly alkaline solutions or administered simultaneously through the same needle during IV infusion	Avoid mixing with alkaline solutions

Primary Drug	Secondary Drug	Effect	Mechanism	Precautions
OPIOIDS ➢ *Analgesics, Opioids*				

PART 10

Drugs to Treat Infections

Ursula Collignon

Primary Drug	Secondary Drug	Effect	Mechanism	Precautions
ANTIBIOTICS				
AMINOGLYCOSIDES				
GENTAMICIN	AGALSIDASE BETA	Possibly ↓ clinical effect of agalsidase beta	Uncertain	Avoid coadministration
AMINOGLYCOSIDES	ANALGESICS—INDOMETHACIN	↑ Amikacin, gentamicin, and vancomycin levels in neonates	Uncertain; indomethacin possibly ↓ renal clearance of these aminoglycosides	Halve the dose of antibiotic. Uncertain if this applies to adults but suggest check levels. Otherwise, use an alternative NSAID
AMINOGLYCOSIDES	**ANTIBIOTICS**			
AMINOGLYCOSIDES	CEPHALOSPORINS	Possible ↑ risk of nephrotoxicity	Additive effect; cephalosporins are rarely associated with interstitial nephritis	Renal function should be carefully monitored
AMINOGLYCOSIDES	COLISTIN	↑ Risk of nephrotoxicity	Additive effect	Renal function should be carefully monitored
NEOMYCIN	PENICILLIN V	↓ Levels of phenoxymethylpenicillin and possible therapeutic failure	↓ Absorption of phenoxymethyl penicillin due to malabsorption syndrome caused by neomycin	Patients should be monitored for efficacy of phenoxymethylpenicillin
AMINOGLYCOSIDES	TEICOPLANIN, VANCOMYCIN	↑ Risk of nephrotoxicity and ototoxicity	Additive effect	Hearing and renal function should be carefully monitored
AMINOGLYCOSIDES	**ANTICANCER AND IMMUNOMODULATING DRUGS**			
AMINOGLYCOSIDES	CICLOSPORIN	↑ Risk of nephrotoxicity	Additive nephrotoxic effects	Monitor renal function
NEOMYCIN	METHOTREXATE—ORAL	↓ Plasma concentrations following oral methotrexate	Oral aminoglycosides ↓ absorption of oral methotrexate by 30%–50%	Separate doses of each drug by at least 2–4 h
AMINOGLYCOSIDES, CAPREOMYCIN, STREPTOMYCIN	PLATINUM COMPOUNDS—CISPLATIN	↑ Risk of renal toxicity and renal failure, and of ototoxicity. The ototoxicity tends to occur when cisplatin is administered early during the course of aminoglycoside therapy	Additive renal toxicity	Monitor renal function prior to and during therapy, and ensure an intake of at least 2 L of fluid daily. Monitor serum potassium and magnesium levels and correct any deficiencies. Most side effects of aminoglycosides are dose related, and it is necessary to ↑ interval between doses and ↓ dose of aminoglycoside if there is impaired renal function

(*Continued*)

Primary Drug	Secondary Drug	Effect	Mechanism	Precautions
ANTIBIOTICS				
AMINOGLYCOSIDES	TACROLIMUS	Risk of renal toxicity	Additive effect	Monitor renal function closely
NEOMYCIN	ANTICOAGULANTS—ORAL	Elevated prothrombin times and ↑ risk of bleeding	The mechanism is not fully understood; however, it is thought that neomycin may ↓ number of vitamin K–producing bacteria in the gastrointestinal tract and/or that the absorption of vitamin K may be ↓ by the neomycin	The INR should be monitored in all patients starting or stopping neomycin therapy. Patients more at risk are those with an inadequate diet
AMINOGLYCOSIDES	**ANTIDIABETIC DRUGS**			
AMINOGLYCOSIDES	ACARBOSE	↑ Postprandial hypoglycemia and ↑ gastrointestinal effects as a result of the concurrent use of acarbose and neomycin	Neomycin is known to cause ↓ blood glucose levels after meals; when used concomitantly with acarbose, this effect may be ↑. Neomycin also exacerbates the adverse gastrointestinal effects caused by acarbose	Blood glucose levels should be closely monitored; if gastrointestinal signs are severe, the dose of acarbose should be ↓.
AMINOGLYCOSIDES	METFORMIN	Risk of hypoglycemia due to ↑ plasma concentrations of metformin	Mechanism uncertain. Metformin does not undergo hepatic metabolism. Renal tubular secretion is the major route of metformin elimination. Aminoglycosides are also principally excreted via the kidney, and nephrotoxicity is an important side effect	Watch/monitor and warn patients about hypoglycemia. ➢ ***For signs and symptoms of hypoglycemia, see Clinical Features of Some Adverse Drug Interactions, Hypoglycemia***
AMINOGLYCOSIDES	ANTIFUNGALS—AMPHOTERICIN	Risk of renal failure	Additive effect	Monitor renal function closely
AMINOGLYCOSIDES	**ANTIVIRALS**			
AMINOGLYCOSIDES	ADEFOVIR DIPIVOXIL	Possible ↑ efficacy and side effects	Competition for renal excretion	Monitor renal function weekly
AMINOGLYCOSIDES	FOSCARNET SODIUM	Possible ↑ nephrotoxicity	Additive side effect	Monitor renal function closely

(Continued)

Primary Drug	Secondary Drug	Effect	Mechanism	Precautions
ANTIBIOTICS				
AMINOGLYCOSIDES	NUCLEOSIDE REVERSE TRANSCRIPTASE INHIBITORS	Possibly ↑ risk of nephrotoxicity	Additive effect	Avoid coadministration if possible; otherwise, monitor renal function weekly
AMINOGLYCOSIDES	BISPHOSPHONATES—SODIUM CLODRONATE	Risk of symptomatic hypocalcemia	Uncertain	Monitor calcium levels closely
AMINOGLYCOSIDES	CARDIAC GLYCOSIDES—DIGOXIN	1. Gentamicin may ↑ plasma concentrations of digoxin 2. Neomycin may ↓ plasma concentrations of digoxin	1. Uncertain; postulated to be due to impaired renal clearance of digoxin 2. Neomycin ↓ absorption of digoxin; this may be offset in some patients by ↓ breakdown of digoxin by intestinal bacterial	1. Monitor digoxin levels; watch for ↑ levels, particularly in diabetics and in the presence of renal insufficiency 2. Monitor digoxin levels; watch for poor response to digoxin
AMINOGLYCOSIDES	DIURETICS—LOOP	↑ Risk of ototoxicity and possible deafness as a result of concomitant use of furosemide and gentamicin	Both furosemide and gentamicin are associated with ototoxicity; this risk is ↑ if they are used together	If used concurrently, patients should be monitored for any hearing impairment
AMINOGLYCOSIDES	MUSCLE RELAXANTS—DEPOLARIZING AND NONDEPOLARIZING	↑ Neuromuscular block	Aminoglycosides ↓ release of ACh at neuromuscular junctions by altering the influx of calcium. It is also thought that it alters the sensitivity of the postsynaptic membrane, with ↓ transmission. These effects are additive to those of the neuromuscular blockers	Monitor neuromuscular blockade closely. Aminoglycosides vary in their potency to block neuromuscular junctions, with neomycin having the highest potency, followed by streptomycin, gentamicin, and kanamycin
AMINOGLYCOSIDES	PARASYMPATHOMIMETICS—NEOSTIGMINE, PYRIDOSTIGMINE	↓ Efficacy of neostigmine and pyridostigmine	Uncertain	Watch for poor response to these parasympathomimetics and ↑ dose accordingly
BETA-LACTAMS				
CEPHALOSPORINS				
CEFPODOXIME, CEFUROXIME	ANTACIDS	↓ Levels of these antibiotics	Antacids that contain aluminum and/or magnesium may bind in stomach and intestines decreasing absorption	Take these cephalosporins at least 2 h after an antacid.

(Continued)

Primary Drug	Secondary Drug	Effect	Mechanism	Precautions
ANTIBIOTICS				
CEPHALOSPORINS	ANALGESICS—INDOMETHACIN	Indomethacin ↑ ceftazidime levels in neonates	Indomethacin ↓ clearance of ceftazidime	The dose of ceftazidime needs to be ↓
CEPHALOSPORINS	ANTIBIOTICS—AMINOGLYCOSIDES	Possible ↑ risk of nephrotoxicity	Additive effect; cephalosporins are rarely associated with interstitial nephritis	Renal function should be carefully monitored
CEPHALOSPORINS	ANTICOAGULANTS—ORAL	Certain cephalosporins (cefaclor, cefixime, ceftriaxone) may ↑ efficacy of oral anticoagulants	These cephalosporins have vitamin K antagonistic activity, which adds to the action of oral anticoagulants	Monitor INR closely; significant ↑ in INR may require vitamin K therapy. If possible, use an alternative cephalosporin
CEPHALOSPORINS	ANTIGOUT DRUGS—PROBENECID	↑ Cephalosporin levels	Uncertain	Watch for ↑ incidence of side effects
CEPHALOSPORINS	H2 RECEPTOR BLOCKERS	↓ Plasma concentrations and risk of treatment failure	↓ Absorption of cephalosporin due to ↑ gastric pH	Avoid concomitant use. If unable to avoid combination, take H2 antagonists at least 2–3 h after the cephalosporin. Consider alternative antibiotic or separate the doses by at least 2 h and give with an acidic drink, e.g., a carbonated drink; ↑ dose may be required
CEPHALOSPORINS	ESTROGENS	Reports of ↓ contraceptive effect	Possibly alteration of bacterial flora necessary for recycling of ethinylestradiol from the large bowel, although not certain in every case	Advise patients to use additional contraception for the period of antibiotic intake and for 1 month after stopping the antibiotic
CEPHALOSPORINS	PROTON PUMP INHIBITORS	Possible ↓ efficacy of cephalosporin	↓ Absorption as ↑ gastric pH	Monitor for ↓ efficacy. Separate doses by at least 2 h. Cefuroxime taken with food (as recommended by manufacturer) is likely to reduce interaction.
OTHER BETA-LACTAMS				
ERTAPENEM, MEROPENEM	ANTIEPILEPTICS—VALPROATE	↓ Valproate levels	Induced metabolism	Monitor levels
MEROPENEM	ANTIGOUT DRUGS—PROBENECID	↑ Meropenem levels	Uncertain	Manufacturers recommend avoiding coadministration

(*Continued*)

Primary Drug	Secondary Drug	Effect	Mechanism	Precautions
ANTIBIOTICS				
IMIPENEM WITH CILASTATIN	ANTIVIRALS—GANCICLOVIR/ VALGANCICLOVIR	↑ Adverse effects (e.g., seizures)	Additive side effects; these drugs can cause seizure activity	Avoid combination if possible; use only if benefit outweighs risk
MACROLIDES				
MACROLIDES	**DRUGS THAT PROLONG THE QT INTERVAL**			
MACROLIDES (ESPECIALLY AZITHROMYCIN, CLARITHROMYCIN, PARENTERAL ERYTHROMYCIN, TELITHROMYCIN)	1. ANTIARRHYTHMICS—amiodarone, disopyramide, procainamide, propafenone 2. ANTIBIOTICS—quinolones (especially moxifloxacin), quinupristin/dalfopristin 3. ANTICANCER AND IMMUNOMODULATING DRUGS—arsenic trioxide 4. ANTIDEPRESSANTS—TCAs, venlafaxine 5. ANTIEMETICS—dolasetron 6. ANTIFUNGALS—fluconazole, posaconazole, voriconazole 7. ANTIHISTAMINES—terfenadine, hydroxyzine, mizolastine 8. ANTIMALARIALS—artemether with lumefantrine, chloroquine, hydroxychloroquine, mefloquine, quinine 9. ANTIPROTOZOALS—pentamidine isethionate 10. ANTIPSYCHOTICS—atypicals, phenothiazines, pimozide 11. BETA-BLOCKERS—sotalol 12. BRONCHODILATORS—parenteral bronchodilators 13. CNS STIMULANTS—atomoxetine	Risk of ventricular arrhythmias, particularly torsades de pointes	Additive effect; these drugs cause prolongation of the QT interval	Avoid coadministration

(Continued)

DRUGS TO TREAT INFECTIONS ANTIBIOTICS Macrolides

Primary Drug	Secondary Drug	Effect	Mechanism	Precautions
ANTIBIOTICS				
MACROLIDES	ANALGESICS—OPIOIDS	Effects of alfentanil ↑ by erythromycin	Erythromycin inhibits metabolism of alfentanil	Be aware that effects of alfentanil (especially when given as an infusion) may be prolonged by erythromycin
AZITHROMYCIN	ANTACIDS	↓ Levels of these antibiotics	↓ Absorption	Take azithromycin at least 1 h before or 2 h after an antacid.
MACROLIDES	**ANTIBIOTICS**			
MACROLIDES	RIFABUTIN	↑ Rifabutin levels	Inhibition of CYP3A4-mediated metabolism of rifabutin	Watch for early features of toxicity of rifabutin (warn patients to report painful eyes)
CLARITHROMYCIN, TELITHROMYCIN	RIFAMPICIN	↓ Levels of these macrolides	Rifampicins induce metabolism of these macrolides	Avoid coadministration for up to 2 weeks after stopping rifampicin
MACROLIDES	**ANTICANCER AND IMMUNOMODULATING DRUGS**			
MACROLIDES	**CYTOTOXICS**			
CLARITHROMYCIN, ERYTHROMYCIN	BUSULFAN	↑ Plasma concentrations of busulfan and ↑ risk of toxicity of busulfan such as veno-occlusive disease and pulmonary fibrosis	Macrolides are inhibitors of CYP3A4. Busulfan clearance may be ↓ by 25%, and the AUC of busulfan may ↑ by 1500 μmol/L	Monitor clinically for veno-occlusive disease and pulmonary toxicity in transplant patients. Monitor busulfan blood levels as AUCs below 1500 μmol/L/min tend to prevent toxicity
ERYTHROMYCIN	DOCETAXEL	↑ Docetaxel levels	Docetaxel is metabolized by enzymes that are moderately inhibited by erythromycin, leading to ↑ levels and possible toxicity	Cautious use or consider use of azithromycin, which has little effect on CYP3A4 and, therefore, is not expected to interact with docetaxel
CLARITHROMYCIN, ERYTHROMYCIN	DOXORUBICIN	↑ Risk of myelosuppression due to ↑ plasma concentrations	Due to ↓ metabolism of doxorubicin by CYP3A4 isoenzymes due to inhibition of those enzymes	Monitor for ↑ myelosuppression, peripheral neuropathy, myalgias, and fatigue

(*Continued*)

Primary Drug	Secondary Drug	Effect	Mechanism	Precautions
ANTIBIOTICS				
CLARITHROMYCIN, ERYTHROMYCIN	IFOSFAMIDE	↓ Plasma concentrations of 4-hydroxyifosfamide, the active metabolite of ifosfamide, and risk of inadequate therapeutic response	Due to inhibition of the isoenzymatic conversion to active metabolites	Monitor clinically the efficacy of ifosfamide and ↑ dose accordingly
CLARITHROMYCIN, ERYTHROMYCIN	IMATINIB	↑ Imatinib levels with ↑ risk of toxicity (e.g., abdominal pain, constipation, dyspnea) and of neurotoxicity (e.g., taste disturbances, dizziness, headache, paresthesia, peripheral neuropathy)	Due to inhibition of CYP3A4-mediated metabolism of imatinib	Monitor for clinical efficacy and for the signs of toxicity listed, along with convulsions, confusion, signs of edema (including pulmonary edema). Monitor electrolytes, liver function, and for cardiotoxicity
CLARITHROMYCIN, ERYTHROMYCIN	IRINOTECAN	↑ Plasma concentrations of SN-38 (>AUC by 100%) and ↑ toxicity of irinotecan, e.g., diarrhea, acute cholinergic syndrome, interstitial pulmonary disease	Due to inhibition of the metabolism of irinotecan by CYP3A4 isoenzymes by macrolides	Peripheral blood counts should be checked before each course of treatment. Monitor lung function. Recommendation is to ↓ dose of irinotecan by 25%
CLARITHROMYCIN, ERYTHROMYCIN	VINCA ALKALOIDS—VINBLASTINE, VINCRISTINE, VINORELBINE	↑ Adverse effects of vinblastine and vincristine	Inhibition of CYP3A4-mediated metabolism. Also inhibition of Pgp efflux of vinblastine	Monitor FBCs. Watch for early features of toxicity (pain, numbness, tingling in the fingers and toes, jaw pain, abdominal pain, constipation, ileus). Consider selecting an alternative drug
MACROLIDES	**HORMONES AND HORMONE ANTAGONISTS**			
CLARITHROMYCIN, ERYTHROMYCIN	TOREMIFENE	↑ Plasma concentrations of toremifene with clarithromycin and erythromycin	Due to inhibition of metabolism of toremifene by the CYP3A4 isoenzymes	Clinical relevance is uncertain. Necessary to monitor for clinical toxicities

(*Continued*)

Primary Drug	Secondary Drug	Effect	Mechanism	Precautions
ANTIBIOTICS				
MACROLIDES	**IMMUNOMODULATING DRUGS**			
CLARITHROMYCIN, ERYTHROMYCIN, TELITHROMYCIN	CICLOSPORIN	↑ Plasma concentrations of ciclosporin, with risk of nephrotoxicity, myelosuppression, neurotoxicity and excessive immunosuppression, with risk of infection and posttransplant lymphoproliferative disease	Inhibition of CYP3A4-mediated metabolism of ciclosporin; these inhibitors vary in potency. Clarithromycin and telithromycin are classified as potent inhibitors	Avoid coadministration with clarithromycin and telithromycin. Consider alternative antibiotics but need to monitor plasma ciclosporin levels to prevent toxicity
CLARITHROMYCIN, ERYTHROMYCIN	CORTICOSTEROIDS	↑ Adrenal suppressive effects of corticosteroids, which may ↑ risk of infections and produce an inadequate response to stress scenarios	Due to inhibition of metabolism of corticosteroids	Monitor cortisol levels and warn patients to report symptoms such as fever and sore throat
CLARITHROMYCIN, ERYTHROMYCIN	SIROLIMUS	↑ Sirolimus levels	Inhibition of metabolism of sirolimus	Avoid coadministration
MACROLIDES	TACROLIMUS	↑ Plasma concentrations of tacrolimus, with risk of toxic effect	Clarithromycin, erythromycin, and telithromycin inhibit CYP3A4-mediated metabolism of tacrolimus. Azithromycin, if at all, mildly inhibits CYP3A4; a marked ↑ in tacrolimus levels is attributed to inhibition of Pgp	Be aware and monitor tacrolimus plasma concentrations
MACROLIDES	ANTICOAGULANTS—ORAL	Occasional episodes of ↑ anticoagulant effect	Uncertain at present	Monitor INR every 2–3 days
MACROLIDES	**ANTIDEPRESSANTS**			
ERYTHROMYCIN	MAOIs—PHENELZINE	Report of fainting and severe hypotension on initiation of erythromycin	Attributed to ↑ absorption of phenelzine due to rapid gastric emptying caused by erythromycin	Be aware

(*Continued*)

Primary Drug	Secondary Drug	Effect	Mechanism	Precautions
ANTIBIOTICS				
MACROLIDES	REBOXETINE	Risk of ↑ reboxetine levels	Possibly inhibition of CYP3A4-mediated metabolism of reboxetine	Avoid coadministration
TELITHROMYCIN	ST. JOHN'S WORT	↓ Telithromycin levels	Due to induction of CYP3A4-mediated metabolism of telithromycin	Avoid coadministration for up to 2 weeks after stopping St. John's wort
ERYTHROMYCIN, CLARITHROMYCIN, TELITHROMYCIN	ANTIDIABETIC DRUGS—REPAGLINIDE	Likely to ↑ plasma concentrations of repaglinide and ↑ risk of hypoglycemic episodes. ↑ risk of gastrointestinal side effects with clarithromycin	Due to inhibition of CYP3A4 isoenzymes, which metabolize repaglinide. These drugs vary in potency as inhibitors (clarithromycin is a potent inhibitor) and ↑ plasma concentrations vary. Clarithromycin ↑ plasma concentrations by 60%. However, the alternative pathway—CYP2C8—is unaffected by these inhibitors	Watch for and warn patients about hypoglycemia. ➢ ***For signs and symptoms of hypoglycemia, see Clinical Features of Some Adverse Drug Interactions, Hypoglycemia***
MACROLIDES	ANTIEMETICS—APREPITANT	↑ Aprepitant levels	Inhibition of CYP3A4-mediated metabolism of aprepitant	Use with caution. Clinical significance unclear; monitor closely
MACROLIDES	**ANTIEPILEPTICS**			
TELITHROMYCIN	BARBITURATES	↓ Levels of these drugs, with risk of therapeutic failure	Induction of hepatic metabolism	1. Avoid coadministration of telithromycin for up to 2 weeks after stopping phenobarbital 2. With the other drugs, monitor for ↓ clinical efficacy and ↑ dose as required
TELITHROMYCIN	CARBAMAZEPINE	↓ Levels of these drugs, with risk of therapeutic failure	Induction of hepatic metabolism	1. Avoid coadministration of telithromycin for up to 2 weeks after stopping carbamazepine 2. With the other drugs, monitor for ↓ clinical efficacy and ↑ dose as required

(Continued)

Primary Drug	Secondary Drug	Effect	Mechanism	Precautions
ANTIBIOTICS				
CLARITHROMYCIN, ERYTHROMYCIN	CARBAMAZEPINE	↑ Carbamazepine levels	Inhibition of metabolism	Monitor carbamazepine levels
TELITHROMYCIN	PHENYTOIN	↓ Levels of these drugs, with risk of therapeutic failure	Induction of hepatic metabolism	1. Avoid coadministration of telithromycin for up to 2 weeks after stopping phenytoin
CLARITHROMYCIN	PHENYTOIN	↑ Phenytoin levels	Inhibited metabolism	Monitor phenytoin levels
ERYTHROMYCIN	VALPROATE	↑ Valproate levels	Inhibited metabolism	Monitor levels
CLARITHROMYCIN, ERYTHROMYCIN, TELITHROMYCIN	ANTIFUNGALS—ITRACONAZOLE, KETOCONAZOLE, VORICONAZOLE	↑ Plasma concentrations of itraconazole, ketoconazole, and voriconazole, and risk of toxic effects	These antibiotics are inhibitors of metabolism of itraconazole by the CYP3A4. Erythromycin is a weaker inhibitor than clarithromycin. The role of clarithromycin and erythromycin as inhibitors of Pgp is not known with certainty. Ketoconazole is a potent inhibitor of Pgp	Monitor LFTs closely. Azithromycin does not cause this effect
ERYTHROMYCIN, CLARITHROMYCIN	ANTIGOUT DRUGS—COLCHICINE	Cases of colchicine toxicity when macrolides added	Uncertain; macrolides may inhibit hepatic metabolism of colchicine. Clarithromycin and erythromycin both inhibit intestinal Pgp, which may ↑ bioavailability of colchicine	Monitor FBC and renal function closely
MACROLIDES	**ANTIMIGRAINE DRUGS**			
MACROLIDES	ERGOT DERIVATIVES	↑ Ergotamine/methysergide levels, with risk of toxicity	Inhibition of CYP3A4-mediated metabolism of the ergot derivatives	Avoid coadministration

(*Continued*)

Primary Drug	Secondary Drug	Effect	Mechanism	Precautions
ANTIBIOTICS				
CLARITHROMYCIN, ERYTHROMYCIN	ALMOTRIPTAN, ELETRIPTAN	↑ Plasma concentrations of almotriptan and eletriptan, with risk of toxic effects, e.g., flushing, sensations of tingling, heat, heaviness, pressure, or tightness of any part of body including the throat and chest, dizziness	Almotriptan is metabolized mainly by CYP3A4 isoenzymes. Most CYP isoenzymes are inhibited by clarithromycin to varying degrees, and since there is an alternative pathway of metabolism by MAOA, the toxicity responses will vary between individuals	Avoid coadministration
CLARITHROMYCIN, ERYTHROMYCIN	ANTIMUSCARINICS—TOLTERODINE	↑ Tolterodine levels	Inhibition of CYP3A4-mediated metabolism	Avoid coadministration (manufacturers' recommendation)
ERYTHROMYCIN	ANTI-PARKINSON'S DRUGS—BROMOCRIPTINE, CABERGOLINE	↑ Bromocriptine and cabergoline levels	Inhibition of metabolism	Monitor BP closely and watch for early features of toxicity (nausea, headache, drowsiness)
ERYTHROMYCIN	ANTIPSYCHOTICS—CLOZAPINE	↑ Clozapine levels, with risk of clozapine toxicity	Clozapine is metabolized by CYPIA2, which is moderately inhibited by erythromycin. Erythromycin is a potent inhibitor of CYP3A4, which has a minor role in the metabolism of clozapine. This may lead to ↓ clearance and therefore ↑ levels of clozapine	Cautious use advised
MACROLIDES	**ANTIVIRALS**			
CLARITHROMYCIN	NNRTIs	1. ↓ Efficacy of clarithromycin but ↑ efficacy and adverse effects of the active metabolite 2. A rash occurs in 46% of patients when efavirenz is given with clarithromycin	1. Uncertain: possibly due to altered CYP3A4-mediated metabolism 2. Uncertain	1. Clinical significance unknown; no dose adjustment is recommended when clarithromycin is coadministered with nevirapine, but monitor LFTs and activity against *Mycobacterium avium intracellulare* complex closely 2. Consider alternatives to clarithromycin for patients on efavirenz

(Continued)

Primary Drug	Secondary Drug	Effect	Mechanism	Precautions
ANTIBIOTICS				
AZITHROMYCIN	PROTEASE INHIBITORS	Risk of ↑ adverse effects of azithromycin with nelfinavir	Possibly involves altered Pgp transport	Watch for signs of azithromycin toxicity
CLARITHROMYCIN, ERYTHROMYCIN	PROTEASE INHIBITORS	Possibly ↑ adverse effects of macrolide with atazanavir, ritonavir (with or without lopinavir), and saquinavir	Inhibition of CYP3A4- and possibly CYP1A2-mediated metabolism. Altered transport via Pgp may be involved. Amprenavir and indinavir are also possibly ↑ by erythromycin	Consider alternatives unless there is *Mycobacterium avium-intracellulare* infection; if combined, ↓ dose by 50% (75% in the presence of renal failure with a creatinine clearance of <30 mL/min)
MACROLIDES	**ANXIOLYTICS AND HYPNOTICS**			
ERYTHROMYCIN, CLARITHROMYCIN, TELITHROMYCIN	MIDAZOLAM, TRIAZOLAM, POSSIBLY ALPRAZOLAM	↑ BZD levels	Inhibition of CYP3A4-mediated metabolism	↓ Dose of BZD by 50%; warn patients not to perform skilled tasks such as driving for at least 10 h after the dose of BZD
MACROLIDES	BUSPIRONE	↑ Buspirone levels	Inhibition of CYP3A4-mediated metabolism	Warn patients to be aware of additional sedation
MACROLIDES	**BRONCHODILATORS**			
MACROLIDES	LEUKOTRIENE RECEPTOR ANTAGONISTS—ZAFIRLUKAST	↓ ZAFIRLUKAST levels	Induction of metabolism. Plasma concentrations may decrease by 40%	Not seen with topical erythromycin
AZITHROMYCIN, CLARITHROMYCIN, ERYTHROMYCIN	THEOPHYLLINE	1. ↑ Theophylline levels 2. Possibly ↓ erythromycin levels when given orally	1. Inhibition of CYP2D6-mediated metabolism of theophylline (macrolides and quinolones—isoniazid not known) 2. ↓ Bioavailability; uncertain mechanism	1. Monitor theophylline levels before, during, and after coadministration 2. Consider an alternative macrolide
MACROLIDES	CALCIUM CHANNEL BLOCKERS	↑ Plasma concentrations of felodipine when coadministered with erythromycin; cases of adverse effects of verapamil (bradycardia and ↓ BP) with both erythromycin and clarithromycin	Erythromycin inhibits CYP3A4-metabolism of felodipine and verapamil. Clarithromycin and erythromycin inhibit intestinal Pgp, which may ↑ bioavailability of verapamil	Monitor PR and BP closely; watch for bradycardia and ↓ BP. Consider ↓ dose of calcium channel blocker during macrolide therapy

(*Continued*)

Primary Drug	Secondary Drug	Effect	Mechanism	Precautions
ANTIBIOTICS				
MACROLIDES	CARDIAC GLYCOSIDES—DIGOXIN	Digoxin concentrations may be ↑ by macrolides	Uncertain; postulated that macrolides inhibit Pgp in both the intestine (↑ bioavailability) and kidney (↓ clearance). It is possible that alterations in intestinal flora may also have a role	Monitor digoxin levels; watch for digoxin toxicity
CLARITHROMYCIN, TELITHROMYCIN	CNS STIMULANTS—MODAFINIL	↑ Plasma concentrations of modafinil, with risk of adverse effects	Due to inhibition of CYP3A4, which has a partial role in the metabolism of modafinil	Be aware. Warn patients to report dose-related adverse effects, e.g., headache, anxiety
ERYTHROMYCIN	DIURETICS—POTASSIUM-SPARING	↑ Eplerenone results in ↑ risk of hypotension and hyperkalemia	Eplerenone is primarily metabolized by CYP3A4; there are no active metabolites. Erythromycin moderately inhibits CYP3A4, leading to ↑ levels of eplerenone	Eplerenone dosage should not exceed 25 mg daily
ERYTHROMYCIN	H2 RECEPTOR BLOCKERS—CIMETIDINE	↑ Efficacy and adverse effects of erythromycin, including hearing loss	↑ Bioavailability	Consider an alternative antibiotic, e.g., clarithromycin. Deafness was reversible with cessation of erythromycin
MACROLIDES	IVABRADINE	1. Risk of arrhythmias with erythromycin 2. Possible ↑ levels with clarithromycin and telithromycin	1. Additive effect 2. Uncertain	Avoid coadministration
MACROLIDES	**LIPID-LOWERING DRUGS**			
MACROLIDES	ATORVASTATIN, SIMVASTATIN	Macrolides may ↑ levels of atorvastatin and simvastatin; the risk of myopathy ↑ >10× when erythromycin is coadministered with a statin	Macrolides inhibit CYP3A4-mediated metabolism of atorvastatin and simvastatin. Also, erythromycin and clarithromycin inhibit intestinal Pgp, which may ↑ bioavailability of statins	Avoid coadministration of macrolides with atorvastatin or simvastatin (temporarily stop the statin if the patient needs macrolide therapy). Manufacturers also recommend that patients are warned to look for the early signs of rhabdomyolysis when other statins are coingested with macrolides

(*Continued*)

DRUGS TO TREAT INFECTIONS ANTIBIOTICS

Primary Drug	Secondary Drug	Effect	Mechanism	Precautions
ANTIBIOTICS				
ERYTHROMYCIN	ROSUVASTATIN	↓ Rosuvastatin levels with erythromycin	Uncertain	Avoid chronic coadministration
ERYTHROMYCIN	ESTROGENS	Reports of ↓ contraceptive effect	Possibly alteration of the bacterial flora necessary for recycling ethinylestradiol from the large bowel, although not certain in every case	Advise patients to use additional contraception for the period of antibiotic intake and for 1 month after stopping the antibiotic
ERYTHROMYCIN	PARASYMPATHOMIMETICS—GALANTAMINE	↑ Galantamine levels	Inhibition of CYP3A4-mediated metabolism of galantamine	Be aware; watch for ↑ side effects from galantamine
ERYTHROMYCIN, CLARITHROMYCIN	PERIPHERAL VASODILATORS—CILOSTAZOL	Cilostazol levels ↑ by erythromycin and possibly clarithromycin	Erythromycin and clarithromycin inhibit CYP3A4-mediated metabolism of cilostazol	Avoid coadministration
MACROLIDES	PHOSPHODIESTERASE TYPE 5 INHIBITORS	↑ Phosphodiesterase type 5 inhibitor levels with erythromycin, and possibly clarithromycin and telithromycin	Inhibition of metabolism	↓ Dose of these phosphodiesterase inhibitors (e.g., start vardenafil at 5 mg)
CLARITHROMYCIN	PROTON PUMP INHIBITORS—OMEPRAZOLE	↑ Efficacy and adverse effects of both drugs	↑ Plasma concentration of both drugs	No dose adjustment recommended. Interaction considered useful for *Helicobacter pylori* eradication
PENICILLINS				
AMPICILLIN	ANESTHETICS—LOCAL—LIDOCAINE SOLUTIONS	Precipitation of drugs, which may not be immediately apparent	A pharmaceutical interaction	Do not mix in the same infusion or syringe
PENICILLIN V	ANTIBIOTICS—NEOMYCIN	↓ Levels of phenoxymethylpenicillin and possible therapeutic failure	↓ Absorption of phenoxymethyl penicillin due to malabsorption syndrome caused by neomycin	Patients should be monitored for efficacy of phenoxymethylpenicillin

(*Continued*)

Primary Drug	Secondary Drug	Effect	Mechanism	Precautions
ANTIBIOTICS				
PENICILLINS	ANTICANCER AND IMMUNOMODULATING DRUGS—METHOTREXATE	↑ Plasma concentrations of methotrexate and risk of toxic effects of methotrexate, e.g., myelosuppression, liver cirrhosis, pulmonary toxicity	Penicillins ↓ renal elimination of methotrexate by renal tubular secretion, which is the main route of elimination of methotrexate. Penicillins compete with methotrexate for renal elimination. Displacement from protein-binding sites may occur and is only a minor contribution to the interaction	Avoid concurrent use. If concurrent use is necessary, monitor clinically and biochemically for blood dyscrasias, liver toxicity, and pulmonary toxicity. Do FBCs and LFTs prior to concurrent treatment
PENICILLINS	ANTICOAGULANTS—ORAL	Occasional episodes of ↑ anticoagulant effect	Uncertain at present	Monitor INR every 2–3 days
PENICILLINS	**ANTIGOUT DRUGS**			
PENICILLINS	ALLOPURINOL	Possible ↑ risk of rash with amoxycillin and ampicillin (over 20% incidence in one study)	Uncertain	Reassure patients that the rash is unlikely to have clinical significance
PENICILLINS	PROBENECID, SULFINPYRAZONE	↑ Penicillin levels	Uncertain	Watch for ↑ incidence of side effects
AMPICILLIN	BETA-BLOCKERS	Plasma concentrations of atenolol were halved by 1 g doses of ampicillin (but not smaller doses)	Uncertain	Monitor BP closely during initiation of therapy with ampicillin
PIPERACILLIN	MUSCLE RELAXANTS—DEPOLARIZING, NONDEPOLARIZING	↑ Effect of muscle relaxants	Piperacillin has some neuromuscular blocking activity	Monitor neuromuscular blockade carefully
AMPICILLIN	ESTROGENS	Reports of ↓ contraceptive effect	Possibly alteration of bacterial flora necessary for recycling ethinylestradiol from the large bowel, although not certain in every case	Advise patients to use additional contraception for the period of antibiotic intake and for 1 month after stopping the antibiotic

(*Continued*)

Primary Drug	Secondary Drug	Effect	Mechanism	Precautions
ANTIBIOTICS				
QUINOLONES				
QUINOLONES	**DRUGS THAT PROLONG THE QT INTERVAL**			
QUINOLONES (ESPECIALLY MOXIFLOXACIN)	1. ANTIARRHYTHMICS—amiodarone, disopyramide, procainamide, propafenone 2. ANTIBIOTICS—macrolides (especially azithromycin, clarithromycin, parenteral erythromycin, telithromycin), quinupristin/dalfopristin 3. ANTICANCER AND IMMUNOMODULATING DRUGS—arsenic trioxide 4. ANTIDEPRESSANTS—TCAs, venlafaxine 5. ANTIEMETICS—dolasetron 6. ANTIFUNGALS—fluconazole, posaconazole, voriconazole 7. ANTIHISTAMINES—terfenadine, hydroxyzine, mizolastine 8. ANTIMALARIALS—artemether with lumefantrine, chloroquine, hydroxychloroquine, mefloquine, quinine 9. ANTIPROTOZOALS—pentamidine isetionate 10. ANTIPSYCHOTICS—atypicals, phenothiazines, pimozide 11. BETA-BLOCKERS—sotalol 12. BRONCHODILATORS—parenteral bronchodilators 13. CNS STIMULANTS—atomoxetine	Risk of ventricular arrhythmias, particularly torsades de pointes	Additive effect; these drugs cause prolongation of the QT interval	Avoid coadministration

(Continued)

Primary Drug	Secondary Drug	Effect	Mechanism	Precautions
ANTIBIOTICS				
QUINOLONES	**ANALGESICS**			
QUINOLONES	NSAIDs	Reports of convulsions when NSAIDs were added to quinolones in those with epilepsy	Unknown	Care in coadministering antiepileptics and NSAIDs in patients with epilepsy
CIPROFLOXACIN	OPIOIDS	1. Effects of methadone ↑ by ciprofloxacin 2. ↓ Levels of ciprofloxacin with opioids	1. Ciprofloxacin inhibits CYP1A2-, CYP2D6-, and CYP3A4-mediated metabolism of methadone 2. Uncertain	1. Watch for ↑ effects of methadone 2. Avoid opioid premedication when ciprofloxacin is used as surgical prophylaxis
QUINOLONES	ANTACIDS	↓ Levels of these antibiotics	↓ Absorption	Separate quinolones and antacids by 2–6 h.
QUINOLONES	**ANTICANCER AND IMMUNOMODULATING DRUGS**			
QUINOLONES	**CYTOTOXICS**			
NALIDIXIC ACID	MELPHALAN	Risk of melphalan toxicity	Uncertain	Avoid coadministration
CIPROFLOXACIN	METHOTREXATE	↑ Plasma concentrations of methotrexate, with risk of toxic effects of methotrexate, e.g., liver cirrhosis, blood dyscrasias, which may be fatal, pulmonary toxicity, stomatitis. Hematopoietic suppression can occur abruptly. Other adverse effects include anorexia, dyspepsia, gastrointestinal ulceration and bleeding, and pulmonary edema	Ciprofloxacin ↓ renal elimination of methotrexate. Ciprofloxacin is known to cause renal failure and interstitial nephritis	Although the toxic effects of methotrexate are more frequent with high doses of methotrexate, it is necessary to do FBC, liver and renal function, tests before starting treatment even with low doses; repeat these tests weekly until therapy is stabilized and thereafter every 2–3 months. Patients should be advised to report symptoms such as sore throat and fever immediately, and also any gastrointestinal discomfort. A profound drop in white cell or platelet counts warrants immediate stoppage of methotrexate therapy and initiation of supportive therapy. Consider a nonreacting antibiotic
CIPROFLOXACIN	PORFIMER	↑ Risk of photosensitivity reactions	Attributed to additive effects	Avoid exposure of skin and eyes to direct sunlight for 30 days after porfimer therapy

(Continued)

Primary Drug	Secondary Drug	Effect	Mechanism	Precautions
ANTIBIOTICS				
QUINOLONES	**IMMUNOMODULATING DRUGS**			
CIPROFLOXACIN	CICLOSPORIN	Ciprofloxacin may ↓ immunosuppressive effect (pharmacodynamic interaction)	Ciprofloxacin ↓ inhibitory effect of ciclosporin on IL-2 production to ↓ immunosuppressive effect	Avoid coadministration
NORFLOXACIN	CICLOSPORIN	↑ Plasma concentrations of ciclosporin, with risk of nephrotoxicity, myelosuppression, neurotoxicity, and excessive immunosuppression, with risk of infection and posttransplant lymphoproliferative disease	Inhibition of CYP3A4-mediated metabolism of ciclosporin; these inhibitors vary in potency	Monitor plasma ciclosporin levels to prevent toxicity. Monitor renal function
NORFLOXACIN	MYCOPHENOLATE	Significant ↓ plasma mycophenolate concentrations	Inhibition of metabolism of mycophenolate	Avoid coadministration
QUINOLONES	ANTICOAGULANTS—ORAL	Occasional episodes of ↑ anticoagulant effect	Uncertain at present	Monitor INR every 2–3 days
CIPROFLOXACIN	ANTIDEPRESSANTS—DULOXETINE	↑ Duloxetine levels, with risk of side effects, e.g., arrhythmias	Inhibition of metabolism of duloxetine	Avoid coadministration
QUINOLONES	**ANTIDIABETIC DRUGS**			
QUINOLONES	ACARBOSE, METFORMIN, NATEGLINIDE, REPAGLINIDE, PIOGLITAZONE, ROSIGLITAZONE, SULFONYLUREAS	↑ Risk of hypoglycemic episodes	Mechanism uncertain. Ciprofloxacin is a potent inhibitor of CYP1A2. Norfloxacin is a weak inhibitor of CYP1A2, but these may inhibit other CYP isoenzymes to varying degrees	Watch for and warn patients about symptoms of hypoglycemia. ➢ ***For signs and symptoms of hypoglycemia, see Clinical Features of Some Adverse Drug Interactions, Hypoglycemia***
LEVOFLOXACIN	INSULIN	Altered insulin requirements	Both hyperglycemia and hypoglycemia	Altered glycemic control requires frequent monitoring

(Continued)

Primary Drug	Secondary Drug	Effect	Mechanism	Precautions
ANTIBIOTICS				
OFLOXACIN	INSULIN	↑ Risk of hypoglycemic episodes	Mechanism for hypoglycemia is not known	Watch for and warn patients about symptoms of hypoglycemia. ➢ ***For signs and symptoms of hypoglycemia, see Clinical Features of Some Adverse Drug Interactions, Hypoglycemia***
CIPROFLOXACIN	ANTIEPILEPTICS—PHENYTOIN	Variable effect on phenytoin levels	Unknown	Monitor phenytoin levels
CIPROFLOXACIN, LEVOFLOXACIN, NALIDIXIC ACID, NORFLOXACIN	ANTIGOUT DRUGS—PROBENECID	↑ Ciprofloxacin, nalidixic acid, and norfloxacin levels	Uncertain	Watch for ↑ incidence of side effects. Moxifloxacin, ofloxacin, and sparfloxacin do not seem to interact and could be used as alternative therapy
QUINOLONES	ANTIMIGRAINE DRUGS—ZOLMITRIPTAN	Possible ↓ plasma concentrations of zolmitriptan, with risk of inadequate therapeutic efficacy	Possibly induced metabolism of zolmitriptan	Be aware of possibility of ↓ response to triptan, and consider ↑ dose if effect is considered to be due to interaction
CIPROFLOXACIN	ANTI-PARKINSON'S DRUGS—ROPINIROLE	↑ Ropinirole levels	Inhibition of CYP1A2-mediated metabolism	Watch for early features of toxicity (nausea, drowsiness)
CIPROFLOXACIN	ANTIPSYCHOTICS—CLOZAPINE, OLANZAPINE	↑ Clozapine levels and possibly ↑ olanzapine levels	Ciprofloxacin inhibits CYP1A2; clozapine is primarily metabolized by CYP1A2, while olanzapine is partly metabolized by it	Watch for the early features of toxicity to these antipsychotics. ↓ dose of clozapine and olanzapine may be required
QUINOLONES	**ANTIVIRALS**			
QUINOLONES	DIDANOSINE	↓ Efficacy of ciprofloxacin and possibly levofloxacin, moxifloxacin, norfloxacin, and ofloxacin with buffered didanosine	Cations in the buffer of didanosine preparation chelate and adsorb ciprofloxacin. Absorption of the other quinolones may be ↓ by the buffered didanosine formulation, which raises gastric pH	Give the antibiotic 2 h before or 6 h after didanosine. Alternatively, consider using the enteric-coated formulation of didanosine, which does not have to be given separately

(*Continued*)

Primary Drug	Secondary Drug	Effect	Mechanism	Precautions
ANTIBIOTICS				
QUINOLONES	FOSCARNET SODIUM	Risk of seizures	Unknown; possibly additive side effect	Avoid combination in patients with past medical history of epilepsy. Consider an alternative antibiotic
QUINOLONES	BRONCHODILATORS—THEOPHYLLINE	1. ↑ Theophylline levels	1. Inhibition of CYP2D6-mediated metabolism of theophylline (macrolides and quinolones—isoniazid not known)	1. Monitor theophylline levels before, during, and after coadministration
CIPROFLOXACIN	CALCIUM	↓ Antibiotic levels	↓ Absorption	Separate doses by at least 2 h
CIPROFLOXACIN, NORFLOXACIN	DAIRY PRODUCTS	↓ Norfloxacin levels, with risk of therapeutic failure	The calcium from dairy products is thought to form an insoluble chelate with norfloxacin, leading to ↓ absorption from the gut	Dairy products should be avoided for 1–2 h before and after taking norfloxacin. Alternatively, moxifloxacin, enoxacin, lomefloxacin, and ofloxacin can be used as alternative therapies as they show minimal interaction
QUINOLONES	DRUG DEPENDENCE THERAPIES—BUPROPION	↑ Risk of seizures. This risk is marked in elderly people, in patients with a history of seizures, with addiction to opiates/cocaine/stimulants, and in diabetics treated with oral hypoglycemics or insulin	Bupropion is associated with a dose-related risk of seizures. These drugs, which lower seizure threshold, are individually epileptogenic. Additive effects occur when they are combined	Extreme caution. The dose of bupropion should not exceed 450 mg/day (or 150 mg/day in those with severe hepatic cirrhosis)
QUINOLONES	IRON—ORAL	↓ Plasma concentrations of these drugs, with risk of therapeutic failure	Iron chelates with and ↓ their absorption	Separate doses of drugs as much as possible and monitor their effects
CIPROFLOXACIN	MUSCLE RELAXANTS—TIZANIDINE	↑ Tizanidine levels	Tizanidine is a substrate for CYP1A2. Ciprofloxacin is a potent inhibitor of CYP1A2 and is thought to inhibit the presystemic metabolism, resulting in ↑ absorption and levels of tizanidine	Avoid coadministration

(*Continued*)

Primary Drug	Secondary Drug	Effect	Mechanism	Precautions
ANTIBIOTICS				
CIPROFLOXACIN	PERIPHERAL VASODILATORS—PENTOXIFYLLINE	Ciprofloxacin may ↑ pentoxifylline levels	Uncertain; likely to be due to inhibition of hepatic metabolism	Warn patients of the possibility of adverse effects of pentoxifylline
CIPROFLOXACIN	SEVELAMER	↓ Plasma concentrations of ciprofloxacin	↓ Absorption	Separate doses as much as possible
CIPROFLOXACIN	SODIUM BICARBONATE	↓ Solubility of ciprofloxacin in the urine, leading to ↑ risk of crystalluria and renal damage	↑ Urinary pH caused by sodium bicarbonate can result in ↓ ciprofloxacin solubility in the urine	If both drugs are used concomitantly, the patient should be well hydrated and monitored for signs of renal toxicity
QUINOLONES	STRONTIUM RANELATE	↓ Levels of these antibiotics	↓ Absorption	Avoid coadministration
QUINOLONES	SUCRALFATE	↓ Levels of these antibiotics	↓ Absorption of these antibiotics	Give the antibiotics at least 2 h before sucralfate
CIPROFLOXACIN	THYROID HORMONES—LEVOTHYROXINE	↓ Levels of levothyroxine and possible therapeutic failure	The mechanism has not been elucidated, the concurrent administration of ciprofloxacin with levothyroxine may interfere with the absorption of levothyroxine and result in lower than expected levels	The interaction may be minimized by separating dosing of the two agents; ciprofloxacin should be taken several hours before or after taking levothyroxine
CIPROFLOXACIN	ZINC	↓ Antibiotic levels	↓ Absorption	Separate doses by at least 2 h
RIFAMYCINS				
RIFAMPICIN	**ANALGESICS**			
RIFAMPICIN	NSAIDs	Rifampicin ↓ diclofenac celecoxib, etoricoxib, and parecoxib levels	Rifampicin ↑ CYP2C9-mediated metabolism of these NSAIDs	Monitor analgesic effects; consider using alternative NSAIDs
RIFAMPICIN	OPIOIDS	↓ Effect of alfentanil, codeine, methadone, and morphine	Rifampicin ↑ the hepatic metabolism of these opioids (alfentanil by CYP3A4, codeine by CYP2D6, morphine unknown). Rifampicin is also known to induce intestinal Pgp, which may ↓ bioavailability of oral morphine	Be aware that alfentanil, codeine, methadone, and morphine doses may need to be ↑

(Continued)

Primary Drug	Secondary Drug	Effect	Mechanism	Precautions
ANTIBIOTICS				
RIFAMPICIN	PARACETAMOL	Rifampicin ↓ paracetamol levels	Rifampicin ↑ glucuronidation of paracetamol	Warn patients that paracetamol may be less effective
RIFAMYCINS	ANTACIDS	↓ Rifamycin levels	↓ Absorption	Separate doses by 2–3 h
RIFAMYCINS	**ANTIARRHYTHMICS**			
RIFAMPICIN	AMIODARONE	↓ Levels of amiodarone	Uncertain, but rifampicin is a known enzyme inducer and may therefore ↑ metabolism of amiodarone	Watch for a poor response to amiodarone
RIFAMPICIN	DISOPYRAMIDE	Disopyramide levels are ↓ by rifampicin	Rifampicin induces hepatic metabolism of disopyramide	Watch for poor response to disopyramide; check serum levels if necessary
RIFAMPICIN	MEXILETINE	Rifampicin ↓ mexiletine levels	Uncertain; postulated that rifampicin may ↑ mexiletine metabolism	Watch for poor response to mexiletine
RIFAMPICIN	PROPAFENONE	Rifampicin may ↓ propafenone levels	Rifampicin may inhibit CYP3A4/1A2-mediated metabolism of propafenone	Watch for poor response to propafenone
RIFAMYCINS	**ANTIBIOTICS**			
RIFAMYCINS	DAPSONE	↓ Levels of dapsone	Rifamycins induce metabolism of dapsone	Watch for poor response to dapsone
RIFAMYCINS	MACROLIDES	1. ↓ Levels of clarithromycin and telithromycin with rifampicin 2. ↑ Rifabutin levels with macrolides	1. Rifampicins induce metabolism of these macrolides 2. Inhibition of CYP3A4-mediated metabolism of rifabutin	1. Watch for poor response to clarithromycin and telithromycin, which may last up to 2 weeks after stopping rifampicin 2. Watch for early features of toxicity of rifabutin; in particular, warn patients to report painful eyes
RIFAMPICIN	QUINUPRISTIN/DALFOPRISTIN	Risk of hepatic toxicity	Additive effect	Monitor LFTs closely
RIFAMYCINS	**ANTICANCER AND IMMUNOMODULATING DRUGS**			
RIFAMYCINS	**CYTOTOXICS**			
RIFAMPICIN	DASATINIB	↓ Dasatinib levels	Rifampicin ↑ metabolism of dasatinib	Avoid coadministration
RIFAMPICIN	ERLOTINIB	↓ Erlotinib levels	Rifampicin ↑ metabolism of erlotinib	Avoid coadministration

(Continued)

Primary Drug	Secondary Drug	Effect	Mechanism	Precautions
ANTIBIOTICS				
RIFAMPICIN	IFOSFAMIDE	↑ Rate of biotransformation to 4-hydroxyifosfamide, the active metabolite, but no change in AUC of 4-hydroxyifosfamide	Due to ↑ rate of metabolism and of clearance due to induction of CYP3A4 and CYP2D6.	Be aware—clinical significance may be minimal or none
RIFAMPICIN	IMATINIB	↓ Imatinib levels	Due to induction of CYP3A4-mediated metabolism of imatinib	Dose adjustments are necessary if concomitant administration is considered absolutely necessary; best, however, to avoid concomitant use
RIFAMPICIN	IRINOTECAN	↓ Plasma concentrations of irinotecan and risk of ↓ therapeutic efficacy. The effects may last for 3 weeks after discontinuation of CYP-inducer therapy	Due to induction of CYP3A4-mediated metabolism of irinotecan	Avoid concomitant use whenever possible; if not, ↑ dose of irinotecan by 50%
RIFAMPICIN	PACLITAXEL	↓ Plasma concentration of paclitaxel and ↓ efficacy of paclitaxel	Due to induction of hepatic metabolism of paclitaxel by the CYP isoenzymes	Monitor for clinical efficacy, and need to ↑ dose if inadequate response is due to interaction
RIFAMPICIN	SUNITINIB	↓ Sunitinib levels	Rifampicin ↑ metabolism of sunitinib	Avoid coadministration
RIFAMPICIN	VINCA ALKALOIDS—VINBLASTINE, VINCRISTINE	↓ Of plasma concentrations of vinblastine and vincristine, with risk of inadequate therapeutic response. Reports of ↓ AUC by 40% and elimination half-life by 35%, and ↑ clearance by 63%, in patients with brain tumors taking vincristine, which could lead to dangerously inadequate therapeutic responses	Due to induction of CYP3A4-mediated metabolism	Monitor for clinical efficacy and ↑ dose of vinblastine and vincristine as clinically indicated; in the latter case, monitor clinically and radiologically for clinical efficacy in patients with brain tumors and ↑ dose to obtain the desired response

(*Continued*)

Primary Drug	Secondary Drug	Effect	Mechanism	Precautions
ANTIBIOTICS				
RIFAMYCINS	**HORMONES AND HORMONE ANTAGONISTS**			
RIFAMPICIN	TAMOXIFEN	↓ Plasma concentrations of tamoxifen and risk of inadequate therapeutic response	Due to induction of metabolism of tamoxifen by the CYP3A isoenzymes by rifampicin	Avoid concurrent use if possible. Otherwise, monitor for clinical efficacy of tamoxifen and ↑ dose of tamoxifen if required
RIFAMYCINS	**IMMUNOMODULATING DRUGS**			
RIFAMYCINS	CICLOSPORIN	↓ Plasma concentrations of ciclosporin, with risk of transplant rejection	Due to induction of CYP3A4-mediated metabolism of ciclosporin by these drugs. The potency of induction varies	Monitor for signs of rejection of transplants. Monitor ciclosporin levels to ensure adequate therapeutic concentrations and ↑ dose when necessary
RIFAMPICIN	CORTICOSTEROIDS	↓ Plasma concentrations of corticosteroids and risk of poor or inadequate therapeutic response, which would be undesirable if used for, e.g., cerebral edema	Due to induction of the hepatic metabolism by the CYP3A4 isoenzymes	Monitor therapeutic response closely—clinically, with ophthalmoscopy and radiologically—and ↑ dose of corticosteroids for desired therapeutic effect
RIFAMPICIN	MYCOPHENOLATE	Significant ↓ plasma mycophenolate concentrations (>60% with rifampicin)	Attributed to induction of glucuronyl transferase	Avoid coadministration
RIFAMPICIN	SIROLIMUS	↓ Sirolimus levels	Induction of CYP3A4-mediated metabolism of sirolimus	Avoid coadministration
RIFAMPICIN	TACROLIMUS	↓ Tacrolimus levels	Induction of CYP3A4-mediated metabolism of tacrolimus	Avoid coadministration
RIFAMPICIN	ANTICOAGULANTS—ORAL	↓ Anticoagulant effect	Rifampicin induces CYP2C9-mediated metabolism of warfarin	Monitor INR closely for at least 1 week after starting rifampicin and up to 5 weeks after stopping it. During coadministration, the warfarin dose may need to be markedly ↑

(Continued)

Primary Drug	Secondary Drug	Effect	Mechanism	Precautions
ANTIBIOTICS				
RIFAMPICIN	**ANTIDIABETIC DRUGS**			
RIFAMPICIN	PIOGLITAZONE, ROSIGLITAZONE	Significant ↓ blood levels of rosiglitazone. Metabolism and clearance is ↑, the latter threefold	Rosiglitazone is metabolized primarily by CYP2C8 with a minor contribution from CYP2C9. Rifampicin is a potent inducer of CYP2C8 and CYP2C9, and ↑ formation of *N*-desmethylrosiglitazone by about 40%	May need to use an alternative drug or ↑ dose of rosiglitazone
RIFAMPICIN	REPAGLINIDE	↓ Plasma concentrations of repaglinide likely. Rifampicin ↓ AUC of repaglinide by 25%	Due to inducing CYP3A4 isoenzymes that metabolize repaglinide. However, the alternative pathway—CYP2C8—is unaffected by these inducers except by rifampicin	The interaction is likely to be most severe with rifampicin. Be aware and monitor for hypoglycemia. ➢ ***For signs and symptoms of hypoglycemia, see Clinical Features of Some Adverse Drug Interactions, Hypoglycemia***
RIFAMPICIN	SULFONYLUREAS	↓ Hypoglycemic efficacy	Plasma levels of sulfonylureas are ↓ by induction of CYP-mediated metabolism	Watch for and warn patients about symptoms of hypoglycemia. ➢ ***For signs and symptoms of hypoglycemia, see Clinical Features of Some Adverse Drug Interactions, Hypoglycemia***
RIFAMPICIN	**ANTIEMETIC**			
RIFAMPICIN	APREPITANT	↓ Aprepitant levels	Induction of CYP3A4-mediated metabolism of aprepitant	Watch for poor response to aprepitant
RIFAMPICIN	5-HT3 ANTAGONISTS—ONDANSETRON, TROPISETRON	↓ Levels of these drugs	Induction of metabolism	Watch for poor response to ondansetron and tropisetron; consider using an alternative antiemetic
RIFAMYCINS	**ANTIEPILEPTICS**			
RIFAMPICIN	BARBITURATES	↓ Levels of these drugs, with risk of therapeutic failure	Induction of hepatic metabolism	Monitor for ↓ clinical efficacy and ↑ their dose as required
RIFABUTIN	CARBAMAZEPINE	↓ Carbamazepine levels	Induction of metabolism	Monitor carbamazepine levels

(*Continued*)

Primary Drug	Secondary Drug	Effect	Mechanism	Precautions
ANTIBIOTICS				
RIFAMPICIN	LAMOTRIGINE	↓ Lamotrigine levels	↑ Metabolism	Monitor levels
RIFAMPICIN, RIFABUTIN	PHENYTOIN	↓ Phenytoin levels	Induced metabolism	Monitor phenytoin levels
RIFAMYCINS	**ANTIFUNGALS**			
RIFAMPICIN, RIFABUTIN, RIFAPENTINE	ITRACONAZOLE, KETOCONAZOLE, POSACONAZOLE, VORICONAZOLE	↓ Levels of these azoles, with significant risk of therapeutic failure. Rifampicin is a very potent inducer that can produce undetectable concentrations of ketoconazole	Rifampicin is a powerful inducer of CYP3A4 and other CYP isoenzymes. Rifabutin is a less powerful inducer but more potent than rifapentine. Rifapentine is an inducer of CYP3A4 and CYP2C8/9. Rifampicin is also a powerful inducer of Pgp, thus ↓ bioavailability of itraconazole	Avoid coadministration of ketoconazole or voriconazole with these drugs. Watch for inadequate therapeutic effects of itraconazole. Higher doses of itraconazole may not overcome this interaction, so consider the use of less lipophilic fluconazole, which is less dependent on CYP metabolism. Avoid coadministration of posaconazole with rifabutin
RIFABUTIN	VORICONAZOLE	↑ Plasma concentrations of rifabutin, with risk of toxic effects of rifabutin (nausea, vomiting). Dangerous toxic effects such as leukopenia and thrombocytopenia may occur	Due to inhibition of metabolism of rifabutin by the CYP3A4 isoenzymes by voriconazole	Avoid concomitant use. If absolutely necessary, close monitoring of FBC and liver enzymes and examination of eyes for uveitis and corneal opacities is necessary
RIFAMPICIN	CASPOFUNGIN	↓ Caspofungin levels, with risk of therapeutic failure	Induction of caspofungin metabolism	↑ Dose of caspofungin to 70 mg daily
RIFAMPICIN	TERBINAFINE	↓ Terbinafine levels	Induction of metabolism	Watch for poor response to terbinafine
RIFAMPICIN	**ANTIHYPERTENSIVES AND HEART FAILURE DRUGS**			
RIFAMPICIN	ACE INHIBITORS	↓ Plasma concentrations and efficacy of imidapril and enalapril	Uncertain; ↓ production of active metabolites has been noted despite rifampicin being an enzyme inducer	Monitor BP at least weekly until stable
RIFAMPICIN	ANGIOTENSIN II RECEPTOR ANTAGONISTS—LOSARTAN	↓ Antihypertensive effect of losartan	Rifampicin induces CYP2C9	Monitor BP at least weekly until stable

(Continued)

Primary Drug	Secondary Drug	Effect	Mechanism	Precautions
ANTIBIOTICS				
RIFAMPICIN	VASODILATOR ANTIHYPERTENSIVES	↓ Bosentan levels	Induction of metabolism	Avoid coadministration
RIFAMYCINS	ANTIMALARIALS—ATOVAQUONE	Both rifampicin and rifabutin ↓ atovaquone levels, although the effect is greater with rifampicin (↓ AUC 50% cf. with 34% rifabutin)	Uncertain because atovaquone is predominantly excreted unchanged via the gastrointestinal route	Avoid coadministration with rifampicin. Take care with rifabutin and watch for poor response to atovaquone
RIFAMPICIN	ANTIMIGRAINE DRUGS—ALMOTRIPTAN	Possible ↓ plasma concentrations of almotriptan, with risk of inadequate therapeutic efficacy	One of the major metabolizing enzymes of almotriptan—CYP3A4 isoenzymes—is induced by rifampicin. As there are alternative metabolic pathways, the effect may not be significant and could vary from individual to individual	Be aware of possibility of ↓ response to triptan and consider ↑ dose if the effect is considered to be due to interaction
RIFAMPICIN	ANTIPROTOZOALS—LEVAMISOLE	↓ Therapeutic efficacy of rifampicin	Levamisole displaces rifampicin from protein-binding sites and ↑ free fraction nearly three times and thus ↑ clearance of rifampicin	Avoid coadministration if possible
RIFABUTIN, RIFAMPICIN	ANTIPSYCHOTICS—ARIPIPRAZOLE, CLOZAPINE, HALOPERIDOL	↓ Levels of these antipsychotics	↑ Metabolism	Watch for poor response to these antipsychotics; consider ↑ dose
RIFAMYCINS	**ANTIVIRALS**			
RIFABUTIN	EFAVIRENZ	Possible ↓ efficacy of rifabutin	↓ Bioavailability	↑ Rifabutin dose by 50% for daily treatment, or double the dose if the patient is on treatment two or three times a week
RIFABUTIN	PROTEASE INHIBITORS	↑ Efficacy and ↑ adverse effects of rifabutin	Inhibition of CYP3A4-mediated metabolism. Nelfinavir also competitively inhibits 2C19	↓ Rifabutin dose by at least 50% when given with amprenavir, indinavir, or nelfinavir, and by 75% with atazanavir, ritonavir (with or without lopinavir), or tipranavir

(Continued)

Primary Drug	Secondary Drug	Effect	Mechanism	Precautions
ANTIBIOTICS				
RIFABUTIN	SAQUINAVIR	↓ Efficacy of saquinavir	Uncertain; probably via altered CYP3A4 metabolism	Avoid coadministration
RIFAMPICIN	EFAVIRENZ	Possible ↓ efficacy of efavirenz	Uncertain	↑ Dose of efavirenz from 600 to 800 mg
RIFAMPICIN	NEVIRAPINE	↓ Efficacy of nevirapine	Uncertain; probable ↑ metabolism of nevirapine	Avoid concomitant use. FDA recommends use only if clearly indicated and monitored closely
RIFAMPICIN	PROTEASE INHIBITORS	↓ Levels of protease inhibitor. Risk of hepatotoxicity with saquinavir	Induction of metabolism	Avoid coadministration
RIFAMPICIN	ZIDOVUDINE	↓ Levels of zidovudine (↓ AUC)	Mechanism-attributed to ↑ clearance of zidovudine	Avoid coadministration
RIFAMPICIN	**ANXIOLYTICS AND HYPNOTICS**			
RIFAMPICIN	BZDs, NOT LORAZEPAM, OXAZEPAM, TEMAZEPAM	↓ BZD levels	Induction of CYP3A4-mediated metabolism	Watch for poor response to these BZDs; consider ↑ dose, e.g., diazepam or nitrazepam 2–3-fold
RIFAMPICIN	BUSPIRONE	↓ Buspirone levels	Induction of CYP3A4-mediated metabolism	Watch for poor response to buspirone; consider ↑ dose
RIFAMPICIN	ZALEPLON, ZOLPIDEM, ZOPICLONE	↓ Levels of these hypnotics	Induction of CYP3A4-mediated metabolism	Watch for poor response to these agents
RIFAMPICIN	BETA-BLOCKERS	↓ Plasma concentrations and efficacy of bisoprolol, carvedilol, celiprolol, metoprolol, and propanolol	Rifampicin induces hepatic enzymes (e.g., CYP2C19), which ↑ metabolism of the beta-blockers; in addition, it may also ↑ Pgp expression	Monitor PR and BP; watch for poor response to beta-blockers
RIFAMPICIN	BRONCHODILATORS—THEOPHYLLINE	↓ Plasma concentrations of theophylline and risk of therapeutic failure	Due to induction of CYP1A2 and CYP3A	May need to ↑ dose of theophylline by 25%

(Continued)

Primary Drug	Secondary Drug	Effect	Mechanism	Precautions
ANTIBIOTICS				
RIFAMPICIN	CALCIUM CHANNEL BLOCKERS	Plasma concentrations of calcium channel blockers may be ↓ by rifampicin	Rifampicin induces CYP3A4-mediated metabolism of calcium channel blockers. It also induces CYP2C9-mediated metabolism of verapamil and induces intestinal Pgp, which may ↓ bioavailability of verapamil	Monitor BP closely; watch for ↓ effect of calcium channel blockers
RIFAMYCINS	**CARDIAC GLYCOSIDES**			
RIFAMPICIN	DIGOXIN	Plasma concentrations of digoxin may be ↓ by rifampicin	Rifampicin seems to induce Pgp-mediated excretion of digoxin in the kidneys	Watch for ↓ response to digoxin, check plasma levels, and ↑ dose as necessary
RIFAMPICIN	DIGITOXIN	Plasma concentrations of digitoxin may be halved by rifampicin	Due to ↑ hepatic metabolism	Watch for poor response to digitoxin
RIFAMPICIN, RIFABUTIN	CNS STIMULANTS—MODAFINIL	↓ Plasma concentrations of modafinil, with possibility of ↓ therapeutic effect	Induction of CYP3A4, which has a partial role in the metabolism of modafinil	Be aware
RIFAMPICIN	DIURETICS—POTASSIUM SPARING	↓ Eplerenone levels	Induction of metabolism	Avoid coadministration
RIFAMPICIN	DRUG DEPENDENCE THERAPIES—BUPROPION	↓ Plasma concentrations of bupropion and lack of therapeutic effect	Induction of CYP2B6	↑ Dose of bupropion cautiously
RIFAMPICIN	GESTRINONE	↓ Gestrinone levels	Induction of metabolism	Watch for poor response to gestrinone
RIFAMPICIN	H2 RECEPTOR BLOCKERS—CIMETIDINE	↓ Efficacy of cimetidine	↑ Metabolism	Change to alternative acid suppression, e.g., rabeprazole, or ↑ dose and/or frequency
RIFAMPICIN	LIPID-LOWERING DRUGS—STATINS	Rifampicin may lower fluvastatin and simvastatin levels	Uncertain	Monitor lipid profile closely; look for poor response to fluvastatin and simvastatin

(Continued)

Primary Drug	Secondary Drug	Effect	Mechanism	Precautions
ANTIBIOTICS				
RIFAMPICIN, RIFABUTIN	ESTROGENS	Marked ↓ contraceptive effect	Induction of metabolism of estrogens	Advise patients to use additional contraception for the period of intake and for 1 month after stopping coadministration of these drugs (4–8 weeks after stopping rifabutin or rifampicin)
RIFAMPICIN, RIFABUTIN	PROGESTOGENS	↓ Progesterone levels, which may lead to a failure of contraception or poor response to treatment of menorrhagia	Possibly induction of metabolism of progestogens	Advise patients to use additional contraception for the period of intake and 1 month after stopping coadministration of these drugs
RIFAMPICIN	TADALAFIL	↓ Tadalafil levels	Probable induction of metabolism	Watch for poor response
RIFAMPICIN	THYROID HORMONES	↓ Levothyroxine levels	Induction of metabolism	Monitor TFTs regularly and consider ↑ dose of levothyroxine
RIFAMPICIN	TIBOLONE	↓ Tibolone levels	Induction of metabolism of tibolone	Watch for poor response to tibolone; consider ↑ dose
SULFONAMIDES				
SULFONAMIDES	ANESTHETICS—GENERAL	↑ Effect of thiopentone but duration of action shortened	Uncertain; possibly displacement from protein-binding sites	Be aware that a smaller dose may be needed
SULFONAMIDES	**ANESTHETICS—LOCAL**			
SULFADIAZINE	LIDOCAINE SOLUTIONS	Precipitation of drugs, which may not be immediately apparent	A pharmaceutical interaction	Do not mix in the same infusion or syringe
SULFONAMIDES	PRILOCAINE	Risk of methemoglobinemia; there is a case report of methemoglobinemia with topical prilocaine in a patient taking sulfonamides	Additive effect	Avoid coadministration

(*Continued*)

Primary Drug	Secondary Drug	Effect	Mechanism	Precautions
ANTIBIOTICS				
SULFONAMIDES	**ANTIARRHYTHMICS**			
CO-TRIMOXAZOLE	AMIODARONE	Risk of ventricular arrhythmias	Uncertain	Avoid coadministration
TRIMETHOPRIM	PROCAINAMIDE	Procainamide levels are ↑ by trimethoprim	Trimethoprim is a potent inhibitor of organic cation transport in the kidney, and the elimination of procainamide is impaired	Watch for signs of procainamide toxicity; ↓ dose of procainamide, particularly in elderly patients
SULFONAMIDES	**ANTIBIOTICS**			
TRIMETHOPRIM	DAPSONE	↑ Levels of both drugs	Mutual inhibition of metabolism	Be aware—watch for ↑ incidence of side effects
SULFONAMIDES	METHENAMINE	Risk of crystalluria	Methenamine is only effective at a low pH, and this is achieved by acidifiers in the formulation. Sulfadiazine crystallizes in an acid environment	Avoid coadministration
SULFONAMIDES	**ANTICANCER AND IMMUNOMODULATING DRUGS**			
SULFONAMIDES	**CYTOTOXICS**			
CO-TRIMOXAZOLE	MERCAPTOPURINE	↑ Risk of bone marrow toxicity	Additive effect	Avoid coadministration
SULFAMETHOXAZOLE/ TRIMETHOPRIM	METHOTREXATE	↑ Plasma concentrations of methotrexate and risk of toxic effects of methotrexate, e.g., myelosuppression, liver cirrhosis, pulmonary toxicity	Sulfamethoxazole displaces methotrexate from plasma protein-binding sites and also ↓ renal elimination of methotrexate. Trimethoprim inhibits dihydrofolate reductase, which leads to additive toxic effects of methotrexate	Avoid concurrent use. If concurrent use is necessary, monitor clinically and biochemically for blood dyscrasias, liver toxicity, renal toxicity, and pulmonary toxicity

(*Continued*)

Primary Drug	Secondary Drug	Effect	Mechanism	Precautions
ANTIBIOTICS				
SULFONAMIDES	METHOTREXATE	↑ Plasma concentrations of methotrexate, with risk of toxic effects of methotrexate, e.g., liver cirrhosis, blood dyscrasias that may be fatal, pulmonary toxicity, stomatitis. Hematopoietic suppression can occur abruptly. Other adverse effects include anorexia, dyspepsia, gastrointestinal ulceration and bleeding, pulmonary edema	The mechanism differs from that caused by sulfamethoxazole–trimethoprim. Sulfonamides such as co-trimoxazole and sulfadiazine are known to cause renal dysfunction—interstitial nephritis, renal failure, which may ↓ excretion of methotrexate. Sulfonamides are also known to compete with methotrexate for renal elimination. Displacement from protein-binding sites of methotrexate is a minor contribution to the interaction	Although the toxic effects of methotrexate are more frequent with high doses of methotrexate, it is necessary to do FBC, liver and renal function tests before starting treatment even with low doses, repeating these tests weekly until therapy is stabilized and thereafter every 2–3 months. Patients should be advised to report symptoms such as sore throat and fever immediately, and also any gastrointestinal discomfort. A profound drop in white cell or platelet counts warrants immediate stoppage of methotrexate therapy and initiation of supportive therapy
SULFONAMIDES	PORFIMER	↑ Risk of photosensitivity reactions	Attributed to additive effects	Avoid exposure of skin and eyes to direct sunlight for 30 days after porfimer therapy
SULFONAMIDES	**ANTICANCER AND IMMUNOMODULATING DRUGS**			
ANTIBIOTICS—CO-TRIMOXAZOLE	AZATHIOPRINE	↑ Risk of leukopenia	Additive effects, as co-trimoxazole inhibits white cell production	Caution. ➢ ***For signs and symptoms of leukopenia, see Clinical Features of Some Adverse Drug Interactions, Immunosuppression, and blood dyscrasias***
CO-TRIMOXAZOLE	CICLOSPORIN	Exacerbates hyperkalemia induced by ciclosporin	Additive effect	Monitor serum potassium levels during coadministration. ➢ ***For signs and symptoms of hyperkalemia, see Clinical Features of Some Adverse Drug Interactions, Hyperkalemia***

(*Continued*)

Primary Drug	Secondary Drug	Effect	Mechanism	Precautions
ANTIBIOTICS				
CO-TRIMOXAZOLE	MYCOPHENOLATE	Exacerbates neutropenia caused by mycophenolate	Additive effect	Monitor blood count closely. ➢ ***For signs and symptoms of neutropenia, see Clinical Features of Some Adverse Drug Interactions, Immunosuppression and blood dyscrasias***
CO-TRIMOXAZOLE	SIROLIMUS	Exacerbates neutropenia caused by sirolimus	Additive effect	Monitor blood count closely. ➢ ***For signs and symptoms of neutropenia, see Clinical Features of Some Adverse Drug Interactions, Immunosuppression and blood dyscrasias***
CO-TRIMOXAZOLE	TACROLIMUS	Exacerbates hyperkalemia induced by tacrolimus	Additive hyperkalemic effects	Monitor electrolytes closely. ➢ ***For signs and symptoms of hyperkalemia, see Clinical Features of Some Adverse Drug Interactions, Hyperkalemia***
SULFONAMIDES, TRIMETHOPRIM	ANTICOAGULANTS—ORAL	↑ Anticoagulant effect	Inhibition of CYP2C9-mediated metabolism of oral anticoagulants	Monitor INR every 2–3 days
SULFONAMIDES	**ANTIDIABETIC DRUGS**			
TRIMETHOPRIM	PIOGLITAZONE, ROSIGLITAZONE	↑ In blood levels of rosiglitazone by nearly 40%	Trimethoprim is a relatively selective inhibitor of CYP2C8	Watch for hypoglycemic events and ↓ dose of rosiglitazone after repeated blood sugar measurements. Warn patients about hypoglycemia. ➢ ***For signs and symptoms of hypoglycemia, see Clinical Features of Some Adverse Drug Interactions, Hypoglycemia***
TRIMETHOPRIM	REPAGLINIDE	↑ Repaglinide levels (by approximately 40%); risk of hypoglycemia	Hepatic metabolism inhibited	Manufacturers do not recommend concurrent use

(Continued)

Primary Drug	Secondary Drug	Effect	Mechanism	Precautions
ANTIBIOTICS				
SULFONAMIDES, TRIMETHOPRIM	ANTIEPILEPTICS—PHENYTOIN	↑ Phenytoin levels	Inhibited metabolism	Monitor phenytoin levels
TRIMETHOPRIM	ANTIHYPERTENSIVES AND HEART FAILURE DRUGS—ACE INHIBITORS	Risk of hyperkalemia when trimethoprim is coadministered with ACE inhibitors in the presence of renal failure	Uncertain at present, but has been linked to sudden death	Avoid concurrent use in the presence of severe renal failure and in the elderly
ANTIBIOTICS—SULFONAMIDES, TRIMETHOPRIM	ANTIMALARIALS—PYRIMETHAMINE	↑ Antifolate effect	Additive effect	Monitor FBC closely; the effect may take a number of weeks to occur
SULFONAMIDES	ANTIPSYCHOTICS—CLOZAPINE	↑ Risk of bone marrow toxicity	Additive effect	Avoid coadministration
SULFONAMIDES	**ANTIVIRALS**			
TRIMETHOPRIM	GANCICLOVIR/ VALGANCICLOVIR	Possibly ↑ adverse effects (e.g., myelosuppression) when trimethoprim is coadministered with ganciclovir or valganciclovir	Small ↑ in bioavailability; possible additive toxicity	Well tolerated in a study. For patients at risk of additive toxicities, use only if benefits outweigh risks, and monitor FBC closely
CO-TRIMOXAZOLE	NUCLEOSIDE REVERSE TRANSCRIPTASE INHIBITORS	↑ Adverse effects	Additive toxicity	↓ Doses as necessary; monitor FBC and renal function closely. Doses of co-trimoxazole used for prophylaxis seem to be tolerated
TRIMETHOPRIM	NUCLEOSIDE REVERSE TRANSCRIPTASE INHIBITORS	Possibly ↑ hematological toxicity	Competition for renal excretion	Monitor FBC and renal function closely
TRIMETHOPRIM, CO-TRIMOXAZOLE	CARDIAC GLYCOSIDES—DIGOXIN	Trimethoprim may ↑ plasma concentrations of digoxin, particularly in elderly people	Uncertain; postulated that trimethoprim ↓ renal clearance of digoxin	Monitor digoxin levels; watch for digoxin toxicity
TRIMETHOPRIM	DIURETICS—POTASSIUM-SPARING	Risk of hyperkalemia when trimethoprim is coadministered with eplerenone	Additive effect	Monitor potassium levels closely
ANTIBIOTICS—CO-TRIMOXAZOLE	LOPERAMIDE	↑ Loperamide levels but no evidence of toxicity	Inhibition of metabolism	Be aware

(Continued)

Primary Drug	Secondary Drug	Effect	Mechanism	Precautions
ANTIBIOTICS				
SULFONAMIDES	ESTROGENS	Reports of ↓ contraceptive effect	Possibly alteration of the bacterial flora necessary for recycling ethinylestradiol from the large bowel, although not certain in every case	Advise patients to use additional contraception for the period of antibiotic intake and for 1 month after stopping the antibiotic
TETRACYCLINES				
TETRACYCLINES	ANTACIDS	↓ Levels of these antibiotics	↓ Absorption	Separate tetracyclines and antacids by 2–3 h
TETRACYCLINES	**ANTICANCER AND IMMUNOMODULATING DRUGS**			
DOXYCYCLINE	CICLOSPORIN	↑ Levels of ciclosporin leading to risk of nephrotoxicity, hepatotoxicity, and possibly neurotoxicity such as hallucinations, convulsions, and coma	The mechanism is not known, but doxycycline is thought to ↑ ciclosporin levels	Concomitant use in transplant patients should be well monitored with frequent assays of ciclosporin levels. In nontransplant patients, renal function should be monitored closely and patients warned about potential side effects such as back pain, flushing, and gastrointestinal upset. The dose of ciclosporin should be ↓ appropriately
DOXYCYCLINE, TETRACYCLINE	METHOTREXATE	↑ Plasma concentrations of methotrexate, with a risk of toxic effects of methotrexate, e.g., liver cirrhosis, blood dyscrasias that may be fatal, pulmonary toxicity, stomatitis. Hematopoietic suppression can occur abruptly. Other adverse effects include anorexia, dyspepsia, gastrointestinal ulceration and bleeding, and pulmonary edema	Tetracyclines destroy the bacterial flora necessary for the breakdown of methotrexate. This results in ↑ free methotrexate concentrations. Tetracyclines are also considered to inhibit the elimination of methotrexate and allow a buildup of methotrexate in the bladder. The effects of the interaction are often delayed	Although the toxic effects of methotrexate are more frequent with high doses of methotrexate, it is necessary to do FBC, liver and renal function tests before starting treatment even with low doses, repeating these tests weekly until therapy is stabilized and thereafter every 2–3 months. The patients should be advised to report symptoms such as sore throat and fever immediately, and also any gastrointestinal discomfort. A profound drop in white cell or platelet counts warrants immediate stoppage of methotrexate therapy and initiation of supportive therapy

(Continued)

Primary Drug	Secondary Drug	Effect	Mechanism	Precautions
ANTIBIOTICS				
TETRACYCLINES	PORFIMER	↑ Risk of photosensitivity reactions	Attributed to additive effects	Avoid exposure of skin and eyes to direct sunlight for 30 days after porfimer therapy
TETRACYCLINE	RETINOIDS	Risk of benign intracranial hypertension with tetracycline	Unknown	Avoid coadministration
TETRACYCLINES	ANTICOAGULANTS—ORAL	Additive effects of warfarin and oxytetracycline, leading to prolongation of the prothrombin time or INR and bleeding	Tetracyclines have been associated with ↓ prothrombin activity, causing hypoprothrombinemia and bleeding. Tetracyclines may also ↓ intestinal flora of the gut, depleting the body of vitamin K2; this may only be significant if the patient's diet is low in vitamin K1	Monitor INR closely and adjust the dose of warfarin accordingly. Patients should be alert for signs of overanticoagulation, bleeding from the gums when brushing their teeth, nosebleeds, unusual bruising, and weakness
DOXYCYCLINE	ANTIEPILEPTICS—BARBITURATES, CARBAMAZEPINE, PHENYTOIN	↓ Doxycycline levels, with risk of therapeutic failure	Induction of hepatic metabolism	Monitor for ↓ clinical efficacy and ↑ dose as required
TETRACYCLINES	ANTIHYPERTENSIVES AND HEART FAILURE DRUGS—ACE INHIBITORS	↓ Plasma concentrations and efficacy of tetracyclines with quinapril	Magnesium carbonate (found in a formulation of quinapril) chelates with tetracyclines in the gut to form a less soluble substance that ↓ absorption of tetracycline	For short-term antibiotic use, consider stopping quinapril for the duration of the course. For long-term use, consider an alternative ACE inhibitor
TETRACYCLINE	ANTIMALARIALS—ATOVAQUONE	↓ Atovaquone levels (40%)	Uncertain	Not clinically significant; combination therapy has been used effectively
TETRACYCLINES	ANTIMIGRAINE DRUGS—ERGOT DERIVATIVES	Cases of ergotism with tetracyclines and ergotamine	Uncertain	Avoid coadministration. If absolutely necessary, advise patients to discontinue treatment immediately if numbness and tingling of the extremities are felt

(Continued)

Primary Drug	Secondary Drug	Effect	Mechanism	Precautions
ANTIBIOTICS				
TETRACYCLINES	ANTIVIRALS—DIDANOSINE	↓ Efficacy of tetracycline, and possibly demeclocycline, doxycycline, lymecycline, minocycline, and oxytetracycline, with buffered didanosine	Absorption may be affected by the buffered didanosine formulation, which ↑ gastric pH	Avoid coadministration with buffered didanosine preparations. Consider changing to enteric-coated didanosine tablets
TETRACYCLINES	CALCIUM	↓ Antibiotic levels	↓ Absorption	Separate doses by at least 2 h
TETRACYCLINES	DAIRY PRODUCTS	↓ Antibiotic levels	↓ Absorption (due to the calcium content of dairy produce)	Separate doses by at least 2 h
TETRACYCLINES	DIURETICS	Possible risk of renal toxicity	Additive effect	Some recommend avoiding coadministration; others advise monitoring renal function closely. Doxycycline is likely to be less of a problem
DOXYCYCLINE	H2 RECEPTOR BLOCKERS	↓ Plasma concentrations and risk of treatment failure	↓ Absorption of doxycycline as ↑ gastric pH	Avoid concomitant use. If unable to avoid combination, take H2 antagonists at least 2–3 h after cephalosporin. Consider an alternative antibiotic or separate the doses by at least 2 h and give with an acidic drink, e.g., carbonated drink; ↑ dose may be required
TETRACYCLINES	IRON—ORAL	1. ↓ Iron levels when iron given orally 2. ↓ Plasma concentrations of tetracycline's with risk of therapeutic failure	1. ↓ Absorption 2. Iron chelates with tetracyclines and ↓ their absorption	1. Separate doses as much as possible—monitor FBC closely 2. Separate doses of other drugs as much as possible and monitor their effect
TETRACYCLINES	KAOLIN	↓ Tetracycline levels	↓ Absorption	Separate doses by at least 2 h
TETRACYCLINE	LIPID-LOWERING DRUGS—ANION EXCHANGE RESINS	↓ Levels of tetracycline and possible therapeutic failure	Tetracycline binds with colestipol and colestyramine in the gut, therefore ↓ its absorption	Dosing should be as separate as possible

(*Continued*)

DRUGS TO TREAT INFECTIONS OTHER ANTIBIOTICS Chloramphenicol

Primary Drug	Secondary Drug	Effect	Mechanism	Precautions
ANTIBIOTICS				
TETRACYCLINES	ESTROGENS	Reports of ↓ contraceptive effect	Possibly alteration of the bacterial flora necessary for recycling ethinylestradiol from the large bowel, although not certain in every case	Advise patients to use additional contraception for the period of antibiotic intake and for 1 month after stopping the antibiotic
TETRACYCLINE	SODIUM BICARBONATE	↓ Tetracycline levels and possible therapeutic failure	It is suggested that when sodium bicarbonate alkalinizes the urine, the renal excretion of tetracycline is ↑.	The interaction can be minimized by separating their dosing by 3–4 h
TETRACYCLINES	STRONTIUM RANELATE	↓ Levels of tetracycline's	↓ Absorption	Avoid coadministration
TETRACYCLINES	SUCRALFATE	↓ Levels of these antibiotics	↓ Absorption of these antibiotics	Give the antibiotics at least 2 h before sucralfate
TETRACYCLINES	TRIPOTASSIUM DICITRATOBISMUTHATE	↓ Levels of tetracyclines	↓ Absorption of tetracyclines	Separate doses by 2–3 h
TETRACYCLINES	ZINC	↓ Antibiotic levels; less of a problem with doxycycline	↓ Absorption	Separate doses by at least 2 h; alternatively, consider giving doxycycline

Primary Drug	Secondary Drug	Effect	Mechanism	Precautions
OTHER ANTIBIOTICS				
CHLORAMPHENICOL				
CHLORAMPHENICOL	ANTICANCER AND IMMUNOMODULATING DRUGS—TACROLIMUS	Toxic blood levels of tacrolimus, usually on the second day of starting chloramphenicol	Attributed to impaired clearance of tacrolimus by chloramphenicol	↓ Dose of nearly 80% of tacrolimus may be required to prevent toxicity. Watch for adverse effects (see below). Monitor tacrolimus plasma concentrations
CHLORAMPHENICOL	ANTICOAGULANTS—ORAL	Occasional episodes of ↑ anticoagulant effect	Uncertain at present	Monitor INR every 2–3 days
CHLORAMPHENICOL	ANTIDIABETIC DRUGS—SULFONYLUREAS	Possibly ↓ hypoglycemic effect of sulfonylureas	Mechanism uncertain. Chloramphenicol is an inhibitor of CYP3A4	Be aware

(Continued)

Primary Drug	Secondary Drug	Effect	Mechanism	Precautions
OTHER ANTIBIOTICS				
CHLORAMPHENICOL	**ANTIEPILEPTICS**			
CHLORAMPHENICOL	BARBITURATES	↓ Levels of chloramphenicol	Induction of hepatic metabolism	1. Avoid coadministration of telithromycin for up to 2 weeks after stopping phenobarbital 2. With the other drugs, monitor for ↓ clinical efficacy, and ↑ their dose as required
CHLORAMPHENICOL	PHENYTOIN	↑ Phenytoin levels	Inhibited metabolism	Monitor phenytoin levels
CHLORAMPHENICOL	ANTIPSYCHOTICS—CLOZAPINE	↑ Risk of bone marrow toxicity	Additive effect	Avoid coadministration
CHLORAMPHENICOL	ANTIVIRALS—STAVUDINE, ZIDOVUDINE	Possible ↑ adverse effects when coadministered with stavudine or zidovudine	Uncertain	Use an alternative antibiotic if possible; otherwise, monitor closely for peripheral neuropathy and check FBC regularly
CHLORAMPHENICOL	CNS STIMULANTS—MODAFINIL	May cause moderate ↑ plasma concentrations of chloramphenicol	Modafinil is a reversible inhibitor of CYP2C19 when used in therapeutic doses	Be aware
CHLORAMPHENICOL	H2 RECEPTOR BLOCKERS—CIMETIDINE	↑ Adverse effects of chloramphenicol, e.g., bone marrow depression	Additive toxicity	Use with caution, monitor FBC regularly
CHLORAMPHENICOL	IRON	↓ Efficacy of iron	Chloramphenicol depresses the bone marrow; this opposes the action of iron	Be aware; monitor FBC and ferritin levels closely
CHLORAMPHENICOL	ESTROGENS	Reports of ↓ contraceptive effect	Possibly alteration of the bacterial flora necessary for recycling ethinylestradiol from the large bowel, although not certain in every case	Advise patients to use additional contraception for the period of antibiotic intake and for 1 month after stopping the antibiotic
CHLORAMPHENICOL	VITAMIN B12	↓ Efficacy of hydroxycobalamin	Chloramphenicol depresses the bone marrow; this opposes the action of vitamin B12	Be aware; monitor FBC and vitamin B12 levels closely

(*Continued*)

Primary Drug	Secondary Drug	Effect	Mechanism	Precautions
OTHER ANTIBIOTICS				
CLINDAMYCIN				
CLINDAMYCIN	MUSCLE RELAXANTS—DEPOLARIZING, NONDEPOLARIZING	↑ Efficacy of these muscle relaxants	Clindamycin has some neuromuscular blocking activity	Monitor neuromuscular blockade carefully
CLINDAMYCIN	ESTROGENS	Reports of ↓ contraceptive effect	Possibly alteration of the bacterial flora necessary for recycling ethinylestradiol from the large bowel, although not certain in every case	Advise patients to use additional contraception for the period of antibiotic intake and for 1 month after stopping the antibiotic
CLINDAMYCIN	PARASYMPATHOMIMETICS—NEOSTIGMINE, PYRIDOSTIGMINE	↓ Efficacy of neostigmine and pyridostigmine	Uncertain	Watch for poor response to these parasympathomimetics and ↑ dose accordingly
COLISTIN				
COLISTIN	**ANTIBIOTICS**			
COLISTIN	AMINOGLYCOSIDES	↑ Risk of nephrotoxicity	Additive effect	Renal function should be carefully monitored
COLISTIN	TEICOPLANIN, VANCOMYCIN	↑ Risk of nephrotoxicity and ototoxicity	Additive effect	Hearing and renal function should be carefully monitored
COLISTIN	**ANTICANCER AND IMMUNOMODULATING DRUGS**			
COLISTIN	CICLOSPORIN	↑ Risk of nephrotoxicity	Additive nephrotoxic effects	Monitor renal function
COLISTIN	PLATINUM COMPOUNDS	↑ Risk of additive renal and ototoxicity. The ototoxicity tends to occur when cisplatin is administered early during the course of aminoglycoside therapy	Additive toxic effects	Monitor renal function and hearing prior to and during therapy, and ensure the intake of at least 2 L of fluid daily. Monitor serum potassium and magnesium levels and correct any deficiencies. Most side effects of aminoglycosides are dose related, and it is necessary to ↑ interval between doses and ↓ dose.

(*Continued*)

Primary Drug	Secondary Drug	Effect	Mechanism	Precautions
OTHER ANTIBIOTICS				
COLISTIN	ANTIFUNGALS—AMPHOTERICIN	Risk of renal failure	Additive effect	Monitor renal function closely
COLISTIN	DIURETICS—LOOP	↑ Risk of ototoxicity and possible deafness as a result of concomitant use of furosemide and colistin	Additive effect	If used concurrently, patients should be monitored for any hearing impairment
COLISTIN	MUSCLE RELAXANTS—DEPOLARIZING, NONDEPOLARIZING	↑ Efficacy of these muscle relaxants	Colistin has some neuromuscular blocking activity	Monitor neuromuscular blockade carefully
COLISTIN	PARASYMPATHOMIMETICS—NEOSTIGMINE, PYRIDOSTIGMINE	↓ Efficacy of neostigmine and pyridostigmine	Uncertain	Watch for poor response to these parasympathomimetics and ↑ dose accordingly
CYCLOSERINE				
CYCLOSERINE	ALCOHOL	Risk of fits	Additive effect; cycloserine can cause fits	Warn patients to drink alcohol minimally while taking cycloserine
CYCLOSERINE	ISONIAZID	Risk of drowsiness and dizziness	Uncertain	Be aware; watch for ↑ sedation
DAPSONE				
DAPSONE	**ANTIBIOTICS**			
DAPSONE	RIFAMYCINS	↓ Levels of dapsone	Rifamycins induce metabolism of dapsone	Watch for poor response to dapsone
DAPSONE	TRIMETHOPRIM	↑ Levels of both drugs	Mutual inhibition of metabolism	Be aware—watch for ↑ incidence of side effects
DAPSONE	ANTICANCER DRUGS—PORFIMER	↑ Risk of photosensitivity reactions	Attributed to additive effects	Avoid exposure of skin and eyes to direct sunlight for 30 days after porfimer therapy
DAPSONE	ANTIGOUT DRUGS	Levels of probenecid may also ↑	Decreased clearance of both drugs	Monitor FBC closely
DAPSONE	ANTIVIRALS—ZIDOVUDINE	Possible ↑ adverse effects when coadministered with zidovudine	Uncertain; possible ↑ bioavailability of zidovudine	Use with caution; monitor for peripheral neuropathy

(Continued)

Primary Drug	Secondary Drug	Effect	Mechanism	Precautions
OTHER ANTIBIOTICS				
DAPTOMYCIN				
DAPTOMYCIN	ANTICANCER DRUGS—CICLOSPORIN	Risk of myopathy	Additive effect	Avoid coadministration
DAPTOMYCIN	LIPID-LOWERING DRUGS—FIBRATES, STATINS	Risk of myopathy	Additive effect	Avoid coadministration
ETHAMBUTOL				
ETHAMBUTOL	ANTIVIRALS—DIDANOSINE	Possibly ↑ adverse effects (e.g., peripheral neuropathy) with didanosine	Additive side effects	Monitor closely for development of peripheral neuropathy, but no dose adjustment is required
FUSIDIC ACID				
FUSIDIC ACID	ANTIVIRALS—PROTEASE INHIBITORS	Possibly ↑ adverse effects	Inhibition of CYP3A4-mediated metabolism of fusidic acid	Avoid coadministration
FUSIDIC ACID	LIPID-LOWERING DRUGS—STATINS	Cases of rhabdomyolysis reported when fusidic acid was coadministered with atorvastatin or simvastatin	Uncertain at present	Monitor LFTs and CK closely; warn patients to report any features of rhabdomyolysis
ISONIAZID				
ISONIAZID	ANALGESICS—PARACETAMOL	Risk of paracetamol toxicity at regular therapeutic doses when coadministered with isoniazid	Uncertain; it seems that the formation of toxic metabolites is ↑ in fast acetylators when isoniazid levels ↓ (i.e., at the end of a dosing period)	There have been cases of hepatic pathology; regular paracetamol should be avoided in those taking isoniazid
ISONIAZID	ANTACIDS	↓ Levels of these antibiotics	↓ Absorption	Separate isoniazid and antacids by 2–3 h
ISONIAZID	ANTIBIOTICS—CYCLOSERINE	Risk of drowsiness and dizziness	Uncertain	Be aware; watch for ↑ sedation
ISONIAZID	ANTIDIABETIC DRUGS	↓ Efficacy of antidiabetic drugs	Isoniazid causes hyperglycemia, the mechanism is uncertain at present	Monitor capillary blood glucose levels closely; ↑ doses of antidiabetic drugs may be needed

(Continued)

Primary Drug	Secondary Drug	Effect	Mechanism	Precautions
OTHER ANTIBIOTICS				
ISONIAZID	**ANTIEPILEPTICS**			
ISONIAZID	CARBAMAZEPINE	↑ Carbamazepine levels	Inhibited metabolism	Monitor carbamazepine levels
ISONIAZID	ETHOSUXIMIDE	Case of ↑ ethosuximide levels with toxicity	Inhibition of metabolism	Watch for early features of ethosuximide toxicity
ISONIAZID	PHENYTOIN	↑ Phenytoin levels	Inhibited metabolism	Monitor phenytoin levels
ISONIAZID	ANTIFUNGALS—ITRACONAZOLE, KETOCONAZOLE, POSACONAZOLE, VORICONAZOLE	↓ Levels of these azoles, with significant risk of therapeutic failure	Isoniazid is a known inhibitor of CYP2E1 and is likely to induce other CYP isoenzymes to varying degrees, usually in a time-dependent manner	Avoid coadministration of ketoconazole or voriconazole with isoniazid. Watch for inadequate therapeutic effects of itraconazole. Higher doses of itraconazole may not overcome this interaction, so consider the use of less lipophilic fluconazole, which is less dependent on CYP metabolism
ISONIAZID	ANTIVIRALS—NUCLEOSIDE REVERSE TRANSCRIPTASE INHIBITORS	↑ Adverse effects with didanosine and possibly stavudine	Additive side effects	Monitor closely for the development of peripheral neuropathy, but no dose adjustment is required
ISONIAZID	ANXIOLYTICS AND HYPNOTICS—DIAZEPAM	↑ Diazepam levels	Inhibited metabolism	Watch for excessive sedation; consider ↓ dose of diazepam
ISONIAZID	BRONCHODILATORS—THEOPHYLLINE	↑ Theophylline levels	Uncertain	Monitor theophylline levels before, during, and after coadministration
LINEZOLID ➢ ***Drugs Acting on the Nervous System, Antidepressants, Monoamine oxidase inhibitors***				
METHENAMINE				
METHENAMINE	ANTIBIOTICS—SULFONAMIDES—SULFADIAZINE	Risk of crystalluria	Methenamine is only effective at a low pH, and this is achieved by acidifiers in the formulation. Sulfadiazine crystallizes in an acid environment	Avoid coadministration

(*Continued*)

Primary Drug	Secondary Drug	Effect	Mechanism	Precautions
OTHER ANTIBIOTICS				
METHENAMINE	DIURETICS—CARBONIC ANHYDRASE INHIBITORS	↓ Efficacy of methenamine	Methenamine is only effective at a low pH; raising the urinary pH ↓ its effect	Avoid coadministration
METHENAMINE	POTASSIUM CITRATE	↓ Efficacy of methenamine	Methenamine is only effective at a low pH; raising the urinary pH ↓ its effect	Avoid coadministration
METHENAMINE	SODIUM BICARBONATE	↓ Efficacy of methenamine	Methenamine is only effective at a low pH; raising the urinary pH ↓ its effect	Avoid coadministration
METRONIDAZOLE				
METRONIDAZOLE	ALCOHOL	Disulfiram-like reaction	Metronidazole inhibits aldehyde dehydrogenase	Avoid coingestion
METRONIDAZOLE	**ANTICANCER AND IMMUNOMODULATING DRUGS**			
METRONIDAZOLE	BUSULFAN	↑ Busulfan levels	Uncertain	Watch for early features of toxicity
METRONIDAZOLE	FLUOROURACIL	↑ Risk of toxic effects of fluorouracil (>27%), e.g., bone marrow suppression, oral ulceration, nausea, and vomiting due to ↑ plasma concentrations of fluorouracil	Metronidazole ↓ clearance of fluorouracil	Avoid coadministration
METRONIDAZOLE	MYCOPHENOLATE	Likely ↓ in plasma concentration of mycophenolate	Theoretically, drugs that alter gastrointestinal flora may ↓ oral bioavailability of mycophenolic acid products by ↓ bacterial hydrolytic enzymes that are responsible for regenerating mycophenolic acid from its glucuronide metabolites following first-pass metabolism	Avoid coadministration

(Continued)

Primary Drug	Secondary Drug	Effect	Mechanism	Precautions
OTHER ANTIBIOTICS				
METRONIDAZOLE	ANTICOAGULANTS—ORAL	↑ Anticoagulant effect	Inhibition of CYP2C9-mediated metabolism of oral anticoagulants	Monitor INR every 2–3 days
METRONIDAZOLE	LITHIUM	↑ Plasma concentrations of lithium, with risk of toxicity	Uncertain; ↓ renal clearance of lithium	Obtain serum lithium levels and serum creatinine before starting metronidazole and continue monitoring serum lithium and creatinine levels until stable.
METRONIDAZOLE	**ANTIEPILEPTICS**			
METRONIDAZOLE	BARBITURATES	↓ Levels of these drugs, with risk of therapeutic failure	Induction of hepatic metabolism. Unlikely with topical metronidazole	1. Avoid coadministration of metronidazole for up to 2 weeks after stopping phenobarbital
METRONIDAZOLE	PHENYTOIN	↑ Phenytoin levels	Inhibited metabolism	Monitor phenytoin levels
METRONIDAZOLE	**ANTIVIRALS**			
METRONIDAZOLE	DIDANOSINE, STAVUDINE	↑ Adverse effects (e.g., peripheral neuropathy) with didanosine and possibly stavudine	Additive effect	Monitor closely for peripheral neuropathy during intensive or prolonged combination
METRONIDAZOLE	PROTEASE INHIBITORS	↑ Adverse effects, e.g., disulfiram-like reaction, flushing, with ritonavir (with or without lopinavir)	Ritonavir and lopinavir oral solutions contain alcohol	Warn patients and give alternative preparation if possible
METRONIDAZOLE	DRUG DEPENDENCE THERAPIES—DISULFIRAM	Report of psychosis	Additive effect; both drugs may cause neurological/psychiatric side effects (disulfiram by inhibiting metabolism of dopamine, metronidazole by an unknown mechanism)	Caution with coadministration. Warn patients and carers to watch for early features
METRONIDAZOLE	H2 RECEPTOR BLOCKERS—CIMETIDINE	↑ Metronidazole levels	Inhibited metabolism	Watch for ↑ side effects of metronidazole
METRONIDAZOLE	ESTROGENS	Reports of ↓ contraceptive effect	Possibly alteration of the bacterial flora necessary for recycling ethinylestradiol from the large bowel, although not certain in every case	Advise patients to use additional contraception for the period of antibiotic intake and for 1 month after stopping the antibiotic

(*Continued*)

Primary Drug	Secondary Drug	Effect	Mechanism	Precautions
OTHER ANTIBIOTICS				
NITROFURANTOIN				
NITROFURANTOIN	ANTACIDS	↓ Levels of these antibiotics	↓ Absorption	Separate nitrofurantoin and antacids by 2–3 h
NITROFURANTOIN	ANTIGOUT DRUGS—PROBENECID, SULFINPYRAZONE	↓ Efficacy of nitrofurantoin in urinary tract infections	↓ Urinary excretion	Watch for poor response to nitrofurantoin
PYRAZINAMIDE				
PYRAZINAMIDE	ANTIGOUT DRUGS	↓ Efficacy of antigout drugs	Pyrazinamide can induce hyperuricemia	Pyrazinamide should not be used in patients with gout
QUINUPRISTIN/DALFOPRISTIN				
QUINUPRISTIN/ DALFOPRISTIN	**DRUGS THAT PROLONG THE QT INTERVAL**			
QUINUPRISTIN/ DALFOPRISTIN	1. ANTIARRHYTHMICS—amiodarone, disopyramide, procainamide, propafenone 2. ANTIBIOTICS—macrolides (especially azithromycin, clarithromycin, parenteral erythromycin, telithromycin), quinolones (especially moxifloxacin) 3. ANTICANCER AND IMMUNOMODULATING DRUGS—arsenic trioxide 4. ANTIDEPRESSANTS—TCAs, venlafaxine 5. ANTIEMETICS—dolasetron 6. ANTIFUNGALS—fluconazole, posaconazole, voriconazole 7. ANTIHISTAMINES—terfenadine, hydroxyzine, mizolastine 8. ANTIMALARIALS—artemether with lumefantrine, chloroquine, hydroxychloroquine, mefloquine, quinine	Risk of ventricular arrhythmias, particularly torsades de pointes	Additive effect; these drugs cause prolongation of the QT interval	Avoid coadministration

(Continued)

Primary Drug	Secondary Drug	Effect	Mechanism	Precautions
OTHER ANTIBIOTICS				
	9. ANTIPROTOZOALS—pentamidine isetionate 10. ANTIPSYCHOTICS—atypicals, phenothiazines, pimozide 11. BETA-BLOCKERS—sotalol 12. BRONCHODILATORS—parenteral bronchodilators 13. CNS STIMULANTS—atomoxetine			
QUINUPRISTIN/ DALFOPRISTIN	ANESTHETICS—LOCAL—LIDOCAINE	Risk of arrhythmias	Additive effect when lidocaine given intravenously	Avoid coadministration of quinupristin/dalfopristin with intravenous lidocaine
QUINUPRISTIN/ DALFOPRISTIN	ANTIBIOTICS—RIFAMPICIN	Risk of hepatic toxicity	Additive effect	Monitor LFTs closely
QUINUPRISTIN/ DALFOPRISTIN	ANTICANCER AND IMMUNOMODULATING DRUGS—CICLOSPORIN	↑ Plasma concentrations of immunosuppressants. ↑ risk of infections and toxic effects of ciclosporin	Due to inhibition of CYP3A4-mediated metabolism of ciclosporin	Monitor renal function prior to concurrent therapy, and blood count and ciclosporin levels during therapy. Warn patients to report symptoms (fever, sore throat) immediately
QUINUPRISTIN/ DALFOPRISTIN	ANTIMIGRAINE DRUGS—ERGOT DERIVATIVES	↑ Ergotamine/ methysergide levels, with risk of toxicity	Inhibition of CYP3A4-mediated metabolism of the ergot derivatives	Avoid coadministration
QUINUPRISTIN/ DALFOPRISTIN	ANXIOLYTICS AND HYPNOTICS—MIDAZOLAM	↑ Midazolam levels	Inhibited metabolism	Watch for excessive sedation; consider ↓ dose of midazolam
QUINUPRISTIN/ DALFOPRISTIN	CALCIUM CHANNEL BLOCKERS	Plasma levels of nifedipine may be ↑ by quinupristin/dalfopristin	Quinupristin inhibits CYP3A4-mediated metabolism of calcium channel blockers	Monitor BP closely; watch for ↓ BP
TEICOPLANIN				
TEICOPLANIN	ANTIBIOTICS—AMINOGLYCOSIDES, COLISTIN, VANCOMYCIN	↑ Risk of nephrotoxicity and ototoxicity	Additive effect	Hearing and renal function should be carefully monitored

(Continued)

Primary Drug	Secondary Drug	Effect	Mechanism	Precautions
OTHER ANTIBIOTICS				
VANCOMYCIN				
VANCOMYCIN	ANTIBIOTICS—AMINOGLYCOSIDES, COLISTIN, TEICOPLANIN	↑ Risk of nephrotoxicity and ototoxicity	Additive effect	Hearing and renal function should be carefully monitored
VANCOMYCIN	**ANTICANCER AND IMMUNOMODULATING DRUGS**			
VANCOMYCIN	CICLOSPORIN	Risk of renal toxicity and ototoxicity	Additive toxic effects	Monitor renal function closely
VANCOMYCIN	PLATINUM COMPOUNDS	↑ Risk of renal toxicity and renal failure, and of ototoxicity	Additive renal toxicity	Monitor renal function and hearing prior to and during therapy, and ensure the intake of at least 2 L of fluid daily. Monitor serum potassium, and magnesium levels, and correct any deficiencies
VANCOMYCIN	TACROLIMUS	Risk of renal toxicity	Additive effect	Monitor renal function closely
VANCOMYCIN	ANTIFUNGALS—AMPHOTERICIN	Risk of renal failure	Additive effect	Monitor renal function closely
VANCOMYCIN	**ANTIVIRALS**			
VANCOMYCIN	ADEFOVIR DIPIVOXIL	Possible ↑ efficacy and side effects	Competition for renal excretion	Monitor renal function weekly
VANCOMYCIN	NUCLEOSIDE REVERSE TRANSCRIPTASE INHIBITORS—TENOFOVIR, ZIDOVUDINE	↑ Adverse effects with zidovudine and possibly tenofovir	Additive toxicity	Monitor FBC and renal function closely (at least weekly)
VANCOMYCIN	DIURETICS—LOOP	Risk of renal toxicity	Additive effect	Monitor renal function closely
VANCOMYCIN (ORAL)	LIPID-LOWERING DRUGS—ANION EXCHANGE RESINS	↓ Vancomycin levels	Inhibition of absorption	Separate doses as much as possible
VANCOMYCIN	MUSCLE RELAXANTS—DEPOLARIZING, NONDEPOLARIZING	1. ↑ Efficacy of these muscle relaxants 2. Possible risk of hypersensitivity reactions	1. Vancomycin has some neuromuscular blocking activity 2. Animal studies suggest an additive effect on histamine release	1. Monitor neuromuscular blockade carefully 2. Be aware
VANCOMYCIN	SYMPATHOMIMETICS	Vancomycin levels are ↓ by dobutamine or dopamine	Uncertain at present	Monitor vancomycin levels closely

Primary Drug	Secondary Drug	Effect	Mechanism	Precautions
ANTIFUNGAL DRUGS				
AMPHOTERICIN				
AMPHOTERICIN	ANESTHETICS—LOCAL—LIDOCAINE AND PROCAINE SOLUTIONS	Precipitation of drugs, which may not be immediately apparent	A pharmaceutical interaction	Do not mix in the same infusion or syringe
AMPHOTERICIN	ANTIBIOTICS—AMINOGLYCOSIDES, COLISTIN, VANCOMYCIN	Risk of renal failure	Additive effect	Monitor renal function closely
AMPHOTERICIN	**ANTICANCER AND IMMUNOMODULATING DRUGS**			
AMPHOTERICIN	CYTOTOXICS—PLATINUM COMPOUNDS	↑ Risk of renal toxicity and renal failure	Additive renal toxicity	Monitor renal function prior to and during therapy, and ensure the intake of at least 2 L of fluid daily. Monitor serum potassium and magnesium levels, and correct any deficiencies
AMPHOTERICIN	**IMMUNOMODULATING DRUGS**			
AMPHOTERICIN	CICLOSPORIN	↑ Risk of nephrotoxicity	Additive nephrotoxic effects	Monitor renal function
AMPHOTERICIN	CORTICOSTEROIDS	Risk of hyperkalemia	Additive effect	Avoid coadministration
AMPHOTERICIN	TACROLIMUS	Risk of renal toxicity	Additive effect	Monitor renal function closely
AMPHOTERICIN	ANTIFUNGALS—FLUCYTOSINE	↑ Flucytosine levels, with risk of toxic effects	Amphotericin causes ↓ renal excretion of flucytosine and ↑ cellular uptake	The combination of flucytosine and amphotericin may be used therapeutically. Watch for early features of flucytosine toxicity (gastrointestinal upset); monitor renal and liver functions closely
AMPHOTERICIN	ANTIPROTOZOALS—PENTAMIDINE ISETIONATE	Risk of arrhythmias	Additive effect	Monitor ECG closely
AMPHOTERICIN	**ANTIVIRALS**			
AMPHOTERICIN	ADEFOVIR DIPIVOXIL	Possible ↑ efficacy and side effects	Competition for renal excretion	Monitor renal function weekly
AMPHOTERICIN	FOSCARNET SODIUM	Possible ↑ nephrotoxicity	Additive side effect	Monitor renal function closely
AMPHOTERICIN	NUCLEOSIDE REVERSE TRANSCRIPTASE INHIBITORS—TENOFOVIR, ZIDOVUDINE	Possibly ↑ adverse effects with tenofovir and zidovudine	Additive toxicity	Avoid if possible; otherwise, monitor FBC and renal function (weekly). ↓ Doses as necessary

(*Continued*)

Primary Drug	Secondary Drug	Effect	Mechanism	Precautions
ANTIFUNGAL DRUGS				
AMPHOTERICIN	CARDIAC GLYCOSIDES—DIGOXIN	Risk of digoxin toxicity due to hypokalemia	Amphotericin may cause hypokalemia	Monitor potassium levels closely. Monitor digoxin levels; watch for digoxin toxicity
AMPHOTERICIN	DIURETICS—LOOP DIURETICS AND THIAZIDES	Risk of hypokalemia	Additive effect	Monitor potassium closely
AZOLES				
AZOLES	**DRUGS THAT PROLONG THE QT INTERVAL**			
FLUCONAZOLE, POSACONAZOLE, VORICONAZOLE	1. ANTIARRHYTHMICS—amiodarone, disopyramide, procainamide, propafenone 2. ANTIBIOTICS—macrolides (especially azithromycin, clarithromycin, parenteral erythromycin, telithromycin), quinolones (especially moxifloxacin), quinupristin/dalfopristin 3. ANTICANCER AND IMMUNOMODULATING DRUGS—arsenic trioxide 4. ANTIDEPRESSANTS—TCAs, venlafaxine 5. ANTIEMETICS—dolasetron 6. ANTIHISTAMINES—terfenadine, hydroxyzine, mizolastine 7. ANTIMALARIALS—artemether with lumefantrine, chloroquine, hydroxychloroquine, mefloquine, quinine 8. ANTIPROTOZOALS—pentamidine isetionate 9. ANTIPSYCHOTICS—atypicals, phenothiazines, pimozide 10. BETA-BLOCKERS—sotalol 11. BRONCHODILATORS—parenteral bronchodilators 12. CNS STIMULANTS—atomoxetine	Risk of ventricular arrhythmias, particularly torsades de pointes	Additive effect; these drugs cause prolongation of the QT interval	Avoid coadministration

(Continued)

Primary Drug	Secondary Drug	Effect	Mechanism	Precautions
ANTIFUNGAL DRUGS				
KETOCONAZOLE	ALISKIREN	Aliskiren levels ↑ due to ketoconazole	Uncertain	Monitor BP and serum potassium at least weekly until stable
FLUCONAZOLE	NSAIDs	Fluconazole ↑ celecoxib and possibly parecoxib levels	Fluconazole inhibits CYP2C9-mediated metabolism of celecoxib and parecoxib	Halve the dose of celecoxib, and start parecoxib at the lowest dose
FLUCONAZOLE, ITRACONAZOLE, KETOCONAZOLE, VORICONAZOLE	OPIOIDS	1. Ketoconazole ↑ effect of buprenorphine 2. Fluconazole and itraconazole ↑ effect of alfentanil 3. Fluconazole and possibly voriconazole ↑ effect of methadone; recognized pharmacokinetic effect but uncertain clinical significance	1. Ketoconazole ↓ CYP3A4-mediated metabolism of buprenorphine 2. ↓ Clearance of alfentanil 3. ↓ Hepatic metabolism	1. The dose of buprenorphine needs to be ↓ (by up to 50%) 2. ↓ Dose of alfentanil 3. Watch for ↑ effects of methadone
ITRACONAZOLE, KETOCONAZOLE	ANTACIDS	↓ Plasma concentration of itraconazole and ketoconazole, with risk of therapeutic failure	Itraconazole absorption in capsule form requires an acidic gastric environment and thus absorption would ↓.	Separate administration of agents that ↓ gastric acidity by 1–2 h. However, absorption of itraconazole liquid solution does not require an acidic environment and could be used instead; it need not be given with food. Fluconazole absorption is not pH dependent, and this is a suitable alternative
ITRACONAZOLE, KETOCONAZOLE, VORICONAZOLE	CLARITHROMYCIN, CLOTRIMAZOLE, ERYTHROMYCIN, TELITHROMYCIN	↑ Plasma concentrations of itraconazole and ketoconazole, and risk of toxic effects	These antibiotics are inhibitors of metabolism of itraconazole by CYP3A4. Erythromycin is a weaker inhibitor than clarithromycin. The role of clarithromycin and erythromycin as inhibitors of Pgp is not known with certainty. Ketoconazole is a potent inhibitor of Pgp	Monitor LFTs closely. Azithromycin is not affected

(*Continued*)

DRUGS TO TREAT INFECTIONS ANTIFUNGAL DRUGS

Primary Drug	Secondary Drug	Effect	Mechanism	Precautions
ANTIFUNGAL DRUGS				
ITRACONAZOLE, KETOCONAZOLE, POSACONAZOLE, VORICONAZOLE	ISONIAZID, RIFAMPICIN, RIFABUTIN, RIFAPENTINE	↓ Levels of these azoles, with significant risk of therapeutic failure. Rifampicin is a very potent inducer that can produce undetectable concentrations of ketoconazole	Rifampicin is a powerful inducer of CYP3A4 and other CYP isoenzymes. Rifabutin is a less powerful inducer but more potent than rifapentine. Rifapentine is an inducer of CYP3A4 and CYP2C8/9. Isoniazid is a known inhibitor of CYP2E1 and is likely to induce other CYP isoenzymes to varying degrees, usually in a time-dependent manner. Rifampicin is also a powerful inducer of Pgp, thus ↓ bioavailability of itraconazole	Avoid coadministration of ketoconazole or voriconazole with these drugs. Watch for inadequate therapeutic effects of itraconazole. Higher doses of itraconazole may not overcome this interaction, so consider use of less lipophilic fluconazole, which is less dependent on CYP metabolism. Avoid coadministration of posaconazole with rifabutin.
VORICONAZOLE	RIFABUTIN	↑ Plasma concentrations of rifabutin, with risk of toxic effects of rifabutin (nausea, vomiting). Dangerous toxic effects such as leukopenia and thrombocytopenia may occur	Due to inhibition of metabolism of rifabutin by the CYP3A4 isoenzymes by voriconazole	Avoid concomitant use. If absolutely necessary, close monitoring of FBC, liver enzymes and examination of eyes for uveitis, and corneal opacities are necessary
AZOLES	**ANTICANCER AND IMMUNOMODULATING DRUGS**			
AZOLES	**CYTOTOXICS**			
ITRACONAZOLE, KETOCONAZOLE	BUSULFAN	↑ Busulfan levels, with risk of toxicity of busulfan, e.g., veno-occlusive disease and pulmonary fibrosis	Itraconazole is a potent inhibitor of CYP3A4. Busulfan clearance may be ↓ by 25% and the AUC of busulfan may ↑ by 1500 μmol/min	Dose adjustments are necessary if concomitant administration is considered absolutely necessary; best, however, to avoid concomitant use. Monitor clinically for veno-occlusive disease and pulmonary toxicity in transplant patients. Monitor busulfan blood levels as an AUC below 1500 μmol/min tends to prevent toxicity

(*Continued*)

Primary Drug	Secondary Drug	Effect	Mechanism	Precautions
ANTIFUNGAL DRUGS				
FLUCONAZOLE, ITRACONAZOLE, KETOCONAZOLE, VORICONAZOLE	DOXORUBICIN	↑ Risk of myelosuppression due to ↑ plasma concentration of doxorubicin	Due to ↓ metabolism of doxorubicin by CYP3A4 isoenzymes owing to inhibition of those enzymes	Monitor for ↑ myelosuppression, peripheral neuropathy, myalgias, and fatigue
FLUCONAZOLE, ITRACONAZOLE, KETOCONAZOLE, VORICONAZOLE	ERLOTINIB	↑ Erlotinib levels	↓ Metabolism of erlotinib	Avoid coadministration
FLUCONAZOLE, ITRACONAZOLE, KETOCONAZOLE, VORICONAZOLE	IFOSFAMIDE	↓ Plasma concentrations of 4-hydroxyifosfamide, the active metabolite of ifosfamide, and risk of inadequate therapeutic response	Due to inhibition of the isoenzymatic conversion to active metabolites	Monitor clinically the efficacy of ifosfamide, and ↑ dose accordingly
FLUCONAZOLE, ITRACONAZOLE, KETOCONAZOLE, VORICONAZOLE	IMATINIB	↑ Plasma concentrations of imatinib, with ↑ risk of toxicity (e.g., abdominal pain, constipation, dyspnea) and neurotoxicity (e.g., taste disturbances, dizziness, headache, paresthesia, peripheral neuropathy)	Due to inhibition of CYP3A4-mediated metabolism of imatinib	Monitor for clinical efficacy and for the signs of toxicity listed, along with convulsions, confusion, and signs of edema (including pulmonary edema). Monitor electrolytes and liver function for cardiotoxicity
FLUCONAZOLE, ITRACONAZOLE, KETOCONAZOLE, VORICONAZOLE	IRINOTECAN	↑ Plasma concentrations of SN-38 (>AUC by 100%) and ↑ toxicity of irinotecan, e.g., diarrhea, acute cholinergic syndrome, interstitial pulmonary disease	Due to inhibition of the metabolism of irinotecan by CYP3A4 isoenzymes by ketoconazole	Peripheral blood counts should be checked before each course of treatment. Monitor lung function. Recommendation is to ↓ dose of irinotecan by 25%
FLUCONAZOLE, ITRACONAZOLE, KETOCONAZOLE, VORICONAZOLE (POSSIBLY POSACONAZOLE)	VINCA ALKALOIDS—VINBLASTINE, VINCRISTINE, VINORELBINE	↑ Adverse effects of vinblastine and vincristine	Inhibition of CYP3A4-mediated metabolism. Also inhibition of Pgp efflux of vinblastine	Monitor FBCs and watch for early features of toxicity (pain, numbness, tingling in the fingers and toes, jaw pain, abdominal pain, constipation, ileus). Consider selecting an alternative drug

(Continued)

Primary Drug	Secondary Drug	Effect	Mechanism	Precautions
ANTIFUNGAL DRUGS				
AZOLES	**HORMONES AND HORMONE ANTAGONISTS**			
AZOLES	TOREMIFENE	↑ Plasma concentrations of toremifene	Due to inhibition of metabolism of toremifene by the CYP3A4 isoenzymes by ketoconazole	Clinical relevance is uncertain. Necessary to monitor for clinical toxicities
AZOLES	**IMMUNOMODULATING DRUGS**			
AZOLES—ITRACONAZOLE, KETOCONAZOLE, VORICONAZOLE	CICLOSPORIN	↑ Plasma concentrations of ciclosporin, with risk of nephrotoxicity, myelosuppression, neurotoxicity, and excessive immunosuppression, with risk of infection and posttransplant lymphoproliferative disease	Inhibition of CYP3A4-mediated metabolism of ciclosporin; these inhibitors vary in potency. Ketoconazole and itraconazole are classified as potent inhibitors. The effect is not clinically relevant with fluconazole	Avoid coadministration with itraconazole or ketoconazole. Consider an alternative azole but need to monitor plasma ciclosporin levels to prevent toxicity
AZOLES—FLUCONAZOLE, ITRACONAZOLE, KETOCONAZOLE, POSACONAZOLE, VORICONAZOLE	CORTICOSTEROIDS	↑ Adrenal suppressive effects of corticosteroids, which may ↑ risk of infections and produce an inadequate response to stress scenarios	Due to inhibition of CYP3A4-mediated metabolism of corticosteroids and inhibition of Pgp (↑ bioavailability of corticosteroids)	Monitor cortisol levels and warn patients to report symptoms such as fever and sore throat
AZOLES	SIROLIMUS	↑ Sirolimus levels	Inhibition of metabolism of sirolimus	Avoid coadministration
AZOLES	TACROLIMUS	↑ Tacrolimus levels	Inhibition of CYP3A4-mediated metabolism of tacrolimus	Monitor clinical effects closely; check levels
FLUCONAZOLE, ITRACONAZOLE, KETOCONAZOLE, MICONAZOLE, VORICONAZOLE	ANTICOAGULANTS—WARFARIN	↑ Anticoagulant effect with azole antifungals. There have been cases of bleeding when topical miconazole (oral gel or pessaries) was used by patients on warfarin. Posaconazole may be a safer alternative	Itraconazole potently inhibits CYP3A4, which metabolizes both *R*-warfarin (also metabolized by CYP1A2) and the more active *S*-warfarin (also metabolized by CYP2C9)	Necessary to monitor the effects of warfarin closely (weekly INR) and to warn patients to report any symptoms of bleeding. ➢ ***For signs and symptoms of overanticoagulation, see Clinical Features of Some Adverse Drug Interactions, Bleeding disorders***

(*Continued*)

Primary Drug	Secondary Drug	Effect	Mechanism	Precautions
ANTIFUNGAL DRUGS				
AZOLES	**ANTIDEPRESSANTS**			
KETOCONAZOLE	MIRTAZAPINE	↑ Mirtazapine levels	Inhibition of metabolism via CYP1A2, CYP2D6, and CYP3A4	Consider alternative antifungals
AZOLES	REBOXETINE	Risk of ↑ reboxetine levels	Possibly inhibition of CYP3A4-mediated metabolism of reboxetine	Avoid coadministration
ITRACONAZOLE, KETOCONAZOLE, MICONAZOLE, FLUCONAZOLE, VORICONAZOLE	TCAs	Possible ↑ plasma concentrations of TCAs	All TCAs are metabolized primarily by CYP2D6. Other pathways include CYP1A2 (e.g., amitriptyline, clomipramine, imipramine), CYP2C9, and CYP2C19 (e.g., clomipramine, imipramine). Ketoconazole and voriconazole are documented inhibitors of CYP2C19. Fluconazole and voriconazole are reported to inhibit CYP2C9	Warn patients to report ↑ side effects of TCAs such as dry mouth, blurred vision, and constipation, which may be an early sign of ↑ TCA levels. In this case, consider ↓ dose of TCA
AZOLES	**ANTIDIABETIC DRUGS**			
KETOCONAZOLE, FLUCONAZOLE, ITRACONAZOLE, VORICONAZOLE	NATEGLINIDE, REPAGLINIDE	Likely to ↑ plasma concentrations of repaglinide and ↑ risk of hypoglycemic episodes	Due to inhibition of CYP3A4-mediated metabolism. These drugs vary in potency as inhibitors (ketoconazole, itraconazole are potent inhibitors) and ↑ plasma concentrations will vary	Watch for and warn patients about symptoms of hypoglycemia. ➢ ***For signs and symptoms of hypoglycemia, see Clinical Features of Some Adverse Drug Interactions, Hypoglycemia***
ITRACONAZOLE, FLUCONAZOLE, MICONAZOLE, VORICONAZOLE	SULFONYLUREAS	↑ Risk of hypoglycemic episodes	Inhibition of CYP2C9-mediated metabolism of these sulfonylureas	Watch for and warn patients about symptoms of hypoglycemia. ➢ ***For signs and symptoms of hypoglycemia, see Clinical Features of Some Adverse Drug Interactions, Hypoglycemia***

(Continued)

DRUGS TO TREAT INFECTIONS ANTIFUNGAL DRUGS

Primary Drug	Secondary Drug	Effect	Mechanism	Precautions
ANTIFUNGAL DRUGS				
KETOCONAZOLE	ANTIEMETICS—APREPITANT	↑ Aprepitant levels	Inhibition of CYP3A4-mediated metabolism of aprepitant	Use with caution. Clinical significance unclear; monitor closely
AZOLES	**ANTIEPILEPTICS**			
FLUCONAZOLE, ITRACONAZOLE, KETOCONAZOLE, VORICONAZOLE	BARBITURATES	↓ Azole levels, with risk of therapeutic failure	Barbiturates induce CYP3A4, which metabolizes itraconazole and the active metabolite of itraconazole. Primidone is metabolized to phenobarbitone	Watch for inadequate therapeutic effects, and ↑ dose of azole if it is due to interaction
MICONAZOLE	BARBITURATES	↑ Phenobarbital levels	Inhibition of metabolism	Be aware; watch for early features of toxicity (e.g., ↑ sedation)
ITRACONAZOLE, KETOCONAZOLE, MICONAZOLE, POSACONAZOLE, VORICONAZOLE	CARBAMAZEPINE, PHENYTOIN	↓ Plasma concentrations of itraconazole and of its active metabolite, ketoconazole, posaconazole, and voriconazole, with risk of therapeutic failure. ↑ phenytoin levels, but clinical significance uncertain. Carbamazepine plasma concentrations are also ↑	These azoles are highly lipophilic, and clearance is heavily dependent upon metabolism by CYP isoenzymes. Phenytoin and carbamazepine are powerful inducers of CYP3A4 and other CYP isoenzymes (CYP2C18/19, CYP1A2); the result is very low or undetectable plasma levels. Phenytoin extensively ↓ AUC of itraconazole by more than 90%. Inhibition of Pgp ↑ bioavailability of carbamazepine	Avoid coadministration of posaconazole or voriconazole with carbamazepine. Watch for inadequate therapeutic effects and ↑ dose of itraconazole. Higher doses of itraconazole may not overcome this interaction. Consider the use of less lipophilic fluconazole, which is less dependent on CYP metabolism. Necessary to monitor phenytoin and carbamazepine levels
ITRACONAZOLE	**ANTIFUNGALS**			
ITRACONAZOLE	KETOCONAZOLE	↑ Itraconazole levels, with risk of toxic effects	Ketoconazole is a potent inhibitor of the metabolism of itraconazole by CYP3A4 and a potent inhibitor of Pgp, which is considered to ↑ bioavailability of itraconazole	Warn patients about toxic effects such as swelling around the ankles (peripheral edema), shortness of breath, loss of appetite (anorexia), and yellow discoloration of the urine and eyes (jaundice). ↓ Dose if due to interaction

(Continued)

Primary Drug	Secondary Drug	Effect	Mechanism	Precautions
ANTIFUNGAL DRUGS				
ITRACONAZOLE	VORICONAZOLE	↓ Levels of itraconazole and of its active metabolite, and significant risk of therapeutic failure	Voriconazole is an inducer of CYP3A4	Watch for inadequate therapeutic effects, and ↑ dose of itraconazole if due to interaction. Higher doses of itraconazole may not overcome this interaction, so consider the use of less lipophilic fluconazole, which is less dependent on CYP metabolism
AZOLES	**ANTIHISTAMINES**			
AZOLES	MIZOLASTINE	↑ Mizolastine levels	Inhibition of metabolism of mizolastine	Avoid coadministration
KETOCONAZOLE, POSACONAZOLE	LORATADINE	↑ Loratadine levels	Inhibition of cytochrome P450, Pgp or both	Avoid coadministration
AZOLES—ITRACONAZOLE	ANTIHYPERTENSIVES AND HEART FAILURE DRUGS—VASODILATOR ANTIHYPERTENSIVES—BOSENTAN	Azole antifungals ↑ bosentan levels	Azoles inhibit CYP3A4 and CYP2C9	Monitor LFTs closely
AZOLES—ITRACONAZOLE	ANTIMIGRAINE DRUGS—5-HT1 AGONISTS	↑ Levels of almotriptan and eletriptan	Inhibited metabolism	Avoid coadministration
ITRACONAZOLE, KETOCONAZOLE	ANTIMUSCARINICS	1. ↓ Ketoconazole levels 2. ↑ Darifenacin, solifenacin and tolterodine levels	1. ↓ Absorption 2. Inhibited metabolism	1. Watch for poor response to ketoconazole 2. Avoid coadministration of ketoconazole and these antimuscarinics
KETOCONAZOLE	ANTIOBESITY DRUGS—RIMONABANT	↑ Rimonabant levels	Ketoconazole inhibits CYP3A4-mediated metabolism of rimonabant	Avoid coadministration
AZOLES	**ANTIVIRALS**			
ITRACONAZOLE, KETOCONAZOLE	PROTEASE INHIBITORS	Possibly ↑ levels of ketoconazole by amprenavir, indinavir, and ritonavir (with or without lopinavir). Conversely, indinavir, ritonavir, and saquinavir levels ↑ by itraconazole and ketoconazole	Inhibition of, or competition for, CYP3A4-mediated metabolism	Use itraconazole with caution and monitor for adverse effects. No dose adjustment is recommended for doses <400 mg/day of ketoconazole

(Continued)

DRUGS TO TREAT INFECTIONS ANTIFUNGAL DRUGS

Primary Drug	Secondary Drug	Effect	Mechanism	Precautions
ANTIFUNGAL DRUGS				
VORICONAZOLE	RITONAVIR	↓ Efficacy of voriconazole	↓ Plasma levels	Avoid coadministration if the dose of ritonavir is 400 mg twice a day or greater. Avoid combining low-dose ritonavir (100 mg twice a day) unless benefits outweigh risks
FLUCONAZOLE, VORICONAZOLE	NNRTIs	Possible ↓ efficacy of azole	↑ CYP3A4-mediated metabolism	Avoid coadministration
AZOLES	**NUCLEOSIDE REVERSE TRANSCRIPTASE INHIBITORS**			
ITRACONAZOLE, KETOCONAZOLE	DIDANOSINE	Possibly ↓ efficacy of ketoconazole and itraconazole with buffered didanosine	Absorption of the ketoconazole and itraconazole may be ↓ by the buffered didanosine formulation, which raises gastric pH	Give the ketoconazole and itraconazole 2 h before or 6 h after didanosine. Alternatively, consider using the enteric-coated formulation of didanosine, which does not have to be given separately
FLUCONAZOLE	ZIDOVUDINE	↑ Zidovudine levels	Inhibition of metabolism	Avoid coadministration
AZOLES	**ANXIOLYTICS AND HYPNOTICS**			
ITRACONAZOLE, KETOCONAZOLE, VORICONAZOLE	BZDs—ALPRAZOLAM, CHLORDIAZEPOXIDE, DIAZEPAM, LORAZEPAM, MIDAZOLAM, OXAZEPAM, TEMAZEPAM	↑ Plasma concentrations of these BZDs, with ↑, a risk of adverse effects. These risks are greater following intravenous administration of midazolam compared with oral midazolam	Itraconazole and ketoconazole are potent inhibitors of phase I metabolism (oxidation and functionalization) of these BZDs by CYP3A4. In addition, a significant ↑ in plasma concentrations following oral midazolam (15 times compared with five times following intravenous use) indicates that the inhibition of Pgp by ketoconazole is important following oral administration	Aim to avoid coadministration. If coadministration is necessary, always start with a low dose and monitor effects closely. Consider use of alternative BZDs that undergo predominantly phase II metabolism by glucuronidation, e.g., flurazepam, quazepam. Fluconazole and posaconazole are unlikely to cause this interaction
ITRACONAZOLE	BUSPIRONE	↑ Buspirone levels	Inhibition of CYP3A4-mediated metabolism	Warn patients to be aware of additional sedation

(Continued)

Primary Drug	Secondary Drug	Effect	Mechanism	Precautions
ANTIFUNGAL DRUGS				
KETOCONAZOLE	ZALEPLON, ZOLPIDEM, ZOPICLONE	↑ Zolpidem levels reported; likely to occur with zaleplon and zopiclone	Inhibition of CYP3A4-mediated metabolism	Warn patients about the risk of ↑ sedation
ITRACONAZOLE, KETOCONAZOLE, POSACONAZOLE	BRONCHODILATORS—THEOPHYLLINE	↑ Theophylline levels, with risk of toxicity, with itraconazole. Unpredictable effect on theophylline levels with ketoconazole	Theophylline is primarily metabolized by CYP1A2. Although azoles are best known as inhibitors of CYP3A4, they also inhibit other CYP isoenzymes to varying degrees	If concurrent use is necessary, monitor theophylline levels at the initiation of itraconazole therapy or on discontinuing therapy. Terbinafine may be a safer alternative
FLUCONAZOLE, ITRACONAZOLE, KETOCONAZOLE, POSACONAZOLE, VORICONAZOLE	CALCIUM CHANNEL BLOCKERS	Plasma concentrations of dihydropyridine calcium channel blockers are ↑ by fluconazole, itraconazole, and ketoconazole. Risk of ↑ verapamil levels with ketoconazole and itraconazole. Itraconazole and possibly posaconazole may ↑ diltiazem levels	The azoles are potent inhibitors of CYP3A4 isoenzymes, which metabolize calcium channel blockers. They also inhibit CYP2C9-mediated metabolism of verapamil. Ketoconazole and itraconazole both inhibit intestinal Pgp, which may ↑ bioavailability of verapamil. Diltiazem is mainly a substrate of CYP3A5 and CYP3A5P1, which are inhibited by itraconazole. 75% of the metabolism of diltiazem occurs in the liver and the rest in the intestine. Diltiazem is a substrate of Pgp (also an inhibitor but unlikely to be significant at therapeutic doses), which is inhibited by itraconazole, resulting in ↑ bioavailability of diltiazem	Monitor PR, BP, and ECG, and warn patents to watch for symptoms/signs of heart failure

(Continued)

Primary Drug	Secondary Drug	Effect	Mechanism	Precautions
ANTIFUNGAL DRUGS				
ITRACONAZOLE	CARDIAC GLYCOSIDES—DIGOXIN	Itraconazole may cause ↑ plasma levels of digoxin; cases of digoxin toxicity have been reported	Itraconazole inhibits Pgp-mediated renal clearance and ↑ intestinal absorption of digoxin	Monitor digoxin levels; watch for digoxin toxicity
ITRACONAZOLE, KETOCONAZOLE	CNS STIMULANTS—MODAFINIL	↑ Plasma concentrations of modafinil, with risk of adverse effects	Due to inhibition of CYP3A4, which has a partial role in the metabolism of modafinil	Be aware. Warn patients to report dose-related adverse effects, e.g., headache, anxiety
KETOCONAZOLE	DIURETICS—POTASSIUM-SPARING DIURETICS AND ALDOSTERONE ANTAGONISTS	↑ Eplerenone levels	Inhibition of metabolism	Avoid coadministration
VORICONAZOLE	ERGOT ALKALOIDS—ERGOTAMINE	↑ Ergotamine/ methysergide levels, with risk of toxicity	Inhibition of metabolism of the ergot derivatives	Avoid coadministration. If absolutely necessary, advise patients to discontinue treatment immediately if numbness and tingling of the extremities are felt
ITRACONAZOLE	GRAPEFRUIT JUICE	Possibly ↓ efficacy	↓ Absorption possibly by inhibition of intestinal CYP3A4, affecting Pgp or lowering duodenal pH	Clinical significance is unknown. The effect of the interaction may vary between capsules and oral liquid preparations
ITRACONAZOLE, KETOCONAZOLE, MICONAZOLE, POSACONAZOLE	H2 RECEPTOR BLOCKERS	↓ Plasma concentrations and risk of treatment failure with azoles	↓ Absorption of these antifungals due to ↑ gastric pH	Avoid concomitant use. If unable to avoid combination, take H2 blockers at least 2–3 h after the antifungal. Use alternative antifungal or separate doses by at least 2 h along with an acidic drink, e.g., a carbonated drink; ↑ dose of antifungal may be required
FLUCONAZOLE, ITRACONAZOLE, KETOCONAZOLE	IVABRADINE	↑ Levels with ketoconazole and possibly fluconazole and itraconazole	Uncertain	Avoid coadministration

(Continued)

Primary Drug	Secondary Drug	Effect	Mechanism	Precautions
ANTIFUNGAL DRUGS				
FLUCONAZOLE, ITRACONAZOLE, KETOCONAZOLE, POSACONAZOLE	LIPID-LOWERING DRUGS—STATINS	Azoles markedly ↑ atorvastatin, simvastatin (both with cases of myopathy reported), and possibly pravastatin. These effects are less likely with fluvastatin and rosuvastatin, although fluconazole may cause moderate rises in their levels	Itraconazole and ketoconazole inhibit CYP3A4-mediated metabolism of these statins; they also inhibit intestinal Pgp, which ↑ bioavailability of statins. Itraconazole may block the transport of atorvastatin due to inhibition of the OATP1B1 enzyme system. Some manufacturers suggest that the small ↑ in plasma levels of pravastatin may be due to ↑ absorption. Voriconazole is an inhibitor of CYP2C9. Fluconazole inhibits CYP2C9 and CYP3A4	Avoid coadministration of simvastatin and atorvastatin with azole antifungals. Care should be taken regarding coadministration of other statins and azoles. Although fluvastatin and rosuvastatin may be considered as alternatives, consider ↓ dose of statin and warn patients to report any features of rhabdomyolysis. Check LFTs and CK regularly
FLUCONAZOLE, ITRACONAZOLE, KETOCONAZOLE, POSACONAZOLE, VORICONAZOLE	ESTROGENS—ORAL CONTRACEPTIVES	The Netherlands Pharmacovigilance Foundation has received reports of pill cycle disturbances 2–3 weeks after the start of the pill cycle, delayed bleeding, and pregnancy. Effects of either or both of estrogen excess and progestogen excess may occur (migraine headaches, thromboembolic episodes, breast tenderness, bloating, weight gain)	The metabolism of oral contraceptives is complex, depending on composition, constituents, and doses. Ethylenestradiol, a common constituent, as well as progestogens are substrates of CYP3A4 that are inhibited by itraconazole. The inhibition of ethinylestradiol and progestogens could lead to effects of estrogen and progestogens excess. Triazole antifungals inhibit biotransformation of steroids, and such an ↑ may cause a delay of withdrawal bleeding	Due to the complex metabolic pathways of oral contraceptives, dependent on constituents, doses, and the reported adverse effects during concomitant use, it is advisable to avoid use of azole antifungals or advise alternative methods of contraception

(*Continued*)

Primary Drug	Secondary Drug	Effect	Mechanism	Precautions
ANTIFUNGAL DRUGS				
KETOCONAZOLE	PARASYMPATHOMIMETICS—GALANTAMINE	↑ Galantamine levels	Inhibition of CYP3A4-mediated metabolism of galantamine	Monitor PR and BP closely, watching for bradycardia and hypotension
FLUCONAZOLE, ITRACONAZOLE, KETOCONAZOLE, MICONAZOLE	PERIPHERAL VASODILATORS—CILOSTAZOL	Fluconazole, itraconazole, ketoconazole, and miconazole ↑ cilostazol levels	These azoles inhibit CYP3A4-mediated metabolism of cilostazol	Avoid coadministration
AZOLES	PHOSPHODIESTERASE TYPE 5 INHIBITORS	↑ Sildenafil, tadalafil, and vardenafil levels	Inhibition of metabolism	↓ dose of these phosphodiesterase inhibitors
AZOLES	**PROTON PUMP INHIBITORS**			
ITRACONAZOLE, KETOCONAZOLE	PROTON PUMP INHIBITORS	Possible ↓ efficacy of the antifungal	↓ Absorption	Monitor for ↓ efficacy; ↑ dose may be required. Separate doses by at least 2 h and give ketoconazole with a cola drink
VORICONAZOLE	OMEPRAZOLE	Possible ↑ efficacy and adverse effects of both drugs	1. Inhibition of voriconazole metabolism via CYP2C19 and CYP3A4 2. Inhibition of metabolism of omeprazole	1. No dose adjustment of voriconazole is recommended 2. Halve the omeprazole dose
ITRACONAZOLE	TOLTERODINE	↑ Tolterodine level. Supratherapeutic levels may cause prolongation of the QT interval	CYP3A4 is the major enzyme involved in the elimination of tolterodine in individuals with deficient CYP2D6 activity (poor metabolizers). Inhibition of CYP3A4 by triazoles in such individuals could cause dangerous ↑ tolterodine levels	Avoid coadministration
CASPOFUNGIN				
CASPOFUNGIN	ANTIBIOTICS—RIFAMPICIN	↓ Caspofungin levels, with risk of therapeutic failure	Induction of caspofungin metabolism	↑ Dose of caspofungin to 70 mg daily

(*Continued*)

Primary Drug	Secondary Drug	Effect	Mechanism	Precautions
ANTIFUNGAL DRUGS				
CASPOFUNGIN	**ANTICANCER AND IMMUNOMODULATING DRUGS**			
CASPOFUNGIN	CICLOSPORIN	1. ↓ Plasma concentrations of ciclosporin, with risk of transplant rejection 2. Enhanced toxic effects of caspofungin and ↑ alanine transaminase levels	1. Due to induction of metabolism of ciclosporin by these drugs. The potency of induction varies 2. Uncertain	1. Monitor for signs of rejection of transplants. Monitor ciclosporin levels to ensure adequate therapeutic concentrations and ↑ dose when necessary 2. Monitor LFTs
CASPOFUNGIN	DEXAMETHASONE	↓ Caspofungin levels, with risk of therapeutic failure	Induction of caspofungin metabolism	↑ Dose of caspofungin to 70 mg daily
CASPOFUNGIN	TACROLIMUS	↓ Tacrolimus levels	Induction of CYP3A4-mediated metabolism of tacrolimus	Avoid coadministration
CASPOFUNGIN	ANTIEPILEPTICS—CARBAMAZEPINE, PHENYTOIN	↓ Caspofungin levels, with risk of therapeutic failure	Induction of caspofungin metabolism	↑ Dose of caspofungin to 70 mg daily
CASPOFUNGIN	ANTIVIRALS—EFAVIRENZ, NEVIRAPINE	↓ Caspofungin levels, with risk of therapeutic failure	Induction of caspofungin metabolism	↑ Dose of caspofungin to 70 mg daily
FLUCYTOSINE				
FLUCYTOSINE	ANTICANCER AND IMMUNOMODULATING DRUGS—CYTARABINE	↓ Flucytosine levels	Uncertain	Watch for poor response to flucytosine
FLUCYTOSINE	ANTIFUNGALS—AMPHOTERICIN	↑ Flucytosine levels, with risk of toxic effects	Amphotericin causes ↓ renal excretion of flucytosine and ↑ cellular uptake	The combination of flucytosine and amphotericin may be used therapeutically. Watch for early features of flucytosine toxicity (gastrointestinal upset); monitor renal and liver functions closely
FLUCYTOSINE	ANTIVIRALS—ZIDOVUDINE	Possibly ↑ adverse effects with zidovudine	Additive toxicity	Avoid if possible; otherwise, monitor FBC and renal function (weekly). ↓ doses as necessary
GRISEOFULVIN				
GRISEOFULVIN	ALCOHOL	Disulfiram-like reaction can occur	Uncertain	Warn patients not to drink alcohol while taking griseofulvin

(Continued)

Primary Drug	Secondary Drug	Effect	Mechanism	Precautions
ANTIFUNGAL DRUGS				
GRISEOFULVIN	ANTICANCER AND IMMUNOMODULATING DRUGS—CICLOSPORIN	↓ Plasma concentrations of ciclosporin (may be as much as 40%) and risk of rejection in patients who have received transplants	Induction of ciclosporin metabolism	Monitor ciclosporin levels closely
GRISEOFULVIN	ANTICOAGULANTS—ORAL	Possible ↓ anticoagulant effect coumarins and phenindione	Unknown	Necessary to monitor the effects of warfarin closely (weekly INR) and to ask/request patients to report any symptoms of bleeding. ➢ ***For signs and symptoms of overanticoagulation, see Clinical Features of Some Adverse Drug Interactions, Bleeding disorders***
GRISEOFULVIN	ANTIDEPRESSANTS—TCAs	Possible ↑ plasma concentrations of TCAs	Inhibition of metabolism	Request/ask patients to report any ↑ side effects of TCAs such as dry mouth, blurred vision, and constipation, which may be an early sign of ↑ TCA levels. In this case, consider ↓ dose of TCA
GRISEOFULVIN	ANTIDIABETIC DRUGS—REPAGLINIDE	↓ Repaglinide levels	Hepatic metabolism induced	Watch for and warn patients about hypoglycemia. ➢ ***For signs and symptoms of hypoglycemia, see Clinical Features of Some Adverse Drug Interactions, Hypoglycemia***
GRISEOFULVIN	ANTIEPILEPTICS—PHENOBARBITONE, PRIMIDONE	↓ Griseofulvin levels	↓ Absorption	Although the effect of ↓ plasma concentrations on therapeutic effect has not been established, concurrent use is preferably avoided
GRISEOFULVIN	BRONCHODILATORS—THEOPHYLLINE	↑ Theophylline levels	Inhibition of metabolism of theophylline	Uncertain clinical significance. Watch for early features of theophylline toxicity

(*Continued*)

Primary Drug	Secondary Drug	Effect	Mechanism	Precautions
ANTIFUNGAL DRUGS				
GRISEOFULVIN	ESTROGENS	↓ Estrogen levels, which may lead to failure of contraception	Induction of metabolism of estrogens	Long-term use of griseofulvin is likely to ↓ effectiveness of oral contraceptives. Patients should be advised to use an alternative method of contraception during griseofulvin therapy and for 1 month after its discontinuation
GRISEOFULVIN	PROGESTOGENS	↓ Progesterone levels, which may lead to a failure of contraception or a poor response to treatment of menorrhagia	Induction of the CYP-mediated metabolism of estrogens	Long-term use of griseofulvin is likely to ↓ effectiveness of oral contraceptives. Patients should be advised to use an alternative method of contraception during griseofulvin therapy and for 1 month after its discontinuation
TERBINAFINE				
TERBINAFINE	ANTIBIOTICS—RIFAMPICIN	↓ Terbinafine levels	Induction of metabolism	Watch for poor response to terbinafine
TERBINAFINE	ANTIDEPRESSANTS—IMIPRAMINE, NORTRIPTYLINE	Possible ↑ plasma concentrations of TCAs	Terbinafine strongly inhibits CYP2D6-mediated metabolism of nortriptyline	Warn patients to report ↑ side effects of TCAs such as dry mouth, blurred vision, and constipation, which may be an early sign of ↑ TCA levels. In this case, consider ↓ dose of TCA
TERBINAFINE	H2 RECEPTOR BLOCKERS—CIMETIDINE	↑ Efficacy and adverse effects of terbinafine	↑ Bioavailability	Consider alternative acid suppression or monitor more closely and consider ↓ dose
TERBINAFINE	ESTROGENS	↓ Estrogen levels, which may lead to failure of contraception	Alteration of the bacterial flora necessary for recycling ethinylestradiol from the large bowel	Patients should be advised to use an alternative method of contraception during terbinafine therapy and for 1 month after its discontinuation
TERBINAFINE	PROGESTOGENS	↓ Progestogen levels, which may lead to a failure of contraception or poor response to treatment of menorrhagia	Induction of the CYP-mediated metabolism of estrogens	Patients should be advised to use an alternative method of contraception during terbinafine therapy and for 1 month after its discontinuation

Primary Drug	Secondary Drug	Effect	Mechanism	Precautions
ANTIMALARIALS				
ARTEMETHER WITH LUMEFANTRINE				
ARTEMETHER WITH LUMEFANTRINE	**DRUGS THAT PROLONG THE QT INTERVAL**			
ARTEMETHER WITH LUMEFANTRINE	1. ANTIARRHYTHMICS—amiodarone, disopyramide, procainamide, propafenone 2. ANTIBIOTICS—macrolides (especially azithromycin, clarithromycin, parenteral erythromycin, telithromycin), quinolones (especially moxifloxacin), quinupristin/dalfopristin 3. ANTICANCER AND IMMUNOMODULATING DRUGS—arsenic trioxide 4. ANTIDEPRESSANTS—TCAs, venlafaxine 5. ANTIEMETICS—dolasetron 6. ANTIFUNGALS—fluconazole, posaconazole, voriconazole 7. ANTIHISTAMINES—terfenadine, hydroxyzine, mizolastine 8. ANTIMALARIALS—chloroquine, hydroxychloroquine, mefloquine, quinine 9. ANTIPROTOZOALS—pentamidine isetionate 10. ANTIPSYCHOTICS—atypicals, phenothiazines, pimozide 11. BETA-BLOCKERS—sotalol 12. BRONCHODILATORS—parenteral bronchodilators 13. CNS STIMULANTS—atomoxetine	Risk of ventricular arrhythmias, particularly torsades de pointes	Additive effect; these drugs cause prolongation of the QT interval	Avoid coadministration
ARTEMETHER WITH LUMEFANTRINE	ANTIARRHYTHMICS—FLECAINIDE	Risk of arrhythmias	Additive effect	Avoid coadministration

(Continued)

Primary Drug	Secondary Drug	Effect	Mechanism	Precautions
ANTIMALARIALS				
ARTEMETHER WITH LUMEFANTRINE	**ANTIDEPRESSANTS**			
ARTEMETHER WITH LUMEFANTRINE	REBOXETINE, SNRIs, TRYPTOPHAN	↑ Artemether/lumefantrine levels, with risk of toxicity, including arrhythmias	Uncertain	Avoid coadministration
ARTEMETHER WITH LUMEFANTRINE	ST. JOHN'S WORT	This antimalarial may cause dose-related dangerous arrhythmias	A substrate mainly consisting of CYP3A4, which may be inhibited by St. John's wort	Manufacturers recommend avoidance of antidepressants
ARTEMETHER WITH LUMEFANTRINE	SSRIs	This antimalarial may cause dose-related dangerous arrhythmias	A substrate consisting mainly of CYP3A4, which may be inhibited by high doses of fluvoxamine and to a lesser degree by fluoxetine	Manufacturers recommend avoidance of antidepressants
ARTEMETHER WITH LUMEFANTRINE	ANTIMALARIALS	Risk of arrhythmias	Additive effect	Avoid coadministration
ARTEMETHER WITH LUMEFANTRINE	ANTIVIRALS—PROTEASE INHIBITORS	↑ Artemether levels	Uncertain; possibly inhibited metabolism	Avoid coadministration
ARTEMETHER WITH LUMEFANTRINE	BETA-BLOCKERS—METOPROLOL	↑ Risk of toxicity	Uncertain	Avoid coadministration
ARTEMETHER WITH LUMEFANTRINE	GRAPEFRUIT JUICE	Possibly ↑ efficacy and adverse effects	↑ Bioavailability; ↓ presystemic metabolism. Constituents of grapefruit juice irreversibly inhibit intestinal cytochrome CYP3A4	Monitor more closely. No ECG changes were seen in the study
ARTEMETHER WITH LUMEFANTRINE	H2 RECEPTOR BLOCKERS—CIMETIDINE	↑ Efficacy and adverse effects of antimalarials	Inhibition of metabolism, some definitely via CYP3A4	Avoid coadministration
ATOVAQUONE				
ATOVAQUONE	**ANTIBIOTICS**			
ATOVAQUONE	RIFAMPICINS	Both rifampicin and rifabutin ↓ atovaquone levels, although the effect is greater with rifampicin (↓ AUC by 50% cf. 34% for rifabutin)	Uncertain because atovaquone is predominantly excreted unchanged via the gastrointestinal route	Avoid coadministration with rifampicin. Take care with rifabutin and watch for poor response to atovaquone

(Continued)

Primary Drug	Secondary Drug	Effect	Mechanism	Precautions
ANTIMALARIALS				
ATOVAQUONE	TETRACYCLINE	↓ Atovaquone levels (40%)	Uncertain	Not clinically significant; combination therapy has been used effectively
ATOVAQUONE	ANTIEMETICS—METOCLOPRAMIDE	↓ Atovaquone levels	Uncertain	Avoid; consider an alternative antiemetic
ATOVAQUONE	ANTIVIRALS—ZIDOVUDINE	Atovaquone ↑ zidovudine levels	Atovaquone inhibits the glucuronidation of zidovudine	Uncertain clinical significance. Monitor FBC, LFTs, and lactate closely during coadministration
ATOVAQUONE	H2 RECEPTOR BLOCKERS—CIMETIDINE	↑ Efficacy and adverse effects of antimalarials	Inhibition of metabolism, some definitely via CYP3A4	Avoid coadministration
CHLOROQUINE/HYDROXYCHLOROQUINE				
CHLOROQUINE/ HYDROXYCHLOROQUINE	**DRUGS THAT PROLONG THE QT INTERVAL**			
CHLOROQUINE/ HYDROXYCHLOROQUINE	1. ANTIARRHYTHMICS—amiodarone, disopyramide, procainamide, propafenone 2. ANTIBIOTICS—macrolides (especially azithromycin, clarithromycin, parenteral erythromycin, telithromycin), quinolones (especially moxifloxacin), quinupristin/dalfopristin 3. ANTICANCER AND IMMUNOMODULATING DRUGS—arsenic trioxide 4. ANTIDEPRESSANTS—TCAs, venlafaxine 5. ANTIEMETICS—dolasetron 6. ANTIFUNGALS—fluconazole, posaconazole, voriconazole 7. ANTIHISTAMINES—terfenadine, hydroxyzine, mizolastine 8. ANTIMALARIALS—artemether with lumefantrine, mefloquine, quinine	Risk of ventricular arrhythmias, particularly torsades de pointes	Additive effect; these drugs cause prolongation of the QT interval	Avoid coadministration

(Continued)

Primary Drug	Secondary Drug	Effect	Mechanism	Precautions
ANTIMALARIALS				
	9. ANTIPROTOZOALS—pentamidine isetionate 10. ANTIPSYCHOTICS—atypicals, phenothiazines, pimozide 11. BETA-BLOCKERS—sotalol 12. BRONCHODILATORS—parenteral bronchodilators 13. CNS STIMULANTS—atomoxetine			
CHLOROQUINE	AGALSIDASE BETA	↓ Efficacy of agalsidase beta	Inhibition of intracellular activity of agalsidase beta	Avoid coadministration—manufacturers' recommendation
CHLOROQUINE	ANTACIDS	↓ Chloroquine levels	↓ Absorption	Separate doses by at least ↓ hours
CHLOROQUINE	CICLOSPORIN	↑ Plasma concentrations of ciclosporin	Likely inhibition of ciclosporin	Monitor renal function weekly
HYDROXYCHLOROQUINE	PORFIMER	↑ Risk of photosensitivity reactions	Attributed to additive effects	Avoid exposure of skin and eyes to direct sunlight for 30 days after porfimer therapy
CHLOROQUINE	ANTIDIARRHEAL DRUGS—KAOLIN	↓ Chloroquine levels	↓ Absorption	Separate doses by at least ↓ hours
CHLOROQUINE	ANTIEPILEPTICS	Risk of seizures	Chloroquine can ↓ seizure threshold	Care with coadministration; ↑ dose of antiepileptic if there is ↑ incidence of fits
CHLOROQUINE	ANTIMALARIALS—MEFLOQUINE	Risk of seizures	Additive effect	Warn patients of the risk; patients should be advised to avoid driving while taking these drugs in combination
CHLOROQUINE	CARDIAC GLYCOSIDES—DIGOXIN	Chloroquine may ↑ plasma concentrations of digoxin	Uncertain at present	Monitor digoxin levels; watch for digoxin toxicity
CHLOROQUINE	DRUG DEPENDENCE THERAPIES—BUPROPION	↑ Risk of seizures. This risk is marked in elderly people, in patients with a history of seizures, with addiction to opiates/cocaine/stimulants, and in diabetics treated with oral hypoglycemics or insulin	Bupropion is associated with a dose-related risk of seizures. These drugs, which lower seizure threshold, are individually epileptogenic. Additive effects occur when they are combined	Extreme caution. The dose of bupropion should not exceed 450 mg/day (or 150 mg/day in patients with severe hepatic cirrhosis)

(Continued)

Primary Drug	Secondary Drug	Effect	Mechanism	Precautions
ANTIMALARIALS				
CHLOROQUINE	H2 RECEPTOR BLOCKERS—CIMETIDINE	↑ Efficacy and adverse effects of chloroquine	Inhibition of metabolism and excretion	Consider ranitidine as an alternative or take cimetidine at least 2 h after chloroquine
CHLOROQUINE	LARONIDASE	↓ Efficacy of laronidase	Uncertain	Avoid coadministration
CHLOROQUINE	PARASYMPATHOMIMETICS	↓ Efficacy of parasympathomimetics	These antimalarials occasionally cause muscle weakness, which may exacerbate the symptoms of myasthenia gravis	Watch for poor response to these parasympathomimetics and ↑ dose accordingly
MEFLOQUINE				
MEFLOQUINE	**DRUGS THAT PROLONG THE QT INTERVAL**			
MEFLOQUINE	1. ANTIARRHYTHMICS—amiodarone, disopyramide, procainamide, propafenone 2. ANTIBIOTICS—macrolides (especially azithromycin, clarithromycin, parenteral erythromycin, telithromycin), quinolones (especially moxifloxacin), quinupristin/dalfopristin 3. ANTICANCER AND IMMUNOMODULATING DRUGS—arsenic trioxide 4. ANTIDEPRESSANTS—TCAs, venlafaxine 5. ANTIEMETICS—dolasetron 6. ANTIFUNGALS—fluconazole, posaconazole, voriconazole 7. ANTIHISTAMINES—terfenadine, hydroxyzine, mizolastine 8. ANTIMALARIALS—artemether with lumefantrine, chloroquine, hydroxychloroquine, quinine 9. ANTIPROTOZOALS—pentamidine isetionate	Risk of ventricular arrhythmias, particularly torsades de pointes	Additive effect; these drugs cause prolongation of the QT interval	Avoid coadministration

(*Continued*)

Primary Drug	Secondary Drug	Effect	Mechanism	Precautions
ANTIMALARIALS				
	10. ANTIPSYCHOTICS—atypicals, phenothiazines, pimozide 11. BETA-BLOCKERS—sotalol 12. BRONCHODILATORS—parenteral bronchodilators 13. CNS STIMULANTS—atomoxetine			
MEFLOQUINE	ANTIEPILEPTICS	↓ Efficacy of antiepileptics	Mefloquine can ↓ seizure threshold	Care with coadministration; ↑ dose of antiepileptic if ↑ incidence of fits
MEFLOQUINE	ANTIMALARIALS—CHLOROQUINE, QUININE	Risk of seizures	Additive effect	Warn patients of the risk; patients should be advised to avoid driving while taking these drugs in combination
MEFLOQUINE	BETA-BLOCKERS	↑ Risk of bradycardia	Mefloquine can cause cardiac conduction disorders, e.g., bradycardia. Additive bradycardic effect. Single case report of cardiac arrest with coadministration of mefloquine and propanolol possibly caused by QT prolongation	Monitor PR closely
MEFLOQUINE	CALCIUM CHANNEL BLOCKERS	Risk of bradycardia	Additive bradycardic effect; mefloquine can cause cardiac conduction disorders, e.g., bradycardia. There is also a theoretical risk of QT prolongation with coadministration of mefloquine and calcium channel blockers	Monitor PR closely
MEFLOQUINE	CARDIAC GLYCOSIDES—DIGOXIN	Risk of bradycardia	Uncertain; probably additive effect; mefloquine can cause AV block	Monitor PR and ECG closely

(Continued)

DRUGS TO TREAT INFECTIONS ANTIMALARIALS Proguanil

Primary Drug	Secondary Drug	Effect	Mechanism	Precautions
ANTIMALARIALS				
MEFLOQUINE	DRUG DEPENDENCE THERAPIES—BUPROPION	↑ Risk of seizures. This risk is prominent in elderly people, in patients with history of seizures, with addiction to opiates/cocaine/stimulants, and in diabetics treated with oral hypoglycemics or insulin	Bupropion is associated with a dose-related risk of seizures. These drugs, which lower seizure threshold, are individually epileptogenic. Additive effects occur when they are combined	Extreme caution. The dose of bupropion should not exceed 450 mg/day (or 150 mg/day in patients with severe hepatic cirrhosis)
MEFLOQUINE	H2 RECEPTOR BLOCKERS—CIMETIDINE	↑ Efficacy and adverse effects of antimalarials	Inhibition of metabolism, some definitely via CYP3A4	Avoid coadministration
MEFLOQUINE	IVABRADINE	Risk of arrhythmias with mefloquine	Additive effect	Monitor ECG closely
PRIMAQUINE				
PRIMAQUINE	ANTIMALARIALS—ARTEMETHER WITH LUMEFANTRINE	Risk of arrhythmias	Additive effect	Avoid coadministration
PRIMAQUINE	H2 RECEPTOR BLOCKERS—CIMETIDINE	↑ Efficacy and adverse effects of antimalarials	Inhibition of metabolism, some definitely via CYP3A4	Avoid coadministration
PRIMAQUINE	MEPACRINE	↑ Primaquine levels	Inhibition of metabolism	Warn patients to report the early features of primaquine toxicity (e.g., gastrointestinal disturbance). Monitor FBC closely
PROGUANIL				
PROGUANIL	ANTACIDS	↓ Proguanil levels	↓ Absorption	Separate doses by at least 4 h
PROGUANIL	ANTIDEPRESSANTS—TCAs	Possible ↑ plasma concentrations of proguanil	Inhibition of CYP2C19-mediated metabolism of proguanil. The clinical significance of this depends upon whether proguanil's alternative pathways of metabolism are also inhibited by coadministered drugs	Warn patients to report any evidence of excessive side effects such as a change in bowel habit or stomatitis

(Continued)

Primary Drug	Secondary Drug	Effect	Mechanism	Precautions
ANTIMALARIALS				
PROGUANIL	**ANTIMALARIALS**			
PROGUANIL	ARTEMETHER WITH LUMEFANTRINE	Risk of arrhythmias	Additive effect	Avoid coadministration
PROGUANIL	PYRIMETHAMINE	↑ Antifolate effect	Additive effect	Monitor FBC closely; the effect may take a number of weeks to occur
PROGUANIL	CNS STIMULANTS—MODAFINIL	May cause moderate ↑ plasma concentrations of these substrates	Modafinil is a reversible inhibitor of CYP2C19 when used in therapeutic doses	Be aware
PROGUANIL	H2 RECEPTOR BLOCKERS—CIMETIDINE	↓ Efficacy of proguanil	↓ Absorption and ↓ formation of active metabolite	Avoid concomitant use. Clinical significance is not established; effectiveness of malarial prophylaxis may be ↓
PYRIMETHAMINE				
PYRIMETHAMINE	ANTIBIOTICS—SULFONAMIDES, TRIMETHOPRIM	↑ Antifolate effect	Additive effect	Monitor FBC closely; the effect may take a number of weeks to occur
PYRIMETHAMINE	ANTIEPILEPTICS—PHENYTOIN	1. ↓ Efficacy of phenytoin 2. ↑ Antifolate effect	1. Uncertain 2. Additive effect	1. Care with coadministration; ↑ dose of antiepileptic if there is ↑ incidence of fits 2. Monitor FBC closely; the effect may take a number of weeks to occur
PYRIMETHAMINE	**ANTIMALARIALS**			
PYRIMETHAMINE	ARTEMETHER WITH LUMEFANTRINE	Risk of arrhythmias	Additive effect	Avoid coadministration
PYRIMETHAMINE	PROGUANIL	↑ Antifolate effect	Additive effect	Monitor FBC closely; the effect may take a number of weeks to occur

(*Continued*)

Primary Drug	Secondary Drug	Effect	Mechanism	Precautions
ANTIMALARIALS				
PYRIMETHAMINE	ANTICANCER AND IMMUNOMODULATING DRUGS—METHOTREXATE	↑ Antifolate effect	Pyrimethamine should not be used alone and is combined with sulfadoxine. Pyrimethamine and methotrexate synergistically induce folate deficiency	Although the toxic effects of methotrexate are more frequent with high doses of methotrexate, it is necessary to do FBC, liver and renal function tests before starting treatment even with low doses, repeating these tests weekly until therapy is stabilized and thereafter every 2–3 months. Patients should be advised to report symptoms such as sore throat and fever immediately, and also any gastrointestinal discomfort. A profound drop in white cell or platelet counts warrants immediate stoppage of methotrexate therapy and initiation of supportive therapy
PYRIMETHAMINE	ANTIVIRALS—ZIDOVUDINE	Possibly ↑ adverse effects with zidovudine	Additive toxicity	Monitor FBC and renal function closely. ↓ Doses as necessary. Use of pyrimethamine as prophylaxis seems to be tolerated
PYRIMETHAMINE	H2 RECEPTOR BLOCKERS—CIMETIDINE	↑ Efficacy and adverse effects of antimalarials	Inhibition of metabolism, some definitely via CYP3A4	Avoid coadministration
QUININE				
QUININE	**DRUGS THAT PROLONG THE QT INTERVAL**			
QUININE	1. ANTIARRHYTHMICS—amiodarone, disopyramide, procainamide, propafenone 2. ANTIBIOTICS—macrolides (especially azithromycin, clarithromycin, parenteral erythromycin, telithromycin), quinolones (especially moxifloxacin), quinupristin/dalfopristin	Risk of ventricular arrhythmias, particularly torsades de pointes	Additive effect; these drugs prolong the QT interval. In addition, quinine inhibits CYP2D6-mediated metabolism of procainamide	Avoid coadministration

(*Continued*)

Primary Drug	Secondary Drug	Effect	Mechanism	Precautions
ANTIMALARIALS				
	3. ANTICANCER AND IMMUNOMODULATING DRUGS—arsenic trioxide 4. ANTIDEPRESSANTS—TCAs, venlafaxine 5. ANTIEMETICS—dolasetron 6. ANTIFUNGALS—fluconazole, posaconazole, voriconazole 7. ANTIHISTAMINES—terfenadine, hydroxyzine, mizolastine 8. ANTIMALARIALS—artemether with lumefantrine, chloroquine, hydroxychloroquine, mefloquine 9. ANTIPROTOZOALS—pentamidine isetionate 10. ANTIPSYCHOTICS—atypicals, phenothiazines, pimozide 11. BETA-BLOCKERS—sotalol 12. BRONCHODILATORS—parenteral bronchodilators 13. CNS STIMULANTS—atomoxetine			
QUININE	ANALGESICS—OPIOIDS	↑ Codeine, fentanyl, pethidine, and tramadol levels	Quinine inhibits CYP2D6	Watch for excessive narcotization
QUININE	FLECAINIDE	Quinine may ↑ flecainide levels	Quinine inhibits CYP2D6-mediated metabolism of flecainide	The effect seems to be slight, but watch for flecainide toxicity; monitor PR and BP closely
QUININE	MEXILETINE	Quinine may ↑ mexiletine levels	Quinine inhibits CYP2D6-mediated metabolism of mexiletine	Monitor PR and BP closely
QUININE	ANTICANCER AND IMMUNOMODULATING DRUGS—PORFIMER	↑ Risk of photosensitivity reactions	Attributed to additive effects	Avoid exposure of skin and eyes to direct sunlight for 30 days after porfimer therapy
QUININE	ANTIMALARIALS—MEFLOQUINE	Risk of seizures	Additive effect	Warn patients of the risk; patients should be advised to avoid driving while taking these drugs in combination

(Continued)

Primary Drug	Secondary Drug	Effect	Mechanism	Precautions
ANTIMALARIALS				
QUININE	ANTI-PARKINSON'S DRUGS—AMANTADINE	↑ Side effects	↓ Renal excretion	Monitor closely for confusion, disorientation, headache, dizziness, and nausea
QUININE	BETA-BLOCKERS	Risk of ↑ plasma concentrations and effects of labetalol, metoprolol, and propranolol; ↑ systemic effects of timolol eye drops	Quinine inhibits CYP2D6, which metabolizes these beta-blockers	Monitor BP at least weekly until stable
QUININE	CARDIAC GLYCOSIDES—DIGOXIN	Plasma concentrations of digoxin may ↑ when it is coadministered with quinine	Uncertain, but seems to be due to ↓ nonrenal (possibly biliary) excretion of digoxin	Monitor digoxin levels; watch for digoxin toxicity
QUININE	H2 RECEPTOR BLOCKERS—CIMETIDINE	↑ Efficacy and adverse effects of antimalarials	Inhibition of metabolism, some definitely via CYP3A4	Avoid coadministration
QUININE	PARASYMPATHOMIMETICS	↓ Efficacy of parasympathomimetics	These antimalarials occasionally cause muscle weakness, which may exacerbate the symptoms of myasthenia gravis	Watch for poor response to these parasympathomimetics and ↑ dose accordingly

Primary Drug	Secondary Drug	Effect	Mechanism	Precautions
OTHER ANTIPROTOZOALS				
This section consists of antiprotozoal drugs. Note that antimalarials are also antiprotozoals but have been described in a separate section. Antibiotics with antiprotozoal activity are not included in this chapter. These include clindamycin, co-trimoxazole/trimethoprim, dapsone, doxycycline, and metronidazole				
LEVAMISOLE				
LEVAMISOLE	ALCOHOL	Risk of a disulfiram-like reaction	Uncertain	Warn patients not to drink while taking levamisole
LEVAMISOLE	ANTIBIOTICS—RIFAMPICIN	↓ Therapeutic efficacy of rifampicin	Levamisole displaces rifampicin from protein-binding sites, ↑ free fraction nearly three times and thus ↑ clearance of rifampicin	Avoid coadministration if possible

(Continued)

Primary Drug	Secondary Drug	Effect	Mechanism	Precautions
OTHER ANTIPROTOZOALS				
LEVAMISOLE	ANTICANCER AND IMMUNOMODULATING DRUGS—FLUOROURACIL	↑ Risk of hepatotoxicity and neurotoxicity despite ↑ Cytotoxic effects	Antiphosphatase activity of levamisole may ↑ fluorouracil cytotoxicity	This combination has been used successfully in the treatment of colon cancer. Monitor FBC and LFTs regularly. Advise patients to report symptoms such as diarrhea, numbness and tingling, and peeling of the skin of the hands and feet (hand–foot syndrome)
LEVAMISOLE	ANTICOAGULANTS—WARFARIN	Possible ↑ anticoagulant effect	Uncertain	Monitor INR closely
LEVAMISOLE	ANTIEPILEPTICS—PHENYTOIN	Possible ↑ phenytoin levels	Uncertain; case report of this interaction when levamisole and fluorouracil were coadministered with phenytoin	Monitor phenytoin levels and ↓ phenytoin dose as necessary
MEBENDAZOLE				
MEBENDAZOLE	ANTIEPILEPTICS—CARBAMAZEPINE, PHENYTOIN	↓ Mebendazole levels	Induction of metabolism	Watch for poor response to mebendazole
MEBENDAZOLE	H2 RECEPTOR BLOCKERS—CIMETIDINE	↑ Mebendazole levels	Inhibition of metabolism	Be aware; cases where this interaction have been used therapeutically
MEPACRINE				
MEPACRINE	ANTIMALARIALS—PRIMAQUINE	↑ Primaquine levels	Inhibition of metabolism	Warn patients to report the early features of primaquine toxicity (e.g., gastrointestinal disturbance). Monitor FBC closely
PENTAMIDINE ISETIONATE				
PENTAMIDINE ISETIONATE	**DRUGS THAT PROLONG THE QT INTERVAL**			
PENTAMIDINE ISETIONATE	1. ANTIARRHYTHMICS—amiodarone, disopyramide, procainamide, propafenone	Risk of ventricular arrhythmias, particularly torsades de pointes	Additive effect; these drugs cause prolongation of the QT interval	Avoid coadministration

(*Continued*)

Primary Drug	Secondary Drug	Effect	Mechanism	Precautions
OTHER ANTIPROTOZOALS				
	2. ANTIBIOTICS—macrolides (especially azithromycin, clarithromycin, parenteral erythromycin, telithromycin), quinolones (especially moxifloxacin), quinupristin/dalfopristin 3. ANTICANCER AND IMMUNOMODULATING DRUGS—arsenic trioxide 4. ANTIDEPRESSANTS—TCAs, venlafaxine 5. ANTIEMETICS—dolasetron 6. ANTIFUNGALS—fluconazole, posaconazole, voriconazole 7. ANTIHISTAMINES—terfenadine, hydroxyzine, mizolastine 8. ANTIMALARIALS—artemether with lumefantrine, chloroquine, hydroxychloroquine, mefloquine, quinine 9. ANTIPSYCHOTICS—atypicals, phenothiazines, pimozide 10. BETA-BLOCKERS—sotalol 11. BRONCHODILATORS—parenteral bronchodilators 12. CNS STIMULANTS—atomoxetine			
PENTAMIDINE	ANTIDIABETIC DRUGS—INSULIN, SULFONAMIDES, NATEGLINIDE, REPAGLINIDE, ACARBOSE	Altered insulin requirement	Attributed to pancreatic beta cell toxicity	Altered glycemic control; need to monitor blood sugar until stable and following withdrawal of pentamidine
PENTAMIDINE ISETIONATE	ANTIFUNGALS—AMPHOTERICIN	Risk of arrhythmias	Additive effect	Monitor ECG closely
PENTAMIDINE ISETIONATE	**ANTIVIRALS**			
PENTAMIDINE ISETIONATE	ADEFOVIR DIPIVOXIL	Possible ↑ efficacy and side effects	Competition for renal excretion	Monitor renal function weekly

(Continued)

Primary Drug	Secondary Drug	Effect	Mechanism	Precautions
OTHER ANTIPROTOZOALS				
PENTAMIDINE ISETIONATE (INTRAVENOUS)	FOSCARNET SODIUM	Risk of hypocalemia	Unclear; possibly additive hypocalcemic effects	Use extreme caution with intravenous pentamidine; monitor serum calcium (correct before the start of treatment), renal function, and for signs of tetany closely. Stop one drug if necessary
PENTAMIDINE ISETIONATE	NUCLEOSIDE REVERSE TRANSCRIPTASE INHIBITORS	↑ Adverse effects with didanosine, tenofovir, and zidovudine	Additive toxicity	Monitor FBC and renal function closely. Consider stopping didanosine while pentamidine is required for *Pneumocystis jiroveci* pneumonia
PENTAMIDINE ISETIONATE	IVABRADINE	Risk of arrhythmias	Additive effect	Monitor ECG closely
TINIDAZOLE				
TINIDAZOLE	ALCOHOL	Risk of a disulfiram-like reaction	Uncertain	Warn patients not to drink alcohol while taking levamisole
TINIDAZOLE	ESTROGENS—COMBINED ORAL CONTRACEPTIVE PILL	Possible ↓ contraceptive effect	Uncertain; possibly due to ↓ absorption resulting from alterations in gut flora	Warn patients to use barrier contraception during and up to 1 month after stopping tinidazole

Primary Drug	Secondary Drug	Effect	Mechanism	Precautions
ANTIVIRALS—ANTIRETROVIRALS				
NONNUCLEOSIDE REVERSE TRANSCRIPTASE INHIBITORS (NNRTIs)				
NNRTIs	**DRUGS THAT PROLONG THE QT INTERVAL**			
RILPIVIRINE	1. ANTIARRHYTHMICS—disopyramide, procainamide 2. ANTIBIOTICS—macrolides (especially azithromycin, clarithromycin, parenteral erythromycin, telithromycin), quinolones (especially moxifloxacin), quinupristin/dalfopristin	Risk of ventricular arrhythmias, particularly torsades de pointes	*Additive effect; these drugs prolong the QT interval*	Manufacturer advises use with caution as limited information is available. When used at 25 mg once daily, rilpivirine did not show a clinically significant effect on QT. If used in combination, monitor ECG and QT interval

(*Continued*)

Primary Drug	Secondary Drug	Effect	Mechanism	Precautions
ANTIVIRALS—ANTIRETROVIRALS				
	3. ANTICANCER AND IMMUNOMODULATING DRUGS—arsenic trioxide 4. ANTIDEPRESSANTS—TCAs, venlafaxine 5. ANTIEMETICS—dolasetron, cisapride 6. ANTIFUNGALS—fluconazole, posaconazole, voriconazole 7. ANTIHISTAMINES—terfenadine, hydroxyzine, mizolastine 8. ANTIMALARIALS—artemether with lumefantrine, chloroquine, mefloquine, quinine 9. ANTIPROTOZOALS—pentamidine isetionate 10. ANTIPSYCHOTICS—atypicals, phenothiazines, pimozide 11. BETA-BLOCKERS—sotalol 12. BRONCHODILATORS—parenteral bronchodilators 13. CNS STIMULANTS—atomoxetine			
NNRTIs	ANALGESICS—OPIOIDS	1. Methadone levels may be significantly ↓ by efavirenz and nevirapine 2. ↓ Bioavailability of buprenorphine and alfentanyl by efavirenz	1. ↑ CYP3A4 and CYP2B6-mediated metabolism of methadone 2. Likely altered metabolism via CYP3A4	Monitor closely for opioid withdrawal, ↑ dose as necessary. **Methadone:** likely to need dose titration of methadone (mean 22% but up to 186% ↑), no dose adjustment expected with etravirine, combination with rilpivirine on a long-term basis may require dose adjustment. **Buprenorphine:** patients did not experience withdrawal. **Alfentanyl:** increased dose of alfentanyl likely in patients on efavirenz

(*Continued*)

Primary Drug	Secondary Drug	Effect	Mechanism	Precautions
ANTIVIRALS—ANTIRETROVIRALS				
RILPIVIRINE	ANTACIDS	↓ Bioavailability of rilpivirine, likely ↓ in efficacy	↓ Absorption due to ↑ gastric pH	Use with caution, give antacid at least 2 h before or 4 h after rilpivirine
ETRAVIRINE	ANTIARRHYTHMICS	Possible ↑ efficacy and ↑ adverse effects	Uncertain	Use with caution and monitor ECG and antiarrhytmic levels if possible
NNRTIs	**ANTIBIOTICS**			
NNRTIs	MACROLIDES—CLARITHROMYCIN	1. ↓ Efficacy of clarithromycin but ↑ efficacy and adverse effects of active metabolite 2. ↑ Plasma levels of etravirine and nevirapine, anticipated ↑ of rilpivirine 3. Rash occurs in 46% of patients when efavirenz is given with clarithromycin	1. Uncertain: possibly due to altered CYP3A4-mediated metabolism 2. Inhibition of metabolism vua CYP3A as clarithromycin destroys the enzyme 3. Uncertain	1. Clinical significance unknown; no dose adjustment is recommended when clarithromycin is coadministered with nevirapine, but monitor LFTs closely. If treating Mycobacterium avium intracellulare complex, choose alternative treatment, e.g., azithromycin as active metabolite is less active against MAC 2. Consider alternatives to clarithromycin for patients on all NNRTIs. No interaction is expected with azithromycin. Erythromycin is expected to interact in a similar way to clarithromycin
NNRTIs	**RIFAMYCINS**			
EFAVIRENZ	RIFABUTIN	Possible ↓ efficacy of rifabutin	↓ bioavailability	↑ Rifabutin dose by 50% for daily treatment, or double the dose if patient is on two or three times a week treatment. Monitor clinical response to treatment closely

(*Continued*)

DRUGS TO TREAT INFECTIONS ANTIVIRALS—ANTIRETROVIRALS

Primary Drug	Secondary Drug	Effect	Mechanism	Precautions
ANTIVIRALS—ANTIRETROVIRALS				
EFAVIRENZ	RIFAMPICIN	Possible ↓ efficacy of efavirenz	Uncertain	For patients >50 kg consider an ↑ dose of efavirenz from 600 to 800 mg daily. Monitor clinical response to treatment closely and monitor for CNS toxicity. Increased dose in patients who lack CYP2B6 metabolizing capacity (homozygous inactive alleles can be up to 50% in African populations) will increase risk of side effects
ETRAVIRINE (WITH BOOSTED PROTEASE INHIBITOR-PI)	RIFABUTIN	1. Possible ↓ efficacy of etravirine 2. Possible increase in rifabutin levels and adverse effects	Likely to be altered metabolism via CYP3A4	Use combination with caution. Monitor closely for clinical response and adverse effects of rifabutin, rifabutin dose should be adjusted according to the PI used. Unboosted PI regimen gives reduced plasma levels of both drugs but combination can be used without dose adjustment of etravirine or rifabutin
ETRAVIRINE	RIFAMPICIN	Possible ↓ efficacy of etravirine	Probable ↑ metabolism of etravirine	Avoid coadministration
NEVIRAPINE	RIFABUTIN	Possible ↑ adverse effects of rifabutin	Likely altered metabolism and interpatient variability	Use with caution, monitor for signs of rifabutin toxicity
NEVIRAPINE	RIFAMPICIN	↓ Efficacy of nevirapine	Uncertain; probable ↑ metabolism of nevirapine	Avoid concomitant use. FDA recommends rifabutin as an alternative. Consider switching to efavirenz regimen. If combination has to be used and patient is already on rifampicin treatment, initiate nevirapine at 200 mg twice daily. Monitor closely. Increased dose in patients lacking CYP2B6 metabolizing capacity (homozygous inactive alleles can be up to 50% in African populations) will only increase risk of side effects e.g., rash, hepatitis

(Continued)

Primary Drug	Secondary Drug	Effect	Mechanism	Precautions
ANTIVIRALS—ANTIRETROVIRALS				
RILPIVIRINE	RIFABUTIN	↓ Efficacy of rilpivirine	Increased metabolism via CYP3A4 due to enzyme induction	When taken in combination, increase dose of rilpivirine from 25 to 50 mg once daily
RILPIVIRINE	RIFAMPICIN	↓ Efficacy of rilpivirine	Increased metabolism via CYP3A4 due to enzyme induction	Avoid coadministration
NNRTIs	**ANTICANCER AND IMMUNOMODULATING DRUGS**			
NNRTIs	**CYTOTOXICS**			
EFAVIRENZ	DOXORUBICIN	↑ Risk of myelosuppression due to ↑ plasma concentrations	Due to ↓ metabolism of doxorubicin by CYP3A4 isoenzymes owing to inhibition of those enzymes	Monitor for ↑ myelosuppression, peripheral neuropathy, myalgias, and fatigue
EFAVIRENZ	IFOSFAMIDE	↓ Plasma concentrations of 4-hydroxyifosfamide, the active metabolite of ifosfamide, and risk of inadequate therapeutic response	Due to inhibition of the isoenzymatic conversion to active metabolites	Monitor clinically the efficacy of ifosfamide and ↑ dose accordingly
EFAVIRENZ	IMATINIB	↑ Imatinib levels with ↑ risk of toxicity (e.g., abdominal pain, constipation, dyspnea) and of neurotoxicity (e.g., taste disturbances, dizziness, headache, paresthesia, peripheral neuropathy)	Due to inhibition of CYP3A4-mediated metabolism of imatinib	Monitor for clinical efficacy and for the signs of toxicity listed, along with convulsions, confusion, and signs of edema (including pulmonary edema). Monitor electrolytes, liver function and for cardiotoxicity
EFAVIRENZ	IRINOTECAN	↑ Plasma concentrations of the metabolite SN-38 (AUC by 100%) and ↑ toxicity of irinotecan, e.g., diarrhea, acute cholinergic syndrome, interstitial pulmonary disease	Due to inhibition of the metabolism of irinotecan by CYP3A4 isoenzymes by efavirenz	Peripheral blood counts should be checked before each course of treatment. Monitor lung function. Recommendation is to ↓ dose of irinotecan by 25%

(Continued)

Primary Drug	Secondary Drug	Effect	Mechanism	Precautions
ANTIVIRALS—ANTIRETROVIRALS				
EFAVIRENZ	VINCA ALKALOIDS	↑ Adverse effects of vinblastine and vincristine	Inhibition of CYP3A4-mediated metabolism. Also inhibition of Pgp efflux of vinblastine	Monitor FBCs and watch for early features of toxicity (pain, numbness, tingling in the fingers and toes, jaw pain, abdominal pain, constipation, ileus). Consider selecting an alternative drug
NNRTIs	**HORMONES AND HORMONE ANTAGONISTS**			
EFAVIRENZ	TOREMIFENE	↑ Plasma concentrations of toremifene	Due to inhibition of metabolism of toremifene by the CYP3A4 isoenzymes by efavirenz	Clinical relevance is uncertain. Necessary to monitor for clinical toxicities
NNRTIs	**IMMUNOMODULATING DRUGS**			
EFAVIRENZ, ETRAVIRINE, NEVIRAPINE	CICLOSPORIN, SIROLIMUS, TACROLIMUS	↓ Efficacy of ciclosporin, sirolimus and tacrolimus	Possibly ↑ CYP3A4-mediated metabolism of ciclosporin and effects on Pgp transport. Not studied for etravirine	Use combination with caution, monitor closely for clinical response, and check immunosuppressant levels for at least 2 weeks when treatment with NNRTIs is started or stopped
NNRTIs	CORTICOSTEROIDS	1. ↑ Adrenal suppressive effects of corticosteroids, which may ↑ risk of infections and produce an inadequate response to stress scenarios 2. Possible ↓ efficacy of rilpivirine and etravirine by dexamethasone	1. Due to inhibition of metabolism of corticosteroids 2. Induction of CYP3A4 by dexamethasone in doses used clinically	Avoid combination of rilpivirine and dexamethasone unless it is part of single dose treatment. Monitor cortisol levels and warn patients to report symptoms such as fever and sore throat
EFAVIRENZ, ETRAVIRINE, NEVIRAPINE	PROTEIN KINASE INHIBITORS—EVEROLIMUS	↓ Efficacy of everolimus	Unknown	Use combination with caution, monitor closely for clinical response when treatment with NNRTIs is started or stopped. Dose increase of everolimus advised with efavirenz and nevirapine, increase by 5 mg on day 4 and day 8 of combined treatment, if combination is stopped, allow a washout period of 3–5 days before reducing dose

(*Continued*)

Primary Drug	Secondary Drug	Effect	Mechanism	Precautions
ANTIVIRALS—ANTIRETROVIRALS				
NNRTIs	**ANTICOAGULANTS**			
RILPIVIRINE	DABIGATRAN	Possible ↑ in plasma levels of dabigatran	Inhibition of Pgp efflux of dabigatran	Use with caution and advise patients to report signs of bruising and bleeding promptly. ➢ **For signs and symptoms of overanticoagulation, see Clinical Features of Some Adverse Drug Interactions, Bleeding disorders**
NEVIRAPINE, ETRAVIRINE, EFAVIRENZ	WARFARIN, ACENOCOUMAROL	↓ Efficacy of warfarin with nevirapine	Altered metabolism. S-warfarin is metabolized by CYP2D6, and R-warfarin is metabolized by CYP3A4	Monitor INR every 3–7 days when starting or altering treatment and adjust dose by 10% as necessary. May need around twofold ↑ in dose with nevirapine
EFAVIRENZ	ANTIDEPRESSANTS—SSRIs	Possible ↓ efficacy with sertraline	CYP2B6 contributes most to the demethylation of sertraline with lesser contributions from CYP2C19, CYP2C9, CYP3A4, and CYP2D6	Watch for therapeutic failure, and advise patients to report persistence or lack of improvement of symptoms of depression. ↑ Dose of sertraline as required, titrating to clinical response
EFAVIRENZ	ANTIDIABETIC DRUGS—REPAGLINIDE	Likely to ↑ plasma concentrations of repaglinide and ↑ risk of hypoglycemic episodes	Due to inhibition of CYP3A4 isoenzymes, which metabolize repaglinide	Watch for and warn patients about hypoglycemia. ➢ **For signs and symptoms of hypoglycemia, see Clinical Features of Some Adverse Drug Interactions, Hypoglycemia**
NNRTIs	**ANTIEPILEPTICS**			
NNRTIs	CARBAMAZEPINE	1. Possible ↓ efficacy of carbamazepine by etravirine and nevirapine 2. ↓ Plasma levels of efavirenz, possible ↓ efficacy of etravirine and efavirenz 3. Possible significant ↓ in plasma levels of rilpivirine, risk of antiviral therapeutic failure	1. ↑ Metabolism via CYP3A4 2. ↑ Metabolism via induction of CYP3A4 and CYP2B6 3. Uncertain	1. Monitor closely, including carbamazepine levels and side effects when initiating or changing treatment 2. Combination with etravirine or efavirenz not recommended. 3. Avoid coadministration

(*Continued*)

Primary Drug	Secondary Drug	Effect	Mechanism	Precautions
ANTIVIRALS—ANTIRETROVIRALS				
EFAVIRENZ, ETRAVIRINE, RILPIVIRINE	PHENYTOIN, PHENOBARBITONE	1. Possible ↑ or ↓ efficacy of antiepileptic with efavirenz 2. Possible ↓ plasma levels of etravirine and rilpivirine	Altered metabolizm via CYP450	Monitor closely. Efavirenz: Monitor antiepileptic levels when starting, stopping, or changing treatment; allow 2 weeks for phenytoin levels to accurately reflect dose changes. Etravirine: combination not recommended. Rilpivirine: avoid coadministration.
NNRTIs	**ANTIFUNGALS**			
NNRTIs	AZOLES	1. Possible ↓ efficacy of itraconazole, ketoconazole and voriconazole 2. ↓ Plasma concentration of posaconazole 3. Possible ↑ in plasma concentration of rilpivirine 4. ↑ In plasma concentration of efavirenz, nevirapine, and etravirine	1. ↑ CYP3A4-mediated metabolism 2. Induction of UDP-G by efavirenz 3 ↓ CYP3A4-mediated metabolism 4. ↓ CYP3A4-mediated metabolism	Avoid coadministration with nevirapine. If nevirapine must be given, use itraconazole but consider a dose increase of itraconazole. If possible, avoid combination of itraconazole or posaconazole and efavirenz. Itraconazole and efavirenz: monitor clinical response closely, dose increase of itraconazole may be required. Voriconazole and efavirenz: increase voriconazole dose to 400 mg twice daily and reduced efavirenz dose by 50% to 300 mg once daily. Fluconazole 200 mg daily and efavirenz 400 mg daily can be combined without dose adjustment. Etravirine and rilpivirine can be used with any azole without dose adjustments of either drug group
EFAVIRENZ, NEVIRAPINE	CASPOFUNGIN	↓ Caspofungin levels, with risk of therapeutic failure	Induction of caspofungin metabolism	↑ Dose of caspofungin to 70 mg daily
EFAVIRENZ	ANTIHISTAMINES—TERFENADINE, ASTEMIZOLE	Risk of ventricular arrhythmias, particularly torsades de pointes	Possible reduced metabolism via CYP3A4	Avoid coadministration, cetirizine is a suitable alternative

(*Continued*)

Primary Drug	Secondary Drug	Effect	Mechanism	Precautions
ANTIVIRALS—ANTIRETROVIRALS				
NNRTIs	**ANTIMALARIALS**			
NNRTIs	LUMEFANTRINE	Possible ↑ plasma levels and ↑ side effects of lumefantrine, e.g., prolonged QT interval	Inhibition of metabolism	Monitor more closely, including ECG
EFAVIRENZ	ATOVAQUONE AND PROGUANIL	↓ Plasma levels of atovaquone and proguanil, risk of therapeutic failure	Uncertain mechanism	Avoid coadministration
ETRAVIRINE	ARTEMETHER WITH LUMEFANTRINE	↓ Levels of artemether and the active metabolite dihydroartemisinin, with risk of therapeutic failure	Uncertain mechanism	Monitor closely, including viral load, CD4 count, and response to antimalarial therapy
EFAVIRENZ, NEVIRAPINE	QUININE	↓ Plasma levels of quinine, ↑ plasma levels of metabolite with possible ↑ adverse effects	Altered metabolism via CYP3A4	Monitor for failure of therapeutic response and for increased side effects
NNRTIs	**ANTIMIGRAINE DRUGS**			
EFAVIRENZ	ERGOT DERIVATIVES	↑ Ergotamine/ methysergide levels, with risk of toxicity	↓ CYP3A4-mediated metabolism of ergot derivatives	Avoid coadministration
EFAVIRENZ	5-HT1 AGONISTS—ALMOTRIPTAN, ELETRIPTAN	↑ Plasma concentrations of almotriptan and eletriptan, and risk of toxic effects, e.g., flushing, sensations of tingling, heat, heaviness, pressure, or tightness of any part of body including the throat and chest, dizziness	Almotriptan and eletriptan are metabolized by CYP3A4 isoenzymes, which may be inhibited by efavirenz. However, since there is an alternative pathway of metabolism by MAOA, the toxicity responses will vary between individuals	The CSM has advised that if chest tightness or pressure is intense, the triptan should be discontinued immediately and the patient investigated for ischemic heart disease by measuring cardiac enzymes and doing an ECG. Avoid concomitant use in patients with coronary artery disease and in those with severe or uncontrolled hypertension
ETRAVIRINE	ANTIPLATELETS—CLOPIDOGREL	Possible ↓ efficacy of clopidogrel	Predicted inhibition of metabolism to clopidogrel's active metabolite	Combination not recommended

(*Continued*)

Primary Drug	Secondary Drug	Effect	Mechanism	Precautions
ANTIVIRALS—ANTIRETROVIRALS				
NNRTIs	**ANTIPSYCHOTICS**			
NNRTIs	ATYPICAL	↓ Efficacy of aripiprazole	↑ CYP3A4-mediated metabolism of aripiprazole	Monitor patient closely and ↑ dose of aripiprazole as necessary, double the dose of aripiprazole may be required
NNRTIs	PIMOZIDE	Possible ↑ efficacy and ↑ adverse effects, e.g., ventricular arrhythmias of pimozide	↓ CYP-3A4-mediated metabolism of pimozide	Avoid coadministration
ANTIVIRALS				
NNRTIs	**ANTIVIRALS FOR HEPATITIS C**			
EFAVIRENZ, NEVIRAPINE	TELAPREVIR	↓ Plasma concentrations of efavirenz and telaprevir possible altered plasma concentrations of nevirapine	↑ CYP3A4-mediated metabolism	If coadministered with efavirenz increase telaprevir to 1125 mg 8-hourly, consider a dose adjustment with nevirapine. No dose adjustment is required for etravirine or rilpivirine
ETRAVIRINE, NEVIRAPINE	BOCEPREVIR	Altered plasma concentrations, ↓ plasma concentrations of boceprevir with etravirine, possible ↓ therapeutic effect	Altered CYP3A4-mediated metabolism	Avoid coadministration with nevirapine, monitor clinical response closely with etravirine
NNRTIs	NNRTIs	1. Possible ↓ plasma levels and ↓ efficacy of etravirine by efavirenz and nevirapine 2. ↓ Plasma levels of efavirenz by nevirapine 3. Possible ↓ efficacy of rilpivirine 4. ↑ Toxicity and antagonistic HIV-1 activity (in vitro) with efavirenz and nevirapine	1. Uncertain 2. Probably increased metabolism 3. Probably increased metabolism of rilpivirine via CYP3A 4. Uncertain	Avoid coadministration. Use of two NNRTIs has not proved beneficial with regard to efficacy or safety. If efavirenz and nevirapine are coadministered, consider ↑ dose of efavirenz to 800 mg once daily

(*Continued*)

Primary Drug	Secondary Drug	Effect	Mechanism	Precautions
ANTIVIRALS—ANTIRETROVIRALS				
NNRTIs	**NRTIs**			
EFAVIRENZ	DIDANOSINE (ENTERIC-COATED), TENOFOVIR	1. A high treatment failure rate is reported when tenofovir, enteric-coated didanosine, and efavirenz are coadministered 2. Possible ↑ adverse effects of efavirenz	1. Unknown 2. Uncertain, possible reduced metabolism of efavirenz if low CYP2B6 activity	Use this combination with caution. Advise patients to report CNS side effects e.g., nightmares, dizziness, a dose reduction of efavirenz may be needed
EFAVIRENZ, NEVIRAPINE	ZIDOVUDINE	1. Possible ↓ efficacy of zidovudine 2. Possible ↑ risk of granulocytopenia with nevirapine	1. Possible ↑ CYP3A4-mediated metabolism of zidovudine 2. Additive side effects	Monitor more closely, including FBC, especially in pediatric patients, those on higher zidovudine doses or those with poor bone marrow reserve
RILPIVIRINE	DIDANOSINE	Possible ↓ efficacy of rilpivirine	Possible reduced absorption if antacids in didanosine formulation ↑ gastric pH, food also affects absorption	Didanosine must be taken on an empty stomach and rilpivirine with food. Take didanosine 2 h before or 4 h after rilpivirine
NNRTIs	**ANTIVIRALS—OTHER**			
NNRTIs	COBICISTAT	1. Possible ↓ plasma levels of cobicistat (not with rilpivirine), risk of treatment failure and resistance 2. Possible ↓ plasma levels of medicines being boosted e.g., protease inhibitor, risk of treatment failure, and resistance 3. Possible increase in plasma levels of nevirapine and rilpivirine	Induction of metabolism via CYP3A	Coadministration with efavirenz, etravirine, or nelfinavir not recommended. If required use with caution, no dose adjustment required with rilpivirne and atazanavir or darunavir/cobicistat combinations

(Continued)

Primary Drug	Secondary Drug	Effect	Mechanism	Precautions
ANTIVIRALS—ANTIRETROVIRALS				
EFAVIRENZ	MARAVIROC	↓ Plasma levels of maraviroc, risk of treatment failure, and resistance	Likely altered metabolism via CYP3A4 and Pgp	If in unboosted PI regimen or with efavirenz alone or in combination with tipranvir/ritonavir, increase maraviroc dose to 600 mg twice daily; if combined with other protease inhibitors or potent CYP3A4 inhibitors, reduce maraviroc to 150 mg twice daily. No interaction expected with nevirapine
EFAVIRENZ, ETRAVIRINE	RALTEGRAVIR	Both increased and decreased plasma levels of raltegravir reported	Altered metabolism	Monitor more closely
ETRAVIRINE	MARAVIROC	1. Possible ↑ bioavailability and ↑ adverse effects of maraviroc	Uncertain	Combination should be used in "boosted" protease inhibitor regimens. Dose adjustment of maraviroc to 150 mg BD required unless fosamprenavir/ritonavir when maraviroc 300 mg BD is required though latter combination is not recommended. Nevirapine can be administered without dose adjustment of either drug
NEVIRAPINE	ELVITEGRAVIR/COBICISTAT	Possible altered plasma levels of all agents	Not studied but altered metabolism via CYP450 likely	Avoid coadadministration
NEVIRAPINE	ZIDOVUDINE	↑ Risk of granulocytopenia	Additive side effects	Monitor closely
PROTEASE INHIBITORS				
NNRTIs	INDINAVIR	Possible ↓ efficacy of indinavir	↑ CYP3A4-mediated metabolism of indinavir	Avoid etravirine and indinavir combination. For others, monitor viral load; with nevirapine ↑ dose of indinavir to 1000 mg 8-hourly, with efavirenz this increase may not be sufficient, no dose adjustment needed for efavirenz or nevirapine when combined with indinavir

(Continued)

Primary Drug	Secondary Drug	Effect	Mechanism	Precautions
ANTIVIRALS—ANTIRETROVIRALS				
NNRTIs	LOPINAVIR AND RITONAVIR	Possible ↓ efficacy of lopinavir/ritonavir	Nevirapine induces metabolism of lopinavir via CYP3A4	Increase of lopinavir/ritonavir dose recommended and monitor drug concentrations with nevirapine. Adults: Use twice daily dosing and increase dose to 533/133 mg (from 3 to 4 caps) or 500/125 mg (5 tabs) or solution from 5 to 6.5 mL. Children: consider dose increase to 300/75 mg/m^2 twice daily taken with food. Monitor viral load closely as this dose ↑ may be insufficient. Monitor LFTs closely. No dose adjustment required with etravirine or rilpivirine
EFAVIRENZ	AMPRENAVIR	Possible ↓ efficacy of amprenavir	Uncertain; ↓ bioavailability of amprenavir	Consider ↑ dose of amprenavir to 1200 mg three times a day, or combine amprenavir 600 mg twice a day with ritonavir 100 mg twice a day
EFAVIRENZ	ATAZANAVIR WITH RITONAVIR	1. ↓ Efficacy of efavirenz 2. Possible ↓ efficacy of atazanavir	↑ CYP3A4-mediated metabolism and Pgp transport of efavirenz and atazanavir	Combination not recommended, if combination is required, increase atazanavir to 400 mg and ritonavir to 200 mg daily and give with efavirenz 600 mg daily
EFAVIRENZ	DARUNAVIR, DARUNAVIR/RITONAVIR	1. ↓ Efficacy of darunavir 2. ↑ Plasma levels and ↑ adverse effects of efavirenz	1. Increased metabolism via CYP3A4 2. Reduced metabolism via CYP3A4	Use with caution and monitor more closely. If used in combination give darunavir 600 mg and ritonavir 100 mg twice daily plus efavirenz 600 mg daily as darunavir/ritonavir 800/100 mg daily may result in treatment failure
EFAVIRENZ	FOSAMPRENAVIR	↓ Efficacy of fosamprenavir	Not studied	Avoid coadministration though an increased dose of fosamprenavir boosted with ritonavir (to 1400/300 mg respectively) can overcome reduction in plasma levels

(*Continued*)

Primary Drug	Secondary Drug	Effect	Mechanism	Precautions
ANTIVIRALS—ANTIRETROVIRALS				
EFAVIRENZ	NELFINAVIR	Possible ↑ efficacy of nelfinavir, with theoretical risk of adverse effects	Small ↑ bioavailability of nelfinavir	No dose adjustment necessary
EFAVIRENZ	RITONAVIR (HIGH DOSE 500 MG BD)	1. ↑ Efficacy and ↑ adverse effects of ritonavir, e.g., dizziness, nausea, paresthesia, and liver dysfunction (with 500 or 600 mg BD dose ritonavir) 2. ↑ Efficacy and ↑ adverse effects of efavirenz	1. ↓ Metabolism of ritonavir; competition for metabolism via CYP3A4. 2. Probably competition for metabolism via CYP3A4 and CYP2B6	Combination with high-dose ritonavir is not well tolerated. Monitor closely, including LFTs. Low-dose ritonavir alone has not been studied
EFAVIRENZ	SAQUINAVIR	↓ Plasma levels of saquinavir and possible ↓ efficacy, risk of treatment failure, ↑ adverse effects, e.g., liver dysfunction (particularly with ritonavir boosted regimen)	↑ CYP3A4-mediated metabolism of saquinavir	Combination not recommended with saquinavir as sole protease inhibitor, always use saquinavir in combination with another agent, e.g., ritonavir, when coadministering with efavirenz and monitor LFTs
ETRAVIRINE	NELFINAVIR	Possible ↑ bioavailability and ↑ adverse effects of nelfinavir	Not studied	Manufacturer of etravirine advises avoid coadministration
ETRAVIRINE	AMPRENAVIR OR FOSAMPRENAVIR/RITONAVIR	Possible ↑ bioavailability and ↑ adverse effects	Likely altered metabolism via CYP2C9 and CYP3A4 and altered transport via Pgp	Dose reduction of amprenavir or fosamprenavir required or fosamprenavir/ritonavir may be required
ETRAVIRINE	TIPRANAVIR/RITONAVIR	↓ Plasma levels of etravirine, ↑ plasma levels of tipranavir	Probably increased metabolism via CYP3A4 and UGT	Avoid concomitant use
ETRAVIRINE	UNBOOSTED PROTEASE INHIBITORS	↓ Plasma levels and efficacy of protease inhibitors	↑ CYP-mediated metabolism	Avoid concomitant use
NEVIRAPINE	AMPRENAVIR	Efficacy of amprenavir predicted to be ↓.	Uncertain; ↓ bioavailability of amprenavir	Monitor viral load
NEVIRAPINE	ATAZANAVIR, ATAZANAVIR/ RITONAVIR	↓ Efficacy of atazanavir, ↑ plasma levels of nevirapine	Atazanavir is a substrate and inhibitor of CYP3A4	Avoid concomitant use

(*Continued*)

Primary Drug	Secondary Drug	Effect	Mechanism	Precautions
ANTIVIRALS—ANTIRETROVIRALS				
NEVIRAPINE	FOSAMPRENAVIR	Possible ↓ plasma levels of fosamprenavir	Probably altered metabolism via CYP3A4 and induction of Pgp	Avoid coadministration unless fosamprenavir is boosted with ritonavir—in that case no dose adjustments are needed
NEVIRAPINE	NELFINAVIR	Possible ↓ efficacy of nelfinavir	Uncertain	Dose adjustment probably not required, although one study suggests ↑ dose of nelfinavir may be required
NEVIRAPINE	SAQUINAVIR	Possible ↓ efficacy, risk of treatment failure of saquinavir	↑ CYP3A4-mediated metabolism of saquinavir	Clinical significance unclear. Different formulations of saquinavir may have different magnitudes of interaction. If boosted with ritonavir, combination can be administered without dose adjustment
RILPIVIRINE	PROTEASE INHIBITORS—BOOSTED AND UNBOOSTED	↑ Plasma levels of rilpivirine	Likely inhibition of metabolism via CYP3A4	No dose adjustment necessary
EFAVIRENZ, ETRAVIRINE, NEVIRAPINE	ANXIOLYTICS AND HYPNOTICS—DIAZEPAM, MIDAZOLAM	↑ Efficacy and ↑ adverse effects, e.g., prolonged sedation	↓ CYP3A4-mediated metabolism of diazepam and midazolam	With all anxiolytics, monitor more closely, especially sedation levels. May need ↓ dose of diazepam or alteration of timing of dose. Avoid coadministration with midazolam and efavirenz. Consider switching to oxazepam or lorazepam as it has no active metabolites and shorter duration of action
EFAVIRENZ, NEVIRAPINE	CALCIUM CHANNEL BLOCKERS—DILTIAZEM	↓ Plasma levels of diltiazem, possible reduced efficacy	↑ Metabolism via CYP3A4	Monitor more closely and adjust dose of diltiazem to clinical response. Other calcium channel blockers metabolized via CYP3A4 are also likely to be affected
ETRAVIRINE	CARDIAC GLYCOSIDES—DIGOXIN	↑ Efficacy and ↑ adverse effects	Possibly due to altered metabolism via Pgp or CYP3A4	No dose adjustment necessary but monitor digoxin levels if toxicity suspected
EFAVIRENZ, NEVIRAPINE	CNS STIMULANTS—MODAFINIL	May ↓ modafinil levels	Induction of CYP3A4, which has a partial role in the metabolism of modafinil	Be aware

(*Continued*)

Primary Drug	Secondary Drug	Effect	Mechanism	Precautions
ANTIVIRALS—ANTIRETROVIRALS				
EFAVIRENZ	DRUG DEPENDENCE THERAPIES—BUPROPION	↓ Plasma concentrations of bupropion	Induction of CYP2B6	Titrate buproprion dose to clinical effect but do not exceed maximum dose
RILPIVIRINE	H2 RECEPTOR BLOCKERS	↓ Bioavailability of rilpivirine, likely ↓ in efficacy	↓ Absorption due to ↑ gastric pH	Use with caution, only dose H2 antagonist once daily at least 4 h after or 12 h before rilpivirine
EFAVIRENZ	GRAPEFRUIT JUICE	Possibly ↑ efficacy and ↑ adverse effects	Inhibition of metabolism via CYP3A4	Monitor more closely
NNRTIs	LIPID-LOWERING DRUGS—STATINS	1. ↓ Levels of atorvastatin, pravastatin, and simvastatin with efavirenz 2. Possible reduced (lovastatin, rosuvastatin, simvastatin) or increased levels (fluvastatin, rosuvastatin) with etravirine 3. ↓ Plasma levels of atorvastatin but ↑ levels of active metabolites with rilpivirine	1. Efavirenz induces CYP3A4 and intestinal Pgp, which may ↓ bioavailability of some statins (including atorvastatin) 2. Likely altered metabolism via CYP3A4 (lovastatin, rosuvastatin, simvastatin) and CYP2C9 (fluvastatin, rosuvastatin) 3. Possibly altered metabolism via CYP enzymes	Monitor lipid profile more closely, titrate doses as necessary. Atorvastatin can be used in combination without initial dose adjustment, including with rilpivirine. No interaction expected with pravastatin
NEVIRAPINE	ESTROGENS—ETHINYLESTRADIOL	Marked ↓ contraceptive effect with nevirapine	Induction of metabolism of estrogens	Avoid coadministration, recommend alternative nonhormonal contraceptives—barrier methods are necessary to prevent transmission of infection. Etravirine and rilpivirine can be used in combination without dose adjustment
ETRAVIRINE	PHOSPHODIESTERASE TYPE 5 INHIBITORS—SILDENAFIL, TADALAFIL, VARDENAFIL	↓ Plasma levels of phosphodiesterase 5 inhibitor	Induction of metabolism via CYP3A4	Dose adjustment may be required, titrate phosphodiesterase inhibitor to clinical effect. No adjustment needed with rilpivirine

(*Continued*)

Primary Drug	Secondary Drug	Effect	Mechanism	Precautions
ANTIVIRALS—ANTIRETROVIRALS				
NEVIRAPINE, EFAVIRENZ	PROGESTOGENS	↓ Efficacy of norethisterone, and levonorgestrel and etonogestrel implants, with risk of contraceptive failure	Uncertain	Avoid coadministration; recommend alternative nonhormonal contraceptives—barrier methods are necessary to prevent transmission of infection. Etravirine can be used in combination without dose adjustment. No pharmacokinetic interaction seen with efavirenz or nevirapine and depot medroxyprogesterone
RILPIVIRINE	PROTON PUMP INHIBITORS	↓ Bioavailability of rilpivirine, likely ↓ in efficacy	↓ Absorption due to ↑ gastric pH	Avoid coadministration
NNRTIs	ST. JOHN'S WORT	↓ Plasma levels of NNRTI and reduced efficacy	Induction of metabolizing enzymes and transport proteins	Avoid coadministration
NUCLEOSIDE REVERSE TRANSCRIPTASE INHIBITORS (NNRTIs)				
NUCLEOSIDE REVERSE TRANSCRIPTASE INHIBITORS	**ANALGESICS**			
TENOFOVIR	NSAIDs	↑ Risk of renal impairment with NSAIDs	Additive side effects	Use with caution. Consider paracetamol with a weak opioid that is needed as an alternative. If coadministered, limit NSAID to a short course
ZIDOVUDINE	NSAIDs	↑ Risk of hematological effects of zidovudine, ↑ risk of bleeding	Additive side effects	If possible avoid coadministration. Consider paracetamol combined with a weak opioid if needed. If combined limit NSAID to a short course <3 days and advise patients to monitor for signs of bleeding or bruising

(Continued)

Primary Drug	Secondary Drug	Effect	Mechanism	Precautions
ANTIVIRALS—ANTIRETROVIRALS				
ABACAVIR, DIDANOSINE (TABLET PREP), STAVUDINE, ZIDOVUDINE	METHADONE	1. ↓ Efficacy of methadone when coadministered with abacavir and possibly with zidovudine 2. ↓ Plasma levels of didanosine and stavudine with long-term methadone 3. ↑ Bioavailability of zidovudine with methadone	1. Uncertain; possibly enzyme induction 2. Possibly reduced absorption 3. Inhibition of glucuronidation	Monitor for opioid withdrawal and consider ↑ dose, monitor clinical response to didanosine; closely consider using GR preparation, monitor for increased zidovudine side effects and toxicity. Changes to stavudine levels not thought to be clinically significant
DIDANOSINE, ZIDOVUDINE	PARACETAMOL	Cases of hepatotoxicity reported when paracetamol was added to either didanosine or zidovudine	Uncertain; possible additive hepatotoxic effect	Monitor liver function regularly during coadministration
NUCLEOSIDE REVERSE TRANSCRIPTASE INHIBITORS	**ANTIBIOTICS**			
NUCLEOSIDE REVERSE TRANSCRIPTASE INHIBITORS	AMINOGLYCOSIDES	Possibly ↑ risk of nephrotoxicity	Additive effect	Avoid coadministration if possible; otherwise, monitor renal function weekly
DIDANOSINE	ETHAMBUTOL	Possibly ↑ adverse effects (e.g., peripheral neuropathy) with didanosine	Additive side effects	Monitor closely for development of peripheral neuropathy, but no dose adjustment required
STAVUDINE, ZIDOVUDINE	CHLORAMPHENICOL	Possible ↑ adverse effects when coadministered with stavudine or zidovudine	Uncertain	Use an alternative antibiotic if possible; otherwise, monitor closely for peripheral neuropathy and check FBC regularly
ZIDOVUDINE	CLARITHROMYCIN	Possible ↓ efficacy of zidovudine	↓ Absorption	Separate doses by 2–4 h
NUCLEOSIDE REVERSE TRANSCRIPTASE INHIBITORS+	CO-TRIMOXAZOLE (TRIMETHOPRIM AND SULFAMETHOXAZOLE)	1. ↑ Adverse effects 2. ↑ Plasma concentration of lamivudine, zalcitabine, and zidovudine	1. Additive toxicity 2. Competition for renal tubular secretion	↓ Doses as necessary; monitor FBC and renal function closely. Coadministration with high dose co-trimoxazole not recommended, if essential monitor for increased lamivudine toxicity. Doses of co-trimoxazole used for prophylaxis seem to be tolerated

(*Continued*)

Primary Drug	Secondary Drug	Effect	Mechanism	Precautions
ANTIVIRALS—ANTIRETROVIRALS				
ZIDOVUDINE	DAPSONE	Possible ↑ adverse effects when coadministered with zidovudine	Uncertain; possible ↑ bioavailability of zidovudine	Use with caution, monitor FBC and for peripheral neuropathy
NUCLEOSIDE REVERSE TRANSCRIPTASE INHIBITORS	ISONIAZID	↑ Adverse effects, including peripheral neuropathy particularly with didanosine and stavudine	Additive side effects	Avoid coadministration with didanosine and stavudine. For others, use with caution, monitor closely for the development of peripheral neuropathy, but no dose adjustment required. If stavudine has to be continued, ensure prophylactic pyridoxine is also given
DIDANOSINE, STAVUDINE	METRONIDAZOLE	↑ Adverse effects (e.g., peripheral neuropathy) with didanosine and possibly stavudine	Additive effect	Monitor closely for peripheral neuropathy during intensive or prolonged combination
DIDANOSINE (BUFFERED TABLETS)	QUINOLONES	↓ Efficacy of ciprofloxacin and possibly levofloxacin, moxifloxacin, norfloxacin, and ofloxacin with buffered didanosine	Cations in the buffer of didanosine preparation chelate and adsorb ciprofloxacin. Absorption of the other quinolones may be ↓ by the buffered didanosine formulation, which also raises gastric pH	Give the antibiotic 2 h before or 6 h after didanosine. Alternatively, consider using the gastroresistant formulation of didanosine, which need not be given separately
DIDANOSINE (BUFFERED TABLETS)	TETRACYCLINES	↓ Efficacy of tetracycline, and possibly demeclocycline, doxycycline, lymecycline, minocycline, and oxytetracycline with buffered didanosine	Absorption may be affected by the buffered didanosine formulation, which raises gastric pH	Avoid coadministration with buffered didanosine preparations. Consider changing to gastroresistant didanosine capsules
NUCLEOSIDE REVERSE TRANSCRIPTASE INHIBITORS	TRIMETHOPRIM	1. Possibly ↑ hematological toxicity 2. ↑ Plasma concentration of lamivudine, zalcitabine and zidovudine	1. Additive toxicity 2. Competition for renal tubular secretion	Monitor FBC and renal function closely, coadministration with high dose co-trimoxazole not recommended, if essential monitor for increased lamivudine toxicity

(*Continued*)

Primary Drug	Secondary Drug	Effect	Mechanism	Precautions
ANTIVIRALS—ANTIRETROVIRALS				
TENOFOVIR, ZIDOVUDINE	VANCOMYCIN	↑ Adverse effects with zidovudine and tenofovir/	Additive toxicity	Avoid coadministration if possible; if not, monitor FBC and renal function closely (at least weekly)
NUCLEOSIDE REVERSE TRANSCRIPTASE INHIBITORS	**CYTOTOXICS**			
TENOFOVIR	CHEMOTHERAPEUTIC REGIMENS FOR LYMPHOMA	↑ Risk of renal toxicity	Additive toxicity	Monitor renal function closely
ZIDOVUDINE	STANDARD CHEMOTHERAPEUTIC REGIMENS	↑ Risk of blood dyscrasias, e.g., neutropenia	Additive toxicity	Substitute zidovudine for an alternative NRTI or consider less myelosuppressive chemotherapy if possible. Monitor closely for neutropenia if combined and ensure patient reports any signs of infection
EMTRICITABINE, LAMIVUDINE	CLADRABINE	Possible therapeutic failure of cladrabine	Competition for intracellular activation via phosphorylation by deoxycytidine kinase	Avoid coadministration
STAVUDINE, ZIDOVUDINE	DOXORUBICIN	1. Possible reduced efficacy of stavudine 2. ↑ Adverse effects when doxorubicin is coadministered with zidovudine	1. Inhibition of activation via phosphorylation 2. Additive toxicity	Use with caution, monitor closely for treatment response and monitor FBC and renal function closely. Adjust doses as necessary
DIDANOSINE, STAVUDINE,	ERLOTINIB AND GEFITINIB	↑ Risk of hematological toxicity	Additive toxicity	Avoid coadministration
DIDANOSINE, STAVUDINE, ZIDOVUDINE	ETOPOSIDE	↑ Risk of hematological toxicity	Additive toxicity	Review for alternative treatment options, consider substitution of an alternative NRTI or antiretroviral
DIDANOSINE, STAVUDINE, ZIDOVUDINE	GEMCITABINE	↑ Risk of hematological and renal toxicity	Additive toxicity	Avoid coadministration with didanosine and stavudine. Monitor renal function closely

(*Continued*)

Primary Drug	Secondary Drug	Effect	Mechanism	Precautions
ANTIVIRALS—ANTIRETROVIRALS				
DIDANOSINE, STAVUDINE, ZIDOVUDINE	HYDROXYCARBAMIDE	1. ↑ Adverse effects, including deaths with didanosine in combination or not with stavudine, and possibly zidovudine, e.g., pancreatitis, heptatotoxicity, and peripheral neuropathy 2. Possible ↑ antiviral efficacy	Additive effects, enhanced antiretroviral activity via ↓ intracellular deoxynucleotides	**Avoid coadministration of triple therapy with didanosine, stavudine, and hydroxycarbamide** as deaths from hepatic failure are most commonly reported with this combination. For other combinations, monitor closely for peripheral neuropathy
DIDANOSINE, STAVUDINE, TENOFOVIR	IRINOTECAN, TOPOTECAN	↑ Adverse effects	Additive toxicity, competition for excretion	Avoid coadministration. Review for alternative treatment options, consider substitution of an alternative NRTI or antiretroviral
DIDANOSINE, STAVUDINE, TENOFOVIR, ZIDOVUDINE	PEMETREXED	↑ Risk of hematological, renal toxicity (particularly with tenofovir)	Additive toxicity, competition for excretion	Avoid coadministration with didanosine and stavudine. Monitor renal function closely, ensure folic acid supplementation especially if co-trimoxazole is co-prescribed
DIDANOSINE, STAVUDINE,	PLATINUM COMPOUNDS	↑ Risk of peripheral neuropathy	Additive toxicity	Review for alternative treatment options, consider substitution of an alternative NRTI or antiretroviral
DIDANOSINE, STAVUDINE,	TAXANES	↑ Risk of peripheral neuropathy	Additive toxicity	Review for alternative treatment options, consider substitution of an alternative NRTI or antiretroviral
DIDANOSINE, STAVUDINE, ZIDOVUDINE	VINCA ALKALOIDS	1. ↑ Risk of peripheral neuropathy particularly with didanosine and stavudine 2. ↑ Adverse effects when vincristine and possibly vinblastine are coadministered with zidovudine	Additive toxicity	Review for alternative treatment options, consider substitution of an alternative NRTI or antiretroviral. Use with caution. Monitor FBC and renal function closely. ↓ Doses as necessary

(*Continued*)

Primary Drug	Secondary Drug	Effect	Mechanism	Precautions
ANTIVIRALS—ANTIRETROVIRALS				
NUCLEOSIDE REVERSE TRANSCRIPTASE INHIBITORS	**IMMUNOMODULATING DRUGS**			
LAMIVUDINE	AZATHIOPRINE	↑ Adverse effects with lamivudine	Unclear	Monitor closely
TENOFOVIR	IL-2	↑ Adverse effects with tenofovir	Uncertain	Avoid if possible, otherwise, monitor renal function weekly
TENOFOVIR	CICLOSPORIN, TACROLIMUS	Possibly ↑ adverse effects	Additive renal toxicity	Monitor renal function
ZIDOVUDINE	INTERFERON	↑ Adverse effects, e.g., lactic acidosis, hepatic decompensation, anemia	Beta interferon inhibits metabolism of zidovudine. Alfa interferon—additive toxicity	Monitor FBC, hepatic and renal function closely. Stop or substitute zidovudine if necessary
DIDANOSINE, STAVUDINE, TENOFOVIR	ANTIDIABETIC DRUGS—METFORMIN	Possible ↑ risk of lactic acidosis	Additive toxicity	Monitor closely
NUCLEOSIDE REVERSE TRANSCRIPTASE INHIBITORS	**ANTIEPILEPTICS**			
DIDANOSINE, STAVUDINE, ZIDOVUDINE	PHENYTOIN	1. Possibly ↑ adverse effects (e.g., peripheral neuropathy) with didanosine, stavudine, and zidovudine 2. Altered phenytoin plasma levels with zidovudine	1. Additive effect 2. Unclear	Monitor closely for peripheral neuropathy during prolonged combination; if on zidovudine, monitor phenytoin levels more closely
ZIDOVUDINE	BARBITURATES/PRIMIDONE	Possible ↓ efficacy; risk of treatment failure of zidovudine	Possibly enzyme induction	Coadminister with caution
ZIDOVUDINE	CARBAMAZEPINE/ OXCARBAZEPINE	Possible ↓ efficacy; risk of treatment failure of zidovudine	Possibly enzyme induction	Coadadminister with caution
ZIDOVUDINE	VALPROATE	↑ Zidovudine levels	Inhibition of metabolism	Watch for early features of toxicity of zidovudine

(*Continued*)

Primary Drug	Secondary Drug	Effect	Mechanism	Precautions
ANTIVIRALS—ANTIRETROVIRALS				
NUCLEOSIDE REVERSE TRANSCRIPTASE INHIBITORS	**ANTIFUNGALS**			
TENOFOVIR, ZIDOVUDINE	AMPHOTERICIN	Possibly ↑ adverse effects with tenofovir and zidovudine	Additive toxicity	Avoid if possible, otherwise, monitor FBC and renal function (weekly). ↓ Doses as necessary
ZIDOVUDINE	AZOLES—FLUCONAZOLE	↑ Zidovudine levels	Inhibition of metabolism	Monitor more closely, especially if for extended course of antifungal treatment, consider a dose reduction of zidovudine
DIDANOSINE (BUFFERED TABLETS)	AZOLES—ITRACONAZOLE, KETOCONAZOLE	Possibly ↓ efficacy of ketoconazole and itraconazole with buffered didanosine	Absorption of ketoconazole and itraconazole may be ↓ by the buffered didanosine formulation, which raises gastric pH	Give the ketoconazole or itraconazole 2 h before or 6 h after didanosine. Alternatively, consider using the enteric-coated formulation of didanosine, which does not have to be given separately
ZIDOVUDINE	FLUCYTOSINE	Possibly ↑ adverse effects with zidovudine	Additive toxicity	Avoid if possible; otherwise, monitor FBC and renal function (weekly). ↓ Doses as necessary
ZIDOVUDINE	RIFAMPICIN	1. ↓ Plasma concentration of zidovudine 2. ↑ Risk of anemia	1. Partially through ↑ glucuronidation 2. Additive toxicity	Manufacturer recommends avoid coadministration but combination is not thought to cause a clinically significant interaction
DIDANOSINE	ALLOPURINOL	↑ Levels of didanosine	Probably altered metabolism via xanthine oxidase	Coadministration not recommended, consider alternative regimens. Watch for early signs of toxicity, especially in patients with renal impairment. A dose reduction of didanosine may be required if combination is essential
ZIDOVUDINE	PROBENECID	↑ Levels of zidovudine, with cases of toxicity	Competition for renal tubular secretion via OATs	Avoid coadministration if possible; if not possible, monitor closely, including LFTs. ↓ Dose of zidovudine

(Continued)

Primary Drug	Secondary Drug	Effect	Mechanism	Precautions
ANTIVIRALS—ANTIRETROVIRALS				
NUCLEOSIDE REVERSE TRANSCRIPTASE INHIBITORS	ANTIHYPERTENSIVES AND HEART FAILURE DRUGS—VASODILATOR ANTIHYPERTENSIVES	Risk of peripheral neuropathy when hydralazine is coadministered with didanosine, stavudine, or zalcitabine	Additive effect; both drugs can cause peripheral neuropathy	Warn patients to report early features of peripheral neuropathy (tingling, weakness, pain); if this occurs, the nucleoside reverse transcriptase inhibitor should be stopped
NUCLEOSIDE REVERSE TRANSCRIPTASE INHIBITORS	**ANTIMALARIALS**			
ZIDOVUDINE	ATOVAQUONE	Atovaquone ↑ zidovudine levels	Atovaquone inhibits glucuronidation of zidovudine	Uncertain clinical significance. Monitor FBC, LFTs, and lactate closely during coadministration. Three-week acute course for pneumocyctis carinii pneumonia (PCP) tolerated but caution with longer treatment
ZIDOVUDINE	PYRIMETHAMINE	Possibly ↑ adverse effects with zidovudine	Additive toxicity	Monitor FBC and renal function closely. ↓ Doses as necessary. Use of pyrimethamine as prophylaxis seems to be tolerated
NUCLEOSIDE REVERSE TRANSCRIPTASE INHIBITORS	ANTIPROTOZOALS—PENTAMIDINE ISETIONATE (IV)	↑ Adverse effects, e.g., pancreatitis with didanosine, tenofovir, and zidovudine	Additive toxicity	Avoid coadministration with tenofovir. For others discontinue NRTI if possible. Monitor FBC, LFTs, and renal function closely. Consider stopping didanosine while pentamidine is required for Pneumocystis jiroveci pneumonia. Nebulized pentamidine not thought to interact significantly
ZIDOVUDINE	BARBITURATES/PRIMIDONE	↑ Adverse effects, e.g., bone marrow suppression	Additive toxicity	Use with caution, monitor more closely, especially FBC
NUCLEOSIDE REVERSE TRANSCRIPTASE INHIBITORS	**ANTIVIRALS—OTHER**			
TENOFOVIR	ADEFOVIR, CIDOFOVIR	↑ Adverse effects	↑ Plasma levels, competition for renal excretion via organic anion transporter	Avoid coadministration

(Continued)

Primary Drug	Secondary Drug	Effect	Mechanism	Precautions
ANTIVIRALS—ANTIRETROVIRALS				
TENOFOVIR, ZALCITABINE	FOSCARNET SODIUM	↑ Adverse effects with tenofovir and possibly zalcitabine	Uncertain; possibly additive toxicity via competition for renal excretion I	Avoid if possible; otherwise, monitor FBC and renal function weekly
NUCLEOSIDE REVERSE TRANSCRIPTASE INHIBITORS	GANCICLOVIR/VALGANCICLOVIR	1. ↑ Adverse effects with tenofovir (renal dysfunction), zidovudine (myelosuppression—severe neutropenia), ↑ plasma levels of didanosine, possible ↑ adverse effects with lamivudine and zalcitabine 2. Possibly ↓ efficacy of ganciclovir by didanosine	1. Uncertain; possibly additive toxicity. Lamivudine and Tenofovir may compete for active tubular secretion in the kidneys. Inhibition of didanosine metabolism via purine nucleoside phosphorlyase-4 2. Uncertain; small ↓ bioavailability	1. Avoid if possible; otherwise, monitor FBC and renal function weekly. It has been suggested that the dose of zidovudine should be halved from 600 to 300 mg daily. Monitor for peripheral neuropathy, particularly with zalcitabine 2. Uncertain clinical significance; if in doubt, consider alternative treatment options. Stavudine does not show any clinical significant interaction
NUCLEOSIDE REVERSE TRANSCRIPTASE INHIBITORS	RIBAVIRIN	1. ↑ Side effects, risk of lactic acidosis, peripheral neuropathy, pancreatitis, hepatic decompensation, and mitochondrial toxicity with didanosine and stavudine. ↑ Risk of anemia, particularly with didanosine, stavudine, and zidovudine, ↑ risk of myelosuppression with zidovudine. Fatal hepatic failure has been reported 2. ↓ Efficacy of lamivudine and possible ↓ efficacy stavudine and zidovudine	1. Additive side effects; ↑ intracellular activation of didanosine 2. ↓ Intracellular activation of lamivudine and possibly stavudine and zidovudine	1. Coadministration with didanosine, stavudine, or zidovudine not recommended. Alter treatment if possible. Use with extreme caution; monitor lactate, FBC, LFTs, and amylase closely. Stop coadministration if peripheral neuropathy occurs. Stavudine and didanosine carry a higher risk 2. Monitor HIV RNA levels; if they ↑, review treatment combination
ABACAVIR	RIBAVIRIN	Risk of poor therapeutic response	Probably competition for phosphorylation	Use with caution, monitor therapeutic response closely when combined with interferon to treat hepatitis C

(*Continued*)

Primary Drug	Secondary Drug	Effect	Mechanism	Precautions
ANTIVIRALS—ANTIRETROVIRALS				
TENOFOVIR, ZIDOVUDINE	TELAPREVIR	1. ↑ Plasma levels of tenofovir by telaprevir 2. ↑ Risk of anemia with zidovudine	1. Altered transport via Pgp (intestinal) 2. Additive toxicity	Use with caution monitor renal function, and for increased side effects of tenofovir, monitor FBC with zidovudine
ZIDOVUDINE	BOCEPREVIR	↑ Risk of anemia	Additive toxicity	Monitor more closely especially if combined with ribavirin
NUCLEOSIDE REVERSE TRANSCRIPTASE INHIBITORS	**NNRTIs**			
DIDANOSINE (ENTERIC-COATED), TENOFOVIR	EFAVIRENZ	1. A high treatment failure rate is reported when tenofovir, enteric-coated didanosine, and efavirenz are coadministered 2. Possible ↑ adverse effects of efavirenz	1. Unknown 2. Uncertain, possible reduced metabolism of efavirenz if low CYP2B6 activity	Use this combination with caution. Advise patients to report CNS side effects e.g., nightmares, dizziness, a dose reduction of efavirenz may be needed
DIDANOSINE	RILPIVIRINE	Possible ↓ efficacy of rilpivirine	Possible reduced absorption if antacids in didanosine formulation ↑ gastric pH, food also affects absorption	Didanosine must be taken on an empty stomach and rilpivirine with food. Take didanosine 2 h before or 4 h after rilpivirine
ZIDOVUDINE	EFAVIRENZ, NEVIRAPINE	1. Possible ↓ efficacy of zidovudine 2. Possible ↑ risk of granulocytopenia with nevirapine	1. Possible ↑ CYP3A4-mediated metabolism of zidovudine 2. Additive side effects	Monitor more closely, including FBC, especially in pediatric patients, those on higher zidovudine doses, or those with poor bone marrow reserve
NUCLEOSIDE REVERSE TRANSCRIPTASE INHIBITORS	**NUCLEOSIDE REVERSE TRANSCRIPTASE INHIBITORS**			
NUCLEOSIDE REVERSE TRANSCRIPTASE INHIBITORS	NUCLEOSIDE REVERSE TRANSCRIPTASE INHIBITORS	↓ Efficacy, high rate of virological failure, viral resistance	Unknown	Avoid combination of lamivudine with tenofovir and abacavir or temofovir and didanosine. Combinations not recommended, clinical experience shows use of one NRTI to give NRTI backbone is preferable rather than combined therapy

(*Continued*)

Primary Drug	Secondary Drug	Effect	Mechanism	Precautions
ANTIVIRALS—ANTIRETROVIRALS				
EMTRICITABINE, STAVUDINE	LAMIVUDINE	Unknown	Unknown	Combination not recommended. Clinical experience shows use of one NRTI to give NRTI backbone is preferable rather than combined therapy
DIDANOSINE	STAVUDINE	↑ Adverse effects, including pancreatitis (fatal and nonfatal), lactic acidosis (in pregnancy, sometimes fatal), ↑ risk of stillbirth and neuropathy (severe in some cases)	Additive effect	Avoid combination in pregnancy and children if possible. Avoid triple combination with hydroxyurea. If used monitor closely, especially for pancreatitis, lactic acidosis, and peripheral neuropathy. Relative risk of neuropathy: stavudine alone 1.39 compared with didanosine; combined use 3.5
DIDANOSINE	TENOFOVIR	1. ↑ Plasma levels of didanosine and ↑ adverse effects, including pancreatitis, lactic acidosis (sometimes fatal), and neuropathy 2. May reduce CD4 count	1. Probably competition for active renal tubular secretion 2. Possibly an intracellular interaction increasing phosphorylation of didanosine	Coadministration not recommended. Not recommended in patients with a high viral load and low CD4 count (enteric-coated and buffered tablets) but 400 mg didanosine has been used. Monitor closely for antiviral efficacy and side effects (pancreatitis, neuropathy, lactic acidosis, renal failure). ↓ dose of didanosine to 250 mg has been tried but high failure rate and emergence of resistance was the result. 1. Do not use in combination as triple therapy with lamivudine is associated with a high level of treatment failure

(*Continued*)

Primary Drug	Secondary Drug	Effect	Mechanism	Precautions
ANTIVIRALS—ANTIRETROVIRALS				
STAVUDINE	ZIDOVUDINE	Possibly ↓ efficacy of stavudine, antagonism (in vivo)	↓ Cellular activation of stavudine. Both are phosphorylated to the active form by thymidine kinase, which preferentially phosphorylates zidovudine, therefore causes ↓ phosphorylation of stavudine	Avoid coadministration
NUCLEOSIDE REVERSE TRANSCRIPTASE INHIBITORS	**PROTEASE INHIBITORS**			
TENOFOVIR	ATAZANAVIR, DARUNAVIR, LOPINAVIR (ALL WITH RITONAVIR)	1. ↓ Efficacy of atazanavir 2. Possible ↑ in plasma levels and ↑ adverse effects of tenofovir by atazanavir, e.g., renal dysfunction 3. ↑ Plasma levels of tenofovir by lopinavir	1. Uncertain; ↓ plasma levels of atazanavir 2. Uncertain 3. Altered transport via Pgp (intestinal)	Use with caution with atazanavir. Monitor renal function and for increased side effects of tenofovir
ABACAVIR, ZIDOVUDINE	LOPINAVIR/RITONAVIR	↓ Plasma levels of abacavir and zidovudine	↓ Plasma levels by ↑ glucuronidation	Avoid coadministration, clinical significance unknown though may be used with dual NRTI in pregnancy
DIDANOSINE (BUFFERED TABLETS)	PROTEASE INHIBITORS	↓ Efficacy of amprenavir, atazanavir, and indinavirar; reduced absorption of these protease inhibitors	Absorption of some protease inhibitors (indinavir) may be affected by the buffered didanosine formulation, which ↑ gastric pH	Separate doses; give indinavir, atazanavir, or ritonavir 2 h before or 2 h afterward. Didanosine should be taken on an empty stomach, advice for protease inhibitors varies: indinavir, empty stomach, atazanavir or ritonavir with food. Alternatively, consider using the gastroresistant formulation of didanosine. No dose adjustment needed with saquinavir/ritonavir

(Continued)

Primary Drug	Secondary Drug	Effect	Mechanism	Precautions
ANTIVIRALS—ANTIRETROVIRALS				
ABACAVIR, ZIDOVUDINE	TIPRANAVIR/RITONAVIR	Possible ↓ efficacy; risk of treatment failure of abacavir or zidovudine	↓ Plasma levels by ↑ glucuronidation	Not recommended unless there are no other available nucleoside reverse transcriptase inhibitors
DIDANOSINE (ENTERIC-COATED)	TIPRANAVIR/RITONAVIR	↓ Plasma levels of didanosine, risk of treatment failure	↓ Absorption	Separate doses by at least 2.5 h
ZIDOVUDINE	ANXIOLYTICS AND HYPNOTICS—BZDs	1. ↑ Adverse effects, including ↑ incidence of headaches when oxazepam is coadministered with zidovudine 2. Possible ↑ adverse effects of zidovudine	1. Uncertain 2. Possibly reduced clearance	Monitor closely
ZALCITABINE, ZIDOVUDINE	H2 RECEPTOR BLOCKERS—CIMETIDINE	↑ Efficacy and adverse effects of zalcitabine	↓ Excretion via inhibition of tubular secretion by OCT2	Clinical significance unclear. Monitor more closely
OTHER DRUGS				
COBICISTAT	ALPHA-BLOCKERS—ALFUZOSIN	↑ Plasma levels	Inhibition of metabolism via CYP3A	Avoid coadministration
HIV ANTIVIRALS—OTHERS	**ANTIARRHYTHMICS**			
COBICISTAT	AMIODARONE	↑ Plasma levels amiodarone	Inhibition of metabolism via CYP3A	Avoid coadministration
COBICISTAT	QUINIDINE	↓ Plasma levels due to ↑ glucuronidation	Inhibition of metabolism via CYP3A	Avoid coadministration
MARAVIROC	DILTIAZEM, VERAPAMIL	Possible ↑ plasma levels diltiazem	Inhibition of metabolism via CYP3A	Avoid coadministration
MARAVIROC	DRONEDARONE	Possible ↑ plasma levels dronedarone	Inhibition of metabolism via CYP3A	Avoid coadministration
HIV ANTIVIRALS	**ANTACIDS**			
DOLUTEGRAVIR	ALUMINUM- OR MAGNESIUM-CONTAINING ANTACIDS	↓ Plasma levels due to ↑ glucuronidation	Chelation of doltegravir with calcium or aluminum ions	Separate doses, take antacids at least 6 h before or 2 h after dolutegravir
ELVITEGRAVIR (RITONAVIR BOOSTED)	ALUMINUM- OR MAGNESIUM-CONTAINING ANTACIDS	↓ Plasma levels of elvitegravir, risk of treatment failure and resistance	Reduced absorption due to chelation of elvitegravir	Separate doses by at least 4 h

(Continued)

Primary Drug	Secondary Drug	Effect	Mechanism	Precautions
ANTIVIRALS—ANTIRETROVIRALS				
RALTEGRAVIR	ALUMINUM- OR MAGNESIUM-CONTAINING ANTACIDS	↓ Plasma concentration of raltegravir, risk of treatment failure	Reduced absorption due to chelation of raltegravir	Avoid coadministration. Calcium-containing antacids can be used as an alternative but separate doses by at least 2 h
HIV ANTIVIRALS	**ANTIBIOTICS**			
COBICISTAT	CLARITHROMYCIN	Possible ↑ plasma levels of clarithromycin	Altered metabolism via CYP3A	Avoid triple combination with atazanavir; with daunavir, dose adjustment may be required
MARAVIROC	MACROLIDES	Possible ↑ plasma levels of maraviroc, risk of toxicity	Inhibition of CYP3A4 by clarithromycin	Reduce dose of maraviroc to 150 mg twice daily
HIV ANTIVIRALS—OTHERS	**ANTICANCER AND IMMUNOMODULATING DRUGS**			
COBICISTAT	CICLOSPORIN, SIROLIMUS, TACROLIMUS	Possible ↑ plasma levels of immunosuppressant	Inhibition of metabolism via CYP3A	Monitor plasma levels of immunosuppressants more closely
MARAVIROC	CICLOSPORIN	Possible ↑ plasma levels of maraviroc	Inhibition of metabolism via CYP3A	Monitor more closely
MARAVIROC	TACROLIMUS	↑ Plasma levels of maraviroc	Inhibition of metabolism via CYP3A	Monitor tacrolimus levels closely, reduced dose likely to be required
HIV ANTIVIRALS—OTHERS	**ANTICOAGULANTS—ORAL**			
COBICISTAT	APIXABAN	Possible ↑ plasma levels of apixaban and ↑ clinical effect	Inhibition of metabolism via CYP3A4	Use with caution, advise patients to report unusual bruising/bleeding, monitor antifactor Xa levels if overanticoagulation suspected
COBICISTAT	DABIGATRAN	Possible altered plasma levels of dabigatran	Altered metabolism via Pgp	Use with caution, advise patients to report unusual bruising/bleeding, monitor through aPTT or dTT if overanticoagulation suspected, consider checking through dabigatran level
COBICISTAT	RIVAROXABAN	Possible altered plasma levels of rivaroxaban	Altered metabolism via CYP3A and Pgp	Coadministration not recommended

(Continued)

Primary Drug	Secondary Drug	Effect	Mechanism	Precautions
ANTIVIRALS—ANTIRETROVIRALS				
HIV ANTIVIRALS—OTHERS	**ANTIEPILEPTICS**			
COBICISTAT	CARBAMAZEPINE, PHENYTOIN, PHENOBARBITONE	1. Possible ↓ plasma levels of cobicistat, risk of treatment failure and resistance 2. Possible ↓ plasma levels of medicines being boosted, e.g., protease inhibitor, risk of treatment failure and resistance	Induction of metabolism via CYP3A	Avoid coadministration
DOLUTEGRAVIR, MARAVIROC	CARBAMAZEPINE/ OXYCARBAMAZEPINE, PHENOBARBITONE, PHENYTOIN	Possible ↓ plasma levels of doltegravir, risk of treatment failure and resistance	Induction of UGT1A1 and CYP3A	Avoid coadministration
HIV ANTIVIRALS—OTHERS	**ANTIFUNGALS**			
ANTIFUNGALS—AZOLES				
COBICISTAT	ITRACONAZOLE, KETOCONAZOLE, AND VORICONAZOLE	1. Possible ↑ plasma levels of both 2. Voriconazole may be increased or decreased	1. Inhibition of metabolism via CYP3A 2. Altered metabolism via CYP3A	Avoid combination with voriconazole, use the rest with caution, maximum dose of itraconazole or ketoconazole is 200 mg/day
ELVITEGRAVIR (COBICISTAT BOOSTED)	AZOLE ANTIFUNGALS—ITRACONASOLE, KETOCONAZOLE AND VORICONAZOLE	Possible ↑ plasma levels of antifungal	Likely via inhibition of CYP3A4	Use with caution, maximum dose of ketoconazole or itraconazole 200 mg/day, consider risk vs. benefit carefully for voraconazole
MARAVIROC	FLUCONAZOLE	Possible ↑ plasma levels of maraviroc, risk of toxicity	Inhibition of CYP3A4 by fluconazole	Use with caution at a dose of maraviroc 300 mg twice daily, monitor for increased side effects
MARAVIROC	ITRACONAZOLE. KETOCONAZOLE	↑ Plasma levels of maraviroc, risk of toxicity	Inhibition of CYP3A4 by ketoconazole	Reduce dose of maraviroc to 150 mg twice daily

(Continued)

DRUGS TO TREAT INFECTIONS ANTIVIRALS—ANTIRETROVIRALS

Primary Drug	Secondary Drug	Effect	Mechanism	Precautions
ANTIVIRALS—ANTIRETROVIRALS				
COBICISTAT	RIFAMPICIN, RIFABUTIN	1. Possible ↓ plasma levels of cobicistat, risk of treatment failure and resistance 2. Possible ↓ plasma levels of medicines being boosted e.g., protease inhibitor, risk of treatment failure and resistance 3. Increased plasma levels of rifabutin active metabolite (25-o-desacetyl-rifabutin), increased risk of side effects e.g., uvetitis	Induction of metabolism via CYP3A	Avoid coadministration with rifampicin, with rifabutin: maximum dose of rifabutin 150 mg three times a week and monitor LFTs closely and for uveitis and neutropenia
DOLUTEGRAVIR	RIFAMPICIN	↓ Plasma levels of doltegravir, risk of treatment failure and resistance	Induction of UGT1A1 and CYP3A	Dose of dolutegravir must be ↑ to 50 mg twice daily; no dose adjustment needed if it is also combined with darunavir, fosamprenavir, or lopinavir, all with ritonavir
ELVITEGRAVIR (COBICISTAT OR RITONAVIR BOOSTED)	RIFABUTIN	1. ↓ Plasma levels of elvitegravir, risk of treatment failure and resistance 2. ↑ Plasma concentration of rifabutin active metabolite (25-o-desacetyl-rifabutin), increased risk of side effects, e.g., uvetitis	1. Induction of metabolism via CYP3A and UGTs 2. Inhibition of CYP3A4 by cobicistat	Coadministration not recommended. If used, rifabutin dose should be 150 mg three times a week
ELVITEGRAVIR	RIFAMPICIN	Possible ↓ plasma levels of elvitegravir, risk of treatment failure and resistance	Altered metabolism	Avoid coadministration
MARAVIROC (AND PROTEASE INHIBITOR)	RIFABUTIN	↑ Plasma levels of maraviroc, risk of toxicity	Altered metabolism via CYP3A	For rifampicin plus tipranavir/ ritonavir combination use maraviroc 300 mg twice daily, for other protease inhibitors reduce dose of maraviroc to 150 mg twice daily

(Continued)

Primary Drug	Secondary Drug	Effect	Mechanism	Precautions
ANTIVIRALS—ANTIRETROVIRALS				
MARAVIROC	RIFAMPICIN	↓ Levels of maraviroc, risk of treatment failure and viral resistance	↑ Metabolism via CYP3A4	Use in triple combination with efavirenz not recommended. With rifampicin alone increase dose of maraviroc to 600 mg twice daily unless also combined with a CYP3A4 inhibitor
RALTEGRAVIR	RIFAMPICIN	↓ Plasma concentration of raltegravir, risk of treatment failure	Induction of metabolism via UGT1A1	Consider rifabutin or rifapentine as alternative therapy or doubling the dose of raltegravir from 400 to 800 mg twice daily, monitor CD4 count and LFTs and for rash, GI and CNS side effects
HIV ANTIVIRALS—OTHERS	**ANTIPLATELETS**			
COBICISTAT	PRASUGREL	↓ Activation of prasugrel, risk of treatment failure	Inhibition of metabolism to active metabolite via CYP3A4	Consider using clopidogrel as an alternative
COBICISTAT	TICAGRELOR	↑ Risk of side effects	Inhibition of metabolism via CYP3A4	Consider using clopidogrel as an alternative
HIV ANTIVIRALS—OTHERS	**ANTIPSYCHOTICS**			
COBICISTAT	PIMOZIDE	↑ Plasma levels	Inhibition of metabolism via CYP3A	Avoid coadministration
COBICISTAT	RISPERIDONE	Possible ↑ plasma levels	Inhibition of metabolism via CYP3A	Dose adjustment may be required
COBICISTAT	BOCEPREVIR	1. Possible ↓ plasma levels of cobicistat, risk of treatment failure and resistance 2. Possible ↓ plasma levels of medicines being boosted, e.g., protease inhibitor, risk of treatment failure and resistance	Induction of metabolism via CYP3A	Combination not recommended
COBICISTAT	SIMEPREVIR	Possible ↑ plasma levels of simeprevir, risk of toxicity	Inhibition of metabolism via CYP3A4	Avoid coadministration

(Continued)

Primary Drug	Secondary Drug	Effect	Mechanism	Precautions
ANTIVIRALS—ANTIRETROVIRALS				
MARAVIROC	BOCEPREVIR, TELAPREVIR	↑ Plasma levels of maraviroc, risk of toxicity	Inhibition of metabolism via CYP3A	Use maraviroc at 150 mg twice daily
HIV ANTIVIRALS—OTHERS	**ANTIVIRALS—HIV OTHERS**			
COBICISTAT	MARAVIROC	↑ Plasma levels maraviroc, risk to toxicity	Inhibition of metabolism via CYP3A	Adjust dose of maraviroc to 150 mg twice daily
ELVITEGRAVIR (WITH RITONAVIR)	MARAVIROC	↑ Plasma levels maraviroc, risk to toxicity	Inhibition of metabolism via CYP3A	Adjust dose of maraviroc to 150 mg twice daily, if elvitegravir alone, no dose adjustment is needed
HIV ANTIVIRALS—OTHERS	**ANTIVIRALS FOR HIV—NNRTIs**			
COBICISTAT	NNRTIs	1. Possible ↓ plasma levels of cobicistat (not with rilpivirine), risk of treatment failure and resistance 2. Possible ↓ plasma levels of medicines being boosted e.g., protease inhibitor, risk of treatment failure and resistance 3. Possible increase in plasma levels of nevirapine and rilpivirine	Induction of metabolism via CYP3A	Coadministration with efavirenz, etravirine, or nelfinavir not recommended. If required use with caution, no dose adjustment required with rilpivirne and atazanavir or darunavir/cobicistat combinations
DOLUTEGRAVIR	NNRTIs	↓ Plasma levels of doltegravir, risk of treatment failure and resistance	Induction of metabolism via UGT1A1 and CYP3A	Etravirine must only be used in combination with atazanavir/ritonavir, darunavir/ritonavir, or lopinavir/ritonavir, with efavirenz and nevirapine, increase dolutegravir dose to 50 mg twice daily, no adjustment needed with rilpivirine
ELVITEGRAVIR	EFAVIRENZ, NEVIRAPINE	Possible ↓ plasma levels of elvitegravir, risk of treatment failure and resistance	Increased metabolism through induction of CYP3A	Coadministration not recommended. Dose adjustment not expected to be required with etravirine and pilpivirine
ELVITEGRAVIR/COBICISTAT	NEVIRAPINE	Possible altered plasma levels of all agents	Not studied but altered metabolism via CYP450 likely	Avoid coadadministration

(*Continued*)

Primary Drug	Secondary Drug	Effect	Mechanism	Precautions
ANTIVIRALS—ANTIRETROVIRALS				
MARAVIROC	EFAVIRENZ	↓ Plasma levels of maraviroc, risk of treatment failure and resistance	Likely altered metabolism via CYP3A4 and Pgp	If in unboosted PI regimen or with efavirenz alone or in combination with tipranvir/ritonavir, increase maraviroc dose to 600 mg twice daily, if combined with other protease inhibitors or potent CYP3A4 inhibitors, reduce maraviroc to 150 mg twice daily. No interaction expected with nevirapine
MARAVIROC	ETRAVIRINE	1. Possible ↑ bioavailability and ↑ adverse effects of maraviroc	Uncertain	Combination should be used in "boosted" protease inhibitor regimens, dose adjustment of maraviroc to 150 mg BD required unless fosamprenavir/ritonavir when maraviroc 300 mg BD is required though later combination not recommended. Nevirapine can be administered without dose adjustment of either drug
RALTEGRAVIR	EFAVIRENZ, ETRAVIRINE	Both increased and decreased plasma levels of raltegravir reported	Altered metabolism	Monitor more closely
HIV ANTIVIRALS—OTHERS	**ANTIVIRALS FOR HIV—NRTIS**			
ADEFOVIR, CIDOFOVIR	TENOFOVIR	↑ Adverse effects	↑ Plasma levels, competition for renal excretion via organic anion transporter	Avoid coadministration
FOSCARNET SODIUM	TENOFOVIR, ZALCITABINE	↑ Adverse effects with tenofovir and possibly zalcitabine	Uncertain; possibly additive toxicity via competition for renal excretion I	Avoid if possible; otherwise, monitor FBC and renal function weekly
HIV ANTIVIRALS—OTHERS	**ANTIVIRALS FOR HIV—PROTEASE INHIBITORS**			
COBICISTAT	ATAZANAVIR, DARUNAVIR	↑ Plasma levels of protease inhibitors	Inhibition of metabolism via CYP3A	Avoid coadministration particularly with other boosted antiretrovirals, e.g., other protease inhibitors or elvitagrevir

(Continued)

Primary Drug	Secondary Drug	Effect	Mechanism	Precautions
ANTIVIRALS—ANTIRETROVIRALS				
DOLUTEGRAVIR	TIPRANAVIR/RITONAVIR	↓ Plasma levels of doltegravir, risk of treatment failure and resistance	Induction of UGT1A1 and CYP3A	Dose of dolutegravir must be 50 mg twice daily, no dose adjustment needed if also combined with darunavir, fosamprenavir, or lopinavir all with ritonavir
ELVITEGRAVIR	ATAZANAVIR/RITONAVIR, LOPINAVIR/RITONAVIR, RITONAVIR (LOW DOSE)	↑ Plasma levels of elvitegravir	Probably involves altered metabolism via CYP3A4, though induction of glucuronidation would reduce levels	Reduce dose of elvitegravir from 150 to 85 mg daily and use atazanavir/ritonavir 300/100 mg. Can be used with darunavir or tipranavir, both with ritonavir without dose adjustment
MARAVIROC	ATAZANAVIR, DARUNAVIR, FOSAMPRENAVIR, INDINAVIR, LOPINAVIR/RITONAVIR, RITONAVIR, SAQUINAVIR, SAQUINAVIR/RITONAVIR	1. ↑ Plasma concentration of maraviroc, risk of toxicity 2. ↓ Levels of amprenavir and ritonavir, risk of treatment failure and viral resistance	Inhibition of metabolism via CYP3A4 and Pgp	Interaction can be combined for therapeutic advantage. Coadministration with fosamprenavir/ritonavir not recommended. With darunavir/ritonavir, lopinavir/ritonavir (400/100 mg), or saquinavir/ritonavir (1000/100 mg), use maraviroc 150 mg twice daily. No dose adjustment needed with tipranavir/ritonavir. Consider dose reduction of maraviroc with atazanavir, indinavir, or saquinavir
MARAVIROC	NELFINAVIR	Possible ↑ plasma levels of maraviroc, risk of toxicity	Inhibition of CYP3A4 by nelfinavir	Use with caution
MARAVIROC	PROTEASE INHIBITOR PLUS NNRTI	↑ Plasma levels of maraviroc, risk of toxicity	Inhibition of metabolism via CYP3A	With tipranvir/ritonavir use maraviroc 600 mg twice daily, for other efavirenz or etravirine/PI, combinations use maraviroc 150 mg twice daily

(Continued)

Primary Drug	Secondary Drug	Effect	Mechanism	Precautions
ANTIVIRALS—ANTIRETROVIRALS				
RALTEGRAVIR	DARUNAVIR/RITONAVIR, FOSAMPRENAVIR/RITONAVIR, TIPRANAVIR/RITONAVIR	1. ↓ Plasma levels of amprenavir and raltegravir, risk of treatment failure 2. ↑ Risk of rash with darunavir	1. Probably increased metabolism via glucuronidation (raltegravir) 2. Additive side effect	1. Avoid coadministration with fosamprenavir or amprenavir 2. Advise patients to report signs of rash, monitor closely. No dose adjustment needed with atazanavir/ritonavir, lopinavir/ritonavir, indinavir, saquinavir, tipranvir/ritonavir
MARAVIROC	ALCOHOL	↑ Plasma levels of alcohol, increased risk of adverse effects	Unknown	Advise patients to be aware of increased effects of alcohol and consider gradual reduction of their alcohol intake
COBICISTAT	BOSENTAN	1. Possible ↓ plasma levels of cobicistat, risk of treatment failure and resistance 2. Possible ↓ plasma levels of medicines being boosted, e.g., protease inhibitor	Induction of metabolism via CYP3A	Combination not recommended
ELVITEGRAVIR	BOSENTAN	↓ Plasma levels of elvitegravir, risk of treatment failure and resistance	Increased metabolism through induction of CYP3A	Coadministration not recommended
MARAVIROC	BOSENTAN	Possible ↓ plasma levels of maraviroc, risk of treatment failure and resistance	Induction of metabolism via CYP3A	Coadministration not recommended
COBICISTAT	BUSPIRONE	Possible ↑ plasma levels of buspirone	Inhibition of metabolism via CYP3A	Use with caution, a reduced dose of buspirone may be required
COBICISTAT	CALCIUM CHANNEL BLOCKERS	Possible ↑ plasma levels	Inhibition of metabolism via CYP3A	Monitor more closely, dose reduction may be required
DOLUTEGRAVIR	CALCIUM SUPPLEMENTS	↓ Plasma levels of doltegravir, risk of treatment failure and resistance	Chelation of doltegravir with calcium ions	Separate doses, take calcium-containing medicines at least 2 h after or 6 h before dolutegravir

(Continued)

Primary Drug	Secondary Drug	Effect	Mechanism	Precautions
ANTIVIRALS—ANTIRETROVIRALS				
COBICISTAT	CISAPRIDE	↑ Plasma levels	Inhibition of metabolism via CYP3A	Avoid coadministration
COBICISTAT	DEXAMETHASONE	Possible ↓ plasma levels of cobicistat, risk of treatment failure and resistance	Induction of metabolism via CYP3A	Use with caution
COBICISTAT	DIGOXIN	↑ Peak plasma levels	Inhibition of transport via Pgp and metabolism via CYP3A	Start with lowest dose, increase slowly and monitor levels
DOLUTEGRAVIR	DOFETILIDE	Possible ↑ plasma concentration of dofetilide, risk of toxicity	Inhibition of transport via OCT2	Avoid coadministration
COBICISTAT	ERGOT ALKALOIDS—DIHYDROERGOTAMINE, ERGOTAMINE, ERGOMETRINE,	↑ Plasma levels	Inhibition of metabolism via CYP3A	Avoid coadministration
COBICISTAT	FLUTICASONE	Possible ↑ plasma concentration from inhaled fluticasone risk of increased steroid exposure and systemic effects	Inhibition of metabolism via CYP3A4	Use with caution if patient on high-dose fluticasone. Monitor closely for signs of corticosteroid toxicity, adrenal suppression, and immunosuppression; review alternatives or ↓ dose as necessary. Short term, low dose or as required use will have less risk of adverse effects. Consider using inhaled beclometasone as an alternative as it is not metabolized via CYP3A4 or mometasone as it has very low systemic bioavailability
DOLUTEGRAVIR	IRON SUPPLEMENTS, MULTIVITAMINS	↓ Plasma levels of doltegravir, risk of treatment failure and resistance	Chelation of doltegravir with calcium or aluminum ions	Separate doses, take supplement at least 2 h after or 6 h before dolutegravir
DOLUTEGRAVIR	METFORMIN	Possible increased plasma concentration of metformin	Inhibition of metformin transport via OCT-2	Monitor for increased side effects of metformin

(Continued)

Primary Drug	Secondary Drug	Effect	Mechanism	Precautions
ANTIVIRALS—ANTIRETROVIRALS				
COBICISTAT	METOPROLOL, TIMOLOL	Possible ↑ plasma levels	Inhibition of metabolism via CYP3A	Monitor more closely, if the patient is already on the beta-blocker, a dose reduction may be required
COBICISTAT	MIDAZOLAM (PO), TRIAZOLAM (PO)	↑ Plasma levels	Inhibition of metabolism via CYP3A	Avoid coadministration. For other sedatives or hypnotics, monitor closely for increased sedation, dose reduction may be required
ENFUVIRTIDE	NIACIN	↑ Risk of injection site reactions, e.g., pain, redness, swelling	Possibly an exaggerated immune response involving Langerhans cells	Advise patients to report ongoing injection site reactions
RALTEGRAVIR	OMEPRAZOLE	Increased plasma concentration of raltegravir	Increased absorption as pH increases	Use with caution, no dose adjustment recommended
ELVITEGRAVIR (COBICISTAT BOOSTED)	ORAL AND TRANSDERMAL CONTRACEPTIVES	↓ Plasma levels of estrogen, ↑ plasma levels of norgestimate—risk of increased progesterone effects	Altered metabolism	Oral contraceptive must contain at least 30 μg ethinylestradiol and norgestimate as the progesterone. Barrier methods are recommended to prevent the transmission of HIV. Review risk benefit particularly in older women or those with additional risk factors for VTE
COBICISTAT	PGE-5 INHIBITORS	↑ Plasma levels	Inhibition of metabolism via CYP3A	Avoid coadministration with sildenafil for PAH, use tadalafil with caution. For erectile dysfunction, maximum dose of sildenafil 25 mg/48 h, vardenafil 2.5 mg/72 h, tadalafil 10 mg/72 h is recommended
COBICISTAT	SALMETEROL	Possible ↑ plasma levels, risk of arrhythmias	Inhibition of metabolism via CYP3A	Coadministration not recommended
COBICISTAT	SIMEPREVIR	Possible ↑ plasma levels	Inhibition of metabolism via CYP3A	Coadministration not recommended
COBICISTAT, DOLUTEGRAVIR, MARAVIROC	ST. JOHN'S WORT	↓ Plasma levels, risk of treatment failure and resistance	Induction of metabolism via CYP3A (all affected) and UGT1A1 (dolutevravir)	Avoid coadministration

(*Continued*)

DRUGS TO TREAT INFECTIONS ANTIVIRALS—ANTIRETROVIRALS Protease inhibitors

Primary Drug	Secondary Drug	Effect	Mechanism	Precautions
ANTIVIRALS—ANTIRETROVIRALS				
COBICISTAT	STATINS	↑ Plasma levels of simvastatin and lovastatin	Inhibition of metabolism via CYP3A	Avoid coadministration. Atorvastatin—combination not recommended, use with caution, start at lowest dose of statin, monitor closely for adverse effects. Pravastatin and rosuvastatin are suitable alternatives
COBICISTAT	TRAZODONE	Possible ↑ plasma levels	Inhibition of metabolism via CYP3A4 and 2D6	Dose adjustment may be required
PROTEASE INHIBITORS				
INDINAVIR	ALITRETINOIN	Possibly ↑ plasma levels	Possibly inhibition of metabolism via CYP3A4	Be aware
RITONAVIR, TIPRANAVIR	AMPHETAMINE AND DERIVATIVES, E.G., METHYLPHENIDATE, DEXAMPHETAMINE	Possibly ↑ plasma levels of amphetamine derivatives	Inhibition of metabolism via CYP2D6	Monitor therapeutic efficacy and adverse effects closely
PROTEASE INHIBITORS	ANESTHETICS—LOCAL	↑ Adverse effects of lidocaine with lopinavir/ritonavir	Uncertain; ↑ bioavailability	Caution; consider using an alternative local anesthetic
ATAZANAVIR/RITONAVIR, DARUNAVIR, FOSAMPRENAVIR/RITONAVIR, LOPINAVIR/RITONAVIR, SAQUINAVIR/RITONAVIR	ANESTHETICS—SYSTEMIC LIDOCAINE	Lidocaine levels may be ↑, increased risk of ventricular arrhythmias	Uncertain but postulated to be due to ↓ metabolism via CYP3A	Avoid combination with saquinavir/ritonavir. For others use with caution, watch closely for lidocaine toxicity, monitor levels; consider ↓ initial lidocaine dose and titrating more slowly

(*Continued*)

Primary Drug	Secondary Drug	Effect	Mechanism	Precautions
ANTIVIRALS—ANTIRETROVIRALS				
PROTEASE INHIBITORS	**ANALGESICS**			
PROTEASE INHIBITORS	NSAIDs—PIROXICAM	Ritonavir ↑ piroxicam levels	Uncertain; ritonavir is known to inhibit CYP2C9, for which NSAIDs are substrates	Avoid coadministration
PROTEASE INHIBITORS	**OPIOIDS**			
PROTEASE INHIBITORS	ALFENTANIL, BUPRENORPHINE, FENTANYL, TRAMADOL	1. Possibly ↑ adverse opioid effects when buprenorphine is coadministered with atazanavir/ritonavir, indinavir, ritonavir, or saquinavir 2. Altered plasma levels of buprenorphine's active metabolite (buprenorphine-3-glucuronide) when coadministered with darunavir/ritonavir, lopinavir/ritonavir, and tipranavir/ritonavir 3. ↑ Plasma levels of alfentanyl (ritonavir, indinavir), and fentanyl (ritonavir)	1. Inhibition of CYP3A4, and CYP2D6 (tramadol), or UGT1A1 by atazanavir (buprenorphine) 2. Possibly induction of glucuronidation (buprenorphine) 3. Inhibition of metabolism via CYP3A4	Buprenorphine for opiod replacement, halve the starting dose and titrate to effect. Patients already on regular buprenorphone should be monitored for sedation, CNS effects, and opioid withdrawal. A dose adjustment may be required, but interaction of darunavir/ritonavir not thought to be clinically significant. For **fentanyl**, give a single injection—monitor sedation and respiratory function closely. If continued use of fentanyl is needed, ↓ dose may be required. Concomitant use of ritonavir and transdermal fentanyl is not recommended
PROTEASE INHIBITORS	CODEINE, DIHYDROCODEINE	↓ Efficacy of codeine and dihydrocodeine when given with ritonavir	Inhibition of CYP2D6-mediated metabolism of codeine to its active metabolites	Use an alternative opioid

(*Continued*)

Primary Drug	Secondary Drug	Effect	Mechanism	Precautions
ANTIVIRALS—ANTIRETROVIRALS				
PROTEASE INHIBITORS	METHADONE, PETHIDINE	1. ↓ Efficacy of methadone, with risk of withdrawal, when coadministered with darunavir/ritonavir, lopinavir/ritonavir, nelfinavir, ritonavir, saquinavir, tipranavir/ritonavir 2. Reduced plasma concentration of pethidine with ritonavir but increased levels of toxic metabolites 3. Risk of cardiac arrhythmias particularly with saquinavir/ritonavir 4. Possible ↓ efficacy of lopinavir	1 and 2. Uncertain; possibly due to induction of CYP3A4 and CYP2D6, ritonavir may induce glucuronidation of methadone 3. Additive side effects 4. Unclear	Avoid coadministration of pethidine and ritonavir or methadone and saquinavir/ritonavir. Monitor ECG and closely for opioid withdrawal, and gradually ↑ dose of methadone as necessary in 10 mg increments over days/week, this advice includes coadministration of methadone with low-dose ritonavir. No significant effect on methadone expected with indinavir or short-term combined use with atazanavir/ritonavir. If protease inhibitor is stopped, methadone dose should be gradually reduced over a few weeks. Morphine and oxycodone are suitable alternatives to pethidine
ATAZANAVIR, INDINAVIR, TIPRANAVIR/RITONAVIR	ANTACIDS	↓ Plasma levels of protease inhibitor	Reduced absorption	Give protease inhibitor 2 h before or 2 h after antacids or buffered medicines
PROTEASE INHIBITORS	ANTIANGINALS—RANOLAZINE	Possibly ↑ plasma levels and adverse effects of ranolazine, e.g., QTc prolongation	Inhibition of metabolism via CYP3A4, CYP2D6, and Pgp	Avoid coadministration
PROTEASE INHIBITORS	**ANTIARRHYTHMICS**			
PROTEASE INHIBITORS	AMIODARONE	Amiodarone levels may be ↑ by protease inhibitors, increased risk of ventricular arrhythmias	Uncertain but postulated to be due to ↓ metabolism of amiodarone via CYP3A	Avoid combination with fosamprenavir/ritonavir, indinavir, ritonavir, saquinavir, and tipranavir/ritonavir. Watch closely for ECG changes and amiodarone toxicity; for patients taking high doses of amiodarone, consider ↓ dose when starting protease inhibitor anti-HIV therapy

(*Continued*)

Primary Drug	Secondary Drug	Effect	Mechanism	Precautions
ANTIVIRALS—ANTIRETROVIRALS				
PROTEASE INHIBITORS	DISOPYRAMIDE	Disopyramide levels may be ↑ by protease inhibitors, possible ↑ side effects	Inhibition of CYP3A4-mediated metabolism of disopyramide	Avoid coadministration with saquinavir. Watch closely for disopyramide toxicity and cardiac and neurological side effects
RITONAVIR, SAQUINAVIR	DRONEDARONE	Dronedarone levels may be ↑ by protease inhibitors, possible ↑ side effects	Probably inhibition of CYP3A4-mediated metabolism of disopyramide	Avoid coadministration
PROTEASE INHIBITORS	FLECAINIDE	Fosamprenavir, ritonavir, and possibly saquinavir and tipranavir/ritonavir ↑ flecainide levels, with risk of ventricular arrhythmias	Uncertain; possibly inhibition of CYP2D6-mediated metabolism of flecainide	Manufacturers recommend avoiding coadministration of flecainide with fosamprenavir, ritonavir, saquinavir, or tipranvir/ritonavir
PROTEASE INHIBITORS	MEXILETINE	Mexiletine levels may be ↑ by ritonavir, possible ↑ side effects	Inhibition of metabolism via CYP2D6, particularly in rapid metabolizers (90% of the population)	Monitor PR, BP, and ECG closely. Watch closely for cardiac and neurological side effects
PROTEASE INHIBITORS	PROPAFENONE	Fosamprenavir, ritonavir, and possibly saquinavir and tipranavir/ritonavir ↑ propafenone levels, with risk of ventricular arrhythmias	Probably inhibition of CYP2D6	Manufacturers recommend avoiding coadministration of propafenone with fosamprenavir, ritonavir, saquinavir, or tipranavir
PROTEASE INHIBITORS	QUINIDINE	Possibly ↑ plasma levels of quinidine, risk of ventricular arrhythmias	Possible inhibition of metabolism via CYP3A	Avoid coadministration
PROTEASE INHIBITORS	**ANTIBIOTICS**			
PROTEASE INHIBITORS	FUSIDIC ACID	Possibly ↑ plasma levels and ↑ adverse effects of both drugs, including rhabdomyolysis	Inhibition of CYP3A4-mediated metabolism of fusidic acid	Avoid coadministration. If unavoidable, monitor closely for muscular adverse events
PROTEASE INHIBITORS	MACROLIDES—AZITHROMYCIN	Risk of ↑ adverse effects of azithromycin with nelfinavir	Possibly involves altered Pgp transport	Watch for signs of azithromycin toxicity

(*Continued*)

DRUGS TO TREAT INFECTIONS ANTIVIRALS—ANTIRETROVIRALS

Primary Drug	Secondary Drug	Effect	Mechanism	Precautions
ANTIVIRALS—ANTIRETROVIRALS				
PROTEASE INHIBITORS	MACROLIDES—CLARITHROMYCIN, ERYTHROMYCIN	Ritonavir, saquinavir, and tipranvir increase levels of clarithromycin and reduce active metabolite, possibly ↑ adverse effects of macrolide with atazanavir, lopinavir/ritonavir, ritonavir, saquinavir (ventricular arrhythmias), and tipranavir. Indinavir and saquinavir are also possibly ↑. ↑ Levels of tipranvir (with ritonavir)	Inhibition of CYP3A4- and possibly CYP1A2-mediated metabolism. Altered transport via Pgp may be involved	Avoid combination with saquinavir/ritonavir, monitor closely for doses >1 g/day with tipranvir/ritonavir. Consider alternatives especially for *H. influenzae* as the 14-OH metabolite is most active. In Mycobacterium avium intracellulare infection if combined, ↓ dose of clarithromycin by 50% (75% in the presence of renal failure with a creatinine clearance of 30 mL/min). With ritonavir do not exceed clarithromycin 1 g/day. Monitor QT interval for increased adverse effects
PROTEASE INHIBITORS	METRONIDAZOLE	↑ Adverse effects, e.g., a disulfiram-like reaction and flushing, with lopinavir/ritonavir, ritonavir, or tipranavir/ritonavir soft capsules	Ritonavir and lopinavir oral solutions and tipranavir/ritonavir soft capsules contain alcohol	Warn patients, and give alternative preparations if possible
ATAZANAVIR, FOSAMPRENAVIR, INDINAVIR, LOPINAVIR, RITONAVIR, SAQUINAVIR	KETOLIDE—TELITHROMYCIN	Possible ↑ in plasma levels and adverse effects	Inhibition of CYP3A4, CYP2D6, and Pgp	Avoid coadministration if there is severe renal and hepatic impairment
RITONAVIR	QUINOLONES—MOXIFLOXACIN	Increased risk of QTc prolongation	Additive side effects	Avoid coadministration or if essential, combine monitor ECG and QTc interval closely
SAQUINAVIR	QUINUPRISTIN/DALFOPRISTIN	Possibly ↑ plasma levels of saquinavir	Inhibition of metabolism via CYP3A4	Monitor closely for saquinavir toxicity

(*Continued*)

Primary Drug	Secondary Drug	Effect	Mechanism	Precautions
ANTIVIRALS—ANTIRETROVIRALS				
PROTEASE INHIBITORS	RIFABUTIN	1. ↑ Plasma levels and adverse effects of rifabutin and some protease inhibitors (Inc darunavir), e.g., uveitis, headache, diarrhea, back pain, leukopenia 2. ↓ Plasma concentration of indinavir, nelfinavir, saquinavir (unboosted)	1. Inhibition of CYP3A4-mediated metabolism of both rifabutin and rifabutin's active metabolite (25-O). Nelfinavir also competitively inhibits CYP2C19 2. Rifabutin induces metabolism via CYP3A4	Coadministration with high dose (600 mg twice daily) ritonavir contraindicated, not recommended with indinavir as appropriate doses not established. For other combinations ↓ rifabutin dose and monitor closely for side effects of rifabutin, including LFTs, neutropenia, uvetis. With atazanavir/ritonavir, fosamprenavir/ritonavir, saquinavir/ritonavir, or tipranavir/ritonavir, reduce rifabutin from 300 mg daily, i.e., by 75% to 150 mg every other day. If not tolerated consider reducing to twice weekly though this may lead to treatment failure. Reduce by at least 50% when given nelfinavir, and by 75% with low-dose ritonavir or tipranavir. With unboosted atazanavir use rifabutin 150 mg daily. Consider monitoring rifabutin and 25-o-desacetyl metabolite levels. Ensure patients know to report eye symptoms and suspected infections promptly
SAQUINAVIR	RIFABUTIN	1. ↑ Plasma levels and adverse effects of rifabutin with atazanavir and indinavir 2. ↓ Efficacy of saquinavir	Uncertain; probably via altered CYP3A4 metabolism	Avoid coadministration

(*Continued*)

Primary Drug	Secondary Drug	Effect	Mechanism	Precautions
ANTIVIRALS—ANTIRETROVIRALS				
PROTEASE INHIBITORS	RIFAMPICIN	1. ↓ Levels of the protease inhibitor, risk of treatment failure 2. ↑ Adverse effects, e.g., hepatotoxicity	1. Induction of metabolism via CYP3A4 2. Additive side effects	Avoid coadministration with protease inhibitors. Ritonavir 600 mg twice daily can be combined as it may not have a clinically relevant interaction with rifampicin but is not well tolerated. Consider rifabutin as alternative. With saquinavir/ritonavir severe hepatotoxicity is possible. If unavoidable increase lopinavir/ritonavir to 400/400 mg twice daily and monitor LFTs and GI function closely
PROTEASE INHIBITORS	**ANTICANCER AND IMMUNOMODULATING DRUGS**			
PROTEASE INHIBITORS	**CYTOTOXICS**			
ATAZANAVIR, INDINAVIR, RITONAVIR, SAQUINAVIR	AXITINIB	Possible ↑ plasma concentrations of axitinib	Uncertain	Reduce dose of axitinib
ATAZANAVIR, INDINAVIR, SAQUINAVIR	CRIZOTINIB	Possible ↑ plasma concentrations of crizotinib	Uncertain	Avoid coadministration
ATAZANAVIR, INDINAVIR, RITONAVIR, SAQUINAVIR, TIPRANAVIR	DASATINIB	Possible ↑ plasma concentrations of dasatinib	Inhibition of metabolism via CYP3A4	
ATAZANAVIR, INDINAVIR, RITONAVIR, SAQUINAVIR	CABAZITAXEL	Reduced response to infection	Uncertain	Avoid coadministration
RITONAVIR	IFOSFAMIDE	↓ Plasma concentrations of 4-hydroxyifosfamide, the active metabolite of ifosfamide, and risk of inadequate therapeutic response	Due to inhibition of the isoenzymatic conversion to active metabolites	Monitor clinically the efficacy of ifosfamide and ↑ dose accordingly

(*Continued*)

Primary Drug	Secondary Drug	Effect	Mechanism	Precautions
ANTIVIRALS—ANTIRETROVIRALS				
RITONAVIR	IMATINIB	↑ Imatinib levels with ↑ risk of toxicity (e.g., abdominal pain, constipation, dyspnea) and of neurotoxicity (e.g., taste disturbances, dizziness, headache, paresthesia, peripheral neuropathy)	Due to inhibition of CYP3A4-mediated metabolism of imatinib	Monitor for clinical efficacy and for the signs of toxicity listed, along with convulsions, confusion, and signs of edema (including pulmonary edema). Monitor electrolytes, liver function and for cardiotoxicity
ATAZANAVIR/RITONAVIR, LOPINAVIR/RITONAVIR, RITONAVIR	IRINOTECAN	↑ Plasma concentrations of SN-38 (AUC by 100%) and ↑ toxicity of irinotecan, e.g., diarrhea, acute cholinergic syndrome, interstitial pulmonary disease	Ritonavir inhibits metabolism of irinotecan by CYP3A4. Atazanavir inhibits metabolism of irinotecan via UGT though ritonavir induces	Peripheral blood counts should be checked before each course of treatment. Monitor lung function. Recommendation is to ↓ dose of irinotecan by 25%
RITONAVIR, SAQUINAVIR	LAPATINIB	Possible ↑ plasma concentrations and adverse effects of lapatinib	Inhibition of metabolism via CYP3A4	Avoid coadministration
RITONAVIR	NILOTINIB	Possible ↑ plasma concentrations and adverse effects of nilotinib	Inhibition of metabolism via CYP3A4	Avoid coadministration
ATAZANAVIR, INDINAVIR, RITONAVIR, SAQUINAVIR	PAZOPANIB	Reduced response to infection	Uncertain	Avoid coadministration
INDINAVIR, LOPINAVIR, RITONAVIR, SAQUINAVIR	RUXOLITINIB	Reduced response to infection	Uncertain	Reduce dose of ruxolitinib by approximately 50%, give twice daily and monitor FBC twice weekly
PROTEASE INHIBITORS	VINCA ALKALOIDS	↑ Adverse effects of vinblastine and vincristine	Probably inhibition of CYP3A4-mediated metabolism, altered transport via Pgp as also inhibition of Pgp efflux of vinblastine	Monitor FBCs; watch for early features of toxicity (pain, numbness, tingling in the fingers and toes, jaw pain, abdominal pain, constipation, ileus). Consider selecting an alternative drug

(*Continued*)

Primary Drug	Secondary Drug	Effect	Mechanism	Precautions
ANTIVIRALS—ANTIRETROVIRALS				
RITONAVIR	VINFLUNINE	Possible ↑ plasma concentrations of vinflunine	Uncertain	Avoid coadministration
PROTEASE INHIBITORS	**HORMONES AND HORMONE ANTAGONISTS**			
RITONAVIR	TAMOXIFEN	Possible ↓ plasma levels of active metabolite, thus reducing therapeutic efficacy	Inhibition of metabolism via CYP2D6	Avoid coadministration
RITONAVIR	TOREMIFENE	↑ Plasma concentrations of toremifene	Due to inhibition of metabolism of toremifene by the CYP3A4 isoenzymes by ritonavir	Clinical relevance is uncertain. Necessary to monitor for clinical toxicities
PROTEASE INHIBITORS	**IMMUNOMODULATING DRUGS**			
PROTEASE INHIBITORS	CICLOSPORIN, SIROLIMUS, TACROLIMUS	↑ Levels with protease inhibitors	Complex. Inhibition of CYP3A4-mediated metabolism of these immunomodulating drugs. Altered transport via Pgp may also be involved	Monitor clinical effects closely and check levels, adjust dose of immunosuppressant as needed, significant dose reductions of tacrolimus required
ATAZANAVIR, DARUNAVIR, INDINAVIR, RITONAVIR, SAQUINAVIR	EVEROLIMUS	Possible ↑ plasma concentrations of everolimus	Predicted inhibition of CYP3A4 metabolism	Avoid coadministration
PROTEASE INHIBITORS	CORTICOSTEROIDS	1. ↑ Plasma levels of betamethasone; dexamethasone; hydrocortisone; prednisolone; triamcinolone; inhaled, intranasal, and rectal budesonide; and inhaled and intranasal fluticasone with lopinavir/ritonavir and ritonavir 2. Possibly ↓ plasma levels of darunavir, indinavir, lopinavir, and saquinavir by dexamethasone	1. Inhibition of CYP3A4-mediated metabolism 2. Increased metabolism via CYP3A4	Avoid combination of budesonide or fluticasone with ritonavir if possible. 1. Monitor closely for signs of corticosteroid toxicity, adrenal suppression and immunosuppression, and ↓ dose as necessary. Steroid withdrawal may need a longer, more gradual reduction. Short-term or low-dose steroid use will have less risk of adverse effects. Consider using inhaled beclometasone as an alternative as it is not metabolized via CYP3A4 2. Use parenteral dexamethasone with caution, monitor CD4 count and viral load more frequently

(*Continued*)

Primary Drug	Secondary Drug	Effect	Mechanism	Precautions
ANTIVIRALS—ANTIRETROVIRALS				
PROTEASE INHIBITORS	DOCETAXEL, PACLITAXEL	↑ Risk of adverse effects of docetaxel and paclitaxel	Inhibition of CYP3A4-mediated metabolism	Use with caution, ritonavir is most commonly implicated. Additional monitoring is required. Monitor FBC weekly
PROTEASE INHIBITORS	DOXORUBICIN	↑ Risk of myelosuppression due to ↑ Plasma concentrations	Due to ↓ metabolism of doxorubicin by CYP3A4 isoenzymes owing to inhibition of those enzymes	Monitor for ↑ myelosuppression, peripheral neuropathy, myalgias, and fatigue
PROTEASE INHIBITORS	IL-2 (ALDESLEUKIN)	↑ Protease inhibitor levels, with risk of toxicity	Aldesleukin induces the formation of IL-6, which inhibits the metabolism of protease inhibitors by the CYP3A4 isoenzymes	Warn patients to report symptoms such as nausea, vomiting, flatulence, dizziness, and rashes. Monitor blood sugar on initiating and discontinuing treatment
PROTEASE INHIBITORS	**ANTICOAGULANTS—ORAL**			
INDINAVIR, RITONAVIR, SAQUINAVIR	DABIGATRAN	Anticoagulant effect may be ↑	Inhibition of transport via Pgp that increases absorption of dabigatran etexilate	Monitor carefully for increased anticoagulant effects, ask patients to observe closely for increased brusing/bleeding and report promptly
PROTEASE INHIBITORS	ACENOCOUMAROL, PHENINDIONE, WARFARIN	1. Anticoagulant effect may be altered (cases of both ↑ and ↓) when ritonavir and possibly saquinavir are given with warfarin 2. Reduced anticoagulant effect with tipranavir/ritonavir after 10 days 3. Possibly ↓ anticoagulant effect when ritonavir and nelfinavir are given with acenocoumarol	1 and 2. Complex interaction. Ritonavir initially inhibits CYP3A4 and CYP2C9, then induces these and CYP1A2 3. Probably competition for metabolism via CYP2C9 (nelfinavir) or CYP2C9 induction (ritnonavir)	Monitor INR closely, adjust anticoagulant doses as needed. Consider alternative anticoagulation
PROTEASE INHIBITORS	APIXABAN	Anticoagulant effect may be ↑.	Altered metabolism via CYP3A4 and transport via Pgp	Avoid coadministration

(Continued)

Primary Drug	Secondary Drug	Effect	Mechanism	Precautions
ANTIVIRALS—ANTIRETROVIRALS				
PROTEASE INHIBITORS	RIVAROXABAN	↑ Plasma levels of rivaroxaban, ↑ risk of overanticoagulation and bleeding	Inhibition of metabolism via CYP3A and Pgp	Avoid coadministration
PROTEASE INHIBITORS	**ANTIDEPRESSANTS**			
PROTEASE INHIBITORS	SSRIs	↑ Adverse effects of fluoxetine, paroxetine, and sertraline when coadministered with lopinavir/ritonavir, ritonavir, or saquinavir. Cardiac and neurological events have been reported, including serotonin syndrome	Ritonavir is associated with the most significant interaction of the protease inhibitors due to potent inhibition of CYP3A, CYP2D6, CYP2C9, CYP2C19, and then induction of CYP3A, 1A2, 2C8, 2C9, 2C19 of isoenzymes	Warn patients to watch for ↑ side effects of SSRIs, monitor ECG and consider ↓ dose of SSRI
DARUNAVIR/RITONAVIR	PAROXETINE, SERTRALINE	↓ Plasma levels of paroxetine and sertraline	Complex. Altered metabolism via CYP2D6 (paroxetine and sertraline) and CYP2C19 and 3A4 (sertraline)	Monitor more closely, may need ↑ dose of SSRI
FOSAMPRENAVIR/ RITONAVIR	PAROXETINE	↓ Plasma levels of paroxetine	Complex. Altered metabolism via CYP2D6	Warn patients to report altered treatment response for depression, watch for reduced efficacy as upward dose titration of paroxetine may be required
PROTEASE INHIBITORS	**TCAs**			
PROTEASE INHIBITORS	AMITRIPTYLINE	↑ Adverse effects when amitriptyline is coadministered with lopinavir/ritonavir, ritonavir or saquinavir, and possibly atazanavir	Inhibition of CYP3A4-mediated metabolism. Amitriptyline is metabolized by a number of enzymes, including CYP1A2, 2C9, 2D6, and CYP3A4; therefore, the effect of protease inhibitors is variable	Avoid coadministration with saquinavir, for other combinations monitor closely

(Continued)

Primary Drug	Secondary Drug	Effect	Mechanism	Precautions
ANTIVIRALS—ANTIRETROVIRALS				
PROTEASE INHIBITORS	AMOXAPINE, CLOMIPRAMINE, DOXEPIN, IMIPRAMINE, NORTRIPTYLINE, TRIMIPRAMINE	Possibly ↑ adverse effects, including ventricular arrhythmias, particularly amoxapine with atazanavir and ritonavir or saquinavir combinations	Inhibition of CYP3A4-mediated metabolism of amoxapine, clomipramine, and doxepin; inhibition of CYP3A4-, CYP2D6-, and CYP2C9-mediated metabolism of imipramine; inhibition of CYP2D6-mediated metabolism of nortriptyline and trimipramine	Monitor closely, including ECG. If QTc >500, stop one of interacting QTc prolonging agents and review therapeutic options, for QTc >470 in women or 440 in men, monitor ECG at least weekly
PROTEASE INHIBITORS	ST. JOHN'S WORT	Markedly ↓ levels and efficacy of protease inhibitors by St. John's wort, risk of viral resistance developing	Possibly ↑ CYP3A4-mediated metabolism of protease inhibitors	Avoid coadministration. Treatment with a protease inhibitor can be initiated without dose adjustment 2 weeks after stopping St. John's wort
RITONAVIR	TRAZODONE	↑ Adverse effects of trazodone, including nausea, dizziness, hypotension, syncope	Probably altered metabolism via CYP3A4 and 2D6	Use with caution; monitor for increased sedation, CVS, and GI side effects
PROTEASE INHIBITORS	**ANTIDIABETIC DRUGS**			
PROTEASE INHIBITORS	INSULIN	↓ Efficacy of insulin	Several mechanisms considered include insulin resistance, impaired insulin-stimulated glucose uptake by skeletal muscle cells, ↓ insulin binding to receptors, and inhibition of intrinsic transport activity of glucose transporters in the body	Necessary to establish baseline values for blood sugar before initiating therapy with a protease inhibitor. Warn patients about hyperglycemia. Atazanavir, darunavir, fosamprenavir, or tipranavir may be safer. ➢ ***For signs and symptoms of hyperglycemia, see Clinical Features of Some Adverse Drug Interactions, Hyperglycemia***
PROTEASE INHIBITORS	NATEGLINIDE, PIOGLITAZONE, REPAGLINIDE	↑ Levels of these antidiabetic drugs	Inhibition of CYP2C9- and CYP3A4-mediated metabolism of nateglinide and CYP3A4-mediated metabolism of pioglitazone and repaglinide	Monitor blood sugar closely

(*Continued*)

Primary Drug	Secondary Drug	Effect	Mechanism	Precautions
ANTIVIRALS—ANTIRETROVIRALS				
PROTEASE INHIBITORS	SULFONYLUREAS	↑ Effect of tolbutamide with ritonavir	Ritonavir is a potent inhibitor of CYP2C9, which metabolizes many sulfonylureas	Watch for hypoglycemia. Warn patients about hypoglycemia ➢ ***For signs and symptoms of hypoglycemia, see Clinical Features of Some Adverse Drug Reactions, Hypoglycemia***
PROTEASE INHIBITORS	ANTIDIARRHEAL DRUGS—LOPERAMIDE	1. ↓ Plasma levels of saquinavir, risk of reduced therapeutic response 2. ↑ Plasma levels of loperamide when loperamide is coingested with ritonavir or saquinavir 3. ↓ Plasma levels of loperamide (tipranavir, tipranavir/ritonavir)	1. Probably altered metabolism via CYP3A4 2. Ritonavir inhibits Pgp and CYP3A4 3. Tipranavir inhibits Pgp	Monitor for clinical effect, adjust dose if necessary. Stop loperamide if there are signs of abdominal distension in HIV patients as toxic megacolon has been reported
PROTEASE INHIBITORS	ANTIEMETICS—APREPITANT	↑ Adverse effects of aprepitant with nelfinavir and lopinavir/ritonavir and ritonavir	Inhibition of CYP3A4-mediated metabolism of aprepitant	Use with caution; clinical significance unclear; monitor closely
PROTEASE INHIBITORS	**ANTIEPILEPTICS**			
LOPINAVIR/RITONAVIR, RITONAVIR	LAMOTRIGINE	↓ Plasma levels of lamotrigine	Increased glucuronidation of lamotrigine	Monitor more closely, take lamotrigine levels within 2 weeks of adjusting therapy. If lopinavir/ritonavir or ritonavir is newly added, increase the dose of antiepileptic
PROTEASE INHIBITORS	PHENOBARBITAL	Possibly ↓ plasma levels of both protease inhibitors and phenobarbital	Increased metabolism of protease inhibitors mainly through induction of CYP3A4, and phenobarbital through CYP2C9 and 2C19	Use with caution. Monitor clinical outcomes closely, including viral load and CD4 count, check phenobarbitone levels and monitor for side effects when initiating or changing treatment

(*Continued*)

DRUGS TO TREAT INFECTIONS ANTIVIRALS—ANTIRETROVIRALS

Primary Drug	Secondary Drug	Effect	Mechanism	Precautions
ANTIVIRALS—ANTIRETROVIRALS				
PROTEASE INHIBITORS	CARBAMAZEPINE	1. Possibly ↑ adverse effects of carbamazepine with protease inhibitors 2. Possibly ↓ plasma levels of protease inhibitors	1. Inhibition of CYP3A4-mediated metabolism of carbamazepine 2. Increased metabolism of protease inhibitors via CYP3A4	Consider alternatives. Combine with caution. Monitor carbamazepine levels and side effects when initiating or changing treatment, monitor CD4 count and viral load closely. Carbamazepine dose may need to be reduced by 25%–50% in combination with darunavir/ritonavir. Lopinavir/ritonavir should always be twice daily; an increased dose of lopinavir may be required
PROTEASE INHIBITORS	PHENYTOIN	1. Possibly ↓ efficacy of phenytoin, with a risk of fits when it is coadministered with fosamprenavir/ritonavir, indinavir, lopinavir/ritonavir, nelfinavir, or ritonavir 2. ↓ Plasma levels of lopinavir (with ritonavir) and possibly darunavir, saquinavir	1. Uncertain; ↓ plasma levels of phenytoin 2. Increased metabolism via CYP450 system	Avoid lopinavir/ritnoavir once daily. Use with caution, a dose increase of lopinavir/ritonavir may be needed. Monitor closely, including CD4 count, viral load, and phenytoin levels;check later weekly when initiating or changing doses. Adjust doses at 7–10-day intervals. Maximum suggested dose adjustment each time is 25 mg
LOPINAVIR/RITONAVIR, RITONAVIR	SODIUM VALPROATE	1. Possible ↓ plasma levels of valproate 2. Possibly ↑ plasma levels of lopinavir	1. Increased glucuronidation of valproate 2. Uncertain	Use with caution, monitor more closely

(*Continued*)

DRUGS TO TREAT INFECTIONS ANTIVIRALS—ANTIRETROVIRALS

DRUGS TO TREAT INFECTIONS ANTIVIRALS—ANTIRETROVIRALS

Primary Drug	Secondary Drug	Effect	Mechanism	Precautions
ANTIVIRALS—ANTIRETROVIRALS				
PROTEASE INHIBITORS	**ANTIFUNGALS—AZOLES**			
PROTEASE INHIBITORS	ITRACONAZOLE, KETOCONAZOLE	Possibly ↑ levels of ketoconazole by atazanavir, darunavir/ritonavir, fosamprenavir, indinavir, tipranvir/ritonavir, ↑ levels by saquinavir and saquinavir/ritonavir and both antifungals by lopinavir/ritonavir and ritonavir. Indinavir, ritonavir, and saquinavir levels are ↑ by itraconazole and ketoconazole, tipranvir/ritonavir are possibly reduced, ↑ darunavir and lopinavir/ritonavir demonstrated with ketoconazole	Inhibition of, or competition for, CYP3A4-mediated metabolism. Altered Pgp transport may affect saquinavir and ritonavir	Use with caution and monitor LFTs and for adverse effects of protease inhibitor and antifungal, e.g., GI; if either combined with indinavir, consider a dose reduction of indinavir from 800 to 600 mg 8-hourly. No dose adjustment required for saquinavir/ritonavir 1000/100 mg twice daily if ketoconazole <= 200 mg/day. Maximum recommended dose of ketoconazole or itraconazole is 200 mg/day
PROTEASE INHIBITORS	VORICONAZOLE	1. ↓ Plasma levels and efficacy of voriconazole and atazanavir. If there is no functional CYP2C19, then increased voriconazole plasma levels can be expected 2. Small reduction in ↓ plasma levels of low-dose ritonavir	Complex. Probably increased metabolism of both via CYP3A4, and voriconazole via 2C9 and 2C19	Avoid coadministration if the dose of ritonavir is 400 mg twice a day or greater. Avoid combining low-dose ritonavir (100 mg once a day) unless benefits outweigh risks. Consider testing for functional CYP2C19 status: in case of one functional allele, monitor closely for poor response to voriconazole and impaired response to protease inhibitor, if there are no functional alleles, monitor for side effects of voriconazole

(*Continued*)

Primary Drug	Secondary Drug	Effect	Mechanism	Precautions
ANTIVIRALS—ANTIRETROVIRALS				
ATAZANAVIR, ATAZANAVIR/ RITONAVIR, FOSAMPRENAVIR	POSACONAZOLE	1. ↑ Plasma levels of protease inhibitors risk of hyperbilirubinemia 2. ↓ Levels of posaconazole (fosamprenavir), risk of treatment failure	1. Uncertain 2. Altered metabolism via Pgp or UGT	Monitor for antifungal efficacy and for increased side effects
PROTEASE INHIBITORS	ANTIHISTAMINES—ASTEMIZOLE, MIZOLASTINE, TERFENADINE	Possibly ↑ adverse effects of antihistamine, including QT prolongation	Inhibition of metabolism via CYP3A4 (all), CYP2D6 (terfenadine), inhibition of transport via Pgp (terfenadine)	Avoid coadministration. Risk is greatest in patients who are also poor CYP2D6 metabolizers
SAQUINAVIR/RITONAVIR	MIZOLASTINE	Possibly ↑ adverse effects, including cardiac arrhythmias	Inhibition of CYP3A4-mediated metabolism	Avoid coadministration
PROTEASE INHIBITORS	**ANTIHYPERTENSIVES AND HEART FAILURE DRUGS**			
PROTEASE INHIBITORS	ALPHA-BLOCKERS	Possible ↑ alfuzosin levels and adverse effects e.g., hypotension with ritonavir	Inhibition of metabolism via CYP3A4	Avoid coadministration
PROTEASE INHIBITORS	VASODILATOR ANTIHYPERTENSIVES	1. ↑ Plasma levels and ↑ adverse effects of bosentan by ritonavir, e.g., headache 2. Possible ↓ in plasma levels of indinavir or atazanavir	1. Inhibition of CYP3A4- and OATP1B1-mediated metabolism of bosentan 2. Uncertain	Coadministration not recommended, monitor closely for bosentan toxicity, including LFTs and for antiviral efficacy. Omit bosentan for 2 days when starting a protease inhibitor other than indinavir or nefinavir. If already on a protease inhibitor, start bosentan at reduced dose and adjust as needed, 62.5 mg daily or alternate day dosing. Use atazanavir with ritonavir
PROTEASE INHIBITORS	**ANTIMALARIALS**			
PROTEASE INHIBITORS	ARTEMETHER WITH LUMEFANTRINE	↑ Artemether levels, darunavir ↑ lumefantrine levels, risk of ventricular arrhythmias	Uncertain; possibly inhibited metabolism via CYP3A4	Use with caution

(Continued)

Primary Drug	Secondary Drug	Effect	Mechanism	Precautions
ANTIVIRALS—ANTIRETROVIRALS				
RITONAVIR BOOSTED PROTEASE INHIBITORS, RITONAVIR	ATOVAQUONE	Possibly ↓ plasma levels of atovaquone	Increased glucuronidation of atovaquone	Avoid coadministration if possible, particularly lopinavir/ritonavir regimen. If essential be alert for possible failure of malaria prophylaxis, increased dose of atovaquone may be required
FOSAMPRENAVIR/RITONAVIR, SAQUINAVIR/RITONAVIR, TIPRANAVIR/RITONAVIR	HALOFANTRINE	1. Possibly ↑ plasma levels of halofantrine 2. Risk of cardiac arrhythmias with saquninavir/ritonavir	Inhibition of metabolism via CYP3A4	Avoid coadministration with saquinavir/ritonavir or low-dose ritonavir, coadministration with other protease inhibitors not recommended
SAQUINAVIR	PIPERAQUINE WITH DIHYDROARTEMISININ	Possibly ↑ adverse effects, including ventricular arrhythmias	Additive side effects	Use with caution, monitor ECG
LOPINAVIR/RITONAVIR, RITONAVIR	PROGUANIL	Possible ↓ plasma levels and efficacy of proguanil	Altered metabolism via CYP2C19	Avoid coadministration if possible, particularly lopinavir/ritonavir regimen. If essential, be alert for possible failure of malaria prophylaxis
PROTEASE INHIBITORS	QUININE	1. ↑ Quinine levels and ↑ risk of toxicity, including ventricular arrhythmias with ritonavir 2. ↓ In plasma levels of quinine with lopinavir/ritonavir	1 and 2. Altered metabolism via CYP3A4 2. Also possible altered glucuronidation	Avoid coadministration with saquinavir, for others, use with caution, monitor therapeutic outcome and ECG
PROTEASE INHIBITORS	**ANTIMIGRAINE DRUGS**			
PROTEASE INHIBITORS	ERGOT ALKALOIDS	↑ Ergotamine/methysergide levels, with risk of toxicity—vasospasm, ischemia	↓ CYP3A4-mediated metabolism of ergot derivatives	Avoid coadministration

(Continued)

Primary Drug	Secondary Drug	Effect	Mechanism	Precautions
ANTIVIRALS—ANTIRETROVIRALS				
PROTEASE INHIBITORS	5-HT1 AGONISTS—ALMOTRIPTAN, ELETRIPTAN	Possibly ↑ plasma levels and ↑ adverse effects when almotriptan or eletriptan is coadministered with indinavir, lopinavir/ritonavir, nelfinavir, or ritonavir	Inhibition of CYP3A4- and possibly CYP2D6-mediated metabolism of eletriptan and CYP3A4-mediated metabolism of almotriptan	Avoid coadministration
PROTEASE INHIBITORS	**ANTIMUSCARINICS**			
PROTEASE INHIBITORS	DARIFENACIN	↑ Adverse effects with atazanavir and possibly with other protease inhibitors	Increased plasma levels as atazanavir reduces darifenacin metabolism via CYP3A4, 2D6, and Pgp	Avoid coadministration
ATAZANAVIR, INDINAVIR, RITONAVIR, SAQUINAVIR	FESTERODINE	↑ Adverse effects	Increased plasma levels, reduces metabolism via CYP3A4 and 2D6	Limit maximum dose of festoterodine to 4 mg daily
RITONAVIR	MIRABEGRON	Possibly ↑ adverse effects	Combination of CYP3A4 inhibition and reduced renal elimination	Reduce dose if mild renal impairment, avoid if severe
PROTEASE INHIBITORS	SOLIFENACIN	↑ Adverse effects with nelfinavir, lopinavir/ritonavir, and ritonavir	Inhibition of CYP3A4-mediated metabolism of solifenacin	Limit maximum dose of solifenacin to 5 mg daily
PROTEASE INHIBITORS	TOLTERODINE	Possibly ↑ adverse effects, including arrythmias with protease inhibitors	Inhibition of CYP2D6- and CYP3A4-mediated metabolism of tolterodine	Avoid coadministration
ATAZANAVIR, RITONAVIR	ANTIPLATELETS—TICAGRELOR	Possibly ↑ levels of ticagrelor	Inhibition of CYP3A4-mediated metabolism of ticagrelor	Avoid coadministration

(*Continued*)

Primary Drug	Secondary Drug	Effect	Mechanism	Precautions
ANTIVIRALS—ANTIRETROVIRALS				
PROTEASE INHIBITORS	**ANTIPSYCHOTICS**			
PROTEASE INHIBITORS	ARIPIPRAZOLE, HALOPERIDOL, CLOZAPINE, PIMOZIDE, QUETIAPINE, RISPERIDONE, SERTINDOLE, THIORIDAZINE	Possibly ↑ levels of antipsychotic and ↑ adverse effects, including hematological abnormalities (clozapine, pimozide), coma (quetiapine), and ventricular arrhythmias (clozapine, haloperidol, pimozide, sertindole, thioridazine)	Inhibition of metabolism mediated by CYP3A4 (quetiapine) and/or CYP2D6 (haloperidol, risperidone, thioridazine). Clozapine affected by inhibition of both enzymes	Avoid coadministration of clozapine with ritonavir or saquinavir, and pimozide, quetiapine, or sertindole with protease inhibitors. Avoid saquinavir with haloperodol or phenothiazines e.g., thioridazine. Use other antipsychotics with caution; ↓ dose may be required. With risperidone, watch closely for extrapyramidal side effects and neuroepileptic malignant syndrome. Monitor baseline ECG and repeat at day 3–4; if QT increases >480 ms or more than 20 ms over baseline, review risk/benefit and consider stopping saquninavir/ritonavir. If baseline QT > 450 ms, avoid coadministration—review for alternative therapy
PROTEASE INHIBITORS	OLANZAPINE	Possibly ↓ efficacy of olanzapine when co-ingested with lopinavir/ritonavir, ritonavir	Possibly ↑ metabolism via CYP1A2 and glucuronyl transferases	Monitor clinical response; ↑ dose as necessary
PROTEASE INHIBITORS	**ANTIVIRALS**			
PROTEASE INHIBITORS	**ANTIVIRALS FOR HEPATITIS C**			
ATAZANAVIR, DARUNAVIR/RITONAVIR, FOSAMPRENAVIR, LOPINAVIR, RITONAVIR	BOCEPREVIR	1. ↓ Plasma concentration of protease inhibitors, possible ↓ efficacy 2. ↓ Plasma concentration of boceprevir with ritonavir	Probably altered metabolism via CYP3A4	Avoid coadministration with darunavir/ritonavir or lopinavir/ritonavir. If combination is essential, monitor viral load and CD4 count closely

(*Continued*)

Primary Drug	Secondary Drug	Effect	Mechanism	Precautions
ANTIVIRALS—ANTIRETROVIRALS				
PROTEASE INHIBITORS	SIMEPREVIR	1. ↑ Plasma concentration of simeprevir, risk of adverse effects 2. Possible altered levels of protease inhibitors	Inhibition of metabolism via CYP3A4	Avoid coadministration
ATAZANAVIR, DARUNAVIR/ RITNAOVIR, FOSAMPRENAVIR/ RITONAVIR, LOPINAVIR/ RITONAVIR, RITONAVIR	TELAPREVIR	↓ Plasma concentration of telaprevir, darunavir and amprenavir, possible ↑ in plasma concentration of atazanavir, risk of hyperbilirubinemia	Probably altered metabolism via CYP3A4	Avoid coadministration unless you are using atazanavir/ ritonavir. If combination essential, monitor viral load and CD4 count closely
PROTEASE INHIBITORS	ANTIVIRALS—FOSCARNET SODIUM	↓ Renal function when coadministered with ritonavir or saquinavir	Uncertain; possibly ↓ renal excretion of foscarnet	Monitor renal function closely
PROTEASE INHIBITORS	**ANTIVIRALS—OTHER**			
ATAZANAVIR, DARUNAVIR	COBICISTAT	↑ Plasma levels of protease inhibitors	Inhibition of metabolism via CYP3A	Avoid coadministration particularly with other boosted antiretrovirals, e.g., other protease inhibitors or Elvitegravir
ATAZANAVIR, DARUNAVIR, FOSAMPRENAVIR, INDINAVIR, LOPINAVIR/ RITONAVIR, RITONAVIR, SAQUINAVIR, SAQUINAVIR/ RITONAVIR	MARAVIROC	1. ↑ Plasma concentration of maraviroc with protease inhibitors, risk of adverse effects 2. ↓ Levels of amprenavir, risk of treatment failure	Inhibition of metabolism via CYP3A4 and Pgp	Interaction can be combined for therapeutic advantage. Coadministration with fosamprenavir/ritonavir not recommended. With darunavir/ ritonavir, lopinavir/ritonavir (400/100 mg), or saquinavir/ ritonavir (1000/100 mg), use maraviroc 150 mg twice daily. No dose adjustment needed with tipranavir/ritonavir. Consider dose reduction of maraviroc with atazanavir or saquinavir

(Continued)

Primary Drug	Secondary Drug	Effect	Mechanism	Precautions
ANTIVIRALS—ANTIRETROVIRALS				
DARUNAVIR/RITONAVIR, FOSAMPRENAVIR/ RITONAVIR, TIPRANAVIR/ RITONAVIR	RALTEGRAVIR	1. ↓ Plasma levels of amprenavir and raltegravir, risk of treatment failure 2. ↑ Risk of rash with darunavir	1. Probably increased metabolism via glucuronidation (raltegravir) 2. Additive side effect	1. Avoid coadministration with amprenavir 2. Advise patients to report signs of rash, monitor closely. No dose adjustment needed with atazanavir/ ritonavir, lopinavir/ritonavir, indinavir, saquinavir, tipranvir/ritonavir
ATAZANAVIR/RITONAVIR, LOPINAVIR/RITONAVIR, RITONAVIR (LOW DOSE)	ELVITEGRAVIR	↑ Plasma levels of elvitegravir	Probably involves altered metabolism via CYP3A4, though induction of glucuronidation would reduce levels	Reduce dose of elvitegravir from 150 to 85 mg daily and use atazanavir/ritonavir 300/100 mg. Can be used with darunavir or tipranvir both with ritonavir without dose adjustment
TIPRANAVIR/RITONAVIR	DOLUTEGRAVIR	↓ Plasma levels of doltegravir, risk of treatment failure and resistance	Induction of UGT1A1 and CYP3A	Dose of dolutegravir must be 50 mg twice daily, no dose adjustment needed if it is also combined with darunavir, fosamprenavir, or lopinavir, all with ritonavir
PROTEASE INHIBITORS	**NNRTIs**			
AMPRENAVIR	EFAVIRENZ	Possible ↓ efficacy of amprenavir	Uncertain; ↓ bioavailability of amprenavir	Consider ↑ dose of amprenavir to 1200 mg three times a day, or combine amprenavir 600 mg twice a day with ritonavir 100 mg twice a day
ATAZANAVIR WITH RITONAVIR	EFAVIRENZ	1. ↓ Efficacy of efavirenz 2. Possible↓ efficacy of atazanavir	↑ CYP3A4-mediated metabolism and Pgp transport of efavirenz and atazanavir	Combination not recommended, if combination is required, increase atazanavir to 400 mg and ritonavir to 200 mg daily and give with efavirenz 600 mg daily
DARUNAVIR, DARINAVIR/ RITONAVIR	EFAVIRENZ	1. ↓ Efficacy of darunavir 2. ↑ Plasma levels and ↑ adverse effects of efavirenz	1. Increased metabolism via CYP3A4 2. Reduced metabolism via CYP3A4	Use with caution monitor more closely. If used in combination give darunavir 600 mg and ritonavir 100 mg twice daily plus efavirenz 600 mg daily as darunavir/ritonavir 800/100 mg daily may result in treatment failure

(Continued)

Primary Drug	Secondary Drug	Effect	Mechanism	Precautions
ANTIVIRALS—ANTIRETROVIRALS				
FOSAMPRENAVIR	EFAVIRENZ	↓ Efficacy of fosamprenavir	Not studied	Avoid coadministration though an increased dose of fosamprenavir boosted with ritonavir (to 1400/300 mg respectively) can overcome reduction in plasma levels
LOPINAVIR/RITONAVIR	EFAVIRENZ	↓ Plasma levels of lopinavir	Efavirenz induces metabolism of lopinavir via CYP3A4	Use twice daily dosing and increase dose of lopinavir/ritonavir soft capsules from 3 to 4 capsules, solution from 5 to 6.5 mL, or tablets from 400/100 to 500/125 mg. Monitor closely as further dose increases may be needed
NELFINAVIR	EFAVIRENZ	Possible ↑ efficacy of nelfinavir, with theoretical risk of adverse effects	Small ↑ bioavailability of nelfinavir	No dose adjustment necessary
RITONAVIR (HIGH DOSE: 500 MG BD)	EFAVIRENZ	↑ Bioavailability of both, ↑ adverse effects, e.g., dizziness, nausea, paresthesia, liver dysfunction	Competition for metabolism via CYP3A4	Combination with high-dose ritonavir is not well tolerated. Monitor closely, including LFTs. Low-dose ritonavir alone has not been studied
SAQUINAVIR	EFAVIRENZ	↓ Plasma levels of saquinavir and possible ↓ efficacy, risk of treatment failure, ↑ adverse effects e.g., liver dysfunction (particularly with ritonavir boosted regimen)	↑ CYP3A4-mediated metabolism of saquinavir	Combination not recommended with saquinavir as sole protease inhibitor, always use saquinavir in combination with another agent, e.g., ritonavir, when coadministering with efavirenz and monitor LFTs
AMPRENAVIR OR FOSAMPRENAVIR/RITONAVIR	ETRAVIRINE	Possible ↑ bioavailability and ↑ adverse effects	Likely altered metabolism via CYP2C9 and CYP3A4 and altered transport via Pgp	Dose reduction of amprenavir or fosamprenavir required or fosamprenavir/ritonavir may be required
NELFINAVIR	ETRAVIRINE	Possible ↑ bioavailability and ↑ adverse effects of nelfinavir	Not studied	Manufacturer of etravirine advises one to avoid coadadministration

(*Continued*)

Primary Drug	Secondary Drug	Effect	Mechanism	Precautions
ANTIVIRALS—ANTIRETROVIRALS				
TIPRANAVIR/RITONAVIR	ETRAVIRINE	↓ Plasma levels of etravirine, ↑ plasma levels of tipranavir	Probably increased metabolism via CYP3A4 and UGT	Avoid concomitant use
UNBOOSTED PROTEASE INHIBITORS	ETRAVIRINE	↓ Plasma levels and efficacy of protease inhibitors	↑ CYP-mediated metabolism	Avoid concomitant use
AMPRENAVIR	NEVIRAPINE	Efficacy of amprenavir predicted to be ↓	Uncertain; ↓ bioavailability of amprenavir	Monitor viral load
ATAZANAVIR, ATAZANAVIR/RITONAVIR	NEVIRAPINE	↓ Efficacy of atazanavir, ↑ plasma levels of nevirapine	Atazanavir is a substrate and inhibitor of CYP3A4	Avoid concomitant use
FOSAMPRENAVIR	NEVIRAPINE	Possible ↓ plasma levels of fosamprenavir	Probably altered metabolism via CYP3A4 and induction of Pgp	Avoid coadministration unless fosamprenavir is boosted with ritonavir—then no dose adjustments are needed
NELFINAVIR	NEVIRAPINE	Possible ↓ efficacy of nelfinavir	Uncertain	Dose adjustment probably not required, although one study suggests ↑ dose may be needed
SAQUINAVIR	NEVIRAPINE	Possible ↓ efficacy; risk of treatment failure of saquinavir	↑ CYP3A4-mediated metabolism of saquinavir	Clinical significance unclear. Different formulations of saquinavir may have different magnitudes of interaction. If boosted with ritonavir, combination can be administered without dose adjustment
INDINAVIR	NNRTIs	Possible ↓ efficacy of indinavir	↑ CYP3A4-mediated metabolism of indinavir, altered metabolism via Pgp is also probable	Avoid etravirine and indinavir combination. For others monitor viral load; with nevirapine ↑ dose of indinavir to 1000 mg 8-hourly, with efavirenz this increase may not be sufficient, no dose adjustment is needed for efavirenz or nevirapine when combined with indinavir

(*Continued*)

Primary Drug	Secondary Drug	Effect	Mechanism	Precautions
ANTIVIRALS—ANTIRETROVIRALS				
LOPINAVIR/RITONAVIR	NNRTIs	Possible ↓ efficacy of lopinavir/ritonavir	Nevirapine induces metabolism of lopinavir via CYP3A4	Increase of lopinavir/ritonavir dose recommended and monitor drug concentrations with nevirapine. Adults: Use twice daily dosing and increase dose to 533/133 mg (from 3 to 4 caps) or 500/125 mg (5 tabs) or solution from 5 to 6.5 mL. Children: consider dose increase to 300/75 mg/m^2 twice daily taken with food. Monitor viral load closely as this dose ↑ may be insufficient. Monitor LFTs closely. No dose is adjustment required with etravirine or rilpivirine
PROTEASE INHIBITORS	**NUCLEOSIDE REVERSE TRANSCRIPTASE INHIBITORS**			
PROTEASE INHIBITORS	DIDANOSINE (BUFFERED)	↓ Efficacy of atazanavir and indinavir	Absorption of some protease inhibitors (indinavir) may be affected by the buffered didanosine formulation, which ↑ gastric pH	Separate doses; give indinavir, atazanavir, or ritonavir 2 h before or 2 h afterward. Didanosine should be taken on an empty stomach, advice for protease inhibitors varies: indinavir, empty stomach; atazanavir or ritonavir with food. Alternatively, consider using the gastroresistant formulation of didanosine. No dose adjustment needed with saquinavir/ritonavir
ATAZANAVIR, DARUNAVIR, LOPINAVIR (ALL WITH RITONAVIR)	TENOFOVIR	1. ↓ Efficacy of atazanavir 2. Possible ↑ in plasma levels and ↑ adverse effects of tenofovir by atazanavir, e.g., renal dysfunction 3. ↑ Plasma levels of tenofovir by lopinavir	1. Uncertain; ↓ plasma levels of atazanavir 2. Uncertain 3. Altered transport via Pgp (intestinal)	Use with caution with atazanavir. Monitor renal function and for increased side effects of tenofovir

(*Continued*)

Primary Drug	Secondary Drug	Effect	Mechanism	Precautions
ANTIVIRALS—ANTIRETROVIRALS				
LOPINAVIR/RITONAVIR	ABACAVIR, ZIDOVUDINE	↓ Efficacy of abacavir and zidovudine	↓ Plasma levels by ↑ glucuronidation	Avoid coadministration, clinical significance unknown though may be used with dual NRTI in pregnancy.
NELFINAVIR	STAVUDINE	Possibly ↑ adverse effects	Uncertain	Warn patients that diarrhea may occur
TIPRANAVIR/RITONAVIR	ABACAVIR, ZIDOVUDINE	Possible ↓ efficacy; risk of treatment failure of abacavir or zidovudine	↓ Plasma levels by ↑ glucuronidation	Not recommended unless there are no other available nucleoside reverse transcriptase inhibitors
TIPRANAVIR/RITONAVIR	DIDANOSINE (ENTERIC-COATED)	↓ Plasma levels of didanosine, risk of treatment failure	↓ Absorption	Separate doses by at least 2.5 h
PROTEASE INHIBITORS	**PROTEASE INHIBITORS**			
ATAZANAVIR	INDINAVIR	↑ Bioavailability and ↑ adverse effects of indinavir; ↑ adverse effects of atazanavir, e.g., hyperbilirubinemia	Inhibition of metabolism via CYP3A4 by atazanavir; inhibition of UDGPT by indinavir	Avoid coadministration
ATAZANAVIR	RITONAVIR (HIGH DOSE)	↑ Plasma concentration and efficacy of atazavir (doses >100 mg ritonavir not studied and likely to ↑ adverse effects of atazanavir, e.g., cardiac effects, hyperbilirubinemia)	Inhibition of CYP3A4-mediated metabolism of atazanavir	Used to therapeutic benefit. Atazanavir 300 mg with ritonavir 100 mg is equivalent to 400 mg atazanavir
ATAZANAVIR	SAQUINAVIR, SAQUINAVIR/RITONAVIR	↑ Efficacy and ↑ adverse effects of saquinavir, ↑ risk of ventricular arrhythmias	Inhibition of CYP3A4-mediated metabolism of saquinavir	Avoid coadministration
ATAZANAVIR	TIPRANAVIR, TIPRANAVIR/RITONAVIR	↑ Plasma concentration of tipranavir or tipranvir/ritonavir, ↓ plasma concentration of atazanavir	Altered metabolism via CYP3A4	Avoid coadministration

(*Continued*)

Primary Drug	Secondary Drug	Effect	Mechanism	Precautions
ANTIVIRALS—ANTIRETROVIRALS				
DARUNAVIR, DARUNAVIR/ RITONAVIR	INDINAVIR	↑ Plasma concentration of both drugs	Inhibition of CYP3A4-mediated metabolism of darunavir	If combination of darunaivir/ ritonavir 400 mg/100 mg with indinavir 800 mg, all twice daily, is not tolerated, reduce indinavir to 600 mg twice daily
DARUNAVIR, DARUNAVIR/ RITONAVIR	LOPINAVIR/RITONAVIR	↓ Plasma concentration of darunavir	Uncertain	Avoid coadministration, required doses have not been established
FOSAMPRENAVIR, FOSAMPRENAVIR/ RITONAVIR	LOPINAVIR/RITONAVIR	↓ Plasma concentration of amprenavir, ↑ lopinavir, ↑ risk of GI side effects and raised triglycerides	Altered metabolism via CYP3A4 (inhibition and induction) and Pgp induction	Avoid coadministration
DARUNAVIR, DARUNAVIR/ RITONAVIR	SAQUINAVIR, SAQUINAVIR/ RITONAVIR	↓ Plasma concentration of darunavir and saquinavir	Uncertain	Avoid coadministration
INDINAVIR	NELFINAVIR	Possibly ↑ efficacy and ↑ adverse effects of both	Inhibition of CYP3A4-mediated metabolism	Suitable doses not yet certain, clinical significance of interaction not established; however, monitor more closely for adverse effects
INDINAVIR	LOPINAVIR/RITONAVIR, RITONAVIR, SAQUINAVIR/ RITONAVIR	↑ Plasma levels of both drugs with ritonavir, ↑ efficacy, and ↑ adverse effects of indinavir. Risk of nephrolithiasis if the dose of indinavir exceeds 800 mg twice a day	Inhibition of CYP3A4-mediated metabolism of indinavir	Indinavir 800 mg with ritonavir 100 mg twice daily may increase side effects. With lopinavir/ ritonavir twice daily, reduce indinavir dose to 600 mg twice daily. Adequate hydration and monitoring are essential. Adults must drink at least 1500 mL/24 h
INDINAVIR	SAQUINAVIR	↑ Plasma concentration of saquinavir, possible ↑ efficacy and ↑ adverse effects	Inhibition of CYP3A4-mediated metabolism	Clinical significance, doses and safety of combination not established. The formulation may affect the interaction. Monitor clinical outcomes and side effects closely
LOPINAVIR/RITONAVIR	SAQUINAVIR	↑ Plasma concentration of saquinavir, ↑ adverse effects ↑ risk of ventricular arrhythmias	Uncertain	Avoid coadministration. If combination cannot be avoided, reduce dose of saquinavir to 1 g with lopinavir/ritnaovir 400/100 mg, all twice daily

(Continued)

Primary Drug	Secondary Drug	Effect	Mechanism	Precautions
ANTIVIRALS—ANTIRETROVIRALS				
NELFINAVIR	RITONAVIR/LOPINAVIR	1. Possibly ↓ efficacy of lopinavir 2. ↑ Efficacy of nelfinavir	1. ↓ Bioavailability of lopinavir and ritonavir 2. Minimal ↑ in plasma levels of nelfinavir and its active metabolites through inhibition of metabolism via CYP3A4	Monitor closely. May need to ↑ doses of lopinavir and ritonavir, an increase of lopinavir/ritonavir to 500/125 mg (tablets) or 522/133 mg (liquid) twice daily has been suggested. Avoid once daily regimens
NELFINAVIR	RITONAVIR	↑ Efficacy and ↑ adverse effects of nelfinavir; unclear effects on ritonavir	Involves CYP450 inhibition and induction. ↑ concentration of nelfinavir and its active metabolite M8	Monitor closely if combination used
NELFINAVIR	SAQUINAVIR, SAQUINAVIR/RITONAVIR	Possibly ↑ efficacy and ↑ adverse effects, e.g., diarrhea	Additive toxicity; ↑ bioavailability. Inhibition of metabolism via CYP3A4	Combination with saquinavir/ritonavir not recommended. If saquinavir alone warn patients of ↑ side effects
RITONAVIR	TIPRANAVIR	Reports of clinical hepatitis and hepatic decompensation, including fatalities	Additive toxicity	Monitor more closely, including LFTs, especially if patients have chronic hepatitis B or C, do not use doses of ritonavir <200 mg twice daily
SAQUINAVIR	RITONAVIR AND LOPINAVIR	Risk of ↑ adverse effects, e.g., life-threatening arrythmias	Inhibition of CYP3A4-mediated metabolism	Avoid coadministration
SAQUINAVIR	RITONAVIR (HIGH DOSE)	↑ Efficacy and ↑ adverse effects of saquinavir, diabetic ketoacidosis, and liver disorders reported, possible additive effect of increase in QT and/or PR interval; no clinically significant interaction for ritonavir	Large ↑ bioavailability of saquinavir via inhibition of CYP3A4 in gut wall and liver	Recommended dose saquinavir 1000 mg with ritonavir 100 mg twice a day. Dose of ritonavir should not exceed 100 mg twice daily
TIPRANAVIR	FOSAMPRENAVIR/RITONAVIR	↓ Plasma levels of fosamprenavir	Altered metabolism via CYP3A4	Avoid coadministration
TIPRANAVIR RITONAVIR	ATAZANAVIR/RITONAVIR	Possibly ↓ efficacy of atazanavir and ↑ toxicity of tipranavir/ritonavir	Inhibition of metabolism via CYP3A4 (atazanavir/ritonavir) and induction by tipranvir/ritonavir	Avoid coadministration, if not possible monitor for side effects and consider monitoring levels of atazanavir

(*Continued*)

Primary Drug	Secondary Drug	Effect	Mechanism	Precautions
ANTIVIRALS—ANTIRETROVIRALS				
TIPRANAVIR RITONAVIR	LOPINAVIR/RITONAVIR	↓ Plasma levels of lopinavir, possibly ↓ efficacy	Possibly induction of metabolism via CYP3A4	Avoid coadministration, if not possible consider monitoring levels of lopinavir
TIPRANAVIR RITONAVIR	SAQUINAVIR/RITONAVIR	↓ Plasma levels of saquinavir, possibly ↓ efficacy	Possibly induction of metabolism via CYP3A4	Avoid coadministration. If not possible consider monitoring saquinavir levels
PROTEASE INHIBITORS	ANXIOLYTICS AND HYPNOTICS—BENZODIAZEPINE, BUSPIRONE	↑ Adverse effects, e.g., prolonged sedation	Inhibition of CYP3A4-mediated metabolism of BZDs and buspirone	Avoid coadministration of protease inhibitors and oral midazolam or triazolam, and alprazolam with indinavir. For IV midazolam consider a dose reduction and intensive monitoring, for other combinations watch closely for ↑ sedation; ↓ dose of sedative as necessary. Some recommend considering substituting long-acting for shorter-acting BZDs with less active metabolites (e.g., lorazepam for diazepam) or less CYP3A4-dependent metabolism
RITONAVIR, SAQUINAVIR, TIPRANAVIR	BETA-BLOCKERS	↑ Adverse effects of carvedilol, metoprolol, propranolol, and timolol ↑ Risk of ventricular arrhythmias with sotalol and saquinavir	Inhibition of CYP2D6-mediated metabolism of these beta-blockers	Avoid coadministration of metoprolol with ritonavir or tipranavir and sotalol with saquinavir. For others use an alternative beta-blocker if possible; if not, monitor closely
RITONAVIR/LOPINAVIR, RITONAVIR, TIPRANAVIR/ RITONAVIR	THEOPHYLLINE	↓ Efficacy	↑ Metabolism via induction of CYP1A2 also altered metabolism via CYP3A4	Monitor clinical response. Measure theophylline levels weekly after starting; ↑ doses may be required
PROTEASE INHIBITORS	CALCIUM CHANNEL BLOCKERS	Plasma concentrations of calcium channel blockers are ↑ by protease inhibitors	Protease inhibitors inhibit CYP3A4-mediated metabolism of calcium channel blockers	Monitor PR, BP, and ECG closely; ↓ dose of calcium channel blocker if necessary (e.g., manufacturers of diltiazem suggest starting at 50% of the standard dose and titrating to effect)

(*Continued*)

DRUGS TO TREAT INFECTIONS ANTIVIRALS—ANTIRETROVIRALS

Primary Drug	Secondary Drug	Effect	Mechanism	Precautions
ANTIVIRALS—ANTIRETROVIRALS				
RITONAVIR BOOSTED PROTEASE INHIBITORS, INDINAVIR, RITONAVIR, SAQUINAVIR	CARDIAC GLYCOSIDES—DIGOXIN	1. Plasma digoxin concentrations may be ↑ 2. ↑ Or ↓ by tipranavir/ritonavir	1. Inhibition of Pgp-mediated renal excretion of digoxin and ↑ intestinal absorption 2. Initial inhibition of Pgp and then induction of Pgp	If already on digoxin, reduce digoxin dose by half and monitor digoxin levels; watch for digoxin toxicity
INDINAVIR, NELFINAVIR, RITONAVIR, SAQUINAVIR	CNS STIMULANTS—MODAFINIL	↑ Plasma concentrations of modafinil, with risk of adverse effects	Due to inhibition of CYP3A4, which has a partial role in the metabolism of modafinil	Be aware. Warn patients to report dose-related adverse effects, e.g., headache, anxiety
PROTEASE INHIBITORS	DIURETICS—POTASSIUM-SPARING—EPLERENONE	Possibly ↑ adverse effects of eplerenone with nelfinavir, lopinavir/ritonavir, ritonavir, and saquinavir	Inhibition of CYP3A4-mediated metabolism of eplerenone	Avoid concomitant use
PROTEASE INHIBITORS	**DRUG DEPENDENCE THERAPIES**			
PROTEASE INHIBITORS	BUPROPION	↓ Levels of bupropion	Probably induction of CYP2B6-mediated metabolism of bupropion with lopinavir, ritonavir, tipranavir	Avoid coadministration. If not possible monitor clinical outcomes closely and do not exceed the maximum recommended dose of bupriprion
SAQUINAVIR	DAPSONE	Increased risk of ventricular arrhythmias	Uncertain	Avoid coadministration
PROTEASE INHIBITORS	DISULFIRAM	↑ Risk of disulfiram reaction with lopinavir/ritonavir and ritonavir solution or tipranavir capsules	Ritonavir and lopinavir/ritonavir oral solutions contain 43% alcohol, tipranavir, i.e., 100 mg ethanol per 250 mg capsule	Warn patients. Consider using lopinavir/ritonavir capsule preparation as an alternative
PROTEASE INHIBITORS	DUTASTERIDE	Possibly ↑ adverse effects of dutasteride with indinavir, lopinavir/ritonavir, or ritonavir	Inhibition of CYP3A4-mediated metabolism of dutasteride	Monitor closely; ↓ dosing frequency if side effects occur

(*Continued*)

Primary Drug	Secondary Drug	Effect	Mechanism	Precautions
ANTIVIRALS—ANTIRETROVIRALS				
RITONAVIR	GALANTAMINE	Possibly ↑ plasma levels and side effects of galantamine, e.g., nausea and vomiting	Possibly inhibition of metabolism via CYP3A4	Monitor more closely
SAQUINAVIR	GARLIC	↓ Plasma levels of saquinavir, risk of treatment failure	Uncertain	Avoid coadministration of garlic capsules
LOPINAVIR/RITONAVIR	GEMFIBROZIL	↓ Plasma levels gemfibrozil	Altered GI absorption	Be aware and monitor for poor response to treatment
SAQUINAVIR (INVIRASE HARD CAPSULES)	GRAPEFRUIT JUICE	Possibly ↑ efficacy	Possibly ↑ bioavailability; ↓ presystemic metabolism. Constituents of grapefruit irreversibly inhibit intestinal cytochrome CYP3A4. Transport via Pgp and MRP-2 efflux pumps is also inhibited	No dose adjustment is advised. Oral bioavailability is very low and is enhanced beneficially with grapefruit juice or grapefruit. Soft gel capsules have greater bioavailability, so they may interact to a lesser degree
ATAZANAVIR/RITONAVIR, SAQUINAVIR	H2 RECEPTOR BLOCKERS	1. ↓ Absorption of a atazanavir 2. Possible ↑ levels of cimetidine and saquinavir	1. ↑ Gastric pH 2. Uncertain mechanism of action on cimetidine	Take atazanavir at least 2 h before or 10 h after the H2 blocker, if doses of H2 blocker > or equivalent to famotidine 40 mg twice daily, consider increasing atazanavir/ritonavir from 300/100 mg to 400/100 mg, increase to this dose automatically if combined with tenofovir and do not increase H2 beyond equivalent of famotidine 40 mg twice daily. No dose adjustment required with lopinavir/ritonavir. In all cases, monitor viral load closely
PROTEASE INHIBITORS	IVABRADINE	↑ Levels of ivabradine with nelfinavir and ritonavir	Inhibition of metabolism via CYP3A4	Avoid coadministration

(*Continued*)

Primary Drug	Secondary Drug	Effect	Mechanism	Precautions
ANTIVIRALS—ANTIRETROVIRALS				
PROTEASE INHIBITORS	**LIPID-LOWERING DRUGS—STATINS**			
PROTEASE INHIBITORS	ATORVASTATIN	↑ Efficacy and ↑ risk of adverse effects of atorvastatin, e.g., myopathy, GI side effects, headache, raised LFTs	Inhibition of CYP3A4-mediated metabolism of atorvastatin	Coadministration with atazanavir/ritonavir, lopinavir/ritonavir, or tipranvir/ritonavir is not recommended. Use with caution. Monitor for atorvastatin toxicity, and monitor LFTs and CK. Inform patients to report muscle pain or weakness and ↓ dose if necessary or start with 10 mg once daily. Use the lowest dose possible to attain the target low-density lipoprotein ↓, if >40 mg/day needed, monitor closely. If combined with fosamprenavir/ritonavir, maximum daily dose is 20 mg for tipranavir/ritonavir 10 mg. Alternatives are pravastatin and fluvastatin
PROTEASE INHIBITORS	LOVASTATIN, SIMVASTATIN	↑ Risk of adverse effects, e.g., myopathy, rhabdomyolysis	Inhibition of CYP3A4-mediated metabolism of these statins	Avoid coadministration. Pravastatin or fluvastatin are suitable alternatives
PROTEASE INHIBITORS	PRAVASTATIN	1. ↑ Plasma levels, ↑ risk of adverse effects, e.g., myopathy (darunavir or lopinavir with ritonavir) 2. ↓ Plasma levels of pravastatin (nelfinavir, saquinavir)	Altered transport via OATP 1B1	Darunavir or lopinavir with ritonavir—start at a low dose and titrate to effect. Nelfinavir or saquinavir—consider dose increase of pravastatin and monitor lipid profile more closely. Inform patients to report muscle pain or weakness
PROTEASE INHIBITORS	ROSUVASTATIN	↑ Plasma levels, ↑ risk of adverse effects, e.g., myopathy	Altered transport, probably inhibition of transport proteins OATP and BCRP	No dose adjustment needed with fosamprenavir/ritonavir, for other combinations avoid coadministration if possible or initiate rosuvastatin at a reduced dose, e.g., 5 mg/day and monitor closely. Maximum suggested dose 10 mg/day with atazanavir or lopinavir

(*Continued*)

Primary Drug	Secondary Drug	Effect	Mechanism	Precautions
ANTIVIRALS—ANTIRETROVIRALS				
RITONAVIR	METOCLOPRAMIDE	Possibly ↑ plasma levels and side effects, e.g., dystonic reactions, oculogyric crisis	Inhibition of metabolism via CYP2D6	Use an alternative if possible, e.g., cyclizine. If not, monitor closely for side effects
PROTEASE INHIBITORS	ESTROGENS	↓ Estrogen plasma levels (ritonavir boosted protease inhibitors, nelfinavir and ritonavir), marked ↓ contraceptive effect, ↑ levels with atazanavir alone, ↑ risk of rash with tipranavir/ritonavir, risk of deranged LFTs (fosamprenavir)	Induction of metabolism of estrogens via CYP3A4 predominates, although metabolism via UGT is also induced. Atazanavir inhibits UGT	Monitor LFTs. Advise patients to use additional contraception for the period of intake and for 1 month after stopping coadministration with protease inhibitors. Barrier methods are necessary to prevent transmission of infection from patients with HIV. If an oral contraceptive is still indicated, at least 50 μg of ethinylestradiol should be given daily. If atazanavir is given alone or if atazanavir/ritonavir is given, 30 μg can be used
SAQUINAVIR, SAQUINAVIR/RITONAVIR	PENTAMIDINE ISETIONATE	Increased risk of ventricular arrhythmias	Uncertain	Avoid coadministration
PROTEASE INHIBITORS	PERIPHERAL VASODILATORS	Amprenavir, indinavir, lopinavir, nelfinavir, ritonavir, and saquinavir ↑ cilostazol levels	These protease inhibitors inhibit CYP3A4-mediated metabolism of cilostazol	Reduce dose of clistazol to 50 mg twice daily
PROTEASE INHIBITORS	PHOSPHODIESTERASE TYPE 5 INHIBITORS—SILDENAFIL, TADALAFIL, VARDENAFIL	↑ Sildenafil, tadalafil and vardenafil levels, ↑ risk of side effects, e.g., headache, GI effects, hypotension and visual changes (common), ventricular arrhythmias (rare) and priapism	Inhibition of CYP3A4- and possibly CYP2C9-mediated metabolism of sildenafil	Avoid coadadministration if the drug is prescribed for pulmonary hypertension. For erectile dysfunction, avoid combining indinavir or ritonavir (low and high dose) and vardenafil, or ritonavir (high dose) or saquinavir and sildenafil, tadalafil, or vardenafil. Use others with caution; monitor BP closely. Suggested starting doses (erectile dysfunction) with low-dose ritonavir: sildenafil 25 mg/48 h, vardenafil 2.5 mg/72 h, or tadalafil 10 mg/72 h

(Continued)

Primary Drug	Secondary Drug	Effect	Mechanism	Precautions
ANTIVIRALS—ANTIRETROVIRALS				
LOPINAVIR/RITONAVIR	PLATELET DISORDERS—ELTROMBOPAG	Possibly ↓ plasma levels of eltrombopag	Uncertain	Monitor more closely
PROTEASE INHIBITORS	PROGESTOGENS—NORETHISTERONE	↑ Adverse effects of norethisterone with amprenavir, atazanavir, and indinavir (all unboosted), small ↑ in bioavailability with tipranavir/ritonavir. Possibly ↓ efficacy and risk of combined oral contraceptive failure with nelfinavir, ritonavir, and other ritonavir boosted protease inhibitors	Probably altered metabolism via CYP450 and UGT	Advise patients to use additional contraception for the period of intake and for 1 month after stopping coadministration with these drugs. Barrier methods are necessary to prevent transmission of infection from patients with HIV. If barrier methods are not possible, a preparation with least 50 mcg of ethinyl estradiol should be used. Watch for early features of toxicity of amprenavir and atazanavir, and adjust the dose accordingly
RITONAVIR	PROGESTERONE RECEPTOR MODULATORS—ULIPRISTAL	Possible reduced contraceptive effect	Uncertain	Avoid coadministration
ATAZANAVIR, DARUNAVIR/RITONAVIR, LOPINAVIR/RITONAVIR, SAQUINAVIR	PROTON PUMP INHIBITORS	1. Possible altered plasma levels of proton pump inhibitors 2. ↓ Plasma levels of atazanavir 3. Possible ↑ levels of saquinavir	1. Complex interactions involving CYP3A4 inhibition and 2C19 induction 2. ↓ Absorption due to due to ↑ gastric pH 3. Uncertain cause	Avoid coadministration. If not possible increase atazanavir/ritonavir to 400/100 mg, do not exceed an equivalent dose of omeprazole 20 mg and monitor closely
INDINAVIR	OMEPRAZOLE	Possibly ↓ efficacy of indinavir	↓ Plasma concentration; uncertain cause	↑ Dose of indinavir from 800 mg three times a day to 1 g three times a day, or preferably add ritonavir 200 mg once daily
SAQUINAVIR/RITONAVIR	OMEPRAZOLE	↑ Levels of saquinavir, risk, e.g., QT prolongation	Uncertain	Avoid coadministration
TIPRANAVIR/RITONAVIR	OMEPRAZOLE/ESOMEPRAZOLE	↓ Plasma levels of proton pump inhibitor	Increased metabolism via CYP 2C19	Avoid coadministration, if not possible consider alternatives or an increased dose of omeprazole may be required

(*Continued*)

Primary Drug	Secondary Drug	Effect	Mechanism	Precautions
ANTIVIRALS—ANTIRETROVIRALS				
ATAZANAVIR/RITONAVIR, LOPINAVIR/RITONAVIR, RITONAVIR, TIPRANAVIR, SAQUINAVIR/RITONAVIR	SALMETEROL	Possibly ↑ plasma levels of salmeterol and ↑ cardiovascular side effects, e.g., QT prolongation, tachycardia	Inhibition of metabolism via CYP3A4	Avoid coadministration in patients with extended QTc interval
PROTEASE INHIBITORS	SYMPATHOMIMETICS	1. Risk of serotonin syndrome when dexamfetamine is administered with ritonavir 2. Indinavir may ↑ phenylpropanolamine levels	1. Protease inhibitors inhibit CYP2D6-mediated metabolism 2. Likely inhibition of phenyl-propanolamine metabolism	1. Avoid coadministration 2. Monitor BP closely; watch for marked ↑ BP
PROTEASE INHIBITORS	THYROID HORMONES	Altered efficacy of levothyroxine by lopinavir/ritonavir or ritonavir and possibly indinavir and nelfinavir	Uncertain; possibly altered metabolism via induction of glucuronosyl transferases	Monitor thyroid function closely, adjust levothyroxine doses as needed
PROTEASE INHIBITORS	**RHEUMATIC DISEASE AND GOUT**			
ATAZANAVIR, DARUNAVIR/RITONAVIR, INDINAVIR, LOPINAVIR/RITONAVIR, RITONAVIR, SAQUINAVIR/RITONAVIR	COLCHICINE	↑ Plasma levels and risk of colchicine toxicity, e.g., neuromuscular events, rhabdomyolysis	Probably inhibition of excretion via Pgp and inhibition of CY3A4	Monitor closely and reduce colchicine dose or omit if combination not tolerated. Combination with lopinavir/ritonavir or tipranvir/ritonavir not recommended
TIPRANAVIR/RITONAVIR	VITAMIN E	Increased risk of bleeding	Uncertain	Avoid coadministration with vitamin E supplements. Monitor for bleeding, advise patients to report any increased bruising or bleeding, review other medication that may increase bleeding risk

(*Continued*)

Primary Drug	Secondary Drug	Effect	Mechanism	Precautions
ANTIVIRALS—ANTIRETROVIRALS				
OTHER				
AMANTADINE is used to treat Parkinson's disease as well as having antiviral activity. It has been included in the Anti-Parkinson's drugs section				
ACICLOVIR, VALACICLOVIR				
ACICLOVIR/VALACICLOVIR	ANTICANCER AND IMMUNOMODULATING DRUGS—1. CICLOSPORIN 2. MYCOPHENOLATE 3. TACROLIMUS	1. ↑ Nephrotoxicity 2. Possible ↑ efficacy 3. ↑ Levels with protease inhibitors	1. Additive side effect 2. Competition for renal excretion 3. Inhibition of CYP3A4-mediated metabolism of tacrolimus	1. Monitor renal function prior to concomitant therapy and monitor ciclosporin levels 2. Monitor renal function particularly if on >4 g valaciclovir; ↓ dose of aciclovir if there is a background of renal failure 3. Monitor clinical effects closely; check levels
ACICLOVIR/VALACICLOVIR	ANTIDEPRESSANTS—LITHIUM	↑ Lithium levels, with risk of toxicity	Possible ↓ renal excretion	Ensure adequate hydration; monitor lithium levels if intravenous aciclovir or >4 g/day valaciclovir is required
ACICLOVIR/VALACICLOVIR	ANTIEPILEPTICS—PHENYTOIN, VALPROATE	↓ Efficacy of phenytoin	Unclear	Warn patients and monitor seizure frequency
ACICLOVIR/VALACICLOVIR	ANTIGOUT DRUGS—PROBENECID	↑ Levels of aciclovir, valaciclovir, and ganciclovir	Competitive inhibition of renal excretion	Care with coadministering probenecid with high-dose antivirals
ACICLOVIR/VALACICLOVIR	BRONCHODILATORS—THEOPHYLLINES	↑ Theophylline levels	Uncertain	Monitor for signs of toxicity and check levels
ACICLOVIR/VALACICLOVIR	H2 RECEPTOR BLOCKERS—CIMETIDINE	↑ Efficacy and adverse effects of antivirals	Competition for renal excretion	Use doses >4 g/day valaciclovir with caution or consider alternative acid suppression. For doses <1 g/day, interaction is not thought to be clinically significant. Studies available only for valaciclovir
GANCICLOVIR/VALGANCICLOVIR	ANTIBIOTICS—1. IMIPENEM WITH CILASTATIN 2. TRIMETHOPRIM	1. ↑ Adverse effects (e.g., seizures) 2. Possibly ↑ adverse effects (e.g., myelosuppression) when trimethoprim is coadministered with ganciclovir or valganciclovir	1. Additive side effects; these drugs can cause seizure activity 2. Small ↑ bioavailability; possible additive toxicity	1. Avoid combination if possible; use only if benefit outweighs risk 2. Well tolerated in one study. For patients at risk of additive toxicities, use only if benefits outweigh risks and monitor FBC closely

(*Continued*)

Primary Drug	Secondary Drug	Effect	Mechanism	Precautions
ANTIVIRALS—ANTIRETROVIRALS				
GANCICLOVIR/ VALGANCICLOVIR	ANTICANCER AND IMMUNOMODULATING DRUGS—1. CICLOSPORIN 2. MYCOPHENOLATE 3. TACROLIMUS	1. ↑ Risk of nephrotoxicity 2. Possible ↑ efficacy 3. Possible ↑ nephrotoxicity/ neurotoxicity	1. Additive nephrotoxic effects 2. Competition for renal excretion 3. Additive side effects	1. Monitor renal function 2. Monitor renal function particularly if on >4 g valaciclovir; ↓ dose of aciclovir if there is a background of renal failure 3. Monitor more closely; check tacrolimus levels
GANCICLOVIR/ VALGANCICLOVIR	ANTIGOUT DRUGS—PROBENECID	↑ Levels of ganciclovir/ valganciclovir	Competitive inhibition of renal excretion	Care with coadministering probenecid with high-dose antivirals
GANCICLOVIR/ VALGANCICLOVIR	ANTIVIRALS—NUCLEOSIDE REVERSE TRANSCRIPTASE INHIBITORS	1. ↑ Adverse effects with tenofovir, zidovudine, and possibly didanosine, lamivudine, and zalcitabine 2. Possibly ↓ efficacy of ganciclovir	1. Uncertain; possibly additive toxicity. Lamivudine may compete for active tubular secretion in the kidneys 2. Uncertain; ↓ bioavailability	1. Avoid if possible, otherwise monitor FBC and renal function weekly. It has been suggested that the dose of zidovudine should be halved from 600 to 300 mg daily. Monitor for peripheral neuropathy, particularly with zalcitabine 2. Uncertain clinical significance; if in doubt, consider alternative cytomegalovirus prophylaxis
ADEFOVIR DIPIVOXIL				
ADEFOVIR DIPIVOXIL	1. ANTIBIOTICS—AMINOGLYCOSIDES, VANCOMYCIN 2. ANTICANCER AND IMMUNOMODULATING DRUGS—CICLOSPORIN, TACROLIMUS 3. ANTIFUNGALS—AMPHOTERICIN 4. ANTIPROTOZOALS—PENTAMIDINE 5. ANTIVIRALS—CIDOFOVIR, FOSCARNET SODIUM, TENOFOVIR	Possible ↑ efficacy and side effects	Competition for renal excretion	Monitor renal function weekly

(Continued)

Primary Drug	Secondary Drug	Effect	Mechanism	Precautions
ANTIVIRALS—ANTIRETROVIRALS				
CIDOFOVIR				
CIDOFOVIR	ANTIDIABETIC DRUGS—METFORMIN	↑ Risk of lactic acidosis	↓ Renal excretion of metformin	Watch for lactic acidosis. The onset of lactic acidosis is often subtle, with symptoms of malaise, myalgia, respiratory distress, and ↑ nonspecific abdominal distress. There may be hypothermia and resistant bradyarrhythmias
CIDOFOVIR	**ANTIVIRALS**			
CIDOFOVIR	ADEFOVIR DIPIVOXIL	Possible ↑ efficacy and side effects	Competition for renal excretion	Monitor renal function weekly
CIDOFOVIR	TENOFOVIR	↑ Adverse effects	↑ Plasma levels; competition for renal excretion via organic anion transporter	Monitor renal function weekly
FOSCARNET SODIUM				
FOSCARNET SODIUM	**ANTIBIOTICS**			
FOSCARNET SODIUM	AMINOGLYCOSIDES	Possible ↑ nephrotoxicity	Additive side effect	Monitor renal function closely
FOSCARNET SODIUM	QUINOLONES	Risk of seizures	Unknown; possibly additive side effect	Avoid combination in patients with past medical history of epilepsy. Consider an alternative antibiotic
FOSCARNET SODIUM	ANTICANCER AND IMMUNOMODULATING DRUGS—CICLOSPORIN	↑ Risk of renal failure	Additive nephrotoxic effects	Monitor renal function
FOSCARNET SODIUM	ANTIFUNGALS—AMPHOTERICIN	Possible ↑ nephrotoxicity	Additive side effect	Monitor renal function closely
FOSCARNET SODIUM	ANTIPROTOZOALS—PENTAMIDINE (INTRAVENOUS)	Risk of hypocalcemia	Unclear; possibly additive hypocalcemic effects	Use extreme caution with intravenous pentamidine; monitor serum calcium (correct before the start of treatment), renal function, and for signs of tetany closely. Stop one drug if necessary
FOSCARNET SODIUM	ADEFOVIR DIPIVOXIL	Possible ↑ efficacy and side effects	Competition for renal excretion	Monitor renal function weekly

(*Continued*)

Primary Drug	Secondary Drug	Effect	Mechanism	Precautions
ANTIVIRALS—ANTIRETROVIRALS				
FOSCARNET SODIUM	NUCLEOSIDE REVERSE TRANSCRIPTASE INHIBITORS—LAMIVUDINE, TENOFOVIR, ZALCITABINE	↑ Adverse effects with tenofovir and possibly lamivudine and zalcitabine	Uncertain; possibly additive toxicity via competition for renal excretion	Avoid if possible; otherwise, monitor FBC and renal function weekly
FOSCARNET SODIUM	PROTEASE INHIBITORS	↓ Renal function when coadministered with ritonavir or saquinavir	Uncertain; possibly ↓ renal excretion of foscarnet	Monitor renal function closely
OSELTAMIVIR	METHOTREXATE	Possible ↑ efficacy/toxicity	Competition for renal excretion	Monitor more closely for signs of immunosuppression. Predicted interaction
RIBAVIRIN				
RIBAVIRIN	ANTIVIRALS—NUCLEOSIDE REVERSE TRANSCRIPTASE INHIBITORS	1. ↑ Side effects; risk of lactic acidosis, peripheral neuropathy, pancreatitis, hepatic decompensation, mitochondrial toxicity, and anemia with didanosine and stavudine 2. ↓ Efficacy of lamivudine	1. Additive side effects; ↑ intracellular activation of didanosine and stavudine 2. ↓ Intracellular activation of lamivudine	1. Not recommended; use with extreme caution. Monitor lactate, LFTs, and amylase closely. Stop coadministration if peripheral neuropathy occurs. Stavudine and didanosine carry a higher risk 2. Monitor HIV RNA levels; if they ↑, review treatment combination
TELBIVUDINE	INTERFERON	Peripheral neuropathy	Unclear	Use with caution

PART 11

Drugs Acting on the Gastrointestinal Tract

Ursula Collignon

1. ANTACIDS
2. ANTIDIARRHEALS
    - CODEINE, DIPHENOXYLATE, MORPHINE—*see Analgesics, Opioids*
    - KAOLIN
    - LOPERAMIDE
3. ANTIEMETICS—*see Drugs Acting on the Nervous System, Antiemetics*
4. ANTIMUSCARINICS—*see Drugs Acting on the Nervous System, Anti-Parkinson's Drugs*
5. DRUGS AFFECTING BILE
    - URSODEOXYCHOLIC ACID
    - CHOLESTYRAMINE—*see Cardiovascular Drugs, Lipid-Lowering Drugs*
6. DRUGS USED TO TREAT INFLAMMATORY BOWEL DISEASE
    - AMINOSALICYLATES—*see Anticancer and Immunomodulating Drugs, Other Immunomodulating Drugs*
    - CORTICOSTEROIDS—*see Anticancer and Immunomodulating Drugs, Other Immunomodulating Drugs*
    - INFLIXIMAB—*see Anticancer and Immunomodulating Drugs, Other Immunomodulating Drugs*
7. H2 RECEPTOR BLOCKERS
8. LAXATIVES
9. PANCREATIN
10. PROTON PUMP INHIBITORS
11. SUCRALFATE
12. TRIPOTASSIUM DICITRATOBISMUTHATE

Primary Drug	Secondary Drug	Effect	Mechanism	Precautions
ANTACIDS				
ANTACIDS	ANALGESICS—NSAIDs	1. Magnesium hydroxide ↑ absorption of ibuprofen, flurbiprofen, mefenamic acid, and tolfenamic acid 2. Aluminum-containing antacids ↓ absorption of these NSAIDs	1. Acidic NSAIDs become more soluble in a more alkaline environment 2. Mechanism uncertain	These effects are ↓ by taking these drugs with food
ANTACIDS	ANTIBIOTICS—AZITHROMYCIN, CEFPODOXIME, CEFUROXIME, ISONIAZID, NITROFURANTOIN, QUINOLONES, RIFAMYCINS, TETRACYCLINES	↓ Levels of these antibiotics	↓ Absorption	Take azithromycin at least 1 h before or 2 h after an antacid. Take these cephalosporins at least 2 h after an antacid. Separate quinolones and antacids by 2–6 h. Separate nitrofurantoin, rifamycins, or tetracyclines and antacids by 2–3 h
ANTACIDS	**ANTICANCER AND IMMUNOMODULATING DRUGS**			
ANTACIDS (LARGE DOSES)	CORTICOSTEROIDS	Prednisone, prednisolone, and dexamethasone absorption ↓	Possibly due to adsorption on to surface of antacid	Consider separating administration
ANTACIDS	LAPATINIB	↓ Lapatinib levels	Solubility reduced at higher pH	Avoid concurrent use
ANTACIDS	MYCOPHENOLATE	↓ Plasma concentrations of mycophenolate (may be 30%)	↓ Absorption	Do not coadminister simultaneously—separate by at least ↓ hours
ANTACIDS	NILOTINIB	↓ Nilotinib levels	Solubility reduced at higher pH	If necessary, antacids can be given separate to nilotinib
ANTACIDS	PENICILLAMINE	↓ Penicillamine levels	↓ Absorption of penicillamine	Avoid coadministration
ANTACIDS	ANTIEPILEPTICS—GABAPENTIN, PHENYTOIN	↓ Levels of these antiepileptics	↓ Absorption	Separate by at least 3 h

(*Continued*)

DRUGS ACTING ON THE GASTROINTESTINAL TRACT ANTACIDS

DRUGS ACTING ON THE GASTROINTESTINAL TRACT ANTACIDS

Primary Drug	Secondary Drug	Effect	Mechanism	Precautions
ANTACIDS				
ANTACIDS	ANTIFUNGALS—AZOLES	↓ Plasma concentration of itraconazole and ketoconazole, with risk of therapeutic failure	Itraconazole absorption in capsule form requires an acidic gastric environment, and thus absorption would be ↓	Separate administration of agents that ↓ gastric acidity by 1–2 h. However, absorption of itraconazole liquid solution does not require an acidic environment; it could be used instead and does not need to be given with food. Fluconazole absorption is not pH dependent, so this is a suitable alternative
ANTACIDS	ANTIHISTAMINES—FEXOFENADINE	↓ Fexofenadine levels	↓ Absorption	Be aware
ANTACIDS	ANTIHYPERTENSIVES AND HEART FAILURE DRUGS—ACE INHIBITORS	↓ Effect, particularly of captopril, fosinopril, and enalapril	↓ Absorption due to ↑ gastric pH	Watch for poor response to ACE inhibitors
ANTACIDS	ANTIMALARIALS—PROGUANIL, CHLOROQUINE	↓ Chloroquine and proguanil levels	↓ Absorption	Separate doses by at least ↓ hours
ANTACIDS	**ANTIPLATELET AGENTS**			
ANTACIDS	ASPIRIN	Antacids may ↓ high-dose aspirin to subtherapeutic levels	Alkalinizing the urine increases aspirin loss in the urine	Monitor salicylate levels when high-dose aspirin therapy is used
ANTACIDS	DIPYRIDAMOLE	Possible ↓ bioavailability of dipyridamole	Dipyridamole tablets require an acidic environment for adequate dissolution; ↑ pH of the stomach impairs dissolution and therefore may ↓ absorption of drug	↑ Dose of dipyridamole or consider using an alternative antiplatelet drug
ANTACIDS	ANTIPSYCHOTICS—PHENOTHIAZINES, SULPIRIDE	↓ Levels of these antipsychotics	↓ Absorption	Separate doses by 2 h (in the case of sulpiride, give sulpiride 2 h after but not before the antacid)
ANTACIDS	**ANTIVIRALS**			
ANTACIDS—ALUMINUM OR MAGNESIUM CONTAINING	DOLUTEGRAVIR	↓ Plasma levels of dolutegravir, risk of treatment failure and resistance	Chelation of dolutegravir with magnesium or aluminum ions	Separate doses, take antacids at least 6 h before or 2 h after dolutegravir

(*Continued*)

Primary Drug	Secondary Drug	Effect	Mechanism	Precautions
ANTACIDS				
ANTACIDS—ALUMINUM OR MAGNESIUM CONTAINING	ELVITEGRAVIR (RITONAVIR BOOSTED)	↓ Plasma levels of elvitegravir, risk of treatment failure and resistance	Reduced absorption due to chelation of elvitegravir	Separate doses by at least 4 h
ANTACIDS—ALUMINUM OR MAGNESIUM CONTAINING	RALTEGRAVIR	↓ Plasma concentration of raltegravir, risk of treatment failure	Reduced absorption due to chelation of raltegravir	Avoid coadministration. Calcium-containing antacids can be used as an alternative, but separate doses by at least 2 h
ANTACIDS CONTAINING MAGNESIUM AND ALUMINUM	BETA-BLOCKERS	↑ Bioavailability of metoprolol and atenolol, which may produce a mild variation in response to both drugs	Variations in absorption of the respective beta-blockers	Clinical significance may be minimal but be aware. Monitor BP at least weekly until stable when initiating antacid therapy. Warn patients to report symptoms of hypotension (light-headedness, dizziness on standing, etc.)
ANTACIDS	BISPHOSPHONATES	↓ Bisphosphonate levels	↓ Absorption	Separate doses by at least 30 min
ANTACIDS CONTAINING ALUMINUM	DEFERASIROX	↓ Levels of deferasirox	↓ Absorption	Avoid coadministration (manufacturers' recommendation)
ANTACIDS	H2-RECEPTOR BLOCKERS	↓ Plasma concentrations and reduced therapeutic effect of H2 blocker	↓ Absorption	Avoid coadministration or take H2 blocker 1–2 h before antacid
ANTACIDS CONTAINING MAGNESIUM	IRON	↓ Iron levels when iron given orally	↓ Absorption	Separate doses as much as possible—monitor FBC closely
ANTACIDS	**LIPID-LOWERING DRUGS**			
ANTACIDS	FIBRATES	Gemfibrozil levels may be ↓ by antacids	Uncertain	Give gemfibrozil 1–2 h before the antacid
ANTACIDS	STATINS	↓ Rosuvastatin levels	Likely reduced absorption. Unclear why other statins not similarly affected	Separate doses by at least 2 h
ANTACIDS	PROTON PUMP INHIBITORS—LANSOPRAZOLE	Possible ↓ efficacy of lansoprazole	↓ Absorption	Separate doses by at least 1 h
ANTACIDS—MAGNESIUM CONTAINING	SODIUM POLYSTYRENE SULFONATE	Cases of metabolic alkalosis	Uncertain; possibly absorption of bicarbonate due to its abnormal neutralization in the stomach	Consider an alternative antacid or administer sodium polystyrene sulfonate as an enema. If both need to be coadministered orally, monitor U&Es and blood gases closely

(Continued)

Primary Drug	Secondary Drug	Effect	Mechanism	Precautions
ANTACIDS				
ANTACIDS—CALCIUM AND MAGNESIUM CONTAINING	TRIENTINE	Possibly ↓ trientine levels	↓ Absorption	Separate doses as much as possible; take antacids after trientine
ANTACIDS CONTAINING ALUMINUM	VITAMIN C	↑ Aluminum levels, with risk of encephalopathy in patients with renal failure	Uncertain; possibly ↑ absorption due to ascorbic acid in the presence of ↓ renal excretion	Avoid coingestion in patients with renal failure

Primary Drug	Secondary Drug	Effect	Mechanism	Precautions
ANTIDIARRHEALS				
CODEINE, DIPHENOXYLATE, MORPHINE—*see Analgesics, Opioids*				
KAOLIN				
KAOLIN	ANTIBIOTICS—TETRACYCLINES	↓ Tetracycline levels	↓ Absorption	Separate doses by at least 2 h
KAOLIN	ANTIMALARIALS—CHLOROQUINE	↓ Chloroquine levels	↓ Absorption	Separate doses by at least ↓ hours
KAOLIN	BETA-BLOCKERS	Possibly ↓ levels of atenolol, propranolol, and sotalol	↓ Absorption	Separate doses by at least 2 h
KAOLIN	CARDIAC GLYCOSIDES—DIGOXIN	Possibly ↓ levels of digoxin	↓ Absorption	Separate doses by at least 2 h
LOPERAMIDE				
LOPERAMIDE	ANTIBIOTICS—CO-TRIMOXAZOLE	↑ Loperamide levels but no evidence of toxicity	Inhibition of metabolism	Be aware
LOPERAMIDE	ANTIVIRALS—PROTEASE INHIBITORS	↑ Risk of adverse effects when loperamide is coingested with ritonavir	Ritonavir inhibits Pgp and CYP3A4	Monitor for clinical effect; consider ↓ dose if necessary. Stop if there are signs of abdominal distension in patients with HIV as toxic megacolon has been reported
LOPERAMIDE	DESMOPRESSIN	↑ Desmopressin levels when given orally	Delayed intestinal transit time ↑ absorption of desmopressin	Watch for early features of desmopressin toxicity (e.g., abdominal pain, headaches)

Primary Drug	Secondary Drug	Effect	Mechanism	Precautions
ANTIEMETICS—see *Drugs Acting on the Nervous System, Antiemetics*				

Primary Drug	Secondary Drug	Effect	Mechanism	Precautions
ANTIMUSCARINICS—see *Drugs Acting on the Nervous System, Anti-Parkinson's Drugs*				

Primary Drug	Secondary Drug	Effect	Mechanism	Precautions
DRUGS AFFECTING BILE				
URSODEOXYCHOLIC ACID				
URSODEOXYCHOLIC ACID	ANTICANCER AND IMMUNOMODULATING DRUGS—CICLOSPORIN	↑ Ciclosporin levels	↑ Absorption	Watch for early features of ciclosporin toxicity; monitor FBC closely
URSODEOXYCHOLIC ACID	LIPID-LOWERING DRUGS—ANION EXCHANGE RESINS	Risk of ↓ absorption of ursodeoxycholic acid	Colestipol and cholestyramine bind with ursodeoxycholic acid in the intestine	Take ursodeoxycholic acid 1 h before or 4–6 h after an anion exchange resin
CHOLESTYRAMINE—see *Cardiovascular Drugs, Lipid-Lowering Drugs*				

Primary Drug	Secondary Drug	Effect	Mechanism	Precautions
DRUGS USED TO TREAT INFLAMMATORY BOWEL DISEASE				
AMINOSALICYLATES—see *Anticancer and Immunomodulating Drugs, Other Immunomodulating Drugs*				
CORTICOSTEROIDS—see *Anticancer and Immunomodulating Drugs, Other Immunomodulating Drugs*				
INFLIXIMAB—see *Anticancer and Immunomodulating Drugs, Other Immunomodulating Drugs*				

Primary Drug	Secondary Drug	Effect	Mechanism	Precautions
H2 RECEPTOR BLOCKERS				
CIMETIDINE, RANITIDINE	ANESTHETICS, LOCAL—LIDOCAINE	↑ Efficacy and adverse effects of lidocaine and bupivacaine, e.g., lightheadedness, paresthesia	Not fully established but likely to be reduced clearance and altered metabolism via CYP enzymes	Uncertain. Consider alternative acid-suppression therapy, or monitor more closely; ↓ dose may be required. No toxicity reported to date with bupivacaine

(Continued)

DRUGS ACTING ON THE GASTROINTESTINAL TRACT H2 RECEPTOR BLOCKERS

Primary Drug	Secondary Drug	Effect	Mechanism	Precautions
H2 RECEPTOR BLOCKERS				
CIMETIDINE	ANESTHETICS, IV—LIDOCAINE	↑ Efficacy and adverse effects.	Not fully established but likely to be reduced clearance and altered metabolism via CYP enzymes	Avoid coadministration, or if essential, monitor closely for symptoms of toxicity, and check lidocaine levels
H2-RECEPTOR BLOCKERS	**ANALGESICS—OPIOIDS**			
CIMETIDINE	ALFENTANIL, FENTANYL, MORPHINE, PETHIDINE, TRAMADOL	↑ Levels and risk of adverse effects including respiratory depression	Inhibition of CYP3A4-mediated metabolism and reduced pethidine clearance	Watch for excessive narcotization; monitor pain, sedation scores, and respiratory rate closely
CIMETIDINE	CODEINE	Cimetidine may ↓ efficacy of codeine	Due to inhibition of enzymatic conversion to active metabolite via CYP2D6	Watch for poor response to codeine. Consider using an alternative opioid or acid-suppression therapy; famotidine, nizatidine, and proton pump inhibitors are not likely to interact significantly
H2-RECEPTOR BLOCKERS	ANTACIDS	↓ Plasma concentrations and reduced therapeutic effect of H2 blocker	↓ Absorption	Avoid coadministration, or take H2 blocker 1–2 h before antacid
H2-RECEPTOR BLOCKERS	**ANTIARRHYTHMICS**			
CIMETIDINE, RANITIDINE	AMIODARONE, FLECAINIDE, MEXILETINE, PROCAINAMIDE, PROPAFENONE	Likely ↑ plasma concentrations of these antiarrhythmics and risk of adverse effects	Cimetidine inhibits CYP2D6-mediated metabolism of flecainide, mexiletine, procainamide, and propafenone. Ranitidine is a much weaker CYP2D6 inhibitor. Cimetidine is a potent inhibitor of organic cation transport in the kidney, impairing renal elimination of procainamide	Monitor PR and BP at least weekly until stable. Warn patients to report symptoms of hypotension (light-headedness, dizziness on standing, etc.). Consider alternative acid-suppression therapy

(*Continued*)

Primary Drug	Secondary Drug	Effect	Mechanism	Precautions
H2 RECEPTOR BLOCKERS				
H2-RECEPTOR BLOCKERS—CIMETIDINE	DOFETILIDE	↑ Dofetilide levels with risk of ↑ QT prolongation	Cimetidine inhibits CYP3A4-mediated metabolism; it also inhibits renal excretion of dofetilide	Avoid coadministration
H2-RECEPTOR BLOCKERS—CIMETIDINE	QUINIDINE	↑ Quinidine levels	Cimetidine inhibits CYP3A4-mediated metabolism. It also reduces renal excretion	Reduce quinidine dose; monitor PR, BP, and ECG closely
H2-RECEPTOR BLOCKERS	**ANTIBIOTICS**			
H2-RECEPTOR BLOCKERS	CEPHALOSPORINS, TETRACYCLINES—DOXYCYCLINE	↓ Plasma concentrations and risk of treatment failure	↓ Absorption of cephalosporin as gastric pH ↑	Avoid concomitant use. Consider an alternative antibiotic. If unable to avoid combination, take H2 antagonists at least 2 h after cephalosporin; giving cephalosporin with an acidic drink, e.g., a carbonated drink, will increase absorption; ↑ dose may be required
CIMETIDINE	CHLORAMPHENICOL	↑ Adverse effects of chloramphenicol, e.g., bone marrow depression	Additive toxicity	Use with caution; monitor FBC regularly
CIMETIDINE	MACROLIDES—ERYTHROMYCIN	↑ Efficacy and adverse effects of erythromycin, including hearing loss	↑ Bioavailability	Consider an alternative antibiotic, e.g., clarithromycin. Deafness has been reversible with cessation of erythromycin
CIMETIDINE	METRONIDAZOLE	↑ Metronidazole levels	Inhibited metabolism	Watch for ↑ side effects of metronidazole
FAMOTIDINE	NORFLOXACIN	↓ Plasma concentrations and risk of treatment failure	Uncertain	Monitor for poor response to antibiotics
CIMETIDINE	RIFAMPICIN	↓ Efficacy of cimetidine	↑ Metabolism	Change to alternative acid-suppression therapy, e.g., rabeprazole, or ↑ dose and/or frequency
H2-RECEPTOR BLOCKERS	**ANTICANCER AND IMMUNOMODULATING DRUGS**			
H2-RECEPTOR BLOCKERS—CIMETIDINE	BENDAMUSTINE	Theoretical risk of ↑ bendamustine levels	CYP1A2 inhibition	Monitor closely

(Continued)

DRUGS ACTING ON THE GASTROINTESTINAL TRACT H2 RECEPTOR BLOCKERS

Primary Drug	Secondary Drug	Effect	Mechanism	Precautions
H2 RECEPTOR BLOCKERS				
CIMETIDINE	BUSULFAN, CARMUSTINE, CHLORAMBUCIL, CYCLOPHOSPHAMIDE, ESTRAMUSTINE, IFOSFAMIDE, LOMUSTINE, THIOTEPA, TREOSULFAN	↑ Adverse effects of cytotoxicity, e.g., myelosuppression	Additive toxicity. Possible minor inhibition of cyclophosphamide metabolism via CYP2C9	Monitor more closely; monitor FBC regularly. Avoid coadministration of cimetidine with cyclophosphamide
CIMETIDINE	CICLOSPORIN	↑ Plasma concentrations of ciclosporin, with risk of nephrotoxicity, myelosuppression, neurotoxicity, and excessive immunosuppression, with risk of infection and posttransplant lymphoproliferative disease	Inhibition of CYP3A4-mediated metabolism of ciclosporin; inhibitors vary in potency; cimetidine is classified as a moderate inhibitor	Avoid coadministration with cimetidine. Consider an alternative H2 blocker but need to monitor plasma ciclosporin and renal function levels to prevent toxicity
CIMETIDINE	CORTICOSTEROIDS	↑ Adrenal suppressive effects of corticosteroids, which may ↑ risk of infections and produce an inadequate response to stress scenarios	Due to inhibition of metabolism of corticosteroids	Monitor cortisol levels, and warn patients to report symptoms such as fever and sore throat
H2-RECEPTOR BLOCKERS	DABRAFENIB	Theoretical risk of ↓ dabrafenib levels	Dabrafenib solubility reduced at higher pH	Avoid concurrent use if possible
FAMOTIDINE	DASATINIB	Possible ↓ dasatinib levels	Famotidine ↑ metabolism of dasatinib	Consider using alternative acid-suppression therapy
CIMETIDINE	DOXORUBICIN	↑ Risk of myelosuppression due to ↑ plasma concentrations	Due to ↓ metabolism of doxorubicin by CYP3A4 isoenzymes due to inhibition of those enzymes	Monitor for ↑ myelosuppression, peripheral neuropathy, myalgias, and fatigue
CIMETIDINE	EPIRUBICIN	↑ Epirubicin levels, with risk of toxicity	Attributed to inhibition of hepatic metabolism of epirubicin by cimetidine	Avoid concurrent treatment, and consider using an alternative H2-receptor blocker, e.g., ranitidine, famotidine
H2-RECEPTOR BLOCKERS	ERLOTINIB	↓ Erlotinib levels	Solubility reduced at higher pH	Avoid concurrent use of H2 antagonists

(Continued)

Primary Drug	Secondary Drug	Effect	Mechanism	Precautions
H2 RECEPTOR BLOCKERS				
CIMETIDINE	EVEROLIMUS	↑ Adverse effects, e.g., thrombocytopenia, hepatotoxicity	Inhibition of metabolism via CYP3A4 and competition with tacrolimus for renal tubular secretion	Consider alternative acid-suppression therapy, e.g., alginate suspension, famotidine, nizatidine, or rabeprazole. Not thought to be clinically significant. Ensure close monitoring of immunosuppressant levels and renal function
CIMETIDINE	FAMPRIDINE	↑ Plasma concentrations	Inhibition of active renal tubular secretion via organic ion transporters	Avoid coadministration
CIMETIDINE	FLUOROURACIL	↑ Fluorouracil levels and altered efficacy of fluorouracil	Inhibition of metabolism and altered action	Monitor more closely. May be of clinical benefit. No additional toxicity was noted in one study
RANITIDINE	GEFITINIB	↓ Gefitinib levels	Solubility reduced at higher pH	Avoid concurrent use of H2 antagonists and simultaneous use of antacids
H2-RECEPTOR BLOCKERS	HISTAMINE	Effects of histamine antagonized	Histamine blockade	Avoid concurrent use
CIMETIDINE	IFOSFAMIDE	↓ Plasma concentrations of 4-hydroxyifosfamide, the active metabolite of ifosfamide, and risk of inadequate therapeutic response	Due to inhibition of the isoenzymatic conversion to active metabolites	Monitor clinically the efficacy of ifosfamide, and ↑ dose accordingly
CIMETIDINE	IMATINIB	↑ Imatinib levels with ↑ risk of toxicity (e.g., abdominal pain, constipation, dyspnea) and of neurotoxicity (e.g., taste disturbances, dizziness, headache, paresthesia, peripheral neuropathy)	Due to inhibition of CYP3A4-mediated metabolism of imatinib	Monitor for clinical efficacy and for the signs of toxicity listed, along with convulsions, confusion, and signs of edema (including pulmonary edema). Monitor electrolytes, liver function, and cardiotoxicity
CIMETIDINE	IRINOTECAN	↑ Plasma concentrations of SN-38 (active metabolite of irinotecan) and ↑ toxicity of irinotecan, e.g., diarrhea, acute cholinergic syndrome, interstitial pulmonary disease	Due to inhibition of the metabolism of irinotecan by CYP3A4 isoenzymes by cimetidine	Peripheral blood counts should be checked before each course of treatment. Monitor lung function. Recommendation is to ↓ dose of irinotecan by 25%

(*Continued*)

DRUGS ACTING ON THE GASTROINTESTINAL TRACT H2 RECEPTOR BLOCKERS

Primary Drug	Secondary Drug	Effect	Mechanism	Precautions
H2 RECEPTOR BLOCKERS				
H2-RECEPTOR BLOCKERS	LAPATINIB	↓ Lapatinib levels	Solubility reduced at higher pH	Avoid concurrent use
CIMETIDINE	MELPHALAN	↓ Plasma concentrations and bioavailability of melphalan by 30% and risk of poor therapeutic response to melphalan	Cimetidine causes a change in gastric pH, which ↓ absorption of melphalan	Avoid concurrent use
H2-RECEPTOR BLOCKERS	NILOTINIB	Possible ↓ absorption of nilotinib	Nilotinib has reduced solubility at higher pH	If combined, give nilotinib 2 h before or 10 h after H2 blocker
H2-RECEPTOR BLOCKERS	PAZOPANIB	Possible ↓ plasma concentrations	Possible ↓ absorption	If combined, give pazopanib 2 h before or 10 h after H2 blocker
CIMETIDINE	RUXOLITINIB	↑ Levels of ruxolitinib	CYP3A4 inhibition	Monitor closely
CIMETIDINE	SIROLIMUS, TACROLIMUS, TEMSIROLIMUS	↑ Adverse effects, e.g., thrombocytopenia, hepatotoxicity	Inhibition of metabolism via CYP3A4 and competition with tacrolimus for renal tubular secretion	Consider alternative acid-suppression therapy, e.g., alginate suspension, famotidine, nizatidine, or rabeprazole. Not thought to be clinically significant. Ensure close monitoring of immunosuppressant levels and renal function
CIMETIDINE	TAMOXIFEN	↓ Plasma concentrations of active metabolite endoxifen	Inhibition of metabolism via CYP2D6 and CYP3A4 by cimetidine	Poorer outcomes for treatment of breast cancer not proven but increasing evidence to avoid combination. Use alternative, e.g., famotidine or nizatidine
CIMETIDINE	TOREMIFENE	↑ Plasma concentrations of toremifene	Due to inhibition of metabolism of toremifene by the CYP3A4 isoenzymes by cimetidine	Clinical relevance is uncertain. Need to monitor for clinical toxicities
CIMETIDINE	VINCA ALKALOIDS	↑ Adverse effects of vinblastine and vincristine	Inhibition of CYP3A4-mediated metabolism. Also inhibition of Pgp efflux of vinblastine	Monitor FBCs, and watch for early features of toxicity (pain, numbness, tingling in the fingers and toes, jaw pain, abdominal pain, constipation, ileus). Consider selecting an alternative drug

(Continued)

Primary Drug	Secondary Drug	Effect	Mechanism	Precautions
H2 RECEPTOR BLOCKERS				
H2-RECEPTOR BLOCKERS	**ANTICOAGULANTS**			
CIMETIDINE, FAMOTIDINE	ANTICOAGULANTS—ORAL	↑ Anticoagulant effect with cimetidine and possibly famotidine	Inhibition of metabolism via CYP1A2, CYP2C9, and CYP2C19	Use alternative acid-suppression therapy, e.g., other H2 antagonist or protein pump inhibitor (not esomeprazole, lansoprazole, or omeprazole), or monitor INR more closely; ↓ dose may be required. Take acid-suppressive drug regularly not PRN if PRN affects INR control
H2-RECEPTOR BLOCKERS	DABIGATRAN	↓ Dabigatran levels	Dabigatran capsules require an acidic environment for dissolution; increasing gastric pH reduces this process	Avoid coadministration
H2-RECEPTOR BLOCKERS	**ANTIDEPRESSANTS**			
CIMETIDINE	MAOIs—MOCLOBEMIDE	↑ Plasma concentrations of moclobemide (by up to 40%)	Inhibition of metabolism	↓ Dose of moclobemide to one-half to one-third of original and then alter as required
CIMETIDINE	MIRTAZAPINE	↑ Efficacy and adverse effects of mirtazapine	Inhibition of metabolism via CYP1A2, CYP2D6, and CYP3A4	Consider alternative acid-suppression therapy, e.g., H2 antagonist (proton pump inhibitors will interact in poor CYP2D6 metabolizers), or monitor more closely for side effects; ↓ dose as necessary
CIMETIDINE	SNRIs—VENLAFAXINE	↑ Efficacy and adverse effects	Inhibition of metabolism	Not thought to be clinically significant, but take care in elderly people and patients with hepatic impairment
CIMETIDINE	SSRIs	↑ Efficacy and adverse effects, e.g., nausea, diarrhea, dyspepsia, dizziness, sexual dysfunction	↑ Bioavailability	Use with caution; monitor for ↑ side effects. ↓ dose may be necessary

(*Continued*)

DRUGS ACTING ON THE GASTROINTESTINAL TRACT H2 RECEPTOR BLOCKERS

Primary Drug	Secondary Drug	Effect	Mechanism	Precautions
H2 RECEPTOR BLOCKERS				
CIMETIDINE	TCAs	↑ Efficacy and adverse effects, e.g., dry mouth, urinary retention, blurred vision, constipation	↓ Metabolism	Use alternative acid-suppression therapy, e.g., famotidine or nizatidine, or monitor more closely and ↓ dose. Rapid hydroxylation may be at ↑ risk
H2-RECEPTOR BLOCKERS	**ANTIDIABETIC DRUGS**			
RANITIDINE	ACARBOSE	↓ Blood levels of ranitidine	Possibly due to ↓ absorption of ranitidine	Be aware
CIMETIDINE, NIZATIDINE	METFORMIN	↑ Level of metformin and risk of lactic acidosis. The onset of lactic acidosis is often subtle with symptoms of malaise, myalgia, respiratory distress, and ↑ nonspecific abdominal distress. There may be hypothermia and persistent bradyarrhythmias	1. Cimetidine competes for renal tubular excretion with metformin that is not metabolized in humans and is not protein bound 2. Nizatidine inhibits MATE2K altering metformin secretion and reabsorption	Requires ↓ metformin dose to be considered or to avoid coadministration
CIMETIDINE	NATEGLINIDE, REPAGLINIDE	Likely to ↑ plasma concentrations of these antidiabetic drugs and ↑ risk of hypoglycemic episodes	Due to inhibition of CYP3A4-mediated metabolism of nateglinide and repaglinide	Watch for and warn patients about hypoglycemia ➢ **For signs and symptoms of hypoglycemia, see Clinical Features of Some Adverse Drug Interactions, Hypoglycemia**
CIMETIDINE, RANITIDINE	SULFONYLUREAS	Altered plasma concentrations of glimepiride, risk of unstable blood sugar control and hypoglycemic episodes with glipizide and glimepiride and of adverse effects with glibenclamide	Cimetidine and ranitidine ↓ renal elimination of glimepiride and ↑ intestinal absorption of glimepiride. Cimetidine also inhibits metabolism via CYP2C9	Avoid coadministration with cimetidine if possible. Consider alternative acid-suppression therapy, e.g., a proton pump inhibitor (not omeprazole), and monitor more closely

(*Continued*)

DRUGS ACTING ON THE GASTROINTESTINAL TRACT H2 RECEPTOR BLOCKERS

Primary Drug	Secondary Drug	Effect	Mechanism	Precautions
H2 RECEPTOR BLOCKERS				
H2-RECEPTOR BLOCKERS	**ANTIEPILEPTICS**			
CIMETIDINE, FAMOTIDINE, RANITIDINE	CARBAMAZEPINE	↑ Plasma concentrations of carbamazepine and risk of adverse effects, including bone marrow depression and skin reactions	Transient inhibition of CYP3A4-mediated metabolism of carbamazepine that may then be countered within a few days via autoinduction by carbamazepine	For cimetidine and carbamazepine, monitor for increased adverse effects though these should subside after about a week; ranitidine appears not to interact with carbamazepine. Nizatidine appears not to interact with antiepileptics
CIMETIDINE, FAMOTIDINE, RANITIDINE	PHENYTOIN	↑ Plasma concentrations of phenytoin, risk of adverse effects, including phenytoin toxicity, bone marrow depression, and skin reactions	Inhibition of phenytoin metabolism via CYP2C9 and CYP2C19	Avoid cimetidine and phenytoin; if no alternative, use low-dose cimetidine <1.2 g/day regularly, and monitor phenytoin levels closely. Famotidine or ranitidine, monitor phenytoin levels more regularly when treatment initiated. Nizatidine appears not to interact with antiepileptics
H2-RECEPTOR BLOCKERS	**ANTIFUNGALS**			
H2-RECEPTOR BLOCKERS	ITRACONAZOLE, KETOCONAZOLE, POSACONAZOLE	1. ↓ Plasma concentrations and risk of treatment failure 2. ↑ Plasma levels of cimetidine by itraconazole	1. ↓ Absorption of these antifungals as gastric pH ↑ 2. Inhibition of Pgp	Avoid concomitant use; use an alternative antifungal. If unable to avoid combination, take H2 blockers at least 2–3 h after antifungals. Separate the doses by at least 2 h, and give with an acidic drink, e.g., a carbonated drink; ↑ dose of the antifungal may be required
CIMETIDINE	TERBINAFINE	↑ Efficacy and adverse effects of terbinafine	↑ Bioavailability	Consider alternative acid-suppression therapy, or monitor more closely and consider ↓ dose
CIMETIDINE, FAMOTIDINE	ANTIGOUTS—PROBENECID	↑ Plasma concentrations of cimetidine or famotidine	↓ Renal tubular secretion	Avoid concomitant use
CIMETIDINE	ANTIHISTAMINES—ASTEMIZOLE, LORATADINE, HYDROXYZINE, MIZOLASTINE, TERFENADINE	↑ Plasma levels, potential to increase in QTc	Inhibition of metabolism	Be aware; manufacturer of mizolastine advises avoiding coadministration. Cimetidine and loratadine were not shown to increase QTc in clinical trials

(Continued)

Primary Drug	Secondary Drug	Effect	Mechanism	Precautions
H2 RECEPTOR BLOCKERS				
H2-RECEPTOR BLOCKERS	ANTIHYPERTENSIVES AND HEART FAILURE DRUGS—ALPHA-BLOCKERS	↓ Efficacy of tolazoline	Uncertain; possibly ↓ absorption	Watch for poor response to tolazoline
H2-RECEPTOR BLOCKERS	**ANTIMALARIALS**			
CIMETIDINE	CHLOROQUINE, HYDROXYCHLOROQUINE, QUININE	↑ Efficacy and adverse effects	Inhibition of metabolism and excretion	Consider alternative H2 blocker, or monitor more closely for adverse effects
CIMETIDINE	ANTIMALARIALS OTHER THAN PROGUANIL	↑ Efficacy and adverse effects of antimalarials	Inhibition of metabolism, some definitely via CYP3A4	Avoid coadministration
H2-RECEPTOR BLOCKERS	**ANTIMIGRAINE DRUGS**			
CIMETIDINE	ERGOT ALKALOIDS	↑ Ergotamine/methysergide levels, with risk of toxicity	Inhibition of metabolism via CYP3A4	Avoid coadministration
CIMETIDINE	5-HT1 AGONISTS—ZOLMITRIPTAN	↑ Efficacy and adverse effects of zolmitriptan, e.g., flushing; sensations of tingling, heat, heaviness, pressure, or tightness of any part of the body, including the throat and chest; dizziness	Inhibition of metabolism via CYP1A2	Consider alternative acid-suppression therapy, e.g., a proton pump inhibitor (not omeprazole or lansoprazole), or monitor more closely, and ↓ maximum dose of zolmitriptan to 5 mg/24 h
CIMETIDINE	ANTI-PARKINSON'S DRUGS—PRAMIPEXOLE, ROPINIROLE	↑ Efficacy and adverse effects of pramipexole and possibly ropinirole	↓ Renal excretion of pramipexole by inhibition of cation transport system; inhibition of CYP1A2-mediated metabolism of ropinirole	Monitor closely; ↓ dose of pramipexole may be required. Adjust the dose of ropinirole as necessary or use alternative acid-suppression therapy, e.g., H2 antagonist or proton pump inhibitor (not omeprazole or lansoprazole)
H2-RECEPTOR BLOCKERS	**ANTIPLATELETS**			
H2-RECEPTOR BLOCKERS—CIMETIDINE	CLOPIDOGREL	Theoretical risk of ↓ efficacy of clopidogrel	Inhibition of CYP2C19-mediated activation of clopidogrel	Consider using an alternative H2-receptor blocker

(Continued)

DRUGS ACTING ON THE GASTROINTESTINAL TRACT H2 RECEPTOR BLOCKERS

Primary Drug	Secondary Drug	Effect	Mechanism	Precautions
H2 RECEPTOR BLOCKERS				
H2-RECEPTOR BLOCKERS	DIPYRIDAMOLE	Possible ↓ bioavailability of dipyridamole	Dipyridamole tablets require an acidic environment for adequate dissolution; ↑ pH of the stomach impairs dissolution and may therefore ↓ absorption of drug	Use M/R preparation of dipyridamole. Consider using an alternative antiplatelet drug or ↑ dose of dipyridamole tablets
CIMETIDINE	ANTIPROTOZOALS—MEBENDAZOLE	↑ Mebendazole levels	Inhibition of metabolism	Be aware; case reports of this interaction has been used therapeutically
CIMETIDINE	ANTIPSYCHOTICS—ASENAPINE, CHLORPROMAZINE, CLOZAPINE, HALOPERIDOL, OLANZAPINE, PERPHENAZINE, RISPERIDONE, SERTINDOLE, THIORIDAZINE, ZUCLOPENTHIXOL	↑ Plasma concentrations of these antipsychotics, with risk of associated adverse effects (see ***Drugs Acting on the Nervous System, Antipsychotics***)	Cimetidine is an inhibitor of CYP3A4 (sertindole, haloperidol, risperidone), CYP2D6 (chlorpromazine, risperidone, zuclopenthixol, thioridazine, perphenazine), and CYP1A2 (asenapine, clozapine, olanzapine, sertindole, haloperidol)	Avoid concomitant use. Choose alternative acid-suppression therapy; nizatidine, famotidine, or rabeprazole likely does not interact significantly
H2-RECEPTOR BLOCKERS	**ANTIVIRALS**			
CIMETIDINE	ACYCLOVIR/VALACYCLOVIR	↑ Efficacy and adverse effects of antivirals	Competition for renal excretion	Use doses of valacyclovir >4 g/day with caution, or consider alternative acid-suppression therapy. For doses <1 g/day, interaction is not thought to be clinically significant. Studies only reported with valacyclovir

(*Continued*)

DRUGS ACTING ON THE GASTROINTESTINAL TRACT H2 RECEPTOR BLOCKERS

DRUGS ACTING ON THE GASTROINTESTINAL TRACT H2 RECEPTOR BLOCKERS

Primary Drug	Secondary Drug	Effect	Mechanism	Precautions
H2 RECEPTOR BLOCKERS				
H2-RECEPTOR BLOCKERS	PROTEASE INHIBITORS—AMPRENAVIR, ATAZANAVIR, SAQUINAVIR	1. ↓ Absorption of a atazanavir 2. Possible ↑ levels of cimetidine and saquinavir	1. ↑ Gastric pH 2. Uncertain mechanism of action on cimetidine	For amprenavir, separate doses by at least 1 h. For atazanavir, dose adjustments are required. If not on tenofovir, limit to famotidine 20 mg b.d. (or equivalent); if a higher dose is required, consider increasing to 400 mg daily and adding ritonavir 100 mg daily. If on tenofovir, increase doses as described and limit to famotidine 40 mg b.d. (or equivalent). Consider TDM, and monitor viral load closely. For saquinavir and fosamprenavir, no dose adjustment needed
H2-RECEPTOR BLOCKERS	RILPIVIRINE	↓ Plasma concentrations	↓ Absorption as gastric pH ↑	Avoid concomitant use. If unable to avoid combination, only use H2 antagonist once daily, and separate by 12 h before or 4 h after rilpivirine. Monitor viral load closely
CIMETIDINE	ZALCITABINE	↑ Efficacy and adverse effects of zalcitabine	↓ Excretion via inhibition of tubular secretion	Clinical significance unclear. Monitor more closely
H2-RECEPTOR BLOCKERS	**ANXIOLYTICS AND HYPNOTICS**			
CIMETIDINE, RANITIDINE	BZDs (NOT LORAZEPAM OR TEMAZEPAM)	↑ Efficacy and adverse effects of BZDs, e.g., sedation	Cimetidine is an inhibitor of CYP3A4, CYP2D6, CYP2C19, and CYP1A2	Not clinically significant for most patients. Conflicting information for some BZDs. Monitor more closely; ↓ dose if necessary
CIMETIDINE	CLOMETHIAZOLE	↑ Efficacy and adverse effects, e.g., sedation, “hangover” effect	Inhibition of metabolism	Monitor closely; ↓ dose may be required
CIMETIDINE	MELATONIN	↑ Plasma concentrations	Inhibition of metabolism via CYP1A2	Be aware
CIMETIDINE	ZALEPLON	↑ Plasma concentrations	Inhibition of metabolism	Monitor closely; ↓ dose may be required

(*Continued*)

Primary Drug	Secondary Drug	Effect	Mechanism	Precautions
H2 RECEPTOR BLOCKERS				
CIMETIDINE	BETA-BLOCKERS	↑ Plasma concentrations and effects of labetalol, metoprolol, and propranolol; possibly systemic effects of timolol eye drops	Cimetidine is an inhibitor of CYP3A4, CYP2D6, CYP2C19, and CYP1A2	Monitor BP and PR, risk of worsening heart failure; monitor these patients more closely. Nebivolol and levels of other CYP2D6 substrates likely to be increased
NIZATIDINE	BETA-BLOCKERS	↑ Bradycardia when nizatidine is added to atenolol. Other beta-blockers have not been studied	Uncertain	Monitor PR when administering nizatidine to patients on beta-blockers
H2-RECEPTOR BLOCKERS	BRONCHODILATORS—THEOPHYLLINE	↑ Efficacy and adverse effects, including seizures. There is conflicting information associated with ranitidine, famotidine, and nizatidine	Inhibition of metabolism via CYP1A2; cimetidine being the most potent inhibitor of the H2 blockers	Use alternative acid-suppression therapy, e.g., a proton pump inhibitor (not omeprazole or lansoprazole), or monitor closely; consider patient variation. Check levels on day 3 and then at 1 week. A 30%–50%, ↓ dose of theophylline may be required. For doses of cimetidine <400 mg/day, the interaction may not be clinically significant
CIMETIDINE, RANITIDINE	CALCIUM CHANNEL BLOCKERS	↑ Levels of calcium channel blockers, especially diltiazem, nifedipine, and isradipine, particularly with cimetidine	Inhibition of CYP3A isoform–mediated metabolism; cimetidine being the most potent inhibitor	Monitor BP and HR closely; be aware of possibility of significant ↓ BP. Consider ↓ dose of diltiazem, nifedipine, and isradipine by up to 50%
FAMOTIDINE	CALCIUM CHANNEL BLOCKERS	Reports of heart failure and ↓ BP when famotidine given with nifedipine	Additive negative inotropic effects	Caution with coadministering famotidine with calcium channel blockers, especially in elderly people
H2-RECEPTOR BLOCKERS	DRUG DEPENDENCE THERAPIES—BUPROPION	↑ Plasma concentrations of cimetidine and ranitidine	Bupropion and its metabolite hydroxybupropion inhibit CYP2D6	Initiate therapy of these drugs at the lowest effective dose
CIMETIDINE, RANITIDINE	**ELIGLUSTAT**	↑ Eliglustat levels	Inhibition of CYP3A4-mediated metabolism	Avoid coadministration in poor metabolizers
CIMETIDINE	MUSCLE RELAXANTS—VECURONIUM	↑ Efficacy of vecuronium	Unclear	Potential for slightly prolonged recovery time (minutes)
CIMETIDINE, RANITIDINE	**NITISINONE**	Possible ↑ nitisinone levels	Inhibition of CYP3A4-mediated metabolism	Monitor carefully

(Continued)

DRUGS ACTING ON THE GASTROINTESTINAL TRACT H2 RECEPTOR BLOCKERS

Primary Drug	Secondary Drug	Effect	Mechanism	Precautions
H2 RECEPTOR BLOCKERS				
CIMETIDINE	PERIPHERAL VASODILATORS—CILOSTAZOL, PENTOXIFYLLINE	Cimetidine ↑ cilostazol and pentoxifylline levels, both reduce pulmonary vasodilation in children	Cimetidine inhibits CYP3A4-mediated metabolism of cilostazol. Antagonism of vasodilation via H2 receptors. Uncertain mechanism for pentoxifylline	Avoid coadministration
CIMETIDINE	PHOSPHODIESTERASE TYPE 5 INHIBITORS—SILDENAFIL	↑ Efficacy and adverse effects of sildenafil	Inhibition of metabolism via CYP3A4	Consider a starting dose of 25 mg of sildenafil
CIMETIDINE	ROFLUMILAST	↑ Plasma levels and adverse effects of roflumilast	Inhibition of metabolism via CYP1A2 and CYP3A4	Monitor closely for adverse effects within the first weeks of treatment as patients may be unable to tolerate combination
FAMOTIDINE	SUCRALFATE	↓ Efficacy of famotidine	↓ Absorption	Take famotidine 2 h before sucralfate
CIMETIDINE	SYMPATHOMIMETICS	↑ Efficacy and adverse effects of sympathomimetics	Unclear	↑ Hypertensive response; ↓ dose may be required. Monitor ECG for tachycardias
CIMETIDINE	THYROID HORMONES	↓ Efficacy of levothyroxine	↓ Absorption	Clinical significance unclear. Monitor requirement for ↑ levothyroxine dose
RANITIDINE	TRIPOTASSIUM DICITRATOBISMUTHATE	↑ Adverse effects of tripotassium dicitratobismuthate	↑ Absorption	Do not use together for more than 16 weeks. Bismuth salicylate and subnitrate do not interact
CIMETIDINE	ULIPRISTAL	Contraceptive effect possibly ↓ (high-dose ulipristal)	Unclear	Avoid coadministration

Primary Drug	Secondary Drug	Effect	Mechanism	Precautions
LAXATIVES				
LAXATIVES—STIMULANT	AMIODARONE	Risk of arrhythmias	Cardiac toxicity directly related to hypokalemia	Manufacturers recommend using alternative laxatives
LAXATIVES	ORLISTAT	↑ Efficacy of laxatives	Additive effect; orlistat may cause soft stools	Start laxatives at low dose and titrate upward as needed

DRUGS ACTING ON THE GASTROINTESTINAL TRACT LAXATIVES

Primary Drug	Secondary Drug	Effect	Mechanism	Precautions
PANCREATIN				
PANCREATIN	ANTIDIABETIC DRUGS—ACARBOSE	Theoretical risk of ↓ efficacy of acarbose	↓ Absorption	Watch for poor response to acarbose; monitor capillary blood glucose level closely
PANCREATIN	IRON	Possible ↓ iron levels when iron is taken orally	↓ Absorption	Watch for poor response to oral iron; monitor FBC closely

Primary Drug	Secondary Drug	Effect	Mechanism	Precautions
PROTON PUMP INHIBITORS				
LANSOPRAZOLE	ANTACIDS	Possible ↓ efficacy of lansoprazole	↓ Absorption	Separate doses by at least 1 h
PROTON PUMP INHIBITORS	**ANTIBIOTICS**			
PROTON PUMP INHIBITORS	CEPHALOSPORINS	Possible ↓ efficacy of cephalosporin	↓ Absorption as gastric pH ↑	Monitor for ↓ efficacy. Separate doses by at least 2 h; take cephalosporin with food
PROTON PUMP INHIBITORS	MACROLIDES—CLARITHROMYCIN	↑ Efficacy and adverse effects of both drugs	↑ Plasma concentration of both drugs	No dose adjustment usually needed. Review severe hepatic impairment, long-term or high-dose treatment. Interaction is considered useful for *Helicobacter pylori* eradication. Not seen with pantoprazole
PROTON PUMP INHIBITORS	**ANTICANCER AND IMMUNOMODULATING DRUGS**			
PROTON PUMP INHIBITORS	BOSUTINIB	↓ Bosutinib levels	pH-dependent solubility of bosutinib	Use short-acting antacids as an alternative, and administer separately to bosutinib
OMEPRAZOLE	CICLOSPORIN	Conflicting information. Possible altered efficacy of ciclosporin	Unclear	Monitor closely. Studies have reported combined use with no significant changes in ciclosporin levels
PROTON PUMP INHIBITORS	DABRAFENIB	Theoretical risk of ↓ dabrafenib levels	Dabrafenib solubility reduced at higher pH	Avoid concurrent use if possible

(Continued)

Primary Drug	Secondary Drug	Effect	Mechanism	Precautions
PROTON PUMP INHIBITORS				
PROTON PUMP INHIBITORS	DASATINIB	↓ Plasma concentration	↓ Absorption as gastric pH ↑	Avoid coadministration. Use an antacid if required, but separate doses by at least 2 h before or after dasatinib administration
PROTON PUMP INHIBITORS	ERLOTINIB	↓ Erlotinib levels	Solubility reduced at higher pH	Avoid concurrent use of proton pump inhibitors antagonists
PROTON PUMP INHIBITORS	GEFITINIB	↓ Gefitinib levels	Solubility reduced at higher pH	Avoid concurrent use of proton pump inhibitors antagonists and simultaneous use of antacids
OMEPRAZOLE	IMATINIB	↑ Plasma concentrations, with risk of toxic effects of these drugs	Imatinib is a potent inhibitor of CYP2C9 isoenzymes, which metabolize these drugs	Watch for the early toxic effects of these drugs. If necessary, consider using alternative acid-suppression therapy while the patient is being given imatinib
PROTON PUMP INHIBITORS	LAPATINIB	↓ Lapatinib levels	Solubility reduced at higher pH	Avoid concurrent use
PROTON PUMP INHIBITORS	METHOTREXATE	Likely ↑ plasma concentrations of methotrexate and ↑ risk of toxic effects, e.g., blood dyscrasias, liver cirrhosis, pulmonary toxicity, renal toxicity	Attributed to omeprazole ↓ renal elimination of methotrexate	Monitor clinically and biochemically for blood dyscrasias and liver, renal, and pulmonary toxicity
PROTON PUMP INHIBITORS	MYCOPHENOLATE	↓ Plasma concentration of mycophenolic acid (active metabolite)	Unclear	Be aware, and monitor for ↓ efficacy though no difference in rejection rates noted in studies
PROTON PUMP INHIBITORS	NILOTINIB	↓ Nilotinib levels	Solubility reduced at higher pH	Caution with concurrent use of proton pump inhibitors
PROTON PUMP INHIBITORS	PAZOPANIB	↓ Plasma concentration	↓ Absorption as gastric pH ↑	Avoid coadministration if possible; otherwise, take pazopanib without food in the evening at the same time as the proton pump inhibitor
PROTON PUMP INHIBITORS	TACROLIMUS	Possible ↑ efficacy and adverse effects of immunosuppression	Altered metabolism from CYP2C19 to CYP3A4 in patients with low CYP2C19 levels	Monitor levels more closely

(Continued)

Primary Drug	Secondary Drug	Effect	Mechanism	Precautions
PROTON PUMP INHIBITORS				
PROTON PUMP INHIBITORS	TACROLIMUS	Possible ↑ efficacy and adverse effects of immunosuppression	Altered metabolism from CYP2C19 to CYP3A4 in patients with low CYP2C19 levels	Monitor tacrolimus levels and renal function more closely; dose adjustment may be needed
PROTON PUMP INHIBITORS—OMEPRAZOLE	TOCILIZUMAB	↓ Levels	Tocilizumab reverses CYP450 isoenzyme suppression by IL-6	Monitor closely and consider dose adjustment
PROTON PUMP INHIBITORS	VANDETANIB	Possible ↓ plasma concentration	↓ Absorption	Manufacturer advises avoiding coadministration
PROTON PUMP INHIBITORS	**ANTICOAGULANTS**			
PROTON PUMP INHIBITORS	ANTICOAGULANTS—ORAL	Possibly ↑ anticoagulant effect particularly when esomeprazole, lansoprazole, or omeprazole is added to warfarin	Omeprazole and lansoprazole induce CYP1A2, which plays a role in the activation of coumarins. Inhibition of anticoagulant metabolism via CYP2C9 and CYP2C19 likely to be involved	Monitor INR more closely. ↓ dose may be required. If values are 10% or 20%–30% over range, omit the dose for 1 or 2 days, respectively, and consider ↓ maintenance dose by 10%. Regular dosing of a proton pump inhibitor is preferable if it affects INR significantly. Not reported with pantoprazole or rabeprazole
PROTON PUMP INHIBITORS	DABIGATRAN	↓ Dabigatran levels	Dabigatran capsules require an acidic environment for dissolution; increasing gastric pH reduces this process	Avoid coadministration
PROTON PUMP INHIBITORS	**ANTIDEPRESSANTS**			
OMEPRAZOLE/ ESOMEPRAZOLE	MAOIs—MOCLOBEMIDE	Possible ↑ efficacy and adverse effects of both drugs	Inhibition of CYP2C19	Monitor more closely. Effect is seen only in extensive CYP2C19 metabolizers; ↓ dose may be required
PROTON PUMP INHIBITORS	SSRIs—FLUVOXAMINE	1. ↓ Fluvoxamine levels with loss of therapeutic efficacy 2. ↑ Plasma concentration of proton pump inhibitor	1. Inhibition of CYP1A2-mediated metabolism by omeprazole 2. Fluvoxamine inhibits metabolism of proton pump inhibitors via CYP2C19	1. Monitor for lack of therapeutic effect of fluvoxamine. When omeprazole is withdrawn, monitor for fluvoxamine toxicity 2. Consider dose reduction of proton pump inhibitor

(*Continued*)

Primary Drug	Secondary Drug	Effect	Mechanism	Precautions
PROTON PUMP INHIBITORS				
OMEPRAZOLE/ ESOMEPRAZOLE	SSRIs—CITALOPRAM/ ESCITALOPRAM	↑ Plasma concentrations	Altered metabolism	Monitor more closely; ↓ dose may be required
PROTON PUMP INHIBITORS	ANTIDIABETIC DRUGS—SULFONYLUREAS	Possible ↑ efficacy and adverse effects of sulfonylurea, e.g., hypoglycemia	Possible ↑ absorption	Monitor capillary blood glucose more closely; ↓ dose may be required
PROTON PUMP INHIBITORS	**ANTIEPILEPTICS**			
PROTON PUMP INHIBITORS	CARBAMAZEPINE	Possible altered efficacy of carbamazepine	Unclear; possibly via ↓ clearance	Use with caution. Monitor carbamazepine levels when starting or stopping therapy, and use the proton pump inhibitor regularly, not PRN. Not reported with pantoprazole or rabeprazole
PROTON PUMP INHIBITORS—OMEPRAZOLE	PHENYTOIN	Possible ↑ efficacy and adverse effects of phenytoin	Unclear; possible altered metabolism via CYP2C19	↓ Dose may be required. Use the proton pump inhibitor regularly, not PRN. Monitor phenytoin levels when starting or stopping treatment. Patients have received omeprazole for 3–5 weeks without altered phenytoin levels. Not reported with pantoprazole or rabeprazole
PROTON PUMP INHIBITORS	**ANTIFUNGALS**			
PROTON PUMP INHIBITORS	ITRACONAZOLE, KETOCONAZOLE, POSACONAZOLE	Possible ↓ efficacy of antifungal	Increased pH ↓ absorption 1. ↓ Absorption of itraconazole and ketoconazole 2. Possible ↓ plasma concentration of posaconazole	1. Monitor for ↓ efficacy and blood levels; ↑ dose may be required. Separate doses by at least 2 h, and give with a carbonated drink; consider itraconazole solution as not affected 2. Manufacturer of posaconazole advises avoiding combination
OMEPRAZOLE/ ESOMEPRAZOLE	VORICONAZOLE	Possible ↑ efficacy and adverse effects of both drugs	1. Inhibition of voriconazole metabolism via CYP2C19 and CYP3A4 2. Inhibition of metabolism of omeprazole	1. No dose adjustment of voriconazole recommended 2. Half omeprazole dose if 40 mg/ day or more

(Continued)

Primary Drug	Secondary Drug	Effect	Mechanism	Precautions
PROTON PUMP INHIBITORS				
OMEPRAZOLE/ ESOMEPRAZOLE	FLUCONAZOLE	Possible ↑ efficacy and adverse effects of omeprazole	Inhibition of metabolism of omeprazole	Be aware
PROTON PUMP INHIBITORS	**ANTIPLATELET AGENTS**			
PROTON PUMP INHIBITORS	DIPYRIDAMOLE	Possible ↓ bioavailability of dipyridamole	Dipyridamole tablets require an acidic environment for adequate dissolution; ↑ pH of the stomach impairs dissolution and may therefore ↓ absorption of the drug	Modified release preparations are not affected or ↑ dose of dipyridamole or consider using an alternative antiplatelet drug
PROTON PUMP INHIBITORS—OMEPRAZOLE	CLOPIDOGREL	↓ Efficacy of clopidogrel	Inhibition of CYP2C19-mediated activation of clopidogrel	Avoid coadministration. Use an alternative proton pump inhibitor
OMEPRAZOLE	ANTIPSYCHOTICS—CLOZAPINE	Possible ↓ efficacy of clozapine	↑ Metabolism via CYP1A2	Clinical significance unclear; monitor more closely
PROTON PUMP INHIBITORS	**ANTIVIRALS**			
PROTON PUMP INHIBITORS	PROTEASE INHIBITORS—ATAZANAVIR, DARUNAVIR/ RITONAVIR, LOPINAVIR/ RITONAVIR	1. Possible altered plasma levels of proton pump inhibitors 2. ↓ Plasma levels of atazanavir	1. Complex interactions involving CYP3A4 inhibition and 2C19 induction 2. ↓ Absorption due to due to ↑ gastric pH	Avoid coadministration. If not possible, increase atazanavir/ ritonavir to 400/100 mg; do not exceed an equivalent dose of omeprazole 20 mg, and monitor closely
PROTON PUMP INHIBITORS	PROTEASE INHIBITORS—SAQUINAVIR	↑ Levels of saquinavir; risk of QT prolongation	Uncertain	Avoid coadministration
OMEPRAZOLE	PROTEASE INHIBITORS—INDINAVIR	Possibly ↓ plasma concentrations and ↓ efficacy of indinavir	Uncertain	↑ Dose of indinavir from 800 mg three times a day to 1 g three times a day, or preferably add ritonavir 200 mg once daily
OMEPRAZOLE/ ESOMEPRAZOLE	PROTEASE INHIBITORS—TIPRANAVIR (BOOSTED WITH RITONAVIR)	↑ Levels of saquinavir; risk of QT prolongation	Uncertain	Avoid coadministration
PROTON PUMP INHIBITORS—OMEPRAZOLE	RALTEGRAVIR	↑ Plasma concentration of raltegravir	Increased absorption as increased pH	Use with caution; no dose adjustment recommended

(*Continued*)

DRUGS ACTING ON THE GASTROINTESTINAL TRACT PROTON PUMP INHIBITORS

Primary Drug	Secondary Drug	Effect	Mechanism	Precautions
PROTON PUMP INHIBITORS				
OMEPRAZOLE/ ESOMEPRAZOLE	ANXIOLYTICS AND HYPNOTICS—BZDs	↑ Efficacy and adverse effects, e.g., prolonged sedation	Inhibition of metabolism via CYP450 (some show competitive inhibition via CYP2C19)	Monitor for ↑ side effects; ↓ dose as necessary. May take longer for patients to recover from interventions or surgical procedures, particularly when BZDs have been used. Consider an alternative proton pump inhibitor, e.g., lansoprazole or pantoprazole
PROTON PUMP INHIBITORS	BETA-BLOCKERS	Risk of ↑ plasma concentrations and effects of propranolol	Omeprazole inhibits CYP2D6- and CYP2C19-mediated metabolism of propanolol	Monitor BP at least weekly until stable
OMEPRAZOLE	CALCIUM CHANNEL BLOCKERS—NIFEDIPINE	Possible ↑ efficacy and adverse effects	Small ↑ of bioavailability possible via ↑ intragastric pH	Unlikely to be clinically significant
PROTON PUMP INHIBITORS	CARDIAC GLYCOSIDES—DIGOXIN	Plasma concentrations of digoxin are possibly ↑ by proton pump inhibitors	Small ↑ of bioavailability, possibly via ↑ intragastric pH or altered intestinal Pgp transport	Be aware; may not be clinically significant unless a poor CYP2C19 metabolizer or high-dose digoxin. Different proton pump inhibitors may interact differently—monitor if changing therapy or doses
PROTON PUMP INHIBITORS	CNS STIMULANTS—MODAFINIL	May cause moderate ↑ in plasma concentrations of the proton pump inhibitor	Modafinil is a reversible inhibitor of CYP2C19 when used in therapeutic doses	Be aware
OMEPRAZOLE	DRUG DEPENDENCE THERAPIES—DISULFIRAM	Possible ↑ adverse effects of disulfiram	Accumulation of metabolites	Monitor closely for ↑ side effects, although patients have received the combination without reported problems
PROTON PUMP INHIBITORS	BISPHOSPHONATES	Possible ↑ efficacy of alendronic acid	Unclear	Consider switching to an alternative, e.g., H2 antagonist
OMEPRAZOLE	HERBAL—GINKGO	↑ Metabolism of omeprazole	Possible reduced effect	Monitor more closely
PROTON PUMP INHIBITORS	LIPID-LOWERING DRUGS—ATORVASTATIN	Possible ↑ efficacy and adverse effects of atorvastatin	Inhibition of Pgp; ↓ first-pass clearance	Monitor closely
PROTON PUMP INHIBITORS	MUSCLE RELAXANTS—VECURONIUM	Possible ↑ efficacy and adverse effects of vecuronium	Unclear	Altered duration of action. May need ↑ recovery time

(*Continued*)

Primary Drug	Secondary Drug	Effect	Mechanism	Precautions
PROTON PUMP INHIBITORS				
PROTON PUMP INHIBITORS	**ESTROGENS**			
PROTON PUMP INHIBITORS	ULIPRISTAL	Possible ↓ efficacy of contraceptive	Unclear	Avoid coadministration
LANSOPRAZOLE	ORAL CONTRACEPTIVES	Possible altered efficacy of contraceptive	Unclear	Clinical significance is uncertain. It would seem to be wise to advise patients to use an alternative form of contraception during and for 1 month after stopping coadministration with lansoprazole
PROTON PUMP INHIBITORS	PERIPHERAL VASODILATORS—CILOSTAZOL	Cilostazol levels are ↑ by omeprazole and possibly lansoprazole	Omeprazole inhibits CYP2C19-mediated metabolism of cilostazol	Avoid concomitant use. U.S. manufacturer advises halving the dose of cilostazol
PROTON PUMP INHIBITORS—OMEPRAZOLE	PIRFENIDONE	↓ Pirfenidone levels	Induction of metabolism of pirfenidone	Manufacturer recommends avoiding coadministration
PROTON PUMP INHIBITORS	SUCRALFATE	Possible ↓ efficacy of omeprazole and lansoprazole	Unclear	Take at least 1 h after sucralfate
LANSOPRAZOLE, OMEPRAZOLE	THEOPHYLLINE	↓ Plasma concentrations of theophylline	Induced CYP1A2-mediated metabolism of theophylline	↑ Dose may be required. Consider using the proton pump inhibitor regularly, not as required. Monitor theophylline levels when starting or stopping treatment

Primary Drug	Secondary Drug	Effect	Mechanism	Precautions
SUCRALFATE				
SUCRALFATE	ANTIBIOTICS—QUINOLONES, TETRACYCLINES	↓ Levels of these antibiotics	↓ Absorption of these antibiotics	Give the antibiotics at least 2 h before sucralfate
SUCRALFATE	ANTICOAGULANTS—ORAL	Possible ↓ anticoagulant effect	↓ Absorption of warfarin	Monitor INR at least weekly until stable
SUCRALFATE	ANTIDEPRESSANTS—AMITRIPTYLINE	Possible ↓ amitriptyline levels	↓ Absorption of amitriptyline	Watch for poor response to amitriptyline

(Continued)

DRUGS ACTING ON THE GASTROINTESTINAL TRACT TRIPOTASSIUM DICITRATOBISMUTHATE

Primary Drug	Secondary Drug	Effect	Mechanism	Precautions
SUCRALFATE				
SUCRALFATE	ANTIEPILEPTICS—PHENYTOIN	↓ Phenytoin levels	↓ Absorption of phenytoin	Give phenytoin at least 2 h after sucralfate
SUCRALFATE	ANTIFUNGALS—KETOCONAZOLE	↓ Ketoconazole levels	↓ Absorption of ketoconazole	Separate doses by at least 2–3 h
SUCRALFATE	ANTIPSYCHOTICS—SULPIRIDE	↓ Sulpiride levels	↓ Absorption of sulpiride	Give sulpiride at least 2 h after sucralfate
SUCRALFATE	BRONCHODILATORS—THEOPHYLLINE	Possibly ↓ theophylline levels (with modified-release preparations)	Possibly ↓ absorption	Watch for poor response to theophylline and monitor levels
SUCRALFATE	CARDIAC GLYCOSIDES—DIGOXIN	Plasma concentrations of digoxin may be ↓ by sucralfate	Uncertain; possibly sucralfate binds with digoxin and ↓ its absorption	Watch for poor response to digoxin
SUCRALFATE	H2-RECEPTOR BLOCKERS—FAMOTIDINE	↓ Efficacy of famotidine	↓ Absorption	Take famotidine 2 h before sucralfate
SUCRALFATE	PROTON PUMP INHIBITORS	Possible ↓ efficacy of omeprazole and lansoprazole	Unclear	Take at least 1 h after sucralfate
SUCRALFATE	THYROID HORMONES	↓ Thyroxine levels	↓ Absorption	Give thyroxine 2–3 h before sucralfate

Primary Drug	Secondary Drug	Effect	Mechanism	Precautions
TRIPOTASSIUM DICITRATOBISMUTHATE				
TRIPOTASSIUM DICITRATOBISMUTHATE	ANTIBIOTICS—TETRACYCLINES	↓ Levels of tetracyclines	↓ Absorption of tetracyclines	Separate doses by 2–3 h
TRIPOTASSIUM DICITRATOBISMUTHATE	H2-RECEPTOR BLOCKERS—RANITIDINE	↑ Adverse effects of tripotassium dicitratobismuthate	↑ Absorption	Do not use together for more than 16 weeks. Bismuth salicylate and subnitrate do not interact
TRIPOTASSIUM DICITRATOBISMUTHATE	PROTON PUMP INHIBITORS—OMEPRAZOLE	↑ Adverse effects of tripotassium dicitratobismuthate	↑ Absorption	Do not use together for more than 16 weeks. Bismuth salicylate and subnitrate do not interact

PART 12

Respiratory Drugs

Simon F.J. Clarke

1. ANTIHISTAMINES
2. ASTHMA PROPHYLAXIS
   - CORTICOSTEROIDS—*see Anticancer and Other Immunomodulating Drugs Section*
   - LEUKOTRIENE RECEPTOR ANTAGONISTS
3. BRONCHODILATORS
   - ANTIMUSCARINICS (IPRATROPIUM, TIOTROPIUM) ➢ *Drugs Acting on the Nervous System, Anti-Parkinson's Drugs*
   - BETA-2 AGONISTS
   - NONSELECTIVE BETA-AGONISTS ➢ *Sympathomimetics Section*—CVS *Chapter*
   - THEOPHYLLINES
4. CYSTIC FIBROSIS THERAPIES—IVACAFTOR
5. DOXAPRAM
6. PHODPHODIESTERASE TYPE 4 INHIBITORS—ROFLUMILAST
7. PIRFENIDONE

Primary Drug	Secondary Drug	Effect	Mechanism	Precautions
ANTIHISTAMINES				
ANTIHISTAMINES	**DRUGS THAT PROLONG THE QT INTERVAL**			
ANTIHISTAMINES—TERFENADINE, HYDROXYZINE, MIZOLASTINE	1. ANTIARRHYTHMICS—ajmaline, amiodarone, azimilide, cibenzoline, disopyramide, dofetilide, dronedarone, ibutilide, procainamide, propafenone, quinidine 2. ANTIBIOTICS—macrolides (especially azithromycin, clarithromycin, parenteral erythromycin, telithromycin), quinolones (especially moxifloxacin), quinupristin/dalfopristin 3. ANTICANCER AND IMMUNOMODULATING DRUGS—arsenic trioxide, bosutinib, crizotinib, dasatinib, eribulin, fingolimod, lapatinib, nilotinib, pazopanib, sunitinib, vandetanib, vemurafenib 4. ANTIDEPRESSANTS—TCAs, venlafaxine 5. ANTIEMETICS—ondansetron 6. ANTIFUNGALS—fluconazole, posaconazole, voriconazole 7. ANTIHYPERTENSIVES—ketanserin 8. ANTIMALARIALS—artemether with lumefantrine, chloroquine, halofantrine, hydroxychloroquine, mefloquine, quinine 9. ANTIPROTOZOALS—pentamidine isetionate 10. ANTIPSYCHOTICS—atypicals, phenothiazines, pimozide 11. ANTIVIRALS—boceprevir, rilpivirine, telaprevir 12. BETA-BLOCKERS—sotalol 13. BRONCHODILATORS—parenteral bronchodilators 14. CNS STIMULANTS—atomoxetine 16. RANOLAZINE	Risk of ventricular arrhythmias, particularly torsades de pointes	Additive effect; these drugs prolong the QT interval. Also, amitriptyline, clomipramine, and desipramine levels may be ↑ by propafenone. Amitriptyline and clomipramine may ↑ propafenone levels. Propafenone and these TCAs inhibit CYP2D6-mediated metabolism of each other	Avoid coadministration

(*Continued*)

RESPIRATORY DRUGS ANTIHISTAMINES

Primary Drug	Secondary Drug	Effect	Mechanism	Precautions
ANTIHISTAMINES				
ANTIHISTAMINES	**DRUGS WITH ANTIMUSCARINIC EFFECTS**			
ANTIHISTAMINES—CHLORPHENAMINE, CYPROHEPTADINE, HYDROXYZINE	1. ANALGESICS—nefopam 2. ANTIARRHYTHMICS—disopyramide, propafenone 3. ANTIDEPRESSANTS—TCAs 4. ANTIEMETICS—cyclizine 5. ANTIMUSCARINICS—atropine, benztropine, cyclopentolate, dicycloverine, flavoxate, homatropine, hyoscine, orphenadrine, oxybutynin, procyclidine, propantheline, tolterodine, trihexyphenidyl, tropicamide 6. ANTI-PARKINSON'S DRUGS—dopaminergics 7. ANTIPSYCHOTICS—phenothiazines, clozapine, pimozide 8. MUSCLE RELAXANTS—baclofen 9. NITRATES—isosorbide dinitrate	↑ Risk of antimuscarinic side effects. **NB ↓ efficacy of sublingual nitrate tablets**	Additive effect; both drugs cause antimuscarinic side effects **Antimuscarinic effects ↓ saliva production, which ↓ dissolution of the tablet**	Warn patients of this additive effect. **Consider changing the formulation to a sublingual nitrate spray**
ANTIHISTAMINES	ALCOHOL	↑ Sedation with sedating antihistamines	Additive effect	Warn patients about this effect
ANTIHISTAMINES	**ANALGESICS**			
ANTIHISTAMINES	OPIOIDS	Promethazine ↑ analgesic and anesthetic effects of opioids However, it has an additive sedative effect	Unknown	Monitor vital signs closely during coadministration
ANTIHISTAMINES	PARACETAMOL	Chlorphenamine, cyclizine, cyproheptadine, and hydroxyzine may slow the onset of action of intermittent-dose paracetamol	Anticholinergic effects delay gastric emptying and absorption	Warn patients that the action of paracetamol may be delayed. This will not be the case when paracetamol is taken regularly
FEXOFENADINE	ANTACIDS	↓ Fexofenadine levels	↓ Absorption	Be aware
ANTIHISTAMINES	**ANTIARRHYTHMICS**			
TERFENADINE, HYDROXYZINE, MIZOLASTINE	FLECAINIDE	Risk of arrhythmias	Additive effect	Avoid coadministration
MIZOLASTINE	MEXILETINE	Risk of arrhythmias	Additive effect	Avoid coadministration

(*Continued*)

Primary Drug	Secondary Drug	Effect	Mechanism	Precautions
ANTIHISTAMINES				
ANTIHISTAMINES	**ANTICANCER AND IMMUNOMODULATING DRUGS**			
ANTIHISTAMINES—ASTEMIZOLE, TERFENADINE	DASATINIB	↑ Levels of these antihistamines	CYP3A4 inhibition	Caution with these CYP3A4 substrates with narrow therapeutic window
ANTIHISTAMINES	HISTAMINE	Effects of histamine antagonized	Histamine blockade	Avoid concurrent use
ALIMEMAZINE (TRIMEPRAZINE), CHLORPHENIRAMINE, PROMETHAZINE	PROCARBAZINE	1. The antimuscarinic effects (dry mouth, urinary retention, blurred vision, gastrointestinal disturbances) are ↑ as are the sedating effects of these older antihistamines 2. Excessive sedation may occur	1. MAOIs cause anticholinergic effects (including antimuscarinic effects), hence the additive effects of both antimuscarinic activity and CNS depression 2. Additive effects on the CNS, although on occasions chlorpheniramine may cause CNS stimulation	Concurrent use is not recommended. If used together, patients should be warned to report any gastrointestinal problems as paralytic ileus has been reported. Also, caution is required when performing activities needing alertness (e.g., driving, using sharp objects). Do not use OTC medications such as nasal decongestants and asthma and allergy remedies without consulting the pharmacist/doctor as these preparations may contain antihistamines
FEXOFENADINE	VEMURAFENIB	Possible ↑ levels of Pgp substrates	Vemurafenib inhibits P-glycoprotein	Be aware. Clinical significance unknown
ANTIHISTAMINES	**ANTIDEPRESSANTS**			
ANTIHISTAMINES	MAOIs	↑ Occurrence of antimuscarinic effects such as blurred vision, confusion (in the elderly), restlessness, and constipation	Additive antimuscarinic effects	Warn patients and carers, particularly those managing elderly patients. See anticholinergic risk scale in appendix

(*Continued*)

Primary Drug	Secondary Drug	Effect	Mechanism	Precautions
ANTIHISTAMINES				
ANTIHISTAMINES—SEDATIVE	MAOIs	Additive depression of CNS ranging from drowsiness to coma and respiratory depression	Synergistic depressant effects on CNS function	Necessary to warn patients, particularly as regards activities that require attention, e.g., driving and using machinery and equipment that could cause self-harm
CYPROHEPTADINE	SSRIs	Antidepressant effect of SSRIs are possibly antagonized by cyproheptadine	Cyproheptadine is an antihistamine with antiserotonergic activity	Be aware
TERFENADINE	SSRIs	Possibility of ↑ terfenadine levels with potential risk of dangerous arrhythmias	These drugs are metabolized mainly by CYP3A4. Fluvoxamine and fluoxetine are inhibitors of CYP3A4 but are relatively weak compared with ketoconazole, which is possibly 100 times more potent as an inhibitor	Avoid coadministration
KETOTIFEN	ANTIDIABETIC DRUGS—METFORMIN	↓ Platelet count	Unknown	Avoid coadministration (manufacturers' recommendation)
ANTIHISTAMINES	**ANTIFUNGALS—AZOLES**			
MIZOLASTINE	AZOLES	↑ Mizolastine levels	Inhibition of metabolism of mizolastine	Avoid coadministration
LORATADINE	KETOCONAZOLE, POSACONAZOLE	↑ loratadine levels	Inhibition of CYP450, Pgp, or both	Avoid coadministration
ANTIHISTAMINES	**ANTIVIRALS**			
ASTEMIZOLE, TERFENADINE	NNRTIs—EFAVIRENZ	Risk of ventricular arrhythmias, particularly torsades de pointes	Possible ↓ metabolism via CYP3A4	Avoid coadministration, cetirizine is a suitable alternative
ASTEMIZOLE, MIZOLASTINE, TERFENADINE	PROTEASE INHIBITORS	Possibly ↑ adverse effects of antihistamine, including QT prolongation	Inhibition of metabolism via CYP3A4 (all) and CYP2D6 (terfenadine), inhibition of transport via Pgp (terfenadine)	Avoid coadministration. Risk is greatest in patients who are also poor CYP2D6 metabolizers

(Continued)

RESPIRATORY DRUGS ANTIHISTAMINES

Primary Drug	Secondary Drug	Effect	Mechanism	Precautions
ANTIHISTAMINES				
ANTIHISTAMINES	ANXIOLYTICS AND HYPNOTICS—SODIUM OXYBATE	Risk of CNS depression—coma, respiratory depression	Additive depression of CNS	Avoid coadministration. Caution even with relatively nonsedating antihistamines (cetirizine, desloratadine, fexofenadine, levocetirizine, loratadine, mizolastine) as they can impair the performance of skilled tasks
ANTIHISTAMINES	**GRAPEFRUIT JUICE**			
FEXOFENADINE	GRAPEFRUIT JUICE	Possibly ↓ efficacy	↓ Absorption possibly by affecting Pgp and direct inhibition of uptake by intestinal OATP-1A2	Clinical significance unclear. No clinically significant changes in ECG parameters were observed in one study
TERFENADINE	GRAPEFRUIT JUICE	Possibly ↑ efficacy and ↑ adverse effects, e.g., torsades de points	Altered metabolism so parent drug accumulates	Avoid concomitant intake
ASTEMIZOLE, LORATADINE, HYDROXYZINE, MIZOLASTINE, TERFENADINE	H2-RECEPTOR BLOCKERS—CIMETIDINE	↑ Plasma levels, potential to increase in QTc	Inhibition of metabolism	Be aware; manufacturer of mizolastine advises avoiding coadministration. Cimetidine and loratadine were not shown to increase QTc in clinical trials

Primary Drug	Secondary Drug	Effect	Mechanism	Precautions
ASTHMA PROPHYLAXIS				
CORTICOSTEROIDS—*see Anticancer and Other Immunomodulating Drugs Section*				
LEUKOTRIENE RECEPTOR ANTAGONISTS				
ZAFIRLUKAST	ANTIPLATELET AGENTS—ASPIRIN	↑ Levels of zafirlukast	Uncertain	Watch for early features of zafirlukast toxicity. Monitor FBC and liver function closely
ZAFIRLUKAST	ANTIBIOTICS—MACROLIDES	↓ Zafirlukast levels	Induction of metabolism	Watch for poor response to zafirlukast

(*Continued*)

Primary Drug	Secondary Drug	Effect	Mechanism	Precautions
ASTHMA PROPHYLAXIS				
ZAFIRLUKAST	ANTICOAGULANTS—ORAL	Zafirlukast ↑ anticoagulant effect	Zafirlukast inhibits CYP2C9-mediated metabolism of warfarin	Monitor INR at least weekly until stable
ZAFIRLUKAST	ANTIDEPRESSANTS—TCAs	Possible ↑ plasma concentrations of zafirlukast	Inhibition of CYP2C9-mediated metabolism of zafirlukast. The clinical significance of this depends upon whether alternative pathways of metabolism are also inhibited by coadministered drugs	Warn patients to report ↑ side effects
MONTELUKAST	ANTIDIABETIC DRUGS—REPAGLINIDE	↑ Repaglinide levels, risk of hypoglycemia	Hepatic metabolism inhibited	Watch for and warn patients about hypoglycemia ➢ ***For signs and symptoms of hypoglycemia, see Clinical Features of Some Adverse Drug Interactions, Hypoglycemia***
MONTELUKAST	ANTIEPILEPTICS—BARBITURATES	↓ Montelukast levels	Induction of metabolism	Watch for poor response to montelukast
ZAFIRLUKAST	BRONCHODILATORS—THEOPHYLLINE	Possibly ↑ theophylline levels. Also possibly ↓ zafirlukast levels	Mutual alteration of metabolism	Be aware; watch for features of theophylline toxicity and measure levels
MONTELUKAST	GRAPEFRUIT JUICE	Montelukast undergoes transport by OATP2B1. GFJ at 5% and 10% (v/v) and orange juice at 10%, ↓ montelukast permeability significantly ~30%	Enteric OATP-mediated drug–grapefruit juice interaction	Clinical relevance of these interactions has not been examined

Primary Drug	Secondary Drug	Effect	Mechanism	Precautions
BRONCHODILATORS				
BRONCHODILATORS	**DRUGS THAT PROLONG THE QT INTERVALS**			
PARENTERAL BRONCHODILATORS	1. ANTIARRHYTHMICS—ajmaline, amiodarone, azimilide, cibenzoline, disopyramide, dofetilide, dronedarone, ibutilide, procainamide, propafenone, quinidine 2. ANTIBIOTICS—macrolides (especially azithromycin, clarithromycin, parenteral erythromycin, telithromycin), quinolones (especially moxifloxacin), quinupristin/dalfopristin 3. ANTICANCER AND IMMUNOMODULATING DRUGS—arsenic trioxide, bosutinib, crizotinib, dasatinib, eribulin, fingolimod, lapatinib, nilotinib, pazopanib, sunitinib, vandetanib, vemurafenib 4. ANTIDEPRESSANTS—TCAs, venlafaxine 5. ANTIEMETICS—ondansetron 6. ANTIFUNGALS—fluconazole, posaconazole, voriconazole 7. ANTIHISTAMINES—terfenadine, hydroxyzine, mizolastine 8. Antihypertensives—ketanserin 9. ANTIMALARIALS—artemether with lumefantrine, chloroquine, halofantrine, hydroxychloroquine, mefloquine, quinine 10. ANTIPROTOZOALS—pentamidine isetionate 11. ANTIPSYCHOTICS—atypicals, phenothiazines, pimozide 12. ANTIVIRALS—boceprevir, rilpivirine, telaprevir 13. BETA-BLOCKERS—sotalol 14. CNS STIMULANTS—atomoxetine 15. RANOLAZINE	Risk of ventricular arrhythmias, particularly torsades de pointes	Additive effect; these drugs prolong the QT interval Also, amitriptyline, clomipramine, and desipramine levels may be ↑ by propafenone Amitriptyline and clomipramine may ↑ propafenone levels Propafenone and these TCAs inhibit CYP2D6-mediated metabolism of each other	Avoid coadministration

(Continued)

Primary Drug	Secondary Drug	Effect	Mechanism	Precautions
BRONCHODILATORS				
ANTIMUSCARINICS (IPRATROPIUM, TIOTROPIUM) ➢ *Drugs Acting on the Nervous System, Anti-Parkinson's Drugs*				
BETA-2 AGONISTS				
TERBUTALINE	ANESTHETICS, GENERAL—HALOTHANE	Cases of arrhythmias when terbutaline coadministered with halothane	Possibly due to sensitization of the myocardium to circulating catecholamines	Risk of cardiac events is higher with halothane. Desflurane is an irritant to the upper respiratory tract, and ↑ secretions can occur; it is best avoided in patients with bronchial asthma. Sevoflurane is nonirritant and unlikely to cause serious adverse effects
BETA-2 AGONISTS	ANALGESICS—NSAIDs	Etoricoxib may ↑ oral salbutamol levels	Etoricoxib inhibits sulfotransferase activity	Monitor PR and BP closely
BETA-2 AGONISTS	ANTIBIOTICS—LINEZOLID	Theoretical risk of hypertensive reactions	Linezolid has weak MAOI properties	Monitor BP closely during coadministration
BETA-2 AGONISTS	ANTICANCER AND IMMUNOMODULATING DRUGS—CORTICOSTEROIDS	Risk of hypokalemia	Additive effect	Monitor blood potassium levels prior to concomitant administration and during therapy (monitor at least daily during parenteral administration). Administer potassium supplements to prevent hypokalemia, which may also be worsened by hypoxia during severe attacks of asthma
BETA-2 AGONISTS	ANTIDEPRESSANTS—MAOIs	↑ Occurrence of headache and hypertensive episodes. Unlikely to occur with moclobemide and selegiline	Due to impaired metabolism of these sympathomimetic amines because of inhibition of MAOI. Moclobemide is involved in the breakdown of serotonin, while selegiline is mainly involved in the breakdown of dopamine	Be aware. Monitor BP closely

(Continued)

Primary Drug	Secondary Drug	Effect	Mechanism	Precautions
BRONCHODILATORS				
BETA AGONISTS	ANTIDIABETIC DRUGS	1. ↑ Risk of hyperglycemia. 2. If administered during pregnancy, there is a risk of hypoglycemia in the fetus, independent of maternal blood glucose levels, ↑ risk of ketoacidosis when administered intravenously	1. By inducing glycogenolysis, beta-adrenergic agonists cause elevation of blood sugar in adults. 2. In the fetus, these agents cause a depletion of fetal glycogen stores	1. Monitor blood sugar closely during concomitant administration until blood sugar levels are stable. 2. Be cautious during use in pregnancy
BETA-2 AGONISTS	ANTIHYPERTENSIVE AND HEART FAILURE DRUGS—CENTRALLY ACTING ANTIHYPERTENSIVES	Cases of ↓ BP when intravenous salbutamol is given with methyldopa	Uncertain at present	Monitor BP closely
SALMETEROL	ANTIVIRALS—COBICISTAT, ATAZANAVIR/RITONAVIR, LOPINAVIR/RITONAVIR, RITONAVIR, TIPRANAVIR, SAQUINAVIR/RITONAVIR	Possibly ↑ plasma levels of salmeterol and ↑ cardiovascular side effects, e.g., QT prolongation, tachycardia	Inhibition of metabolism via CYP3A4	Coadministration not recommended
BETA-2 AGONISTS	BETA-BLOCKERS	Nonselective beta-blockers (e.g., propanolol) ↓ or prevent the bronchodilator effect of beta-2 agonists	Nonselective beta-blockers antagonize the effect of beta-2 agonists on bronchial smooth muscle	Avoid coadministration
SALBUTAMOL	BETAHISTINE	↓ Or prevents the bronchodilator effect	Betahistine causes bronchoconstriction	Avoid coadministration
BETA-2 AGONISTS	**BRONCHODILATORS**			
BETA-2 AGONISTS	THEOPHYLLINE	Risk of hypokalemia	Additive effect. The CSM notes that this effect occurs with beta-2 agonists, theophyllines, and corticosteroids, all of which may be given during severe asthma; hypoxia exacerbates this effect	Coadministration is useful for the management of severe asthma. Monitor blood potassium levels prior to concomitant administration and during therapy (monitor 1–2 hourly during parenteral administration). Administer potassium supplements to prevent hypokalemia, which may also be worsened by hypoxia during severe asthma attacks

(Continued)

Primary Drug	Secondary Drug	Effect	Mechanism	Precautions
BRONCHODILATORS				
BETA AGONISTS	ANTIDIABETIC DRUGS	1. ↑ Risk of hyperglycemia. 2. If administered during pregnancy, there is a risk of hypoglycemia in the fetus, independent of maternal blood glucose levels, ↑ risk of ketoacidosis when administered intravenously	1. By inducing glycogenolysis, beta-adrenergic agonists cause elevation of blood sugar in adults. 2. In the fetus, these agents cause a depletion of fetal glycogen stores	1. Monitor blood sugar closely during concomitant administration until blood sugar levels are stable. 2. Be cautious during use in pregnancy.
SALBUTAMOL	IPRATROPIUM BROMIDE	A few reports of acute closed-angle glaucoma when nebulized ipratropium and salbutamol were coadministered	Ipratropium dilates the pupil, which ↓ drainage of aqueous humor, while salbutamol ↑ production of aqueous humor	Warn patients to prevent the solution/mist entering the eye. Use extreme caution in coadministering these bronchodilators by the nebulized route in patients with a history of acute closed-angle glaucoma
BETA-2 AGONISTS	CARDIAC GLYCOSIDES—DIGOXIN	1. Hypokalemia may exacerbate digoxin toxicity 2. Salbutamol may ↓ digoxin levels (by 16%–22%) after 10 days of concurrent therapy	1. Beta-2 agonists may cause hypokalemia 2. Uncertain	1. Monitor potassium levels closely 2. Clinical significance is uncertain. Useful to monitor digoxin levels if there is a clinical indication of ↓ response to digoxin
SALBUTAMOL	CNS STIMULANTS—ATOMOXETINE	↑ Risk of arrhythmias with parenteral salbutamol	Additive effect	Avoid coadministration of atomoxetine with parenteral salbutamol
BETA-2 AGONISTS	DIURETICS—CARBONIC ANHYDRASE INHIBITORS, LOOP, AND THIAZIDES	Risk of hypokalemia	Additive effects	Monitor blood potassium levels prior to concomitant administration and during therapy. Administer potassium supplements to prevent hypokalemia

(Continued)

Primary Drug	Secondary Drug	Effect	Mechanism	Precautions
BRONCHODILATORS				
SALBUTAMOL	EPHEDRA	Risk of marked ↑ heart rate and of BP	Additive effect; ephedra causes vasoconstriction	The U.S. FDA has banned products containing ephedra. Warn patients on salbutamol to avoid traditional remedies containing ephedra
BAMBUTEROL	MUSCLE RELAXANTS—SUXAMETHONIUM	↑ Effect of suxamethonium	Bambuterol is an inhibitor of pseudocholinesterase, which hydrolyzes suxamethonium	Be cautious of prolonged periods of respiratory muscle paralysis, and monitor respiration closely until complete recovery
SALBUTAMOL	YOHIMBINE	↑ Risk of CNS stimulation	Uncertain; yohimbine may cause ↑ dopamine levels	Warn patients taking salbutamol to avoid remedies containing yohimbine
NONSELECTIVE BETA-AGONISTS ➢ *Sympathomimetics Section*—CVS *Chapter*				
THEOPHYLLINES				
THEOPHYLLINE	**ANESTHETICS—GENERAL**			
THEOPHYLLINE	HALOTHANE	Case reports of arrhythmias	Possibly due to sensitization of the myocardium to circulating catecholamines	Risk of cardiac events is higher with halothane. Desflurane is an irritant to the upper respiratory tract, and ↑ secretions can occur; it is best avoided in patients with bronchial asthma. Sevoflurane is nonirritant and unlikely to cause serious adverse effects
THEOPHYLLINE	KETAMINE	Risk of fits	Uncertain	A careful risk–benefit assessment should be made before using ketamine. However, there are significant benefits for the use of ketamine to anesthetize patients for the emergency management of life-threatening asthma

(*Continued*)

Primary Drug	Secondary Drug	Effect	Mechanism	Precautions
BRONCHODILATORS				
AMINOPHYLLINE	PROCAINE SOLUTIONS	Precipitation of drugs, which may not be immediately apparent	A pharmaceutical interaction	Do not mix in the same infusion or syringe
THEOPHYLLINE	**ANTIARRHYTHMICS**			
THEOPHYLLINE	ADENOSINE	↓ Efficacy of adenosine	Theophylline and other xanthines are adenosine receptor antagonists	Watch for poor response to adenosine; higher doses may be required
THEOPHYLLINE	AMIODARONE	Theophylline levels may be ↑ by amiodarone (single case report of theophylline levels doubling)	Uncertain; amiodarone probably inhibits the metabolism of theophylline	Watch for theophylline toxicity; monitor theophylline levels regularly until stable
THEOPHYLLINE	MEXILETINE	Theophylline levels may be ↑ by mexiletine; cases of theophylline toxicity have been reported	Mexiletine inhibits CYP1A2-mediated metabolism of theophylline	↓ Theophylline dose (by up to 50%). Monitor theophylline levels and watch for toxicity
THEOPHYLLINE	MORACIZINE	↓ Plasma concentrations of theophylline and risk of therapeutic failure	Due to induction of microsomal enzyme activity	May need to ↑ dose of theophylline by 25%
THEOPHYLLINE	PROPAFENONE	Case reports of ↑ theophylline levels with toxicity when propafenone was added	Uncertain at present	Watch for signs of theophylline toxicity
THEOPHYLLINE	**ANTIBIOTICS**			
THEOPHYLLINE	ISONIAZID, MACROLIDES (azithromycin, clarithromycin, erythromycin, telithromycin), QUINOLONES	1. ↑ Theophylline levels. 2. Possibly ↓ erythromycin levels when given orally	1. Inhibition of CYP2D6-mediated metabolism of theophylline (macrolides and quinolones—isoniazid not known) 2. ↓ Bioavailability; uncertain mechanism	1. Monitor theophylline levels before, during, and after coadministration 2. Consider alternative macrolide
THEOPHYLLINE	RIFAMPICIN	↓ Plasma concentrations of theophylline and risk of therapeutic failure	Due to induction of CYP1A2 and CYP3A3	May need to ↑ dose of theophylline by 25%

(Continued)

Primary Drug	Secondary Drug	Effect	Mechanism	Precautions
BRONCHODILATORS				
THEOPHYLLINE	**ANTICANCER AND IMMUNOMODULATING DRUGS**			
THEOPHYLLINE	ADALIMUMAB	Possible ↓ levels of theophylline	Reversal of CYP450 suppression by adalimumab. Theophylline has a narrow therapeutic index	Monitor closely; dose adjustment may be needed
THEOPHYLLINE	ANAKINRA	Possible ↓ levels of theophylline	Reversal of CYP450 suppression by adalimumab. Theophylline has a narrow therapeutic index	Monitor closely; dose adjustment may be needed
THEOPHYLLINE	AXITINIB	Possible ↑ levels of theophylline	Axitinib inhibits CYP1A2	Caution with concurrent use
THEOPHYLLINE	CORTICOSTEROIDS	Risk of hypokalemia	Additive effect. The CSM notes that this effect occurs with beta-2 agonists, theophyllines, and corticosteroids, all of which may be given during severe asthma; hypoxia exacerbates this effect	Monitor blood potassium levels prior to concomitant administration and during therapy (monitor at least daily during parenteral administration). Administer potassium supplements to prevent hypokalemia, which may also be worsened by hypoxia during severe attacks of asthma
THEOPHYLLINE	GOLIMUMAB	Possible ↓ levels of theophylline	Induction of metabolism	Monitor closely; dose adjustment may be needed
THEOPHYLLINE	INFLIXIMAB	Possible ↓ levels of theophylline	Reversal of CYP450 suppression by adalimumab. Theophylline has a narrow therapeutic index	Monitor closely; dose adjustment may be needed
THEOPHYLLINE	INTERFERON ALFA	↑ Theophylline levels	Inhibition of theophylline metabolism	Monitor theophylline levels before, during, and after coadministration
THEOPHYLLINE	LOMUSTINE	Single case report of thrombocytopenia and bleeding	Inhibition of platelet phosphodiesterase activity by theophylline	Be aware. Clinical significance uncertain

(*Continued*)

RESPIRATORY DRUGS BRONCHODILATORS

Primary Drug	Secondary Drug	Effect	Mechanism	Precautions
BRONCHODILATORS				
THEOPHYLLINE	METHOTREXATE	Possible ↑ theophylline levels	Possibly inhibition of CYP2D6-mediated metabolism of theophylline	Monitor clinically for toxic effects, and advise patients to seek medical attention if they have symptoms suggestive of theophylline toxicity. Measure theophylline levels before, during, and after coadministration
THEOPHYLLINE	PIXANTRONE	Theoretical risk of ↑ theophylline levels	Pixantrone inhibits CYP1A2	Manufacturer advises close monitoring
THEOPHYLLINE	TOCILIZUMAB	↓ Levels	Tocilizumab reverses CYP450 isoenzyme suppression by IL-6	Monitor closely and consider dose adjustment
THEOPHYLLINE	**ANTIDEPRESSANTS**			
THEOPHYLLINE INCLUDES CAFFEINE	LITHIUM	↓ Plasma levels of lithium and risk of therapeutic failure	Theophylline ↑ renal clearance of lithium	May need to ↑ dose of lithium by 60%
THEOPHYLLINE	ST. JOHN'S WORT	↓ Theophylline levels	Inhibition of CYP1A2-mediated metabolism of theophylline	Avoid coadministration
THEOPHYLLINE	SSRIs—FLUVOXAMINE	Fluvoxamine is a potent inhibitor of CYP1A2, fluoxetine is less potent, and paroxetine and sertraline are weak inhibitors	Consider an alternative antidepressant, e.g., escitalopram and citalopram, which are not currently known to cause any inhibition	Fluvoxamine is a potent inhibitor of CYP1A2, fluoxetine is less potent, and paroxetine and sertraline are weak inhibitors
THEOPHYLLINE	TCAs	Possible ↑ theophylline levels	Inhibition of CYP1A2- and CYP2D6-mediated metabolism of theophylline. The clinical significance of this depends upon whether theophylline's alternative pathways of metabolism are also inhibited by coadministered drugs	Warn patients to report any ↑ side effects of theophylline, and monitor PR and ECG carefully

(*Continued*)

Primary Drug	Secondary Drug	Effect	Mechanism	Precautions
BRONCHODILATORS				
THEOPHYLLINE	ANTIEPILEPTICS—BARBITURATES, CARBAMAZEPINE	↓ Theophylline levels. Possibly ↓ carbamazepine and phenytoin levels	Due to induction of microsomal enzyme activity. Theophylline ↓ absorption of phenytoin	May need to ↑ dose of theophylline by 25%. Monitor for inadequate therapeutic response to carbamazepine and phenytoin. Measure levels of these drugs
THEOPHYLLINE	PHENYTOIN	1. ↓ Levels of theophylline with risk of therapeutic failure 2. Phenytoin levels may be ↓ by theophylline	1. Induction of hepatic metabolism 2. Uncertain; theophylline ↓ absorption of phenytoin	1. Monitor for ↓ clinical efficacy and ↑ their dose as required. May need to ↑ dose of theophylline by 25% 2. Monitor phenytoin levels when coadministered with theophylline
THEOPHYLLINE	**ANTIFUNGALS**			
THEOPHYLLINE	AZOLES—ITRACONAZOLE, KETOCONAZOLE	↑ Theophylline levels, with risk of toxicity with itraconazole Unpredictable effect on theophylline levels with ketoconazole	Theophylline is primarily metabolized by CYP1A2. Although azoles are best known as inhibitors of CYP3A4, they also inhibit other CYP isoenzymes to varying degrees	If concurrent use is necessary, monitor theophylline levels on initiation and discontinuation of itraconazole therapy. Other azoles or terbinafine may be a safer alternative
THEOPHYLLINE	GRISEOFULVIN	↑ Theophylline levels	Inhibition of metabolism of theophylline	Uncertain clinical significance. Watch for early features of theophylline toxicity
THEOPHYLLINE	**ANTIGOUT DRUGS**			
THEOPHYLLINE	ALLOPURINOL	May ↑ theophylline levels	Probable inhibition of theophylline metabolism	Watch for early features of toxicity of theophylline (headache, nausea). Monitor theophylline levels when starting or increasing allopurinol
THEOPHYLLINE	SULFINPYRAZONE	↓ Theophylline levels	Due to ↑ demethylation and hydroxylation and thus ↑ clearance of theophylline	May need to ↑ dose of theophylline by 25%

(Continued)

Primary Drug	Secondary Drug	Effect	Mechanism	Precautions
BRONCHODILATORS				
THEOPHYLLINE	**ANTIVIRALS**			
THEOPHYLLINE	ACYCLOVIR/VALACYCLOVIR	↑ Theophylline levels	Uncertain	Monitor for signs of toxicity and check levels
THEOPHYLLINE	INDINAVIR	Possibly ↑ efficacy	Inhibition of metabolism via CYP3A4, but mainly metabolized via CYP1A2, which is not inhibited	Not thought to be clinically significant; however, monitor levels more closely in unstable patients
THEOPHYLLINE	RITONAVIR (± LOPINAVIR)	↓ Efficacy	↑ Metabolism via induction of CYP1A2; also altered metabolism via CYP3A4	Monitor clinical response; measure levels weekly after starting; ↑ doses may be required
THEOPHYLLINE	ANXIOLYTICS AND HYPNOTICS—benzodiazepines	↓ Therapeutic effect of benzodiazepines	Benzodiazepines ↑ CNS concentrations of adenosine, a potent CNS depressant, while theophylline blocks adenosine receptors	Larger doses of diazepam are required to produce desired therapeutic effects such as sedation. Discontinuation of theophylline without ↓ the dose of benzodiazepines ↑ risk of sedation and respiratory depression
THEOPHYLLINE	BETA-BLOCKERS—PROPRANOLOL	↑ Plasma levels of theophylline with propranolol	Propranolol exerts a dose-dependent inhibitory effect on the metabolism of theophylline	Monitor theophylline levels during propranolol coadministration
THEOPHYLLINE	BRONCHODILATORS—BETA-2 AGONISTS	Risk of hypokalemia	Additive effect. The CSM notes that this effect occurs with beta-2 agonists, theophyllines, and corticosteroids, all of which may be given during severe asthma; hypoxia exacerbates this effect	Coadministration is useful for the management of severe asthma. Monitor blood potassium levels prior to concomitant administration and during therapy (monitor 1–2 hourly during parenteral administration). Administer potassium supplements to prevent hypokalemia, which may also be worsened by hypoxia during severe attacks of asthma

(*Continued*)

Primary Drug	Secondary Drug	Effect	Mechanism	Precautions
BRONCHODILATORS				
THEOPHYLLINE	**CALCIUM CHANNEL BLOCKERS**			
THEOPHYLLINE	DILTIAZEM, VERAPAMIL	↑ Theophylline levels with diltiazem and verapamil. Mostly not clinically significant but two case reports of theophylline toxicity with verapamil	Uncertain but thought to be due to inhibition of CYP1A2-mediated metabolism of theophylline	Be aware of the small possibility of theophylline toxicity when commencing calcium channel blockers; check levels if any problems occur, and consider either ↓ the dose of theophylline or using an alternative calcium channel blocker
THEOPHYLLINE	NIFEDIPINE	Clinically nonsignificant ↓ theophylline levels with nifedipine, but case reports of theophylline toxicity after starting nifedipine	Uncertain; probably due to alterations in either the metabolism or volume of distribution of theophylline	Be aware of the small possibility of theophylline toxicity when commencing calcium channel blockers; check levels if any problems occur, and consider either ↓ the dose of theophylline or using an alternative calcium channel blocker
THEOPHYLLINE	CNS STIMULANTS—MODAFINIL	May cause ↓ theophylline levels	Modafinil is a moderate inducer of CYP1A2 in a concentration-dependent manner	Be aware; watch for poor response to theophylline and measure levels
THEOPHYLLINE	DIURETICS—CARBONIC ANHYDRASE INHIBITORS, LOOP, AND THIAZIDES	Risk of hypokalemia	Additive effects	Monitor blood potassium levels prior to concomitant administration and during therapy. Administer potassium supplements to prevent hypokalemia
THEOPHYLLINE	DOXAPRAM	Reports of ↑ muscle tone and CNS excitation	Uncertain	Be aware

(Continued)

Primary Drug	Secondary Drug	Effect	Mechanism	Precautions
BRONCHODILATORS				
THEOPHYLLINE	**DRUG DEPENDENCE THERAPIES**			
THEOPHYLLINE	BUPROPION	1. ↑ Theophylline levels 2. ↑ Risk of seizures. This risk is marked in elderly people, patients with a history of seizures, with addiction to opiates/cocaine/stimulants, and diabetics treated with oral hypoglycemics or insulin	1. Smoking induces mainly CYP1A2 and CYP2E1. Thus, deinduction takes place following the cessation of smoking 2. Bupropion is associated with a dose-related risk of seizures. These drugs, which lower seizure threshold, are individually epileptogenic. Additive effects occur when they are combined	1. Be aware, particularly with drugs with a narrow therapeutic index (See Appendix B). Monitor clinically and biochemically (e.g., INR, plasma theophylline levels) 2. Extreme caution. The dose of bupropion should not exceed 450 mg/day (or 150 mg/day in patients with severe hepatic cirrhosis)
THEOPHYLLINE	DISULFIRAM	↑ Theophylline levels	Disulfiram ↓ theophylline clearance by inhibiting hydroxylation and demethylation	Monitor theophylline levels before, during, and after coadministration
THEOPHYLLINE	GRAPEFRUIT JUICE	Possibly ↓ efficacy	Unclear. ↓ Bioavailability (significant from 1 to 4 h)	Avoid concomitant intake if slow-release theophylline preparations are used. Monitor levels and clinical state weekly if the intake of grapefruit is altered
THEOPHYLLINE	H2 RECEPTOR BLOCKERS—CIMETIDINE, FAMOTIDINE, NIZATIDINE, RANITIDINE	↑ Efficacy and adverse effects, including seizures. There is conflicting information associated with ranitidine, famotidine, and nizatidine	Inhibition of metabolism via CYP1A2, cimetidine being the best known inhibitor	Use alternative acid suppression, e.g., an H2 antagonist or proton pump inhibitor (not omeprazole or lansoprazole), or monitor closely; there is considerable patient variation. Check levels on day 3 and then at 1 week. A 30%–50% ↓ dose of theophylline may be required. For doses <400 mg/day, the interaction may not be clinically significant

(Continued)

Primary Drug	Secondary Drug	Effect	Mechanism	Precautions
BRONCHODILATORS				
THEOPHYLLINE	LEUKOTRIENE RECEPTOR ANTAGONISTS—ZAFIRLUKAST	Possibly ↑ theophylline levels. Also possibly ↓ zafirlukast levels	Mutual alteration of metabolism	Be aware; watch for features of theophylline toxicity and measure levels
THEOPHYLLINE	MUSCLE RELAXANTS—PANCURONIUM	Antagonism of neuromuscular block	Uncertain	Larger doses of pancuronium may be needed to obtain the desired muscle relaxation during anesthesia; other nondepolarizing muscle relaxants do not seem to be affected
THEOPHYLLINE	ESTROGENS	↑ Theophylline levels	↓ Clearance of theophylline in a dose-dependent manner	Be aware; watch for features of theophylline toxicity and measure levels
THEOPHYLLINE	PERIPHERAL VASODILATORS—PENTOXIFYLLINE	Possibly ↑ theophylline levels	Uncertain; possibly competitive inhibition of theophylline metabolism (pentoxifylline is also a xanthine derivative)	Warn patients of the possibility of adverse effects of theophylline; monitor levels if necessary
THEOPHYLLINE	PHOSPHODIESTERASE INHIBITORS—ENOXIMONE	Theophylline may ↓ efficacy of enoximone	Possibly competitive inhibition of phosphodiesterases	Be aware; watch for poor response to enoximone
THEOPHYLLINE	PROTON PUMP INHIBITORS—LANSOPRAZOLE, OMEPRAZOLE	↓ Plasma concentrations of theophylline	Induced CYP1A2-mediated metabolism of theophylline	↑ Dose may be required. Consider using the proton pump inhibitor regularly, not as required. Monitor theophylline levels when starting or stopping treatment
THEOPHYLLINE	SUCRALFATE	Possibly ↓ theophylline levels (with modified-release preparations)	Possibly ↓ absorption	Watch for poor response to theophylline and monitor levels
THEOPHYLLINE	**SYMPATHOMIMETICS**			
THEOPHYLLINE	INDIRECTLY ACTING SYMPATHOMIMETICS	↑ Incidence of side effects of theophylline (without a change in its serum concentrations) when coadministered with ephedrine	Uncertain	Avoid coadministration. Warn patients to avoid OTC remedies containing ephedrine

(Continued)

RESPIRATORY DRUGS BRONCHODILATORS

RESPIRATORY DRUGS CYSTIC FIBROSIS THERAPIES—IVACAFTOR

Primary Drug	Secondary Drug	Effect	Mechanism	Precautions
BRONCHODILATORS				
THEOPHYLLINE	DIRECTLY ACTING SYMPATHOMIMETICS	Case report of marked tachycardia when dobutamine was given to a patient already taking theophylline	Uncertain	Carefully titrate the dose of dobutamine in patients taking theophylline therapy
THEOPHYLLINE	THYROID HORMONES	Altered theophylline levels (↑ or ↓) when thyroid status is altered therapeutically	Uncertain	Monitor theophylline levels closely during changes in treatment of abnormal thyroid function. Watch for early features of theophylline toxicity

Primary Drug	Secondary Drug	Effect	Mechanism	Precautions
CYSTIC FIBROSIS THERAPIES—IVACAFTOR				
IVACAFTOR	**ANTIBIOTICS**			
IVACAFTOR	MACROLIDES—CLARITHROMYCIN, ERYTHROMYCIN, TELITHROMYCIN	↑ Ivacaftor levels	Inhibition of CYP3A4-mediated metabolism of ivacaftor	Manufacturers recommend reducing ivacaftor dose to 150 mg 2×/week (150 mg od with erythromycin)
IVACAFTOR	RIFAMPICIN, RIFABUTIN	↓ Ivacaftor levels	Induction of CYP3A4-mediated metabolism of ivacaftor	Manufacturers advise against coadministration
IVACAFTOR	ANTICANCER AND OTHER IMMUNOMODULATING DRUGS—CICLOSPORIN, TACROLIMUS	Possible increased ciclosporin and tacrolimus levels	Pgp inhibition	Caution with concurrent use
IVACAFTOR	ANTICOAGULANTS—WARFARIN	Theoretical risk of ↑ warfarin levels	Ivacaftor inhibits CYP2C9 that metabolizes warfarin	Monitor INR closely until stable
IVACAFTOR	ANTIDEPRESSANTS—ST. JOHN'S WORT	↓ Ivacaftor levels	Induction of CYP3A4-mediated metabolism of ivacaftor	Manufacturers advise against coadministration
IVACAFTOR	ANTIEPILEPTICS—CARBAMAZEPINE, FOSPHENYTOIN, PHENYTOIN	↓ Ivacaftor levels	Induction of CYP3A4-mediated metabolism of ivacaftor	Manufacturers advise against coadministration
IVACAFTOR	ANTIFUNGALS—FLUCONAZOLE, ITRACONAZOLE, KETOCONAZOLE, POSACONAZOLE, VORICONAZOLE	↑ Ivacaftor levels	Inhibition of CYP3A4-mediated metabolism of ivacaftor	Manufacturers recommend reducing ivacaftor dose to 150 mg 2×/week (150 mg od with fluconazole)

(*Continued*)

Primary Drug	Secondary Drug	Effect	Mechanism	Precautions
CYSTIC FIBROSIS THERAPIES—IVACAFTOR				
IVACAFTOR	ANTIHYPERTENSIVES AND HEART FAILURE DRUGS—BOSENTAN	↓ Ivacaftor levels	Induction of CYP3A4-mediated metabolism of ivacaftor	Manufacturers advise avoiding coadministration
IVACAFTOR	**ANTIVIRALS**			
IVACAFTOR	BOCEPREVIR, COBICISTAT, NELFINAVIR, RITONAVIR, SAQUINAVIR, TELAPREVIR	↑ Ivacaftor levels	Inhibition of CYP3A4-mediated metabolism of ivacaftor	Manufacturers recommend reducing ivacaftor dose to 150 mg 2×/week
IVACAFTOR	EFAVIRENZ	↓ Ivacaftor levels	Induction of CYP3A4-mediated metabolism of ivacaftor	Manufacturers advise avoiding coadministration
IVACAFTOR	ANXIOLYTICS AND HYPNOTICS—MIDAZOLAM	Possible ↑ midazolam levels	Ivacaftor possibly inhibits CYP3A4-mediated metabolism of midazolam	Monitor levels of sedation closely
IVACAFTOR	CARDIAC GLYCOSIDES—DIGOXIN	Plasma digoxin concentrations may be ↑ by ivacaftor	Uncertain; probably due to inhibition of Pgp-mediated renal excretion of digoxin and ↑ intestinal absorption	Monitor digoxin levels; watch for digoxin toxicity

Primary Drug	Secondary Drug	Effect	Mechanism	Precautions
DOXAPRAM				
DOXAPRAM	BRONCHODILATORS—THEOPHYLLINE	Reports of ↑ muscle tone and CNS excitation	Uncertain	Be aware
DOXAPRAM	SYMPATHOMIMETICS	Risk of ↑ BP	Uncertain at present	Monitor BP closely

Primary Drug	Secondary Drug	Effect	Mechanism	Precautions
PHODPHODIESTERASE TYPE 4 INHIBITORS—ROFLUMILAST				
ROFLUMILAST	ANTIBIOTICS—RIFAMPICIN	↓ Efficacy of roflumilast	Induction of CYP3A4- and 1A2-mediated metabolism of roflumilast and its active metabolite	Monitor for poor response and increase dose as necessary
ROFLUMILAST	ANTIEPILEPTICS—CARBAMAZEPINE, PHENOBARBITAL, PHENYTOIN	↓ Efficacy of roflumilast	Induction of CYP3A4- and 1A2-mediated metabolism of roflumilast and its active metabolite	Monitor for poor response and increase dose as necessary

(Continued)

RESPIRATORY DRUGS PHODPHODIESTERASE TYPE 4 INHIBITORS—ROFLUMILAST

Primary Drug	Secondary Drug	Effect	Mechanism	Precautions
PHODPHODIESTERASE TYPE 4 INHIBITORS—ROFLUMILAST				
ROFLUMILAST	H2-RECEPTOR BLOCKERS—CIMETIDINE	↑ Plasma levels and adverse effects of roflumilast	Inhibition of metabolism via CYP1A2 and CYP3A4	Monitor closely for adverse effects within first weeks of treatment as patients may be unable to tolerate combination

Primary Drug	Secondary Drug	Effect	Mechanism	Precautions
PIRFENIDONE				
PIRFENIDONE	ANTIARRHYTHMICS—AMIODARONE, PROPAFENONE	↑ Pirfenidone levels	Inhibition of metabolism of pirfenidone	Manufacturer recommends avoiding coadministration
PIRFENIDONE	**ANTIBIOTICS**			
PIRFENIDONE	QUINOLONES—CIPROFLOXACIN, ENOXACIN	↑ Pirfenidone levels	Inhibition of CYP1A2-mediated metabolism of pirfenidone	Manufacturer recommends avoiding coadministration
PIRFENIDONE	RIFAMPICIN	↓ Pirfenidone levels	Induction of metabolism of pirfenidone	Manufacturer recommends avoiding coadministration
PIRFENIDONE	ANTIDEPRESSANTS—FLUVOXAMINE	↑ Pirfenidone levels	Inhibition of CYP1A2-mediated metabolism of pirfenidone	Manufacturer recommends avoiding coadministration
PIRFENIDONE	GRAPEFRUIT JUICE	↑ Pirfenidone levels	Inhibition of metabolism of pirfenidone	Manufacturer recommends avoiding coadministration
PIRFENIDONE	PROTON PUMP INHIBITORS—OMEPRAZOLE	↓ Pirfenidone levels	Induction of metabolism of pirfenidone	Manufacturer recommends avoiding coadministration

PART 13

Metabolic Drugs

Simon F.J. Clarke

1. AGALSIDASE
2. ELIGLUSTAT
3. LARONIDASE
4. NITISINONE
5. PENICILLAMINE—*see Anticancer and Immunomodulating Drugs, Other Immunomodulating Drugs*
6. SAPROPTERIN
7. SODIUM PHENYLBUTYRATE
8. TRIENTINE

Primary Drug	Secondary Drug	Effect	Mechanism	Precautions
AGALSIDASE				
AGALSIDASE	ANTIARRHYTHMICS—AMIODARONE	↓ Clinical effect of agalsidase	Uncertain	Avoid coadministration
AGALSIDASE	ANTIBIOTICS—GENTAMICIN	Possibly ↓ clinical effect of agalsidase	Uncertain	Avoid coadministration
AGALSIDASE	ANTIMALARIALS—CHLOROQUINE	↓ Efficacy of agalsidase	Inhibition of intracellular activity of agalsidase beta	Avoid coadministration—manufacturers' recommendation

Primary Drug	Secondary Drug	Effect	Mechanism	Precautions
ELIGLUSTAT				
Eliglustat is Contraindicated in Patients Already Taking A Combination of CYP2D6 and 3A4 Inhibitors				
ELIGLUSTAT	**ANTIARRHYTHMICS**—QUINIDINE	↑ Eliglustat levels	Inhibition of CYP2D6-mediated metabolism	Reduce dose to 85 mg od
ELIGLUSTAT	**ANTIBIOTICS**			
ELIGLUSTAT	MACROLIDES—CLARITHROMYCIN, ERYTHROMYCIN, ROXITHROMYCIN, TELITHROMYCIN	↑ Eliglustat levels	Inhibition of CYP3A4-mediated metabolism	Reduce dose to 85 mg od in extensive metabolizers. Avoid coadministration in intermediate and poor metabolizers. Roxithromycin is a weak inhibitor of CYP3A4; it should be avoided in poor metabolizers
ELIGLUSTAT	RIFAMPICIN	↓ Eliglustat levels	Induction of CYP3A4-mediated metabolism	Avoid coadministration
ELIGLUSTAT	ANTICOAGULANTS—DABIGATRAN	↑ Dabigatran levels	Inhibition of Pgp	Reduce dose of dabigatran; warn patients to report bleeding
ELIGLUSTAT	**ANTIDEPRESSANTS**			
ELIGLUSTAT	FLUOXETINE, PAROXETINE	↑ Eliglustat levels	Inhibition of CYP2D6-mediated metabolism	Reduce dose to 85 mg od
ELIGLUSTAT	FLUVOXAMINE, NEFAZODONE	↑ Eliglustat levels	Inhibition of CYP3A4-mediated metabolism	Nefazodone: reduce dose to 85 mg od in extensive metabolizers. Avoid coadministration in intermediate and poor metabolizers Fluvoxamine is a weak inhibitor of CYP3A4; it should be avoided in poor metabolizers

(*Continued*)

Primary Drug	Secondary Drug	Effect	Mechanism	Precautions
ELIGLUSTAT				
ELIGLUSTAT	ST. JOHN'S WORT	↓ Eliglustat levels	Induction of CYP3A4-mediated metabolism	Avoid coadministration
ELIGLUSTAT	TCAs—AMITRIPTYLINE, IMIPRAMINE, NORTRIPTYLINE	↑ Levels of these antidepressants	Inhibition of CYP2D6-mediated metabolism	Avoid coadministration
ELIGLUSTAT	ANTIEMETICS—APREPITANT	↑ Eliglustat levels	Inhibition of CYP3A4-mediated metabolism	Reduce dose to 85 mg od in extensive metabolizers. Avoid coadministration in intermediate and poor metabolizers
ELIGLUSTAT	ANTIEPILEPTICS—CARBAMAZEPINE, BARBITURATES, PHENYTOIN	↓ Eliglustat levels	Induction of CYP3A4-mediated metabolism	Avoid coadministration
ELIGLUSTAT	**ANTIFUNGALS**			
ELIGLUSTAT	KETOCONAZOLE, FLUCONAZOLE, POSACONAZOLE, VORICONAZOLE	↑ Eliglustat levels	Inhibition of CYP2A4-mediated metabolism	Reduce dose to 85 mg od
ELIGLUSTAT	TERBINAFINE	↑ Eliglustat levels	Inhibition of CYP2D6-mediated metabolism	Reduce dose to 85 mg od in extensive metabolizers. Avoid coadministration in intermediate and poor metabolizers
ELIGLUSTAT	ANTIGOUT DRUGS—COLCHICINE	↑ Colchicine levels	Inhibition of Pgp	Reduce dose of colchicine; watch for adverse effects
ELIGLUSTAT	ANTIOBESITY DRUGS—LORCASERIN	↑ Eliglustat levels	Inhibition of CYP2D6-mediated metabolism	Reduce dose to 85 mg od in extensive metabolizers. Avoid coadministration in intermediate and poor metabolizers
ELIGLUSTAT	ANTIPSYCHOTICS—CHLOERPROMAZINE, PERPHENAZINE	↑ Levels of these antipsychotics	Inhibition of CYP2D6-mediated metabolism	Reduce doses of these antipsychotics; titrate to effect
ELIGLUSTAT	ANTIVIRALS—COBICISTAT, PROTEASE INHIBITORS	↑ Eliglustat levels	Inhibition of CYP3A4-mediated metabolism	Reduce dose to 85 mg od in extensive metabolizers. Avoid coadministration in intermediate and poor metabolizers
ELIGLUSTAT	BETA-BLOCKERS—METOPROLOL	↑ Metoprolol levels	Inhibition of CYP2D6-mediated metabolism	Reduce dose of metoprolol; monitor PR and BP closely
ELIGLUSTAT	CALCIUM CHANNEL BLOCKERS—DILTIAZEM, VERAPAMIL	↑ Eliglustat levels	Inhibition of CYP3A4-mediated metabolism	Reduce dose to 85 mg od in extensive metabolizers. Avoid coadministration in intermediate and poor metabolizers
ELIGLUSTAT	CARDIAC GLYCOSIDES—DIGOXIN	↑ Digoxin levels	Inhibition of Pgp	Reduce dose of digoxin by 30%. Monitor digoxin levels

(*Continued*)

Primary Drug	Secondary Drug	Effect	Mechanism	Precautions
ELIGLUSTAT				
ELIGLUSTAT	CINACALCET	↑ Eliglustat levels	Inhibition of CYP2D6-mediated metabolism	Reduce dose to 85 mg od
ELIGLUSTAT	CONIVAPTAN	↑ Eliglustat levels	Inhibition of CYP3A4-mediated metabolism	Reduce dose to 85 mg od in extensive metabolizers. Avoid coadministration in intermediate and poor metabolizers
ELIGLUSTAT	DRUG DEPENDENCY THERAPIES—BUPROPION	↑ Eliglustat levels	Inhibition of CYP2D6-mediated metabolism	Reduce dose to 85 mg od
ELIGLUSTAT	GRAPEFRUIT JUICE	↑ Eliglustat levels	Inhibition of CYP3A4-mediated metabolism	Avoid coadministration
ELIGLUSTAT	H2-RECEPTOR BLOCKERS—CIMETIDINE, RANITIDINE	↑ Eliglustat levels	Inhibition of CYP3A4-mediated metabolism	Avoid coadministration in poor metabolizers
ELIGLUSTAT	LIPID-LOWERING DRUGS—LOMITAPIDE	↑ Eliglustat levels	Inhibition of CYP3A4-mediated metabolism	Avoid coadministration in poor metabolizers
ELIGLUSTAT	RANOLAZINE	↑ Eliglustat levels	Inhibition of CYP3A4-mediated metabolism	Avoid coadministration in poor metabolizers

Primary Drug	Secondary Drug	Effect	Mechanism	Precautions
LARONIDASE				
LARONIDASE	ANESTHETICS—LOCAL—PROCAINE	Possibly ↓ efficacy of laronidase	Uncertain	Avoid coadministration
LARONIDASE	ANTIMALARIALS—HYDROXYCHLOROQUINE CHLOROQUINE	↓ Efficacy of laronidase	Uncertain	Avoid coadministration

Primary Drug	Secondary Drug	Effect	Mechanism	Precautions
NITISINONE				
NITISINONE	**ANTIBIOTICS**			
NITISINONE	MACROLIDES—CLARITHROMYCIN, ERYTHROMYCIN, ROXITHROMYCIN, TELITHROMYCIN	Possible ↑ nitisinone levels	Inhibition of CYP3A4-mediated metabolism	Monitor carefully

(Continued)

METABOLIC DRUGS NITISINONE

Primary Drug	Secondary Drug	Effect	Mechanism	Precautions
NITISINONE				
NITISINONE	RIFAMPICIN	Possible ↓ nitisinone levels	Induction of CYP3A4-mediated metabolism	Avoid coadministration
NITISINONE	**ANTIDEPRESSANTS**			
NITISINONE	FLUVOXAMINE, NEFAZODONE	Possible ↑ nitisinone levels	Inhibition of CYP3A4-mediated metabolism	Monitor carefully
NITISINONE	ST. JOHN'S WORT	Possible ↓ nitisinone levels	Induction of CYP3A4-mediated metabolism	Avoid coadministration
NITISINONE	ANTIEMETICS—APREPITANT	Possible ↑ nitisinone levels	Inhibition of CYP3A4-mediated metabolism	Monitor carefully
NITISINONE	ANTIEPILEPTICS—CARBAMAZEPINE, BARBITURATES, PHENYTOIN	Possible ↓ nitisinone levels	Induction of CYP3A4-mediated metabolism	Avoid coadministration
NITISINONE	**ANTIFUNGALS**			
NITISINONE	KETOCONAZOLE, FLUCONAZOLE, POSACONAZOLE, VORICONAZOLE	Possible ↑ nitisinone levels	Inhibition of CYP3A4-mediated metabolism	Monitor carefully
NITISINONE	ANTIVIRALS—COBICISTAT, PROTEASE INHIBITORS	Possible ↑ nitisinone levels	Inhibition of CYP3A4-mediated metabolism	Monitor carefully
NITISINONE	CALCIUM CHANNEL BLOCKERS—DILTIAZEM, VERAPAMIL	Possible ↑ nitisinone levels	Inhibition of CYP3A4-mediated metabolism	Monitor carefully
NITISINONE	CONIVAPTAN	Possible ↑ nitisinone levels	Inhibition of CYP3A4-mediated metabolism	Monitor carefully
NITISINONE	GRAPEFRUIT JUICE	Possible ↑ nitisinone levels	Inhibition of CYP3A4-mediated metabolism	Monitor carefully
NITISINONE	H2-RECEPTOR BLOCKERS—CIMETIDINE, RANITIDINE	Possible ↑ nitisinone levels	Inhibition of CYP3A4-mediated metabolism	Monitor carefully
NITISINONE	LIPID-LOWERING DRUGS—LOMITAPIDE	Possible ↑ nitisinone levels	Inhibition of CYP3A4-mediated metabolism	Monitor carefully
NITISINONE	RANOLAZINE	Possible ↑ nitisinone levels	Inhibition of CYP3A4-mediated metabolism	Monitor carefully

Primary Drug	Secondary Drug	Effect	Mechanism	Precautions
PENICILLAMINE—see ***Anticancer and Immunomodulating Drugs, Other immunomodulating drugs***				

METABOLIC DRUGS NITISINONE

Primary Drug	Secondary Drug	Effect	Mechanism	Precautions
SAPROPTERIN				
SAPROPTERIN	ANTICANCER AND IMMUNOMODULATING DRUGS—METHOTREXATE	Predicted ↓ sapropterin levels	Inhibition of dihydropteridine reductase, which reduces the regeneration of sapropterin by this enzyme	Caution with concurrent use
SAPROPTERIN	VASODILATOR ANTIHYPERTENSIVES	↑ Hypotensive effect	Additive hypotensive effect	Monitor BP at least weekly until stable. Warn patients to report symptoms of hypotension (light-headedness, dizziness on standing, etc.)
SAPROPTERIN	NITRATES	↑ Hypotensive effect	Additive hypotensive effect	Monitor BP at least weekly until stable. Warn patients to report symptoms of hypotension (light-headedness, dizziness on standing, etc.)

Primary Drug	Secondary Drug	Effect	Mechanism	Precautions
SODIUM PHENYLBUTYRATE				
SODIUM PHENYLBUTYRATE	ANTIGOUT DRUGS—PROBENECID	Possibly ↑ sodium phenylbutyrate levels	Possibly ↓ excretion of the conjugation product of sodium phenylbutyrate	Watch for signs of sodium phenylbutyrate toxicity. Monitor FBC, U&Es, and ECG
SODIUM PHENYLBUTYRATE	CORTICOSTEROIDS, HALOPERIDOL, VALPROATE	Possibly ↓ efficacy of sodium phenylbutyrate	These drugs are associated with ammonia levels	Avoid coadministration

Primary Drug	Secondary Drug	Effect	Mechanism	Precautions
TRIENTINE				
TRIENTINE	ANTACIDS—CALCIUM AND MAGNESIUM—CONTAINING	Possibly ↓ trientine levels	↓ Absorption	Separate doses as much as possible; take antacids after trientine
TRIENTINE	IRON–ORAL	↓ Iron levels when iron is given orally	↓ Absorption	Separate doses by at least 2 h—monitor FBC closely
TRIENTINE	ZINC	↓ Zinc and trientine levels	Mutually ↓ absorption	Separate doses by at least 2 h

PART **14**

Obstetrics and Gynecology

Gregory Ian Giles and Simon F.J. Clarke

1. DANAZOL
2. ERGOMETRINE ➢ *Drugs Acting on the Nervous System, Antimigraine Drugs*
3. GESTRINONE
4. MIFEPRISTONE
5. ESTROGENS
6. OXYTOCIN
7. PROGESTOGENS
8. PROSTAGLANDINS
   - ALPROSTADIL—*see Urological Drugs Section*
   - DINOPROSTONE
9. RALOXIFENE
10. TIBOLONE
11. ULIPRISTAL

Primary Drug	Secondary Drug	Effect	Mechanism	Precautions
DANAZOL				
DANAZOL	**ANTICANCER AND IMMUNOMODULATING DRUGS**			
DANAZOL	CICLOSPORIN	↑ Plasma concentrations of ciclosporin, with risk of toxic effects	Inhibition of ciclosporin metabolism	Watch for toxic effects of ciclosporin
DANAZOL	EVEROLIMUS	Possible ↑ everolimus levels	CYP3A4 inhibition	Caution with concurrent use
DANAZOL	SIROLIMUS	Possible ↑ sirolimus levels	CYP3A4 inhibition	Caution with concurrent use
DANAZOL	TACROLIMUS	Cases of ↑ tacrolimus levels	Uncertain	Watch for early features of tacrolimus toxicity
DANAZOL	TEMSIROLIMUS	Possible ↑ temsirolimus levels	CYP3A4 inhibition	Caution with concurrent use
DANAZOL	ANTICOAGULANTS—WARFARIN	Possible ↓ anticoagulant effect	Uncertain	Monitor INR at least weekly until stable
DANAZOL	ANTIEPILEPTICS—CARBAMAZEPINE	↑ Plasma concentrations of carbamazepine, with risk of toxic effects	Inhibition of carbamazepine metabolism	Watch for toxic effects of carbamazepine
DANAZOL	LIPID-LOWERING DRUGS—LOVASTATIN, SIMVASTATIN	↑ Levels of simvastatin and lovastatin, ↑ risk of adverse effects such as myopathy	Inhibition of CYP3A4-mediated metabolism of simvastatin and lovastatin	Manufacturers advise avoiding coadministration of simvastatin and danazol. It would seem sensible to also avoid coadministration of danazol and lovastatin
DANAZOL	ESTROGENS	↓ Efficacy of both danazol and estrogen contraceptives	Uncertain; possibly competition for same receptors	Use alternative forms of contraception

Primary Drug	Secondary Drug	Effect	Mechanism	Precautions
ERGOMETRINE ➢ *Drugs Acting on the Nervous System, Antimigraine Drugs*				
GESTRINONE				
GESTRINONE	1. ANTIBIOTICS—RIFAMPICIN	↓ Gestrinone levels	Induction of metabolism	Watch for poor response to gestrinone
GESTRINONE	ANTICOAGULANTS—WARFARIN	Possible ↓ anticoagulant effect	Uncertain	Monitor INR at least weekly until stable
GESTRINONE	ANTIEPILEPTICS—BARBITURATES, CARBAMAZEPINE, PHENYTOIN	↓ Gestrinone levels	Induction of metabolism	Watch for poor response to gestrinone
GESTRINONE	ESTROGENS	Theoretical risk of ↓ efficacy of both gestrinone and estrogen contraceptives	Uncertain; possibly competition for the same receptors	Use alternative forms of contraception

OBSTETRICS AND GYNECOLOGY GESTRINONE

Primary Drug	Secondary Drug	Effect	Mechanism	Precautions
MIFEPRISTONE				
MIFEPRISTONE	ANALGESICS—NSAIDs	↓ Efficacy of mifepristone	NSAIDs have an antiprostaglandin effect	Avoid coadministration
MIFEPRISTONE	**ANTIBIOTICS**			
MIFEPRISTONE	MACROLIDES—ERYTHROMYCIN	Theoretical risk of ↑ levels of mifepristone	Inhibition of CYP3A4-mediated metabolism of mifepristone	Warn patients of possible ↑ in side effects (nausea, vomiting, diarrhea, uterine cramps)
MIFEPRISTONE	RIFAMPICIN	Theoretical risk of ↓ levels of mifepristone	Induction of CYP3A4-mediated metabolism of mifepristone	Watch for poor response to mifepristone
MIFEPRISTONE	ANTICANCER AND OTHER IMMUNOMODULATING DRUGS—CORTICOSTEROIDS	Reduced effects of corticosteroids	Antiglucocorticoid activity of mifepristone	Avoid concurrent use Monitor closely if necessary
MIFEPRISTONE	ANTIDEPRESSANTS—ST. JOHN'S WORT	Theoretical risk of ↓ levels of mifepristone	Induction of CYP3A4-mediated metabolism of mifepristone	Watch for poor response to mifepristone
MIFEPRISTONE	ANTIEPILEPTICS—CARBAMAZEPINE, PHENOBARBITAL, PHENYTOIN	Theoretical risk of ↓ levels of mifepristone	Induction of CYP3A4-mediated metabolism of mifepristone	Watch for poor response to mifepristone
MIFEPRISTONE	ANTIFUNGALS—ITRACONAZOLE, KETOCONAZOLE	Theoretical risk of ↑ levels of mifepristone	Inhibition of CYP3A4-mediated metabolism of mifepristone	Warn patients of possible ↑ in side effects (nausea, vomiting, diarrhea, uterine cramps)
MIFEPRISTONE	ANTIPLATELET AGENTS—ASPIRIN	↓ Efficacy of mifepristone	Antiprostaglandin effect of aspirin antagonizes the action of mifepristone	Avoid coadministration
MIFEPRISTONE	GRAPEFRUIT JUICE	Theoretical risk of ↑ levels of mifepristone	Inhibition of CYP3A4-mediated metabolism of mifepristone	Warn patients of possible ↑ in side effects (nausea, vomiting, diarrhea, uterine cramps)

Primary Drug	Secondary Drug	Effect	Mechanism	Precautions
ESTROGENS				
ESTROGENS	**ANALGESICS**			
ESTROGENS	NSAIDs	Etoricoxib may ↑ ethinylestradiol levels	Etoricoxib inhibits sulfotransferase activity	Consider using a formulation with a lower dose of ethinylestradiol

(*Continued*)

Primary Drug	Secondary Drug	Effect	Mechanism	Precautions
ESTROGENS				
ESTROGENS	OPIOIDS	Effect of morphine may be ↓ by combined oral contraceptives	↑ Hepatic metabolism of morphine	Be aware that the morphine dose may need to be ↑. Consider using an alternative opioid such as pethidine
ESTROGENS	**ANTIBIOTICS**			
ESTROGENS	AMPICILLIN, CEPHALOSPORINS, CHLORAMPHENICOL, CLINDAMYCIN, ERYTHROMYCIN, METRONIDAZOLE, SULFONAMIDES	Reports of ↓ contraceptive effect	Possibly alteration of the bacterial flora necessary for recycling ethinylestradiol from the large bowel, although not certain in every case	Advise patients to use additional contraception for the period of antibiotic intake and for 1 month after stopping the antibiotic
ESTROGENS	RIFABUTIN, RIFAMPICIN	Marked ↓ contraceptive effect	Induction of metabolism of estrogens. Modafinil is moderate inducer of CYP1A2 in a concentration-dependent manner	Advise patients to use additional contraception for the period of intake and for 1 month after stopping coadministration of these drugs (4–8 weeks after stopping rifabutin or rifampicin)
ESTROGENS	**ANTICANCER AND IMMUNOMODULATING DRUGS**			
ESTROGENS	CICLOSPORIN, TACROLIMUS	1. Risk of gynecomastia. 2. Possibly ↑ plasma concentrations of these immunomodulating drugs	1. Inhibition of 2-hydroxylation or 17-oxidation of estradiol in the liver, causing ↑ estradiol pool in the body 2. Inhibition of metabolism	1. Watch for gynecomastia and warn patients 2. Monitor blood levels of these drugs; warn patients to report symptoms such as fever and sore throat
ESTROGENS	CORTICOSTEROIDS	Possibly ↑ plasma concentrations of these immunomodulating drugs	Inhibition of metabolism	Monitor blood levels of these drugs; warn patients to report symptoms such as fever and sore throat
ORAL CONTRACEPTIVES	CRIZOTINIB	Possible ↓ contraceptive effect	Induction of PXR and CAR-regulated enzymes	Use barrier contraceptive
ORAL CONTRACEPTIVES	DABRAFENIB	Possible ↓ efficacy of hormonal contraceptives	Dabrafenib induces CYP3A4/CYP2Cs/CYP2B6	Manufacturer recommends alternative contraceptive methods
COMBINED ORAL CONTRACEPTIVE	LENALIDOMIDE	Theoretical ↑ risk of thromboembolic events	Additive	Contraception must be used as drug is a teratogen, but UK manufacturer advises avoiding combined hormonal contraceptive

(*Continued*)

OBSTETRICS AND GYNECOLOGY ESTROGENS

Primary Drug	Secondary Drug	Effect	Mechanism	Precautions
ESTROGENS				
HRT	LENALIDOMIDE	Possible ↑ risk of thromboembolic events	Additive	Caution with concurrent use
ESTROGENS	MYCOPHENOLATE	Possible altered efficacy of contraceptive	Unclear	Clinical significance uncertain. It would seem to be wise to advise patients to use an alternative form of contraception during and for 1 month after stopping coadministration of these drugs
COMBINED ORAL CONTRACEPTIVE	THALIDOMIDE	Theoretical ↑ risk of thromboembolic events	Additive	Contraception must be used as thalidomide is a teratogen, but UK manufacturer advises avoiding combined hormonal contraceptive
HRT	THALIDOMIDE	Possible ↑ risk of thromboembolic events	Additive	Caution with concurrent use
ORAL CONTRACEPTIVES	TOCILIZUMAB	↓ Levels	Tocilizumab reverses CYP450 isoenzyme suppression by IL-6	Monitor closely and consider dose adjustment
ESTROGENS—ORAL CONTRACEPTION	VEMURAFENIB	Possible ↓ efficacy of contraception	CYP3A4 induction	Alternative contraception may be required
ESTROGENS	ANTICOAGULANTS—ORAL	↑ Anticoagulant effect	Uncertain at present	Estrogens are usually not recommended in patients with a history of thromboembolism; if they are used, monitor INR closely
ESTROGENS	ANTIDEPRESSANTS—ST. JOHN'S WORT	Marked ↓ contraceptive effect	Induction of metabolism of estrogens. Modafinil is a moderate inducer of CYP1A2 in a concentration-dependent manner	Advise patients to use additional contraception for the period of intake and for 1 month after stopping coadministration of these drugs. Avoid coadministration of estrogens with St. John's wort
ESTROGENS	ANTIDIABETIC DRUGS	Altered glycemic control	Uncertain at present	Monitor blood glucose closely
ESTROGENS	ANTIEMETICS—APREPITANT	Possible altered efficacy of contraceptive	Unclear	Clinical significance uncertain. It would seem to be wise to advise patients to use an alternative form of contraception during and for 1 month after stopping coadministration of these drugs

(*Continued*)

Primary Drug	Secondary Drug	Effect	Mechanism	Precautions
ESTROGENS				
ESTROGENS	**ANTIEPILEPTICS—LAMOTRIGINE**			
ESTROGENS	BARBITURATES, CARBAMAZEPINE, OXCARBAZEPINE, PHENYTOIN, TOPIRAMATE	Marked ↓ contraceptive effect	Induction of metabolism of estrogens. Modafinil is a moderate inducer of CYP1A2 in a concentration-dependent manner	Advise patients to use additional contraception for the period of intake and for 1 month after stopping coadministration of these drugs
ESTROGENS	LAMOTRIGINE	↓ Lamotrigine levels	↑ Metabolism	Monitor levels
ESTROGENS	**ANTIFUNGALS**			
ESTROGENS—ORAL CONTRACEPTIVES	FLUCONAZOLE, ITRACONAZOLE, KETOCONAZOLE, POSACONAZOLE, VORICONAZOLE	The Netherlands Pharmacovigilance Foundation received reports of pill cycle disturbances 2–3 weeks after the start of the pill cycle, delayed bleeding, and pregnancy. Effects of either or both of estrogen excess and progestogen excess may occur (migraine headaches, thromboembolic episodes, breast tenderness, bloating, and weight gain)	The metabolism of oral contraceptives is complex, dependent on composition, constituents, and doses. Ethylene estradiol, a common constituent, and progestogens are substrates of CYP3A4, which are inhibited by itraconazole. The inhibition of ethinylestradiol and progestogens could lead to effects of estrogen and progestogen excess. Triazole antifungals inhibit the biotransformation of steroids, and such an ↑ may cause delay of withdrawal bleeding	Due to the complex metabolic pathways of oral contraceptives, dependent on constituents, doses, and the reported adverse effects during concomitant use, it is advisable to avoid the use of azole antifungals and advise alternative methods of contraception
ESTROGENS	GRISEOFULVIN, TERBINAFINE	Marked ↓ contraceptive effect	Induction of metabolism of estrogens. Modafinil is moderate inducer of CYP1A2 in a concentration-dependent manner	Advise patients to use additional contraception for the period of intake and for 1 month after stopping coadministration of these drugs (4–8 weeks after stopping rifabutin or rifampicin)

(Continued)

Primary Drug	Secondary Drug	Effect	Mechanism	Precautions
ESTROGENS				
ESTROGENS	**ANTIHYPERTENSIVES AND HEART FAILURE DRUGS**			
ESTROGENS	ANTIHYPERTENSIVES AND HEART FAILURE DRUGS	↓ Hypotensive effect	Estrogens cause sodium and fluid retention	Monitor BP at least weekly until stable; the routine prescription of estrogens in patients with ↑ BP is not advisable
ESTROGENS	VASODILATOR ANTIHYPERTENSIVES—BOSENTAN	↓ Estrogen levels, which may lead to failure of contraception or poor response to treatment of menorrhagia	Possibly induction of metabolism of estrogens	1. <2 month course of bosentan: advise patients to use additional contraception for the period of intake and for 1 month after stopping coadministration with these drugs 2. For long-term use, consider alternative contraceptive methods
ESTROGENS	VASODILATOR ANTIHYPERTENSIVES—DIAZOXIDE	Risk of hyperglycemia when diazoxide is coadministered with combined oral contraceptives	Additive effect; both drugs have a hyperglycemic effect	Monitor blood glucose closely, particularly with diabetics
ESTROGENS	ANTI-PARKINSON'S DRUGS—ROPINIROLE, SELEGILINE	↑ Levels of ropinirole and selegiline	Inhibition of metabolism (possibly *N*-demethylation)	Watch for early features of toxicity (nausea, drowsiness) when starting estrogens in a patient stabilized on these dopaminergics. Conversely, watch for a poor response to them if estrogens are stopped
ESTROGENS	ANTIPROTOZOALS—TINIDAZOLE	Reports of ↓ contraceptive effect	Possibly alteration of the bacterial flora necessary for recycling ethinylestradiol from the large bowel, although not certain in every case	Advise patients to use additional contraception for the period of antibiotic intake and for 1 month after stopping the antibiotic
ESTROGENS	**ANTIVIRALS**			
ESTROGENS—ORAL AND TRANSDERMAL CONTRACEPTIVES	ELVITEGRAVIR (COBICISTAT BOOSTED)	↓ Plasma levels of estrogen, ↑ plasma levels of norgestimate—risk of increased progesterone effects	Altered metabolism	Oral contraceptive must contain at least 30 μg ethinylestradiol and norgestimate as the progesterone. Barrier methods are recommended to prevent the transmission of HIV. Review the risk and benefit particularly in older women or those with additional risk factors for VTE

(*Continued*)

Primary Drug	Secondary Drug	Effect	Mechanism	Precautions
ESTROGENS				
ESTROGENS	NELFINAVIR, NEVIRAPINE, RITONAVIR	↓ Estrogen plasma levels (ritonavir boosted protease inhibitors, nelfinavir, and ritonavir), marked ↓ contraceptive effect, ↑ levels with atazanavir alone, ↑ risk of rash with tipranavir/ritonavir, risk of deranged LFTs (fosamprenavir)	Induction of metabolism of estrogens. Modafinil is a moderate inducer of CYP1A2 in a concentration-dependent manner	Advise patients to use additional contraception for the period of intake and for 1 month after stopping coadministration of these drugs. Barrier methods are necessary to prevent transmission of infection from patients with HIV
ESTROGENS	ANXIOLYTICS AND HYPNOTICS—BZDs, MEPROBAMATE	Possible altered efficacy of contraceptive; reports of breakthrough bleeding when BZDs or meprobamate were coadministered with oral contraceptives	Unclear	Clinical significance uncertain. It would seem to be wise to advise patients to use an alternative form of contraception during and for 1 month after stopping coadministration of these drugs
ESTROGENS	BETA-BLOCKERS	↓ Hypotensive effect	Estrogens cause sodium and fluid retention	Monitor BP at least weekly until stable; the routine prescription of estrogens in patients with ↑ BP is not advisable
ESTROGENS	BRONCHODILATORS—THEOPHYLLINE	↑ Theophylline levels	↓ Clearance of theophylline in a dose-dependent manner	Be aware; watch for features of theophylline toxicity and measure levels
ESTROGENS	**CALCIUM CHANNEL BLOCKERS**			
ESTROGENS	CALCIUM CHANNEL BLOCKERS	↓ Hypotensive effect	Estrogens cause sodium and fluid retention	Monitor BP at least weekly until stable; the routine prescription of estrogens in patients with ↑ BP is not advisable
ESTROGENS	NICARDIPINE, NISOLDIPINE, VERAPAMIL	Risk of gynecomastia	Inhibition of 2-hydroxylation or 17-oxidation of estradiol in the liver, causing ↑ estradiol pool in the body	Watch for gynecomastia and warn patients

(Continued)

OBSTETRICS AND GYNECOLOGY ESTROGENS

Primary Drug	Secondary Drug	Effect	Mechanism	Precautions
ESTROGENS				
ESTROGENS	CNS STIMULANTS—MODAFINIL	Marked ↓ contraceptive effect	Induction of metabolism of estrogens. Modafinil is a moderate inducer of CYP1A2 in a concentration-dependent manner	Advise patients to use additional contraception for the period of intake and for 1 month after stopping coadministration of these drugs (4–8 weeks after stopping rifabutin or rifampicin). Barrier methods are necessary to prevent transmission of infection from patients with HIV. Avoid coadministration of estrogens with St. John's wort
ESTROGENS	DANAZOL	↓ Efficacy of both danazol and estrogen contraceptives	Uncertain; possibly competition for the same receptors	Use alternative forms of contraception
ESTROGENS	DIURETICS—SPIRONOLACTONE	Risk of gynecomastia	Inhibition of 2-hydroxylation or 17-oxidation of estradiol in the liver, causing ↑ estradiol pool in the body	Watch for gynecomastia and warn patients
ESTROGENS	GESTRINONE	Theoretical risk of ↓ efficacy of both gestrinone and estrogen contraceptives	Uncertain; possibly competition for same receptors	Use alternative forms of contraception
ESTROGENS—ESTRADIOL, POSSIBLY ETHINYLESTRADIOL	GRAPEFRUIT JUICE	↑ Efficacy and ↑ adverse effects of estrogens	Oral administration only, ↑ bioavailability, and ↓ presystemic metabolism. Constituents of grapefruit juice irreversibly inhibit intestinal CYP3A4. Transport via Pgp and MRP-2 efflux pumps is also inhibited	Monitor for ↑ side effects
ESTROGENS	LIPID-LOWERING DRUGS—ANION EXCHANGE RESINS	Colesevelam and probably ↓ absorption of combined oral contraceptives. Theoretical risk of contraceptive failure	Anion-binding resins bind oral contraceptives in the intestine	Giving the oral contraceptive 4 h before the anion exchange resin should minimize this effect
ESTROGENS	NITRATES	↓ Hypotensive effect	Estrogens cause sodium and fluid retention	Monitor BP at least weekly until stable; the routine prescription of estrogens in patients with ↑ BP is not advisable

(*Continued*)

Primary Drug	Secondary Drug	Effect	Mechanism	Precautions
ESTROGENS				
ESTROGENS	PROTON PUMP INHIBITORS—LANSOPRAZOLE	Possible altered efficacy of contraceptive; reports of breakthrough bleeding when BZDs or meprobamate were coadministered with oral contraceptives	Unclear	Clinical significance uncertain. It would seem to be wise to advise patients to use an alternative form of contraception during and for 1 month after stopping coadministration of these drugs
ESTROGENS	SOMATROPIN	Possible ↓ efficacy of somatropin	Uncertain	↑ Dose of somatropin may be needed

Primary Drug	Secondary Drug	Effect	Mechanism	Precautions
OXYTOCIN				
OXYTOCIN	ANESTHETICS—GENERAL	Report of arrhythmias and cardiovascular collapse when halothane was given to patients taking oxytocin	Uncertain; possibly an additive effect. High-dose oxytocin may cause hypotension and arrhythmias	Monitor PR, BP, and ECG closely; give oxytocin in the lowest possible dose. Otherwise, consider using an alternative inhalational anesthetic
OXYTOCIN	SYMPATHOMIMETICS	Risk of ↑ BP when oxytocin is coadministered with ephedrine, metaraminol, norepinephrine, or pseudoephedrine	Additive vasoconstriction	Monitor PR, BP, and ECG closely; start inotropes at a lower dose

Primary Drug	Secondary Drug	Effect	Mechanism	Precautions
PROGESTOGENS				
PROGESTOGENS	ANTIEMETICS—APREPITANT	↓ Progestogen levels, with risk of contraceptive failure	Uncertain	Advise patients to use an alternative form of contraception during and for 1 month after discontinuing the aprepitant
PROGESTOGENS	**ANALGESICS**			
PROGESTOGENS	NSAIDs	↑ Risk of hyperkalemia	Drospirenone (component of the Yasmin brand of combined contraceptive pill) is a progestogen derived from spironolactone that can cause potassium retention	Monitor serum potassium weekly until stable and then every 6 months

(Continued)

Primary Drug	Secondary Drug	Effect	Mechanism	Precautions
PROGESTOGENS				
PROGESTOGENS	ANALGESICS—OPIOIDS	Gestodene ↑ effect of buprenorphine	Gestodene ↓ CYP3A4-mediated metabolism of buprenorphine	The dose of buprenorphine needs to be ↓ (by up to 50%)
PROGESTOGENS	ANTIBIOTICS—RIFABUTIN, RIFAMPICIN	↓ Progesterone levels, which may lead to failure of contraception or poor response to treatment of menorrhagia	Possibly induction of metabolism of progestogens	Advise patients to use additional contraception for the period of intake and for 1 month after stopping coadministration with these drugs
PROGESTOGENS	ANTICANCER AND IMMUNOMODULATING DRUGS—CICLOSPORIN	↑ Plasma concentrations of ciclosporin	Inhibition of metabolism of ciclosporin	Monitor blood ciclosporin concentrations. Monitor renal function prior to concurrent therapy. Be aware that infections in immunocompromised patients carry a serious threat to life
PROGESTOGENS	ANTICOAGULANTS—ORAL	↓ Anticoagulant effect	Uncertain at present	Monitor INR closely
PROGESTOGENS	ANTIDEPRESSANTS—ST. JOHN'S WORT	↓ Progesterone levels, which may lead to failure of contraception or poor response to treatment of menorrhagia	Possibly induction of metabolism of progestogens	Advise patients to use additional contraception for the period of intake and for 1 month after stopping coadministration with these drugs. Avoid coadministration of progestogens with St. John's wort
PROGESTOGENS	ANTIDIABETIC DRUGS	Altered glycemic control	Uncertain at present	Monitor blood glucose closely
PROGESTOGENS	ANTIEPILEPTICS—BARBITURATES, CARBAMAZEPINE, OXCARBAZEPINE, PHENYTOIN, TOPIRAMATE	↓ Progesterone levels, which may lead to failure of contraception or poor response to treatment of menorrhagia	Possibly induction of metabolism of progestogens	Advise patients to use additional contraception for the period of intake and for 1 month after stopping coadministration with these drugs
PROGESTOGENS	ANTIEPILEPTICS—LAMOTRIGINE	↓ Lamotrigine levels	↑ Metabolism	Monitor level
PROGESTOGENS	ANTIFUNGALS—GRISEOFULVIN, TERBINAFINE	↓ Progesterone levels, which may lead to failure of contraception or poor response to treatment of menorrhagia	Possibly induction of metabolism of progestogens	Advise patients to use additional contraception for the period of intake and for 1 month after stopping coadministration with these drugs

(*Continued*)

Primary Drug	Secondary Drug	Effect	Mechanism	Precautions
PROGESTOGENS				
PROGESTOGENS	**ANTIHYPERTENSIVES AND HEART FAILURE DRUGS**			
PROGESTOGENS	ACE INHIBITORS, ANGIOTENSIN II RECEPTOR ANTAGONISTS	↑ Risk of hyperkalemia	Drospirenone (component of the Yasmin brand of combined contraceptive pill) is a progestogen derived from spironolactone that can cause potassium retention	Monitor serum potassium weekly until stable and then every 6 months
PROGESTOGENS	VASODILATOR ANTIHYPERTENSIVES—BOSENTAN	↓ Progesterone levels, which may lead to failure of contraception or poor response to treatment of menorrhagia	Possibly induction of metabolism of progestogens	1. <2 month course of bosentan: advise patients to use additional contraception for the period of intake and for 1 month after stopping coadministration with these drugs 2. For long-term use, consider alternative contraceptive methods
PROGESTOGENS	ANTI-PARKINSON'S DRUGS—SELEGILINE	↑ Selegiline levels	Inhibition of metabolism	Watch for early features of toxicity (nausea, drowsiness) when starting progestogens in a patient stabilized on these dopaminergics. Conversely, watch for a poor response to them if progestogens are stopped
PROGESTOGENS—ORAL AND TRANSDERMAL CONTRACEPTIVES	ANTIVIRALS—ELVITEGRAVIR (COBICISTAT BOOSTED)	↓ Plasma levels of estrogen, ↑ plasma levels of norgestimate—risk of increased progesterone effects	Altered metabolism	Oral contraceptive must contain at least 30 μg ethinylestradiol and norgestimate as the progesterone. Barrier methods are recommended to prevent the transmission of HIV. Review the risk and benefit particularly in older women or those with additional risk factors for VTE

(*Continued*)

OBSTETRICS AND GYNECOLOGY PROGESTOGENS

Primary Drug	Secondary Drug	Effect	Mechanism	Precautions
PROGESTOGENS				
PROGESTOGENS	ANTIVIRALS—PROTEASE INHIBITORS	1. ↓ Progesterone levels with amprenavir, nelfinavir, nevirapine, and ritonavir, which may lead to failure of contraception or poor response to treatment of menorrhagia 2. ↑ Adverse effects with amprenavir and atazanavir	1. Possibly induction of metabolism of progestogens 2. Uncertain	Advise patients to use additional contraception for the period of intake and for 1 month after stopping coadministration with these drugs. Barrier methods are necessary to prevent transmission of infection from patients with HIV 2. Watch for early features of toxicity of amprenavir and atazanavir, and adjust the dose accordingly
PROGESTOGENS	DIURETICS—POTASSIUM-SPARING	↑ Risk of hyperkalemia	Drospirenone (component of some brands of combined contraceptive pill) is a progestogen derived from spironolactone that can cause potassium retention	Monitor serum potassium weekly until stable, then every 6 months
PROGESTOGENS	LIPID-LOWERING DRUGS—ANION EXCHANGE RESINS	Colesevelam and probably ↓ absorption of combined oral contraceptives. Theoretical risk of contraceptive failure	Anion-binding resins bind oral contraceptives in the intestine	Giving the oral contraceptive 4 h before the anion exchange resin should minimize this effect

Primary Drug	Secondary Drug	Effect	Mechanism	Precautions
PROSTAGLANDINS				
ALPROSTADIL—*see Urological Drugs Section*				
DINOPROSTONE				
DINOPROSTONE	ANALGESICS—NSAIDs	Theoretical risk of ↓ efficacy of dinoprost; not confirmed in clinical studies	Antagonism of effect	UK manufacturers recommend stopping NSAIDs before administering dinoprostone. U.S. manufacturer does not give this advice
DINOPROSTONE	ANTIPLATELETS—ASPIRIN	Theoretical risk of ↓ efficacy of dinoprost; not confirmed in clinical studies	Antagonism of effect	UK manufacturers recommend stopping aspirin (in analgesic doses) before administering dinoprostone. U.S. manufacturer does not give this advice

Primary Drug	Secondary Drug	Effect	Mechanism	Precautions
RALOXIFENE				
RALOXIFENE	ANTICOAGULANTS—ORAL	Possible ↓ anticoagulant, effect which may take several weeks to develop	Uncertain at present	Monitor INR closely for several weeks
RALOXIFENE	ANTIVIRALS—FAMCICLOVIR	Possible ↓ efficacy of famciclovir	Inhibition of metabolism to the active metabolite of famciclovir	Watch for poor response to famciclovir
RALOXIFENE	LIPID-LOWERING DRUGS—ANION EXCHANGE RESINS	Raloxifene levels may be ↓ by cholestyramine	Cholestyramine interrupts the enterohepatic circulation of raloxifene	Avoid coadministration

Primary Drug	Secondary Drug	Effect	Mechanism	Precautions
TIBOLONE				
TIBOLONE	ANTIBIOTICS—RIFAMPICIN	↓ Tibolone levels	Induction of metabolism of tibolone	Watch for poor response to tibolone; consider ↑ dose
TIBOLONE	ANTICANCER AND OTHER IMMUNOMODULATING DRUGS—TAMOXIFEN	↓ Efficacy of tamoxifen with risk of recurrence of breast cancer	Tibolone has estrogenic effects that oppose the effects of tamoxifen	Avoid coadministration
TIBOLONE	ANTIEPILEPTICS—BARBITURATES, CARBAMAZEPINE, PHENYTOIN	↓ Tibolone levels	Induction of metabolism of tibolone	Watch for poor response to tibolone; consider ↑ dose
TIBOLONE	THYROID HORMONES	Case reports of ↓ efficacy of levothyroxine	Uncertain	Separate doses by 12 h—monitor thyroid function closely for at least 6 months

Primary Drug	Secondary Drug	Effect	Mechanism	Precautions
ULIPRISTAL				
ULIPRISTAL	ANTICOAGULANTS—DABIGATRAN	↑ Dabigatran levels	Inhibition of Pgp	Avoid coadministration
ULIPRISTAL	PROTEASE INHIBITORS—RITONAVIR	Possible ↓ contraceptive effect	Uncertain	Avoid coadministration
ULIPRISTAL	H2-RECEPTOR BLOCKERS—CIMETIDINE	Contraceptive effect possibly ↓ (high-dose ulipristal)	Unclear	Avoid coadministration
ULIPRISTAL	PROTON PUMP INHIBITORS	Possible ↓ efficacy of contraceptive	Unclear	Avoid coadministration

OBSTETRICS AND GYNECOLOGY ULIPRISTAL

PART 15

Drugs Used to Treat the Urinary System

Simon F.J. Clarke

1. DRUGS USED FOR URINARY RETENTION
   - ALPHA-BLOCKERS—*see Cardiovascular Drugs, Antihypertensives, and Heart Failure Drugs*
   - DUTASTERIDE, FINASTERIDE
   - PARASYMPATHOMIMETICS—*see Drugs Acting on the Nervous System, Drugs Used to Treat Neuromuscular Diseases and Movement Disorders*
2. DRUGS USED FOR URINARY INCONTINENCE
   - ANTIMUSCARINICS—*see Drugs Acting on the Nervous System, Anti-Parkinson's Drugs*
   - DESMOPRESSIN—*see Other Endocrine Drugs*
   - DULOXETINE—*see Drugs Acting on the Nervous System, Antidepressants*
   - MIRABEGRON
3. DRUGS USED FOR ERECTILE DYSFUNCTION
   - ALPROSTADIL
   - PHOSPHODIESTERASE TYPE 5 INHIBITORS

Primary Drug	Secondary Drug	Effect	Mechanism	Precautions
DRUGS USED FOR URINARY RETENTION				
ALPHA-BLOCKERS—see *Cardiovascular Drugs, Antihypertensives, and Heart Failure Drugs*				
DUTASTERIDE, FINASTERIDE				
DUTASTERIDE, FINASTERIDE	ANTIVIRALS—PROTEASE INHIBITORS	Possibly ↑ adverse effects of dutasteride with indinavir or ritonavir (with or without lopinavir)	Inhibition of CYP3A4-mediated metabolism of dutasteride	Monitor closely; ↓ dosing frequency if side effects occur
DUTASTERIDE, FINASTERIDE	CALCIUM CHANNEL BLOCKERS	Plasma concentrations of dutasteride may ↑ when it is coadministered with diltiazem or verapamil	Uncertain but postulated that it may be due to inhibition of CYP3A4-mediated metabolism of dutasteride	Watch for side effects of dutasteride
DUTASTERIDE, FINASTERIDE	TESTOSTERONE	↑ Testosterone levels when testosterone administered orally	↑ Bioavailability	May be used therapeutically
PARASYMPATHOMIMETICS—see *Drugs Acting on the Nervous System, Drugs Used to Treat Neuromuscular Diseases and Movement Disorders*				

Primary Drug	Secondary Drug	Effect	Mechanism	Precautions
DRUGS USED FOR URINARY INCONTINENCE				
ANTIMUSCARINICS (DARIFENACIN, FESOTERODINE, FLAVOXATE, OXYBUTYNIN, PROPANTHELINE, PROPIVERINE, SOLIFENACIN, TOLTERODINE, TROSPIUM)—see *Drugs Acting on the Nervous System, Anti-Parkinson's Drugs*				
DESMOPRESSIN—see *Other Endocrine Drugs*				
DULOXETINE—see *Drugs Acting on the Nervous System, Antidepressants*				
MIRABEGRON				
MIRABEGRON	ANTIARRHYTHMICS—FLECAINIDE, PROPAFENONE	↑ Flecainide and propafenone levels	Mirabegron inhibits CYP2D6. These drugs have a narrow therapeutic index	Manufacturer advises caution in coadministration. Warn patients to report symptoms such as dizziness, chest pain, or palpitations

(*Continued*)

Primary Drug	Secondary Drug	Effect	Mechanism	Precautions
DRUGS USED FOR URINARY INCONTINENCE				
MIRABEGRON	ANTIDEPRESSANTS—TRICYCLICS	↑ TCA levels	Mirabegron inhibits CYP2D6. These drugs have a narrow therapeutic index	Manufacturer advises caution in coadministration. Warn patients to report symptoms such as drowsiness, dizziness, or palpitations
MIRABEGRON	CARDIAC GLYCOSIDES—DIGOXIN	↑ Digoxin levels	Mirabegron inhibits Pgp	Monitor digoxin levels

Primary Drug	Secondary Drug	Effect	Mechanism	Precautions
DRUGS USED FOR ERECTILE DYSFUNCTION				
ALPROSTADIL				
ALPROSTADIL	ANTIHYPERTENSIVES AND HEART FAILURE DRUGS, BETA-BLOCKERS, CALCIUM CHANNEL BLOCKERS, NITRATES	↑ Hypotensive effect	Additive hypotensive effect	Monitor BP at least weekly until stable. Warn patients to report symptoms of hypotension (light-headedness, dizziness on standing, etc.)
ALPROSTADIL	PERIPHERAL VASODILATORS—MOXISYLYTE	Risk of priapism if intracavernous alprostadil is given with moxisylyte	Additive effect	Avoid coadministration
PHENTOLAMINE—*see Cardiovascular Drugs, Antihypertensives and Heart Failure Drugs, Alpha-Blockers*				
PHOSPHODIESTERASE TYPE 5 INHIBITORS				
PHOSPHODIESTERASE TYPE 5 INHIBITORS	**ANTIBIOTICS**			
PHOSPHODIESTERASE TYPE 5 INHIBITORS	MACROLIDES	↑ Phosphodiesterase type 5 inhibitor levels with erythromycin, and possibly clarithromycin and telithromycin	Inhibition of metabolism	↓ Dose of these phosphodiesterase type 5 inhibitors (e.g., start vardenafil at 5 mg)
TADALAFIL	RIFAMPICIN	↓ Tadalafil levels	Probable induction of metabolism	Watch for poor response

(Continued)

Primary Drug	Secondary Drug	Effect	Mechanism	Precautions
DRUGS USED FOR ERECTILE DYSFUNCTION				
PHOSPHODIESTERASE TYPE 5 INHIBITORS	**ANTICANCER AND IMMUNOMODULATING DRUGS**			
PHOSPHODIESTERASE TYPE 5 INHIBITORS—SILDENAFIL	CICLOSPORIN	↑ Plasma concentrations of ciclosporin, with risk of adverse effects	Competitive inhibition of CYP3A4-mediated metabolism of ciclosporin	Be aware. Sildenafil is taken intermittently and is unlikely to be of clinical significance unless concomitant therapy is long term
PHOSPHODIESTERASE TYPE-5 INHIBITORS—SILDENAFIL	TACROLIMUS	Increased sildenafil levels, reduction in blood pressure	Uncertain	Start on lower dose of sildenafil if needed
PHOSPHODIESTERASE TYPE 5 INHIBITORS	ANTIFUNGALS—AZOLES	↑ Sildenafil, tadalafil, and vardenafil levels	Inhibition of metabolism	↓ Dose of these phosphodiesterase type 5 inhibitors
PHOSPHODIESTERASE TYPE 5 INHIBITORS	**ANTIHYPERTENSIVES AND HEART FAILURE DRUGS**			
PHOSPHODIESTERASE TYPE 5 INHIBITORS	ALPHA-ADRENERGIC BLOCKERS	Risk of marked ↓ BP	Additive hypotensive effect	Avoid coadministration if possible (manufacturers particularly mention tadalafil). If others must be administered with alpha blockers, warn patients about the clinical features of orthostatic hypotension
SILDENAFIL	VASODILATOR ANTIHYPERTENSIVES—BOSENTAN	↓ Sildenafil levels	Probable induction of metabolism	Watch for poor response
PHOSPHODIESTERASE TYPE 5 INHIBITORS	**ANTIVIRALS**			
PHOSPHODIESTERASE TYPE 5 INHIBITORS	COBICISTAT	↑ Plasma levels	Inhibition of metabolism via CYP3A	Avoid coadministration with sildenafil for PAH, use tadalafil with caution. For erectile dysfunction, maximum dose of sildenafil 25 mg/48 h, vardenafil 2.5 mg/72 h, and tadalafil 10 mg/72 h

(Continued)

Primary Drug	Secondary Drug	Effect	Mechanism	Precautions
DRUGS USED FOR ERECTILE DYSFUNCTION				
PHOSPHODIESTERASE TYPE 5 INHIBITORS	PROTEASE INHIBITORS	↑ Sildenafil, tadalafil, and vardenafil levels	Inhibition of CYP3A4- and possibly CYP2C9-mediated metabolism of sildenafil	Avoid coadministration if for pulmonary hypertension. For erectile dysfunction, avoid combining indinavir or ritonavir (low and high dose) and vardenafil, or ritonavir (high dose) or saqunavir and sildenafil, tadalafil, or vardenafil. Use others with caution; monitor BP closely. Suggested starting doses (erectile dysfunction) with low. dose ritonavir: sildenafil 25 mg/48 h, vardenafil 2.5 mg/72 h, or tadalafil 10 mg/72 h
PHOSPHODIESTERASE TYPE 5 INHIBITORS—SILDENAFIL, TADALAFIL, VARDENAFIL	NNRTIs—ETRAVIRINE	↓ Plasma levels of phosphodiesterase 5 inhibitor	Induction of metabolism via CYP3A4	Dose adjustment may be required, titrate phosphodiesterase inhibitor to clinical effect. No adjustment needed with rilpivirine
PHOSPHODIESTERASE TYPE 5 INHIBITORS	CALCIUM CHANNEL BLOCKERS	↑ Hypotensive action, particularly with sildenafil and vardenafil	Additive effect; phosphodiesterase type 5 inhibitors cause vasodilatation	Warn patients of the small risk of postural ↓ BP

(*Continued*)

Primary Drug	Secondary Drug	Effect	Mechanism	Precautions
DRUGS USED FOR ERECTILE DYSFUNCTION				
PHOSPHODIESTERASE TYPE 5 INHIBITORS (E.G., SILDENAFIL, TADALAFIL, VARDENAFIL)	GRAPEFRUIT JUICE	Possibly ↑ efficacy and ↑ adverse effects, e.g., hypotension	Small ↑ in bioavailability, ↑ variability in pharmacokinetics, i.e., interindividual variations in metabolism	Safest to advise against intake of grapefruit juice for at least 48 h prior to intending to take any of these preparations. When necessary, the starting dose of sildenafil should not exceed 25–50 mg and that of tadalafil 10 mg. Avoid coadministration with vardenafil
PHOSPHODIESTERASE TYPE 5 INHIBITORS—SILDENAFIL	H2 RECEPTOR BLOCKERS—CIMETIDINE	↑ Efficacy and adverse effects of sildenafil	Inhibition of metabolism via CYP3A4	Consider a starting dose of 25 mg of sildenafil
PHOSPHODIESTERASE TYPE 5 INHIBITORS	NICORANDIL	Risk of severe ↓ BP	Additive effect	Avoid coadministration
PHOSPHODIESTERASE TYPE 5 INHIBITORS	NITRATES	Risk of severe ↓ BP and precipitation of myocardial infarction	Additive effect	Avoid coadministration
PHOSPHODIESTERASE TYPE 5 INHIBITORS	POTASSIUM CHANNEL ACTIVATORS	↑ Hypotensive effect	Both drugs have vasodilating properties	Monitor BP closely
URINARY ALKALINIZATION—SODIUM BICARBONATE	ANESTHETICS—LOCAL—PROCAINE SOLUTIONS	Precipitation of drugs, which may not be immediately apparent	A pharmaceutical interaction	Do not mix in the same infusion or syringe
URINARY ALKALINIZATION—AMMONIUM CHLORIDE, SODIUM BICARBONATE	ANTIARRHYTHMICS—AMIODARONE, FLECAINIDE, QUINIDINE	Urinary alkalinization ↑ levels of these antiarrhythmics	These antiarrhythmics excretion ↓ in the presence of an alkaline urine; they exist in predominantly nonionic form, which is more readily reabsorbed from the renal tubules	Monitor PR and BP closely

(*Continued*)

Primary Drug	Secondary Drug	Effect	Mechanism	Precautions
DRUGS USED FOR ERECTILE DYSFUNCTION				
URINARY ALKALINIZATION—SODIUM BICARBONATE	**ANTIBIOTICS**			
SODIUM BICARBONATE	CIPROFLOXACIN	↓ Solubility of ciprofloxacin in the urine, leading to ↑ risk of crystalluria and renal damage	Any ↑ urinary pH caused by sodium bicarbonate can result in ↓ ciprofloxacin solubility in the urine	If both drugs are used concomitantly, the patient should be well hydrated and be monitored for signs of renal toxicity
SODIUM BICARBONATE	TETRACYCLINE	↓ Tetracycline levels and possible therapeutic failure	↑ Is suggested when sodium bicarbonate alkalinizes the urine, the renal excretion of tetracycline	The interaction can be minimized by administering the doses 3–4 h apart
URINARY ALKALINIZATION—SODIUM BICARBONATE ACETAZOLAMIDE	ANTICANCER AND IMMUNOMODULATING DRUGS—METHOTREXATE	Increased urinary excretion of methotrexate	Methotrexate has increased solubility in alkaline fluids	Interaction normally used therapeutically to reduce toxicity
URINARY ALKALINIZATION—SODIUM BICARBONATE	ANTIDEMENTIA DRUGS—MEMANTINE	Possible ↑ memantine levels	↓ Renal excretion	Watch for early features of memantine toxicity
URINARY ALKALINIZATION—POTASSIUM ACETATE, POTASSIUM CITRATE, SODIUM BICARBONATE, AND SODIUM CITRATE	ANTIDEPRESSANTS—LITHIUM	↓ Plasma concentrations of lithium, with risk of lack of therapeutic effect	Due to ↑ renal excretion of lithium	Monitor clinically and by measuring blood lithium levels to ensure adequate therapeutic efficacy
URINARY ALKALINIZATION—SODIUM BICARBONATE	MUSCLE RELAXANTS—NONDEPOLARIZING MIVACURIUM	Inactivation of mivacurioum in the presence of an alkaline environment—pH > 8.5. In the presence of an alkaline solution, there is a risk that mivacurium may be inactivated and a free acid precipitated	Mivacurium injection is acidic (pH 3.5–5.5) and should not be mixed in the same syringe with highly alkaline solutions or administered simultaneously through the same needle during i.v. infusion	Avoid mixing with alkaline solutions
URINARY ALKALINIZATION—SODIUM BICARBONATE	SYMPATHOMIMETICS—EPHEDRINE, PSEUDOEPHEDRINE	Possibly ↑ ephedrine/pseudoephedrine levels	Alkalinizing the urine ↓ excretion of these sympathomimetics	Watch for early features of toxicity (tremor, insomnia, tachycardia)

PART 16

Drugs of Abuse

Lakshman Delgoda Karalliedde and Janaka Karalliedde

1. CANNABIS
2. AMPHETAMINES
3. METHYLENEDIOXYMETHAMPHETAMINE (MDMA, ECSTASY)
4. COCAINE
5. HEROIN ➢ *Analgesics, Opioids*
6. HALLUCINOGENS
7. GAMMA-HYDROXYBUTYRIC ACID ➢ *Drugs Acting on the Nervous System, Anxiolytics and Hypnotics*
8. AMYL NITRITE

Primary Drug	Secondary Drug	Effect	Mechanism	Precautions
CANNABIS				
There are more than 60 psychoactive constituents of cannabis that contribute to its effects; these are called cannabinoids, the most important of which is delta-9-tetrahydrocannabinol. This is the most widely used illicit drug. The U.S. FDA has approved it for chemotherapy-related nausea and vomiting, and for loss of appetite and weight loss associated with HIV/AIDS. Buccal spray from the whole cannabis plant has been developed in Canada for the treatment of neuropathic pain associated with multiple sclerosis. The active constituents—cannabinoids (there are others)—are highly protein bound and are metabolized by CYP2C9 and CYP3A4. Any form of smoking induces CYP1A2; also it may cause inhibition/induction of CYP3A4. Acute adverse effects include psychomotor impairment, dysphoria, anxiety, paranoia, tachycardia, flushing, and nausea.				
CANNABIS	ANESTHETICS—LOCAL—LIDOCAINE	Unpredictable changes in plasma concentrations. Risk of toxicity or therapeutic failure with intravenous lidocaine	Induction or inhibition of CYP3A4-mediated metabolism by cannabis. It is not yet known whether the effects are dependent on the degree of cannabis consumption	Be aware. Watch for signs of toxicity, especially when cannabis use abruptly changes
CANNABIS	ANALGESICS—OPIOIDS—ALFENTANIL, FENTANYL, METHADONE, CODEINE, DEXTROMETHORPHAN	Unpredictable changes in plasma concentration. Risk of toxicity or therapeutic failure, particularly of drugs with a narrow therapeutic index	Induction or inhibition of CYP3A4-mediated metabolism by cannabis. It is not yet known whether the effects are dependent on the degree of cannabis consumption	Be aware. Watch for signs of toxicity, especially when cannabis use abruptly changes
CANNABIS	**ANTIARRHYTHMICS**			
CANNABIS	AMIODARONE	Unpredictable changes in plasma concentration. Risk of toxicity or therapeutic failure, particularly of drugs with a narrow therapeutic index	Induction or inhibition of CYP3A4-mediated metabolism by cannabis. It is not yet known whether the effects are dependent on the degree of cannabis consumption	Be aware. Watch for signs of toxicity especially when cannabis use abruptly changes
CANNABIS	PROPAFENONE	Unpredictable changes in plasma concentration. Risk of toxicity or therapeutic failure, particularly of drugs with a narrow therapeutic index	Induction or inhibition of CYP3A4-mediated metabolism by cannabis. It is not yet known whether the effects are dependent on the degree of cannabis consumption	Be aware. Watch for signs of toxicity especially when cannabis use abruptly changes

(*Continued*)

DRUGS OF ABUSE CANNABIS

DRUGS OF ABUSE CANNABIS

Primary Drug	Secondary Drug	Effect	Mechanism	Precautions
CANNABIS				
CANNABIS	ANTIBIOTICS—MACROLIDES—ERYTHROMYCIN	Unpredictable changes in plasma concentration. Risk of toxicity or therapeutic failure, particularly of drugs with a narrow therapeutic index	Induction or inhibition of CYP3A4-mediated metabolism by cannabis. It is not yet known whether the effects are dependent on the degree of cannabis consumption	Be aware. Watch for signs of toxicity especially when cannabis use abruptly changes
CANNABIS	**ANTICANCER AND IMMUNOMODULATING DRUGS**			
CANNABIS	CYTOTOXICS—CYCLOPHOSPHAMIDE, DOXORUBICIN, IFOSFAMIDE, LOMUSTINE, VINCA ALKALOIDS	Unpredictable changes in plasma concentration. Risk of toxicity or therapeutic failure, particularly of drugs with a narrow therapeutic index	Induction or inhibition of CYP3A4-mediated metabolism by cannabis. It is not yet known whether the effects are dependent on the degree of cannabis consumption	Be aware. Watch for signs of toxicity, especially when cannabis use abruptly changes
CANNABIS	HORMONES AND HORMONE ANTAGONISTS—TAMOXIFEN	Unpredictable changes in plasma concentration. Risk of toxicity or therapeutic failure, particularly of drugs with a narrow therapeutic index	Induction or inhibition of CYP3A4-mediated metabolism by cannabis. It is not yet known whether the effects are dependent on the degree of cannabis consumption	Be aware. Watch for signs of toxicity, especially when cannabis use abruptly changes
CANNABIS	IMMUNOMODULATING DRUGS—CICLOSPORIN, CORTICOSTEROIDS	Unpredictable changes in plasma concentration. Risk of toxicity or therapeutic failure, particularly of drugs with a narrow therapeutic index	Induction or inhibition of CYP3A4-mediated metabolism by cannabis. It is not yet known whether the effects are dependent on the degree of cannabis consumption	Be aware. Watch for signs of toxicity, especially when cannabis use abruptly changes
CANNABIS	ANTICOAGULANTS—WARFARIN	Unpredictable changes in plasma concentration. Cannabinoids are highly protein bound, raising the potential for interactions with other highly protein bound drugs such as warfarin	1. Induction or inhibition of CYP3A4-mediated metabolism by cannabis. It is not yet known whether the effects are dependent on the degree of cannabis consumption 2. Induction of CYP1A2-mediated metabolism by any form of smoking. Foods (e.g., broccoli, cabbage, Brussels sprouts, chargrilled meat) also induce this isoenzyme	Be aware. Monitor INR closely, especially when cannabis use abruptly changes

(Continued)

Primary Drug	Secondary Drug	Effect	Mechanism	Precautions
CANNABIS				
CANNABIS	**ANTIDEPRESSANTS**			
CANNABIS	LITHIUM	May ↑ plasma concentrations of lithium	Mechanism uncertain	Be aware and measure plasma lithium levels if indicated by clinical observations
CANNABIS	**SSRIs**			
CANNABIS	FLUOXETINE	Report of mania	Mechanism uncertain and may not be due to an interaction	Unclear whether this was a specific interaction, or caused by fluoxetine alone. In clinical practice, cannabis and SSRIs are frequently used together with negligible adverse effects-proposed interaction is rare
CANNABIS	FLUVOXAMINE	↓ Levels, with risk of therapeutic failure	Induction of CYP1A2-mediated metabolism by any form of smoking. Foods (e.g., broccoli, cabbage, Brussels sprouts, chargrilled meat) also induce this isoenzyme	Watch for poor response to fluvoxamine; conversely, watch for toxic effects if a previously heavy cannabis user stops smoking
CANNABIS	SERTRALINE, VENLAFAXINE	Unpredictable changes in plasma concentration. Risk of toxicity or therapeutic failure, particularly of drugs with a narrow therapeutic index	Induction or inhibition of CYP3A4-mediated metabolism by cannabis. It is not yet known whether the effects are dependent on the degree of cannabis consumption	Be aware. Watch for signs of toxicity, especially when cannabis use abruptly changes
CANNABIS	**TCAs**			
CANNABIS	AMITRIPTYLINE, CLOMIPRAMINE, DESIPRAMINE, IMIPRAMINE, NORTRIPTYLINE	↑ Risk of tachycardia. Heart rate may ↑ to 100–160 beats/min, with some records of 300 beats/min resistant to verapamil therapy	Due to beta-adrenergic effects of cannabis coupled with the anticholinergic effect of tricyclic antidepressants	Onset is variable, typically within 1 h of administration. Patients receiving treatment with anticholinergic medication and use cannabis are advised to monitor their heart rate

(Continued)

Primary Drug	Secondary Drug	Effect	Mechanism	Precautions
CANNABIS				
CANNABIS	**OTHER ANTIDEPRESSANTS**			
CANNABIS	MIRTAZAPINE	↓ Levels, with risk of therapeutic failure	Induction of CYP1A2-mediated metabolism by any form of smoking. Foods (e.g., broccoli, cabbage, Brussels sprouts, chargrilled meat) also induce this isoenzyme	Watch for poor response to mirtazapine; conversely, watch for toxic effects if a previously heavy cannabis user stops smoking
CANNABIS	ANTIEMETICS—ONDANSETRON	↓ Levels, with risk of therapeutic failure	Induction of CYP1A2-mediated metabolism by any form of smoking. Foods (e.g., broccoli, cabbage, Brussels sprouts, chargrilled meat) also induce this isoenzyme	Watch for poor response to ondansetron; conversely, watch for toxic effects if a previously heavy cannabis user stops smoking
CANNABIS	ANTIHISTAMINES—BROMPHENIRAMINE, CHLORPHENIRAMINE	May increase side effects of antihistamines e.g. dizziness, drowsiness, and difficulty concentrating. Some may experience impairment in thinking and judgment	Additive effects on CNS	Avoid or limit the use of alcohol. Avoid driving or operating hazardous machinery until you know how the medications affect you
CANNABIS	ANTIMUSCARINICS—ATROPINE, FLAVOXATE, HYOSCINE, OXYBUTYNIN, TOLTERODINE	↑ Risk of tachycardia. Smoking cannabis alone ↑s heart rate by ~20 beats /min. Addition of antimuscarinic (atropine) increase heart rate by 50 beats per min	Anti-muscarinic effect added to cannabis mediated ↑ via adrenergic receptors as latter response is prevented by propranolol	Ask patients about cannabis use if they present with otherwise unexplained tachycardias while taking these drugs
CANNABIS	ANTIOBESITY DRUGS—RIMONABANT	↓ Most effects of cannabis that are due to its activity at central cannabinoid receptor	Rimonabant is a selective antagonist at central cannabinoid receptors, and thus the effects of either drug may be ↓.	Be aware
CANNABIS	ANTI-PARKINSON'S DRUGS—PROCYCLIDINE, TRIHEXYPHENIDYL (BENZHEXOL)	↑ Risk of tachycardia. Cannabis can worsen existing symptoms e.g. apathy and depression in Parkinson's disease. Psychosis can be caused by Parkinson's medicines and can also be caused by marijuana. The combined risk is unknown	Additive effects with antimuscarinics used in Parkinson's disease. Claims for therapeutic benefit in Parkinson's require further study	Ask patients about cannabis use if they present with otherwise unexplained tachycardias while taking these drugs

(Continued)

Primary Drug	Secondary Drug	Effect	Mechanism	Precautions
CANNABIS				
CANNABIS	ANTIPSYCHOTICS—CHLORPROMAZINE, CLOZAPINE, OLANZAPINE, HALOPERIDOL	↓ Plasma levels of these antipsychotics (plasma concentrations of clozapine may be halved), with the risk of therapeutic failure	Induction of CYP1A2-mediated metabolism by any form of smoking. Foods (e.g., broccoli, cabbage, Brussels sprouts, chargrilled meat) also induce this isoenzyme	Watch for poor response to these antipsychotics. Conversely, watch for toxic effects of these antipsychotics if a previously heavy cannabis user stops smoking (case report of confusion associated with raised blood levels of clozapine when the user stopped both tobacco and cannabis)
CANNABIS	ANTIVIRALS—PROTEASE INHIBITORS—INDINAVIR, NELFINAVIR, NEVIRAPINE, RITONAVIR, SAQUINAVIR	Cannabis may cause ↓ plasma concentrations of protease inhibitors, particularly indinavir and nelfinavir	Cannabis may cause inhibition or induction of CYP3A4 isoenzymes, which metabolize these protease inhibitors	Be aware. Regular monitoring of viral indicators is necessary
CANNABIS	ANXIOLYTICS AND HYPNOTICS—BZDs—ALPRAZOLAM, DIAZEPAM, MIDAZOLAM, TRIAZOLAM	Unpredictable changes in plasma concentration. Risk of toxicity or therapeutic failure, particularly of drugs with a narrow therapeutic index	Induction or inhibition of CYP3A4-mediated metabolism by cannabis. It is not yet known whether the effects are dependent on the degree of cannabis consumption	Be aware. Watch for signs of toxicity, especially when cannabis use abruptly changes
CANNABIS	BETA-BLOCKERS—PROPRANOLOL	↓ Levels, with risk of therapeutic failure	Induction of CYP1A2-mediated metabolism by any form of smoking. Foods (e.g., broccoli, cabbage, Brussels sprouts, chargrilled meat) also induce this isoenzyme	Watch for poor response to propranolol; conversely, watch for toxic effects if a previously heavy cannabis user stops smoking
CANNABIS	BRONCHODILATORS—THEOPHYLLINE	↓ Theophylline levels, with risk of therapeutic failure (theophylline has a narrow therapeutic range)	Induction of CYP1A2-mediated metabolism by any form of smoking; smoking both tobacco and cannabis is likely to produce a greater effect than the use of either drug alone. Foods (e.g., broccoli, cabbage, Brussels sprouts, chargrilled meat) also induce this isoenzyme. Although cannabis is considered to cause bronchodilatation, regular smoking leads to poorer respiratory function	Watch for poor response to theophylline; consider monitoring theophylline levels if a previously heavy cannabis user stops smoking, because of the risk of toxic effects. Regular cannabis users may require higher theophylline doses. Cessation of cannabis use may increase theophylline clearance

(*Continued*)

DRUGS OF ABUSE CANNABIS

Primary Drug	Secondary Drug	Effect	Mechanism	Precautions
CANNABIS				
CANNABIS	**CALCIUM CHANNEL BLOCKERS**			
CANNABIS	DILTIAZEM, FELODIPINE, NIFEDIPINE, NIMODIPINE, NISOLDIPINE	Unpredictable changes in plasma concentration. Risk of toxicity or therapeutic failure, particularly of drugs with a narrow therapeutic index	Induction or inhibition of CYP3A4-mediated metabolism by cannabis. It is not yet known whether the effects are dependent on the degree of cannabis consumption	Be aware. Watch for signs of toxicity, especially when cannabis use abruptly changes
CANNABIS	VERAPAMIL	Unpredictable changes in plasma concentration. Risk of toxicity or therapeutic failure, particularly of drugs with a narrow therapeutic index	1. Induction of CYP1A2-mediated metabolism by any form of smoking. Foods (e.g., broccoli, cabbage, Brussels sprouts, chargrilled meat) also induce this isoenzyme. 2. Induction or inhibition of CYP3A4-mediated metabolism by cannabis. It is not yet known whether the effects are dependent on the degree of cannabis consumption	Watch for poor response to verapamil; conversely, watch for toxic effects if a previously heavy cannabis user stops smoking
CANNABIS	**DRUG DEPENDENCE THERAPIES**			
CANNABIS	BUPROPION	Unpredictable changes in plasma concentration. Risk of toxicity or therapeutic failure, particularly of drugs with a narrow therapeutic index	Induction or inhibition of CYP3A4-mediated metabolism by cannabis. It is not yet known whether the effects are dependent on the degree of cannabis consumption	Be aware. Watch for signs of toxicity, especially when cannabis use abruptly changes
CANNABIS	DISULFIRAM	Risk of hypomania	Mechanism uncertain and may be due to the presence of adulterants	Be aware

(*Continued*)

Primary Drug	Secondary Drug	Effect	Mechanism	Precautions
CANNABIS				
CANNABIS	DRUGS OF ABUSE—COCAINE	Quickens the onset of effects of cocaine and ↑ bioavailability of cocaine, leading to enhanced subjective effects of cocaine (e.g., euphoria), and ↑ heart rate and other cardiac effects such as ischemia	Attributed to cannabis-induced vasodilatation of the nasal mucosa, which leads to ↑ absorption of cocaine	Be aware. May be the cause of ischemic cardiac pain in young adults
CANNABIS	ECHINACEA AND OTHER IMMUNOSTIMULANTS	May ↓ immunostimulant effects	The cannabinoid receptor is considered to mediate immunosuppressant effects and is currently being investigated in the development of novel immunosuppressants	Be aware
CANNABIS	ESTROGENS—ETHINYLESTRADIOL	Unpredictable changes in plasma concentration. Risk of toxicity or therapeutic failure, particularly of drugs with a narrow therapeutic index	Induction or inhibition of CYP3A4-mediated metabolism by cannabis. It is not yet known whether the effects are dependent on the degree of cannabis consumption	Be aware. Watch for signs of toxicity, especially when cannabis use abruptly changes
CANNABIS	PHOSPHODIESTERASE TYPE 5 INHIBITORS—SILDENAFIL	Report of myocardial infarction	Both drugs have been independently linked to myocardial infarction. However, the exact mechanism is uncertain	Be aware
CANNABIS	PROGESTOGENS	Unpredictable changes in plasma concentration. Risk of toxicity or therapeutic failure, particularly of drugs with a narrow therapeutic index	Induction or inhibition of CYP3A4-mediated metabolism by cannabis. It is not yet known whether the effects are dependent on the degree of cannabis consumption	Be aware. Watch for signs of toxicity, especially when cannabis use abruptly changes
CANNABIS	PROTON PUMP INHIBITORS—OMEPRAZOLE, LANSOPRAZOLE	Unpredictable changes in plasma concentration. Risk of toxicity or therapeutic failure, particularly of drugs with a narrow therapeutic index	Induction or inhibition of CYP3A4-mediated metabolism by cannabis. It is not yet known whether the effects are dependent on the degree of cannabis consumption	Be aware. Watch for signs of toxicity, especially when cannabis use abruptly changes

DRUGS OF ABUSE CANNABIS

Primary Drug	Secondary Drug	Effect	Mechanism	Precautions
AMPHETAMINES				
Amphetamines are available in various forms. It is metabolized primarily by CYP2D6. There is a salt form—methylamphetamine ("speed")—and a free base form ("base"), which looks like a damp or oily paste and a crystalloid form ("ice" or "crystal meth") and is taken orally or intranasally ("snorting"), or injected intravenously. Primary mode of action is ↑ release of dopamine. It also inhibits dopamine metabolism and its reuptake, and ↑ release of norepinephrine and serotonin. Toxic effects include restlessness, tremor, anxiety, irritability, insomnia, psychosis, aggression, sweating, palpitations, chest pain, ↑ blood pressure, shortness of breath, and headache. In Australia, methamphetamine is the second most commonly used illicit drug after cannabis, with almost 10% of the population having tried it. Methamphetamine produces similar effects to amphetamine, but at smaller doses, it produces prominent CNS effects.				
AMPHETAMINES METHAMPHETAMINE, MDMA	ETHANOL	Increase serum concentrations of MDMA by 9%–15%	Alcohol may slow methamphetamine metabolism	Need to warn users
AMPHETAMINES	ALPHA-BLOCKERS	Antagonism of hypotensive effect	Due to ↑ release of norepinephrine	Need to warn users
AMPHETAMINES	ANALGESICS—OPIOIDS—ALFENTANIL, FENTANYL, PROPOXYPHENE	↑ Plasma concentrations of amphetamine, with risk of toxic effects	Due to inhibition of CYP2D6-mediated metabolism of amphetamine	Need to warn users
AMPHETAMINES	ANTIARRHYTHMICS—AMIODARONE	↑ Plasma concentrations of amphetamine, with risk of toxic effects	Due to inhibition of CYP2D6-mediated metabolism of amphetamine	Need to warn users
AMPHETAMINES	QUINIDINE	↑ Plasma concentrations of amphetamine, with risk of toxic effects	Due to inhibition of CYP2D6-mediated metabolism of amphetamine	Need to warn users
AMPHETAMINES	**ANTIDEPRESSANTS**			
AMPHETAMINES	MAOIs	Risk of severe and life-threatening hypertension. The risk is greatest with nonselective MAOIs	MAOI is an enzyme that metabolizes dopamine, norepinephrine, and other amines	Need to warn users
AMPHETAMINES	SSRIs	↑ Plasma concentrations of amphetamine, with risk of toxic effects	Due to inhibition of CYP2D6-mediated metabolism of amphetamine	Need to warn users
AMPHETAMINES	TCAs	Risk of severe and life-threatening hypertension and arrhythmias. May give false–positive urine tests for amphetamines	Additive effects on cardiovascular system due to enhanced noradrenergic activity	Need to warn users

(*Continued*)

Primary Drug	Secondary Drug	Effect	Mechanism	Precautions
AMPHETAMINES				
AMPHETAMINES	VENLAFAXINE	Risk of severe and life-threatening hypertension and arrhythmias	Additive effects on cardiovascular system due to enhanced noradrenergic activity	Need to warn users
AMPHETAMINES	ANTIMIGRAINE DRUGS—ERGOT ALKALOIDS	↑ Risk of ergotism, usually beginning as numbness and tingling of the extremities	Additive peripheral vasoconstriction	Need to warn users
AMPHETAMINES	ANTIVIRALS—RITONAVIR	↑ Plasma concentrations of amphetamine, with risk of toxic effects	Due to inhibition of CYP2D6-mediated metabolism of amphetamine	Need to warn users
AMPHETAMINES	BRONCHODILATORS—BETA-2 AGONISTS	↑ Risk of tachycardia, arrhythmias, and hypertension	Additive effect on target organ receptors (myocardium, blood vessels)	Need to warn users
AMPHETAMINES	H2 RECEPTOR BLOCKERS—CIMETIDINE	↑ Plasma concentrations of amphetamine, with risk of toxic effects	Due to inhibition of CYP2D6-mediated metabolism of amphetamine	Need to warn users
AMPHETAMINES	SYMPATHOMIMETICS	Risk of severe and life-threatening hypertension and arrhythmias	Additive effects on cardiovascular system due to enhanced noradrenergic activity	Need to warn users
AMPHETAMINES	URINARY ALKALINIZERS	Alkaline urine increases amounts of unionized amphetamine, which then permits increased tubular reabsorption	This effect may increase the half-life from 7–12 h to 18–34 h for methamphetamine or from 7 to 16–31 h for MDMA	Depending on the situation, some amphetamine users may find this a beneficial effect, whereas others may find it problematic

Primary Drug	Secondary Drug	Effect	Mechanism	Precautions
METHYLENEDIOXYMETHAMPHETAMINE (MDMA, ECSTASY)				

This is "ecstasy," which is structurally related to amphetamine and the hallucinogen mescaline. It is metabolized by a range of CYP isoenzymes, mainly CYP2D6.

It produces a massive ↑ in serotonin release via its effects on the serotonin transporter. MDMA damages brain serotonergic neurons, and functional sequelae (verbal and visual memory problems) may persist even after long periods of abstinence.

Adverse effects are related to excessive CNS and cardiovascular system stimulation (similar to amphetamines). Others are due to excess serotonin—jaw clenching, tooth grinding. There is growing evidence that MDMA may be hepatotoxic; theoretically, concurrent use with potentially hepatotoxic medication, for example, methotrexate may increase the risk of adverse hepatic effects.

Importantly, most MDMA tablets contain other potentially toxic substances, for example, ephedrine, dextromethorphan.

(*Continued*)

DRUGS OF ABUSE METHYLENEDIOXYMETHAMPHETAMINE (MDMA, ECSTASY)

DRUGS OF ABUSE METHYLENEDIOXYMETHAMPHETAMINE (MDMA, ECSTASY)

Primary Drug	Secondary Drug	Effect	Mechanism	Precautions
METHYLENEDIOXYMETHAMPHETAMINE (MDMA, ECSTASY)				
MDMA	**ANALGESICS (OPIOIDS)**			
MDMA	CODEINE, FENTANYL, METHADONE, MEPERIDINE, PENTAZOCINE, D-PROPOXYPHENE, TRAMADOL	↑ Risk of serotonin syndrome	Tramadol produces analgesia by an opioid effect and by the enhancement of serotonergic and adrenergic pathways. The phenylpiperidine series of opioids (meperidine, tramadol, methadone, fentanyl, D-propoxyphene) are very weak serotonin reuptake inhibitors. Codeine is also a substrate of CYP2D6	Need to warn users. ➢ ***For signs and symptoms of serotonin toxicity, see clinical features of some adverse drug interactions, serotonin toxicity, and serotonin syndrome***
MDMA	ALFENTANIL, FENTANYL, PROPOXYPHENE	↑ Plasma concentrations of MDMA, with risk of toxic effects	Due to inhibition of CYP2D6-mediated metabolism of MDMA	Need to warn users
MDMA	ANTIARRHYTHMICS—AMIODARONE	↑ Plasma concentrations of MDMA, with risk of toxic effects	Due to inhibition of CYP2D6-mediated metabolism of MDMA	Need to warn users
MDMA	**ANTIDEPRESSANTS**			
MDMA	ANTIDEPRESSANTS	Risk of hyponatremia, particularly where dehydration may occur, such as long periods of dancing. The CSM has advised that hyponatremia should be considered in all patients who develop drowsiness, confusion, or convulsions while taking an antidepressant	Hyponatremia (usually in elderly people and possibly due to inappropriate secretion of ADH) has been associated with all types of antidepressants, more frequently with SSRIs. Additive effect	Be aware and measure serum electrolytes when there is clinical suspicion
MDMA	DULOXETINE	↑ Risk of serotonin syndrome	Duloxetine inhibits the reuptake of both serotonin and norepinephrine and is metabolized by CYP1A2 and CYP2D6	Need to warn users. ➢ ***For signs and symptoms of serotonin toxicity, see clinical features of some adverse drug interactions, serotonin toxicity, and serotonin syndrome***

(*Continued*)

Primary Drug	Secondary Drug	Effect	Mechanism	Precautions
METHYLENEDIOXYMETHAMPHETAMINE (MDMA, ECSTASY)				
MDMA	MAOIs	Risk of severe and life-threatening hypertension. Risk is greatest with nonselective MAOIs. At least four deaths have been reported following the ingestion of MDMA and moclobemide. Another death was reported after phenelzine coingestion	MAO is an enzyme that metabolizes dopamine, norepinephrine, and other amines	Need to warn users
MDMA	SSRIs	↑ Risk of serotonin syndrome	Additive effect; ↑ release by MDMA and inhibition of reuptake by SSRIs causes increased brain concentrations of serotonin	Need to warn users. ➢ ***For signs and symptoms of serotonin toxicity, see clinical features of some adverse drug interactions, serotonin toxicity, and serotonin syndrome***
MDMA	TRYPTOPHAN	Tryptophan administration produces poor therapeutic response and adverse effects as passage across the blood–brain barrier is impaired in users and ex-users	5-HTP is a necessary precursor for the brain to produce more serotonin, and MDMA use depletes a person's natural serotonin levels. MDMA can also inhibit tryptophan hydroxylase and the parent compound cannot easily cross the blood–brain barrier	Need to warn users. ➢ ***For signs and symptoms of serotonin toxicity, see clinical features of some adverse drug interactions, serotonin toxicity, and serotonin syndrome***
MDMA	ANTIMIGRAINE DRUGS—5-HT1 Agonists	↑ Risk of serotonin syndrome	Triptans cause direct stimulation of 5-HT receptors, while MDMA causes ↑ release of serotonin	Need to warn users. ➢ ***For signs and symptoms of serotonin toxicity, see clinical features of some adverse drug interactions, serotonin toxicity, and serotonin syndrome***

(Continued)

DRUGS OF ABUSE METHYLENEDIOXYMETHAMPHETAMINE (MDMA, ECSTASY)

Primary Drug	Secondary Drug	Effect	Mechanism	Precautions
METHYLENEDIOXYMETHAMPHETAMINE (MDMA, ECSTASY)				
MDMA	ANTIVIRALS—RITONAVIR	↑ Plasma concentrations of MDMA, with risk of toxic effects. Several cases are reported where concurrent use of MDMA and ritonavir produced serious, sometimes fatal interactions. One death after using methamphetamine and amyl nitrate. In one case, serum concentrations of MDMA were 10-times higher than expected given the dose ingested	Due to inhibition of CYP2D6-mediated metabolism of MDMA	Need to warn users
MDMA	DRUG DEPENDENCE THERAPIES—BUSPIRONE	Markedly ↑ risk of serotonin syndrome	Buspirone is a direct stimulant of 5-HT receptors (5-HT1A)	Need to warn users. ➢ ***For signs and symptoms of serotonin toxicity, see clinical features of some adverse drug interactions, serotonin toxicity, and serotonin syndrome***
MDMA	H2 RECEPTOR BLOCKERS—CIMETIDINE	↑ Plasma concentrations of MDMA, with risk of toxic effects	Due to inhibition of CYP2D6-mediated metabolism of MDMA	Need to warn users

Primary Drug	Secondary Drug	Effect	Mechanism	Precautions
COCAINE				

Cocaine has a number of actions that are as follows:

- It blocks sodium channels, which gives it its local anesthetic properties.
- It increases dopamine (and possibly serotonin), which produces euphoria associated with increased energy, reduced fatigue, and heightened mental alertness. It is highly addictive.
- It has both alpha- and beta-adrenergic effects leading to ↑ heart rate, BP, and cardiac output, and vasoconstriction. This produces an increased oxygen demand with a reduced oxygen supply, which can produce cardiac chest pain even in the presence of normal coronary arteries.
- It enhances platelet aggregation and is atherogenic (leading to narrowed coronary arteries with regular use), which can cause myocardial infarction.

In the United States, cocaine is classified as a schedule II drug, meaning it has a high potential for abuse but can be administered by a physician for legitimate medical uses. By prescription, it is available in the United States as a solution for local mucosal anesthesia. Cocaine is most commonly abused by snorting, smoking, or injecting the drug. It can also be rubbed onto mucous membranes.

(Continued)

Primary Drug	Secondary Drug	Effect	Mechanism	Precautions
COCAINE				
COCAINE				
COCAINE	**ANTIDEPRESSANTS**			
COCAINE	MAOIs INCLUDING ISOCARBOXAZID, LINEZOLID, MOCLOBEMIDE, PHENELZINE, PROCARBAZINE, RASAGILINE, SELEGILINE, TRANYLCYPROMINE	Hypertensive crisis	Due to ↓ metabolism of vasoactive amines following inhibition of enzyme monoamine oxidase	Need to warn users
COCAINE	SSRIs—FLUOXETINE	↓ Euphoria of cocaine	Mechanism uncertain	Need to warn users
COCAINE	TCAs	Increased risk of seizures	Additive effects due to lowered seizure threshold. Cocaine poses the greatest risk for drug-induced seizures	Need to warn users
COCAINE	ANTIEPILEPTICS—CARBAMAZEPINE	Concurrent use of cocaine and carbamazepine may lead to large elevations in blood pressure and heart rate	Uncertain; effect is not consistently reported	Need to warn users
COCAINE	ANTIPSYCHOTICS—PHENOTHIAZINES	Increased risk of seizures	Additive effects due to lowered seizure threshold. Cocaine poses the greatest risk for drug-induced seizures	Need to warn users
COCAINE	BETA-BLOCKERS	Risk of hypertensive crisis	Cocaine produces both alpha- and beta-adrenergic agonist effects; selective beta-blockade leads to unopposed alpha agonism (vasoconstriction)	Need to warn users
COCAINE	BRONCHODILATORS—THEOPHYLLINE	Increased risk of seizures	Additive effects due to lowered seizure threshold. Cocaine poses the greatest risk for drug-induced seizures	Need to warn users
COCAINE	NICOTINE	Since nicotine, like cocaine, is a risk factor for cardiac disease, it is thought that smoking may increase the incidence of cardiac complications arising from cocaine use	Cocaine and nicotine produce a synergistic effect on dopamine release in the reward areas of the brain. Cocaine and nicotine may also exert synergistic effects on myocardial oxygen supply, arterial pressure, cardiac contractility, and atherogenesis	Need to warn users

DRUGS OF ABUSE AMYL NITRITE

Primary Drug	Secondary Drug	Effect	Mechanism	Precautions
HEROIN ➢ ***Analgesics, Opioids***				

Primary Drug	Secondary Drug	Effect	Mechanism	Precautions
HALLUCINOGENS				
LSD—“acid”; psilocybin—magic mushrooms; mescaline—peyote cactus Most hallucinogens act on the serotonergic system				
HALLUCINOGENS	ANTIDEPRESSANTS—LITHIUM, MAOIs, SSRIs, TCAs	Chronic use is considered to ↑ subjective effects of LSD	Uncertain	Be aware

Primary Drug	Secondary Drug	Effect	Mechanism	Precautions
GAMMA-HYDROXYBUTYRIC ACID—***see Drugs Acting on the Nervous System, Anxiolytics and Hypnotics***				

Primary Drug	Secondary Drug	Effect	Mechanism	Precautions
AMYL NITRITE				
AMYL NITRITE	SILDENAFIL	Risk of potentially fatal hypotension	Additive effects on blood vessels	Avoid concurrent use

PART 17

Miscellaneous

Lakshman Delgoda Karalliedde, Janaka Karalliedde, and Seneka Abeyratne

1. Miscellaneous Pharmaceuticals
2. Minerals and Vitamins
3. Alcohol
4. Fruit Juices
5. Herbs

Primary Drug	Secondary Drug	Effect	Mechanism	Precautions
MISCELLANEOUS PHARMACEUTICALS				
ANAGRELIDE				
ANAGRELIDE	DABIGATRAN	Theoretical ↑ risk of bleeding	Additive effect; both drugs have the potential to cause bleeding	Warn patients to report early evidence of bleeding
ANAGRELIDE	ANTICOAGULANTS ANTIPLATELETS (CLOPIDOGREL, ASPIRIN) NSAIDs CILOSTAZOL MILRINONE SSRIs MELATONIN	↑ Risk of bleeding	Additive effects on coagulation e.g., ↓ platelets, ↓ coagulationfactors, Melatonin ↑ prothrombin time.	Monitor coagulation profiles, e.g., INR. Warnpatients to report easy bruising (e.g., bleeding whilst brushing teeth), nose bleeds, etc.
ANAGRELIDE	CIPROFLOXACIN FLUVOXAMINE ONDANSETRON THEOPHYLLINE Other CYP1A2 inhibitors	↑ Adverse effects of anagrelide. May result in QT prolongation	Primarily metabolized by CYP1A2 to the active metabolite, 3-hydroxy-anagrelide, which is subsequently metabolized by CYP1A2 to the inactive metabolite. ~ 35 to 75% of the interindividual variability in CYP1A2 activity is due to genetic factors. Caution with any inhibitor of CYP1A2	Warn patients re dizziness, palpitations, diarrhoea. Do not drive, use machinery, or activities that requires alertness. Limit alcoholic beverages.
ANAGRELIDE	OMEPRAZOLE	↓ Effect of anagrelide	Inducer of CYP1A2 metabolism.	Monitor platelet counts to ensure therapeutic efficay
CINACALCET				
CINACALCET	ANTICANCER AND IMMUNOMODULATING DRUGS—GEFITINIB	Increased levels of gefitinib	CYP2D6 inhibition	Monitor closely
CINACALCET	BUPROPION	↑ Plasma concentrations of these substrates, with risk of toxic effects	Bupropion and its metabolite hydroxybupropion inhibit CYP2D6	Initiate therapy of these drugs, particularly those with a narrow therapeutic index, at the lowest effective dose. Interaction is likely to be important with substrates for which CYP2D6 is considered the only metabolic pathway (e.g., hydrocodone, oxycodone, desipramine, paroxetine, chlorpheniramine, mesoridazine, alprenolol, amphetamines, atomoxetine)

(*Continued*)

Primary Drug	Secondary Drug	Effect	Mechanism	Precautions
MISCELLANEOUS PHARMACEUTICALS				
CINACALCET	ELIGLUSTAT	↑ Eliglustat levels	Inhibition of CYP2D6-mediated metabolism	Reduce dose to 85 mg od
CINACALCET	AZOLE ANTIFUNGALS, ERYTHROMYCIN	↑ Effects of cinacalcet. Symptoms of low blood calcium levels (e.g. burning, numbness, or tingling; muscle aches, cramps, pain, spasms, or weakness; seizures).	Cinacalet ↓ blood Ca2+. Cinacalcet is extensively metabolized by primarily 3A4, 2D6 and 1A2 (e.g., ketoconazole, erythromycin, itraconazole)	Measure serum-Ca2+ before initiation of treatment and within 1 week after starting treatment. Do not use in patients with low blood Ca2+. Dose adjustments of cinacalcet may be necessary, and parathyroid hormone (PTH) and serum calcium concentrations should be closely monitored on initiation and discontinuation of therapy with a strong CYP3A4 inhibitor
CINACALCET	CARVEDILOL, FLECAINIDE, METOPROLOL, THIORIDAZINE, TCAs, VINBLASTINE	↑ Side effects of these drugs when used with cinacalcet	Cinacalcet is a strong inhibitor of CYP2D6 that metabolizes flecainide, vinblastine, thioridazine, and most TCAs.	Dose adjustment of concomitant medications that are predominantly metabolized by CYP2D6 and have a narrow therapeutic index
COLONY-STIMULATING FACTORS				
COLONY-STIMULATING FACTORS	BLEOMYCIN	Increased risk of pulmonary toxicity	Unknown	Monitor pulmonary function more closely
G-CSF	CYCLOPHOSPHAMIDE	Increased risk of pulmonary toxicity	Unknown	Monitor pulmonary function more closely
G-CSF	TOPOTECAN	↓ Response to G-CSF	Uncertain	Adived to delay G-CSF for 24 hr after completing topotecan therapy.
COLONY-STIMULATING FACTORS—FILGRASTIM	FLUOROURACIL	Possible ↑ risk of neutropenia	Uncertain	Monitor FBC regularly
DEFERASIROX				
DEFERASIROX	ANTICANCER AND IMMUNOMODULATING DRUGS—PACLITAXEL	Possible interaction with paclitaxel	Effects on CYP2C8	Caution with concurrent use

(*Continued*)

Primary Drug	Secondary Drug	Effect	Mechanism	Precautions
MISCELLANEOUS PHARMACEUTICALS				
DEFERASIROX	ANTIDIABETICS—REPAGLINIDE	Increased risk of hypoglycemia	Plasma concentration of repaglinide increased	Monitor blood glucose levels closely if used concomitantly
DEFERASIROX	BISPHOSPHONATES	May increase risk of gastrointestinal bleeds	Both drugs can cause GI bleeding	Avoid concomitant prescribing
DEFASIROX	Bile acid sequestrants e.g., cholestyramine, colesevelam, colestipol	↓ Blood levels of defarsirox	Uncertain, probably ↓ absorption	Avoid concomitant use. If unavoidable, start with ↑ dose of defasirox
DEFASIROX	Aluminum-containing preparations	↓ Blood levels of defarsirox	Uncertain, probably ↓ absorption	Avoid concomitant use. If unavoidable, start with ↑ dose of defasirox
DEFASIROX	SUBSTRATES OF CYP3A4 (See CYP Table)	↓ Blood concentrations of these substrates	Deferasirox may induce CYP3A4	Closely monitor for therapeutic efficacy of substrates
DEFASIROX	CYP2C8 SUBSTRATE (e.g., repaglinide and paclitaxel) See CYP Table	↑ Blood concentrations of these substrates	Deferasirox inhibits CYP2C8	Decrease dose of substrates whilst monitoring for therapeutic efficacy
DEFASIROX	CYP1A2 SUBSTRATE DRUGS- See CYP Table	↑ Blood concentrations of these substrates	Deferasirox inhibits CYP1A2	Avoid the concomitant use of theophylline or other CYP1A2 substrates with a narrow therapeutic index (e.g., tizanidine)
DEFASIROX	DRUGS INDUCING UDP-GLUCURONYLTRANSFERASE (UGT) METABOLISM, e.g., RIFAMPICIN, PHENYTOIN, PHENOBARBITAL, RITONAVIR	↓ Efficacy of Defasirox	Deferasirox is a substrate of UGT1A1 and to a lesser extent UGT1A3.	↑ Of initial dose is often necessary and monitor therapeutic response
DEFEROXAMINE				
DEFEROXAMINE	PROCHLORPERAZINE	Reports of coma (metabolic encephalopathy) when prochlorperazine is given with deferoxamine	Uncertain	Avoid coadministration; patients have been unconscious for 48–72 hours
DEFEROXAMINE	ASCORBIC ACID	Apparent risk of cataract and of heart disease	Uncertain	Warn patients to abstain from herbs and vitamin preparations with vitamin C
DEFEROXAMINE	GALLIUM CITRATE- Ga-67	↓ Effect of Gallium citrate	Uncertain	Dose adjustments are often required for gallium citrate
DEFEROXAMINE	VIGABATRIN	Prolonged use of both drugs may cause vision loss	Uncertain	Routine vision testing required during vigabatrin therapy

(Continued)

Primary Drug	Secondary Drug	Effect	Mechanism	Precautions
MISCELLANEOUS PHARMACEUTICALS				
ELTROMBOPAG				
ELTROMBOPAG	**ANTICANCER AND IMMUNOMODULATING DRUGS**			
ELTROMBOPAG	AZATHIOPRINE	May result in higher than desired platelet counts in patients with ITP	Additive	Monitor closely
ELTROMBOPAG	METHOTREXATE	Possible increased methotrexate levels	Inhibition of OATPB1 and BCRP. Methotrexate is primarily a substrate of OATP1B1	Caution with concurrent use
ELTROMBOPAG	TOPOTECAN	Possible increased topotecan levels	Inhibition of BCRP	Caution with concurrent use
ELTROMBOPAG	ANTIVIRALS—LOPINAVIR/ RITONAVIR	Possibly ↓ plasma levels of eltrombopag	Uncertain; possible antagonism of eltrombopag	Monitor more closely
ELTROMBOPAG	STATINS	↑ Levels of rosuvastatin, atorvastatin, cerivastatin, and possibly other statins. ↑ Risk of rhabdomyolysis.	Eltromobag is an inhibitor of OATP 1B1 that metabolizes rosuvastatin (an OATP1B1 substrate) was accompanied by a twofold increase in plasma rosuvastatin	Warn patients to report immediately unexplained muscle pain, tenderness, or weakness especially if these symptoms are accompanied by fever or dark colored urine. Especially if these symptoms are accompanied by fever or dark colored urine. Dose of concomitant statins (rosuvastatin, pravastatin, simvastatin, and lovastatin) should be reduced
ELTROMBOPAG	BRENTUMIXAB VEDOTIN, TERIFLUNOMIDE INTERFERON-BETA-1b	↑ Risk of liver dysfunction/ failure. Teriflunomide likely to remain in blood for a prolonged period after the last dose, interactions with other drugs may occur after stopping	Additive effect	Avoid or limit the use of alcohol. Warn patients and watch for early signs of liver failure-e.g., fever, chills, joint pain or swelling, unusual bleeding or bruising, skin rash, itching, loss of appetite, fatigue, nausea, vomiting, abdominal pain, dark colored urine, light colored stools, and/or yellowing of the skin or eyes.

(*Continued*)

Primary Drug	Secondary Drug	Effect	Mechanism	Precautions
MISCELLANEOUS PHARMACEUTICALS				
ELTROMBOPAG	Products with MAGNESIUM, ALUMINUM, CALCIUM, IRON, and/or OTHER MINERALS reduce its effectiveness.	↓ Efficacy of Eltrombopag	Interferes with the absorption of eltrombopag. Systemic exposure is ↑ in people of East Asian descent (population-based PK model).	Separate the dosing of eltrombopag and mineral preparations by at least 4 hours. ↓ Initial dose to 25 mg/day in those of East Asian descent
ELTROMBOPAG	SULFASALAZINE	↑ Effects of sulfasalazine		Adjust dose if toxic effects of sulfasalazine occur
ELTROMBOPAG	VALSARTAN OLMESARTAN	↑ Effects and blood levels of valsartan, olmesartan	Inhibition of substrates of OATP1B1	Adjust dose if toxic effects of valsartan occur.
ELTROMBOPAG	ACETAMINOPHEN, BENZYLPENICILLIN, BOSENTAN, DOXORUBICIN, EZETIMIBE, GLYBURIDS, CIPRFLOXACIN, FLUVOXAMINE, GEMFIBROZIL,TRIMETHOPRIM	↑ Risk of adverse effects of Eltrombopag, attributed to ↓ metabolism/elimination	Eltrombopag is metabolized by liver P450- isoenzymes CYP1A, CYP2C8, and UGT 1A1 and UGT1A3 as major pathways. Inhibition of metabolic pathways	Warn patients to report nausea, vomiting, menorrhagia, myalgia, numbness and tingling of extremities during concurrent therapy.
ELTROMBOPAG	OMEPRAZOLE, RIFAMPIN	↓ Efficacy of Eltrombopag	Attributed to ↑ metabolism	Dose increases of eltromobag may be required.
ELTROMBOPAG	IMATINIB, IRINOTECAN, LAPATINIB, MEGLITINIDES (E.G., NATEGLINIDE, REPAGLINIDE), MITOXANTRONE, CODEINE, NSAIDs, OLMESARTAN, EZETIMIBE, GLYBURIDE	↑ Risk of side effects by eltrombopag	Potentiate substrates of OATP1B1 (bosentan, ezetimibe, glyburide, repaglinide, rifampin) or BCRP (e.g., imatinib, irinotecan, lapatinib, mitoxantrone, sulfasalazine, topotecan);	Be aware and warn patients re toxic effects of these drugs when coadministered with eltrombopag. Monitor and consider ↓ their doses.
EPOETINS				
EPOETINS	ANTICANCER AND IMMUNOMODULATING DRUGS			
EPOETINS	LENALIDOMIDE	Increased risk of thromboembolic events	Additive	Caution with concurrent use; risk is greater when dexamethasone is also used
EPOETINS	THALIDOMIDE	Possible increased thromboembolic risk	Additive	Monitor closely Consider thromboprophylaxis; risk is greater when dexamethasone is also used

(Continued)

Primary Drug	Secondary Drug	Effect	Mechanism	Precautions
MISCELLANEOUS PHARMACEUTICALS				
EPOETINS	DICHLORPHENAMIDE	↓ Potassium	Additive effects	Monitor serum K+ closely as this is a potentially serious interaction
EPOETINS	METHYL TESTOSTERONE, TESTOSTERONE, DANAZOL, OXANDROLONE	↑ Effect of epoetin	Pharmacodynamic interaction. Interaction is less severe with testosterone	Dose reduction of epoetin is often necessary
EPOETINS	CICLOSPORIN	↑ BP. Ciclosporin levels are affected	Epoetin alfa affects red blood cells, it may alter the blood levels of ciclosporin	Check blood pressure and ciclosporin levels as frequently as possible until stable.
EPOETINS	C1 ESTERASE INHIBITORS (Human) CONESTAT ALPHA	↑ Risk of thromboembolism	Additive effect	Avoid concurrent use. When used, monitor closely.
EPOETINS	POMALIDOMIDE	↑ Risk of thromboembolism	Additive effect	Avoid concurrent use. When used, monitor closely.
ROMIPLOSTIM				
ROMIPLOSTIM	AZATHIOPRINE	May result in higher than desired platelet counts in patients with ITP	Additive	Monitor closely
FOLIC ACID—*See Folinic Acid, Anticancer, and Immunomodulating Section*				
METHOXSALEN	**ANTICANCER AND OTHER IMMUNOMODULATING DRUGS**			
METHOXSALEN	CICLOSPORIN	Slight increase in ciclosporin levels	Methoxsalen is a furocoumarin and potent inhibitor of cytochrome P450 (both the liver and intestine). Ciclosporin is metabolized by this enzyme in liver and intestine	General significance uncertain. Be aware of interaction
METHOXSALEN	TEGAFUR	Possible increased levels of tegafur	Tegafur metabolized by CYP2A6. Methoxasalen is a potent inhibitor of CYP2A6	Clinical relevance remains to be determined. Caution with concurrent use

(*Continued*)

Primary Drug	Secondary Drug	Effect	Mechanism	Precautions
MISCELLANEOUS PHARMACEUTICALS				
METHOXSALEN	ISOTRETINON AMINOLEVULINIC ACID–TOPICAL TCAs, STATINS SULFASALAZIN TETRACYCLINES, AMIODARONE, THIAZIDE's, CHLORPROMAZINE CHLORTHALIDONE, QUINOLES TORSEMIDE TRIAMTERENE ETHACRYNIC ACID FLUPHENAZINE GRISEOFULVIN INDAPAMIDE LAMOTRIGINE METHOTREXATE METALAZONE NALIDIXIC ACID	↑ Sensitivity to sunlight	Additive effect Methoxsalen is a naturally occurring substance that is reactive to light. Acts by enhancing the body's sensitivity to ultraviolet light A.	Avoid exposure to sunlight or artificial UV rays (sunlamps or tanning beds. Use a topical sunblock and UVA-absorbing sunglasses for the 24 hour following treatment with methoxsalen
POLYSTYRENE SULFONATE RESINS				
POLYSTYRENE SULFONATE RESINS	NON-ABSORBABLE CATION DONATING ANTACIDS AND LAXATIVES, E.G., MAGNESIUM HYDROXIDE, ALUMINUM HYDROXIDE, ALUMINUM CARBONATE	Systemic alkalosis. Case of grand mal seizure reported in patient with chronic hypocalcemia of renal failure given Sodium Polystyrene Sulfonate with magnesium hydroxide as a laxative. Intestinal obstruction due to concretions of aluminum hydroxide when used in combination. Antacids ↓ resin's potassium exchange capability.	Acts in large intestine, which excretes potassium ions to a greater degree than does the small intestine.	Use only in patients with normal bowel function. Magnesium hydroxide should not be administered with Sodium Polystyrene Sulfonate. Monitor for hypokalemia. See Hypokalemia–introductory section
POLYSTYRENE SULFONATE RESINS	SORBITOL	Cases of intestinal necrosis (may be fatal), and other serious GI adverse events (bleeding, ischemic colitis, perforation) reported		
POLYSTYRENE SULFONATE RESINS	LITHIUM, THYROXINE	↓ Levels of lithium and thyroid hormone preparations. Risk of therapeutic failure	↓ Absorption by resin	Monitor lithium and thyroid hormone levels.

(Continued)

Primary Drug	Secondary Drug	Effect	Mechanism	Precautions
MISCELLANEOUS PHARMACEUTICALS				
SEVELAMER				
SEVELAMER	QUINOLNES, CICLOSPORIN, LEVOTHYROXINE, NALIDIXIC ACID, FUROSEMIDE	↓ Absorption	Sevelamar is used to bind phosphate. Also binds to several other medications.	Separate doses
SEVELAMER	**ANTICANCER AND IMMUNOMODULATING DRUGS**			
SEVELAMER	MYCOPHENOLATE	↓ Plasma concentrations of mycophenolate	Attributed to binding of mycophenolate to calcium free phosphate binders	Separate administration by at least 2 h
SEVELAMER	TACROLIMUS	Possible reduced tacrolimus absorption	Sevelamer binds tacrolimus in gut	Avoid giving drugs at same time and monitor closely
TRANEXAMIC ACID, OTHER INTRAVENOUS ANTIFIBRINOLYTICS	RETINOIDS—TRETINOIN	Increased risk of fatal thrombotic complications in acute promyelocytic leukemia	Additive	Caution with concurrent use
TRANEXAMIC ACID	ESTROGEN PREPARATIONS ESTRADIOL (TOPICAL), NORETHIDRONE, LEVONORGESTREL OSPEMIFENE, CHLOROTRIANISENE TAMOXIFEN RALOXIFENE TOREMIFENE QUINESTROL TRETINON	↑ Risk of blood clots		Do not coadminsiter-Depo-Provera Contraceptive (medroxyprogesterone) levonorgestral.
TRANEXAMIC ACID	AMINOCAPROIC ACID, APROTONIN	↑ Risk of thrombosis	Additive or synergistic pharmacodynamic effects	Concomitant administration of antifibrinolytic agents with other hemostatic agents should be avoided. Consult manufacturer's product labeling for recommended dosing intervals between products.

Primary Drug	Secondary Drug	Effect	Mechanism	Precautions
MINERALS AND VITAMINS				
MORE COMMONLY PRESCRIBED MINERALS AND VITAMINS				
CALCIUM				
CALCIUM	ANALGESICS—ASPIRIN	May ↓ calcium levels in blood and body	Attributed to aspirin ↑ excretion	Be aware
CALCIUM	ANTIBIOTICS—QUINOLONES (CIPROFLOXACIN) TETRACYCLINES	↓ Antibiotic levels	↓ Absorption due to formation of unabsorbable chelates	Separate doses by at least 2 h
CALCIUM	**ANTICANCER AND IMMUNOMODULATING DRUGS**			
CALCIUM	CORTICOSTEROIDS	↓ Calcium levels	↓ Intestinal absorption and ↑ excretion	Separate doses as much as possible
CALCIUM AND DAIRY PRODUCTS	ESTRAMUSTINE	↓ Plasma concentrations of estramustine and risk of poor therapeutic response	Due to ↓ absorption of estramustine due to the formation of a calcium phosphate complex	Administer estramustine 1 h before or 2 h after dairy products or calcium supplements
CALCIUM	**ANTIEPILEPTIC DRUGS**			
CALCIUM	ANTIEPILEPTIC DRUGS	↓ Plasma/body concentrations of calcium	A direct ↓ effect on absorption and also by ↓ vitamin D	Be aware
CALCIUM SALTS; OR ENTERAL FEEDING PRODUCTS (TUBE FEEDING)	PHENYTOIN	↓ Phenytoin levels	↓ Absorption	Separate administration of phenytoin and enteral feeding products by at least 2 h
CALCIUM SUPPLEMENTS	ANTIVIRALS—DOLUTEGRAVIR	↓ Plasma levels of dolutegravir, risk of treatment failure, and resistance	Chelation of dolutegravir with calcium ions	Separate doses, take calcium containing medicines at least 2 h after or 6 h before dolutegravir
CALCIUM	BISPHOSPHONATES	↓ Bisphosphonate levels	↓ Absorption	Separate doses by at least 30 min
CALCIUM	CARDIAC GLYCOSIDES—DIGOXIN	Risk of cardiac arrhythmias with large intravenous doses of calcium	Uncertain. It is known that calcium levels directly correlate with the action of digoxin; therefore, high levels, even if transient, may increase the chance of toxicity	It is recommended that the parenteral administration of calcium should be avoided in patients taking digoxin. If this is not possible, administer calcium slowly and in small aliquots

(Continued)

Primary Drug	Secondary Drug	Effect	Mechanism	Precautions
MINERALS AND VITAMINS				
CALCIUM	DIURETICS—THIAZIDES	Risk of hypercalcemia with high-dose calcium	↓ Renal excretion of calcium by thiazides	Monitor calcium levels closely
CALCIUM	FLUORIDE	↓ Efficacy of fluoride	↓ Absorption	Separate doses by 2–3 h
CALCIUM	IRON—ORAL	↓ Iron levels when iron is given orally. Possibly ↓ calcium levels	↓ Absorption. These two minerals compete for absorption	Separate doses as much as possible; monitor FBC closely. Monitor plasma calcium levels
CALCIUM COMPOUNDS	SYMPATHOMIMETICS	Parenteral calcium administration may ↓ positive inotropic effects of epinephrine and dobutamine	Uncertain; postulated that calcium modulates signal transmission from the receptor	Monitor BP closely; watch for poor response to these inotropes
CALCIUM	THYROID HORMONES—LEVOTHYROXINE	↓ Levothyroxine levels	↓ Absorption due to formation of unabsorbable chelates	Separate doses by at least ↓ hours. Monitor TFTs regularly and consider ↑ dose of levothyroxine
CALCIUM	ZINC	↓ Efficacy of zinc	Unknown	Separate doses by 2–3 h
FLUORIDE				
FLUORIDE	CALCIUM	↓ Efficacy of fluoride	↓ Absorption	Separate doses by 2 h
IRON				
IRON	LEVOFLOXACIN	↓ Plasma/body levels of iron	↓ Absorption due to formation of unabsorbable chelates	Separate oral intake by at least 2 h
IRON-CONTAINING COMPOUNDS	ANTI-PARKINSON'S DRUGS—LEVODOPA, METHYLDOPA	↓ Plasma concentrations of methyldopa (peak levels ↓ by 55%) and levodopa, with risk of therapeutic failure	Iron preparations impair the absorption of methyldopa and levodopa	Be aware and separate oral intake by at least 2 h
IRON SUPPLEMENTS	ANTIVIRALS—DOLUTEGRAVIR	↓ Plasma levels of dolutegravir, risk of treatment failure, and resistance	Chelation of dolutegravir with calcium or iron ions	Separate doses, take supplement at least 2 h after or 6 h before dolutegravir
IRON—ORAL	ZINC	↓ Iron levels when iron is given orally	↓ Absorption	Separate doses as much as possible—monitor FBC closely
MAGNESIUM				
MAGNESIUM (PARENTERAL)	ANESTHETICS—LOCAL—PROCAINE SOLUTIONS	Precipitation of drugs, which may not be immediately apparent	A pharmaceutical interaction	Do not mix in the same infusion or syringe

(Continued)

Primary Drug	Secondary Drug	Effect	Mechanism	Precautions
MINERALS AND VITAMINS				
MAGNESIUM	ANALGESICS—ASPIRIN	May ↓ effects of magnesium in the body	Attributed to an antagonistic effect; mechanism is uncertain	Be aware
MAGNESIUM (PARENTERAL)	CALCIUM CHANNEL BLOCKERS	Case reports of profound muscular weakness when nifedipine was given with parenteral magnesium	Both drugs inhibit calcium influx across cell membranes, and magnesium promotes the movement of calcium into the sarcoplasmic reticulum; this results in muscular paralysis	Do not administer calcium channel blockers during parenteral magnesium therapy
MAGNESIUM (PARENTERAL)	MUSCLE RELAXANTS—DEPOLARIZING, NONDEPOLARIZING	↑ Efficacy of these muscle relaxants, with risk of prolonged neuromuscular blockade	Additive effect; magnesium inhibits ACh release and ↓ postsynaptic receptor sensitivity	Monitor nerve blockade closely
MAGNESIUM	HORMONE REPLACEMENT THERAPY	May cause magnesium depletion	Mg levels tend to ↓ during menopause. Risk–benefit ratios need to be considered on an individual basis as there are suggestions that magnesium can counteract the alleged ↑ risk of heart attacks and strokes in patients on hormone replacement therapy	Be aware
MAGNESIUM	ORAL CONTRACEPTIVES	May cause magnesium depletion	Oral contraceptives tend to increase copper levels, which when high results in ↓ magnesium levels	Be aware
MAGNESIUM	PENICILLAMINE	May cause magnesium depletion	Penicillamine ↓ absorption of several minerals, including magnesium	Be aware and separate the oral intake. Parenteral magnesium is unlikely to be affected
POTASSIUM				
Warn patients to avoid salt substitutes that contain potassium. OTC preparations of minerals and vitamins are unlikely to contain a potentially harmful content of potassium. However, a quarter of a teaspoon of salt substitute with potassium may contain 650 mg of potassium, compared with a prescription potassium tablet of 20 mEq, which contains 750 mg.				
POTASSIUM	POTASSIUM SUPPLEMENTS	Risk of hyperkalemia	Additive effect	Avoid coadministration

(*Continued*)

Primary Drug	Secondary Drug	Effect	Mechanism	Precautions
MINERALS AND VITAMINS				
POTASSIUM	**ANALGESICS**			
POTASSIUM	ASPIRIN	Risk of hypokalemia	Aspirin is considered to ↑ excretion of potassium	Be aware, particularly in people on long-term aspirin therapy, although it is uncertain whether 75–100 mg doses of aspirin cause significant effects
POTASSIUM	NSAIDs	↑ Risk of hyperkalemia	Additive effect	➢ ***For signs and symptoms of hyperkalemia, see clinical features of some adverse drug interactions, hyperkalemia***
POTASSIUM CITRATE	ANTIBIOTICS—METHENAMINE	↓ Methenamine levels	Citrate alkalinizes the urine, which ↑ excretion of methenamine	Avoid coadministration
POTASSIUM	**ANTICANCER AND IMMUNOMODULATING DRUGS**			
POTASSIUM	CICLOSPORIN	↑ Risk of hyperkalemia	Additive effect	➢ ***For signs and symptoms of hyperkalemia, see clinical features of some adverse drug interactions, hyperkalemia***
POTASSIUM	CORTICOSTEROIDS	Risk of hypokalemia	Most corticosteroids (cortisone, prednisone) ↑ loss of potassium	Be aware and monitor serum potassium levels, particularly in patients on long-term therapy with steroids
POTASSIUM	TACROLIMUS	Risk of hyperkalemia	Additive effect	Monitor potassium levels closely
POTASSIUM	ANTIHYPERTENSIVES AND HEART FAILURE DRUGS—ACE INHIBITORS, ANGIOTENSIN II RECEPTOR ANTAGONISTS	↑ Risk of hyperkalemia	Retention of potassium by ACE inhibitors and additional intake of potassium	Monitor serum potassium daily
POTASSIUM	DIURETICS—POTASSIUM-SPARING	Risk of hyperkalemia	Additive effect	Monitor potassium levels closely
POTASSIUM	LAXATIVES	Long-term use of laxatives may cause hypokalemia. Laxatives may cause ↓ plasma/body concentrations of several minerals	Due to ↑ intestinal loss of potassium. Long-term use may cause ↓ absorption of several minerals	Be aware

(*Continued*)

Primary Drug	Secondary Drug	Effect	Mechanism	Precautions
MINERALS AND VITAMINS				
VITAMINS				
VITAMINS—A, D, E, K, BETA-CAROTENE	ORLISTAT	↓ Absorption of the fat-soluble vitamins	Inhibition of pancreatic lipase by orlistat	Be aware that efficacy of these vitamins may be reduced, e.g., osteoporosis in postmenopausal women
VITAMIN A	RETINOIDS	Risk of vitamin A toxicity	Additive effect; tretinoin is a form of vitamin A	Avoid coadministration
VITAMIN B3 (NIACIN)	ENFUVIRTIDE	↑ Risk of injection site reactions, e.g., pain, redness, swelling	Possibly an exaggerated immune response involving Langerhans cells	Advise patients to report ongoing injection site reactions
VITAMIN B6	ANTIEPILEPTICS—PHENOBARBITONE, PHENYTOIN	↓ Plasma concentrations of these antiepileptics	Uncertain	Watch for poor response to these antiepileptics if large doses of vitamin B6 are given
VITAMIN B6	ANTI-PARKINSON'S DRUGS—LEVODOPA	↓ Efficacy of levodopa (in the absence of a dopa decarboxylase inhibitor)	A derivative of vitamin B6 is a cofactor in the peripheral conversion of levodopa to dopamine, which ↓ amount available for conversion in the CNS. DOPA decarboxylase inhibitors inhibit this peripheral reaction	Avoid coadministration of levodopa with vitamin B6; coadministration of vitamin B6 with co-beneldopa or co-careldopa is acceptable
VITAMIN B12	ANTIBIOTICS—CHLORAMPHENICOL	↓ Efficacy of hydroxycobalamin	Chloramphenicol depresses the bone marrow; this opposes the action of vitamin B12	Be aware; monitor FBC and vitamin B12 levels closely
VITAMIN C	ANTACIDS CONTAINING ALUMINUM	↓ Aluminum levels, with risk of encephalopathy in patients with renal failure	Uncertain; possibly ↑ absorption due to the ascorbic acid in the presence of ↓ renal excretion	Avoid coingestion in patients with renal failure
VITAMIN C	ASPIRIN	May ↓ vitamin C levels	Attributed to aspirin "blocking" the absorption of vitamin C. Aspirin has been found to ↑ elimination of vitamin C and all B vitamins	Be aware

(*Continued*)

Primary Drug	Secondary Drug	Effect	Mechanism	Precautions
MINERALS AND VITAMINS				
VITAMIN D—CALCITRIOL	ANTICANCER AND IMMUNOMODULATING DRUGS—CORTICOSTEROIDS	Possible antagonism of activity by corticosteroids	Antagonism of increased calcium absorption by calcitriol	Be aware of interaction
VITAMIN D	ANTIEPILEPTICS—PHENYTOIN, CARBAMAZEPINE, PRIMIDONE, BARBITURATES	↓ Efficacy of vitamin D	Attributed to induction of vitamin D metabolism	Be aware; consider ↑ dose of vitamin D
VITAMIN D	BISPHOSPHONATES	May cause hypercalcemia	Both drugs increase calcium levels	Monitor calcium and phosphorus levels
VITAMIN D	CARDIAC GLYCOSIDES—DIGOXIN	Theoretical risk of cardiac arrhythmias if hypercalcemia occurs due to vitamin D therapy	Uncertain; it is known that calcium levels directly correlate with the action of digoxin; therefore, high levels, even if transient, may ↑ the chance of toxicity	Monitor serum calcium levels closely
VITAMIN D	DIURETICS—THIAZIDES	Risk of hypercalcemia with vitamin D	↓ Renal excretion of calcium by thiazides	Monitor calcium levels closely
VITAMIN D	MAGNESIUM	↑ Plasma concentrations of magnesium	Due to ↑ absorption	Be aware
VITAMIN E	ANTICOAGULANTS—ORAL	Case of ↑ anticoagulant effect	Uncertain	Monitor INR closely for 1–2 weeks after starting and stopping vitamin E
OTHER MINERAL–DRUG INTERACTIONS				
ANTACIDS	COPPER	↓ Plasma concentration of copper	Most antacids will ↓ absorption of copper	If antacids are used in the long term, consider copper supplements of 1–2 mg/day
ANTIBIOTICS				
AZITHROMYCIN	MAGNESIUM	↓ Plasma/body concentrations of magnesium	Due to ↓ absorption	Be aware
CIPROFLOXACIN	MINERALS—CALCIUM, MAGNESIUM, IRON	↓ Plasma/body levels of calcium, magnesium and iron	↓ Absorption due to formation of unabsorbable chelates	Separate oral intake by at least 2 h

(*Continued*)

Primary Drug	Secondary Drug	Effect	Mechanism	Precautions
MINERALS AND VITAMINS				
CIPROFLOXACIN	ZINC	1. ↓ Antibiotic levels with zinc; 2. ↓ Plasma/body levels of zinc	1. ↓ Absorption 2. ↓ Absorption due to formation of unabsorbable chelates	Separate doses by at least 2 h
ETHAMBUTOL	COPPER	↓ Plasma concentration of copper	Ethambutol binds to copper	Be aware and separate oral intake by at least 2 h
LEVOFLOXACIN	MAGNESIUM	↓ Plasma/body levels of magnesium	↓ Absorption due to formation of unabsorbable chelates	Separate oral intake by at least 2 h
NITROFURANTOIN	MAGNESIUM	↓ Plasma/body concentrations of magnesium	Due to ↓ absorption	Be aware
OFLOXACIN	MINERALS—IRON, ZINC	↓ Absorption of iron and zinc	Due to formation of unabsorbable chelates	Separate oral intake by at least 2 h
TETRACYCLINES	CALCIUM, MAGNESIUM, IRON	↓ Plasma/body levels of calcium, magnesium and iron	↓ Absorption due to formation of unabsorbable chelates	Separate oral intake by at least 2 h
TETRACYCLINES	ZINC	1. ↓ Antibiotic levels with zinc; doxycycline is less of a problem than the other tetracyclines 2. ↓ Plasma/body levels of zinc	1. ↓ Absorption 2. ↓ Absorption due to formation of unabsorbable chelates	Separate doses by at least 2 h
ANTICANCER AND IMMUNOMODULATING DRUGS				
CORTICOSTEROIDS	SELENIUM, CHROMIUM	↓ Selenium and chromium levels	Attributed to ↑ loss of selenium and chromium	Be aware
PREDNISONE, CORTISONE	ZINC, CALCIUM, CHROMIUM, MAGNESIUM, SELENIUM	↓ Plasma/body concentrations of these minerals	Attributed to ↑ loss and/or ↓ absorption	Be aware and monitor plasma concentrations of these minerals; provide supplements
PENICILLAMINE	IRON AND OTHER MINERALS	↓ Plasma concentrations of several minerals	Due to formation of unabsorbable chelates	Separate oral intake by at least 2 h
PENICILLAMINE	ZINC	↓ Penicillamine and zinc levels	Mutual ↓ absorption	Avoid coadministration
ANTICOAGULANTS—WARFARIN	MAGNESIUM, IRON, ZINC	↓ Plasma/body concentrations of magnesium, iron and zinc	Due to ↓ absorption	Be aware
ANTIDIABETIC DRUGS				
GLIPIZIDE	MAGNESIUM	↓ Plasma/body concentrations of magnesium	Due to ↓ absorption	Be aware

(Continued)

Primary Drug	Secondary Drug	Effect	Mechanism	Precautions
MINERALS AND VITAMINS				
HYPOGLYCEMIC DRUGS	CHROMIUM	Chromium supplements may ↑ risk of hypoglycemia	Chromium is necessary for the production of insulin	Be aware
ANTIEPILEPTICS				
CARBAMAZEPINE PHENYTOIN BARBITURATES PRIMIDONE	COPPER AND ZINC	↓ Plasma concentrations of copper and zinc	Attributed to ↓ absorption	Be aware
VALPROIC ACID	SELENIUM	↓ Selenium levels	Uncertain	Be aware
ANTIGOUT DRUGS—ALLOPURINOL	COPPER	↓ Plasma concentration of copper	Allopurinol chelates copper	Be aware and separate oral intake by at least 2 h
ANTIPSYCHOTIC DRUGS—CLOZAPINE	SELENIUM	↓ Selenium levels	Uncertain	Be aware
ANTIVIRALS—ZIDOVUDINE	ZINC	↓ Plasma/body concentrations of zinc	Due to ↓ absorption	Be aware
H2 RECEPTOR BLOCKERS	COPPER AND IRON, ZINC AND CALCIUM	↓ Plasma and body concentrations of copper, iron, zinc, and calcium	As a class, H2 antagonists act as free radical scavengers and cause depletion of calcium, iron, and zinc. Cimetidine in particular binds to copper and iron, and these minerals are not made available for free radical production	Be aware and separate oral intake by 2 h
LIPID-LOWERING DRUGS—CHOLESTYRAMINE, COLESTIPOL	IRON	↓ Plasma/body concentrations of iron	Due to ↓ absorption	Be aware and do an FBC at least 2-weekly if on long-term therapy. Separate oral intake by 2 h
PROTON PUMP INHIBITORS	IRON	↓ Plasma concentrations of iron	Proton pump inhibitors inhibit the absorption of iron	Consider use of parenteral iron in patients on proton pump inhibitors treatment
TRIENTINE	ZINC	↓ Zinc and trientine levels	Mutually ↓ absorption	Separate doses by at least 2 h

Primary Drug	Secondary Drug	Effect	Mechanism	Precautions
ALCOHOL				
Alcohol is an ingredient in many OTC and even some prescription medicines. The amounts are modest in most cases, but a few reach concentrations of 40% or 50% proof. Cough and cold elixirs are the most likely sources, but some vitamin "tonics" and laxatives also contain alcohol.				
ALCOHOL	**ANALGESICS**			
ALCOHOL	ASPIRIN	Alleged ↑ effects of alcohol after relatively innocuous amounts of wine, beer, etc., which made it popular among users; the effects are, however, unproven. One study found that aspirin taken an hour before drinking a modest amount of alcohol (one and a half drinks) raised levels in the bloodstream by 26%. ↑ Risk of gastric irritation	A study suggested the presence of alcohol dehydrogenase in the stomach of some men, which was inactivated by aspirin. Additive irritant effects on gastric mucosa	Be aware. The FDA has considered the probability of inactivation of stomach alcohol dehydrogenase as "not dangerous"
ALCOHOL	OPIOIDS	↑ Sedation. Report of hypotension with codeine	Additive effect	Warn patients
ALCOHOL	**ANTIBIOTICS**			
ALCOHOL	CEPHALOSPORINS	Disulfiram-like reaction, with flushing, wheezing, breathing difficulties, nausea, and vomiting with some cephalosporins. This potentially dangerous interaction can come on right away, or it may be delayed by as much as a few days	It is considered that a reactive metabolite probably inactivates alcohol dehyrogenase	Do not consume alcohol for 3 days following stopping the antibiotic
ALCOHOL	CYCLOSERINE	Risk of fits	Additive effect; cycloserine can cause fits	Warn patients to drink alcohol only minimally while taking cycloserine
ALCOHOL	METRONIDAZOLE	Disulfiram-like reaction. Unsteadiness, and incoordination caused by metronidazole may be aggravated by alcohol	Metronidazole inhibits aldehyde dehydrogenase. Additive side effects	Avoid coingestion
ALCOHOL	TETRACYCLINE	Likely ↓ efficacy of antibiotic	Uncertain	Be aware

(*Continued*)

Primary Drug	Secondary Drug	Effect	Mechanism	Precautions
ALCOHOL				
ALCOHOL	**ANTICANCER AND IMMUNOMODULATING DRUGS**			
ALCOHOL	METHOTREXATE	↑ Risk of liver damage/toxicity	Additive liver toxicity	Be aware; advocate abstinence. Monitor liver function
ALCOHOL	PROCARBAZINE	May cause a disulfiram-like reaction, additive depression of the CNS, and postural hypotension	Some alcoholic beverages (beer, wine, ale) contain tyramine, which may induce hypertensive reactions	Avoid coadministration
ALCOHOL	TRABECTEDIN	Increased risk of hepatotoxicity	Additive	Avoid alcohol consumption
ALCOHOL	ANTICOAGULANTS—ORAL	Fluctuations in anticoagulant effect in heavy drinkers or patients with liver disease who drink alcohol	Alcohol may reduce the half-life of oral anticoagulants by inducing hepatic enzymes. Also, they may alter the hepatic synthesis of clotting factors	Caution should be taken when prescribing oral anticoagulants to alcoholics, particularly those who binge drink or have liver damage
ALCOHOL	**ANTIDEPRESSANTS**			
ALCOHOL	MAOIs	Additive depression of CNS ranging from drowsiness to coma and respiratory depression	Synergistic depressant effects on CNS function	Necessary to warn patients, particularly regard activities that require attention, e.g., driving or using machinery and equipment that could cause self-harm
ALCOHOL	SSRIs	↑ Risk of sedation	Additive CNS depressant effects. Acute ingestion of alcohol inhibits CYP2D6 and CYP2C19, whereas chronic use induces CYP2E1 and CYP3A4	Be aware and caution against excessive alcohol intake
ALCOHOL	TCAs, MIRTAZAPINE	↑ Sedation	Additive effect	Warn patients about this effect
ALCOHOL	**ANTIEPILEPTICS**			
ALCOHOL	BARBITURATES	↑ Sedation	Additive sedative effect	Warn patients about this effect
ALCOHOL	PHENYTOIN	↑ Phenytoin levels and risk of toxic effects of phenytoin. Daily alcohol use can decrease your blood levels of phenytoin, and ↑ increase risk of seizures	Uncertain	Warn patients re alcohol consumption
ALCOHOL	TOPIRAMATE	↑ Sedation	Additive sedative effect	Warn patients about this effect

(*Continued*)

Primary Drug	Secondary Drug	Effect	Mechanism	Precautions
ALCOHOL				
ALCOHOL	**ANTIDIABETIC DRUGS**			
ALCOHOL	ANTIDIABETIC DRUGS	Tends to mask signs of hypoglycemia and ↑ risk of hypoglycemic episodes	Inhibits glucose production and release from many sources including the liver	Watch for and warn patients about symptoms of hypoglycemia ➢ ***For signs and symptoms of hypoglycemia, see clinical features of some adverse drug interactions, hypoglycemia***
ALCOHOL	METFORMIN	Enhanced effect of metformin and ↑ risk of lactic acidosis. May cause a disulfiram-like interaction	Alcohol is known to potentiate the effect of metformin on lactate metabolism. It inhibits glucose production and release from many sources, including the liver	The onset of lactic acidosis is often subtle with symptoms of malaise, myalgia, respiratory distress, and ↑ nonspecific abdominal distress. There may be hypothermia and resistant bradyarrhythmias
ALCOHOL	**ANTIFUNGALS**			
ALCOHOL	GRISEOFULVIN	A disulfiram-like reaction can occur	Uncertain	Warn patients not to drink alcohol while taking griseofulvin
ALCOHOL	KETOCONAZOLE	May ↑ risk of liver damage. Symptoms of nausea, headache, flushing, and discomfort (similar to a disulfiram-type reaction) may occur	Additive liver toxicity	Be aware
ALCOHOL	**ANTIHISTAMINES**			
ALCOHOL	ANTIHISTAMINES	↑ Sedation with sedating antihistamines	Additive effect	Warn patients about this effect. Remember that cold medicines as well as allergy pills may well contain antihistamines
ALCOHOL	CIMETIDINE, RANITIDINE	Alleged ↑ effects of alcohol after relatively innocuous amounts of wine, beer, etc., which made it popular among users; the effect is, however, unproven	A study suggested the presence of alcohol dehydrogenase in the stomach of some men, which was inactivated by cimetidine and ranitidine	Be aware. The FDA has considered the probability of inactivation of stomach alcohol dehydrogenase as "not dangerous"

(*Continued*)

Primary Drug	Secondary Drug	Effect	Mechanism	Precautions
ALCOHOL				
ALCOHOL	**ANTIHYPERTENSIVES AND HEART FAILURE DRUGS**			
ALCOHOL	ANTIHYPERTENSIVES AND HEART FAILURE DRUGS	1. Acute alcohol ingestion may ↑ hypotensive effects 2. Chronic moderate or heavy drinking ↓ hypotensive effects	1. Additive hypotensive effect 2. Chronic alcohol excess is associated with hypertension	Monitor BP closely as unpredictable responses can occur. Advise patients to drink alcohol only in moderation and to avoid large variations in the amount of alcohol drunk
ALCOHOL	ALPHA-BLOCKERS	↑ Levels of both alcohol and indoramin prazosin occur with concurrent use	Uncertain	Warn patients about the risk of ↑ sedation dizziness
ALCOHOL	CENTRALLY ACTING ANTIHYPERTENSIVES	Clonidine and moxonidine may exacerbate the sedative effects of alcohol, particularly during initiation of therapy	Uncertain	Warn patients of this effect, and advise them to avoid driving or operating machinery if they suffer from sedation
ALCOHOL	RESERPINE	↑ Effects of both reserpine and alcohol	Reserpine has CNS effects, while alcohol may act as a vasodilator hypotensive	Avoid concomitant use
ALCOHOL	ANTIMUSCARINICS—ATROPINE, GLYCOPYRRONIUM	↑ Sedation	Additive effect	Warn patients about this effect, and advise them not to drink while taking these antimuscarinics
ALCOHOL	**ANTIPROTOZOALS**			
ALCOHOL	LEVAMISOLE	Risk of a disulfiram-like reaction	Uncertain	Warn patients not to drink alcohol while taking levamisole
ALCOHOL	TINIDAZOLE	Risk of a disulfiram-like reaction	Uncertain	Warn patients not to drink alcohol while taking tinidazole
ALCOHOL	ANTIPSYCHOTICS	Risk of excessive sedation	Additive effect	Warn patients of this effect, and advise them to drink alcohol only in moderation
ALCOHOL	ANTIVIRALS—MARAVIROC	↑ Plasma levels of alcohol, increased risk of adverse effects	Unknown	Advise patients to be aware of increased effects of alcohol and consider gradual reduction of their alcohol intake

(*Continued*)

Primary Drug	Secondary Drug	Effect	Mechanism	Precautions
ALCOHOL				
CNS DEPRESSANTS—INCLUDING ALCOHOL	ANXIOLYTICS AND HYPNOTICS	↑ Sedation	Additive effect	Warn patients to be aware of this added effect
ALCOHOL	BETA-BLOCKERS	Acute alcohol ingestion may ↑ hypotensive effects. Chronic moderate or heavy drinking ↓ hypotensive effects. Might cause higher blood alcohol levels from modest amounts of alcohol	Additive hypotensive effect. Mechanism underlying the opposite effect with chronic intake is uncertain. A study suggested the presence of alcohol dehydrogenase in the stomach of some men, which was inactivated by propranolol	Monitor BP closely as unpredictable responses can occur. Advise patients to drink alcohol only in moderation and to avoid large variations in the amount of alcohol drunk. The FDA has considered the probability of inactivation of stomach alcohol dehydrogenase as “not dangerous”
ALCOHOL	BETA-CAROTENE (a precursor to vitamin A and a popular antioxidant supplement)	↑ Risk of liver damage	Alcohol combined with beta-carotene led to more liver damage than was produced by alcohol exposure alone	Be aware
ALCOHOL	BROMOCRIPTINE	↑ Risk of severe side effects if alcohol is taken at the same time. (e.g., nausea, stomach pain, dizziness)	Uncertain	Be aware
ALCOHOL	CALCIUM CHANNEL BLOCKERS	1. Acute alcohol ingestion may ↑ hypotensive effects. Chronic moderate or heavy drinking ↓ hypotensive effects 2. Verapamil may ↑ peaked serum concentration and prolong the effects of alcohol	1. Additive hypotensive effect with acute alcohol excess. Chronic alcohol excess is associated with hypertension 2. Uncertain at present, but presumed to be due to inhibition of the hepatic metabolism of alcohol, a mechanism similar to that with cimetidine, ranitidine, and aspirin	1. Monitor BP closely as unpredictable responses can occur. Advise patients to drink alcohol only in moderation and to avoid large variations in the amount of alcohol drunk 2. Warn patients about potentiation of the effects of alcohol, particularly the risks to driving

(*Continued*)

Primary Drug	Secondary Drug	Effect	Mechanism	Precautions
ALCOHOL				
ALCOHOL	DIURETICS—THIAZIDES	1. Acute alcohol ingestion may ↑ hypotensive effects 2. Chronic moderate/heavy drinking ↓ hypotensive effect	1. Additive hypotensive effect 2. Chronic alcohol excess is associated with hypertension	Monitor BP closely as unpredictable responses can occur. Advise patients to drink only in moderation and avoid large variations in the amount of alcohol drunk
ALCOHOL	**DRUG DEPENDENCE THERAPIES**			
ALCOHOL	BUPROPION	Rare reports of adverse neuropsychiatric events, including report of seizures. ↓ alcohol tolerance	Uncertain	Warn patients to avoid or minimize alcohol intake during bupropion treatment
ALCOHOL	DISULFIRAM	Disulfiram reaction	See drugs acting on the nervous system	Do not coadminister. Disulfiram must not be given within 12 h of ingestion of alcohol. This reaction could occur even with the small amounts of alcohol found in cough syrup or cold remedies
ALCOHOL	LOFEXIDINE	↑ Sedation	Additive effect	Warn patients of risk of excessive sedation
ALCOHOL	MINERALS IRON, ZINC, MAGNESIUM, SELENIUM, CADMIUM	Regular intake of alcohol could cause depletion of iron, zinc, magnesium, and selenium. Alcoholic drinks such as wine and whisky may have high or potentially toxic contents of the toxic element cadmium	Attributed to ↓ absorption or ↓ intake of nutrients	Be aware. Monitor cadmium levels as well as plasma levels of other minerals
ALCOHOL	MUSCLE RELAXANTS—BACLOFEN, METHOCARBAMOL, TIZANIDINE	↑ Sedation	Additive effect	Warn patients; advise them to drink alcohol only in moderation and not to drive if they have drunk any alcohol while taking these muscle relaxants

(*Continued*)

Primary Drug	Secondary Drug	Effect	Mechanism	Precautions
ALCOHOL				
ALCOHOL	NITRATES, NITROGLYCERIN	↑ Risk of postural ↓ BP when GTN is taken with alcohol	Additive effect; both are vasodilators	Warn patients about the risk of feeling faint. Advise them to drink alcohol only in moderation and to avoid binge drinking
ALCOHOL	PARACETAMOL	↑ Risk of liver damage. Might cause higher blood alcohol levels from modest amounts of alcohol, as with aspirin, cimetidine, ranitidine, propranolol, and verapamil	Paracetamol tends to cause greater toxicity in chronic alcoholics with malnutrition or diseased livers. A study suggested the presence of alcohol dehydrogenase in the stomach of some men, which could be inactivated by paracetamol	Be aware, particularly when toxic doses of paracetamol have been taken. The FDA has considered the probability of inactivation of stomach alcohol dehydrogenase as "not dangerous"
ALCOHOL	POTASSIUM CHANNEL ACTIVATORS	Acute alcohol ingestion may ↑ hypotensive effects. Chronic moderate or heavy drinking ↓ hypotensive effects	Additive hypotensive effect. Mechanism underlying the opposite effect with chronic intake is uncertain	Monitor BP closely as unpredictable responses can occur. Advise patients to drink alcohol only in moderation and to avoid large variations in the amount of alcohol drunk
ALCOHOL	VITAMIN C (large doses, e.g., 1000 mg)	May ↑ elimination of alcohol, but this is unproven	Uncertain	Unlikely to be of clinical significance

FRUIT JUICES

Fruit juices that are known to have potential to cause interactions by altering the metabolism of pharmaceuticals.

Grapefruit Juice (*Citrus paradisi*)

Grapefruit juice (GFJ) has a number of actions on drug metabolism and distribution.

1. Decrease intestinal CYP3A4 activity, reducing first-pass metabolism.
   a. It can enhance systemic drug exposure by up to 1400%.
   b. Inhibition is localized largely in the gut with little effect on hepatic CYP3A4.
   c. It has little effect on the pharmacokinetics of an intravenously administered substrate.
   d. It has little effect on the elimination half-life of an orally administered substrate.
2. Inhibition of the efflux transporter Pgp, thus increasing the bioavailability of several drugs. Whether or not GFJ modulates intestinal Pgp activity remains controversial.
3. Inhibition of enteric OATP activity.
4. Onset of interaction can occur within 30 min of drinking a single glass of juice.
5. Inhibition can last up to 3 days following the last administration of GFJ.
6. One whole grapefruit or 200 mL of juice is sufficient to cause enough of an increase in the concentrations of active drugs to have an effect on the body, and therefore could cause side effects.
7. If a drug has low inherent oral bioavailability from presystemic metabolism by CYP3A4 or efflux transport by Pgp and the potential to produce serious overdose toxicity, avoidance of GFJ entirely during pharmacotherapy appears mandatory.

Primary Drug	Secondary Drug	Effect	Mechanism	Precautions
GRAPEFRUIT JUICE				
GRAPEFRUIT JUICE	**ANALGESICS**			
GRAPEFRUIT JUICE	NSAIDS—DICLOFENAC	Although low doses (1 mg/kg) of grapefruit juice did not potentiate the effect of diclofenac, higher doses ↑ anti-inflammatory effect (as assessed by an effect on rat's paw edema)	Diclofenac undergoes phenyl hydroxylation catalyzed by CYP2C9 and CYP3A4. High dose of grapefruit juice possibly ↑ effects by inhibiting CYP3A4	Be aware as all the effects of diclofenac, including toxic effects, may ↑
GRAPEFRUIT JUICE	**OPIOIDS**			
GRAPEFRUIT JUICE	METHADONE	↑ Plasma concentrations and ↑ risk of adverse effects. Interaction is considered to be of rapid onset but of minor clinical significance	Methadone is metabolized by intestinal CYP3A4, which is inhibited by grapefruit juice	Prudent to be aware and warn users and carers of rapid onset of drowsiness, difficulty in breathing
GRAPEFRUIT JUICE	MORPHINE	Grapefruit juice ↑ morphine antinociception. Gradually ↓ CSF and blood concentrations following repeated treatment with morphine	Grapefruit juice is considered to ↑ intestinal absorption of morphine due to inhibition of Pgp, which also probably contributes to ↓ CSF concentrations	This interaction is unlikely to be of clinical significance, but be aware. Warn patients, carers to report any difficulty in breathing, excessive drowsiness
GRAPEFRUIT JUICE	**ANTIARRHYTHMICS**			
GRAPEFRUIT JUICE	AMIODARONE	Markedly ↑ plasma concentrations of amiodarone (AUC >50%, maximum concentration >84%). Possibly ↓ effect of amiodarone (↓ in P–R and QTc intervals). This could lead to ↓ therapeutic effect due to ↓ production of active metabolite	Due to inhibition of CYP3A4-mediated metabolism of amiodarone by grapefruit juice, which results in near-complete inhibition of the production of N-desethylamiodarone (DEA, the active and major metabolite of amiodarone)	Warn patients to avoid grapefruit juice; if amiodarone becomes less effective, ask the patient about grapefruit juice. **Torsade de pointes reported with high volumes of GFJ**
GRAPEFRUIT JUICE	AMLODIPINE	↑ Plasma amlodipine levels (AUC ↑ by 116%, maximum concentration ↑ by 115%) but no adverse hemodynamic (no changes in PR, heart rate) effects. Unlikely to be clinically significant	There is report of pharmacokinetic interaction between amlodipine and grapefruit in healthy volunteers (maximum concentration and AUC were significantly higher when amlodipine 5 mg was administered with grapefruit compared with water)	Considering the interindividual variation in the pharmacokinetics of amlodipine, the possible interaction between amlodipine and grapefruit juice cannot be neglected in the clinical setting even though the interaction does not seem to be of great clinical significance in human volunteer studies

(*Continued*)

Primary Drug	Secondary Drug	Effect	Mechanism	Precautions
GRAPEFRUIT JUICE				
GRAPEFRUIT JUICE	DISOPYRAMIDE	Possibly ↓ effect of disopyramide	Likely to be due to inhibited CYP3A4-mediated metabolism of disopyramide	Monitor ECG and side effects more closely
GRAPEFRUIT JUICE	DRONEDARONE	↑ Levels of dronedarone	Grapefruit juice inhibits CYP 3A4-mediated metabolism of dronedarone	Warn patient to avoid grapefruit juice while taking dronedarone
GRAPEFRUIT JUICE	DOFETILIDE	Risk of ↑ dofetilide levels with risk of ↑ QT prolongation	Grapefruit juice inhibits CYP3A4-mediated metabolism of dofetilide	Avoid coadministration
GRAPEFRUIT JUICE	PROPAFENONE	Grapefruit juice may ↑ propafenone levels	Grapefruit juice inhibits CYP2D6-mediated metabolism of propafenone	Advice patient to avoid grapefruit juice
GRAPEFRUIT JUICE	QUINIDINE	Absorption of quinidine is delayed (e.g., from 1.6 to 3.3 h) by grapefruit juice in a dose-dependent manner	Possibly due to effects on intestinal CYP3A4	Be aware. Avoid concomitant use. Torsade de pointes reported with high volumes of GFJ
GRAPEFRUIT JUICE	ANTIBIOTICS—CLARITHROMYCIN, ERYTHROMYCIN	Significant delay in onset of action of clarithromycin (↑ from 82 to 148 min). ↑ Plasma concentrations of erythromycin (maximum concentration ↑, AUC ↑ 1.5-fold)	Due to inhibition of absorption attributed to effect on Pgp	The interaction is unlikely to cause clinically relevant ↓ antimicrobial activity of clarithromycin Telithromycin is unlikely to be affected by grapefruit juice. Be aware
GRAPEFRUIT JUICE	**ANTICANCER AND IMMUNOMODULATING DRUGS**			
GRAPEFRUIT JUICE	**CYTOTOXICS**			
GRAPEFRUIT JUICE	AXITINIB	Increased levels of axitinib	CYP3A4/5 inhibition	Manufacturer advises avoid concurrent use with strong CYP3A4/5 inhibitors if possible. If concurrent use is necessary, dose adjustment is recommended
GRAPEFRUIT JUICE	BOSUTINIB	Increased bosutinib levels	CYP3A inhibition	Manufacturer advises avoid concurrent use. If not possible, interruption of therapy or dose reduction should be considered

(Continued)

Primary Drug	Secondary Drug	Effect	Mechanism	Precautions
GRAPEFRUIT JUICE				
GRAPEFRUIT JUICE	CRIZOTINIB	Possible increased crizotinib levels	CYP3A inhibition	Manufacturer advises avoid concurrent use
GRAPEFRUIT JUICE	DASATINIB	Possible increased dasatinib levels	CYP3A4 inhibition	Avoid concurrent use
GRAPEFRUIT JUICE	DOCETAXEL	↑ Docetaxel levels	Inhibition of CYP3A4-mediated metabolism of docetaxel	Warn patients to avoid grapefruit juice
GRAPEFRUIT JUICE	DOXORUBICIN	↑ Risk of myelosuppression due to ↑ plasma concentrations	Due to ↓ metabolism of doxorubicin by CYP3A4 isoenzymes owing to an inhibition of those enzymes	Monitor for ↑ myelosuppression, peripheral neuropathy, myalgias, and fatigue
GRAPEFRUIT JUICE	ERLOTINIB	Possible slightly increased erlotinib levels	CYP3A4 inhibition	Caution with concurrent use
GRAPEFRUIT JUICE	ETOPOSIDE	↓ In plasma concentrations of etoposide (AUC ↓ 1.32-fold). Clinical significance is uncertain. Possibly ↓ efficacy	↓ Bioavailability. Unclear	Interindividual variability is considerable. Be aware. Advise patients to ↓ intake of foods and beverages containing bioflavonoids. Monitor therapeutic effects closely
GRAPEFRUIT JUICE	EVEROLIMUS	Possible increased everolimus levels	CYP3A4 inhibition	Caution with concurrent use
GRAPEFRUIT JUICE	IFOSFAMIDE	↓ Plasma concentrations of 4-hydroxyifosfamide, the active metabolite of ifosfamide, and risk of inadequate therapeutic response	Due to inhibition of the isoenzymatic conversion to active metabolites	Monitor the efficacy of ifosfamide clinically and ↑ dose accordingly
GRAPEFRUIT JUICE	IMATINIB	Possible increased imatinib levels	CYP3A4 inhibition	Avoid concurrent use
GRAPEFRUIT JUICE	IRINOTECAN	↑ Plasma concentrations of SN-38 (active metabolite of irinotecan) and ↑ toxicity of irinotecan, e.g., diarrhea, acute cholinergic syndrome, interstitial pulmonary disease	Due to inhibition of metabolism of irinotecan by CYP3A4 isoenzymes by grapefruit juice	Peripheral blood counts should be checked before each course of treatment. Monitor lung function. Recommendation is to ↓ dose of irinotecan by 25%
GRAPEFRUIT JUICE	LAPATINIB	Possible increased lapatinib levels	CYP3A4 inhibition	Avoid concurrent use
GRAPEFRUIT JUICE	NILOTINIB	Increased nilotinib levels	CYP3A4 inhibition	Avoid concurrent use
GRAPEFRUIT JUICE	PAZOPANIB	Possible increased pazopanib levels	CYP3A4 inhibition	Avoid concurrent use
GRAPEFRUIT JUICE	PONATINIB	Possible increased ponatinib levels	CYP3A4 inhibition	Caution with concurrent use. Consider dose reduction

(Continued)

MISCELLANEOUS GRAPEFRUIT JUICE

Primary Drug	Secondary Drug	Effect	Mechanism	Precautions
GRAPEFRUIT JUICE				
GRAPEFRUIT JUICE	REGORAFENIB	Predicted increased regorafenib levels	CYP3A4 inhibition	Manufacturer advises avoid concurrent use
GRAPEFRUIT JUICE	SUNITINIB	Possible increased sunitinib levels	CYP3A4 inhibition	Avoid concurrent use
GRAPEFRUIT JUICE	VINBLASTINE, VINCRISTINE	↑ Adverse effects of vinblastine and vincristine	Inhibition of CYP3A4-mediated metabolism. Also inhibition of intestinal Pgp efflux of vinblastine. Quercetin constituent of grapefruit juice enhances the phosphorylation of Pgp	Advice patients to ↓ intake foods and beverages containing bioflavonoids. Monitor FBC and watch for early features of toxicity (pain, numbness, tingling in the fingers and toes, jaw pain, abdominal pain, constipation, paralytic ileus). Consider selecting an alternative drug
GRAPEFRUIT JUICE	**HORMONES AND HORMONE ANTAGONISTS**			
GRAPEFRUIT JUICE	TAMOXIFEN	Likely interaction	Due to inhibition of CYP3A4-mediated metabolism of tamoxifen. Clinical significance is not yet known as the interaction has not been scientifically tested	Be aware. Advise patients to ↓ intake of foods and beverages containing bioflavonoids
GRAPEFRUIT JUICE	TOREMIFENE	↑ Plasma concentrations of toremifene	Inhibition of CYP3A4-mediated metabolism of toremifene	Clinical relevance is uncertain. Necessary to monitor for clinical toxicities
GRAPEFRUIT JUICE	**IMMUNOMODULATING DRUGS**			
GRAPEFRUIT JUICE	CICLOSPORIN	↑ Plasma concentrations of ciclosporin, with risk of nephrotoxicity, myelosuppression, neurotoxicity, excessive immunosuppression, and posttransplant lymphoproliferative disease	Inhibition of CYP3A4-mediated metabolism of ciclosporin; these inhibitors vary in potency. Grapefruit juice is classified as a potent inhibitor	Avoid grapefruit juice while taking ciclosporin
GRAPEFRUIT JUICE	CORTICOSTEROIDS	↑ Adrenal suppressive effects of corticosteroids, which may ↑ risk of infections and produce an inadequate response to stress scenarios (e.g., septic shock). However, studies have shown only moderate ↑ plasma concentrations of methylprednisolone and minimal or no changes with prednisolone	Due to inhibition of metabolism of corticosteroids	Monitor cortisol levels and warn patients to report symptoms such as fever and sore throat

(*Continued*)

Primary Drug	Secondary Drug	Effect	Mechanism	Precautions
GRAPEFRUIT JUICE				
GRAPEFRUIT JUICE	EVEROLIMUS	Possible increased everolimus levels	CYP3A4 inhibition	Caution with concurrent use
GRAPEFRUIT JUICE	SIROLIMUS, TACROLIMUS	Possibly ↑ efficacy and ↑ adverse effects	Possibly ↑ bioavailability via inhibition of intestinal CYP3A4 and effects of Pgp	Avoid coadministration
GRAPEFRUIT JUICE	ANTICOAGULANTS—ORAL	↑ Efficacy and ↑ adverse effects of warfarin, e.g., ↑ INR, hemorrhage	Unclear. Possibly via inhibition of intestinal CYP3A4	Monitor INR more closely. Avoid concomitant use if unstable INR
GRAPEFRUIT JUICE	**ANTIDEPRESSANTS**			
GRAPEFRUIT JUICE	FLUVOXAMINE, SERTRALINE	Possibly ↑ efficacy and ↑ adverse effects due to ↑ plasma concentrations	Possibly ↓ metabolism	Clinical significance unclear
GRAPEFRUIT JUICE	CLOMIPRAMINE	↑ Risk of clomipramine toxicity. Not known whether ↑ plasma concentration is sustained	Clomipramine metabolism involves several CYP isoenzymes (e.g., CYP1A2, CYP3A4, ↓ CYP2D6)	Be aware
GRAPEFRUIT JUICE	ANTIDIABETIC DRUGS—REPAGLINIDE	Possibly ↑ repaglinide levels	Due to inhibition of CYP3A4 isoenzymes, which metabolize repaglinide	Uncertain if clinically significant. May need to monitor blood glucose more closely
GRAPEFRUIT JUICE	ANTIEPILEPTICS—CARBAMAZEPINE	↑ In plasma concentrations of carbamazepine (AUC ↑ 1.4-fold, maximum concentration ↑), which is of clinical significance because of the narrow therapeutic index of carbamazepine; thus, toxic effects are likely. ↑ Efficacy and ↑ adverse effects	Grapefruit juice irreversibly inhibits intestinal CYP3A4. Transport via Pgp and MRP-2 efflux pumps is also inhibited	Monitor for ↑ side effects/toxicity and check carbamazepine levels weekly. If levels or control of fits are variable, remove grapefruit and grapefruit juice from the diet
GRAPEFRUIT JUICE	**ANTIFUNGALS**			
GRAPEFRUIT JUICE	ITRACONAZOLE	Coadministration of grapefruit juice ↓ AUC and maximum concentration of itraconazole by 47% and 35%, respectively	↓ Absorption, possibly by inhibition of intestinal CYP3A4, affecting Pgp or lowering duodenal pH. Effect appears to be greater in females	Clinical significance is unknown. The effect of the interaction may vary between capsules and oral liquid preparations
GRAPEFRUIT JUICE	IVABRADINE	↑ Levels with grapefruit juice	Reduced CYP3A4 mediated metabolism of ivabradine	Avoid coadministration

(Continued)

MISCELLANEOUS GRAPEFRUIT JUICE

Primary Drug	Secondary Drug	Effect	Mechanism	Precautions
GRAPEFRUIT JUICE				
GRAPEFRUIT JUICE	**ANTIHISTAMINES**			
GRAPEFRUIT JUICE	ASTEMIZOLE	Likely ↑ in cardiotoxicity. Likely ↑ in QTc interval	Due to effects of grapefruit juice on CYP isoenzymes and Pgp	Do not coadminister as there are suitable alternatives that are less harmful, e.g., loratadine, cetirizine, desloratadine
GRAPEFRUIT JUICE	FEXOFENADINE	↓ Plasma concentrations of fexofenadine (AUC <2.7-fold, maximum concentration <2.1-fold). Risk of lack of therapeutic effects. Possibly ↓ efficacy	↓ Absorption, possibly by affecting Pgp and direct inhibition of uptake by intestinal OATP1A2	Clinical significance unclear. No clinically significant changes in ECG parameters were observed in the study. Suitable alternatives are available
GRAPEFRUIT JUICE	RUPATADINE	↑ Risk of cardiac toxicity due to threefold ↑ plasma concentrations of rupatadine	Due to effects of grapefruit juice on CYP isoenzymes and Pgp	Do not coadminister as there are suitable alternatives that are less harmful, e.g., loratadine, cetirizine, desloratadine
GRAPEFRUIT JUICE	TERFENADINE	Statistically ↑ QT interval prolongation, hence the risk of cardiac toxicity. ↑ in AUC, maximum concentration and ↑ max. Two-fold ↑ half-life. Possibly ↑ efficacy and ↑ adverse effects, e.g., torsade de pointes	Altered metabolism so the parent drug accumulates. Due to effects of grapefruit juice on CYP isoenzymes and Pgp	Avoid concomitant intake. Suitable alternatives that are less harmful are available, e.g., loratadine (which is also metabolized by CYP2D6), cetirizine, desloratadine. This is despite a report that no significant cardiotoxicity is likely in normal subjects
GRAPEFRUIT JUICE	**ANTIHYPERTENSIVE AND HEART FAILURE DRUGS**			
GRAPEFRUIT JUICE	ALISKIREN	↓ Aliskiren levels	Possibly inhibition of enteric OATP-mediated uptake by GFJ could account for the reduced exposure	Monitor BP closely
GRAPEFRUIT JUICE	ALPHA-BLOCKERS—SILODOSIN, TAMSULOSIN	↑ Silodosin and tamsulosin levels	Inhibition of metabolism (UGT2B7 and CYP3A4)	Avoid grapefruit juice while taking silodosin and tamsulosin

(Continued)

Primary Drug	Secondary Drug	Effect	Mechanism	Precautions
GRAPEFRUIT JUICE				
GRAPEFRUIT JUICE	**ANTIMALARIALS**			
GRAPEFRUIT JUICE	ARTEMETHER (WITH LUMEFANTRINE)	↑ Plasma concentrations of artemether (AUC by 2.5-fold, maximum concentration > twofold). There were no signs of bradycardia or evidence of QTc prolongation	Very likely to be due to inhibition of intestinal CYP3A4 by grapefruit juice, which suggests a role for the presystemic metabolism of artemether	Monitor more closely. No ECG changes were seen in the study. Be aware
GRAPEFRUIT JUICE	CHLOROQUINE	↑ Plasma concentrations of chloroquine (AUC ↑ 1.3-fold, ↑ maximum concentration). The interaction has not been studied in patients with malaria	Due to inhibition of metabolism of chloroquine	Be aware
GRAPEFRUIT JUICE	HALOFANTRINE	Markedly ↑ plasma concentrations of halofantrine (AUC ↑ 2.8-fold, maximum concentration ↑ 3.2-fold). Maximum QTc prolongation was ↑ from 17 to 31 ms, thus giving a risk of cardiotoxicity	Due to inhibition of metabolism of CYP3A4-mediated metabolism of halofantrine	Do not coadminister because of QTc interval prolongation effects
GRAPEFRUIT JUICE	QUININE	Report of ↓ heart rate and PR that returned to normal 4–6 h after intake of quinine. Not considered to be clinically significant	Due to inhibition of metabolism of CYP3A4-mediated metabolism. However, metabolism of quinine is predominantly hepatic and thus unaffected by grapefruit juice	Be aware
GRAPEFRUIT JUICE	**ANTIMIGRAINE DRUGS**			
GRAPEFRUIT JUICE	ERGOT ALKALOIDS—ERGOTAMINE	Possibly ↑ efficacy and ↑ adverse effects, e.g., vasospasm, ergotism, peripheral vasoconstriction, gangrene	Oral administration only. ↑ bioavailability; ↓ presystemic metabolism. Constituents of grapefruit juice and grapefruit irreversibly inhibit intestinal cytochrome CYP3A4. Transport via Pgp and MRP-2 efflux pumps is also inhibited	Monitor for ↑ side effects; stop intake of grapefruit preparations if side effects occur

(*Continued*)

MISCELLANEOUS GRAPEFRUIT JUICE

Primary Drug	Secondary Drug	Effect	Mechanism	Precautions
GRAPEFRUIT JUICE				
GRAPEFRUIT JUICE	5-HT1 AGONISTS—ALMOTRIPTAN, ELETRIPTAN	↑ Plasma concentrations of almotriptan and eletriptan, with risk of toxic effects, e.g., flushing, sensations of tingling, heat, heaviness, pressure or tightness of any part of body including the throat and chest, dizziness	Almotriptan and eletriptan are metabolized mainly by CYP3A4 isoenzymes. Most CYP isoenzymes are inhibited by grapefruit juice to varying degrees, and since there is an alternative pathway of metabolism by MAOA, toxicity responses vary between individuals	The CSM has advised that if chest tightness or pressure is intense, the triptan should be discontinued immediately and the patient investigated for ischemic heart disease by measuring cardiac enzymes and doing an ECG. Avoid concomitant use in patients with coronary artery disease and in those with severe or uncontrolled hypertension
GRAPEFRUIT JUICE	ANTIMUSCARINICS—DARIFENACIN, FESOTERODINE, SOLIFENACIN	↑ Levels of darifenacin and fesoterodine	Inhibition of metabolism	Avoid grapefruit juice while taking these antimuscarinics
GRAPEFRUIT JUICE	ANTIOBESITY DRUGS—SIBUTRAMINE	Possibly ↑ efficacy and ↑ adverse effects, e.g., higher BP and raised heart rate	Unclear	Monitor PR and BP
GRAPEFRUIT JUICE	**ANTPROTOZOALS**			
GRAPEFRUIT JUICE	ALBENDAZOLE	↑ Plasma levels of albendazole by nearly threefold. Risk of toxic effects of albendazole	Albendazole is metabolized by intestinal CYP3A4, which is inhibited by grapefruit juice	Monitor for toxic effects of albendazole. Side effects that occur with a frequency of ~1% include jaundice, abdominal pain, nausea, vomiting, headache, and dizziness
GRAPEFRUIT JUICE	PRAZIQUANTEL	Marked ↑ in plasma concentrations of praziquantel (AUC ↑ 2.5-fold, maximum concentration ↑ threefold). In human liver, maximum concentration ↑ 1.6-fold and AUC 1.9-fold	Possibly via a role of Pgp—inhibition of Pgp may ↑ plasma concentrations	Be aware and watch for toxic effects of praziquantel. Toxicity is rare but includes liver toxicity-monitor liver function (transaminases)—warn re jaundice, dark urine and other symptoms of liver dysfunction
GRAPEFRUIT JUICE	**ANTIPLATELETS**			
GRAPEFRUIT JUICE	CLOPIDOGREL	↓ Peak plasma concentration (C_{max}) of the active metabolite of clopidogrel to 13% of the control, AUC from 0 to 3h to 14% of the control	No significant effect on parent clopidogrel. GFJ markedly ↓ the platelet-inhibitory effect of clopidogrel	Concomitant use of grapefruit juice may impair the efficacy of clopidogrel. Use of GFJ is best avoided during clopidogrel therapy

(*Continued*)

Primary Drug	Secondary Drug	Effect	Mechanism	Precautions
GRAPEFRUIT JUICE				
GRAPEFRUIT JUICE	TICAGRELOR	↑ Ticagrelor exposure by more than twofold, ↑ and prolonged ticagrelor antiplatelet effect. ↑ the mean C_{max} of ticagrelor by about 70% and more than doubled its AUC	Inhibition of the first-pass metabolism of ticagrelor is the principal mechanism of the observed mainly at intestinal levels	Clinically important. Risk of adverse effects—dyspnea and hyperuricemia. Do not coadminister
GRAPEFRUIT JUICE	ANTIPSYCHOTICS—PIMOZIDE	Possibly ↑ efficacy and ↑ adverse effects. Interaction may occur rapidly, but clinical significance is uncertain	Not evaluated in clinical trials	Avoid concomitant use. No interaction was observed with haloperidol
GRAPEFRUIT JUICE	**ANTIVIRALS**			
GRAPEFRUIT JUICE	EFAVIRENZ	Possibly ↑ efficacy and ↑ adverse effects	Unclear	Monitor more closely
GRAPEFRUIT JUICE	MARAVIROC	Substrate of CYP3A and P-glycoprotein	Used with other medicines to treat HIV	Stop taking maraviroc and call your doctor right away if you develop yellow eyes or skin, dark urine, vomiting, or abdominal pain. Let your doctor know right away if you develop nausea, fever, flu-like symptoms, or fatigue, but continue taking your maraviroc
GRAPEFRUIT JUICE	RILPIVIRINE	↑ Rilpivirine levels	Inhibition of intestinal CYP3A by GFJ	Warn patients to report adverse effects of rilpivirine (e.g., headache, nausea, and sleep problems
GRAPEFRUIT JUICE	SAQUINAVIR (invirase hard capsules)	Possibly ↑ efficacy with oral (and not when administered intravenous) preparations. The AUC of oral saquinavir ↑ by 50%, but maximum concentration, ↑ max and terminal half-life were not significantly altered in one study	Possibly ↑ bioavailability; ↓ presystemic metabolism. Constituents of grapefruit juice and grapefruit irreversibly inhibit intestinal cytochrome CYP3A4. Transport via Pgp and MRP-2 efflux pumps is also inhibited	No dose adjustment is advised. Oral bioavailability is very low and is enhanced beneficially with grapefruit juice or grapefruit. Soft gel capsules have greater bioavailability so may interact to a lesser degree. No dose adjustments are recommended by manufacturers for indinavir

(Continued)

Primary Drug	Secondary Drug	Effect	Mechanism	Precautions
GRAPEFRUIT JUICE				
GRAPEFRUIT JUICE	**ANXIOLYTICS AND HYPNOTICS**			
GRAPEFRUIT JUICE	BUSPIRONE—ORAL	Significant ↑ pharmacodynamic effects. AUC ↑ 9.2-fold and maximum concentration 4.3-fold, with ↑ in T_{max}. Possibly ↑ efficacy and ↑ adverse effects, e.g., sedation, CNS depression	Possibly ↑ bioavailability; ↓ presystemic metabolism. Constituents of grapefruit juice irreversibly inhibit intestinal cytochrome CYP3A4. Transport via Pgp and MRP-2 efflux pumps is also inhibited	Avoid concomitant use. Be particularly vigilant in elderly patients or those with impaired liver function. Consider an alternative, e.g., temazepam
GRAPEFRUIT JUICE	BZDs—MIDAZOLAM, TRIAZOLAM, QUAZEPAM, DIAZEPAM, ALPRAZOLAM	A slight but statistically significant ↑ drowsiness due to a 1.5-fold ↑ in AUC and a 1.3-fold ↑ in maximum concentration with triazolam that was accompanied by a ↑ in reaching peak effects (from 1.6 to 2.5 h). There is ↑ AUC, maximum concentration and ↑ max of quazepam and its active metabolite 2-oxoquazepam. No change is seen in psychomotor function with alprazolam, while with diazepam there was ↑ maximum concentration. With midazolam, there was minor ↑ reaction time (and minor ↑ digital symbol substitution test results)	With alprazolam, due to its inherent high bioavailability, grapefruit juice is unlikely to produce a significant change, in contrast to midazolam and triazolam. There is less contribution to presystemic metabolism by intestinal CYP3A4 for alprazolam. Grapefruit juice caused ↓ CYP3A12 activity in the liver and ↑ CYP3A12 activity in the intestine when tested with diazepam. This was attributed to the bergamottin constituent of grapefruit juice	Alprazolam is probably the BZD least affected by grapefruit juice, although many consider that the effect of grapefruit juice on midazolam is unlikely to be clinically important with 300 mL of juice. ↑ Plasma concentrations of diazepam are considered to be clinically insignificant—be aware of impaired cognition
GRAPEFRUIT JUICE	**BETA-BLOCKERS**			
GRAPEFRUIT JUICE	CELIPROLOL	Very likely to be ineffective therapeutically due to a great ↓ plasma concentrations (AUC ↓ by 85% and maximum concentration by 95%)	Attributed mainly to marked ↓ absorption. This may be due to physicochemical factors or due to an inhibition of drug uptake transporters	Do not coadminister
GRAPEFRUIT JUICE	TALINOLOL	Significant risk of ↓ therapeutic effects	Talinolol is a substrate of Pgp, and less than 1% is metabolized in the liver. However, inhibition by grapefruit juice of an intestinal uptake process other than Pgp is considered likely	Do not coadminister

(Continued)

Primary Drug	Secondary Drug	Effect	Mechanism	Precautions
GRAPEFRUIT JUICE				
GRAPEFRUIT JUICE	BRONCHODILATORS—THEOPHYLLINES	Possibly ↓ efficacy	Unclear. ↓ bioavailability (significant from 1 to ↓ hours)	Avoid concomitant intake if slow-release theophylline preparations are used. Monitor levels and clinical state weekly if intake of grapefruit is altered
GRAPEFRUIT JUICE	**CALCIUM CHANNEL BLOCKERS**			
GRAPEFRUIT JUICE	CALCIUM CHANNEL BLOCKERS	↑ Bioavailability of felodipine and nisoldipine (with reports of adverse effects), and ↑ bioavailability of isradipine, lacidipine, lercanidipine, nicardipine, nifedipine, nimodipine, and verapamil (without reported adverse clinical effects)	Postulated that flavonoids in grapefruit juice (and possibly Seville oranges and limes) inhibit intestinal (but not hepatic) CYP3A4. They also inhibit intestinal Pgp, which may ↑ the bioavailability of verapamil	Avoid concurrent use of felodipine and nisoldipine and grapefruit juice
GRAPEFRUIT JUICE	CARDIAC GLYCOSIDES—DIGOXIN	Possible ↑ efficacy and ↑ adverse effects	Possibly via altered absorption	Most patients were unaffected. Consider if unexpected bradycardia or heart block with digoxin. Rationale is based on the theoretical concept that digoxin is a substrate of Pgp
GRAPEFRUIT JUICE	CISAPRIDE	↑ Plasma concentrations and likely ↑ risk of adverse effects (e.g., cardiotoxicity, QT prolongation, torsade de pointes)	↑ Oral bioavailability and slight but significant ↑ elimination half-life	Although a study in volunteers did not show any changes in heart rate, PR or QT prolongation, avoid concurrent use
GRAPEFRUIT JUICE	ELIGLUSTAT	↑ Eliglustat levels	Inhibition of CYP3A4-mediated metabolism	Avoid coadministration
GRAPEFRUIT JUICE	LIPID-LOWERING DRUGS—ATORVASTATIN, SIMVASTATIN	↑ Levels of simvastatin; slight rise with atorvastatin. ↑ risk of adverse effects such as myopathy	Constituent of grapefruit juice inhibits CYP3A4-mediated metabolism of simvastatin	Patients taking simvastatin and atorvastatin should avoid grapefruit juice
GRAPEFRUIT JUICE	MIFEPRISTONE	Theoretical risk of ↑ levels of mifepristone	Inhibition of CYP3A4-mediated metabolism of mifepristone	Warn patients of possible ↑ in side effects (nausea, vomiting, diarrhea, uterine cramps)

(Continued)

Primary Drug	Secondary Drug	Effect	Mechanism	Precautions
GRAPEFRUIT JUICE				
GRAPEFRUIT JUICE	MONTELUKAST	Montelukast undergoes transport by OATP2B1. GFJ at 5% and 10% (v/v), and orange juice at 10%, ↓ montelukast permeability significantly ~30%	Enteric OATP-mediated drug-GFJ interaction	Clinical relevance of these interactions has not been examined
GRAPEFRUIT JUICE	NICOTINE	Significant ↑ renal clearance of nicotine	Grapefruit juice inhibits the formation of cotinine from nicotine, ↑ renal clearance of cotinine and ↓ plasma concentrations of cotinine by 15%	Be aware in patients using varying forms of nicotine replacement therapy for stopping smoking
GRAPEFRUIT JUICE	NITISINONE	Possible ↑ nitisinone levels	Inhibition of CYP3A4-mediated metabolism	Monitor carefully
GRAPEFRUIT JUICE	ESTROGENS—ESTRADIOL, POSSIBLY ETHINYL ESTRADIOL	↑ Efficacy and ↑ adverse effects	Oral administration only. ↑ bioavailability; ↓ presystemic metabolism. Constituents of grapefruit juice and grapefruit irreversibly inhibit intestinal cytochrome CYP3A4. Transport via Pgp and MRP-2 efflux pumps is also inhibited	Monitor for ↑ side effects
GRAPEFRUIT JUICE	PHOSPHODIESTERASE TYPE 5 INHIBITORS (e.g., sildenafil, tadalafil, vardenafil)	Possibly ↑ efficacy and ↑ adverse effects, e.g., hypotension	Small ↑ bioavailability. ↑ variability in pharmacokinetics, i.e., interindividual variations in metabolism	Safest to advise against intake of grapefruit juice for at least 48 h prior to intending to take any of these preparations. When necessary, the starting dose of sildenafil should not exceed 25–50 mg and that of tadalafil 10 mg. Avoid coadministration with vardenafil
GRAPEFRUIT JUICE	PIRFENIDONE	↑ Pirfenidone levels	Inhibition of metabolism of pirfenidone	Manufacturer recommends avoiding coadministration

Cranberry Juice (*Vaccinium macrocarpon*)

In vitro studies have shown that cranberry juice is an inhibitor of CYP enzymes and at higher amounts as potent as ketoconazole (CYP3A) and fluconazole (CYP2C9). In contrast, no significant inhibition has been seen in vivo observations with the exception of a single report on midazolam, where there was a moderate increase in the AUC of midazolam in subjects pretreated with cranberry juice. Further studies are needed to ascertain if any significant interactions occur.

Pomegranate Juice (*Punica granatum*)

Human in vitro and rat in vivo studies suggested that pomegranate juice can inhibit enteric CYP3A activity (carbamazepine epoxidation). Although volunteer studies have not found any significant interactions recent anecdotal reports have suggested an interaction between pomegranate juice and warfarin, as assessed by an increase in INR. One case report involving rosuvastatin, which undergoes minimal metabolism, described rhabdomyolysis possibly due to an interaction with pomegranate juice. Again, further studies are needed to ascertain if any significant interactions occur.

Pomelo Juice (*Citrus maxima*)

The pomelo or pummelo is a citrus fruit native to Asia. Juice prepared from some species of pomelo has been reported to contain furanocoumarins in concentrations comparable to those in grapefruit juice. There is no clinical evidence of any significant clinical effect.

Apple Juice

Quercetin, known to be present in apples (*Malus domestica*) and apple juice, inhibits OATP1A2-mediated fexofenadine uptake and OATP1A2- and OATP2B1-mediated bromosulfophthalein uptake. The highest concentration of juice inhibited activity by >85% relative to water. Clinical studies are needed to identify any significant interactions.

Orange Juice

Hesperidin, a major component of orange juice, is a flavonoid glycoside with a molecular structure similar to that of naringin. Hesperidin has been shown to inhibit OATP1A2-mediated uptake of fexofenadine in vitro, similar to that of naringin. Orange juice contains trace amounts of furanocoumarins. Orange juice (10%, v/v) inhibited both SULTs, by >95% (SULT1A1) and 20% (SULT1A3). The orange juice components, tangeretin and nobiletin (both at 10 μM), were the most potent single components, inhibiting SULT1A1 almost completely and SULT1A3 by ~20%.

There is some evidence from volunteer studies that interactions may occur but further studies are needed.

Herbal Drug	Allopathic Drug	Clinical Effects	Probable Mechanism of Interaction	Precautions
HERBS				
HERBAL DRUGS				
Herbs that may ↑ risk of bleeding				
1. Arnica 2. Bilberry leaf 3. Black cohosh 4. Boldo 5. *Capsicum* spp. (chili pepper) 6. Chamomile 7. Chinese wolfberry (*Lycium barbarum*) 8. Clove 9. Cranberry juice 10. Curbicin (containing pumpkin seed—*Cucurbita pepo*) 11. Dan shen (*Salvia miltiorrhiza*) 12. Devil's claw 13. Dong quai 14. Evening primrose oil 15. Fenugreek 16. Feverfew 17. Garlic (*Allium sativum*) 18. Ginger 19. Ginkgo biloba 20. Ginseng 21. Goldenseal 22. Horse chestnut	1. Aspirin 2. Clopidogrel 3. Ticlopidine 4. Dipyridamole 5. Warfarin 6. Heparin	May cause easy bruising and excessive bleeding from minor injuries. Reports of hemorrhage with concomitant use of warfarin and dan shen. INR may not always be altered. Case report with ginseng of normal coagulation studies during postoperative bleeding	• Antiplatelet effect (bilberry leaf, evening primrose, garlic, ginger, gingko biloba, ginseng). Clove contains eugenol derivatives, which inhibit platelets • Inhibit the metabolizing isoenzyme (CYP2C9) of warfarin (cranberry juice, dan shen, ginseng, lycium, soy/soya) • Coumarin constituents (black cohosh, chamomile, fenugreek, horse chestnut, sweet melilot, tonka beans, sweet woodruff). Naturally occurring coumarins are only weakly anticoagulant, but improper storage causes the production of dicoumarol by microbial transformation. Woodruff may contain constituents of warfarin • ↑ Fibrinolytic activity (capsicum) • Unknown mechanisms (arnica, boldo, cucurbita, devil's claw, dong quai, kangen-karyu, papaya, saw palmetto) • ↓ Vitamin K absorption (senna) • Other: tamarind ↑ bioavailability of aspirin. Meadow sweet and willow bark contain salicylates leading to ↑ effects of aspirin. Feverfew is considered to inhibit the release of serotonin from platelets	Inform physicians if either drug is introduced. Avoid changes in dosage of the herb. Monitor INR closely. If maintenance of the desired INR is difficult, avoid the herb. Monitor for ↑ tendency to bleed (petechiae, bruising, bleeding). Avoid concomitant use if possible

(*Continued*)

Herbal Drug	Allopathic Drug	Clinical Effects	Probable Mechanism of Interaction	Precautions
HERBS				
23. Kangen-karyu (a mixture containing dan shen, saussurea root, cnidium, cyperus rhizomes) 24. Lycium 25. Melilot (sweet clover) 26. Papaya 27. Prickly ash 28. Quassia 29. Saw palmetto 30. Senna 31. Soy/soya 32. Tonka beans 33. Sweet woodruff 34. Tamarind 35. Umbelliferae 36. Willow 37. Woodruff				
Herbs that may ↓ anticoagulant or antiplatelet effects				
1. Asian ginseng 2. Avocado 3. American ginseng 4. Goldenseal 5. Green tea 6. Psyllium seed (*Plantago psyllium*) 7. Ispaghula husk 8. Yarrow	1. Aspirin 2. Clopidogrel 3. Ticlopidine 4. Dipyridamole 5. Warfarin 6. Heparin	May ↓ effect of warfarin with ↓ INR, ↓ antiplatelet effects and antithrombotic effects	• ↓ Absorption of warfarin (avocado, psyllium seed, ispaghula husk) • Unknown (ginseng, goldenseal) • Contains vitamin K, which antagonizes the action of warfarin (green tea). Poyphenols in tea (consumed in larger quantities) may inhibit the absorption of warfarin. Yarrow has been found to be a coagulant in vivo	Inform physicians if either drug is introduced. Avoid changes in dosage of the herb. Monitor INR closely. If maintenance of the desired INR is difficult, avoid the herb. Avoid concomitant use if possible
Herbs that may ↑ sedation				

(*Continued*)

Herbal Drug	Allopathic Drug	Clinical Effects	Probable Mechanism of Interaction	Precautions
HERBS				
1. Bai zhi 2. Calamus 3. Catnip 4. Elecampane 5. Jamaican dogwood 6. German chamomile 7. Hops 8. Kava kava 9. Passion flower 10. Valerian	BZDs and barbiturates 1. Alprazolam 2. Clobazam 3. Clonazepam 4. Diazepam 5. Midazolam 6. Nitrazepam 7. Triazolam 8. Quazepam 9. Flunitrazepam 10. Phenobarbitone 11. Primidone	↑ Sedative effects	• Inhibits the metabolizing enzyme CYP3A4 (bai zhi, German chamomile) • Contains additive sedative action. May possess the ability to mediate GABA (catnip, German chamomile, hops, kava kava, passion flower, valerian)	Avoid driving and actions that need fine movements if either drug is added. ↓ dose of the herb if the patient is excessively sleepy
Herbs that may ↓ sedative action of sedatives				
1. Ginkgo biloba	BZDs and barbiturates as mentioned earlier	May antagonize the sedative action of these drugs	Induces the metabolizing enzyme CYP3A4: gingko weakly induces CYP2D6, which metabolizes alprazolam	Avoid concomitant use if possible. If the sedative action is impaired, discontinue the herb
Herbs that may ↓ blood levels of anti-HIV drugs				
1. Garlic 2. Ginger 3. Milk thistle	1. Indinavir 2. Lamivudine 3. Amprenavir 4. Saquinavir 5. Nelfinavir 6. Lopinavir 7. Efavirenz 8. Nevirapine	↓ Blood levels of these drugs. Blood levels of saquinavir may be ↓ by garlic and ginger. Milk thistle ↓ blood levels of indinavir. Garlic ↑ gastrointestinal side effects of ritonavir	• Induces metabolizing enzymes (CYP3A4). Garlic and ginger ↓ blood levels of saquinavir • Unknown mechanism (milk thistle) • Induction of transport protein Pgp (St. John's wort)	Avoid concomitant use
Herbs that may ↑ blood levels of anti-HIV drugs				
1. *Piper longum* 2. *Hypoxis hemerocallidea*	1. Nevirapine	↑ Blood levels, with potential risk of side effects	• Inhibits metabolizing CYP450 isoenzyme (nevirapine) • Inhibits both CYP3A4 and Pgp (*Hypoxis hemerocallidea*)	If either drug is introduced, monitor closely for side effects
Herbs that may ↑ effects of drugs used in blood sugar control				

(*Continued*)

Herbal Drug	Allopathic Drug	Clinical Effects	Probable Mechanism of Interaction	Precautions
HERBS				
1. *Angelica dahurica* 2. Aloe 3. Asian ginseng 4. Bai zhi 5. Garlic 6. Gingko biloba 7. Guarana 8. Karela (bitter melon) 9. Ma huang (*Ephedra sínica*) 10. Neem 11. Rosemary 12. Sage 13. Milk thistle	1. Tolbutamide 2. Metformin 3. Glimepiride 4. Glipizide 5. Glyburide 6. Insulin 7. Pioglitazone 8. Nateglinide 9. Repaglinide	May ↑ serum insulin levels (rosemary ↑ insulin in rats)	• ↓ Absorption of sugar (aloe) • Unknown (Asian ginseng, garlic, karela, neem) • Inhibits CYP2E1 isoenzyme (bai zhi). Gingko biloba induces metabolism of tolbutamide) • May ↑ serum insulin level (rosemary T insulin in rats)	Monitor blood glucose regularly when either drug is introduced. Once the blood sugar has been stabilized, avoid sudden changes of doses of either form of drug. Use alternative antidiabetic drugs metabolized less through CYP2E1 (pioglitazone, rosiglitazone, netoglitazone, repaglinide) when indicated. Avoid using longer-acting oral hypoglycemic drugs such as glibenclamide, especially in elderly people. Report symptoms such as light-headedness, lethargy and sweating to the physician
Herbs that may ↓ effects of drugs used in blood sugar control				
1. Guar gum	1. Metformin 2. Glibenclamide	May lead to ↑ blood sugar levels	• ↓ Absorption of metformin and glibenclamide	Avoid concomitant use. Monitor blood sugar closely if either drug is introduced
Herbs that may ↑ blood levels of antiepileptic medications or ↑ potency of antiepileptic medications				
1. *Piper longum* 2. *Piper nigrum* 3. Willow 4. Valerian 5. Passion flower 6. Kava 7. Shankapushpi	1. Phenytoin 2. Carbamazepine 3. Valproate 4. Lamotrigine 5. Gabapentin	↑ Phenytoin levels, which may lead to ↑ side effects. Valerian, passion flower and kava kava may theoretically potentiate antiepileptic drugs as animal experiments have revealed antiseizure activity. Valerian constituents inhibit breakdown of GABA and enhance BZD binding, which could potentiate the effects of carbamazepine	• Inhibition of transport (Pgp) and metabolizing enzymes (CYP2C9 and CYP3A4). Piperine found in *Piper nigrum* (black pepper) and *Piper longum* ↑ bioavailability of phenytoin • Displaces from protein binding (salicylate contained in willow displaces phenytoin from binding sites) • Passion flower contains chrysin, which is a partial agonist at GABA receptors and shows antiseizure effects	Closely monitor for side effects of phenytoin if *Piper nigrum* is introduced. Avoid sudden withdrawal of the herb after stabilization to avoid breakthrough seizures

(*Continued*)

Herbal Drug	Allopathic Drug	Clinical Effects	Probable Mechanism of Interaction	Precautions
HERBS				
Herbs that may ↓ plasma levels of antiepileptic drugs or ↓ seizure threshold				
1. Borage oil 2. Ginkgo biloba 3. Evening primrose oil 4. Plantain 5. Sage 6. Shankapushpi 7. Guarana, cola (contain caffeine) 8. Volatile oils, e.g., rosemary, sage, hyssop, fennel	1. Valproate 2. Carbamazepine	↓ Valproate and carbamazepine levels and may precipitate seizures. Evening primrose oil and borage oil contain gamolenic acid, which is reported to ↓ seizure threshold. Report of tonic–clonic seizures in subjects without a prior history of epilepsy after using essential oils transdermally and orally	• Unknown mechanism (ginkgo biloba ↓ valproate levels) • ↓ Seizure threshold (evening primrose oil, shankhapushpi) • Plantain ↓ absorption of valproate • Caffeine is known to ↓ seizure threshold and exacerbate seizures in animals. Volatile oils contain epileptogenic compounds (e.g., cineole, camphor, fenchone), which can be absorbed through the skin during aromatherapy. Sage is known to cause seizures in large doses	Avoid concomitant use if possible. Avoid eating plantains 30 min before and after carbamazepine. Avoid concomitant use of St. John's wort, especially in patients with poor seizure control. Avoid driving and work with machinery if either drug is introduced
Herbs that may ↑ cardiac glycoside effects or levels				
1. Adonis 2. Aloe 3. Ashwagandha 4. Asian ginseng 5. Broom 6. Cascara 7. Dan shen (*Salvia miltiorrhiza*) 8. Devil's claw 9. Echinacea 10. Ginger 11. Ginkgo biloba 12. Ginseng 13. Ginseng (Siberian) 14. Hawthorn 15. Kyushin 16. Liquorice 17. Plantain 18. Oleander 19. Rhubarb 20. Squill 21. Uzara root	1. Digoxin 2. Digitoxin 3. Ouabain 4. Deslanoside	May worsen the adverse effects of cardiac glycosides. May give rise to falsely ↑ or ↓ digoxin levels	• Contains cardiac glycosides or cardioactive substances (adonis, broom, devil's claw, ginger, hawthorn, oleander, squill) • Lowers serum potassium (aloe, cascara, liquorice, rhubarb) • Interferes with digoxin assay using fluorescence polarization immunoassay (ashwagandha, ginseng and Siberian ginseng falsely elevate, Asian ginseng and dan shen ↑ or ↓ levels) • Inhibits Pgp (echinacea, ginkgo biloba) • ↑ Levels due to unknown mechanism (ginseng)	Avoid the concomitant use of herbs that contain cardiac glycosides with these drugs. Monitor serum potassium and administer potassium supplements orally if indicated. Take drugs 1 h before or 2 h after herbal products. Avoid taking ashwagandha and Asian ginseng at least a week before digoxin assay

(*Continued*)

Herbal Drug	Allopathic Drug	Clinical Effects	Probable Mechanism of Interaction	Precautions
HERBS				
Herbs that may ↓ cardiac glycoside levels				
1. Guar gum 2. Senna	1. Digoxin 2. Digitoxin 3. Ouabain 4. Deslanoside	May lower therapeutic effect	• May lower the absorption of these drugs (guar gum, senna) • Induces Pgp (St. John's wort)	Avoid concomitant use. Monitor for worsening of therapeutic effects if the herb is introduced. If used concomitantly, take herbs at least 1 h before or after these drugs
Herbs that may ↑ antibiotic blood levels				
1. *Piper nigrum* and *Piper longum*	1. Amoxicillin 2. Cefotaxime 3. Rifampicin 4. Erythromycin 5. Telithromycin	↑ Blood levels of these antibiotics	• Attributed to inhibition of metabolism and of Pgp, e.g., *Piper longum*	Be aware that toxic effects of antibiotics may occur, particularly when the prescriber/dispenser is unaware of the intake of herbal medicines
Herbs that may ↓ antibiotic blood levels				
1. Dandelion 2. Fennel 3. Guar gum 4. Khat 5. Yohimbine	1. Ciprofloxacin 2. Amoxicillin 3. Penicillin 4. Tetracycline	↓ Blood levels may potentially ↓ Antibacterial activity	• Unknown mechanism (dandelion ↓ ciprofloxacin levels in rats; khat ↓ absorption and thus blood levels of ampicillin and amoxicillin, possibly due to the formation of a tannin–antibiotic complex; guar gum ↓ absorption of penicillin) • Other mechanism (yohimbine chelates tetracyclines). Fennel extracts are considered to chelate with ciprofloxacin	Be aware. Discontinue the herb during the course of antibiotic therapy. Penicillins should be taken on an empty stomach
Herbs that may ↓ immunosuppressant effects				

(*Continued*)

Herbal Drug	Allopathic Drug	Clinical Effects	Probable Mechanism of Interaction	Precautions
HERBS				
1. Astragalus 2. Echinacea 3. Liquorice 4. Milk thistle 5. Neem 6. Sea buckthorn	1. Ciclosporin 2. Azathioprine 3. Methotrexate 4. Tacrolimus 5. Daclizumab 6. Cyclophosphamide	Possibility of graft rejection	• ↓ Blood level; unknown mechanism (astralagus) • Other mechanisms: alkylamides from echinacea modulate tumor necrosis factor-alpha-mRNA expression in human monocytes/macrophages via the cannabinoid type-2 receptor • Unknown mechanism (milk thistle is known to ↓ cyclosporine levels; neem ↓ effects of azathioprine, prednisolone, and daclizumab; sea buckthorn may ↓ effects of cyclophosphamide) • Induces metabolizing enzymes, CYP3A4 and Pgp (St. John's wort ↓ ciclosporin and tacrolimus levels)	Avoid concomitant use of the herb
Herbs that may ↑ immunosuppressant effects				
1. Black cohosh 2. *Geum chiloense* 3. Liquorice	1. Cisplatin 2. Azathioprine 3. Ciclosporin 4. Prednisolone	↑ Cytotoxaic properties. Geum ↑ plasma ciclosporin levels six–eightfold	• Unknown mechanism (black cohosh) • Inhibits metabolizing enzymes. Glycyrrhizin present in liquorice inhibits the metabolizing enzyme of prednisolone, 11 beta-hydroxysteroid dehydrogenase, which converts the active metabolite to an inactive form. ↓ clearance of prednisolone in healthy individuals	Be aware. Advice is to avoid echinacea with immunosuppressants
Herbs that may ↓ effects of anticancer medication				
1. Aloe 2. Soy/soya 3. Red clover 4. Kava kava 5. Ginseng 6. Garlic 7. Echinacea 8. Beta-carotene 9. Quercetin	1. Cisplatin 2. Tamoxifen	Lower the anticancer activity of these drugs. Most oncolytic drugs have a narrow therapeutic window	• Red clover and soya contain estrogenic isoflavonoids. Unknown mechanism with aloe • Induces the metabolizing enzyme (soy induces CYP isoenzymes that metabolize tamoxifen)	It is best to avoid the concomitant use of herbs with hormonal effects (includes dong quai, chasteberry, black cohosh) in patients with hormone-dependent cancers, e.g., breast cancer

(*Continued*)

Herbal Drug	Allopathic Drug	Clinical Effects	Probable Mechanism of Interaction	Precautions
HERBS				
Herbs that may ↑ effects of anticancer medication				
1. Black cohosh 2. Caffeine 3. Evening primrose oil 4. *Scutellaria baicalensis* 5. Starflower (borage)	1. Docetaxel 2. Paclitaxel 3. Doxorubicin 4. Tamoxifen 5. Cisplatin 6. Vinorelbine	↑ Cytotoxic properties	• Unknown mechanism (black cohosh). Caffeine ↑ cytotoxic effects of cisplatin; wogonin present in *Scutellaria* enhances etoposide-induced apoptosis. Gamolenic acid found in evening primrose oil and borage potentiated the in vitro toxicity of paclitaxel and vinorelbine, attributed to an unsaturated fatty acid as modulators of tumor cell chemosensitivity	Be aware and avoid concomitant use
Herbs that may interact with MAOIs				
1. Anise 2. Asian ginseng 3. Cereus 4. Ephedra 5. Ginseng 6. Parsley 7. Shepherd's purse 8. Verbena (vervain) 9. Capsicum	1. Phenelzine 2. Tranylcypromine 3. Moclobemide	May cause ↑ blood pressure with anise and ephedra. ↑ risk of side effects such as psychosis and hallucinations with Asian ginseng. Headache, tremulousness, and manic episodes have been reported with ginseng and phenelzine	• Unknown mechanism (anise, Asian ginseng) • Inhibits metabolism of ephedra (MAOIs inhibit the metabolism of ephedra)	Avoid concomitant use
Herbs that may ↑ effects of diuretics				
1. Aloe 2. Comfrey 3. Couch grass 4. Dandelion 5. Elder 5. Guar gum 6. Liquorice 7. Nettle 8. Rhubarb	1. Bendroflumethiazide 2. Bumetanide 3. Chlortalidone 4. Hydrochlorothiazide 5. Indapamide 6. Furosemide 7. Torasemide	Low body potassium, which may give rise to lethargy and muscle weakness	• ↑ Potassium loss from the gut (aloe, liquorice) • Possess diuretic properties (dandelion, elder, nettle, rhubarb)	Avoid concomitant use. Provide potassium supplements orally. Use a potassium-sparing diuretic such as spironolactone or amiloride
Herbs that may ↓ effects of diuretics				

(*Continued*)

Herbal Drug	Allopathic Drug	Clinical Effects	Probable Mechanism of Interaction	Precautions
HERBS				
1. Ginkgo biloba 2. Ginseng	1. Bendroflumethiazide 2. Bumetanide 3. Chlortalidone 4. Hydrochlorothiazide 5. Torasemide	Poor blood pressure control and diuresis	• Unknown (ginkgo biloba ↓ effect of thiazide diuretics; ginseng) • ↓ Absorption (guar gum has been shown to ↓ absorption of bumetanide)	Avoid concomitant use of the herb if blood pressure control is poor
Herbs that may interfere with antihypertension medication				
1. Betel nut 2. *Piper longum*/*Piper nigrum* 3. Black cohosh 4. Capsicum 5. Cowslip 6. Ginkgo biloba 7. Ginseng (American, Asian) 8. Hawthorn 9. Indian snakeroot 10. Liquorice (*Glycyrrhiza glabra*) 11. Parsley	1. Beta-blockers (atenolol, acebutolol, bisoprolol, carvedilol, esmolol, labetalol, metoprolol, nadolol, nebivolol, pindolol, sotalol, timolol) 2. Calcium channel blockers (amlodipine, diltiazem, felodipine, isradipine, lacidipine, nicardipine, nifedipine, nimodipine, nisoldipine, verapamil) 3. ACE inhibitors and angiotensin II receptor blockers (captopril, lisinopril, enalapril, verapamil, losartan, candesartan)	Has been known to worsen bradycardia and hypotension. May worsen cough associated with ACE inhibitors	• Betel nut causes bradycardia and hawthorn ↓ blood pressure through unknown mechanisms • Piperine, a constituent of black pepper and other species (e.g., *Piper nigrum*), ↑ bioavailability of propranolol. Indian snakeroot was found to contain a "reserpine"-like constituent • Inhibits the metabolizing enzymes. *Piper longum* inhibits CYP1A1 and CYPA2, which metabolize propranolol. Ginkgo inhibits metabolism of nifedipine, nicardipine (CYP3A4) and propranolol (CYP1A2) enzymes. Ginseng inhibits CYP3A4 and ↑ nifedipine levels. Goldenseal inhibits losartan's metabolizing enzyme. Grapefruit inhibits the metabolizing enzyme (CYP3A4) of felodipine, nicardipine, nifedipine, nisoldipine or nitrendipine. Grapefruit juice may also inhibit the metabolism of verapamil and losartan • Unknown (black cohosh) • Other mechanisms (capsicum depletes substance P; cowslip has demonstrated hypotensive properties in animals)	Inform physicians if either drug is introduced. Avoid sudden changes of the herb dose. Monitor PR and blood pressure closely if either drug is introduced. Discontinue the herb if side effects worsen. Use alternative antihypertensive medications if possible (e.g., replace beta-blockers and calcium channel blockers with ACE inhibitors or angiotensin II receptor blockers if bradycardia is worsened, and replace ACE inhibitors with angiotensin II receptor blockers if cough is worsened)
Herbs that may ↓ effect of antihypertension medication				

(*Continued*)

Herbal Drug	Allopathic Drug	Clinical Effects	Probable Mechanism of Interaction	Precautions
HERBS				
1. Broom 2. Ephedra 3. Glycyrrhizin (liquorice) 4. Ma huang 5. Sage 6. Yohimbe	The antihypertensive drugs mentioned earlier	Poor control of hypertension	• Causes peripheral vasoconstriction (broom) • Contains vasoconstrictive alkaloids (ephedrine). Ma huang (a constituent of slimming pills, decongestants, and antiasthma drugs) contains ephedrine • Pseudoaldosteronism (glycyrrhizin causes pseudaldosteronism and antagonizes the effect of ACE inhibitors) • Yohimbe bark contains yohimbine, which is a presynaptic alpha-2 adrenoceptor agonist (and possibly an MAOI)	Avoid concomitant use
Herbs that may ↑ effect of antiarrhythmic medication				
1. Adonis 2. Guarana 3. Liquorice 4. Milk thistle 5. Scopolia 6. Squill	1. Quinidine 2. Amiodarone 3. Adenosine 4. Procainamide	May cause ↑ adverse effects of quinidine and amiodarone. ↑ Risk of prolonged QT interval on ECG	• Additive inotropic effects of the constituent cardiac glycosides of the herb (adonis and squill) • Inhibits metabolizing enzymes (grapefruit juice inhibits CYP3A4, which metabolizes amiodarone and quinidine; milk thistle inhibits the metabolizing enzyme of amiodarone [CYP3A4]) • Unknown (liquorice, scopolia)	Avoid concomitant use. Monitor for side effects of amiodarone if the herb is introduced. Inform physicians if used concomitantly. Monitor QT interval
Herbs that may ↓ effect of antiarrhythmic medication				
1. Guar gum	1. Adenosine	↓ Blood levels and therapeutic effects	• Unknown	Be aware
Herbs that may ↑ effects of antidepressant medication				

(Continued)

Herbal Drug	Allopathic Drug	Clinical Effects	Probable Mechanism of Interaction	Precautions
HERBS				
1. Broom 2. Ginkgo biloba 3. Scopolia 4. Yohimbine	1. TCAs (e.g., amitriptyline, nortriptyline, clomipramine) 2. SSRIs (e.g., fluvoxamine, fluoxetine, paroxetine) 3. Venlafaxine 4. Trazodone	May develop cardiac arrhythmias and side effects such as dryness of the mouth, retention of urine, and tachycardia; ↑ sedation	• Broom contains cardioactive alkalamines such as sparteine • Inhibits metabolizing enzymes • Anticholinergic properties (hyoscine present in scopolia may worsen side effects of TCAs additive antimuscarinic effects) • Yohimbine alone can cause hypertension, but lower doses cause hypertension when combined with TCAs • Unknown mechanism (ginkgo ↑ sedative effects of trazodone) • St. John's wort inhibits the uptake of serotonin and thereby ↑ serotonin levels	Avoid concomitant use. An SSRI may be a better alternative to be used with broom
Herbs that may ↑ effects of antipsychotic medication				
1. Betel nut 2. Caffeine 3. Ephedra 4. Ginkgo biloba 5. Hops 6. Kava kava 7. Valerian	1. Phenothiazines (e.g., chlorpromazine, promazine, levomepromazine, pericyazine, pipotiazine, fluphenazine, perphenazine, trifluoperazine) 2. Clozapine 3. Lithium 4. Haloperidol 5. Risperidone	Worsening of side effects such as slowness, stiffness and tremor. ↑ Blood levels. A single case report of priapism induced by a ginkgo–risperidone combination. Hyperthermia	• Unknown mechanism (betel nut worsens the side effects of flupentixol and fluphenazine). Ginkgo may ↑ haloperidol effects. Kava kava ↑ side effects of haloperidol and risperidone • Inhibits metabolizing enzymes (caffeine inhibits CYP1A2, which metabolizes clozapine). Inhibition of CYP by ginkgo ↑ alpha-1 effects of risperidone. Valerian may worsen the sedative properties of haloperidol. Hops and phenothiazine have been associated with hyperthermia in dogs • Worsens the cardiovascular effects of phenothiazines (ephedra)	Be aware. Discontinue the herb if the side effects of these drugs ↑
Herbs that may ↓ effects of antipsychotic medication				

(*Continued*)

Herbal Drug	Allopathic Drug	Clinical Effects	Probable Mechanism of Interaction	Precautions
HERBS				
1. Caffeine 2. Chaste tree 3. Green tea 4. Plantain (*Plantain orata*, *Plantain psyllium*) 5. Ispaghula (psyllium)	1. Lithium 2. Phenothiazines (e.g., chlorpromazine, promazine, levomepromazine, pericyazine, pipotiazine, fluphenazine, perphenazine, trifluphenazine) 3. Clozapine	↓ Blood lithium levels with ↓ clinical effects with ispaghula and psyllium. ↓ effects of phenothiazines. Herbal diuretics contained in a mixture of juniper, buchu, horsetail, corn silk, bearberry, parsley, bromelain, and paprika caused lithium toxicity	• Unknown mechanism (caffeine). • Contains dopamine agonists (chaste tree). • Induction of metabolizing enzymes (green tea may induce CYP1A2, which metabolizes clozapine). • ↓ Absorption from the gut (plantain, psyllium, and ispaghula may ↓ absorption of lithium, or preparations may have high sodium content in the form of sodium bicarbonate to aid their dispersal in water before ingestion). Herbal diuretics are weak compared with their allopathic counterparts. This may be due to diuresis or other factors, e.g., enzyme inhibition	Be aware. Caffeine withdrawal may precipitate lithium toxicity, so avoid sudden caffeine withdrawal. Avoid concomitant use if possible
Herbs that may interact with melatonin				
1. Ashwagandha 2. Celery 3. Chamomile 4. German chamomile 5. Goldenseal 6. Hops 7. Kava kava 8. Valerian	1. Melatonin	May cause ↑ sedation	Unknown mechanism	Be aware
Herbs that may ↑ risk of theophylline adverse effects				
1. *Piper longum* 2. Caffeine 3. Capsicum 4. Dan shen 5. Ephedra 6. Green tea 7. Guarana 8. Squill	1. Theophylline	↑ Plasma level of theophylline and may potentiate side effects. Ephedra, caffeine, squill, and green tea may worsen tachycardia and palpitation	• Inhibition of CYP 450 enzymes (*Piper longum*, dan shen) • Additive sympathetic stimulation (caffeine, ephedra, green tea, guarana) • May ↑ absorption (capsicum) • Unknown mechanism (squill)	Inform physicians if either drug is introduced. Avoid sudden changes of the herb dose. Discontinue the herb if side effects worsen

(*Continued*)

Herbal Drug	Allopathic Drug	Clinical Effects	Probable Mechanism of Interaction	Precautions
HERBS				
Herbs that may interfere with general anesthetic medication				
1. Black cohosh 2. Kava kava 3. Ginkgo 4. Ginseng 5. Garlic 6. Goldenseal 7. Ma huang 8. Echinacea 9. Aloe 10. Ephedra 11. Sage 12. Sassafras 13. Valerian 14. Wild carrot	Anesthetic medication, including drugs used in premedication, induction, maintenance of anesthesia, muscle relaxation, analgesia (intra- and postoperative), bleeding, and recovery	These effects are attributed to herbs that may have sedating properties (e.g., valerian, kava kava) or cause ↑ bleeding (e.g., garlic, ginger, gingko), or those that may cause changes in blood pressure (often unpredictable), e.g., black cohosh, ma huang, ephedra. Also mentioned are herbs that may interfere with healing (e.g., echinacea). Aloe vera ↓ prostaglandin synthesis and inhibits aggregations of platelets, while sevoflurane inhibits thromboxane A2 formation, resulting in ↑ blood loss.	Herbal preparations are known to • ↑ Intra- and postoperative bleeding • ↑ CNS effects of drugs used in anesthesia • Cause unpredictable changes in blood pressure and PR • Cause unpredictable effects on the excretions of drugs used during anesthesia	The American Society of Anesthesiologists has recommended that all herbal medications be stopped 2–3 weeks prior to an elective surgical procedure. Employ stringent measures related to discontinuing ginkgo, ginseng, and garlic because of ↑ risk of bleeding. Discontinue black cohosh 2 weeks before surgery. Inform the anesthetist before the procedure
Herbs that may ↑ side effects of lipid-lowering agents				
1. Goldenseal	1. Atorvastatin 2. Simvastatin 3. Lovastatin	↑ Blood levels of atorvastatin (grapefruit juice) and lovastatin (goldenseal), with ↑ Risk of side effects (e.g., muscle pain due to rhabdomyolysis)	• Possibly through inhibition of Pgp. Also through the inhibition of CYP3A4. Goldenseal inhibits CYP3A4	Avoid concomitant use. Report muscle pain to physicians. Suitable alternatives are pravastatin, rosuvastatin, and fluvastatin, which interact less with Pgp. Pravastatin and rosuvastatin are mainly excreted unchanged, and fluvastatin (CYP2C9) is not metabolized through CYP3A4
Herbs that may interfere with ACh receptor antagonists				

(*Continued*)

Herbal Drug	Allopathic Drug	Clinical Effects	Probable Mechanism of Interaction	Precautions
HERBS				
1. Areca nut	1. Procyclidine (used to control extrapyramidal—parkinsonian—with antipsychotic medications)	Caused severe rigidity and jaw tremor. This is an established and clinically significant interaction	• Procyclidine is an antimuscarinic agent, i.e., antagonizes the effects of ACh in one set of ACh receptors. Thus, herbal products used culturally with effects similar to ACh, e.g., areca nut, will produce enhanced effects at other—nicotinic receptors to produce adverse effects	Avoid chewing betel nut (also found in prepared "pan masala")
Herbs that may ↑ effects of antipsychotic medication				
1. Betel nut 2. Caffeine 3. Ephedra 4. Ginkgo biloba 5. Hops 6. Kava kava 7. Valerian	1. Phenothiazines (e.g., chlorpromazine, promazine, levomepromazine, pericyazine, pipotiazine, fluphenazine, perphenazine, trifluphenazine) 2. Clozapine 3. Lithium 4. Haloperidol 5. Risperidone	Worsen side effects such as slowness, stiffness and tremor. ↑ Blood levels. A single case report of priapism induced by a ginkgo–risperidone combination. Hyperthermia	• Unknown mechanism (betel nut worsens the side effects of flupentixol and fluphenazine) • Ginkgo may ↑ haloperidol effects. Kava kava ↑ side effects of haloperidol and risperidone • Inhibits metabolizing enzymes (caffeine inhibits CYP1A2, which metabolizes clozapine). Inhibition of CYP by ginkgo ↑ alpha-1 effects of risperidone. Valerian may worsen the sedative properties of haloperidol. Hops and phenothiazine have been associated with hyperthermia in dogs • Worsens the cardiovascular effects of phenothiazines (ephedra)	Be aware. Discontinue the herb if the side effects of these drugs ↑
Herbs that may ↓ effects of antipsychotic medication				
1. Caffeine 2. Chaste tree 3. Green tea 4. Plantain	1. Lithium 2. Phenothiazines (e.g., chlorpromazine, promazine, levomepromazine, pericyazine, pipotiazine, fluphenazine, perphenazine, trifluphenazine) 3. Clozapine	↓ Blood lithium levels with ↓ clinical effects. ↓ Effects of phenothiazines	• Unknown mechanism (caffeine) • Contains dopamine agonists (chaste tree) • Induction of metabolizing enzymes (green tea may induce CYP1A2, which metabolizes clozapine) • ↓ Absorption from the gut (plantain may ↓ absorption of lithium)	Be aware. Caffeine withdrawal may precipitate lithium toxicity, so avoid sudden caffeine withdrawal. Avoid concomitant use if possible

(Continued)

Herbal Drug	Allopathic Drug	Clinical Effects	Probable Mechanism of Interaction	Precautions
HERBS				
Herbs that may ↓ effect of theophylline				
1. St. John's wort 2. Royal jelly	1. Theophylline	↓ Theophylline levels and risk of therapeutic failure	• Due to activation of metabolizing CYP1A2 enzymes, which metabolize theophylline	Discontinue St. John's wort if the therapeutic effects of theophylline ↓
Herbs that may interact with phosphodiesterase inhibitors used for impotence				
1. Grapefruit juice 2. Squill	1. Sildenafil 2. Tadalafil 3. Vardenafil	↑ Blood levels of the medication, leading to serious vasodilatation. ↑ Risk of cardiac arrhythmia	• Inhibits CYP3A4, which metabolizes these drugs (grapefruit juice) • Unknown mechanism (squill)	Avoid concomitant use. Avoid the combination of grapefruit juice and nitrates with these medications
Herbs that may ↑ adverse effects of lipid-lowering agents				
1. Grapefruit juice 2. Goldenseal	1. Atorvastatin 2. Simvastatin 3. Lovastatin	↑ Blood levels of atorvastatin (grapefruit juice) and lovastatin (goldenseal) with ↑ risk of side effects (e.g., muscle pain due to rhabdomyolysis)	• Possibly through inhibition of Pgp. Also through inhibition of CYP3A4 (grapefruit juice). Goldenseal inhibits CYP3A4	Avoid concomitant use. Report muscle pain to physicians. Suitable alternatives are pravastatin, rosuvastatin, and fluvastatin, which interact less with Pgp. Pravastatin and rosuvastatin are mainly excreted unchanged, while fluvastatin (CYP2C9) is not metabolized through CYP3A4
Herbs that may ↓ effects of lipid-lowering agents				
1. St. John's wort	1. Atorvastatin 2. Simvastatin 3. Lovastatin	↓ Blood levels and lipid-lowering effect	• Induction of metabolizing CYP3A4 enzymes, which metabolize simvastatin	Avoid concomitant use if possible. Monitor response to simvastatin closely. Avoid sudden changes of the herb dosage
Herbs that may interfere with oral contraceptive medication				
1. St. John's wort 2. Red clover 3. Saw palmetto	1. Oral contraceptives	Failure of contraception. Theoretically, saw palmetto could interfere with oral contraception and hormone replacement therapy	St. John's wort preparations induce metabolizing CYP3A4 enzymes and glycoprotein drug transporters of these medications	Avoid concomitant use. Use an alternative contraceptive methods (barrier methods) if the herb is introduced

(Continued)

Herbal Drug	Allopathic Drug	Clinical Effects	Probable Mechanism of Interaction	Precautions
HERBS				
Herbs that may cause additive hepatotoxicity				
1. Echinacea	1. Hepatotoxic drugs, e.g., anabolic steroids 2. Amiodarone 3. Methotrexate 4. Ketoconazole	Risk of additive hepatotoxicity	• Use of echinacea for over 8 weeks can cause hepatotoxicity	Be aware and use drugs with a potential to cause hypertonicity cautiously, monitoring clinically and biochemically for any early signs of hepatic dysfunction
Herbs that may cause additive endocrine effects				
1. Ginseng 2. Saw palmetto 3. Kelp 4. Sage	1. Corticosteroids 2. Estrogens 3. Androgens (e.g., finasteride, flutamide) 4. Thyroid replacement therapy	Risk of additive/antagonistic hormonal effects. Kelp may interfere with thyroid therapy. Saw palmetto interferes with male hormones and estrogen-containing therapies	• Additive/antagonistic hormonal effects. Kelp is a source of iodine. Sage may increase TSH levels	Be aware
Herbs that may ↓ absorption of coadministered drugs				
1. St. John's wort 2. Saw palmetto	1. Iron	↓ Absorption of coadministered iron	• Due to tannic acid content	Be aware and separate oral intake by at least 2 h
Herbs that may interfere with drugs used in the treatment of migraine				
1. Feverfew	1. Antimigraine drugs, e.g., sumatriptan	↑ Risk of episodes of tachycardia and hypertension (may be dangerous)	The parthenolide constituent of feverfew has been shown to inhibit the release of serotonin and prostaglandins. Sumatriptan is an SSRI	Avoid concomitant use
Herbs that may interfere with drugs used in the treatment of Alzheimer's disease				
	1. Donepezil 2. Galantamine 3. Memantine	May ↑ anticholinergic effects	Sage possesses some anticholinergic effects, such as that on sweating	Be aware

PART 18

Over-the-Counter/Online Drugs and Remedies

Lakshman Delgoda Karalliedde, Janaka Karalliedde, and Seneka Abeyratne

CONTENTS

18.1 INTRODUCTION

18.1.1 Over-the-Counter Medications

More OTC drugs have been introduced to encourage self-care for minor ailments and for patients to take greater responsibility for their own health. This section gives an overview of the constituents of OTC drugs that could be involved in adverse drug interactions.

Also considered are drugs available for purchase online. An important difference between OTC drugs and those available online is that approval for drugs available OTC has undergone a rather rigorous assessment by regulatory bodies such as the Medicines and Healthcare products Regulatory Agency in the United Kingdom, while drugs available online include products that are available only on prescription in the United Kingdom (e.g., diazepam, sildenafil) as well as a wide range of hallucinogens and similar drugs affecting the CNS, which are often illegal in a particular country or state (as in the United States).

18.1.2 Online Medications

The US Food and Drug Administration Consumer Health Information Web page (www.fda.gov/consumer) warns consumers about the possible dangers of buying medicines over the Internet. This provides the opportunity for drug interactions to occur that may not be reported, especially with traditional remedies, or may not be detected because of the anonymity that consumers desire when purchasing drugs online. In addition, any increase in the number of preparations taken by an individual, including medications of varying composition bought from multiple online sites, increases the likelihood of potential interactions. The delay in identifying these potential interactions may have severe, even life-threatening consequences.

In simple terms, "rogue websites" often sell unapproved drugs. In the United States, the FDA states that counterfeit drugs (fake or copycat products) may

- Be contaminated with dangerous ingredients
- Not provide the desired therapeutic response
- Cause serious side effects
- Contain the wrong active ingredient
- Be made with the wrong amount of active ingredient (varying from no active ingredient to too much) and be packaged in phoney packaging that looks legitimate

In addition, many online drugs also contain glucose, sodium, and potassium as constituents, so patients with diabetes, renal impairment, and heart failure should take extra-precautions when using these drugs.

Some sites that offer prescription drugs without prescription provide assurances of free medical consultations and the services of experienced, trusted, fully licensed pharmacists. However, the range of drugs available online (some sites offering over 1000 medications) causes severe concerns associated with adverse drug interactions as they include benzodiazepines (e.g., alprazolam, lorazepam), antidepressants (escitalopram, fluoxetine), antimigraine drugs (e.g., sibutramine), hypnotics (e.g., Zolpidem), sildenafil, injectable testosterone, human growth hormone, and drugs used in the treatment of asthma, skin disorders (e.g., psoriasis), and fungal infections (e.g., itraconazole). The patient's past medical history and current drug armamentarium may also not be fully taken into account.

The United Kingdom's Medicines Control Agency investigated 24 British websites as, under the Medicines Act of 1968, it is illegal to sell prescription drugs to an individual without a prescription. Unfortunately, as many online pharmacies operate internationally, the Medicines Control Agency has no jurisdiction abroad.

18.1.3 Traditional and Herbal Remedies

More and more traditional medicines and nutritional supplements are available. Such preparations have the potential for serious drug interactions (e.g., St. John's wort, grapefruit juice, ginseng, ephedra, garlic). Furthermore, traditional medicines in particular may contain heavy metals (e.g., mercury, lead, arsenic) or adulterants (which may be banned in the country of use, e.g., fenfluramine, phenylbutazone).

This résumé is intended to warn consumers in particular and also to make doctors and pharmacists aware of the likelihood that people seeking prescriptions or medications will take drugs from online pharmacies and possibly not reveal them to either the doctor or the pharmacist. **It is important for health-care professionals to ask specifically whether the patient uses drugs bought online, as well as asking about prescribed medicines, OTC drugs and supplements, and traditional and herbal remedies.**

The following is an overview of interactions that may occur with OTC drugs. The OTC drugs are classified following the classification used in the September 2008 edition of *Guide to OTC Medicines and Diagnostics.*

18.1.4 Analgesics

There is a common perception among the general public that analgesics are harmless; therefore, they may not realize that there is potential for interactions, for example,

- Drugs that cause additive adverse effects on the gastric mucosa, kidney, or liver (e.g., **aspirin, NSAIDs**)
- Dangerous interactions with antidepressants (e.g., **MAOIs**) may also occur (from opioids such as **codeine** and **dextromethorphan** in several cough and flu remedies)
- Inadvertent overdose may occur if OTC analgesics or analgesic-containing "cold cures" are taken in addition to prescribed analgesics especially paracetamol (acetaminophen)

18.2 EXAMPLES OF INTERACTIONS THAT MAY OCCUR WITH COMMONLY AVAILABLE OTC DRUGS

18.2.1 Analgesics

18.2.1.1 NSAIDs

- **Antacids**—decrease the absorption of NSAIDs.
- **Other NSAIDs**—risk of overdose if the patient already taking regular NSAID does not realize that the new drug is also a NSAID; an additive irritant effect on the gastric mucosa and a risk of renal impairment.
- **Anticoagulants**—a risk of catastrophic hemorrhage from the gastric mucosa.
- **Antigout drugs** (e.g., probenecid and sulfinpyrazone)—decrease the uricosuric effect.
- **Methotrexate**, which is used for several disease states such as rheumatoid arthritis (where OTC analgesics are often taken to relieve pain) or malignant disease, as a cytotoxic (where pain relief also becomes important)—increased methotrexate levels may occur, with risk of toxicity.
- **Drugs** used to treat heart failure and high blood pressure—a decreased effect of these drugs because NSAIDs cause fluid retention.
- **Antiepileptics**—aspirin may cause an elevation and even toxic effects of phenytoin and valproate.
- **Antidiabetic drugs**—high-dose aspirin may cause hypoglycemia, which may add to the effect of the drugs used to treat diabetes mellitus, thus increasing the risk of hypoglycemic episodes.

For full details of the potential interactions, see

- Aspirin—cardiovascular drugs, antiplatelets
- NSAIDs—analgesics, non-steroidal anti-inflammatory drugs

18.2.1.2 Paracetamol (Acetaminophen)

The biggest risk with OTC paracetamol is inadvertent overdose when patients take multiple OTC remedies without realizing that they contain paracetamol.

- The absorption of paracetamol is decreased by anion exchange resins (**cholestyramine**).
- In contract, some drugs used to control nausea and vomiting, such as **metoclopramide** and **domperidone**, hasten the absorption of paracetamol.

For full details of potential interactions, see

- Analgesics, paracetamol

18.2.1.3 Opioids

Several OTC pain relievers and antitussives contain opioids such as codeine, dextromethorphan or pholcodine, which can cause additive depression of the CNS when used with other sedative drugs:

- **Alcohol**
- **Antihistamines**, which are both prescribable and found in OTC cold and flu preparations, and as treatment for travel sickness
- **Anxiolytics** and **hypnotics**—"sleeping tablets" such as benzodiazepines or "Z" drugs
- **Antidepressants**
- **Antipsychotics**

These interactions impair the performance of tasks that require attention and quick reflexes (e.g., driving motor vehicles and using machinery or sharp instruments). It is necessary to warn consumers in order to prevent injury to themselves and others.

In addition, dextromethorphan is a substrate of CYP2B6 (minor), CYP2C8/9 (minor), CYP2C19 (minor), CYP2D6 (major), CYP2E1 (minor), and CYP3A4 (minor), and inhibits CYP2D6 (weak effect).

For full details of potential interactions, see

- Analgesics, opioids

18.2.2 Antihistamines

OTC drugs available for treating allergies usually contain the following:

- ***Sedating antihistamines*** (promethazine, e.g., Phenergan; chlorphenamine, e.g., Allercalm, Allerief, Hayleve, Haymine, Piriton, Pollenase; diphenhydramine, e.g., Histergan), which may impair tasks requiring attention (e.g., driving, using machinery). Increased sedation may occur if these drugs are taken with other **sedatives**, including **alcohol**.

- ***Nonsedating antihistamines*** (loratidine, e.g., Clarityn; cetirizine, e.g., Benadryl, Piriteze, Zirtek; clemastine), which can cause dangerous arrhythmias with antifungal agents (**itraconazole, ketoconazole**), antibiotics (**erythromycin, clarithromycin**), and drugs, are used to counteract acidity (e.g., **H2 antagonists**—for cimetidine).

For full details of potential interactions, see

- Respiratory drugs, antihistamines

18.3 COLD REMEDIES

18.3.1 Symptomatic Relief for Coryza

These may contain a mixture of active ingredients including

- Paracetamol (acetaminophen), NSAIDs, opioids, antihistamines (as mentioned earlier).
- ***Caffeine,*** which may cause tremor or arrhythmias.
- ***Sympathomimetics*** (pseudoephedrine, e.g., Sudafed; phenylephrine, e.g., Fenox; oxymetazoline, e.g., Lemsip, Otrivine, Vicks). **They should not be used if taking antidepressants, particularly MAOIs and TCAs**, because of the risk of life-threatening episodes of high blood pressure (hypertensive crisis) and adverse effects on the CNS. These drugs also need to be used cautiously by patients with heart disease and those on treatment for high blood pressure.

18.3.2 Medications to Treat a Sore Throat

OTC drugs available may contain

- ***NSAIDs***—see preceding text
- ***Local anesthetics***, for example, benzocaine and lidocaine—see anesthetic drugs, anesthetics—local
- ***Antiseptics*** such as amylmetacresol, hexylresorcinol, chlorhexidine, benzalkonium chloride, cetylpyridinium, and dequalinium

18.4 DRUGS ACTING ON THE GASTROINTESTINAL TRACT

18.4.1 Antacids

These include

- Aluminum-containing products, for example, Alu-cap, AlternaGel, Amphojel, and Basaljel
- Aluminum and magnesium combinations, for example, Gelusil, Maalox, Mylanta, and Riopan. Sucralfate (e.g., Carafate), which is an antiulcer preparation, also contains aluminum
- Calcium-containing products such as Caltrate, Citrucel, Os-Cal, PhosLo, Titralac, and Tums
- Magnesium-containing products, for example, Almora, citrate of magnesium, Mag-Ox 400, Milk of Magnesia, Slow-Mag, and Uro-Mag

The aforementioned preparations are also referred to as drugs containing divalent and trivalent cations (which also includes preparations containing iron).

Antacids essentially produce the following changes in the stomach:

- ***Alter the pH within the stomach.*** This may alter the dissolution of some drug formulations, reducing their absorption.

- ***Bind to other drugs*** that are administered within 1 or 2 h of the antacid. This process results in reduced availability of the co-administered drug for absorption. For example, the chelation of tetracyclines (e.g., **tetracycline, doxycycline**) will decrease their absorption by up to 90%.
- ***Precipitation*** occurs with drugs such as **quinine** with aluminum and magnesium hydroxide preparations, which results in a decreased absorption of quinine. Also the absorption of fluoroquinolones (e.g., **ciprofloxacin, norfloxacin, ofloxacin, enoxacin, perfloxacin**) will be decreased by 60%–75% if they are co-administered with divalent and trivalent cations. Patients are recommended not to take these divalent and trivalent cationic preparations until fluoroquinolone therapy is discontinued. If concomitant intake is absolutely necessary, the intake of the two drugs should be separated by at least 2 h:
  - Drugs acting on the gastrointestinal tract, antacids
  - Drugs to treat infections, antibiotics sections
  - Miscellaneous, minerals
- ***Alkalinization of the urine*** may occur with rapidly absorbed antacids (e.g., sodium bicarbonate), which can affect elimination of other drugs:
  - Urology drugs, urinary alkalinizers

Inadvertent *overdosing of potassium bicarbonate–containing* indigestion preparations has led to severe metabolic alkalosis and unconsciousness needing intensive care management (Gawarammana et al., 2007). The extraordinarily large intake in that case was certainly not of suicidal intent and can be attributed to insufficient information/knowledge for consumers regarding the dosages, adverse effects, and precautions related to OTC drugs.

18.4.2 H2 Receptor Antagonists

This group of drugs (e.g., cimetidine) is used to relieve gastric acidity and dyspepsia. Cimetidine may cause inhibition of metabolism of a large number of drugs as it inhibits multiple CYP isoenzymes. This will increase the levels of substrates of these enzymes with a risk of producing toxic effects, for example

- Anticoagulants such as **warfarin**
- Antiepileptics, for example, **phenytoin** and **carbamazepine**
- **Theophylline**

Conversely, H2 receptor blockers may reduce the absorption of certain drugs, for example

- Antimalarials—**proguanil**
- **Dipyridamole**—an antiplatelet drug used in patients who have had a stroke, to reduce the risk of further strokes

For full details of potential interactions, see drugs acting on the gastrointestinal tract, antacids.

18.4.3 Antidiarrheal Preparations

The OTC drugs available may contain

- ***Opioids*** such as morphine and codeine—see preceding text.
- ***Adsorbents***, for example, kaolin. Kaolin can reduce the absorption and efficacy of other drugs, notably drugs acting on the heart, such as **digoxin** and **beta-blockers**.

See drugs acting on the gastrointestinal tract, antidiarrheals.

18.4.4 Drugs to Treat Constipation

The main adverse drug interactions are associated with abuse, which leads to hypokalemia and in some instances to decreased absorption of other orally administered drugs.

18.4.5 Drugs for Irritable Bowel Syndrome

OTC drugs available may contain

- Anticholinergic antimuscarinics, such as hyoscine

See drugs acting on the nervous system, anti-Parkinson's drugs.

18.5 DRUGS FOR PREVENTION OF HEART DISEASE

The OTC drugs available are

- ***Aspirin*** (usually enteric coated in 75 mg doses)—see preceding text
- ***Statins*** (simvastatin)

The most serious adverse effect of simvastatin is myopathy, which rarely may progress to rhabdomyolysis. Abnormalities of liver function may also occur. These effects are dose dependent, and a number of drugs and foods may inhibit the metabolism of simvastatin, thereby increasing its toxicity, for example

- **Grapefruit juice**
- **Macrolides**

These should be avoided in patients taking simvastatin.

For full details of potential interactions, see cardiovascular drugs, lipid-lowering drugs.

18.6 DRUGS ACTING ON THE CENTRAL NERVOUS SYSTEM

- Hypnotics "sleeping tablets"
  - OTC drugs available may contain sedating **antihistamines**—see preceding text.
- Travel sickness medications
  The OTC drugs available may contain
  - ***Antihistamines***—see preceding text
  - Hyoscine

Hyoscine has antimuscarinic side effects that may add to the effect of a wide range of prescribable medications such as **TCAs**. Also, the antimuscarinic effect may reduce the efficacy of sublingual **GTN** tablets.

For full details of potential interactions, see drugs acting on the nervous system, anti-Parkinson's drugs.

18.7 TOPICAL FORMULATIONS

Systemic absorption is usually not significant in normal conditions; however, excessive absorption may occur, for example

- If applied on damaged skin
- If too much is applied
- If the area is covered with bandages
- If applied on erythematous skin (such as in the presence of cellulitis, burns, in excessively hot conditions)

18.7.1 Topical Analgesics May Contain

- ***Salicylates*—*see cardiovascular drugs, antiplatelets***
- ***NSAIDs*—*see analgesics, non-steroidal anti-inflammatory drugs***
- ***Belladonna* alkaloids**, for example, hyoscyamine—see drugs acting on the nervous system, anti-Parkinson's drugs section

18.7.2 Antifungals May Contain Azoles

These decrease the metabolism of a wide range of drugs including

- **Warfarin.**
- **Sulfonylureas.**
- **Phenytoin.**
- **Antihistamines, for example**, astemizole, terfenadine (high concentrations of these two drugs would cause life-threatening ventricular arrhythmias with torsades des pointes).
- **Theophylline.**
- The diuretic **hydrochlorothiazide**, which decreases the metabolism of fluconazole and may cause toxic effects of fluconazole.
- The antibiotic **rifampicin**, which increases the metabolism of fluconazole and thus reduces its efficacy.

See drugs to treat infections, antifungal drugs.

18.8 NUTRITIONAL SUPPLEMENTS

OTC drugs available include the following vitamins:

- A—retinol
- B1—thiamin
- B2—riboflavin
- B6—pyridoxine
- B12—cyanocobalamine
- Nicotinic acid—a constituent of the vitamin B complex
- Folic acid—a constituent of the vitamin B complex, whose concentrations and activity can be decreased by **antiepileptics**
- C—ascorbic acid, the absorption of which is reduced by **aspirin**
- D—calciferol, levels of which are reduced by **phenytoin**
- E—tocopherol
- K—phytomenadione

For full details of potential interactions, see Miscellaneous, Minerals section.

Minerals and electrolytes are also available in OTC preparations:

- Iodine, which increases the risk of hypothyroidism
- Iron
- Calcium
- Magnesium
- Potassium
- Phosphorus
- Zinc

Potassium supplements are associated with an increased risk of hyperkalemia with **ACE inhibitors** and **potassium-sparing diuretics**. Salt substitutes (which may be recommended for patients with hypertension) contain potassium, so patients taking ACE inhibitors should be advised not to use salt substitutes.

For full details of potential interactions, see Cardiovascular Drugs, Antihypertensive and Heart Failure Drugs, Diuretics.

INFORMATION SOURCE

Chemist and Druggist. *Guide to OTC Medicines and Diagnostics: For Pharmacists and Pharmacy Assistants*, 33rd edn. Tonbridge, U.K.: CMPMedica, 2008.

Gawarammana IB, Coburn J, Greene S, Dargan PI, and Jones AL. Severe hypokalaemic metabolic alkalosis following ingestion of gaviscon®. Clin Toxicol. 2007; 45: 176–178.

APPENDIX A: Factors Associated with Drug Effects

Simon F.J. Clarke, Lakshman Delgoda Karalliedde, and Ursula Collignon

A.1 SYSTEMIC DRUG AVAILABILITY

Following absorption from the gut, a proportion of the dose may be eliminated by the liver before reaching the systemic circulation. **This presystemic or first-pass elimination is determined by the hepatic clearance or extraction for the compound**. Some examples of drugs with high and low hepatic extraction.

A.1.1 Bioavailability

Bioavailability is the proportion of an extravascular dose (enteral, intranasal, buccal/sublingual) that enters the circulation. Note that this does not equate to the dose that reaches the target organ because many drugs are bound to proteins (primarily to albumin and/or α-1-acid-glycoprotein) in plasma and tissues. It is the free, unbound concentration of the drug that is distributed to act on the target structures (receptors, bacteria) and is eliminated.

A.1.2 Extraction Ratios

High Extraction Ratio	Low Extraction Ratio
Dependent on blood flow and hepatocyte function	Dependent on hepatocyte function only
1. Antidepressants	1. NSAIDs
2. Chlorpromazine/haloperidol	2. Diazepam
3. Calcium-channel blockers	
4. Morphine	
5. Glyceryl trinitrate	
6. Levodopa	
7. Propranolol	

A.1.3 First-Pass Metabolism

In general, if a drug has a high first-pass metabolism through the liver, one can expect a marked increase in its concentration if it is taken with another drug that inhibits metabolism. Whether or not this change in concentration is clinically significant is related to the factors affecting the concentration–effect relationship.

Examples of drugs that undergo first-pass metabolism by CYP3A4 include

1. Very high first-pass metabolism: buspirone, ergotamine, lovastatin, nimodipine, saquinavir, and simvastatin
2. High first-pass metabolism: estradiol, atorvastatin, felodipine, indinavir, isradipine, nicardipine, propafenone, and tacrolimus
3. Intermediate first-pass metabolism: amiodarone, carbamazepine, carvedilol, cisapride, cyclosporin, diltiazem, ethinylestradiol, etoposide, losartan, midazolam, nifedipine, nelfinavir, ondansetron, pimozide, sildenafil, triazolam, and verapamil

A.2 PHARMACOKINETICS

Pharmacokinetics describes the relationship between drug dosing and drug concentration–time profile in the body (i.e., what the body does to the drug).

A.3 PHARMACODYNAMICS

Pharmacodynamics describes the relationship between concentration and both the wanted and unwanted effects (i.e., what the drug does to the body).

The total exposure is described as the area under the concentration–time curve (AUC) (i.e., the total amount of drug absorbed).

A.4 ENTEROHEPATIC CIRCULATION

Following metabolism, compounds are excreted directly into the bile, or reenter the systemic circulation and are excreted as polar metabolites or conjugates by the kidney. When excreted in the bile (mainly glucuronidated drugs), the compound enters the biliary duct system and is secreted into the upper small intestine. Throughout the ileum, these conjugated bile salts (some with drugs attached to them) are reabsorbed and transported back to the liver via the portal circulation. **This is known as enterohepatic circulation**. Each bile salt is reused approximately 20 times and often repeatedly in the same digestive phase. Thus, compounds may reach high hepatic concentrations resulting in significant hepatotoxicity. Extensive enterohepatic cycling occurs with colchicine, phenytoin, leflunomide, and tetracycline antibiotics.

APPENDIX B: Factors Associated with Interactions

Simon F.J. Clarke, Lakshman Delgoda Karalliedde, and Ursula Collignon

B.1 "ON-TARGET AND OFF-TARGET" TOXICITY AND INTERACTIONS

Drug toxicity results from the inhibition or activation of a therapeutic target by a drug or from an interaction between a drug and a target protein different from the therapeutic target of the drug. In the former, "on-target" toxicity, an example is excessive bleeding from high doses of warfarin. In "off-target" toxicity, an example is statin-induced myopathy.

B.2 POLYPHARMACY

B.2.1 Synopsis of King's Fund Report (London)

In the past 10 years, the average number of items prescribed for each person per year in England has increased by 53.8%, from 11.9 in 2001 to 18.3 in 2011. A Scottish study of more than 300,000 patients found that between 1995 and 2010, the proportion of patients receiving five or more drugs increased from 12% to 22% and the proportion receiving 10 or more drugs rose from 1.9% to 5.8%. For older people, the figures are even higher, with 1 in 6 patients over the age of 65 receiving 10 or more drugs (Polypharmacy: a necessary evil. BMJ 2013; 347).

- For many people, appropriate polypharmacy will extend life expectancy and improve quality of life. Their medicines' use will be optimized and prescribed according to best evidence.
- In problematic polypharmacy, there can be an increased risk of drug interactions and adverse drug reactions, together with impaired adherence to medication and quality of life for patients.
- Many clinical trials and practice guidelines do not consider polypharmacy in the context of multimorbidity. It is important that pragmatic clinical trials are conducted that include patients with multimorbidity and polypharmacy.
- Patients with multimorbidity could have all their long-term conditions reviewed in one visit by a clinical team responsible for coordinating their care.
- Patients may struggle with complex drug regimens; their perspective on medicine-taking must be taken into account when prescribing.

B.3 NARROW THERAPEUTIC RANGE/INDEX

Drugs with a narrow therapeutic range (NTR) have little difference between therapeutic and toxic doses or the associated blood or plasma concentrations (i.e., exposures). Generally, toxicity is considered to be serious toxicity, not symptomatic reversible toxicity (most drugs have diverse adverse effects within the therapeutic range). CYP substrates with an NTR have a high risk of adverse drug interactions when coadministered with CYP inhibitors.

Classic examples of NTR drugs include

- Aminoglycoside antibiotics—gentamicin and tobramycin
- Anticoagulants—warfarin (where a modest increase from the titrated [INR-monitored] concentration can cause major bleeding) and heparin
- Anticonvulsants—carbamazepine, phenytoin, and valproic acid

- Antidepressants—lithium and tricyclics
- Aspirin
- Conjugated estrogens and esterified estrogens
- Ciclosporin
- Digoxin, procainamide, and quinidine
- Hypoglycemic agents
- Statins—lovastatin and simvastatin can cause myopathy leading to rhabdomyolysis, a rare but life-threatening condition, if taken with a strong CYP3A inhibitor (mibefradil, removed from the US market) and can cause ↑ in blood levels
- Levothyroxine sodium
- Theophylline
- Drugs with concentration-related QT effects (cisapride, astemizole, dofetilide) where a previously tolerated dose could become toxic with a doubling of serum concentration
- Most cytotoxic oncologic drugs

APPENDIX C: Foods Implicated in Potentially Severe Interactions

Lakshman Delgoda Karalliedde, Janaka Karalliedde, and Seneka Abeyratne

C.1 FOOD AND PRODUCTS RICH IN VITAMIN K (AFFECTS ANTICOAGULANTS)

Alfalfa tablets, broccoli, Brussels sprouts, cabbage, cauliflower (raw), green leafy vegetables (spinach, collard greens), green tea, liver, soybean, vegetable oils (canola, soybean), watercress.

C.2 FOODS WITH HIGH CONTENT OF TYRAMINE (ASSOCIATED WITH INTERACTIONS WITH MAOIs)

Ale, avocados, bananas, beans (lima, butter, bean pods), caviar, cheese (especially aged), chocolate, coffee, figs, fish (smoked or pickled), processed meat (bologna, fermented meat, salami, pepperoni, summer sausage, liver [beef or chicken]), raspberries, raisins, sour cream, soy beans, tofu, wines (especially red), yeast, yoghurt.

APPENDIX D: Clinical Drug Development

Lakshman Delgoda Karalliedde and Janaka Karalliedde

Trials used in the development are divided into three phases:

- Phase I: Escalating doses of single and multiple doses are administered, typically to healthy volunteers, and the goal is to determine pharmacokinetics (PK) and side effects.
- Phase II: The aim is to confirm signs of efficacy and evaluate different doses and schedules.
- Phase III: The efficacy of the drug is compared with currently used therapy or placebo.

The quantitative assessment of the potential for a drug to be involved in a drug–drug interaction uses a variety of models (basic models, mechanistic static models, physiologically based pharmacokinetic [PBPK] models) and appropriately designed pharmacokinetic studies performed in early phases of drug development. Information from in vitro studies and in vivo investigations can be used for PBPK model construction and refinement. If potential drug–drug interactions are identified based on in vitro and/or in vivo studies, sponsors should design further studies or collect information to determine

1. Whether additional studies are needed to better quantify the effect and to examine the effects of weaker inhibitors (early studies usually examine strong inhibitors) on the investigational drugs as substrates and effects of investigational drugs (as inhibitors) on a range of substrates
2. Whether dosage adjustments or other prescribing modifications (e.g., additional safety monitoring or contraindications) are needed based on the identified interaction(s) to avoid undesired consequences

Drug interaction information is used along with information about exposure–response relationships in the general population and specific populations, to help predict the clinical consequences of drug–drug interactions.

Population pharmacokinetic (PopPK) analyses: Data obtained from large-scale clinical studies that include sparse or intensive blood sampling help characterize the clinical impact of known or newly identified interactions and determine recommendations for dosage modifications for the investigational drug as a substrate. PopPK evaluations may also detect unsuspected drug–drug interactions and provide further evidence of absence of a drug–drug interaction, when supported by prior evidence and mechanistic data.

Clinical drug–drug interaction studies performed using healthy volunteers will predict findings in the patient population for which the drug is intended. Safety considerations often preclude the use of healthy subjects in studies of certain drugs. The extent of drug interactions (inhibition or induction) may be different depending on the subjects' genotype for the specific enzyme or transporter being evaluated. Subjects lacking the major polymorphic clearance pathway will show reduced total metabolism or transport and an alternative pathway becomes quantitatively more important, and the alternative pathway should be understood and studied appropriately. Thus, phenotype or genotype determinations to identify genetically determined metabolic or transporter polymorphisms are important when evaluating effects on enzymes or transporters with polymorphisms, such as CYP2D6, CYP2C19, CYP2C9, UGT1A1, and OATP1B1 (SLCO1B1). A viable alternative is to consider powering the study for the genotype status that is likely to have the highest potential for interaction.

APPENDIX E: Assessments of Manifestations of DDIs

Simon F.J. Clarke and Ursula Collignon

E.1 ANTICHOLINERGIC RISK SCALE

(Rudolph JI et al. *Arch Intern Med*. 2008;168(5):508–513)

1. Anticholinergic effects are associated with impaired cognition, dizziness, and risk of falls particularly in frail adults.
2. Link to mortality with the increasing number and potency of anticholinergics.
3. Significant morbidity can occur from other anticholinergic effects such as dry mouth, dry eyes, urinary retention, and constipation.
4. The higher the score, the more likely that the patient will suffer anticholinergic effects (e.g., ARS score 3 associated with ≥2 anticholinergic effects in 70% elderly patients).

Three Points	Two Points	One Point
Amitriptyline	Amantadine	Carbidopa/levodopa
Atropine	Baclofen	Entacapone
Benztropine	Cetirizine	Haloperidol
Carisoprodol	Cimetidine	Methocarbamol
Chlorphenamine	Clozapine	Metoclopramide
Chlorpromazine	Cyclobenzaprine	Mirtazapine
Cyproheptadine	Desipramine	Paroxetine
Dicyclomine	Loperamide	Pramipexole
Diphenhydramine	Loratadine	Quetiapine
Fluphenazine	Nortriptyline	Ranitidine
Hydroxyzine	Olanzapine	Risperidone
Hyoscyamine	Prochlorperazine	Selegiline
Imipramine	Pseudoephedrine	Trazodone
Meclizine	Tolterodine	Ziprasidone
Oxybutynin		
Perphenazine		
Promethazine		
Thioridazine		
Thiothixene		
Tizanidine		
Trifluoperazine		

E.2 DRUG-INDUCED LIVER INJURY

Drug-induced liver injury (DILI) is probably the most common cause for termination of clinical trials of new drugs (~33%) and the main cause for withdrawal of clinical drugs from the market. The observed incidence of symptomatic hepatic adverse drug reactions is 8 in 100,000. Idiosyncratic DILI causes 13% of acute liver failure in the United States with 75% of patients dying or requiring liver transplantation. Though the pathogenesis of DILI remains uncertain, there is a genetic association for a few drugs. Flucloxacillin is associated with cholestatic hepatitis (incidence of 8.5 in every 100,000 new users 1–45 days after the start of the drug); 80-fold higher risk of flucloxacillin is attributed to a human leukocyte antigen gene polymorphism.

APPENDIX F: Triptan Sensations

Lakshman Delgoda Karalliedde and Janaka Karalliedde

Seen with drugs used to treat migraine.

Common sensations of tingling, heat, pain, heaviness, or tightness in any part of the body, including chest and throat, flushing, dizziness, feeling of weakness, drowsiness, fatigue, nausea, vomiting, dry mouth, and transient increase in BP occur during the use of triptans. Rash is infrequent. Rare is the occurrence of angina, MI and death, arrhythmias, stroke, seizures, ischemic colitis, and hypersensitivity reactions, including anaphylaxis. There is no evidence that any triptan is safer than another, although the response to each agent can vary considerably between patients.

APPENDIX G: Assessment of Severity of Liver Disease

Chulananda Goonasekera

G.1 CHILD–TURCOTTE–PUGH CLASSIFICATION

Parameter	1 Point	2 Points	3 Points
Serum albumin (g/dL)	>3.5	2.8–3.5	<2.8
Serum bilirubin (mg/dL)	1–2	2–3	<3
Prothrombin time (seconds above control)	1–4	4–10	>10
Ascites	Absent	Slight	Moderate
Encephalopathy grade	0	1–2	3–4
Total number of points	5–6	7–9	>9
Child–Turcotte–Pugh classification	A (mild)	B (moderate)	C (severe)

G.2 MELD/PELD CALCULATOR

The MELD/PELD Calculator is a utility that allows you to enter hypothetical or actual parameters and calculate a MELD or PELD score for an individual patient.

The MELD/PELD Calculator provided on this site uses the specific formulas approved by the OPTN/UNOS Board of Directors and used for the allocation of livers by the OPTN match system. The MELD score calculation uses the following: serum creatinine (mg/dL) * bilirubin (mg/dL) * INR. For candidates on dialysis, defined as having 2 or more dialysis treatments within the prior week, or candidates who have received 24 h of CVVHD within the prior week will have their serum creatinine level automatically set to 4.0 mg/dL. The MELD Calculator is used for candidates who are 12 years and older. After entering the laboratory values, you may calculate the score by clicking Calculate. The MELD score displays in the MELD Score field. You may also calculate a score by simply tabbing into the MELD Score field. The PELD score calculation uses the following: albumin (g/dL), bilirubin (mg/dL), INR, growth failure (based on gender, height, and weight), age at listing. The PELD Calculator is used for candidates who are under 12 years old. After entering the laboratory values, you may calculate the score by clicking Calculate. The PELD score displays in the PELD Lab Value field. You can also calculate a score by simply tabbing into the PELD Lab Value field.

The MELD score is calculated using the following formula:

$$\text{MELD Score} = 0.957 \times \text{Loge(creatinine mg/dL)} + 0.378 \times \text{Loge(bilirubin mg/dL)} + 1.120 \times \text{Loge(INR)} + 0.6431$$

Multiply the score by 10 and round to the nearest whole number. Laboratory values less than 1.0 are set to 1.0 for the purposes of the MELD score calculation. At the July 2001 meeting of the Liver and Intestinal Organ Transplantation Committee, the committee agree to 0.643 points for etiology to all patients in order to make the MELD score comparable to previously published data.

G.3 MELD/PELD CALCULATOR DOCUMENTATION

The maximum serum creatinine considered within the MELD score equation is 4.0 mg/dL (e.g., if you enter 4.3 for serum creatinine, the formula will calculate 0.957 × Loge(4.0) for the serum creatinine portion of the MELD formula).

APPENDIX H: Prescribing Guidelines for Elderly Patients

Andrea Corsonello and Giuseppe Maltese

The FORTA (Fit fOR The Aged) list—medications are rated in four categories:

1. Clear benefit
2. Proven but limited efficacy or some safety concerns
3. Questionable efficacy or safety profile—consider alternative
4. Clearly avoid and find alternative

The ratings are based on the individual patient's indication for the medication. Developed in Germany, it has undergone consensus validation with a panel of care of the elderly physicians though its impact on clinical outcomes is still uncertain.

Health Care Financing Administration: The US Centers for Medicare and Medicaid Services studied drug utilization on eight prescription drug classes (digoxin, calcium-channel blockers, ACE inhibitors, H2 receptor antagonists, NSAIDs, benzodiazepines, antipsychotics, and antidepressants) and four types of prescribing problems (inappropriate dosage, inappropriate duration of therapy, duplication of therapies, and potential for drug–drug interactions). It revealed that 19% of 2508 community dwelling older adults were using one or more medications inappropriately; NSAIDs and benzodiazepines were the drug classes with the most potential problems.

The Screening Tool of Older Person's Prescriptions (STOPP) is introduced in 2008. STOPP and Beers criteria overlapped in several areas. STOPP includes consideration of drug–drug interactions and duplication of drugs within a class.

TTB (Time to Benefit), defined as the time to significant benefit observed in trials of people treated with a drug compared to controls, can be estimated from data from randomized controlled trials. Such information, not currently available, may in the future help guide decision-making for specific drug prescribing in individual patients.

APPENDIX I: Factors Affecting Efficacy of Anti-Infective Agents

Niroshini Manthri Giles and Lakshman Delgoda Karalliedde

Antibiotic efficacy depends on both the concentration of free drug at the site of action and the duration it is present there. The relative importance of each of these factors varies between different antibiotics.

I.1 TIME DEPENDENT, NONCONCENTRATION DEPENDENT

Antimicrobial effect is defined by the cumulative percentage of time over a 24-h period that the free (or unbound) antimicrobial concentration exceeds the minimum inhibitory concentration (MIC) (f.T > MIC), e.g., beta-lactams, some of the macrolides, and clindamycin.

When the concentration of the drug exceeds a certain MIC to achieve killing, increasing the concentration of the drug further has no effect. Critical factor is the amount of time the drug concentration exceeds the MIC at the site of the infection. For effective bactericidal activity against resistant organisms, the drug concentration must exceed the MIC for more than 40%–50% of the dosing interval. Effectiveness is greatest when the drug concentration exceeds the MIC for more than 60%–70% of the dosing interval. Efficacy varies by antimicrobial class. For example, amoxicillin- and amoxicillin/clavulanate-associated killing is found when serum concentrations exceed the MIC for only 30% of the dosing interval. Thus, for time-dependent killing, the goal of therapy is to maximize the duration of drug exposure.

I.2 CONCENTRATION-DEPENDENT ANTIMICROBIAL EFFECT

This is defined by the peak concentration in a dosing interval divided by the MIC (C_{max}/MIC). The usual target is a C_{max}/MIC that exceeds 8–10. The PK/PD parameters, C_{max}/MIC or AUC/MIC ratio, logically correlates with their activity, e.g., aminoglycosides, azalides, daptomycin, fluoroquinolones, ketolides, some macrolides, and vancomycin. Bacterial killing is more rapid when the peak serum concentration (or area under the curve, AUC) is appreciably above the MIC. Thus, the AUC-to-MIC ratio is a good parameter for predicting the efficacy of these antimicrobials.

The change of drug in plasma (A_{cAG}) with time (t) was determined by nonrenal elimination described by k_{nr}, renal elimination dependent on $CL_{CR(t)}$, and the tubular fraction reabsorbed (f_{reabs}). The model was used to simulate dosing regimens, and it could be shown that administering aminoglycosides in the middle of the day (1:30 PM) resulted in the lowest aminoglycoside nephrotoxicity.

I.3 CONCENTRATION AND TIME-DEPENDENT

Antimicrobial effect is defined by the AUC_{0-24h} over a 24-h period divided by the MIC (AUC_{0-24h}/MIC), e.g., fluoroquinolones, tigecycline, linezolid, and glycopeptides.

- **MIC** is the "lowest drug concentration that completely inhibits visible growth of microorganisms under the conditions of their use."
- **AUC** is the area under the concentration–time curve.
- C_{max} is the highest concentration reached (the peak).
- **f** is introduced to indicate that the free, unbound fraction of the drug was used in the calculations.
- $T_{>MIC}$ is the cumulative percentage of a 24 h period that the concentration is above MIC.

Changes in PK during the time course of infection will consequently affect the antibacterial effect and thus are important to consider in the evaluation of PK/PD relationships.

I.4 ANTIMICROBIAL RESISTANCE

The World Health Organization has labeled this critical issue as one of the three greatest threats to human health. The overwhelming prevalence of resistant gram-positive organisms has resulted in the development of several potent and efficacious antimicrobials in the forms of linezolid, daptomycin, tigecycline, and ceftaroline to battle infections caused by methicillin-resistant *Staphylococcus aureus* or vancomycin-resistant Enterococci. Tigecycline and ceftaroline are broad-spectrum antimicrobials that exhibit activity against gram-negative pathogens as well. However, there is an absence of new antimicrobials with novel mechanisms of action and narrow spectrum of activity against resistant gram-negative pathogens. This deficiency necessitates heightened assessment of PK/PD characteristics of ubiquitous antimicrobials that are used both broadly and specifically for nosocomial gram-negative infections: beta-lactams (i.e., piperacillin/tazobactam, cefepime) and carbapenems (i.e., meropenem, doripenem).

APPENDIX J: Assessments of Obesity

Lakshman Delgoda Karalliedde and H.M.U. Amila Jayasinghe

The BMI is calculated as weight in kilograms (kg) divided by height in meters squared (m^2). It is generally accepted that an ideal BMI ranges from 20 to 25. In children, BMI is calculated by multiplying the child's weight in pounds by 705 and then dividing this figure with the child's height in inches twice. BMI of 25–29.9 kg/m^2 is overweight. BMI of 30–34.9 kg/m^2 is obese (grade I). BMI of 35–39.9 kg/m^2 is obese (grade II). BMI of ≥40 kg/m^2 is obese (grade III) or morbidly obese—with a real and imminent threat to health. Exceptions are those who are very muscular with great mass of muscle, not necessarily with excess of fat.

Waist-to-hip ratio (WHR) is an indicator of abdominal fat that is considered a more accurate predictor for cardiovascular risk than BMI in different ethnic populations and in those aged over 75 years. The acceptable upper limit is 0.90 for men and 0.85 for women.

Clinicians must be aware of what "weight" to use to calculate dosage:

$$\text{Total body weight (TBW)} = \text{actual weight}$$

The formulae developed by Devine are used to estimate lean body mass (LBM). Ideal body weight (IBW) is a calculated estimate of LBM adjusted for gender and height. Devine went on to develop IBW calculations for men and women for medical purposes. These equations are commonly used today for dosing of specific medications such as acyclovir. This approach is beneficial since LBM is not readily measured in obesity. IBW may be underestimated in the obese when using the Devine equation. Body surface area (BSA) is also a classification of body size. Calculating BSA involves the use of body weight and height. Two formulae commonly used to calculate BSA are the DuBois and Mosteller equations.